The GALE ENCYCLOPEDIA of SURGERY

A GUIDE FOR PATIENTS AND CAREGIVERS

VOLUME

3

P-Z

ANTHONY J. SENAGORE, M.D., EXECUTIVE ADVISOR
CLEVELAND CLINIC FOUNDATION

GALE®

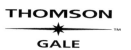

THOMSON
✶
GALE™

Detroit • New York • San Diego • San Francisco • Cleveland • New Haven, Conn. • Waterville, Maine • London • Munich

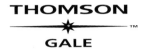

THOMSON

GALE

Gale Encyclopedia of Surgery: A Guide for Patients and Caregivers

Anthony J. Senagore MD, Executive Adviser

Project Editor
Kristine Krapp

Editorial
Stacey L. Blachford, Deirdre Blanchfield, Madeline Harris, Chris Jeryan, Jacqueline Longe, Brigham Narins, Mark Springer, Ryan Thomason

Editorial Support Services
Andrea Lopeman, Sue Petrus

Indexing
Synapse

Illustrations
GGS Inc.

Permissions
Lori Hines

Imaging and Multimedia
Leitha Etheridge-Sims, Lezlie Light, Dave Oblender, Christine O'Brien, Robyn V. Young

Product Design
Michelle DiMercurio, Jennifer Wahi

Manufacturing
Wendy Blurton, Evi Seoud

LIBRARY OF CONGRESS CATALOGING-IN-PUBLICATION DATA

Gale encyclopedia of surgery : a guide for patients and caregivers / Anthony J. Senagore, [editor].
    p. cm.
        Includes bibliographical references and index.
        ISBN 0-7876-7721-3 (set : hc) — ISBN 0-7876-7722-1 (v. 1) — ISBN 0-7876-7723-X (v. 2) — ISBN 0-7876-9123-2 (v. 3)
        Surgery—Encyclopedias. 2. Surgery—Popular works. I. Senagore, Anthony J., 1958-

RD17.G34 2003
617'.91'003—dc22   2003015742

CONTENTS

List of Entries vii

Introduction xiii

Contributors xv

Entries

Volume 1: A-F **1**

Volume 2: G-O **557**

Volume 3: P-Z **1079**

Glossary 1577

Organizations Appendix 1635

General Index 1649

LIST OF ENTRIES

A

Abdominal ultrasound
Abdominal wall defect repair
Abdominoplasty
Abortion, induced
Abscess incision and drainage
Acetaminophen
Adenoidectomy
Admission to the hospital
Adrenalectomy
Adrenergic drugs
Adult day care
Ambulatory surgery centers
Amniocentesis
Amputation
Anaerobic bacteria culture
Analgesics
Analgesics, opioid
Anesthesia evaluation
Anesthesia, general
Anesthesia, local
Anesthesiologist's role
Angiography
Angioplasty
Anterior temporal lobectomy
Antianxiety drugs
Antibiotics
Antibiotics, topical
Anticoagulant and antiplatelet drugs
Antihypertensive drugs
Antinausea drugs
Antiseptics
Antrectomy
Aortic aneurysm repair
Aortic valve replacement

Appendectomy
Arteriovenous fistula
Arthrography
Arthroplasty
Arthroscopic surgery
Artificial sphincter insertion
Aseptic technique
Aspirin
Autologous blood donation
Axillary dissection

B

Balloon valvuloplasty
Bandages and dressings
Bankart procedure
Barbiturates
Barium enema
Bedsores
Biliary stenting
Bispectral index
Bladder augmentation
Blepharoplasty
Blood donation and registry
Blood pressure measurement
Blood salvage
Bloodless surgery
Bone grafting
Bone marrow aspiration and biopsy
Bone marrow transplantation
Bone x rays
Bowel resection
Breast biopsy
Breast implants
Breast reconstruction

Breast reduction
Bronchoscopy
Bunionectomy

C

Cardiac catheterization
Cardiac marker tests
Cardiac monitor
Cardiopulmonary resuscitation
Cardioversion
Carotid endarterectomy
Carpal tunnel release
Catheterization, female
Catheterization, male
Cephalosporins
Cerebral aneurysm repair
Cerebrospinal fluid (CSF) analysis
Cervical cerclage
Cervical cryotherapy
Cesarean section
Chest tube insertion
Chest x ray
Cholecystectomy
Circumcision
Cleft lip repair
Club foot repair
Cochlear implants
Collagen periurethral injection
Colonoscopy
Colorectal surgery
Colostomy
Colporrhaphy
Colposcopy
Colpotomy

Complete blood count
Cone biopsy
Corneal transplantation
Coronary artery bypass graft
  surgery
Coronary stenting
Corpus callosotomy
Corticosteroids
Craniofacial reconstruction
Craniotomy
Cricothyroidotomy
Cryotherapy
Cryotherapy for cataracts
CT scans
Curettage and electrosurgery
Cyclocryotherapy
Cystectomy
Cystocele repair
Cystoscopy

D

Death and dying
Debridement
Deep brain stimulation
Defibrillation
Dental implants
Dermabrasion
Dilatation and curettage
Discharge from the hospital
Disk removal
Diuretics
Do not resuscitate order (DNR)

E

Ear, nose, and throat surgery
Echocardiography
Elective surgery
Electrocardiography
Electroencephalography
Electrolyte tests
Electrophysiology study of the heart
Emergency surgery
Endolymphatic shunt

Endoscopic retrograde
  cholangiopancreatography
Endoscopic sinus surgery
Endotracheal intubation
Endovascular stent surgery
Enhanced external counterpulsation
Enucleation, eye
Epidural therapy
Episiotomy
Erythromycins
Esophageal atresia repair
Esophageal function tests
Esophageal resection
Esophagogastroduodenoscopy
Essential surgery
Exenteration
Exercise
Extracapsular cataract extraction
Eye muscle surgery

F

Face lift
Fasciotomy
Femoral hernia repair
Fetal surgery
Fetoscopy
Fibrin sealants
Finding a surgeon
Finger reattachment
Fluoroquinolones
Forehead lift
Fracture repair

G

Gallstone removal
Ganglion cyst removal
Gastrectomy
Gastric acid inhibitors
Gastric bypass
Gastroduodenostomy
Gastroenterologic surgery
Gastroesophageal reflux scan
Gastroesophageal reflux surgery

Gastrostomy
General surgery
Gingivectomy
Glossectomy
Glucose tests
Goniotomy

H

Hair transplantation
Hammer, claw, and mallet toe
  surgery
Hand surgery
Health care proxy
Health history
Heart surgery for congenital defects
Heart transplantation
Heart-lung machines
Heart-lung transplantation
Hemangioma excision
Hematocrit
Hemispherectomy
Hemoglobin test
Hemoperfusion
Hemorrhoidectomy
Hepatectomy
Hip osteotomy
Hip replacement
Hip revision surgery
Home care
Hospices
Hospital services
Hospital-acquired infections
Human leukocyte antigen test
Hydrocelectomy
Hypophysectomy
Hypospadias repair
Hysterectomy
Hysteroscopy

I

Ileal conduit surgery
Ileoanal anastomosis
Ileoanal reservoir surgery

Ileostomy
Immunoassay tests
Immunologic therapies
Immunosuppressant drugs
Implantable cardioverter-
    defibrillator
In vitro fertilization
Incision care
Incisional hernia repair
Informed consent
Inguinal hernia repair
Intensive care unit
Intensive care unit equipment
Intestinal obstruction repair
Intravenous rehydration
Intussusception reduction
Iridectomy
Islet cell transplantation

K

Kidney dialysis
Kidney function tests
Kidney transplantation
Knee arthroscopic surgery
Knee osteotomy
Knee replacement
Knee revision surgery
Kneecap removal

L

Laceration repair
Laminectomy
Laparoscopy
Laparoscopy for endometriosis
Laparotomy, exploratory
Laryngectomy
Laser in-situ keratomileusis (LASIK)
Laser iridotomy
Laser posterior capsulotomy
Laser skin resurfacing
Laser surgery
Laxatives
Leg lengthening/shortening

Limb salvage
Lipid tests
Liposuction
Lithotripsy
Liver biopsy
Liver function tests
Liver transplantation
Living will
Lobectomy, pulmonary
Long-term care insurance
Lumpectomy
Lung biopsy
Lung transplantation
Lymphadenectomy

M

Magnetic resonance imaging
Mammography
Managed care plans
Mastoidectomy
Maze procedure for atrial
    fibrillation
Mechanical circulation support
Mechanical ventilation
Meckel's diverticulectomy
Mediastinoscopy
Medicaid
Medical charts
Medical errors
Medicare
Meningocele repair
Mentoplasty
Microsurgery
Minimally invasive heart surgery
Mitral valve repair
Mitral valve replacement
Modified radical mastectomy
Mohs surgery
Multiple-gated acquisition
    (MUGA) scan
Muscle relaxants
Myelography
Myocardial resection
Myomectomy
Myringotomy and ear tubes

N

Necessary surgery
Needle bladder neck suspension
Nephrectomy
Nephrolithotomy, percutaneous
Nephrostomy
Neurosurgery
Nonsteroidal anti-inflammatory
    drugs
Nursing homes

O

Obstetric and gynecologic surgery
Omphalocele repair
Oophorectomy
Open prostatectomy
Operating room
Ophthalmologic surgery
Orchiectomy
Orchiopexy
Orthopedic surgery
Otoplasty
Outpatient surgery
Oxygen therapy

P

Pacemakers
Pain management
Pallidotomy
Pancreas transplantation
Pancreatectomy
Paracentesis
Parathyroidectomy
Parotidectomy
Patent urachus repair
Patient confidentiality
Patient rights
Patient-controlled analgesia
Pectus excavatum repair
Pediatric concerns
Pediatric surgery

Pelvic ultrasound
Penile prostheses
Pericardiocentesis
Peripheral endarterectomy
Peripheral vascular bypass surgery
Peritoneovenous shunt
Phacoemulsification for cataracts
Pharyngectomy
Phlebography
Phlebotomy
Photocoagulation therapy
Photorefractive keratectomy (PRK)
Physical examination
Planning a hospital stay
Plastic, reconstructive, and
    cosmetic surgery
Pneumonectomy
Portal vein bypass
Positron emission tomography (PET)
Post-surgical pain
Postoperative care
Power of attorney
Preoperative care
Preparing for surgery
Presurgical testing
Private insurance plans
Prophylaxis, antibiotic
Pulse oximeter
Pyloroplasty

Q

Quadrantectomy

R

Radical neck dissection
Recovery at home
Recovery room
Rectal prolapse repair
Rectal resection
Red blood cell indices
Reoperation
Retinal cryopexy
Retropubic suspension

Rhinoplasty
Rhizotomy
Robot-assisted surgery
Root canal treatment
Rotator cuff repair

S

Sacral nerve stimulation
Salpingo-oophorectomy
Salpingostomy
Scar revision surgery
Scleral buckling
Sclerostomy
Sclerotherapy for esophageal
    varices
Sclerotherapy for varicose veins
Scopolamine patch
Second opinion
Second-look surgery
Sedation, conscious
Segmentectomy
Sentinel lymph node biopsy
Septoplasty
Sex reassignment surgery
Shoulder joint replacement
Shoulder resection arthroplasty
Sigmoidoscopy
Simple mastectomy
Skin grafting
Skull x rays
Sling procedure
Small bowel resection
Smoking cessation
Snoring surgery
Sphygmomanometer
Spinal fusion
Spinal instrumentation
Spirometry tests
Splenectomy
Stapedectomy
Stereotactic radiosurgery
Stethoscope
Stitches and staples
Stress test
Sulfonamides

Surgical instruments
Surgical oncology
Surgical team
Sympathectomy
Syringe and needle

T

Talking to the doctor
Tarsorrhaphy
Telesurgery
Tendon repair
Tenotomy
Tetracyclines
Thermometer
Thoracic surgery
Thoracotomy
Thrombolytic therapy
Thyroidectomy
Tonsillectomy
Tooth extraction
Tooth replantation
Trabeculectomy
Tracheotomy
Traction
Transfusion
Transplant surgery
Transurethral bladder resection
Transurethral resection of the
    prostate
Tubal ligation
Tube enterostomy
Tube-shunt surgery
Tumor marker tests
Tumor removal
Tympanoplasty
Type and screen

U

Umbilical hernia repair
Upper GI exam
Ureteral stenting
Ureterosigmoidoscopy
Ureterostomy, cutaneous

Urinalysis
Urinary anti-infectives
Urologic surgery
Uterine stimulants

V

Vagal nerve stimulation

Vagotomy
Vascular surgery
Vasectomy
Vasovasostomy
Vein ligation and stripping
Venous thrombosis prevention
Ventricular assist device
Ventricular shunt
Vertical banded gastroplasty
Vital signs

W

Webbed finger or toe repair
Weight management
White blood cell count and
    differential
Wound care
Wound culture
Wrist replacement

PLEASE READ—
IMPORTANT INFORMATION

The *Gale Encyclopedia of Surgery* is a medical reference product designed to inform and educate readers about a wide variety of surgeries, tests, drugs, and other medical topics. The Gale Group believes the product to be comprehensive, but not necessarily definitive. While the Gale Group has made substantial efforts to provide information that is accurate, comprehensive, and up-to-date, the Gale Group makes no representations or warranties of any kind, including without limitation, warranties of merchantability or fitness for a particular purpose, nor does it guarantee the accuracy, comprehensiveness, or timeliness of the information contained in this product. Readers should be aware that the universe of medical knowledge is constantly growing and changing, and that differences of medical opinion exist among authorities.

INTRODUCTION

The *Gale Encyclopedia of Surgery: A Guide for Patients and Caregivers* is a unique and invaluable source of information for anyone who is considering undergoing a surgical procedure, or has a loved one in that situation. This collection of 465 entries provides in-depth coverage of specific surgeries, diagnostic tests, drugs, and other related entries. The book gives detailed information on 265 surgeries; most include step-by-step illustrations to enhance the reader's understanding of the procedure itself. Entries on related topics, including anesthesia, second opinions, talking to the doctor, admission to the hospital, and preparing for surgery, give lay readers knowledge of surgery practices in general. Sidebars provide information on who performs the surgery and where, and on questions to ask the doctor.

This encyclopedia minimizes medical jargon and uses language that laypersons can understand, while still providing detailed coverage that will benefit health science students.

Entries on surgeries follow a standardized format that provides information at a glance. Rubrics include:

Definition
Purpose
Demographics
Description
Diagnosis/Preparation
Aftercare
Risks
Normal results
Morbidity and mortality rates
Alternatives
Resources

Inclusion criteria

A preliminary list of surgeries and related topics was compiled from a wide variety of sources, including professional medical guides and textbooks, as well as consumer guides and encyclopedias. Final selection of topics to include was made by the executive adviser in conjunction with the Gale editor.

About the Executive Adviser

The Executive Adviser for the *Gale Encyclopedia of Surgery* was Anthony J. Senagore, MD, MS, FACS, FASCRS. He has published a number of professional articles and is the Krause/Lieberman Chair in Laparoscopic Colorectal Surgery, and Staff Surgeon, Department of Colorectal Surgery at the Cleveland Clinic Foundation in Cleveland, Ohio.

About the contributors

The essays were compiled by experienced medical writers, including physicians, pharmacists, nurses, and other health care professionals. The adviser reviewed the completed essays to ensure that they are appropriate, up-to-date, and medically accurate. Illustrations were also reviewed by a medical doctor.

How to use this book

The **Gale Encyclopedia of Surgery** has been designed with ready reference in mind.

- Straight **alphabetical arrangement** of topics allows users to locate information quickly.
- **Bold-faced terms** within entries and **See also terms** at the end of entries direct the reader to related articles.
- **Cross-references** placed throughout the encyclopedia direct readers from alternate names and related topics to entries.
- A list of **Key terms** is provided where appropriate to define unfamiliar terms or concepts.
- A sidebar describing **Who performs the procedure and where it is performed** is listed with every surgery entry.
- A list of **Questions to ask the doctor** is provided wherever appropriate to help facilitate discussion with the patient's physician.

Introduction

- The **Resources** section directs readers to additional sources of medical information on a topic. Books, periodicals, organizations, and internet sources are listed.
- A **Glossary** of terms used throughout the text is collected in one easy-to-use section at the back of book.
- A valuable **Organizations appendix** compiles useful contact information for various medical and surgical organizations.
- A comprehensive **General index** guides readers to all topics mentioned in the text.

Graphics

The *Gale Encyclopedia of Surgery* contains over 230 full-color illustrations, photos, and tables. This includes over 160 step-by-step illustrations of surgeries. These illustrations were specially created for this product to enhance a layperson's understanding of surgical procedures.

Licensing

The Gale Encyclopedia of Surgery is available for licensing. The complete database is provided in a fielded format and is deliverable on such media as disk or CD-ROM. For more information, contact Gale's Business Development Group at 1-800-877-GALE, or visit our website at www.gale.com/bizdev.

CONTRIBUTORS

Laurie Barclay, M.D.
Neurological Consulting Services
Tampa, FL

Jeanine Barone
Nutritionist, Exercise Physiologist
New York, NY

Julia R. Barrett
Science Writer
Madison, WI

Donald G. Barstow, R.N.
Clinical Nurse Specialist
Oklahoma City, OK

Mary Bekker
Medical Writer
Willow Grove, PA

Mark A. Best, MD, MPH, MBA
Associate Professor of Pathology
St. Matthew's University
Grand Cayman, BWI

Maggie Boleyn, R.N., B.S.N.
Medical Writer
Oak Park, MIn

Susan Joanne Cadwallader
Medical Writer
Cedarburg, WI

Diane Calbrese
Medical Sciences and Technology Writer
Silver Spring, MD

Richard H. Camer
Editor
International Medical News Group
Silver Spring, MD

Rosalyn Carson-DeWitt, M.D.
Medical Writer
Durham, NC

Lisa Christenson, PhD
Science Writer
Hamden, CT

Rhonda Cloos, RN
Medical Writer
Austin, TX

Angela Costello
Medical writer
Cleveland, OH

Esther Csapo Rastegari, RN, BSN, EdM
Medical Writer
Holbrook, MA

L. Lee Culvert, BS, Biochemistry
Health Writer
Alna, ME

Tish Davidson, AM
Medical Writer
Fremont, CA

Lori De Milto
Medical Writer
Sicklerville, NJ

Victoria E. DeMoranville
Medical Writer
Lakeville, MA

Altha Roberts Edgren
Medical Writer
Medical Ink
St. Paul, MN

Lorraine K. Ehresman
Medical Writer
Northfield, Quebec, Canada

L. Fleming Fallon, Jr., MD, DrPH
Professor of Public Health
Bowling Green State University
Bowling Green, OH

Paula Ford-Martin
Freelance Medical Writer
Warwick, RI

Janie Franz
Freelance Journalist
Grand Forks, ND

Rebecca J. Frey, PhD
Freelance Medical Writer
New Haven, CT

Debra Gordon
Medical Writer
Nazareth, PA

Jill Granger, M.S.
Sr. Research Associate
Dept. of Pathology
University of Michigan Medical Center
Ann Arbor, MI

Laith F. Gulli, M.D.
M.Sc., M.Sc.(MedSci), M.S.A., Msc.Psych, MRSNZ
FRSH, FRIPHH, FAIC, FZS
DAPA, DABFC, DABCI
Consultant Psychotherapist in Private Practice
Lathrup Village, MI

Stephen John Hage, AAAS, RT(R), FAHRA
Medical Writer
Chatsworth, CA

Maureen Haggerty
Medical Writer
Ambler, PA

Robert Harr, MS, MT (ASCP)
Associate Professor and Chair
Department of Public and Allied Health
Bowling Green State University
Bowling Green, OH

Dan Harvey
Medical Writer
Wilmington, DE

Katherine Hauswirth, APRN
Medical Writer
Deep River, CT

Caroline Helwick
Medical Writer
New Orleans, LA

Lisette Hilton
Medical Writer
Boca Raton, FL

René A. Jackson, RN
Medical Writer
Port Charlotte, FL

Nadine M. Jacobson, RN
Medical Writer
Takoma Park, MD

Randi B. Jenkins, BA
Copy Chief
Fission Communications
New York, NY

Michelle L. Johnson, M.S., J.D.
Patent Attorney and Medical Writer
ZymoGenetics, Inc.
Seattle, WA

Paul A. Johnson, Ed.M.
Medical Writer
San Diego, CA

Cindy L. A. Jones, Ph.D.
Biomedical Writer
Sagescript Communications
Lakewood, CO

Linda D. Jones, BA, PBT (ASCP)
Medical Writer
Asheboro, NY

Crystal H. Kaczkowski, MSc.
Health Writer
Chicago, IL

Beth A. Kapes
Medical Writer
Bay Village, OH

Jeanne Krob, M.D., F.A.C.S.
Physician, Writer
Pittsburgh, PA

Monique Laberge, PhD
Sr. Res. Investigator
Dept. of Biochemistry & Biophysics, School of Medicine
University of Pennsylvania
Philadelphia, PA

Richard H. Lampert
Senior Medical Editor
W.B. Saunders Co.
Philadelphia, PA

Victor Leipzig, Ph.D.
Biological Consultant
Huntington Beach, CA

Lorraine Lica, PhD
Medical Writer
San Diego, CA

John T. Lohr, Ph.D.
Assistant Director, Biotechnology Center
Utah State University
Logan, UT

Jennifer Lee Losey, RN
Medical Writer
Madison Heights, MI

Jacqueline N. Martin, MS
Medical Writer
Albrightsville, PA

Nancy F. McKenzie, PhD
Public Health Consultant
Brooklyn, NY

Mercedes McLaughlin
Medical Writer
Phoenixville, CA

Christine Miner Minderovic, BS, RT, RDMS
Medical Writer
Ann Arbor, MI

Mark A. Mitchell, M.D.
Freelance Medical Writer
Bothell, WA

Erika J. Norris, MD, MS
Medical Writer
Oak Harbor, WA

Teresa Norris, R.N.
Medical Writer
Ute Park, NM

Debra Novograd, BS, RT(R)(M)
Medical Writer
Royal Oak, MI

Jane E. Phillips, PhD
Medical Writer
Chapel Hill, NC

J. Ricker Polsdorfer, M.D.
Medical Writer
Phoenix, AZ

Elaine R. Proseus, M.B.A./T.M., B.S.R.T., R.T.(R)
Medical Writer
Farmington Hills, MI

Robert Ramirez, B.S.
Medical Student
University of Medicine & Dentistry of New Jersey
Stratford, NJ

Martha S. Reilly, OD
Clinical Optometrist/ Medical Freelance Writer
Madison, WI

Toni Rizzo
Medical Writer
Salt Lake City, UT

Richard Robinson
Freelance Medical Writer
Sherborn, MA

Nancy Ross-Flanigan
Science Writer
Belleville, MI

Belinda Rowland, Ph.D.
Medical Writer
Voorheesville, NY

Laura Ruth, Ph.D.
*Medical, Science, & Technology
   Writer*
Los Angeles, CA

Kausalya Santhanam, Ph.D.
Technical Writer
Branford, CT

Joan Schonbeck
Medical Writer
Nursing Department
Massachusetts Department of
   Mental Health
Marlborough, MA

Stephanie Dionne Sherk
Freelance Medical Writer
University of Michigan
Ann Arbor, MI

Lee A. Shratter, MD
Consulting Radiologist
Kentfield, CA

Jennifer Sisk
Medical Writer
Havertown, PA

Allison J. Spiwak, MSBME
Circulation Technologist
The Ohio State University
Columbus, OH

Kurt Sternlof
Science Writer
New Rochelle, NY

Margaret A Stockley, RGN
Medical Writer
Boxborough, MA

Dorothy Stonely
Medical Writer
Los Gatos, CA

Bethany Thivierge
Biotechnical Writer/Editor
Technicality Resources
Rockland, ME

Carol Turkington
Medical Writer
Lancaster, PA

Samuel D. Uretsky, Pharm.D.
Medical Writer
Wantagh, NY

Ellen S. Weber, M.S.N.
Medical Writer
Fort Wayne, IN

Barbara Wexler
Medical Writer
Chatsworth, CA

Abby Wojahn, RN, BSN, CCRN
Medical Writer
Milwaukee, WI

Kathleen D. Wright, R.N.
Medical Writer
Delmar, DE

Mary Zoll, Ph.D.
Science Writer
Newton Center, MA

Michael V. Zuck, Ph.D.
Medical Writer
Boulder, CO

Pacemaker implantation *see* **Pacemakers**

Pacemakers

Definition

A pacemaker is a surgically implanted electronic device that regulates a cardiac arrhythmia.

Pacemakers are most frequently prescribed when the heartbeat decreases under 60 beats per minute at rest (severe symptomatic bradycardia). They are also used in some cases to slow a fast heart rate over 120 beats per minute at rest (tachycardia).

Demographics

The population for pacemaker implant is not limited by age, sex, or race. Over 100,000 pacemakers are implanted per year in the United States. The occurrence is more frequent in the elderly with over 85% of implants received by those over age 65. A history of myocardial infarction (heart attack), congenital defect, or cardiac transplant also increases the likelihood of pacemaker implant.

Description

Approximately 500,000 Americans have an implantable permanent pacemaker device. A pacemaker implantation is performed under local anesthesia in a hospital by a surgeon assisted by a cardiologist. An insulated wire called a lead is inserted into an incision above the collarbone and guided through a large vein into the chambers of the heart. Depending on the configuration of the pacemaker and the clinical needs of the patient, as many as three leads may be used in a pacing system. Current pacemakers have a double, or bipolar, electrode attached to the end of each lead. The electrodes deliver an electrical charge to the heart to regulate heartbeat. They are positioned on the areas of the heart that require stimulation.

The leads are then attached to the pacemaker device, which is implanted under the skin of the patient's chest.

Patients undergoing surgical pacemaker implantation usually stay in the hospital overnight. Once the procedure is complete, the patient's **vital signs** are monitored and a **chest x ray** is taken to ensure that the pacemaker and leads are properly positioned.

Modern pacemakers have sophisticated programming capabilities and are extremely compact. The smallest weigh less than 13 grams (under half an ounce) and are the size of two stacked silver dollars. The actual pacing device contains a pulse generator, circuitry programmed to monitor heart rate and deliver stimulation, and a lithium iodide battery. Battery life typically ranges from seven to 15 years, depending on the number of leads the pacemaker is configured with and how much energy the pacemaker uses. When a new battery is required, the unit can be exchanged in a simple outpatient procedure.

A temporary pacing system is sometimes recommended for patients who are experiencing irregular heartbeats as a result of a recent heart attack or other

Pacemaker

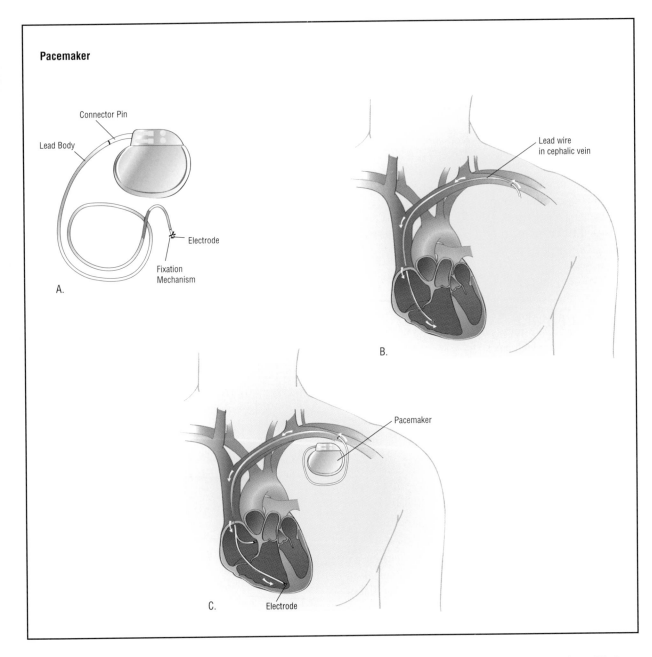

Connector Pin

Lead Body

Electrode

Fixation
Mechanism

A.

Lead wire
in cephalic vein

B.

Pacemaker

C.   Electrode

To place a pacemaker, a lead wire is inserted into the cephalic vein of the shoulder and fed into the heart chambers (B). An electrode is implanted in the heart muscle of the lower chamber, and the device is attached (C). *(Illustration by Argosy.)*

acute medical condition. The implantation procedure for the pacemaker leads is similar to that for a permanent pacing system, but the actual pacemaker unit housing the pulse generator remains outside the patient's body. Temporary pacing systems may be replaced with a permanent device at a later date.

Diagnosis/Preparation

Patients being considered for pacemaker implantation will undergo a full battery of cardiac tests, including an electrocardiogram (ECG) or an electrophysiological study or both, to fully evaluate the bradycardia or tachycardia.

The symptoms of fatigue and lightheadedness that are characteristic of bradycardia can also be caused by a number of other medical conditions, including anemia. Certain prescription medications can also slow the heart rate. A doctor should take a complete medical history and perform a full physical work-up to rule out all non-cardiac causes of bradycardia.

Patients are advised to abstain from eating six to eight hours before the surgical procedure. The patient is usually given a sedative to help him or her relax for the procedure. An intravenous (IV) line will also be inserted into a vein in the patient's arm before the procedure begins in case medication or blood products are required during the insertion.

Aftercare

After an implant without complications the patient can expect a hospital stay of one to five post-procedure days. Pacemaker patients should schedule a follow-up visit with their cardiologist approximately six weeks after the surgery. During this visit, the doctor will make any necessary adjustments to the settings of the pacemaker. Pacemakers are programmed externally with a handheld electromagnetic device. Pacemaker batteries must be checked regularly. Some pacing systems allow patients to monitor battery life through a special telephone monitoring service that can read pacemaker signals.

Patients with cardiac pacemakers should not undergo a **magnetic resonance imaging** (MRI) procedure. Devices that emit electromagnetic waves (including magnets) may alter pacemaker programming or functioning. A 1997 study found that cellular phones often interfere with pacemaker programming and cause irregular heart rhythm. However, advances in pacemaker design and materials have greatly reduced the risk of pacemaker interference from electromagnetic fields.

Risks

Because pacemaker implantation is an invasive surgical procedure, internal bleeding, infection, hemorrhage, and embolism are all possible complications. Infection is more common in patients with temporary pacing systems. Antibiotic therapy given as a precautionary measure can reduce the risk of pacemaker infection. If infection does occur, the entire pacing system may have to be removed.

The placing of the leads and electrodes during the implantation procedure also presents certain risks for the patient. The lead or electrode could perforate the heart or cause scarring or other damage. The electrodes can also cause involuntary stimulation of nearby skeletal muscles.

A complication known as pacemaker syndrome develops in approximately 7% of pacemaker patients with single-chamber pacing systems. The syndrome is characterized by the low blood pressure and dizziness that are symptomatic of bradycardia. It can usually be corrected by the implantation of a dual-chamber pacing system.

QUESTIONS TO ASK THE DOCTOR

- How many pacemaker implants has the physician performed?
- What type of pacemaker will be implanted, univentricular or biventricular, and how many of the specific procedure has the physician performed?
- How long will the expected hospital stay be?
- What precautions should be taken in the weeks following discharge from the hospital?
- What precautions will need to taken in day to day activities following pacemaker implant?
- When can normal daily, such as driving, **exercise** and work, activities be initiated?
- What will indicate that the pacemaker is failing and when should emergency care be sought?
- How long will the battery function and when should treatment to replace the device be sought?
- Is there special documentation I will need for air travel during security screenings?
- Will there be notification of manufacturer recalls?

Normal results

Pacemakers that are properly implanted and programmed can correct a patient's arrhythmia and resolve related symptoms.

Morbidity and mortality rates

In the United States, patients experience complications in 3.3% and 3.8% of cases, with those over 65 years of age demonstrating a slightly higher complication rate of 6.1%. The most common complications include lead dislodgement, pneumothorax (collapsed lung), and cardiac perforation. The risk of death is less then 0.5% throughout the course of the hospital stay.

Resources

BOOKS

DeBakey, Michael E. and Antonio Gotto Jr. *The New Living Heart.* Holbrook, MA: Adams Media Corporation, 1997.

KEY TERMS

Electrocardiogram (ECG)—A recording of the electrical activity of the heart. An ECG uses externally attached electrodes to detect the electrical signals of the heart.

Electrophysiological study—A test that monitors the electrical activity of the heart in order to diagnose arrhythmia. An electrophysiological study measures electrical signals through a cardiac catheter that is inserted into an artery in the leg and guided up into the atrium and ventricle of the heart.

Embolism—A blood clot, air bubble, or clot of foreign material that blocks the flow of blood in an artery. When an embolism blocks the blood supply to a tissue or organ, the tissue the artery feeds dies (infarction). Without immediate and appropriate treatment, an embolism can be fatal.

Magnetic resonance imaging (MRI)—An imaging technique that uses a large circular magnet and radio waves to generate signals from atoms in the body. These signals are used to construct images of internal structures.

PERIODICALS

Gregoratas, Gabriel, et al. "ACC/AHA Guidelines for Implantation of Pacemakers and Antiarrhythmia Devices." *Journal of the American College of Cardiology* 31 (April 1998): 1175–209.

Link, Mark S, et al. "Complications of Dual Chamber Pacemaker Implantation in the Elderly." *Journal of Interventional Cardiac Electrophysiology* 2 (1998): 175–179.

ORGANIZATIONS

American Heart Association. 7320 Greenville Ave. Dallas, TX 75231. (214) 373-6300. <http://www.americanheart.org>.

Paula Anne Ford-Martin
Allison J. Spiwak, MSBME

Packed cell volume *see* **Hematocrit**

Packed red blood cell volume *see* **Hematocrit**

Pain management

Definition

If pain can be defined as a highly unpleasant, individualized experience of one of the body's defense mechanisms indicating an injury or problem, pain management encompasses all interventions used to understand and ease pain, and, if possible, to alleviate the cause of the pain.

Purpose

Pain serves to alert a person to potential or actual damage to the body. The definition for damage is quite broad: pain can arise from injury as well as disease. After the message is received and interpreted, further pain can be counterproductive. Pain can have a negative impact on a person's quality of life and impede recovery from illness or injury, thus contributing to escalating health care costs. Unrelieved pain can become a syndrome in its own right and cause a downward spiral in a person's health and outlook. Managing pain properly facilitates recovery, prevents additional health complications, and improves an individual's quality of life.

Yet, the experiencing of pain is a completely unique occurrence for each person, a complex combination of several factors other than the pain itself. It is influenced by:

• Ethnic and cultural values. In some cultures, tolerating pain is related to showing strength and endurance. In others, it is considered punishment for misdeeds.

• Age. This refers to the concept that grownups never cry.

• Anxiety and stress. This is related to being in a strange, fearful place such as a hospital, and the fear of the unknown consequences of the pain and the condition causing it, which can all combined to make pain feel more severe. For patients being treated for pain, knowing the duration of activity of an analgesic leads to anxiety about the return of pain when the drug wears off. This anxiety can make the pain more severe.

• Fatigue and depression. It is known that pain in itself can actually cause depression. Fatigue from lack of sleep or the illness itself also contribute to depressed feelings.

Precautions

The perception of pain is an individual experience. Health care providers play an important role in understanding their patients' pain. All too often, both physicians and nurses have been found to incorrectly assess the severity of pain. A study reported in the *Journal of Advanced Nursing* evaluated nurses' perceptions of a select group of white American and Mexican-American women patients' pain following gallbladder surgery. Objective assessments of each patient's pain showed little difference between the perceived severities for each group. Yet, the nurses involved in the study consistently rated all patients' pain as less than the patients reported, and with equal consistency, believed that better-educated women born in the United States were suffering more than less-educated Mexican-American women. Nurses from a northern European background were more apt to minimize the severity of pain than nurses from eastern and southern Europe or Africa. The study indicated how health care staff, and especially nursing staff, need to be aware of how their own background and experience contributes to how they perceive a person's pain.

In a 1990 study reported in the journal *Pain*, nurses were found to overestimate the severity of pain in patients with severe burns. In most other studies, nurses and physicians ascribe a lower pain severity than do patients.

Description

Before considering pain management, a review of pain definitions and mechanisms may be useful. Pain is the means by which the peripheral nervous system (PNS) warns the central nervous system (CNS) of injury or potential injury to the body. The CNS comprises the brain and spinal cord, and the PNS is composed of the nerves that stem from and lead into the CNS. PNS includes all nerves throughout the body, except the brain and spinal cord. Pain is sometimes categorized by its site of origin, either cutaneous (originating in the skin of subcutaneous tissue, such as a shaving nick or paper cut), deep somatic pain (arising from bone, ligaments and tendons, nerves, or veins and arteries), or visceral (appearing as a result of stimulation of pain receptor nerves around organs such as the brain, lungs, or those in the abdomen).

A pain message is transmitted to the CNS by special PNS nerve cells called nociceptors, which are distributed throughout the body and respond to different stimuli depending on their location. For example, nociceptors that extend from the skin are stimulated by sensations such as pressure, temperature, and chemical changes.

When a nociceptor is stimulated, neurotransmitters are released within the cell. Neurotransmitters are chemicals found within the nervous system that facilitate nerve cell communication. The nociceptor transmits its signal to nerve cells within the spinal cord, which conveys the pain message to the thalamus, a specific region in the brain.

Once the brain has received and processed the pain message and coordinated an appropriate response, pain has served its purpose. The body uses natural painkillers, called endorphins, to derail further pain messages from the same source. However, these natural painkillers may not adequately dampen a continuing pain message. Also, depending on how the brain has processed the pain information, certain hormones such as prostaglandins may be released. These hormones enhance the pain message and play a role in immune system responses to injury, such as inflammation. Certain neurotransmitters, especially substance P and calcitonin gene-related peptide, actively enhance the pain message at the injury site and within the spinal cord.

Pain is generally divided into two additional categories: acute and chronic. Nociceptive pain, or the pain that is transmitted by nociceptors, is typically called acute pain. This kind of pain is associated with injury, headaches, disease, and many other conditions. Response to acute pain is made by the sympathetic nervous system (the nerves responsible for the fight-or-flight response of the body). It normally resolves once the condition that precipitated it is resolved.

Following some disorders, pain does not resolve. Even after healing or a cure has been achieved, the brain continues to perceive pain. In this situation, the pain may be considered chronic. Chronic pain is within the province of the parasympathetic nervous system, and the changeover occurs as the body attempts to adapt to the pain. The time limit used to define chronic pain typically ranges from three to six months, although some health care professionals prefer a more flexible definition, and consider chronic pain as pain that endures beyond a normal healing time. The pain associated with cancer; persistent and degenerative conditions; and neuropathy, or nerve damage, is included in the chronic category. Also, unremitting pain that lacks an identifiable physical cause such as the majority of cases of low back pain may be considered chronic. The underlying biochemistry of chronic pain appears to be different from regular nociceptive pain.

It has been hypothesized that uninterrupted and unrelenting pain can induce changes in the spinal cord. In the past, severing a nerve's connection to the CNS has treated intractable pain. However, the lack of any sensory information being relayed by that nerve can cause pain transmission in the spinal cord to go into overdrive, as evidenced by the phantom limb pain experienced by amputees. Evidence is accumulating that unrelenting pain or the complete lack of nerve signals increases the number of pain receptors in the spinal cord. Nerve cells in the spinal cord may also begin secreting pain-amplifying neurotransmitters independent of actual pain signals from the body. Immune chemicals, primarily cytokines, may play a prominent role in such changes.

Managing pain

Considering the different causes and types of pain, as well as its nature and intensity, management can require an interdisciplinary approach. The elements of this approach include treating the underlying cause of pain, pharmacological and non-pharmacological therapies, and some invasive (surgical) procedures.

Treating the cause of pain underpins the idea of managing it. Injuries are repaired, diseases are diagnosed, and certain encounters with pain can be anticipated and treated prophylactically (by prevention). However, there are no guarantees of immediate relief from pain. Recovery can be impeded by pain and quality of life can be damaged. Therefore, pharmacological and other therapies have developed over time to address these aspects of disease and injury.

PHARMACOLOGICAL OPTIONS. General guidelines developed by the World Health Organization (WHO) have been developed for pain management. These guidelines operate upon the following three-step ladder approach:

• Mild pain is alleviated with **acetaminophen** or a nonsteroidal anti-inflammatory drug (NSAID). NSAIDs and acetaminophen are available as over-the-counter and prescription medications, and are frequently the initial pharmacological treatment for pain. These drugs can also be used as adjuncts to the other drug therapies that might require a doctor's prescription. NSAIDs include **aspirin**, ibuprofen (Motrin, Advil, Nuprin), naproxen sodium (Aleve), and ketoprofen (Orudis KT). These drugs are used to treat pain from inflammation and work by blocking production of pain-enhancing neurotransmitters. Acetaminophen is also effective against pain, but its ability to reduce inflammation is limited. NSAIDs and acetaminophen are effective for most forms of acute (sharp, but of a short duration) pain.

• Mild to moderate pain is eased with a milder opioid medication, plus acetaminophen or NSAIDs. Opioids are both actual opiate drugs such as morphine and codeine, and synthetic drugs based on the structure of opium. This drug class includes drugs such as oxycodon, methadone, and meperidine (Demerol). They provide pain relief by binding to specific opioid receptors in the brain and spinal cord.

• Moderate to severe pain is treated with stronger opioid drugs, plus acetaminophen or NSAIDs. Morphine is sometimes referred to as the gold standard of palliative care as it is not expensive, can be given by starting with smaller doses and gradually increased, and is highly effective over a long period of time. It can also be given by a number of different routes, including by mouth, rectally, or by injection.

Although antidepressant drugs were developed to treat depression, it has been discovered that they are also effective in combating chronic headaches, cancer pain, and pain associated with nerve damage. Antidepressants that have been shown to have analgesic (pain-reducing) properties include amitriptyline (Elavil), trazodone (Desyrel), and imipramine (Tofranil). Anticonvulsant drugs share a similar background with antidepressants. Developed to treat epilepsy, anticonvulsants were found to relieve pain as well. Drugs such as phenytoin (Dilantin) and carbamazepine (Tegretol) are prescribed to treat the pain associated with nerve damage.

Close monitoring of the effects of pain medications is required in order to assure that adequate amounts of medication are given to produce the desired pain relief. When a person is comfortable with a certain dosage of medication, oncologists typically convert to a long-acting version of that medication. Transdermal fentanyl patches (Duragesic) are a common example of a long-acting opioid drug often used for cancer pain management. A patch containing the drug is applied to the skin and continues to deliver the drug to the person for typically three days. Pumps are also available that provide an opioid medication upon demand when the person is experiencing pain. By pressing a button, they can release a set dose of medication into an intravenous solution or an implanted catheter. Another mode of administration involves implanted catheters that deliver pain medication directly to the spinal cord. Because these pumps offer the patient some degree of control over the amount of analgesic administered, the system, commonly called patient controlled analgesia (PCA), reduces the level of anxiety about availability of pain medication. Delivering drugs in this way can reduce side effects and increase the effectiveness of the drug. Research is underway to develop toxic substances that act selectively on nerve cells that carry pain messages to the brain. These substances would kill the selected cells and thus stop transmission of the pain message.

NON-PHARMACOLOGICAL OPTIONS. Pain treatment options that do not use drugs are often used as adjuncts to, rather than replacements for, drug therapy. One of the benefits of non-drug therapies is that an individual can take a more active stance against pain. Relaxation techniques such as yoga and meditation are used to focus the brain elsewhere than on the pain, decrease muscle tension, and reduce stress. Tension and stress can also be reduced through biofeedback, in which an individual consciously attempts to modify skin temperature, muscle tension, blood pressure, and heart rate.

Participating in normal activities and exercising can also help control pain levels. Through physical therapy, an individual learns beneficial exercises for reducing stress, strengthening muscles, and staying fit. Regular **exercise** has been linked to production of endorphins, the body's natural painkillers.

Acupuncture involves the insertion of small needles into the skin at key points. Acupressure uses these same key points, but involves applying pressure rather than inserting needles. Both of these methods may work by prompting the body to release endorphins. Applying heat or being massaged are very relaxing and help reduce stress. Transcutaneous electrical nerve stimulation (TENS) applies a small electric current to certain parts of nerves, potentially interrupting pain signals and inducing release of endorphins. To be effective, use of TENS should be medically supervised.

INVASIVE PROCEDURES. There are three types of invasive procedures that may be used to manage or treat pain: anatomic, augmentative, and ablative. These procedures involve surgery, and certain guidelines should be followed before carrying out a procedure with permanent effects. First, the cause of the pain must be clearly identified. Next, surgery should be done only if noninvasive procedures are ineffective. Third, any psychological issues should be addressed. Finally, there should be a reasonable expectation of success.

Anatomic procedures involve correcting the injury or removing the cause of pain. Relatively common anatomic procedures are decompression surgeries such as repairing a herniated disk in the lower back or relieving the nerve compression related to carpal tunnel syndrome. Another anatomic procedure is neurolysis, also called a nerve block, which involves destroying a portion of a peripheral nerve.

Augmentative procedures include electrical stimulation or direct application of drugs to the nerves that are transmitting the pain signals. Electrical stimulation works on the same principle as TENS. In this procedure, instead of applying the current across the skin, electrodes are implanted to stimulate peripheral nerves or nerves in the spinal cord. Augmentative procedures also include implanted drug-delivery systems. In these systems, catheters are implanted in the spine to allow direct delivery of drugs to the CNS.

Ablative procedures are characterized by severing a nerve and disconnecting it from the CNS. However, this method may not address potential alterations within the spinal cord. These changes perpetuate pain messages and do not cease, even when the connection between the sensory nerve and the CNS is severed. With growing understanding of neuropathic pain and development of less invasive procedures, ablative procedures are used less frequently. However, they do have applications in select cases of peripheral neuropathy, cancer pain, and other disorders.

Preparation

Prior to beginning management, pain is thoroughly evaluated. Pain scales or questionnaires are used to at-

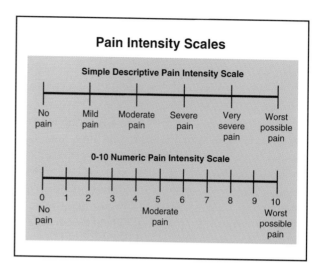

Pain intesity scales used with patients to describe their pain. *(Public domain.)*

tach an objective measure to a subjective experience. Objective measurements allow health care workers to better understand the pain being suffered by the patient. Evaluation also includes physical examinations and diagnostic tests to determine underlying causes. Some evaluations require assessments from several viewpoints, including neurology, psychiatry and psychology, and physical therapy. If pain is due to a medical procedure, management consists of anticipating the type and intensity of associated pain and managing it preemptively.

Nurses or physicians often take what is called a pain history. This will help to provide important information that can help health care providers to better manage the patient's pain. A typical pain history includes the following questions:

• Where is the pain located?

• On a scale of 1 to 10, with 1 indicating the least pain, how would the person rate the pain being experienced?

• What does the pain feel like?

• When did (or does) the pain start?

• How long has the person had it?

• Is the person sometimes free of pain?

• Does the person know of anything that triggers the pain, or makes it worse?

• Does the person have other symptoms (nausea, dizziness, blurred vision, etc.) during or after the pain?

• What pain medications or other measures has the person found to help in easing the pain?

• How does the pain affect the person's ability to carry on normal activities?

KEY TERMS

Acute—Referring to pain in response to injury or other stimulus that resolves when the injury heals or the stimulus is removed.

Central nervous system (CNS)—The part of the nervous system that includes the brain and the spinal cord.

Chronic—Referring to pain that endures beyond the term of an injury or painful stimulus. Can also refer to cancer pain, pain from a chronic or degenerative disease, and pain from an unidentified cause.

Iatrogenic—Resulting from the activity of the physician.

Neuropathy—Nerve damage.

Neurotransmitter—Chemicals within the nervous system that transmit information from or between nerve cells.

Nociceptor—A nerve cell that is capable of sensing pain and transmitting a pain signal.

Non-pharmacological—Referring to therapy that does not involve drugs.

Parasympathetic nervous system—That part of the autonomic nervous system consisting of nerves that arise from the cranial and sacral regions and function in opposition to the sympathetic nervous system.

Peripheral nervous system (PNS)—Nerves that are outside of the brain and spinal cord.

Pharmacological—Referring to therapy that relies on drugs.

Stimulus—A factor capable of eliciting a response in a nerve.

Sympathetic nervous system—That portion of the autonomic nervous system consisting of nerves that originate in the thoracic and lumbar spinal cord and function in opposition to the parasympathetic nervous system.

• What does it mean to the person that he or she is experiencing pain?

Aftercare

An assessment by nursing staff as well as other health care providers should be made to determine the effectiveness of the pain management interventions employed. There are objective, measurable signs and symptoms of pain that can be looked for. The goal of good pain management is the absence of these signs. Signs of acute pain include:

• rise in pulse and blood pressure
• more rapid breathing
• perspiring profusely, clammy skin
• taut muscles
• more tense appearance, fast speech, very alert
• unusually pale skin
• dilated pupils of the eye

    Signs of chronic pain include:

• lower pulse and blood pressure
• changeable breathing pattern
• warm, dry skin
• nausea and vomiting
• slow speech in monotone

• inability, or difficulty in getting out of bed and doing activities
• constricted pupils of the eye

When these signs are absent and the patient appears to be comfortable, health care providers can consider their interventions to have been successful. It is also important to document interventions used, and which ones were successful.

Risks

Owing to toxicity over the long term, some drugs can only be used for acute pain or as adjuncts in chronic pain management. NSAIDs have the well-known side effect of causing gastrointestinal bleeding, and long-term use of acetaminophen has been linked to kidney and liver damage. Other drugs, especially narcotics, have serious side effects such as constipation, drowsiness, and nausea. Serious side effects can also accompany pharmacological therapies; mood swings, confusion, bone thinning, cataract formation, increased blood pressure, and other problems may discourage or prevent use of some **analgesics**.

Non-pharmacological therapies carry little or no risks. However, it is advised that individuals recovering from serious illness or injury consult with the health care providers or physical therapists before making use of adjunct therapies. Invasive procedures carry risks similar to other surgical procedures, such as infection, reaction to anesthesia, and iatrogenic (injury as a result of treatment) injury.

A traditional concern about narcotics use has been the risk of promoting addiction. As narcotic use continues over time, the body becomes accustomed to the drug and adjusts normal functions to accommodate to its presence. Therefore, to elicit the same level of action, it is necessary to increase dosage over time. As dosage increases, an individual may become physically dependent on narcotic drugs.

However, physical dependence is different from psychological addiction. Physical dependence is characterized by discomfort if drug administration suddenly stops, while psychological addiction is characterized by an overpowering craving for the drug for reasons other than pain relief. Psychological addiction is a very real and necessary concern in some instances, but it should not interfere with a genuine need for narcotic pain relief. However, caution must be taken with people who have a history of addictive behavior.

Normal results

Effective application of pain management techniques reduces or eliminates acute or chronic pain. This treatment can improve an individual's quality of life and aid in recovery from injury and disease.

Resources

BOOKS

Kozier, Barbara, Glenora Erb, Kathleen Blais, and Judith M. Wilkinson. *Fundamentals of Nursing, Concepts, Process and Practice,* 5th edition. Redwood City, CA: Addison-Wesley, 1995.

Salerno, Evelyn, and Joyce S. Willens, eds. *Pain Management Handbook: An Interdisciplinary Approach.* St. Louis: Mosby, 1996.

PERIODICALS

Choiniere, M., R. Melzack, N. Girard, J. Rondeau, and M. J. Paquin. "Comparisons between Patients' and Nurses' Assessment of Pain and Medication Efficacy in Severe Burn Injuries." *Pain* 40, no.2 (February 1990): 143–52.

Everett, J. J., D. R. Patterson, J. A. Marvin, B. Montgomery, N. Ordonez, and K. Campbell. "Pain Assessment from Patients with Burns and Their Nurses." *Journal of Burn Care Rehabilitation* 15, no.2 (Mar–Apr 1994): 194–8.

McPherson, M. L., C. D. Ponte, and R. M. Respond (eds.). "Profiles in Pain Management." *Journal of the American Pharmacists Association* (June 2003).

ORGANIZATIONS

American Chronic Pain Association. P.O. Box 850, Rocklin, CA 95677-0850. (916) 632-0922. <http://members.tripod.com/~widdy/acpa.html>.

American Pain Society. 4700 West Lake Ave., Glenview, IL 60025. (847) 375-4715. <http://www.ampainsoc.org>.

National Chronic Pain Outreach Association, Inc. P.O. Box 274, Millboro, VA 24460- 9606. (540) 597-5004.

OTHER

What We Know About Pain. National Institute of Dental Research, National Institute of Health, Bethseda, MD 20892. (301) 496-4261.

Joan M. Schonbeck
Sam Uretsky, PharmD

Pain relievers *see* **Analgesics**

Pallidotomy

Definition

Pallidotomy is the destruction of a small region of the brain, the globus pallidus internus, in order to treat some of the symptoms of Parkinson's disease.

Purpose

The symptoms of Parkinson's disease (PD) include rigidity, slowed movements, and tremor, along with postural instability and a variety of non-motor symptoms (i.e., symptoms not involving movement). These symptoms are due to degeneration of a small portion of the brain called the substantia nigra, the cells of which secrete the chemical dopamine that influences cells in another brain region called the globus pallidus internus (GPi). Together with other brain regions, these two structures take part in complex control loops that govern certain aspects of movement and, when substantia nigra cells degenerate, these loops are disrupted and movements become unregulated, producing the symptoms of Parkinson's disease.

The effects of dopamine on the brain can be mimicked by the drug levodopa: levodopa therapy is the mainstay of PD treatment in its early stages. Unfortunately, levodopa becomes less effective over time, and also produces unwanted and uncontrolled movements called dyskinesias. This may occur after five to 10 years or more of successful levodopa treatment. Once a patient can no longer be treated effectively with levodopa, surgery is considered as a management option. Pallidotomy is one of the main surgical options for treatment of advanced PD.

The effect of dopamine on the cells of the GPi is to suppress them by preventing them from firing. Pallidoto-

WHO PERFORMS THE PROCEDURE AND WHERE IS IT PERFORMED?

Pallidotomy is performed in the hospital by a neurosurgeon, in coordination with the patient's neurologist.

my mimics this action by permanently destroying the GPi cells. It may seem odd that the treatment for degeneration of one brain area is to destroy another, but in the absence of dopamine, the GPi cells are overactive, and therefore, eliminating them is an appropriate treatment.

The GPi has two halves that control movements on opposites sides: right controls left, left controls right. Unilateral (one-sided) pallidotomy may be used if symptoms are markedly worse on one side or the other, or if the risks from bilateral (two-sided) pallidotomy are judged to be too great.

Demographics

Parkinson's disease affects approximately one million Americans. The peak incidence is approximately at age 62, but young-onset PD can occur as early as age 40. Because young-onset patients live with their disease for so many more years, they are more likely to become candidates for surgery than older-onset patients. In addition, younger patients tend to do better with surgery and suffer fewer adverse effects from the surgery. Approximately 5% of older PD patients receive one form or another of PD surgery; many more develop the symptoms for which surgery may be effective, but either develop them at an advanced age, making surgery inadvisable, or decide the risks of surgery are not worth the potential benefit, or do not choose surgery for some other reason.

Description

Pallidotomy requires the insertion of a long needle-like probe deep into the brain through a hole in the top of the skull. In order to precisely locate the GPi target, and to ensure the probe is precisely placed in the target, a "stereotactic frame" is used. This device is a rigid frame attached to the patient's head, providing an immobile three-dimensional coordinate system, which can be used to precisely track the location of the GPi and the movement of the probe.

For unilateral pallidotomy, a single "burr hole" is made in the top of the skull; bilateral pallidotomy re-

quires two holes. A strong topical anesthetic is used to numb the shaved area before this hole is drilled. Since there are no pain receptors in the brain, there is no need for deeper anesthetic. In addition, the patient must remain awake in order to report any sensory changes during the surgery. The lesion made in the GPi is very close to the optic tract that carries visual information from the eyes to the rear of the brain. Visual changes may indicate the probe is too close to this region.

Once the burr hole is made, the surgeon inserts a microelectrode probe, which is used to more precisely locate the GPi. Electrical stimulation of the brain through the electrode can help determine exactly which structure is being stimulated. This is harmless, but may cause twitching, light flashes, or other sensations. A contrast dye may also be injected into the spinal fluid, which allows the surgeon to visualize the brain's structure using one or more imaging techniques. During the procedure, the patient will be asked to make various movements to assist in determining the location of the electrode.

When the proper target is located, the electrode tip is briefly heated, carefully destroying the surrounding tissue to about the size of a pearl. If bilateral pallidotomy is being performed, the localizing and lesioning will be repeated on the other side.

Diagnosis/Preparation

Pallidotomy is performed in patients with Parkinson's disease who are still responsive to levodopa, but who have developed disabling drug treatment complications known as motor fluctuations, including rapid wearing off of drug effect, unpredictable "off states" (times of low levodopa levels in the blood), and disabling dyskinesias. Those who are very elderly, demented, or with other significant medical conditions that would be compromised by surgery are usually not candidates for pallidotomy.

The surgical candidate should discuss all the surgical options with the neurologist before deciding on pallidotomy. A full understanding of the risks and potential benefits must be understood before consenting to the surgery.

The patient will undergo a variety of medical tests, and one or more types of neuroimaging procedures, including **magnetic resonance imaging** (MRI), computed tomography (CT) scanning, **angiography** (imaging the brain's blood vessels), and ventriculography (imaging the brain's ventricles). On the day of the surgery, the stereotactic frame will be fixed to the patient's head. First, a local anesthetic is applied at the four sites where the frame's pins contact the head; there may nonetheless be some initial discomfort. A final MRI is done with the frame in place to help set the coordinates of the GPi in relation to the frame.

The patient will receive a mild sedative to ease the anxiety of the procedure.

Aftercare

The procedure requires several hours. Some centers perform pallidotomy as an outpatient procedure, sending the patient home the same day. Most centers keep the patient overnight or longer for observation. Patients will feel improved movement immediately. Medications may be adjusted somewhat to accommodate the changes in symptoms.

Risks

The key to successful outcome in pallidotomy is extremely precise placement of the electrode. While there are several controversies in the field of PD surgery, all experts agree that risks are reduced in procedures performed by the most experienced neurosurgeons.

Hemorrhage in the brain is a possible complication, as is infection. There are small but significant risks of damage to the optic tract, which can cause visual deficits. Speech impairments may also occur, including difficulty retrieving words and slurred speech. Some cognitively fragile patients may become even more impaired after surgery.

Normal results

Pallidotomy improves the motor ability of patients, especially during "off" periods. Studies show the procedure generally improves tremor, rigidity, and slowed movements by 25–60%. Dyskinesias typically improve by 75% or more. Improvements from unilateral pallidotomy are primarily on the side opposite the surgery. Balance does not improve, nor do non-motor symptoms such as drooling, constipation, and orthostatic hypotension (lightheadedness on standing).

Morbidity and mortality rates

Among the best surgeons, the risk of serious morbidity or mortality is 1–2%. Hemorrhage may occur in 2–6%, visual field deficits in 0–6%, and weakness in 2–8%. Most patients gain weight after surgery.

Alternatives

Patients whose symptoms are well managed by drugs are not recommended for surgery, and significant effort will usually be made to adjust medications to control symptoms before surgery is considered.

Thalamotomy, surgery to the thalamus, was recommended in the past to control tremor. It is rarely per-

---

QUESTIONS TO ASK THE DOCTOR

- How many pallidotomies has the neurosurgeon performed?
- What is the surgeon's own rate of serious complications?
- Would **deep brain stimulation** of the subthalamic nucleus be appropriate for me?
- How will my medications change after the operation?

---

formed today, and few centers would consider thalamotomy for any patient unless tremor was the only troubling and uncontrolled symptom.

Deep-brain stimulation (DBS) of the GPi is an alternative treatment in widespread use, as is DBS of another brain region, the subthalamic nucleus. Both procedures use permanemtly implanted, programmable electrodes to deliver a very small, continuous electric current to the target region. This has the same effect as a lesion, but is adjustable. DBS of the subthalamic nucleus typically produces better symtomatic results that either DBS to the GPi or pallidotomy. However, both forms of DBS carry the risk of long-term complications from the implanted hardware, as well as other risks.

See also Deep brain stimulation.

Resources

BOOKS

Jahanshahi, M., and C. D. Marsden. *Parkinson's Disease: A Self-Help Guide.* New York: Demos Medical Press, 2000.

ORGANIZATIONS

National Parkinson's Disease Foundation. <http://www.npf.org>. WE MOVE. <http://www.wemove.org>.

Richard Robinson

Pancreas removal *see* **Pancreatectomy**

Pancreas transplantation

Definition

Pancreas transplantation is a surgical procedure in which a diseased pancreas is replaced with a healthy

---

pancreas that has been obtained from an immunologically compatible cadavear or living donor.

Purpose

The pancreas secretes insulin that regulates glucose (blood sugar) metabolism. Patients with type I diabetes have experienced partial or complete damage to the insulin-producing beta cells of the pancreas. Consequently, they are unable to generate sufficient insulin to control blood glucose levels. Long-term uncontrolled high blood glucose levels can cause damage to every system of the body, so type I patients must inject insulin to do the work of the beta cells. Pancreas transplantation allows the body to once again make and secrete its own insulin, and establishes insulin independence for these individuals.

Demographics

It is estimated that over one million people in the United States have type 1 diabetes mellitus (also called insulin-dependant diabetes or juvenile diabetes). Among these individuals, the best candidates for pancreas transplantation are typically:

- between the ages of 20 and 40
- those who have extreme difficulty regulating their glucose levels with insulin therapy (a condition called brittle diabetes)
- those who have few secondary complications of diabetes
- those who are in good cardiovascular health

A pancreas-only transplant is an uncommon procedure, with only 163 procedures occurring in the United States in 2001. More common is the combined kidney-pancreas transplant, which was performed on 885 patients the same year. An additional 305 patients received a PAK, or pancreas after kidney transplant, according to the United Network for Organ Sharing (UNOS).

Description

Once a donor pancreas is located and tissue typing deems it compatible, the patient is contacted and prepared for surgery. Blood tests, a **chest x ray**, and an electrocardiogram (ECG) are performed and an intravenous (IV) line is started for fluid and medication administration. Once the transplant procedure is ready to start, general anesthesia is administered.

The surgeon makes an incision under the ribs and locates the pancreas and duodenum. The pancreas and duodenum (part of the small intestine) are removed. The new pancreas and duodenum are then connected to the patient's duodenum, and the blood vessels are sutured together to restore blood flow to the new pancreas. The patient's original pancreas is left in place.

Replacing the duodenum allows the pancreas to drain into the gastrointestinal system. The transplant can also be done creating bladder drainage. Bladder drainage makes it easier to monitor organ rejection because pancreatic secretions can be measured in the patient's urine. Once the new pancreas is in place, the abdomen and skin are sutured closed. This surgery is often done at the same time as kidney **transplant surgery**.

Diagnosis/Preparation

After the patient and doctor have decided on a pancreas transplant, a complete immunological study is performed to match the patient to a donor. An extensive medical history and **physical examination** is performed, including radiological exams, blood and urine tests, and psychological evaluation. Once the patient is approved for transplant, he or she will be placed on the United

Network for Organ Sharing (UNOS) Organ Center waiting list. The timing of surgery depends on the availability of a donated living or cadaver organ.

Aftercare

Patients receiving a pancreas transplantation are monitored closely for organ rejection. The average hospital stay is three weeks, and it takes about six months to recover from surgery. Patients will take **immunosuppressant drugs** for the rest of their lives.

Risks

Diabetes and poor kidney function greatly increase the risk of complications from anesthesia during surgery. Organ rejection, excessive bleeding, and infection are other major risks associated with this surgery.

The reason simultaneous kidney-pancreas transplants and pancreas after kidney transplants are performed more frequently than pancreas only transplants is the relative risk of immunosuppressant drugs in people with diabetes. People with type I diabetes are already at risk for autoimmune problems, are more prone to infections, and have a complicated medical history that makes suppressing the immune system unadvisable.

On the other hand, diabetes is also the number one cause of chronic kidney failure, or end-stage renal disease (ESRD), which makes this group more likely to eventually require a kidney transplant for survival. In those patients with diabetes who will receive or are already receiving immunosuppressive treatment for a life-saving kidney transplant, a pancreas transplant can return their ability to self-produce insulin.

Patients with type I diabetes considering pancreas transplantation alone must weigh the risks and benefits of the procedure and decide with their doctors whether life-long treatment with immunosuppressive drugs is preferable to life-long insulin dependence.

Normal results

In a successful transplant, the pancreas begins producing insulin, bringing the regulation of glucose back under control. Natural availability of insulin prevents the development of additional complications associated with diabetes, including kidney damage, vision loss, and nerve damage. Many patients report an improved quality of life.

Morbidity and mortality rates

In their 2002 Annual Report, the Organ Procurement and Transplant Network (OPTN) reported that the patient survival rate for pancreas transplant alone was 98.6% after one year and 86% after three years. Survival

KEY TERMS

Cadaver organ—A pancreas, kidney, or other organ from a brain-dead organ donor.

Duodenum—The section of the small intestine immediately after the stomach.

rates for pancreas-kidney transplant recipients were 95.1% after one year and 89.2% after three years.

Alternatives

Innovations in islet cell transplants, a procedure that involves transplanting a culture of the insulin-producing islet cells of a healthy pancreas to a patient with type I diabetes, have increased the frequency of this procedure. The Edmonton Protocol, a type of islet cell transplant developed in 1999 by Dr. James Shapiro at the University of Alberta (Canada), uses a unique immunosuppressant drug regimen that has dramatically improved success rates of the islet transplant procedure. As of early 2003, the Edmonton Protocol was still considered investigational in the United States, and a number of clinical trials were ongoing.

Resources

PERIODICALS

Norton, Patrice. "Pancreatic Human Islet Cells Offer Alternative to Pancreas Transplant." *Family Practice News.* 33 (January 2003): 14.

Reddy, K.S. et al. "Long-term survival following simultaneous kidney-pancreas transplantation versus kidney transplantation alone in patients with type 1 diabetes mellitus and renal failure." *American Journal of Kidney Disease* 41 (February 2003): 464–70.

ORGANIZATIONS

American Diabetes Association. 1701 North Beauregard Street, Alexandria, VA 22311. (800) 342-2383. <http://www.diabetes.org>.

United Network for Organ Sharing (UNOS). 700 North 4th St., Richmond, VA 23219. (888) 894-6361. <http://www.transplantliving.org>.

Tish Davidson, A.M.
Paula Anne Ford-Martin

Pancreatectomy

Definition

A pancreatectomy is the surgical removal of the pancreas. A pancreatectomy may be total, in which case the entire organ is removed, usually along with the spleen, gallbladder, common bile duct, and portions of the small intestine and stomach. A pancreatectomy may also be distal, meaning that only the body and tail of the pancreas are removed, leaving the head of the organ attached. When the duodenum is removed along with all or part of the pancreas, the procedure is called a pancreaticoduodenectomy, which surgeons sometimes refer to as "Whipple's procedure." Pancreaticoduodenectomies are increasingly used to treat a variety of malignant and benign diseases of the pancreas. This procedure often involves removal of the regional lymph nodes as well.

Purpose

A pancreatectomy is the most effective treatment for cancer of the pancreas, an abdominal organ that secretes digestive enzymes, insulin, and other hormones. The thickest part of the pancreas near the duodenum (a part of the small intestine) is called the head, the middle part is called the body, and the thinnest part adjacent to the spleen is called the tail.

While surgical removal of tumors in the pancreas is the preferred treatment, it is only possible in the 10–15% of patients who are diagnosed early enough for a potential cure. Patients who are considered suitable for surgery usually have small tumors in the head of the pancreas (close to the duodenum, or first part of the small intestine), have jaundice as their initial symptom, and have no evidence of metastatic disease (spread of cancer to other sites). The stage of the cancer will determine whether the pancreatectomy to be performed should be total or distal.

A partial pancreatectomy may be indicated when the pancreas has been severely injured by trauma, especially injury to the body and tail of the pancreas. While such surgery removes normal pancreatic tissue as well, the long-term consequences of this surgery are minimal, with virtually no effects on the production of insulin, digestive enzymes, and other hormones.

Chronic pancreatitis is another condition for which a pancreatectomy is occasionally performed. Chronic pancreatitis—or continuing inflammation of the pancreas that results in permanent damage to this organ—can develop from long-standing, recurring episodes of acute (periodic) pancreatitis. This painful condition usually results from alcohol abuse or the presence of gallstones. In most patients with the alcohol-induced disease, the pancreas is widely involved, therefore, surgical correction is almost impossible.

Description

A pancreatectomy can be performed through an open surgery technique, in which case one large incision is made, or it can be performed laparoscopically, in which case the surgeon makes four small incisions to insert tube-like **surgical instruments**. The abdomen is filled with gas, usually carbon dioxide, to help the surgeon view the abdominal cavity. A camera is inserted through one of the tubes and displays images on a monitor in the **operating room**. Other instruments are placed through the additional tubes. The laparoscopic approach allows the surgeon to work inside the patient's abdomen without making a large incision.

If the pancreatectomy is partial, the surgeon clamps and cuts the blood vessels, and the pancreas is stapled and divided for removal. If the disease affects the splenic artery or vein, the spleen is also removed.

If the pancreatectomy is total, the surgeon removes the entire pancreas and attached organs. He or she starts by dividing and detaching the end of the stomach. This part of the stomach leads to the small intestine, where the pancreas and bile duct both attach. In the next step, he removes the pancreas along with the connected section of the small intestine. The common bile duct and the gallbladder are also removed. To reconnect the intestinal tract, the stomach and the bile duct are then connected to the small intestine.

During a pancreatectomy procedure, several tubes are also inserted for **postoperative care**. To prevent tissue fluid from accumulating in the operated site, a temporary drain leading out of the body is inserted, as well as a **gastrostomy** or g-tube leading out of the stomach in order to help prevent nausea and vomiting. A jejunostomy or j-tube may also be inserted into the small intestine as a pathway for supplementary feeding.

Diagnosis/Preparation

Patients with symptoms of a pancreatic disorder undergo a number of tests before surgery is even considered. These can include ultrasonography, x ray examinations, computed tomography scans (CT scan), and **endoscopic retrograde cholangiopancreatography** (ERCP), a specialized imaging technique to visualize the ducts that carry bile from the liver to the gallbladder. Tests may also include **angiography**, another imaging technique used to visualize the arteries feeding the pancreas, and needle aspiration cytology, in which cells are drawn from areas suspected to contain cancer. Such tests are required to establish a correct diagnosis for the pancreatic disorder and in the planning the surgery.

Since many patients with pancreatic cancer are undernourished, appropriate nutritional support, sometimes by tube feedings, may be required prior to surgery.

Some patients with pancreatic cancer deemed suitable for a pancreatectomy will also undergo chemotherapy and/or radiation therapy. This treatment is aimed at shrinking the tumor, which will improve the chances for successful surgical removal. Sometimes, patients who are not initially considered surgical candidates may respond so well to chemoradiation that surgical treatment becomes possible. Radiation therapy may also be applied during the surgery (intraoperatively) to improve the patient's chances of survival, but this treatment is not yet in routine use. Some studies have shown that intraoperative radiation therapy extends survival by several months.

Patients undergoing distal pancreatectomy that involves removal of the spleen may receive preoperative medication to decrease the risk of infection.

Aftercare

Pancreatectomy is major surgery. Therefore, extended hospitalization is usually required with an average hospital stay of two to three weeks.

Some pancreatic cancer patients may also receive combined chemotherapy and radiation therapy after surgery. This additional treatment has been clearly shown to enhance survival rates.

After surgery, patients experience pain in the abdomen and are prescribed pain medication. Follow-up exams are required to monitor the patient's recovery and remove implanted tubes.

A total pancreatectomy leads to a condition called pancreatic insufficiency, because food can no longer be normally processed with the enzymes normally produced by the pancreas. Insulin secretion is likewise no longer possible. These conditions are treated with pancreatic enzyme replacement therapy, which supplies digestive enzymes; and with insulin injections. In some case, distal pancreatectomies may also lead to pancreatic insufficiency, depending on the patient's general health condition before surgery and on the extent of pancreatic tissue removal.

QUESTIONS TO ASK THE DOCTOR

- What do I need to do before surgery?
- What type of anesthesia will be used?
- How long will it take to recover from the surgery?
- When can I expect to return to work and/or resume normal activities?
- What are the risks associated with a pancreatectomy?
- How many pancreatectomies do you perform in a year?
- Will there be a scar?

Risks

There is a fairly high risk of complications associated with any pancreatectomy procedure. A recent Johns Hopkins study documented complications in 41% of cases. The most devastating complication is postoperative bleeding, which increases the mortality risk to 20–50%. In cases of postoperative bleeding, the patient may be returned to surgery to find the source of hemorrhage, or may undergo other procedures to stop the bleeding.

One of the most common complications from a pancreaticoduodenectomy is delayed gastric emptying, a condition in which food and liquids are slow to leave the stomach. This complication occurred in 19% of patients in the Johns Hopkins study. To manage this problem, many surgeons insert feeding tubes at the original operation site, through which nutrients can be fed directly into the patient's intestines. This procedure, called enteral nutrition, maintains the patient's nutrition if the stomach is slow to recover normal function. Certain medications, called promotility agents, can help move the nutritional contents through the gastrointestinal tract.

The other most common complication is pancreatic anastomotic leak. This is a leak in the connection that the surgeon makes between the remainder of the pancreas and the other structures in the abdomen. Most surgeons handle the potential for this problem by checking the connection during surgery.

Normal results

After a total pancreatectomy, the body loses the ability to secrete insulin, enzymes, and other substances; therefore, the patient has to take supplements for the rest of his/her life.

KEY TERMS

Chemotherapy—A treatment of cancer with synthetic drugs that destroy the tumor either by inhibiting the growth of the cancerous cells or by killing the cancer cells.

Computed tomography (CT) scan—An imaging technique that creates a series of pictures of areas inside the body, taken from different angles. The pictures are created by a computer linked to an x ray machine.

Endoscopic retrograde cholangiopancreatography (ERCP)—A procedure to x ray the ducts (tubes) that carry bile from the liver to the gallbladder and from the gallbladder to the small intestine.

Laparoscopy—In this procedure, a laparoscope (a thin, lighted tube) is inserted through an incision in the abdominal wall to determine if the cancer is within the pancreas only or has spread to nearby tissues and if it can be removed by surgery later. Tissue samples may be removed for biopsy.

Magnetic resonance imaging (MRI)—A procedure in which a magnet linked to a computer is used to create detailed pictures of areas inside the body.

Pancreas—A large gland located on the back wall of the abdomen, extending from the duodenum (first part of the small intestine) to the spleen. The pancreas produces enzymes essential for digestion,

and the hormones insulin and glucagon, which play a role in diabetes.

Pancreaticoduodenectomy—Removal of all or part of the pancreas along with the duodenum. Also known as "Whipple's procedure" or "Whipple's operation."

Pancreatitis—Inflammation of the pancreas, either acute (sudden and episodic) or chronic, usually caused by excessive alcohol intake or gallbladder disease.

Positron emission tomography (PET) scan—A PET scan creates a picture showing the location of tumor cells in the body. A substance called radionuclide dye is injected into a vein, and the PET scanner rotates around the body to create the picture. Malignant tumor cells show up brighter in the picture because they are more active and take up more dye than normal cells.

Radiation therapy—A treatment using high-energy radiation from x ray machines, cobalt, radium, or other sources.

Ultrasonogram—A procedure where high-frequency sound waves that cannot be heard by human ears are bounced off internal organs and tissues. These sound waves produce a pattern of echoes which are then used by the computer to create sonograms, or pictures of areas inside the body.

Patients usually resume normal activities within a month. They are asked to avoid heavy lifting for six to eight weeks following surgery and not to drive as long as they take narcotic medication.

When a pancreatectomy is performed for chronic pancreatitis, the majority of patients obtain some relief from pain. Some studies report that one-half to three-quarters of patients become free of pain.

Morbidity and mortality rates

The mortality rate for pancreatectomy has decreased in recent years to 5–10%, depending on the extent of the surgery and the experience of the surgeon. A study of 650 patients at Johns Hopkins Medical Institution, Baltimore, found that only nine patients, or 1.4%, died from complications related to surgery.

Unfortunately, pancreatic cancer is the most lethal form of gastrointestinal malignancy. However, for a highly selective group of patients, a pancreatectomy offers a chance for cure, especially when performed by experienced surgeons. The overall five-year survival rate for patients who undergo pancreatectomy for pancreatic cancer is about 10%; patients who undergo pancreaticoduodenectomy have a 4–5% survival at five years. The risk for tumor recurrence is thought to be unaffected by whether the patient undergoes a total pancreatectomy or a pancreaticoduodenectomy, but is increased when the tumor is larger than 1.2 in (3 cm) and the cancer has spread to the lymph nodes or surrounding tissue.

Alternatives

Depending on the medical condition, a **pancreas transplantation** may be considered as an alternative for some patients.

See also Pancreas transplantation.

Resources

BOOKS

Bastidas, J. Augusto, and John E. Niederhuber. "The Pancreas." In *Fundamentals of Surgery*. Edited by John E. Niederhuber. Stamford: Appleton & Lange, 1998.

Mayer, Robert J. "Pancreatic Cancer." In *Harrison's Principles of Internal Medicine*. Edited by Anthony S. Fauci, et al. New York: McGraw-Hill, 1997.

PERIODICALS

Cretolle, C., C. N. Fekete, D. Jan, et al. "Partial elective pancreatectomy is curative in focal form of permanent hyperinsulinemic hypoglycaemia in infancy: A report of 45 cases from 1983 to 2000." *Journal of Pediatric Surgery* 37 (February 2002): 155–158.

Lillemoe, K. D., S. Kaushal, J. L. Cameron, et al. "Distal pancreatectomy: indications and outcomes in 235 patients." *Annals of Surgery* 229 (May 1999): 698–700.

McAndrew, H. F., V. Smith, and L. Spitz. "Surgical complications of pancreatectomy for persistent hyperinsulinaemic hypoglycaemia of infancy." *Journal of Pediatric Surgery* 38 (January 2003): 13–16.

Patterson, E. J., M. Gagner, B. Salky, et al. "Laparoscopic pancreatic resection: single-institution experience of 19 patients." *Journal of the American College of Surgeons* 193 (September 2001): 281–287.

ORGANIZATIONS

American College of Gastroenterology. 4900 B South 31st St., Arlington, VA 22206. (703) 820-7400. <http://www.acg.gi.org>.

American Gastroenterological Association (AGA). 4930 Del Ray Avenue, Bethesda, MD 20814. (301) 654-2055. <http://www.gastro.org>.

National Cancer Institute (NCI). NCI Public Inquiries Office, Suite 3036A, 6116 Executive Boulevard, MSC8322 Bethesda, MD 20892-8322. (800) 422-6237. <http://www.cancer.gov>.

OTHER

NIH CancerNet: Pancreatic Cancer Homepage. [cited July 1, 2003]. <http://www.cancer.gov/cancerinfo/types/pancreatic>.

Caroline A. Helwick
Monique Laberge, Ph.D.

Paracentesis

Definition

Paracentesis is a minimally invasive procedure using a needle to remove fluid from the abdomen.

Purpose

There are two reasons to take fluid out of the abdomen. One is to analyze it for diagnostic purposes; the other is to relieve pressure. Liquid that accumulates in the abdomen is called ascites. Ascites seeps out of organs for several reasons related either to disease in the organ or fluid pressures that are changing.

Liver disease

All the blood flowing through the intestines passes through the liver on its way back to the heart. When progressive disease such as alcohol damage or hepatitis destroys enough liver tissue, the scarring that results shrinks the liver and constricts blood flow. Such scarring of the liver is called cirrhosis. Pressure builds in the intestinal blood circulation, slowing flow and pushing fluid into the surrounding tissues. Slowly the fluid accumulates in areas with the lowest pressure and greatest capacity. The free space around abdominal organs receives the greatest amount. This space is called the peritoneal space because it is enclosed by a thin membrane called the peritoneum. The peritoneum wraps around nearly every organ in the abdomen, providing many folds and spaces for the fluid to gather.

Infections

Peritonitis is an infection of the peritoneum that can develop in several ways. Many abdominal organs contain germs that do not occur elsewhere in the body. If they spill their contents into the peritoneum, infection is the result. Infection changes the dynamics of body fluids, causing them to seep into tissues and spaces. The gall bladder, the stomach, any part of the intestine, and most especially the appendix—all cause peritonitis when they leak or rupture. Tuberculosis can infect many organs in the body; it is not confined to the lungs. Tuberculous peritonitis causes ascites.

Other inflammations

Peritoneal fluid is not just produced by infections. An inflamed pancreas, called pancreatitis, can cause a massive sterile peritonitis when it leaks its digestive enzymes into the abdomen.

Cancer

Any cancer that begins in or spreads to the abdomen can leak fluid. One particular tumor of the ovary that leaks fluid and results in fluid accumulation is called Meigs' syndrome.

Kidney disease

Since the kidneys are intimately involved with the body's fluid balance, diseases of the kidney often cause excessive fluid to accumulate. Nephrosis and nephrotic syndrome are the general terms for diseases that cause the kidneys to retain water and promote its movement into body tissues and spaces.

Heart failure

The ultimate source of fluid pressure in the body is the heart, whose pumping generates blood pressure. All other pressures in the body are related to blood pressure. As the heart starts to fail, blood backs up, waiting to be pumped. This increases pressure in the veins leading to the heart, particularly below it where gravity is also pulling blood down. The extra fluid from heart failure is first noticed in the feet and ankles, where gravitational effects are most evident. In the abdomen, the liver swells first, then it and other abdominal organs start to leak.

Pleural fluid

The other major body cavity (besides the abdomen) is the chest. The tissue in the chest corresponding to the peritoneum is called the pleura, and the space contained within the pleura, between the ribs and the lungs, is called the pleural space. Fluid is often found in both cavities, and fluid from one cavity can find its way into the other.

Fluid that accumulates in the abdomen creates abnormal pressures on organs in the abdomen. Digestion is hindered; blood flow is slowed. Pressure upward on the chest from fluid-filled organs compromises breathing. The kidneys function poorly in the presence of such external pressures and may even fail.

Description

During paracentesis, special needles puncture the abdominal wall, being careful not to hit internal organs. If fluid is needed only for analysis, less than 7 oz (200 ml) are removed. If pressure relief is an additional goal, many quarts may be removed. Rapid removal of large amounts of fluid can cause blood pressure to drop suddenly. For this reason, the physician will often leave a tube in place so that fluid can be removed slowly, giving the system time to adapt.

A related procedure called culpocentesis removes ascitic fluid from the very bottom of the abdominal cavity through the back of the vagina. This is used most often to diagnose female genital disorders like ectopic pregnancy, which may bleed or exude fluid into the peritoneal space.

Fluid is sent to the laboratory for testing, where cancer and blood cells can be detected, infections identified, and chemical analysis can direct further investigations.

KEY TERMS

Ascites—Fluid in the abdomen.

Ectopic pregnancy—A pregnancy occurring outside the womb that often ruptures and requires surgical removal.

Hepatitis—An inflammation of the liver.

Aftercare

An adhesive bandage and perhaps a single stitch close the insertion site. Nothing more is required.

Risks

Risks are negligible. It is remotely possible that an organ could be punctured and bleed or that an infection could be introduced.

Normal results

A diagnosis of the cause and/or relief from accumulated fluid pressure are the expected results. Fluid will continue to accumulate until the cause is corrected. Repeat procedures may be needed.

Resources

BOOKS

Chung, Raymond T. and Daniel K. Podolsky. "Cirrhosis and its Complications." In *Harrison's Principles of Internal Medicine*, edited by Eugene Braunwald, et al. New York: McGraw-Hill, 2001.

Henry, J. B. *Clinical Diagnosis and Management by Laboratory Methods*. 20th ed. Philadelphia, PA: W. B. Saunders Company, 2001.

OTHER

Lehrer, Jennifer K. *Abdominal tap—paracentesis*. National Institutes of Health. January 1, 2003 [cited April 4, 2003]. <http://www.nlm.nih.gov/medlineplus/encyclopedia.html>.

"Paracentesis." American Thoracic Society. April, 2003 [cited April 4, 2003]. <http://www.thoracic.org/assemblies/cc/ccprimer/infosheet10.html>.

J. Ricker Polsdorfer, MD
Mark A. Best, MD

Paralytic ileus *see* **Intestinal obstruction repair**

Parathyroid gland removal *see* **Parathyroidectomy**

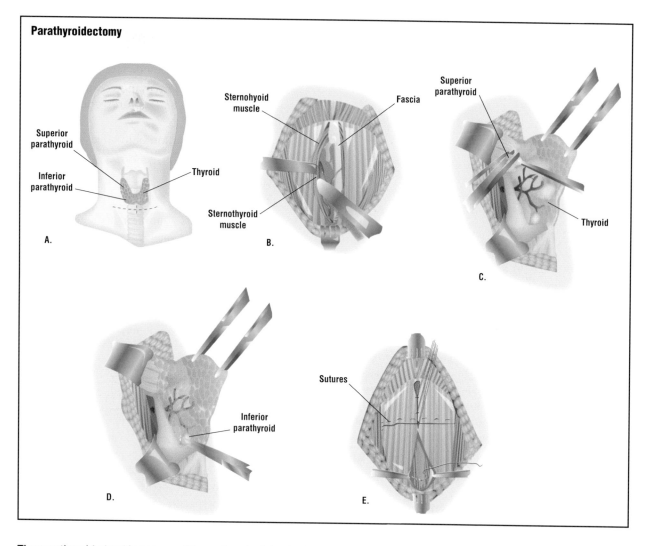

Parathyroidectomy

Superior parathyroid
Inferior parathyroid
Thyroid
A.

Sternohyoid muscle
Fascia
Sternothyroid muscle
B.

Superior parathyroid
Thyroid
C.

Inferior parathyroid
D.

Sutures
E.

The parathryoid gland is accessed through an incision in the neck (A). Muscles and connecting tissues, or fascia, are cut open (B). The thyroid gland is exposed, and the superior (C) and inferior parathyroid glands are removed (D). The muscle layers are stitched (E), and the wound closed. *(Illustration by GGS Inc.)*

Parathyroidectomy

Definition

Parathyroidectomy is the removal of one or more parathyroid glands. A person usually has four parathyroid glands, although the exact number may vary from three to seven. The glands are located in the neck, in front of the Adam's apple, and are closely linked to the thyroid gland. The parathyroid glands regulate the balance of calcium in the body.

Purpose

Parathyroidectomy is usually performed to treat hyperparathyroidism (abnormal over-functioning of the parathyroid glands).

Demographics

The number of parathyroidectomy procedures has risen due to routine measurement of calcium in the blood. Incidence rates vary between 25 and 50 per 100,000 persons. The number of procedures in females is approximately twice that of males. The incidence of parathyroidectomy rises after age 40.

Description

The operation begins when an anesthesiologist administers general anesthesia. The surgeon makes an incision in the front of the neck where a tight-fitting necklace would rest. All of the parathyroid glands are identified. The surgeon then identifies the diseased gland or glands, and confirms the diagnosis by sending a piece of the gland(s) to the pathology department for immediate microscopic examination. The diseased glands are then removed, and the incision is closed and covered with a dressing.

Parathyroidectomy patients usually stay overnight in the hospital after the operation. Some patients remain hospitalized for one or two additional days.

Diagnosis/Preparation

Prior to the operation, the diagnosis of hyperparathyroidism should be confirmed using lab tests. Occasionally, physicians order computed tomography scans (**CT scans**), ultrasound exams, or **magnetic resonance imaging** (MRI) tests to determine the total number of parathyroid glands, and their location prior to the procedure.

Parathyroidectomy should only be performed when other non-operative methods have failed to control a person's hyperparathyroidism.

Preparation is similar to other surgical procedures requiring general anesthetic. The patient is not allowed any food or drink by mouth after midnight the night before surgery. He or she should ask the physician for specific directions regarding preparation for surgery, including food, drink, and medication intake.

Aftercare

The incision should be watched for signs of infection. In general, no special **wound care** is required.

The calcium level is monitored during the first 48 hours after the operation by obtaining frequent blood samples for laboratory analysis.

Most individuals require only two or three days of hospitalization to recover from the operation. They can usually resume most of their normal activities within one to two weeks.

Risks

The major risk of parathyroidectomy is injury to the recurrent laryngeal nerve (a nerve that lies very near the

parathyroid glands and serves the larynx or voice box). If this nerve is injured, the voice may become hoarse or weak.

Occasionally, too much parathyroid tissue is removed, and a person may develop hypoparathyroidism (under-functioning of the parathyroid glands). If this occurs, he or she will require daily calcium supplements.

In some cases, the surgeon is unable to locate all of the parathyroid glands, and cannot remove them in one procedure. A fifth or sixth gland may be located in an aberrant place such as the chest (ectopic parathyroid). If this occurs, the hyperparathyroidism may not be corrected with one operation, and a second procedure may be required to find all of the patient's remaining parathyroid gland tissue.

Normal results

The surgery progresses normally if the diseased parathyroid glands are located and removed from the neck region.

Morbidity and mortality rates

Hematoma formation (collection of blood under the incision) is a possible complication of any operative procedure. However, in procedures that involve the neck it is of particular concern because a rapidly enlarging hematoma can obstruct the airway.

Infection of the surgical incision may occur, as it may in any operative procedure, but this is uncommon in parathyroidectomy.

Before the function of the parathyroid gland was understood, people undergoing a **thyroidectomy** often died

KEY TERMS

Anesthesiologist—A physician who specializes in anesthetizing persons for operations or other medical procedures.

Ectopic parathyroid tissue—Parathyroid tissue located in an abnormal place.

Hyperparathyroidism—Abnormal over-functioning of the parathyroid glands.

Hypoparathyroidism—Abnormal under-functioning of the parathyroid glands.

Otolaryngologist—A surgeon who treats people with abnormalities in the head and neck regions of the body.

Recurrent laryngeal nerve—A nerve that lies very near the parathyroid glands, and serves the larynx or voice box.

due to the lack of calcium in their blood caused by removal of the parathyroid glands. This is not a problem today.

Alternatives

There is no safe or reliable alternative to removal of the parathyroid glands for the treatment of hyperparathyroidism. Oral phosphates can lower serum calcium levels, but the long-term use of this approach is not well understood.

See also Thyroidectomy.

Resources

BOOKS

Bilezikan, J.P., R. Marcus, M. Levine. *The Parathyroids* 2nd Edition. St. Louis: Academic Press, 2001.

Bland, K.I, W.G. Cioffi, M.G. Sarr. *Practice of General Surgery.* Philadelphia: Saunders, 2001.

Randolph, G. *Surgery of Thyroid and Parathyroid Glands.* St. Louis: Elsevier, 2002.

Schwartz, S.I., J.E. Fischer, F.C. Spencer, G.T. Shires, J.M. Daly. *Principles of Surgery* 7th edition. New York: McGraw Hill, 1998.

Townsend C., K.L. Mattox, R.D. Beauchamp, B.M. Evers, D.C. Sabiston *Sabiston Review of Surgery* 3rd Edition. Philadelphia: Saunders, 2001.

PERIODICALS

Awad, S.S., J. Miskulin, N. Thompson. "Parathyroid Adenomas versus Four-gland Hyperplasia as the Cause of Primary Hyperparathyroidism in Patients with Prolonged Lithium Therapy." *World Journal of Surgery* 27, no.4 (2003): 486-8.

Genc, H., E. Morita, N.D. Perrier, D. Miura, P. Ituarte, Q.Y. Duh, O.H. Clark. "Differing Histologic Findings after Bilateral and Focused Parathyroidectomy." *Journal of the American College of Surgery* 196, no.4 (2003): 535-40.

Goldstein, R.E., D. Billheimer, W.H. Martin, K. Richards. "Sestamibi Scanning and Minimally Invasive Radioguided Parathyroidectomy without Intraoperative Parathyroid Hormone Measurement." *Annals of Surgery* 237, no.5 (2003): 722-31.

Miccoli, P., P. Berti, G. Materazzi, G. Donatini. "Minimally Invasive Video Assisted Parathyroidectomy (MIVAP)." *European Journal of Surgical Oncology* 29, no.2 (2003): 188-90.

ORGANIZATIONS

American College of Surgeons. 633 North St. Clair Street, Chicago, IL 60611-32311. (312) 202-5000, fax: (312) 202-5001. <http://www.facs.org>, E-mail: <postmaster@facs.org>.

American Medical Association. 515 N. State Street, Chicago, IL 60610. (312) 464-5000. <http://www.ama-assn.org>.

American Academy of Otolaryngology-Head and Neck Surgery. One Prince St., Alexandria, VA 22314-3357. (703) 836-4444. <http://www.entnet.org/index2.cfm>.

American Osteopathic College of Otolaryngology-Head and Neck Surgery. 405 W. Grand Avenue, Dayton, OH 45405. (937) 222-8820 or (800) 455-9404, fax (937) 222-8840. Email: <info@aocoohns.org>.

Association of Thyroid Surgeons. 717 Buena Vista St., Ventura, CA 93001. Fax: (509) 479-8678. <info@thyroidsurgery.org>.

OTHER

Columbia University Medical Center. [cited May 5, 2003] <http://cpmcnet.columbia.edu/dept/thyroid/parasurgHP.html>.

Mayo Clinic. [cited May 5, 2003] <http://www.mayoclinic.org/checkup/02mar-parathyroid.html>.

Ohio State University. [cited May 5, 2003] <http://www.acs.ohio-state.edu/units/osuhosp/patedu/ Materials/PDF Docs/surgery/thyroid.pdf>.

University of California-San Diego. [cited May 5, 2003] <http://www-surgery.ucsd.edu/ent/PatientInfo/th_parathyroid.html>.

University of Wisconsin. [cited May 5, 2003] <http://www.surgery.wisc.edu/general/patients/endocrine.shtml>.

L. Fleming Fallon, Jr., M.D., Dr.PH.

Paravaginal surgery *see* **Needle bladder neck suspension**

Parkinson's surgery *see* **Deep brain stimulation**

Parotid gland removal *see* **Parotidectomy**

Parotidectomy

Definition

Parotidectomy is the removal of the parotid gland, a salivary gland near the ear.

Purpose

The parotid gland is the largest of the salivary glands. There are two parotid glands, one on each side of the face, just below and to the front of the ear. A duct through which saliva is secreted runs from each gland to the inside of the cheek.

The main purpose of parotidectomy is to remove abnormal growths (neoplasms) that occur in the parotid gland. Parotid gland neoplasms may be benign (approximately 80%) or malignant. Tumors may spread from other areas of the body, entering the parotid gland by way of the lymphatic system.

Demographics

Benign parotid gland growths usually appear after the age of 40. Malignant growths most often affect women over the age of 60, while benign tumors affect both sexes equally. Cancer of the salivary glands accounts for only 1% of all cancers, and 7% of all head and neck cancers.

Description

During surgery, two different areas of the parotid gland are identified: the superficial lobe and the deep lobe. Superficial parotidectomy removes just the superficial lobe, while total parotidectomy removes both lobes.

The patient is first placed under general anesthesia to ensure that no pain is experienced and that all muscles remain relaxed. An incision is made directly to the front or back of the ear and down the jaw line. The skin is folded back to expose the parotid gland. The

---

WHO PERFORMS THE PROCEDURE AND WHERE IS IT PERFORMED?

Parotidectomy is performed in a hospital **operating room**, usually by an otolaryngologist, a medical doctor who specializes in the treatment of diseases that affect the ear, nose, throat, and other structures of the head and neck.

---

various facial nerves are identified and protected during the surgery so as to avoid permanent facial paralysis or numbness. A superficial or total parotidectomy is then performed, depending on the type and location of the tumor. If the tumor has spread to involve the facial nerve, the operation is expanded to include parts of the bone behind the ear (mastoid) to remove as much tumor as possible. Before the incision is closed, a drain is inserted into the area to collect any leaking saliva, if a superficial parotidectomy was performed. The procedure typically takes from two to five hours to complete, depending on the extent of surgery and the skill of the surgeon.

Diagnosis/Preparation

A complete **physical examination** and medical history is performed, as are diagnostic tests to help the surgeon better plan for the surgery. Some tests that may be performed include computed tomography (CT) scan, **magnetic resonance imaging** (MRI), and fine-needle aspiration biopsy (using a thin needle to withdraw fluid and cells from the growth).

Aftercare

After surgery, the patient will remain in the hospital for one to three days. The incision site will be watched closely for signs of infection and heavy bleeding (hemorrhage). The incision site should be kept clean and dry until it is completely healed. If the patient has difficulty smiling, winking, or drinking fluids, the physician should be contacted immediately. These are signs of facial nerve damage.

Risks

There are a number of complications that are associated with parotidectomy. Facial nerve paralysis after minor surgery should be minimal. After major surgery, a graft is attempted to restore nerve function to facial muscles. Salivary fistulas can occur when saliva collects in the incision site or drains through the incision. Recurrence of cancer is the single most important consideration for patients who have undergone parotidectomy. Long-term survival rates are largely dependent on the tumor type and the stage of tumor development at the time of the operation.

Other risks include hematoma (collection of blood under the skin) and infection. The most common long-term complication of parotidectomy is redness and sweating in the cheek, known as Frey's syndrome. Rarely, paralysis may extend throughout all the branches of the facial nervous system.

Normal results

Although some facial numbness or weakness is normal immediately following parotidectomy, these symptoms usually subside within a few months, with most patients regaining full function within one year. Return of a benign tumor is very rare.

Morbidity and mortality rates

There is a 25–50% risk of temporary facial weakness following parotidectomy, and a 1–2% risk of permanent weakness. Frey's syndrome may be experienced by up to 90% of patients to some extent and causes perspiration on that side of the face with eating. There is very little or no risk of mortality associated with the surgery. The survival rate of malignant parotid gland tumors depends on their size, location, extension, and if metastasis has occurred. The 10-year survival rate ranges from 32% to 83%.

Alternatives

A benign parotid neoplasm may be managed expectantly (i.e., adhering to a period of watchful waiting) so that the growth is of a larger size before it is removed (the risk of facial nerve damage increases with each subsequent parotidectomy). There is generally no alternative to surgical treatment of parotid gland neoplasms, although radiation therapy may be recommended after the procedure in the case of malignant tumors.

Resources

PERIODICALS

Califano, Joseph, and David W. Eisele. "Benign Salivary Gland Neoplasms." *Otolaryngology Clinics of North America* 32, no. 5 (October 1, 1999): 861–73.

Carlson, Grant W. "The Salivary Glands: Embryology, Anatomy, and Surgical Applications." *Surgical Clinics of North America* 80, no. 1 (February 1, 2000): 261–73.

Sinha, Uttam, and Matthew Ng. "Surgery of the Salivary Glands." *Otolaryngology Clinics of North America* 32, no. 5 (October 1, 1999): 887–906.

ORGANIZATIONS

American Academy of Otolaryngology. One Prince St., Alexandria, VA 22314-3357. (703) 836-4444. <http://www.entnet.org>.

OTHER

Gordon, Ashley D. "Parotid Tumors, Benign." *eMedicine,* December 27, 2001 [cited April 7, 2003] <http://www.emedicine.com/plastic/topic371.htm>.

Johns, Michael M. "Salivary Gland Neoplasms." *eMedicine,* May 17, 2002 [cited April 7, 2003] <http://www.emedicine.com/ent/topic679.htm>.

Shelato, Dwight. *The Patient's Forum on Tumors of the Parotid Gland,* [cited April 7, 2003] <http://patientsforum.com>.

Mary K. Fyke
Stephanie Dionne Sherk

Patella removal *see* **Kneecap removal**

Patent ductus arteriosis repair *see* **Heart surgery for congenital defects**

Patent urachus repair

Definition

Patent urachus repair is surgery to correct a urachus (a tube that connects the fetal bladder to the umbilical cord) that fails to close after birth.

Purpose

A patent urachus is an anomaly, and repair is recommended for these defects occurring at birth.

Demographics

The condition occurs three times more often in male infants than in females.

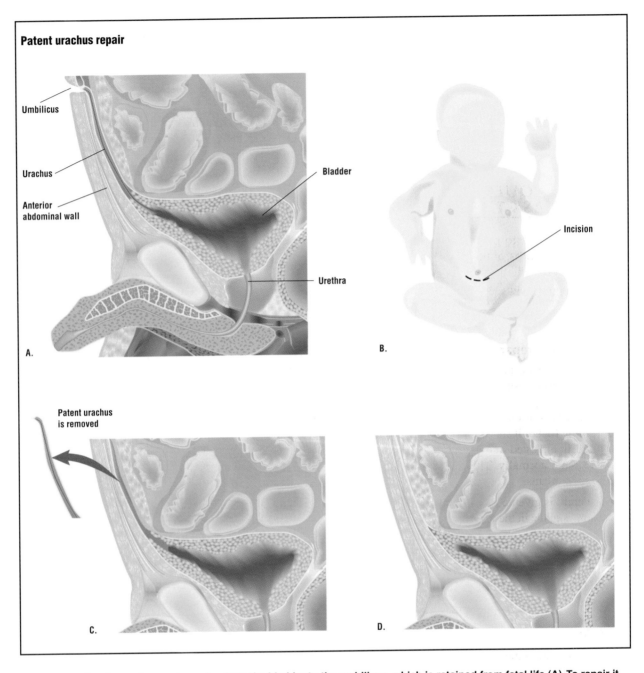

Patent urachus repair

A. Umbilicus
Urachus
Anterior abdominal wall
Bladder
Urethra

B. Incision

Patent urachus is removed

C.

D.

A patent urachus is an abnormal opening from the bladder to the umbilicus, which is retained from fetal life (A). To repair it, an incision is made in the baby's abdomen (B). The patent urachus is removed (C), and the opening to the bladder is closed (D). *(Illustration by GGS Inc.)*

Description

As fetal development progresses, the urachus, a tube that can measure from 1.2–3.9 in (3–10 cm) long and 0.3–0.4 in (8–10 mm) in diameter, forms, extending from the front dome of the bladder to the umbilicus. Following birth, the tube, adjacent to the umbilical ligaments, closes and itself becomes ligament. Should this closure fail, it may result in several types of urachal rem-nants. If the urachus remains completely open, it is known as a patent urachus. This type of abnormality makes up 50% of all urachal anomalies.

If the urachus remains open all the way to the bladder, there is the danger that bacteria will enter the bladder through the open tube and cause infection. For this reason, the patent urachus of the infant must be re-moved.

Diagnosis/Preparation

This anomaly occurs as an isolated event or in association with prune-belly syndrome, in which there is continuous drainage of urine from the umbilicus. If urine freely discharges through the umbilicus, the patent urachus is rarely found. It should be suspected, however, if a local cord is enlarged and affected with edema, or is slow to slough normally. The condition customarily is diagnosed in infants.

The child is given a general anesthetic, after which an incision is made in the lower abdomen.

Aftercare

Surgery for patent urachus repair may require several days' hospitalization, during which infants can be fed as normal.

Risks

Risks are the same as for those patients receiving any anesthesia: a reaction to medication and/or breathing problems. There is also the risk of bladder infection or bladder leaks. In the latter case, a catheter is put in place until the bladder heals.

Normal results

The outcomes of patent urachus repair in infants are excellent, as a rule, and most children recover rapidly.

Morbidity and mortality rates

Patent urachal anomalies do not usually cause significant morbidity or mortality. However, adenocarcino-

ma has been reported in adults with urachal remnants, presumably from chronic inflammation and infection. Patency is noted in only 2% of adults.

Alternatives

Sometimes more conservative treatment than surgery is advised, with radical excision reserved for persistent or recurring cases. Because the urachus may not completely close at birth, but may close within the first few months of the infant's life, observation may be advised before moving forward with surgery.

Resources

BOOKS

Campbell, Meredith F. and Patrick C. Walsh, eds. *Campbell's Urology,* 8th ed. Philadephia: W.B. Saunders Company, 2002.

PERIODICALS

Razvi, S., R. Murphy, E. Shlasko, and C. Cunningham-Rundles. "Delayed Separation of the Umbilical Cord Attributable to Urachal Anomalies." *NIH/NLM MEDLINE* 108, no.2 (August 1, 2001): 493–494.

Nancy McKenzie, PhD

Patient-controlled analgesia

Definition

Patient-controlled analgesia (PCA) is a means for the patient to self-administer **analgesics** (pain medications) intravenously by using a computerized pump, which introduces specific doses into an intravenous line.

Purpose

The purpose of PCA is improved pain control. The patient receives immediate delivery of pain medication without the need for a nurse to administer it. The patient controls when the medication is given. More importantly, PCA uses more frequent but smaller doses of medication, and thus provides more even levels of medication within the patient's body. Syringe-injected **pain management** by a nurse requires larger doses of medication given less frequently. Larger doses peak shortly after administration, often causing undesirable side effects such as nausea and difficulty in breathing. Their pain-suppressing effects also often wear off before the next dose is scheduled.

Description

PCA uses a computerized pump, which is controlled by the patient through a hand-held button that is connected to the machine. The pump usually delivers medications in small regular doses, and it can be programmed to issue a large initial dose and then a steady, even flow. The PCA pump can deliver medicine into a vein (intravenously, the most common method), under the skin (subcutaneously), or between the dura mater and the skull (epidurally).

When the patient feels the need for medication, the patient presses a button similar to a nurse call button. When this button is pressed, some sound (usually a beep) is heard, indicating that the pump is working properly and that the button was pressed correctly. The pump delivers the medication through an intravenous line, a plastic tube connected to a needle inserted into a vein. Glucose and other medications can also be administered through intravenous lines, along with analgesics.

The medications most commonly used in PCA pumps are synthetic, opium-like pain-relievers (opioids), usually morphine and meperidine (Demerol).

The pump may be set to deliver a larger initial dose of the prescribed drug. The health-care provider sets the pump to deliver a specified dose, determined by the physician, on demand with a lockout time (for example, 1 mg of morphine on demand, but not more frequently than one dose every six minutes). If the patient presses the button before six minutes have elapsed, the pump will not dispense the medication. The pump also generates a record that the health personnel can access. An around-the-clock, even dose may also be set. The practitioner sets a total limit for an hour (or any other period) that takes into account the initial dose, the demand doses, and the around-the-clock doses. The pump's internal computer calculates all these amounts, makes a record of the requests it received and those it refused, and also keeps inventory of the medication being administered, which warns the staff when the supply is getting low.

An example of how a nurse might program the pump might be for a patient who has a prescription for a maximum of 11 mg of morphine an hour. The nurse sets the machine to deliver 1 mg at the beginning of the hour, and 1 mg on demand with a six-minute lockout. There are 10 six-minute periods in an hour, so the patient can request and receive 10 mg over that hour.

Using a PCA pump requires that the patient understand how the system works and has the physical strength to press the button. Therefore, PCA should not be offered to patients who are confused, unresponsive, or paralyzed. Patients with neurologic disease or head injuries in whom narcotics would mask neurologic changes are not eligible for PCA. Patients with poor kidney or lung function are usually not good candidates for PCA, unless they are monitored very closely.

PCA may be used by children as young as seven years old. It has proven safe and successful in such children in the control of postoperative pain, sickle-cell pain, and pain associated with bone-marrow transplantation. In all cases, the child should manage the PCA pump himself or herself. As morphine can slow breathing in young patients, the blood oxygen levels of children must be closely monitored.

In addition, PCA has been found safe for nursing mothers after a **cesarean section**. Very small amounts of morphine do pass into the milk of breastfeeding mothers, but it has not proved harmful to infants.

Preparation

When preparing for PCA, the nurse must assess the patient to determine whether PCA is appropriate and then must set the total dose and the timing of the doses as prescribed by the physician. Since there is only a small amount of drug administered (3,000 doses at 10 mg each weigh less than 1 oz total), it is not sufficient fluid to keep the tubing and the needle from clogging and the contents from coagulating. Therefore, the drug must be put in a solution (flush solution) that will flow through the tube and needle easily, and permit rapid administration. The flush solution also keeps the line open for administration of other medications or in case the patient has a reaction to the pain medications. For example, a patient may have a reaction to morphine and would need counteractive medication immediately. The flush solution can also keep the patient from becoming dehydrated. In addition, many painkillers that are prescribed (such as morphine sulfate) are solid crystals at room temperature and need to be dissolved in some fluid to be absorbed by the body.

When entering the settings into the PCA system, the nurse must pay close attention to the physician's orders to ensure that the correct medication is used, that the concentration of the drug in the flushing solution is correct, that the dose of the drug itself is correct, that the lockout time is appropriate, and that the total hourly limit is properly entered into the pump's computerized controls. To eliminate the risk of incorrect programming, many institutions have adopted policies that require verification by a registered nurse (RN) to witness for all programming. That is, everything must be checked by two nurses, and both must sign the written record.

Another important aspect of PCA is patient education. The settings on the PCA pump must be explained to patients so that they understand how and when medications will be available. The nurse should observe patients as they first start using the button, should ensure that the equipment is functioning properly, and be clear that the patients understand their role in the process and are carrying it out correctly.

Whenever opium-like painkillers are administered to the elderly patient, it must be remembered that older adults may be more susceptible to the side effects of narcotics because the heart, liver, and kidneys of the elderly function less efficiently than those of younger patients. The elderly may also clear the narcotic out of their system at a slower pace. If the pump's timing device is calibrated for a younger person's rate of elimination, the elderly patient could accidentally receive an overdose. Doses for such elderly patients should be calculated more conservatively.

Normal results

The goal of patient-controlled analgesia is managed pain control, enhanced by a stable and constant level of the pain medication in the body. The patient is able to rest better and breathe more deeply. Since the patient is comfortable, he or she is more able to participate in activities that would enhance recovery. PCA also gives the patient in the hospital some control in an unfamiliar and uncomfortable situation. When administered properly, and with watchful assessment by health care providers, PCA can be a safe alternative to traditional methods of relieving pain.

Interestingly enough, studies have shown that when patients control their pain medication, most use less medication overall than patients who have nurse-administered painkillers.

Risks

Problems that may occur with PCA include allergic reactions to the medications and adverse side effects such as nausea, a dangerous drop in the rate and effectiveness of breathing, and excessive sedation. The PCA device must be monitored frequently to prevent tamper-

KEY TERMS

Analgesia—A medicine that relieves pain.

Epidural—Between the vertebrae and the dura mater of the spinal cord. Analgesia is introduced into this space anywhere along the spinal column.

Intravenous—Within a vein, usually meaning something introduced into a vein such as an injection.

Lockout time—The minimum amount of time (usually expressed in minutes) after one dose of pain medication on demand is given before the patient is allowed to receive the next dose on demand.

Opioid—A synthetic drug resembling opium or alkaloids of opium.

Respiratory depression—Decreased rate (number of breaths per minute) and depth (how much air is inhaled with each breath) of breathing.

Subcutaneous—Under the skin, as in an injection under the skin.

ing. Even sophisticated devices that monitor themselves and sound an alarm should be checked often, since no machine is perfect. Ineffective pain control must be assessed to determine whether the problem stems from inadequate dosage or from inability, or unwillingness, of the patient to carry out his or her own pain management.

Resources

BOOKS

Lehne, Richard A. *Pharmacology for Nursing Care,* 3rd edition. Philadelphia: W. B. Saunders Company, 1998.

PERIODICALS

Baka, Nour-Eddine. "Colostrum Morphine Concentrations during Postcesarean Intravenous Patient-controlled Analgesia." *Journal of the American Medical Association* 287, no. 12 (March 27, 2002): 1508.

Ellis, Jacqueline A., Renee Blouin, and Jean Lockett. "Patient-Controlled Analgesia: Optimizing the Experience." *Clinical Nursing Research* 8, no. 3 (August 1999): 283–294.

"Give a PCA Pump to Patients in Pain." *ED Nursing* 5, no 2 (December 2001): 27.

"Patient Controlled Analgesia for Children." *CareNotes* (December 2001).

ORGANIZATIONS

American Association of Nurse Anesthetists/AANA. 222 South Prospect Avenue, Park Ridge, IL 60068-4001. (847) 692-

7050; Fax: (847) 692-6968. E-mail: <info@aana.com>. Web site: <http://www.aana.com>.

American Association of Nurse Anesthetists/AANA, Federal Government Affairs Office. 412 1st Street, SE, Suite 12, Washington, DC 20003. (202) 484-8400; Fax: (202) 484-8408. E-mail: <info@aanadc.com>.

American Society of PeriAnesthesia Nurses/ASPAN. 10 Melrose Avenue, Suite 110, Cherry Hill, NJ 08003-3696. (877) 737-9696; Fax: (856) 616-9601. E-mail: <aspan@aspan.org>. <http://www.aspan.org>.

American Society of Anesthesiologists/ASA. 520 North Northwest Highway, Park Ridge, IL 60068-2573. (847) 825-5586; Fax: (847) 825-1692. E-mail: <mail@asahq.org>.

The National Hospice and Palliative Care Organization/ NHPCO. 1700 Diagonal Road, Suite 300, Alexandria, VA 22314. (703) 837-1500. E-mail: <info@nhpco.org>.

Janie F. Franz
Jennifer Lee Losey, RN

Patient charts *see* **Medical charts**

Patient confidentiality

Definition

Confidentiality is the right of an individual to have personal, identifiable medical information kept private. Such information should be available only to the physician of record and other health care and insurance personnel as necessary. As of 2003, patient confidentiality was protected by federal statute.

Purpose

The passage of federal regulations (the Health Insurance Portability and Accountability Act of 1996) was prompted by the need to ensure privacy and protection of personal records and data in an environment of electronic medical records and third-party insurance payers.

Description

Patient confidentiality means that personal and medical information given to a health care provider will not be disclosed to others unless the individual has given specific permission for such release.

Because the disclosure of personal information could cause professional or personal problems, patients rely on physicians to keep their medical information private. It is rare for medical records to remain completely

sealed, however. The most benign breach of confidentiality takes place when clinicians share medical information as case studies. When this data is published in professional journals the identity of the patient is never divulged, and all identifying data is either eliminated or changed. If this confidentiality is breached in any way, patients may have the right to sue.

The greatest threat to medical privacy, however, occurs because most medical bills are paid by some form of health insurance, either private or public. This makes it difficult, if not impossible, to keep information truly confidential. Health records are routinely viewed not only by physicians and their staffs, but by the employees of insurance companies, medical laboratories, public health departments, researchers, and many others. If an employer provides health insurance, the employer and designated employees may have access to employee files.

The Health Insurance Portability and Accountability Act (HIPAA) of 1996 requires all professionals and organizations to guard the privacy of their patients and customers. Individuals must provide written consent for any and all releases of medical or health-related information. Employees at all levels are required to maintain confidentiality. Similar policies have been in place for some time. This was a requirement of the Joint Commission on Accreditation of Healthcare Organizations (JCAHO) to maintain accreditation. All confidentiality releases must identify the types of information that can be released, the people or groups that have been permitted access to the information, and limit the length of time for which the release is valid.

Before the enactment of HIPAA, despite having voluntary safeguards, patient confidentiality had eroded with the almost-complete dominance of health-maintenance organizations and other types of third-party payers. Confidentiality is essential for a good relationship between patient and practitioner, whose duty to keep information private stems from the Hippocratic Oath. If personal information is disseminated without the patient's permission, it can erode confidence in the medical profession and expose health care professionals to legal action.

Physicians are increasingly being sued by patients whose information has been released without their permission. Even though the plaintiffs do not always prevail, the costs of legal action are burdensome to both sides.

Each state and the federal government have enacted laws to protect the confidentiality of health care information generally, with particular attention paid to information about communicable diseases and mental health. For example, through the 1960s substance and alcohol abuse were treated as mental illnesses, with patient confidentiality determined by the laws in each state, since at the time the state was responsible for mental health care and treatment.

In the early 1970s, however, the rising numbers of those needing substance abuse treatment came to the attention of the federal government, because drug-related activity, including the treatment for substance abuse, could be the basis for criminal prosecution on a federal level. Congress concluded that this might stop individuals needing treatment from seeking it. HIPAA was enacted to provide a strict confidentiality law and limit disclosure of information that could reveal a patient's identity.

Confusion ensued when practitioners who were treating substance abusers were required to follow two practices for patient confidentiality. One set of requirements was mandated by the state. The federal government dictated the other. With the varying degrees of protection provided by state mental health laws, the confusion increased. While all states specify exceptions to confidentiality, few have spelled out the necessary elements of valid consent for disclosure of mental health information. Some states presently allow disclosure of the following types of mental health information without patient consent:

• to other treatment providers

• to health care services payers or other sources of financial assistance to the patient

• to third parties that the mental health professional feels might be endangered by the patient

• to researchers

• to agencies charged with oversight of the health care system or the system's practitioners

• to families under certain circumstances

• to law enforcement officials under certain circumstances

• to public health officials

Prior to 2003, providers had become increasingly concerned that these exceptions are not addressed uniformly, particularly when providers and payers conducted business across state lines. This resulted in open-ended disclosures that specify neither the parties to whom disclosure is to be made nor the specific information allowed to be revealed.

Both the ethical and the legal principles of confidentiality are rooted in a set of values regarding the relationship between caregiver and patient. It is essential that a patient trust a caregiver so that a warm and accepting relationship may develop. This is particularly true in a mental health treatment.

Normal results

The Health Insurance Portability and Accountability Act of 1996 was enacted to address the issue of patient confidentiality. Full implementation of HIPAA regulations began in April 2003. If individuals and organizations having patient data adhere to the requirements of HIPAA, patient confidentiality will be enhanced.

HIPAA provides a uniform set of guidelines that apply to all providers and organizations. HIPAA requirements are not affected by state boundaries.

See also Informed consent; Patient rights.

Resources

BOOKS

Carter P. I. *HIPAA Compliance Handbook 2003*. Gaithersburg, Maryland: Aspen, 2002.
Hubbard, M. W., K. E. Glover, and C. P. Hartley. *HIPAA Policies and Procedures Desk Reference*. Chicago: American Medical Association, 2003.
Pabrai, U. A. *Getting Started with HIPAA* Boston: Premier Press, 2003.
Radford, Roger. *Informed Consent*. Booklocker.com, 2002.

PERIODICALS

Cole A. and K. Oxtoby. "Patient power." *Nursing Times* 98 (2002: 22–25.
Landrum, S. E. "Patients' rights and responsibilities." *Journal of the Arkansas Medical Society* 99 (2003): 222–223.
Rosenbaum, S. "Managed care and patients' rights." *Journal of the American Medical Association* 289 (2003): 906–907.
Sugarman, J. "Missing the informed in consent." *Anesthesia and Analgesia* 96 (2003): 319–320.

ORGANIZATIONS

American Academy of Family Physicians. 11400 Tomahawk Creek Parkway, Leawood, KS 66211-2672. (913) 906-6000. <http://www.aafp.org>. <fp@aafp.org>.
American College of Physicians. 190 N Independence Mall West, Philadelphia, PA 19106-1572. (800) 523-1546, ext. 2600. (215) 351-2600. <http://www.acponline.org>.
American Medical Association. 515 N. State Street, Chicago, IL 60610. (312) 464-5000. <http://www.ama-assn.org>.
National Patient Advocate Foundation. 753 Thimble Shoals Blvd, Suite A, Newport News, VA 23606. (800) 532-5274. <http://www.npaf.org>. <action@npaf.org>.

OTHER

American Psychological Association. [cited March 21, 2003] <http://www.apa.org/practice/senate_compromises.html>.
HIPAA website. [cited March 24, 2003]. <http://www.hipaa.org>.
National Academy of Sciences. [cited March 21, 2003]. <http://www.nap.edu/readingroom/books/for/index.html>
Persons United Limiting Substandards and Errors in Health Care (P.U.L.S.E.). [cited March 21, 2003]. <http://www.pulseamerica.org>.

KEY TERMS

HIPAA—Health Insurance Portability and Accountability Act of 1996.

Joint Commission on Accreditation of Healthcare Organizations (JCAHO)—The accrediting organization that evaluates virtually all U.S. health care organizations and programs. Accreditation is maintained with onsite surveys every three years; laboratories are surveyed every two years.

Stanford University. [cited March 21, 2003]. <http://www.stanford.edu/class/siw198q/websites/HearingMar01/bill.html>.

U.S. House or Representatives, Democratic Staff or the Energy and Commerce Committee. [cited March 21, 2003]. <http://www.house.gov/commerce_democrats/pbor/107pborsummary.htm>.

L. Fleming Fallon, Jr., MD, DrPH

Patient rights

Definition

Patient rights encompass legal and ethical issues in the provider-patient relationship, including a person's right to privacy, the right to quality medical care without prejudice, the right to make informed decisions about care and treatment options, and the right to refuse treatment.

Purpose

The purpose of delineating patient rights is to ensure the ethical treatment of persons receiving medical or other professional health care services. Without exception, all persons in all settings are entitled to receive ethical treatment.

Description

Many issues comprise the rights of patients in the medical system, including a person's ability to sue a health plan provider; access to emergency and specialty care, diagnostic testing, and prescription medication without prejudice; confidentiality and protection of patient medical information; and continuity of care.

Health care reform led to an emergence of health maintenance organizations (HMOs) and other managed health care plans. The rapid change in medical care moved health care decision making from medical professionals to business entities, a move many consider to be detrimental to the health care industry in general. Establishing a patient's bill of rights has been the response to this concern. The Bipartisan Patient Protection Act of 2001 has been debated and passed by the U.S. Senate and the U.S. House of Representatives and signed into law.

At issue, besides basic rights of care and privacy, is the education of patients concerning what to expect of their health care facility and its providers. These basic rights include the right to:

• participate in the development and implementation in the plan of care

• be treated with respect and dignity

• be informed about condition, treatment options, and the possible results and side effects of treatment

• refuse treatment in accordance with the law, and receive information about the consequences of refusal

• quality health care without discrimination because of race, creed, gender, religion, national origin, or source of payment

• privacy and confidentiality, which includes access to medical records upon request

• personal safety

• know the identity of the person treating the patient, as well as any relationship between professionals and agencies involved in the treatment

• informed consent for all procedures

• information, including the medical records by the patient or by the patient's legally authorized representative and hospital charges, except for **Medicaid** and general assistance

• consultation and communication

• complain or compliment without the fear of retaliation or compromise of access or quality of care

The patient is also expected to meet a fair share of responsibility by following the plan of care, providing complete and accurate health information, and communicating comprehension of instructions on procedures and treatment. The patient is further responsible for consequences of refusal of treatment, of not following the rules and regulations of a hospital, and of not being considerate of others' rights. The patient is also responsible for providing assurance that financial obligations of care are met.

The American Hospital Association provides an informal bill of rights for patients who are hospitalized, which informs patients that they have the right to refuse any procedure or medication that is prescribed, and that states that full information should be provided by the attending physician if the patient has expressed doubts or concerns.

Persons United Limiting Substandards and Errors in Health Care (PULSE), a non-profit organization concerned with patient education and improving communication within the health care system, encourages the partnership of health care professionals and patients. A patient who is educated about his or her own medical condition can work together with health care providers regarding treatment decisions.

New federal privacy rules, beyond the proposed patient bill of rights, give patients additional control over private medical information. Patients have the right to examine their own medical records and to amend them if necessary. In practice, medical personnel have often been reluctant to part with patient records, even when requested by the patients themselves. While health care providers and patients assume that medical records are private, the widespread use of computer transmissions opens the potential for seriously compromising **patient confidentiality**. Regulations recently imposed by the federal government are aimed at protecting patient records by creating limits on the methods in which medical information is shared. Direct authorization from a patient must be gained before information may be released. Criminal and civil penalties may be imposed for a privacy violation. Intentional disclosure of private information can bring a $50,000 fine and a one-year prison term. Penalties for selling medical information are higher. These rules became enforceable in February 2003.

Alternatives

Not all individuals or organizations agree with the new regulations. Some complain that they are too restrictive, while others maintain that they are not restrictive enough. The Joint Commission on Accreditation of Healthcare Organizations (JCAHO) cites complexity and cost factors as major problems, and that the full extent of the impact caused by the ruling was not adequately considered when it passed in 2003. Government estimates are that it will cost taxpayers $17.6 billion over 10 years to comply with the privacy regulations. Critics of the regulations imply that the cost will be more than triple the estimate, and that billable hours for attorneys specializing in the complexities of the regulations will skyrocket, thus resulting in even higher costs of patient care.

See also Do not resuscitate order; Medical charts; Patient confidentiality.

Resources

BOOKS

Radford, Roger. *Informed Consent.* Booklocker.com, 2002.

PERIODICALS

Cole, A., and K. Oxtoby. "Patient Power." *Nursing Times* 98, no.51 (2002): 22–25.
Landrum, S. E. "Patients' Rights and Responsibilities." *Journal of the Arkansas Medical Society* 99, no.7 (2003): 222–223.
Rosenbaum, S. "Managed Care and Patients' Rights." *Journal of the American Medical Association* 289, no.7 (2003): 906–907.
Sugarman, J. "Missing the Informed in Consent." *Anesthesia and Analgesia* 96, no.2 (2003): 319–320.

ORGANIZATIONS

American Academy of Family Physicians. 11400 Tomahawk Creek Parkway, Leawood, KS 66211-2672. (913) 906-6000. E-mail: <fp@aafp.org>. <http://www.aafp.org>.
American College of Physicians. 190 N Independence Mall West, Philadelphia, PA 19106-1572. (800) 523-1546, x2600, or (215) 351-2600. <http://www.acponline.org>.
American Medical Association. 515 N. State Street, Chicago, IL 60610. (312) 464-5000. <http://www.ama-assn.org>.
National Patient Advocate Foundation. 753 Thimble Shoals Blvd, Suite A, Newport News, VA 23606. 800-532-5274. E-mail: <action@npaf.org>. <http://www.npaf.org>.

OTHER

American Psychological Association. [cited March 2, 2003] <http://www.apa.org/practice/senate_compromises.html>.
Persons United Limiting Substandards and Errors in Health Care (P.U.L.S.E.). [cited March 2, 2003] <//www.pulseamerica.org/>.
Stanford University. [cited March 2, 2003] <http://www.stanford.edu/class/siw198q/websites/HearingMar01/bill.html>.
U.S. House or Representatives, Democratic Staff or the Energy and Commerce Committee. [cited March 2, 2003. <http://www.house.gov/commerce_democrats/pbor/107pborsummary.htm>.

L. Fleming Fallon, Jr, MD, DrPH

PCA *see* **Patient-controlled analgesia**
PCNL *see* **Nephrolithotomy, percutaneous**
PCV *see* **Hematocrit**

Pectus excavatum repair

Definition

Pectus excavatum repair, also called "funnel chest repair" or "chest deformity repair," is a type of surgery performed to correct pectus excavatum, a deformity of the front of the chest wall with depression of the breast-

Pectus excavatum repair

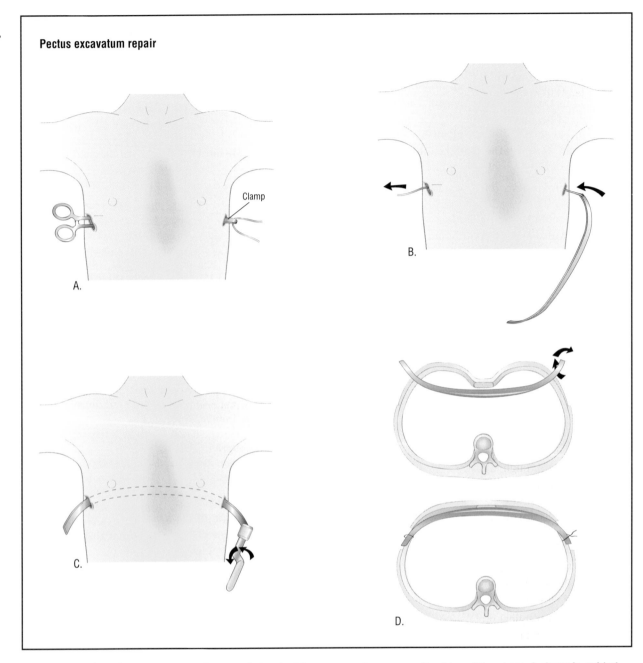

In a minimally invasive pectus excavatum repair, two incisions are made on opposite sides of the chest. A clamp is guided beneath the sternum to create a tunnel for the bar (A), which is then fed through (B). The bar is turned over to push the sternum out (C and D) and attached to the ribcage. *(Illustration by Argosy.)*

bone (sternum) and rib (costal) cartilages. It is sometimes associaated with Marfan or Poland syndromes.

Purpose

The chest consists of the rib cage and sternum, which protect the upper-abdominal cavity and its contents. Pectus excavatum, also called "funnel chest" or "depressed sternum" is a deformity that is usually diagnosed shortly after birth. In some people, it is not visible until they are older. The exact cause is not known, but it is believed to be due to overgrowth of the rib cartilage connected to the sternum, which results in the sternum being pushed backward toward the spine. Most people have no symptoms, but if the breastbone is pushed back far enough, heart and lung function may be affected. The purpose of pectus excavatum repair surgery is to correct the deformity to improve physical appearance, posture, and breathing.

Demographics

In the United States, pectus excavatum is the most common chest wall deformity observed in children, occurring more commonly in boys than in girls. Pectus excavatum tends to run in families. The funnel chest usually progresses as the child grows, often showing a dramatic deterioration during the puberty growth spurt.

Pectus excavatum repair is technically easiest to perform in preadolescent children, and the recovery is faster. However, almost half of the patients undergoing the operation are teenagers. Repair is rarely performed on children under eight years of age. In recent years, a large number of adults over the age of 21 years have undergone repair with equally good results as those observed with children.

Description

Pectus excavatum repair is always performed with the patient under general anesthesia. An epidural catheter is inserted for the management of pain after the operation. The surgeon makes two incisions over the sternum, on either side of the chest, for insertion of a curved steel bar or strut under the sternum. He or she proceeds to remove the deformed cartilages. The rib lining is left in place to allow renewed cartilage growth. The sternum is then repositioned, and the metal strut is placed behind it and brought out through the muscles and skin for future attachment to a brace, which will stay in place six to 12 weeks. The metal strut is fixed to the ribs on either side, and the incisions are closed and dressed. A small steel grooved plate may be used at the end of the bar to help stabilize and fix the bar to the rib. A blood **transfusion** is not required during surgery. The surgeon may insert a temporary chest tube to re-expand the lung if the lining of the lung is entered.

A variety of surgical procedures are available to repair pectus excavatum.

Nuss procedure

A common technique is the Nuss procedure, developed in 1987 by Dr. Donald Nuss, a pediatric surgeon at Children's Hospital of the The King's Daughters and Eastern Virginia Medical School in Norfolk, Virginia. The procedure is minimally invasive, and results in very little blood loss and short recovery times.

Leonard procedure

Another surgical approach that drastically reduces the time required for surgery is the Leonard procedure, developed by Dr. Alfred Leonard, a Minneapolis thoracic

and pediatric surgeon. This operation does not violate the chest, and is combined with a bracing technique.

Diagnosis/Preparation

A pediatrician diagnoses pectus excavatum after observing a child when he or she inhales, exhales, and rests. The pediatrician also calculates the depth of the chest from front to back using x rays of the chest to determine whether the diameter is shorter than average, as is the case with funnel chest. The heart is usually larger and displaced to the left. The pediatrician also evaluates lung capacity using **exercise** tests and lung scans that can reveal mismatched lungs.

Other diagnostic tests may include:

- Electrocardiogram (ECG or EKG). This test records the electrical activity of the heart, and shows abnormal rhythms (arrhythmias or dysrhythmias).

- Echocardiogram (echo). This test evaluates the structure and function of the heart by using sound waves recorded on an electronic sensor that yields a moving picture of the heart and its valves.

Before surgery, a bone density test is performed to ensure that the patient does not have soft bones that would deform again right after the surgery. After a complete **health history** is taken, a patient whose condition is considered severe enough to warrant surgery is sent for a CT scan and further evaluation of his or her pulmonary function.

Because of the great variablity of pectus excavatum among those who have it, custom-made bars (or braces) must be used. The brace is a light vest to which the deformity-correcting wire will be attached at surgery. Patients are fitted with the brace prior to surgery.

Aftercare

Usual recovery time in the hospital is four to five days. Attention is paid to post-operative **pain management**. The patient is encouraged to breathe deeply, and receives assistance with movement (to avoid dislodging

QUESTIONS TO ASK THE DOCTOR

- Can exercises correct pectus excavatum?

- How is pectus excavatum surgery performed?

- Should everyone with pectus excavatum have surgery?

- What surgical procedures does the doctor use?

- How many pectus excavatum surgeries does the physician perform each year?

the bar). After discharge, the patient slowly resumes a normal, but restricted, activity level. Most children are able to return to school in two to three weeks, with exercise restrictions for six weeks (no physical education classes, heavy lifting, or athletics).

The pectus excavatum support bar is removed under general anesthesia two to four years after insertion, usually on an outpatient basis. In most cases, patients are able to leave the hospital within one to two hours after bar removal.

Risks

Risks associated with pectus excavatum repair include those normally associated with the administration of anesthesia (such as adverse reactions to medications and breathing problems), and risks associated with any surgery (such as bleeding and infection). Specific pectus excavatum surgery risks may include lung collapse (pneumothorax) and the recurrence of the funnel chest. Bar displacement may occasionally require repositioning.

Normal results

Pectus excavatum repair, in almost all instances, restores the ability of patients to participate in full activities, even strenuous activities and athletics. Also, there is a marked improvement in the patient's self image.

Morbidity and mortality rates

According to the National Institutes of Health (NIH), excellent results (95–98%) are reported over a lengthy follow-up time of 25 years. Long-term follow-up (over 15 years) shows that the Nuss procedure provides excellent results with less than 5% recurrence of the deformity after the bar is removed.

KEY TERMS

Marfan syndrome—A condition occasionally associated with chest wall deformities, in which the patients have a characteristic tall, thin appearance, and cardiac and great vessel abnormalities.

Pectus carinatum—A chest wall deformity characterized by a protrusion of the sternum.

Pectus excavatum—A chest wall deformity in which the chest wall takes on a sunken appearance.

Poland syndrome—A condition associated with chest wall deformities in which varying degrees of underdevelopment of one side of the chest and arm may occur.

Sternum—The breastbone. It connects with ribs one to seven on either side of the chest.

Alternatives

Mild cases of pectus excavatum may respond to an exercise and posture physiotherapy program. Many patients with rounded shoulders and a slouching posture have benefited from these techniques, with or without additional surgical correction. However, body-building exercises usually result in worsening of cosmetic appearance due to the enhancement of the pectoral muscles.

Resources

BOOKS

Pearson, F. G. *Thoracic Surgery*. Philadelphia: W. B. Saunders Co., 2002.

Ravitch, M. M. *Congenital Deformities of the Chest Wall and Their Operative Correction*. Philadelphia: W. B. Saunders Co., 1977.

PERIODICALS

Engum, S., F. Rescorla, K. West, T. Rouse, L.R. Scherer, and J. Grosfeld. "Is the Grass Greener? Early Results of the Nuss Procedure." *Journal of Pediatric Surgery* 35 (2000): 246-51.

Genc, A., and O. Mutaf. "Polytetrafluoroethylene Bars in Stabilizing the Reconstructed Sternum for Pectus Excavatum Operations in Children." *Chest* 110 (July 2002): 54-7.

Hebra, A., B. Swoveland, M. Egbert, E.P. Tagge, K. Georgeson, H.B. Othersen, and D. Nuss. "Outcome Analysis of Minimally Invasive Repair of Pectus Excavatum: Review of 251 Cases." *Journal of Pediatric Surgery* 35 (2000): 252-7.

Jacobs, J. P., J.A. Quintessenza, V.O. Morell, L.M. Botero, H.M. van Gelder, and C. I. Tchervenkov. "Minimally Invasive Endoscopic Repair of Pectus Excavatum." *European Journal of Cardiothoracic Surgery* 21 (2002): 869-83.

ORGANIZATIONS

American Pediatric Surgical Association (APSA). 60 Revere Drive, Suite 500, Northbrook, IL 60062. (847) 480-9576. <www.eapsa.org>.

Southern Thoracic Surgical Association. 633 N. Saint Clair St., Suite 2320, Chicago, IL, 60611-3658. (800) 685-7872. <www.stsa.org/>.

OTHER

"Pectus Excavatum Repair." *BestHealth*. <www.besthealth.com/surgery/PectusExcavatumRepair_1.html>.

Monique Laberge, Ph.D.

Pediatric concerns

Definition

Pediatric concerns refers to those issues that are unique to the care of children when surgery and hospitalization are involved.

Description

Children are not just little adults. When dealing with children medically, it is important to keep in mind the stage of their physical growth and development; their emotional development; and their maturity level. There are many different kinds of pediatric surgeries and procedures. A pediatric hospital is planned around the special needs of children and their families. All of the staff, including doctors (pediatric surgeons, pediatric anesthesiologists, pediatric radiologists), nurses, and technical support, have special training in pediatrics. Children's hospitals have specific expertise in pediatric problems and special programs for children who are ill or injured.

Helping a child prepare for surgery

When parents are helping their child prepare for surgery, it is important to realize that, no matter how mature the child may act, he or she still needs to be treated differently than adults. Some children find it comforting to know exactly what will happen, when, and how, all in great detail. Others do not want much detail. They may need just an overview of what to expect, keeping just one step ahead of what will be done to them. The particular level of a child's development will determine the specific concerns.

For example, the biggest fear for infants and toddlers is being away from their parents. Parents should stay with the child as much as possible, and ensure that basic needs (such as eating, play, or sleeping) are met, both at home and in the hospital. Preschoolers also fear being away from the parents, but, additionally, they see hospitalization as a punishment and fear bodily harm. In this case, parents should, again, stay with the child as much as possible, and start talking to them at home about the coming operation to help reassure them. For the hospital stay, parents should bring the child's favorite blanket and/or toys, pictures from home, and maybe music tapes.

For school-age children, the biggest fears are needles and pain. Parents can help by giving them information about their body and how it works, and vaguely explain that the doctor will fix them, but parents should not use language like "cut, incision, open you up, make a hole, etc." To make the hospital feel more familiar, parents can bring pictures and music tapes and/or videos from home. By adolescence, children are worried about the loss of independence, being separated from their peers, and being different (i.e., a change in their appearance). For teenagers at this stage of development, it is extremely important to explain an illness or hospitalization to them in terms that they can understand, using examples to which they can relate, and allow them to be involved in decisions, if possible. The parents should encourage them to ask questions.

What to expect at the hospital

Being in a hospital and undergoing surgery is scary and stressful for a child. Hospitalization disrupts their normal routines. If the staff behaves in a trusting, nurturing way, the child may become comfortable enough to return to some normal behaviors. Trust is important to all ages of children. If a procedure will hurt, it is important to be honest and let them know what to expect. Children can only learn to trust the staff if the staff is honest with them and treats them with respect.

Books and videos developed for children that explain about going to the hospital can be helpful. Some hospitals provide programs for children to come and visit before hospitalization, so that children will already be familiar with the hospital environment when they are admitted. Play is a child's way of expressing emotion, especially under difficult situations. Play can serve as a distracter as well as a means by which surgery and hospitalization can be explained to children. Dolls or stuffed animals can be used to walk young children through what they will be experiencing. Hospital play areas will often have toys that represent hospital equipment, so that a procedure can be explain with the use of props. For example, there may be pretend casts and bandages that a child can put on a stuffed animal. How children play can also serve as an insight for parents and staff as to understand how their children are feeling about what is happening to them. As children express their concerns through play, parents and staff can then address those concerns. Play is therapeutic for children, helping them feel safer in an unfamiliar environment, and should be considered an essential element in preparing for a child's hospital stay. Play areas help to make a strange place feel comfortable, both for the child as well as for the parents. Play areas also provide a relaxed area for parents to be with their child, a friendly home-like environment where nurturing can take place.

Unfortunately, some surgeries are not planned. Emergency situations are always more stressful, both because they are unexpected and because they are often more serious. Children take their cue on how to behave from those around them. When parents are noticeably concerned, children's anxiety levels rise. Parents should remain as calm as possible to be fully present for their children.

Parents should expect to be able to be with their children most of the time. For most day surgeries, parents can stay with their child until he or she is asleep, and then can be waiting in the **recovery room** when the child is waking up after the procedure is completed. Some facilities provide pullout beds for parents to spend the night with their children, and may even have a small kitchen where they can prepare food to eat in their child's room.

Qualified staff should be available to help parents work through their concerns and anxiety. Parents with more than one child may sometimes need to leave their hospitalized child completely in the hands of hospital staff as they attend to their other children at home. Many facilities have volunteers who can stay with children when their parents need to leave the hospital.

What to look for in health care for a child

While those hospitals designed especially for children are a wonderful resource, other hospitals that care for patients of all ages will often provide comparable care. If the surgery allows for time to select a surgeon and hospital, things to look for include:

- surgeons and physicians who are board certified in pediatrics
- staff with special training in pediatrics
- equipment designed for pediatric use
- a separate wing or floor for children
- child life specialists on staff
- play rooms and toys that can be brought into a child's room

A pediatric hospital or wing will have equipment that is smaller, better suited to the child's size. Bandages

KEY TERMS

Child life specialist—A person who has had specific training in the care of children, including understanding growth and development specific to each age range and how to talk to children of different ages.

Pediatrics—The medical specialty of caring for children.

Separation anxiety—A fear of being separated from a parent or loved one; a normal developmental process, occurring at certain points in a young child's life.

may have pictures of cartoon characters on them; there may be paintings of characters from children's movies on the walls.

Staff will usually have had special training to understand what issues are important to children at different stages of development. They should use language that is adapted to explain what is happening to the child in ways that make sense to them. For example, instead of just asking a child to blow, they may ask them to imagine that they are blowing out candles on a birthday cake. All of these techniques help to make the hospital a more familiar and friendlier place, putting the child at ease and helping to lessen anxiety.

Resources

BOOKS

Hautzig, Deborah, Dan Elliott, Joseph Mathieu, and Joe Mathieu. *A Visit to the Sesame Street Hospital: Featuring Jim Henson's Sesame Street Muppets.* London: Random House, 1985.

Rogers, Fred. *Going to the Hospital.* New York: Penguin Books for Young Readers, 1997.

ORGANIZATIONS

The Nemours Foundation. <http://kidshealth.org>.

Esther Csapo Rastegari, RN, BSN, EdM

Pediatric surgery

Definition

Pediatric surgery is a specialized field of surgery for the treatment of conditions that can be surgically corrected in a baby, child, or adolescent.

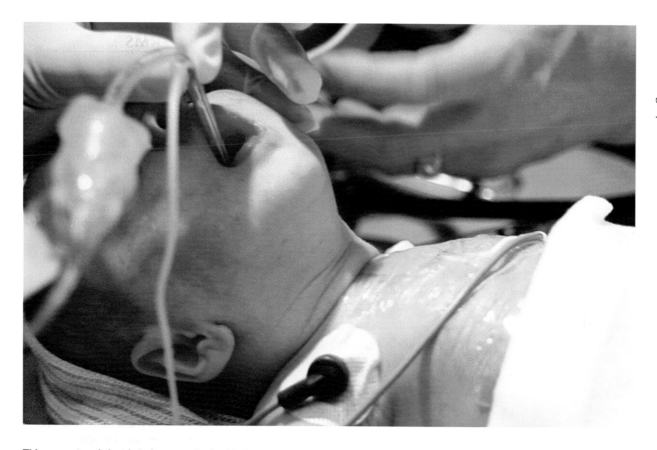

This premature infant is being anesthetized before undergoing surgery. *(Custom Medical Stock Photo. Reproduced by permission.)*

Purpose

The purpose of pediatric surgery varies with the procedure. In general, the purpose is to surgically correct a congenital condition, disease, traumatic injury, or other disorder in the pediatric patient.

Demographics

Pediatric surgeons provide treatment for young patients—newborns up through late adolescence.

Description

Pediatric surgery is the surgical branch that uses operative techniques to correct certain pediatric conditions (i.e., congenital abnormalities, tumors, chronic diseases, and traumatic injuries). There are different specialties within the field that include:

- pediatric **general surgery**
- pediatric otolaryngology (ear, nose, and throat)
- pediatric ophthalmology (eye)
- pediatric urology (urogenital system)
- pediatric orthopedic (bone) surgery

- pediatric neurological (brain and spinal cord) surgery
- pediatric plastic (reconstructive and cosmetic) surgery

The American Academy of Pediatrics has established specific guidelines for referral to subspecialists. The pediatric patient has special considerations that differentiate him or her, both physically and psychologically, from an adult. A neonate (newborn) poses great challenge in surgical treatment since the tiny structures and immature organ systems may not cope with disease-induced stress and the physical demands of a major operative procedure. A newborn infant may still be developing key bodily functions, or may have special requirements. Key areas of concern in the newborn include:

- cardiovascular (heart) system
- thermoregulation (temperature requirements of 73°F [22.8°C])
- pulmonary (lung) function
- renal (kidney) function
- immature immunity and liver
- special requirements for fluid, electrolyte (necessary elements such as sodium, potassium, and calcium) and nutrition

The pediatric surgeon must take into account the special requirements unique to the young surgical patient. The pediatric surgeon is trained to treat the entire spectrum of surgical illnesses. The following is an overview (with symptoms) of the more common pediatric conditions that require surgery typically performed by the pediatric surgeon.

Alimentary tract obstruction

Obstruction of the alimentary tract (tubes of digestion extending from the mouth to the anus) is characterized by four cardinal symptoms:

- abdominal distention (an abdomen that becomes large and appears swollen)
- bilious vomiting (due to bile in the stomach)
- maternal polyhydramnios (excess amniotic fluid in the amniotic sac, greater than 2,000 ml) before birth
- failure to pass meconium (dark green or black sticky excretion passed via the newborn's rectum) in the first 24 hours of life

ESOPHAGEAL ATRESIA AND TRACHEOESOPHAGEAL FISTULA. This is a congenital deformity of the esophagus (the tube that passes food from the mouth to the stomach). Symptoms include severe respiratory distress (the neonate cannot breathe) and excessive salivation. Other clinical signs include cyanosis (bluish discoloration of the skin due to oxygen deprivation), choking, and coughing.

PYLORIC ATRESIA AND RELATED CONDITIONS. Pyloric atresia is a condition that occurs when the pyloric valve, located between the stomach and duodenum, fails to open. Food cannot pass out of the stomach, resulting in vomiting clear gastric juice at attempted feedings. Maternal polyhydramnios is present before birth in more than 60% of cases.

Other areas of the colon (duodenum, jejunum, ileum) can be obstructed during development, with symptoms present at birth. Most of these disorders share the four cardinal symptoms of alimentary obstruction.

INTUSSUSCEPTION. Intussusception accounts for 50% of intestinal obstruction in patients who are three months to one year of age. Eighty percent of cases are observed by the child's second birthday. The cause of intussusception is not known, and it is more common in males who are well nourished and apparently healthy. The symptoms include a sudden onset of abdominal pain characterized by episodic screaming and drawing up of the legs. In 60% of patients, vomiting and blood in the stool are common findings (either bright red or occult [hidden] blood). Typically, the bowel movements look like currant jelly, consisting of mucus and blood mixed together. Currant jelly stool is the most common clinical observation for patients with intussusception. During

physical examination, patients will exhibit abdominal distention, and in 65% of cases there is a sausage-shaped mass that can be felt in the upper right portion of the abdomen toward the mid-abdomen. Ultrasound studies are a reliable method of diagnosis.

FAILURE TO PASS MECONIUM. Failure to pass meconium (meconium ileus) is associated with cystic fibrosis (a genetic disorder), colonic obstruction (colonic atresia), meconium plug syndrome, and aganglionic megacolon (also called Hirschsprung's disease, a congenital absence of the nerves that provide gastrointestinal tract mobility).

Anorectal anomalies

There are many different types of anorectal anomalies common to male and female neonates, as well as deformities that are gender-specific since involvement of genitalia can occur. The surgery for these cases is complicated, and must be performed by an experienced pediatric surgeon. Complications of these procedures could result in permanent problems.

Necrotizing enterocolitis (NEC)

NEC affects 1–2% of patients admitted to a neonatal **intensive care unit**. It is a life-threatening illness characterized by abdominal distention, bilious vomiting, lethargy, fever, occult (not obvious) or gross (clearly seen) rectal bleeding. Additionally, affected patients may exhibit signs of hypothermia (temperature less than 96.5°F or 35.8°C), bradycardia (slow heart rate), abdominal mass (felt during palpation), oliguria, jaundice, and episodes of breathlessness (apnea). Survival of NEC surgery can be expected for 60–70% of patients.

Abdominal wall defects

Omphalocele is a defect that involves protrusion of abdominal contents into an external sac. This disorder occurs in one per 5,000 births. More than 50% of omphalocele patients have serious genetic deformities involving these body systems: cardiovascular (heart), musculoskeletal (muscle and bones), genitourinary (genital and bladder systems), and central nervous (brain and spinal cord). The overall survival rate for infants with omphalocele varies, and depends on defect size, other associated genetic abnormalities, and age of newborn. (Many infants with omphalocele are premature.) Approximately 33% of patients with omphaloceles do not survive.

GASTROSCHISIS. Gastroschisis is a defect in the abdominal wall to the side (lateral) of the umbilicus. It usually occurs to the right of an intact normal umbilical cord. The cause is unknown. The bowel protrudes to the outside of the abdomen during intrauterine life (while the embryo is developing inside the uterus). The amniotic fluid has an irritating effect on the exposed bowel, and causes infection of the bowels. The problem can be detected by ultrasound studies during pregnancy. Some pediatric surgeons and obstetricians recommend **cesarean section** (early elective delivery) to spare bowel trauma. The newborn patients typically require surgery, tube feedings for three to four weeks, and hospitalization for several weeks. The current survival rate for infants with gastroschisis is greater than 90%.

Congenital diaphragmatic hernia (CDH)

CDH can be diagnosed by the fourth month of pregnancy via ultrasound studies. Of the infants with congenital diaphragmatic hernia (CDH), 44–66% have other congenital abnormalities as a result of developmental malformations. Anatomically, patients with CDH have a defect in development that allows a communication between the chest and abdomen. Through this defect, the abdominal contents enter the lung cavity and interfere with normal lung development. The incidence is approximately one per 2,200 live births, and males are more commonly affected than females. Usually the infants are full-term, and the defect occurs on the left side in the majority—88%—of patients.

Treatment is extensive, and usually requires three major areas:

• stabilization of patient and preoperative preparation

• operative treatment

• postoperative respiratory, metabolic, circulatory, and nutritional supportive measures

Postoperatively, the infant is monitored in the neonatal intensive care setting. The postoperative period is more critical if a lung is severely underdeveloped.

Pyloric stenosis (PS)

Pyloric stenosis is an obstruction in the intestine due to a larger-than-normal size of the muscle fibers of the pylorus (lower stomach opening). Pyloric stenosis is a common hereditary condition that affects males more than females, and occurs in one per 750 births. The typical symptoms include a progressive, often projectile, vomiting after attempted feedings. The gastric vomitus (bloody in 80% of patients) usually begins during the second and third week of life, and increases in force and frequency. Typically, the infant fails to gain weight, and the number of bowel movements and rate of urination decreases.

Physical examination is usually helpful in establishing a diagnosis. Palpation of the enlarged muscle fibers can be felt as an olive-shaped mass located in the midline approximately one-third to one-half of the distance

from the umbilicus to the xiphoid (end of the breast bone), when the stomach is empty. Careful abdominal examination and palpation can usually identify the pyloric mass in 85% of cases.

Gastroesophageal reflux

Gastroesophageal reflux (GER) is a common disorder in infancy, and usually disappears by the baby's first birthday. The largest group of patients with clinically significant GER are those who have neurologic impairment. Symptoms often include vomiting, repeated lung infections (from aspirating gastric contents during regurgitation of foodstuffs), and delayed gastric emptying. The success rate with infants who have procedures necessary to correct GER is over 90%.

Meckel's diverticulum

Meckel's diverticulum occurs in approximately 2% of the U.S. population. The diverticulum is an outgrowth of intestine is located in a portion of the intestines called the ileum. Symptoms of obstruction are more often observed in infants, and bleeding is more common in patients after age four.

Intestinal polyps

Juvenile polyps are usually present between the ages of four and 14 years, and tend to be inflammatory. The most common symptom of intestinal polyps is rectal bleeding, which is commonly due to a solitary polyp (80% of cases). Diagnosis can be done by proctosigmoidoscopy, which allows visualization of 85% of polyps.

Acute appendicitis

Acute appendicitis is a relatively common surgical emergency that is misdiagnosed in 28% of patients due to a broad spectrum of symptoms that can confuse the clinician. The classic clinical symptom of acute appendicitis is the onset of pain in the middle region of the abdomen that is followed by anorexia, nausea, and vomiting. The pain is persistent and radiates to the right lower abdomen, becoming more intense and localized. The physical and abdominal examinations must be carefully and accurately performed. Patients with acute appendicitis usually have an increased white blood cell (cells that fight infection) count.

Once the diagnosis is established, the child is prepared for surgery. Preoperative **antibiotics** are started at least one-half hour before the operation. If the appendix is perforated (ruptured), complications can occur as a result of kidney (renal) failure, seizures due to fever, and gram-negative sepsis (an infection that enters the bloodstream and interferes with life-saving chemical reactions). Patients who are very young, or those who were misdiagnosed and incurred long delays in treatment, are susceptible to death.

Inflammatory bowel diseases

Some cases (approximately 25%) of inflammatory bowel disease are found in persons younger than 20 years of age. Two types can occur, Crohn's disease and ulcerative colitis.

The diagnosis of inflammatory bowel disease is usually based on presenting clinical symptoms, laboratory analysis results, endoscopic appearance, and radiologic findings. Approximately 50–60% of patients have bloody diarrhea, severe cramping, abdominal pain, and urgency.

CROHN'S DISEASE. The symptoms of Crohn's disease includes cramping abdominal pain, diarrhea, and

strictures (constriction) resulting from bowel obstruction. Removal of diseased portions in children with Crohn's disease may be temporarily beneficial, but recurrence after surgical removal occurs in about 50% of cases within four years. Chronic symptoms may remain into adult life, making long-term follow-up essential.

ULCERATIVE COLITIS. Ulcerative colitis is limited to the colon. A surgical procedure known as colectomy is curative, and indicated for intractable disease (64% of patients). Colectomy is the removal of the entire colon, or the inflamed part of it.

Biliary tract disorders

A variety of biliary tract conditions may be present at birth, some requiring surgical correction.

NEONATAL JAUNDICE. Neonatal jaundice is common, and results from an immature system not capable of some basic biochemical reactions. Food intake can help speed these reactions, which usually resolves the condition within seven to 10 days. Jaundice that persists for over two weeks is abnormal, and could be caused by over 30 possible disorders.

BILIARY ATRESIA. Biliary atresia is a disease that causes inflammation of the ducts within the biliary system, resulting in fibrosis of these ducts. The incidence of biliary atresia is one per 15,000 live births, and is more common in females. Time is critical, and most patients must have surgery by two months of life. Approximately 25–30% of patients who receive early operative intervention have long-term successful outcomes. Some patients may require **liver transplantation**, and 85–90% of these patients survive.

CHOLELITHIASIS. Gallbladder obstruction in infants and young children is usually caused by pigmented (colored) stones resulting from blood disorders. Removal of the gallbladder (laparoscopic **cholecystectomy**) is the treatment of choice.

Trauma

Accidents are the leading cause of death in children between the ages of one and 15 years, and accounts for 50% of all deaths in the pediatric age group. More than half of these deaths are due to motor vehicle accidents, followed by falls, bicycle injuries, drowning, burns, child abuse, and birth trauma. Head trauma is the single most common organ associated with traumatic death. Within recent years, the number of fatalities related to the use of firearms and violence has increased.

More than 20 million children each year sustain injuries requiring treatment. These injuries account for 100,000 cases of permanent pediatric disability. Response to trauma in pediatric patients is significantly different from older patients. Pediatric patients require special attention concerning temperature regulation, blood volume, metabolic rate and requirements, and airway maintenance. Other special pediatric considerations include response to stress, communication difficulties, psychological trauma, a different pediatric trauma score system, smaller airway diameter, and increased risk of aspirating gastric contents (which could cause pneumonia). Pediatric trauma patients should have access to appropriate pre-hospital transportation, and must receive medical attention in a pediatric trauma center capable of providing the complex level of care necessary for serious pediatric trauma situations.

Neck masses

Neck masses during infancy and childhood may be caused by tumors or infections, or they may be congenital. Lymphadenitis is an infection of a lymph node that becomes enlarged and tender. Most cases are resolved by treating the primary source of infection (i.e., middle ear infection and tonsillitis). Some inflamed nodes may require an incision and drainage of infection.

Hernias

INGUINAL HERNIA AND HYDROCELE. Inguinal (groin) hernia is the most frequent disorder requiring surgery in the pediatric age group. Clinically, a right-sided inguinal hernia is more common in males (60% of cases), and there is a familial tendency. The incidence is higher in full-term infants (3.5–5%). Full-term infants and older children (without underlying diseases) can receive surgical repair in an outpatient setting. An inguinal hernia may result in herniation of the scrotum, and a communicating hydrocele (hernia with a small connection to the peritoneal cavity).

UMBILICAL HERNIA. Umbilical hernia is a defect of the umbilical ring, and is more common in females and African American children. Spontaneous involution occurs in 80% of cases. Larger defects may be observed for several years without complications, and their spontaneous resolution is possible. If the umbilical hernia persists, patients may develop feeding intolerance, pain, and local skin breakdown.

Undescended testes

Undescended testes are observed in 1–2% of full-term males. Approximately 30% of preterm males may have an undescended testis. Undescended testis in premature infants may descend by the first year of life, and observation is often the treatment during that time.

KEY TERMS

Atresia—Thinning or narrowing of a passageway.

Large intestine—The portion of the colon that includes the cecum; ascending, transverse, and descending sigmoid colon; rectum; and anal canal.

Oliguria—Decreased urine production.

Pediatric aged patient—The pediatric aged patient encompasses several periods during development. The first four weeks after birth are callled the neonatal period. The first year after birth is called infancy, and childhood is from 13 months until puberty (between the ages of 12 and 15 years in girls and 13 and 16 years in boys).

Polyp—A tumor mass, generally benign and capable of surgical removal.

Pylorus—The area that controls food passage from the stomach to the first part of the small intestine (duodenum).

Small intestine—The part of the intestines that consists of the duodenum, jejunum, and ileum.

Tumors

Wilm's tumor (nephroblastoma) is a tumor in the kidneys that forms during embryonic development. The tumor is due to a genetic abnormality; and approximately 80% of children are diagnosed between one and five years of age. In about 75–95% of cases, the patient has an abdominal mass that is detected by a parent during bathing. Blood in the urine (hematuria) occurs in 10–15% of cases, and high blood pressure (hypertension) is present in 20–25% of cases. Hypertension is the result of the tumor compressing the kidney in a specific area, causing it to release a chemical called renin, which elevates blood pressure. During physical examination, the Wilm's tumor is a smooth, round, hard, nontender flank mass. The treatment of Wilm's tumor depends on its stage, and may include surgery, chemotherapy, or radiotherapy.

Resources

BOOKS

Townsend, Courtney. *Sabiston Textbook of Surgery* 16th ed. St. Louis: W. B. Saunders Company, 2001.

PERIODICALS

Coran, A. "American Academy of Pediatrics: Guidelines for Referral to Pediatric Surgical Specialists." *Pediatrics* 110, no.1 (July 2002).

Okada P. J., B. Hicks. "Pediatric Surgical Emergencies: Neonatal Surgical Energencies." *Clinical Pediatric Emergency Medicine* 3, no.1 (March 2002:).

ORGANIZATIONS

The American Pediatric Surgical Association. 60 Revere Drive Suite 500 Northbrook, Il 60062. (847) 480-9576. Fax: (847) 480-9282 E-mail: eapsa@eapsa.org.

Laith Farid Gulli, M.D.,M.S.
Nicole Mallory, M.S.,PA-C
Abraham F. Ettaher,M.D.
Robert Ramirez, B.S.

PEG tube insertion *see* **Gastrostomy**

Pelvic ultrasound

Definition

Pelvic ultrasound is a procedure in which high-frequency sound waves create images of the pelvic organs. The sound waves are projected into the pelvis, and measure how they reflect—or echo—back from the different tissues.

Purpose

Ultrasound is a preferred method of examining the pelvis, and functions as an extension of a **physical examination**, particularly for obese patients. It is a common initial step after physical examination when a patient complains of pelvic pain or abnormal vaginal bleeding. The procedure is performed routinely during pregnancy and examinations to determine the cause of infertility. Ultrasound has the ability to detect the size and shape of pelvic organs, such as the bladder, and is useful in evaluating the cause of bladder dysfunction. In women, pelvic ultrasound is used to examine the uterus, ovaries, cervix, and vagina. In general, ultrasound can detect inflammation, free fluid, cysts (abnormal fluid-filled spaces), and tumors in the pelvic region.

A primary use of pelvic ultrasound is during pregnancy. In early pregnancy (about five to seven weeks), ultrasound may determine the size of the fetus to confirm the suspected due date, detect multiple fetuses, or confirm that the fetus is alive (viable). Ultrasound is particularly useful in distinguishing between intrauterine (within the uterus) and ectopic (outside the uterus) pregnancies. Toward the middle of the pregnancy (about 16–20 weeks), the procedure can confirm fetal growth, reveal defects in the anatomy of the fetus, and check the placenta and amniotic fluid. Toward the end of pregnancy, it may be used to evaluate fetal size, position, growth, or to check the placenta.

Doctors may use ultrasound to guide the biopsy needle during **amniocentesis** and chorionic villus sampling. The imaging allows precise placement of the long needle that is inserted into the patient's uterus to collect cells from the placenta or amniotic fluid.

Description

Depending on the goal of the procedure, a pelvic ultrasound can also be called a bladder ultrasound, pelvic gynecologic sonogram, or obstetric sonogram. Ultrasound examinations are usually done in a doctor's office, clinic, or hospital setting. Typically, the patient will lie on an examination table with the pelvis exposed. Special gel is applied to the area to make sure that there is no air between the hand-held transducer and the skin, and to facilitate transducer movement. The physician or technologist guides the transducer over the abdomen. The transducer both creates and receives the echoes of the high-frequency sound waves (usually in the range of 3.5–10.0 megahertz). An ultrasound scan reveals the shape and densities of organs and tissues. By performing repeated scans over time, much like the frames of a movie, ultrasound can also reveal movement, such as the motions of a fetus. This technique is called real-time ultrasound.

Using a computerized tool, called a caliper, the ultrasound technologist can measure various structures shown in the image. For example, the length of the upper thigh bone (femur) or the distance between the two sides of the skull can indicate the age of the fetus.

Ultrasound technology has been safely used in medical settings for over 30 years, and several significant extensions to the procedure have made it even more useful. A specially designed transducer probe can be placed in the vagina to provide better ultrasound images. This transvaginal or endovaginal scan is particularly useful in early pregnancy or in cases where ectopic pregnancy is suspected. It is also routinely used to provide better anatomic delineation of the endometrium and pelvic masses. In men, transrectal scans, where the probe is placed in the rectum, are done to check the prostate. Doppler ultrasound has the ability to follow the flow of blood through veins and arteries, and can be useful in detecting disorders such as abnormal blood flow associated with ovarian torsion (a twisted blood supply that causes pelvic pain). Color enhancement is particularly useful in Doppler imaging, where shades of red signify flow away from the transducer and shades of blue signify flow toward it.

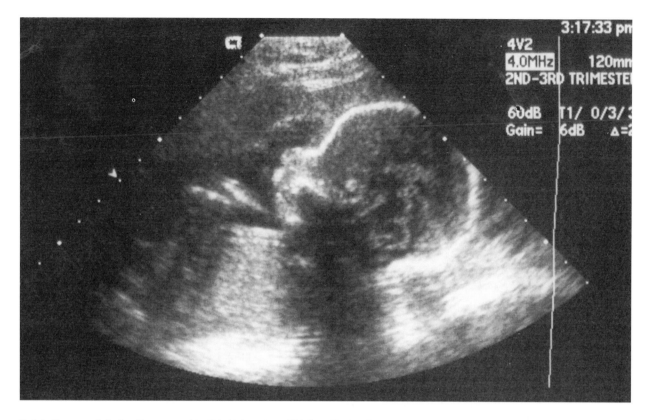

Fetal ultrasound during the second to third trimester. *(Brigham Narins. Reproduced by permission.)*

Hysterosonography is another variant ultrasound procedure. It involves the injection of saline solution into the uterus during an endovaginal scan. The saline distends the uterine cavity (or endometrium) and simplifies the identification of polyps, fibroids, and tumors. The saline outlines the lesion, making it easier to find and evaluate. Hysterosonography can also be used in the testing of patency (openness) of the fallopian tubes during infertility evaluations.

Preparation

Before undergoing a pelvic ultrasound, the patient may be asked to drink several glasses of water and to avoid urinating for about one hour prior to exam time. When the bladder is full, it forms a convenient path, called an acoustic window, for the ultrasonic waves. A full bladder is not necessary for an endovaginal examination, sometimes making it a preferred choice in emergency situations. Women usually empty their bladders completely before an endovaginal exam.

Aftercare

For a diagnostic ultrasound, the lubricating gel applied to the abdomen is wiped off at the end of the procedure and the patient can immediately resume normal activities.

Risks

Ultrasound carries with it almost no risk for complications.

Normal results

A normal scan reveals no abnormalities in the size, shape, or density of the organs scanned. During pregnancy, a normal scan reveals a viable fetus of expected size and developmental stage. Although ultrasound is an extremely useful tool, it cannot detect all problems in the pelvic region. If a tumor or other lesion is very small or if it is masked by another structure, it may not be detected. When used during pregnancy, patients should be advised that ultrasound does not reveal all fetal abnormalities. Additionally, the reliability of ultrasound readings can depend on the skill of the technologist or physician performing the scan.

An abnormal scan may show the presence of inflammation, cysts, tumors, or abnormal blood flow patterns. These results may suggest further diagnostic procedures, or surgical or pharmacological treatment. Obstetrical ultrasound examinations may alter the anticipated due date or detect abnormalities or defects in the fetus. This information may reveal that the fetus cannot survive on its

KEY TERMS

Acoustic window—Area through which ultrasound waves move freely.

Amniocentesis—A procedure where a needle is inserted through the pregnant woman's abdomen and into the uterus to withdraw a sample of amniotic fluid surrounding the fetus.

Chorionic villus sampling—A procedure where a needle is inserted into the placenta to withdraw a sample of the placenta's inner wall cells surrounding the fetus.

Ectopic pregnancy—A pregnancy where the fertilized egg becomes implanted somewhere other than in the uterus; if in a fallopian tube it is called a tubal pregnancy.

Real-time—A type of ultrasound that takes multiple images over time in order to record movement, or the observations obtained while scanning (rather than obtained by looking at films after the procedure).

Sonographer—A technologist or physician who uses an ultrasound unit to takes ultrasound images of patients.

Transducer—The handheld part of the ultrasound unit that produces the ultrasound waves and receives the ultrasound echos.

Ultrasound—Sound above what can be heard by the human ear, generally above 20,000 Hz (cycles per second).

own after birth, or that it will require extensive treatment or care. The technologist performing the ultrasound should consult with a radiologist or other physician if any questionable results appear.

Resources

BOOKS

Sanders, Roger C. *Clinical Sonography: A Practical Guide.* Boston: Little, Brown and Company, 1998.

PERIODICALS

Galen, Barbara A. "Diagnostic Imaging: An Overview." *Primary Care Practice* 3 (September/October 1999).

Jorizzo, J. "Sonohysterography: The Next Step in the Evaluation of the Abnormal Endometrium." *Radiographics* 117 (Oct. 1999).

Kaakagi, Y. "Sonography of Obstetric and Gynecologic Emergencies: Part II, Gynecologic Emergencies." *American Journal of Roetgenology* 661 (Mar. 2000).

Wooldridge, Leslie. "Ultrasound Technology and Bladder Dysfunction." *American Journal of Nursing Supplement* 100 (June 2000).

ORGANIZATIONS

American Institute of Ultrasound in Medicine. 14750 Sweiter Lane, Suite 100, Laurel, MD 20707-5906. (301) 498-4100 or (800) 638-5352. <http://www.aium.org>.

American Registry of Diagnostic Medical Sonographers (ARDMS). 600 Jefferson Plaza, Suite 360, Rockville, MD 20852-1150. (301) 738-8401 or (800) 541-9754. <http://www.ardms.org>.

OTHER

Valley, Verna T. "Ultrasonography, Pelvic." *Emedicine.* January 17, 2001. [cited May 6, 2001] <http://www.emedicine.com/emerg/topic622.htm>.

Michelle L. Johnson, M.S., J.D.
Lee A. Shratter, M.D.

Penile implant surgery *see* **Penile prostheses**

Penile prostheses

Definition

Penile prostheses are semi-rigid or inflatable devices that are implanted into penises to alleviate impotence.

Purpose

The penis is composed of one channel for urine and semen, and three compartments with tough, fibrous walls containing erectile tissue. With appropriate stimulation, the blood vessels that lead out of these compartments constrict, trapping blood. Blood pressure fills and hardens the compartments producing an erection of sufficient firmness to perform sexual intercourse. Additional stimulation leads to ejaculation, where semen is pumped out of the urethra. When this system fails, erectile dysfunction or impotence (failure to create and maintain an erection) occurs.

Impotence can be caused by a number of conditions, including diabetes, spinal cord injury, prolonged drug abuse, and removal of the prostate gland. If the medical condition is irreversible, a penile prosthesis may be considered. Men whose impotence is caused by psychological problems are not recommended for implant surgery.

Demographics

Recently, it has been reported that surgeons insert approximately 20,000 penile implants into American

Penile prostheses

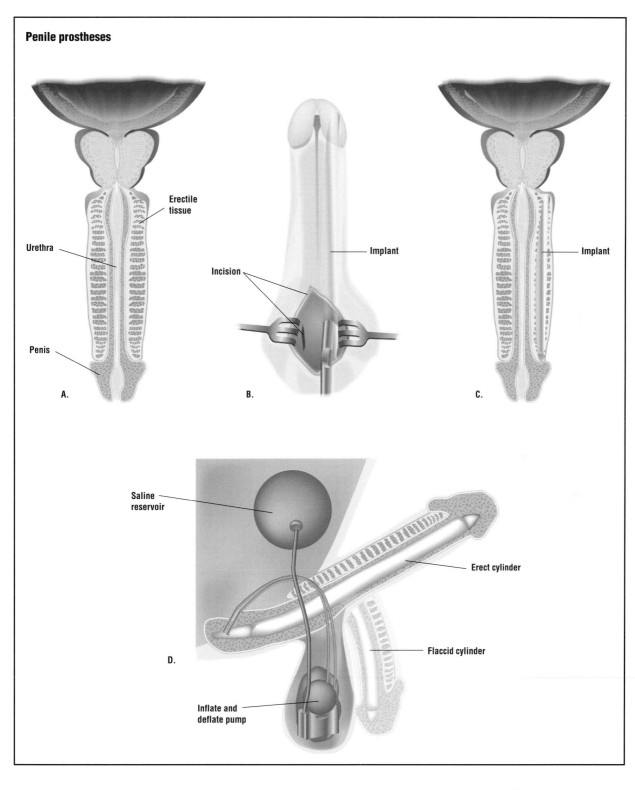

An incision is made at the base of the penis to implant a prosthesis in an area of erectile tissue (B and C). Once in place, a pump placed in the scrotum can be used to inflate and deflate the implant when an erection is desired (D). *(Illustration by GGS Inc.)*

men yearly. The most common device is a multi-component inflatable implant (approximately 45% of all implants). Semi-rigid rods account for about 35% of the implants. Self-contained devices comprise approximately 20% of implants.

Description

Penile implant surgery is conducted on persons who have exhausted all other areas of treatment. Semi-rigid devices consist of two rods that are easier and less expensive to implant than the inflatable cylinders. Once implanted, the semi-rigid device needs no follow-up adjustments; however, it produces a penis that constantly remains semi-erect. Inflatable cylinders produce a more natural effect. Men using them are able to simulate an erection via a pump located in the scrotum.

With a surgical patient under general anesthesia, the device is inserted into the erectile tissue of the penis through an incision in the fibrous wall. In order to insert the pump for the inflatable implant, incisions are made in the abdomen and the perineum (area between the anus and the genitals). A fluid reservoir is placed into the groin, and the pump is placed in the scrotum. The cylinders, reservoir, and pump are connected by tubes and tested before the incisions are closed.

Diagnosis/Preparation

Surgery always requires a patient who is adequately informed about the procedure's risks and benefits. The sexual partner should also be involved in the discussion. Prior to surgery, the region undergoes antibacterial cleansing and is shaved.

Aftercare

To minimize swelling, ice packs are applied to the penis for the first 24 hours following surgery. The incision sites are cleansed daily to prevent infection. Pain relievers may be taken.

Risks

With any implant, there is a slightly greater risk of infection than with simple surgery. The implant may irritate the penis and cause continuous pain. The inflatable prosthesis may need follow-up surgery to repair leaks in the reservoir or to reconnect the tubing.

Normal results

Successful implantation of a penile prosthesis solves some problems related to impotence. After healing from the surgical procedure, men with a penile prosthesis can resume normal sexual activities.

Morbidity and mortality rates

On a purely technical basis, morbidity associated with a surgically implanted penile implants is relatively uncommon, and is usually due to a post-surgical infection or to mechanical failure of the implanted device. Experts feel that personal dissatisfaction with a penile implant procedure is more common, and is usually due to unreasonable or inappropriate expectations for the procedure. Mortality is quite rare.

Alternatives

Medication (sildenafil citrate [Viagra]) is useful for some men with erectile dysfunction. The medication must be prescribed and monitored by a physician.

Impotence caused psychological factors can usually be treated with appropriate counseling and therapy.

Creams are available for purchase. Most experts agree that these cannot reverse physiological impotence.

Most experts consider mechanical rings that prevent blood flow out of a penis to be dangerous, and advise against their use.

See also Open prostatectomy.

Resources

BOOKS

Bland, K.I., W.G. Cioffi, M.G. Sarr. *Practice of General Surgery.* Philadelphia: Saunders, 2001.

Campbell, M.F., P.C. Walsh, A.B. Restik. *Campbell's Urology,* 8th ed. Philadelphia: Saunders, 2002.

Grace, P.A., A. Cuschieri, D. Rowley, N. Borley, A. Darzi. *Clinical Surgery,* 2nd ed. Londin, 2003.

Hanna, P.M., S.B. Malkowicz, and A.J. Wein. *Clinical Manual of Urology,* 3rd ed. New York: McGraw Hill, 2001.

Schwartz S.I., J.E. Fischer, F.C. Spencer, G.T. Shires, J.M. Daly. *Principles of Surgery,* 7th ed. New York: McGraw Hill, 1998.

Townsend C, K.L. Mattox, R.D. Beauchamp, B.M. Evers, D.C. Sabiston. *Sabiston's Review of Surgery,* 3rd ed. Philadelphia: Saunders, 2001.

PERIODICALS

Carson, C.C. "Penile Prostheses: Are They Still Relevant?" *British Journal of Urology International* 91, no.3 (2003): 176-7.

Carson, C.C. "Therapeutic Strategies for Managing Erectile Dysfunction: A Step-care Approach." *Journal of the American Osteopathic Medical Association* 102, no.12 Suppl 4 (2002): S12-18.

Montague, D.K., K.W. Angermeier. "Current Status of Penile Prosthesis Implantation." *Current Urology Reports* 1, no.4 (2002): 291-6.

Rees, R.W., J. Kalsi, S. Minhas, J. Peters, P. Kell, D.J. Ralph. "The Management of Low-flow Priapism with the Immediate Insertion of a Penile Prosthesis." *British Journal of Urology International* 90, no.9 (2002): 893-7.

ORGANIZATIONS

American Board of Surgery. 1617 John F. Kennedy Boulevard, Suite 860, Philadelphia, PA 19103. (215) 568-4000. Fax: (215) 563-5718. <http://www.absurgery.org>.

American Board of Urology. 2216 Ivy Road, Suite 210, Chaarlottesviille, VA 22903. (434) 979-0059. <http://www.abu.org> .

American College of Surgeons. 633 North St. Clair Street, Chicago, IL 60611-32311. (312) 202-5000. Fax: (312) 202-5001. E-mail: <postmaster@facs.org>. <http://www.facs.org>.

American Foundation for Urologic Disease. 1128 North Charles Street, Baltimore, MD 21201. (800) 242-2383. <http://www.afud.org> .

American Medical Association. 515 N. State Street, Chicago, IL 60610. (312) 464-5000. <http://www.ama-assn.org>.

American Urological Association. 1120 North Charles Street, Baltimore, MD 21201. (410) 727-1100. <http://www.auanet.org>.

KEY TERMS

General anesthesia—Deep sleep induced by a combination of medicines that allows surgery to be performed.

Genital—Sexual organ.

Perineum—Area between the anus and genitals.

Scrotum—The external pouch containing the male reproductive glands (testes) and part of the spermatic cord.

OTHER

Cornell University. [cited May 5, 2003] <http://www.cornel-lurology.com/cornell/ sexualmedicine/ed/implant.shtml>.

Ohio State University Medical Center. [cited May 5, 2003] <http://www.acs.ohio-state.edu/units/osuhosp/patedu/Materials/PDFDocs/procedure/impo-imp.pdf>.

Phoenix5. [cited May 5, 2003] <http://www.phoenix5.org/sexaids/implants/surgerydiags.html>.

University of California-Davis Medical Center. [cited May 5, 2003] <http://www.ucdmc.ucdavis.edu/ucdhs/health/a-z/15Impotence/doc15procedures.html>.

L. Fleming Fallon, Jr., M.D., Dr.PH.

Percutaneous nephrolithotomy *see* **Nephrolithotomy, percutaneous**

Percutaneous transluminal angioplasty *see* **Angioplasty**

Pericardiocentesis

Definition

A procedure performed with a needle to remove fluid for diagnostic or therapeutic purposes from the tissue covering the heart (pericardial sac).

Purpose

The heart is surrounded by a membrane covering called the pericardial sac. The sac consists of two layers, the parietal (outer) and visceral (inner) layer, and normally contains a small amount of fluid to cushion and lubricate the heart as it contracts and expands. When too much fluid gathers in the pericardial cavity, the space between the pericardium and the outer layers of the heart, a condition known as pericardial effusion occurs. Abnormal amounts of fluid may result from:

• pericarditis, infection caused by inflammation of the pericardial sac

• trauma, such as an abnormal collection of blood due to an accident

• surgery or invasive heart procedures

• heart attack (myocardial infarction) or congestive heart failure, which occurs when the heart looses its pumping capability due to a heart condition

• kidney (renal) failure

• cancer (producing malignant effusions)

The rate of pericardial fluid accumulation is important. If fluid accumulation develops slowly, then problems with blood flow will not develop until fluid retention becomes massive. Blood can also enter the pericardial sac (hemopericardium) due to trauma, blood-thinning medications, or disease. When there is rapid or excessive build-up of fluid or blood in the pericardial cavity, the resulting compression on the heart impairs the pumping action of the vascular system (a condition called cardiac tamponade). Pericardiocentesis can be used in such an emergency situation to remove the excess accumulations of blood or fluid from the pericardial sac. For diagnostic purposes, pericardiocentesis may be advised in order to obtain fluid samples from the sac for laboratory analysis.

Prior to the discovery of **echocardiography**, pericardiocentesis was a risky procedure. The clinician had to insert a long needle below the breastbone into the pericardial sac without internal visualization. This blind approach was associated with damage to the lungs, coronary arteries, myocardium, and liver. However, with direct visualization using echocardiography, pericardiocentesis can now be performed with minor risk. Some risk is still associated with the procedure since it is considered an invasive measure.

Demographics

Cardiac tamponade and pericarditis are two primary complications that require intervention with pericardiocentesis. Cardiac tamponade has an incidence of two in 10,000 the general U.S. population. Approximately 2% of cases are attributed to injuries that penetrate the chest. Pericarditis is more common in males than females with a ratio of seven to three. In young adults, pericarditis is usually caused by HIV infection or a trauma injury. Malignancy or renal failure are the main causes of this disorder in the elderly.

Description

The patient should sit with the head elevated 30-40 degrees. This is done to maximize fluid drainage. A site close to the pericardial sac is chosen, and if time permits the patient is sedated. The puncture site is cleaned with an antiseptic iodine solution, and the area is shaved and anesthetized with lidocaine (a local anesthetic). A long cardiac needle is inserted under the xiphoid (the bottom of the breastbone) approach on the left side of the heart using guided imagery into the chest wall until the needle reaches the pericardial sac. Usually, the patient may experience a sensation of pressure when the tip of the needle penetrates the pericardial sac. When guided imagery confirms correct placement, fluid is aspirated from the sac.

If the procedure is performed for diagnostic purposes, aspirated fluid can be collected in specimen vials and sent for pathological analysis (i.e. for cancer cell detection in cases where malignant effusion is suspected), or the fluid is just removed if the procedure was performed urgently (i.e. cardiac tamponade). For therapeutic cases, a pericardial catheter may be attached and fixed into position to allow for continuous drainage. When the needle is removed, pressure is applied for five minutes at the puncture site to stop the bleeding, and the site is bandaged.

Diagnosis/Preparation

The typical symptom associated with patients requiring pericardiocentesis is chest pain, usually indicative of severe effusion. Patients with cardiac tamponade commonly have dyspnea (difficulty breathing) and those with an infection may have fever. Some patients may have a hoarse voice from compression of a nerve called the recurrent laryngeal nerve; the pericardial sac may be so large that it pushes or compresses neighboring anatomical structures. Physical symptoms may vary, dependent both on size and the rate of filling of the pericardial effusion. Patients can also present with the following physical symptoms:

• tachycardia, an increased heart rate

- tachypnea, an increase in breathing rate
- jugular vein enlargement
- narrow pulse pressure (pulsus paradoxus)
- pericardial friction rub
- elevated central venous pressure
- hiccups from esophageal compression
- Ewart's sign (dull sound when the doctor taps the chest, tactile fremitus, egobronchophony)

The procedure can be performed in an emergency room, ICU, or at the bedside. Before the procedure patients should have an echocardiogram and basic blood analysis. No special dietary restrictions are required for pericardiocentesis. The patient will receive an IV line for sedation or other necessary medications and an electrocardiogram (ECG) to monitor cardiac activity. The patient must lie flat on the table, with the body elevated to a 60-degree angle. If the test is elective, then food and water restriction is recommended for six hours before the test. For infants and children, preparation depends on the child's age, level of trust, and previous exposure to this or similar procedures.

Aftercare

The puncture site, or if a catheter is fixed in place, the catheter site, should be inspected regularly for signs of infection such as redness or swelling. **Vital signs** such as blood pressure and pulse are monitored following the procedure.

Risks

Pericardiocentesis is an invasive procedure and therefore has associated risks. Complications are possible, but have become less common due to guided imaging techniques that improved the past blind approach. Possible risks include:

- puncture of the myocardium, the outer muscle layer of the heart

- puncture of a coronary artery, a blood vessel that supplies blood to heart muscle
- myocardial infarction (heart attack)
- needle induced arrhythmias (irregular heartbeats)
- pneumopericardium, air entry into the pericardial sac
- infection of the pericardial membranes (pericarditis)
- accidental puncture of the stomach, lung, or liver

Normal results

Normal pericardial fluid is clear to straw colored. During pathological examination normal pericardial fluid does not contain blood, cancer cells, or bacteria. In most individuals, a small amount of fluid (10–50 ml) is in the pericardial sac to cushion the heart. Pericardial fluid volumes over 50 ml suggest pericardial effusion. The presence of microorganisms (such as *Staphylococcus aureus*) in aspirated pericardial fluid indicates bacterial pericarditis. Blood in pericardial fluid can be seen in patients with cancer; cardiac rupture, which can occur with myocardial infarction; or hemorrhage due to traumatic injury or accident.

Morbidity and mortality rates

The success of pericardiocentesis has greatly improved with the use of guided imagery during the procedure. Only about 5% of patients will experience a major complication as a result of pericardiocentesis. Cardiac tamponade is fatal in almost all cases unless the excess fluid in the pulmonary sac is removed.

Resources

BOOKS

Behrman, Richard. *Nelson Textbook of Pediatrics*, 16th ed. Philadelphia: W. B. Saunders Company, 2000.

Braunwald, Eugene. *Heart Disease: A Textbook of Cardiovascular Medicine*, 6th ed. Philadelphia: W. B. Saunders, 2001.

Cecil, Russell, J. Claude Bennett, and Lee Goldman, eds. *Cecil Textbook of Medicine*, 21st ed. Philadelphia: W. B. Saunders Company, 2001.

Gunn, Veronica, and Christian Nechyba, eds. *The Harriet Lane Handbook: A Manual for the Pediatric House Officers*, 16th ed. Philadelphia: W. B. Saunders Company, 2002.

Marx, J. *Rosen's Emergency Medicine: Concepts and Clinical Practice*, 5th ed. St. Louis: Mosby, Inc., 2002.

Roberts, James. *Clinical Procedures in Emergency Medicine*, 3rd ed. Philadelphia: W. B. Saunders Company, 1998.

PERIODICALS

A.D.A.M., Inc. "Pericardiocentesis." January 31, 2003 [cited June 26, 2003]. University of Pennsylvania Health System. <http://www.pennhealth.com/ency/article/003872.htm>.

Desai, K., et al. "Pericardiocentesis." eMedicine.com. April 25, 2002 [cited June 26, 2003]. <http://www.emedicine.com/med/topic3560.htm>.

Laith Farid Gulli,, MD, MS
Alfredo Mori,, MBBS
Abraham F. Ettaher,, MD
Robert Ramirez,, BS

Peripheral endarterectomy

Definition

A peripheral endarterectomy is the surgical removal of fatty deposits, called plaque, from the walls of arteries other than those of the heart and brain. The surgery is performed when plaque blocks an artery and obstructs the flow of blood and oxygen to other parts of the body, most commonly the legs but also the arms, kidneys, or intestines. The peripheral arteries most often treated with endarterectomy are those that supply the legs, especially the aortoiliac arteries in the pelvic area. Other arteries that may be treated with endarterectomy include the femoral arteries in the groin, the renal arteries that supply the kidneys, and the superior mesenteric arteries that supply the intestines.

Purpose

Endarterectomy surgeries are performed to treat advanced peripheral arterial disease (PAD). PAD most often occurs as a result of atherosclerosis, a condition characterized by the gradual build up of fats, cholesterol, cellular waste, calcium, and other substances on the inner walls of large and medium-sized arteries. Plaque, the hardened, waxy substance that results from this build up, can cause narrowing (stenosis) of an artery and block the flow of blood and oxygen. Peripheral endarterectomies are performed to reopen blocked arteries and to restore blood flow in the body (revascularization), helping to prevent heart attack, stroke, the **amputation** of a limb, organ failure, or death.

Demographics

People who have been diagnosed with PAD caused by atherosclerosis are at high risk of arterial blockage (occlusion) and are candidates for peripheral endarterectomy. Occlusive arterial disease is found in 15 to 20% of men and women older than age 70. When found in people younger than 70, it occurs more often in men than in women, particularly in those who have ever smoked or who have diabetes. Women with PAD live longer than men with the same condition, which accounts for the equal incidence in older Americans. African-Americans have been shown to be at greater risk for arterial occlusion than other racial groups in the United States.

Description

PAD is a progressive occlusive disease of the arteries, common in older people who have ever smoked or who have diabetes. Although there are other forms of arterial disease that affect peripheral arteries (Buerger's disease, Raynaud's disease, and acrocyanosis), PAD in most people is caused by widespread artherosclerosis, the accumulation of plaque on the inner lining (endothelium) of the artery walls. Most commonly, occlusive PAD develops in the legs, including the femoral arteries that supply the thighs with blood or in the common iliac arteries, which are branches of the lower abdominal aorta that also supply the legs. The arteries that supply the shoulders and arms are less commonly affected. Branches of the aorta that deliver blood to the kidneys, the infrarenal aorta and renal arteries, can become narrowed as a result of artherosclerosis, but are only rarely blocked suddenly and completely, a condition requiring immediate surgery. Even more rare is blockage of the branches that supply the liver and spleen.

The development of atherosclerosis and PAD is influenced by heredity and also by lifestyle factors, such as dietary habits and levels of **exercise**. The risk factors for atherosclerosis include:

- high levels of blood cholesterol and triglycerides
- high blood pressure
- cigarette smoking or exposure to tobacco smoke
- diabetes, types I and II
- obesity
- inactivity, lack of exercise
- family history of early cardiovascular disease

Just as coronary artery disease (CAD) can cause a heart attack when plaque blocks the arteries of the heart, or blockage in the carotid artery leading to the brain can cause a stroke, blockage of the peripheral arteries can create life-threatening conditions. When peripheral arteries have become narrowed by plaque accumulation (atheroma), the flow of oxygen-carrying blood to the arms, legs, or body organs will be interrupted, which can cause cell death from lack of oxygen (ischemia) and nutrition. Normal growth and cell repair cannot take place, which can lead to gangrene in the limbs and subsequent amputation. When blood flow is blocked to internal organs, such as the kidneys or intestines, the result of tissue death can be the shutdown of the affected organ system and systemic (whole body) poisoning from waste accumulation. Death can result if **emergency surgery** is not performed to correct the blockage.

In some cases, the body will attempt to change the flow of blood when a portion of an artery is blocked by plaque. Smaller arteries around the blockage will begin to take some of the blood flow. This adaptation of the body (collateral circulation) is one reason for a lack of symptoms in some people who actually have PAD. Symptoms usually occur when the blockage is over 70% or when complete blockage occurs as a result of a piece of plaque breaking off and blocking the artery. Blockage in the legs, for example, will reduce or cut off circulation, causing painful cramping in the legs during walking

WHO PERFORMS THE PROCEDURE AND WHERE IS IT PERFORMED?

Peripheral endarterectomy is performed in a hospital **operating room** by a vascular surgeon.

(intermittent claudication) and pain in the feet during rest, especially during the night. When an artery gradually becomes narrowed by plaque, the symptoms are not as severe as when sudden, complete blockage occurs. Sudden blockage does not offer time for collateral vessels to develop and symptoms can be equally sudden and dramatic. Possible symptoms of reduced blood flow in the most typically affected arteries include:

- Arteries of the arms and legs: Gradual blockage creates muscle aches and pain, cramping, and sensations of tiredness or numbness; sudden blockage may cause severe pain, coldness and numbness. A leg or arm may become blue (cyanotic) from lack of oxygen. No pulse will be felt. Paralysis may occur.
- Lower aorta, femoral artery, and common iliac arteries: Gradual narrowing causes intermittent claudication affecting the buttocks and thighs. Men may become impotent. Sudden blockage will cause both legs to become painful, pale, and cold. No pulse will be felt. Legs may become numb. The feet may become painful, infected, or even gangrenous when gradual or complete blockage limits or cuts off circulation
- Renal arteries: Gradual narrowing may produce no symptoms and no change in kidney function. Sudden, complete blockage may cause sudden pain in the side and bloody urine. This is an emergency situation.
- Superior mesenteric artery: Gradual narrowing causes steady, severe pain in the middle of the abdomen about 30 to 60 minutes after a meal. Nutrients are lost and weight loss is common. Sudden, complete blockage causes severe abdominal pain, vomiting, and the urge to move the bowels. Blood pressure falls, intestinal gangrene may develop, and the patient may go into shock. This is an emergency situation.

Sudden, complete occlusion of an artery can also happen when a clot (thrombus) forms in an already narrowed artery. Clot formation (thrombosis) can occur anywhere in the body and travel to a narrowed portion of an affected artery and become lodged (embolism), blocking blood flow. Clots can sometimes be dissolved with anticoagulant drug therapy. When this therapy is not effective or a life-threatening blockage occurs suddenly, clots can be surgically removed using thromboendarterectomy, a procedure similar to peripheral endarterectomy.

Early treatment for PAD may include medical treatment to reduce the underlying causes: lowering cholesterol, lowering blood pressure, stopping smoking, increasing exercise, and reducing the likelihood of clot formation. Clot-dissolving drugs (thrombolytic drugs) may also be used to remove a clot medically rather than to perform surgery. When these measures are not effective, or an artery becomes completely blocked, peripheral endarterectomy may be performed to remove the blockage (see also **angioplasty** and **peripheral vascular bypass surgery**). Treatment of risk factors must continue, because surgery only corrects the immediate problem, not the underlying causes.

Peripheral endarterectomy works best in narrow areas like the leg where the artery can be easily accessed, or when there is complete blockage of an artery by an atheroma that is short in length. Endarterectomy does not work as well for smaller arteries lower in the leg or in the foot or arm. Drug therapy, **angiography**, stent placement, or surgical bypass may be used to treat blockages of the arteries in these areas.

Patients undergoing peripheral endarterectomy will typically be given general anesthesia. The surgery is an open surgical procedure in which a vascular surgeon makes a relatively large incision in the outer skin to access the obstructed artery being treated. In order to perform the surgery, the blood that normally flows through the artery must first be rerouted through a tube connecting the blood vessels below and above the surgical site. The surgeon will

then cut the obstructed artery lengthwise and will use surgical tools to clean away the accumulation of plaque. The hard, waxy substance comes out fairly easily, sometimes in a single piece. The artery will then be sutured closed or patched with a piece of a vein, usually from the patient's leg, to enlarge the repaired artery and prevent later narrowing from post-operative scarring. The entire procedure will take about one hour if there are no complications.

Diagnosis/Preparation

A complete patient history is essential to diagnosis, particularly information about family members who may have had diabetes or early cardiovascular disease. Symptoms will be important diagnostic indicators, letting the physician know what areas of the body may have reduced blood flow. Blood pressure will be taken in the arms and legs. Pulses will be measured in the arms, armpits, wrists, groin, ankles, and behind the knees. This will show where blockages may exist, since the pulse below a blockage is usually absent. Additionally, a **stethoscope** will be used to listen for abnormal sounds in the arteries that may indicate narrowing. Blood flow procedures may be performed, including:

- Doppler ultrasonography—direct measurement of blood flow and rates of flow, sometimes performed in conjunction with stress testing (exercise between tests).
- Angiography—an x ray procedure that provides clear images of the affected arteries before surgery is performed.
- Blood tests—routine tests such as cholesterol and glucose, as well as tests to help identify other causes of narrowed arteries, such as inflammation, thoracic outlet syndrome, high homocycteine levels, or arteritis.
- Spiral computed tomography (CT angiography) or magnetic resonance angiography (MRI)—less invasive forms of angiography.

If ultrasonography or angiography procedures were not performed earlier to diagnose arterial blockage, these tests will be performed before surgery to evaluate the amount of plaque and the extent and exact location of narrowing. **Aspirin** therapy or other clot-prevention medication may be prescribed before surgery. Any underlying medical condition, such as high blood pressure, heart disease, or diabetes will be treated prior to peripheral endarterectomy to help get the best result from the surgery. Upon **admission to the hospital**, routine blood and urine tests will be performed.

Aftercare

After the peripheral endarterectomy, the patient's blood pressure, temperature, and heart rate will be monitored in a hospital **recovery room** for an hour or more, and the surgical site will be checked regularly. The patient will then be transferred to a concentrated care unit to be observed for any sign of complications. The total hospital stay may be two to three days. When the patient returns home, activities can be resumed gradually. Walking and strenuous activity may be restricted, especially if surgery was performed on the groin or leg. During recuperation, the patient may be given pain medication as needed and clot-prevention (anticoagulant) medication. Patients will be advised to reduce the risk factors for artherosclerosis in order to avoid repeat narrowing or blockage of the arteries. Repeat stenosis (restenosis) has been shown to occur frequently in people who do not make the necessary changes in lifestyle, such as changes in diet, exercise, and quitting smoking. The benefits of the surgery may only be temporary if underlying disease, such as artherosclerosis, high blood pressure, or diabetes, is not also treated.

Risks

The risks associated with peripheral endarterectomy primarily involve the underlying conditions that led to blockage of arteries in the first place. Embolism is the most serious post-operative risk; a clot or piece of tissue from the endarterectomy site that may travel to the heart, brain, or lungs can cause heart attack, stroke, or death. Restenosis, the continuing build-up of plaque, can occur within months to years after surgery if risk factors are not controlled. Other complications may include:

- reactions to anesthesia
- breathing difficulties
- changes in blood pressure
- nerve injury
- post-operative bleeding

Normal results

The outcomes of peripheral endarterectomy as a treatment for arterial blockage are usually good. Blood flow can be restored quickly to relieve symptoms and help prevent heart attack, stroke, organ failure, or limb amputation.

Morbidity and mortality rates

Morbidity and mortality depend upon the artery involved, the extent of the blockage, and the patient's overall condition, which directly influences response to the surgery. Time is also a factor. In cases of sudden and complete blockage of the mesenteric arteries, for example, only immediate surgery can save the person's life.

KEY TERMS

Atheroma—A collection of plaque (lesion) blocking a portion of an artery.

Atherosclerosis (arteriosclerosis)—A process of thickening and hardening of large and medium-sized arteries as a result of fatty deposits on their inner linings.

Ischemia—An inadequate blood supply (circulation) in an area of the body when arteries in the area are blocked.

Peripheral arterial disease (PAD)—An occlusive disease of the arteries most often caused by progressive artherosclerosis.

Peripheral endarterectomy—The surgical removal of fatty deposits, called plaque, from the walls of arteries other than those of the heart and brain.

Plaque—A collection of wax-like fatty deposits on the insides of artery walls.

Restenosis—The repeat narrowing of blood vessels that may occur after surgical removal of plaque when preventive measures are not taken.

Revascularization—Retoring normal blood flow (circulation) in the body's vascular (veins and arteries) system.

Stenosis—The narrowing of a blood vessel.

Although death does not frequently occur during peripheral endarterectomy surgery, patients with widespread atherosclerosis and PAD have been shown to have increased morbidity and mortality associated with coronary artery disease, because of the common risk factors, such as cigarette smoking, high blood pressure, and diabetes. PAD patients with diabetes are shown to represent 50% of all amputations. However, only a small percentage of patients undergoing peripheral endarterectomy will suffer limb loss or associated disability and reduced quality of life.

Alternatives

Peripheral endarterectomy removes plaque directly from blocked arteries; there is no alternative way to mechanically remove plaque. However, there are alternative ways to prevent plaque build-up and reduce the risk of narrowing or blocking the peripheral arteries. Certain vitamin deficiencies in older people, for example, are known to promote high levels of homocysteine, an amino acid that contributes to atherosclerosis and a higher risk for PAD. Some nutritional supplements and alternative therapies that are recommended to help promote good vascular health include:

• Folic acid can help lower homocysteine levels and increase the oxygen-carrying capacity of red blood cells.

• Vitamins B_6 and B_{12} can lower homocycteine levels.

• Antioxidant vitamins C and E work together to promote healthy blood vessels and improve circulation.

• Angelica, an herb that contains coumadin, a recognized anticoagulant, may help prevent clot formation in the blood.

• Essential fatty acids, as found in flax seed and other oils, can help reduce blood pressure and cholesterol, and maintain elasticity of blood vessels.

• Chelation therapy may be used to break up plaque and improve circulation.

Resources

BOOKS

Cranton, Elmer MD., ed. *Bypassing Bypass Surgery: Chelation Therapy: A Non-Surgical Treatment for Reversing Arteriosclerosis, Improving Blocked Circulation, and Slowing the Aging Process.* Hampton Roads Pub. Co., 2001.

McDougal, Gene. *Unclog Your Arteries: How I Beat Artherosclerosis.* 1st Books Library, Nov 2001.

ORGANIZATIONS

American Heart Association (AHA). 7272 Greenville Ave., Dallas, TX 75231. (800) 242-8721. <http://www.americanheart.org>.

Vascular Disease Foundation. 3333 South Wadsworth Blvd. B104-37, Lakewood, CO 80227. (303) 949-8337; (866) PADINFO (723-4636). <http://www.vdf.org>.

OTHER

Hirsch, Alan T. MD. "Occlusive Peripheral Arterial Disease." *The Merck Manual of Medicine.* Home Edition [cited July 7, 2003]. <http://www.merck.com/pubs>.

"Patient Information: Frequently Asked Questions." Peripheral Vascular Surgery Society [cited July 7, 2003]. <http://www.pvss.org>.

L. Lee Culvert

Peripheral vascular bypass surgery

Definition

A peripheral vascular bypass, also called a lower extremity bypass, is the surgical rerouting of blood flow around an obstructed artery that supplies blood to the legs and feet. This surgery is performed when the build-up of fatty deposits (plaque) in an artery has blocked the normal flow of blood that carries oxygen and nutrients to the lower extremities. Bypass surgery reroutes blood from above the obstructed portion of an artery to another vessel below the obstruction.

A bypass surgery is named for the artery that will be bypassed and the arteries that will receive the rerouted blood. The three common peripheral vascular bypass surgeries are:

• Aortobifemoral bypass surgery, which reroutes blood from the abdominal aorta to the two femoral arteries in the groin.

• Femoropopliteal bypass (fem-pop bypass) surgery, which reroutes blood from the femoral artery to the popliteal arteries above or below the knee.

• Femorotibial bypass surgery, which reroutes blood between the femoral artery and the tibial artery.

A substitute vessel or graft must be used in bypass surgeries to reroute the blood. The graft may be a healthy segment of the patient's own saphenous vein (autogenous graft), a vein that runs the entire length of the thigh. A synthetic graft may be used if the patient's saphenous vein is not healthy or long enough, or if the vessel to be bypassed is a larger artery that cannot be replaced by a smaller vein.

Purpose

Peripheral vascular bypass surgery is performed to restore blood flow (revascularization) in the veins and arteries of people who have peripheral arterial disease (PAD), a form of peripheral vascular disease (PVD). People with PAD develop widespread hardening and narrowing of the arteries (atherosclerosis) from the gradual build-up of plaque. In advanced PAD, plaque accumulations (atheromas) obstruct arteries in the lower abdomen, groin, and legs, blocking the flow of blood, oxygen, and nutrients to the lower extremities (legs and feet). Rerouting blood flow around the blockage is one way to restore circulation. It relieves symptoms in the legs and feet, and helps avoid serious consequences such as heart attack, stroke, limb **amputation**, or death.

Demographics

Approximately 8–10 million people in the United States have PAD caused by atherosclerosis. These people are at high risk of arterial occlusion, and are candidates for peripheral vascular bypass surgery. Occlusive arterial disease is found in 15–20% of men and women older

Peripheral vascular bypass surgery

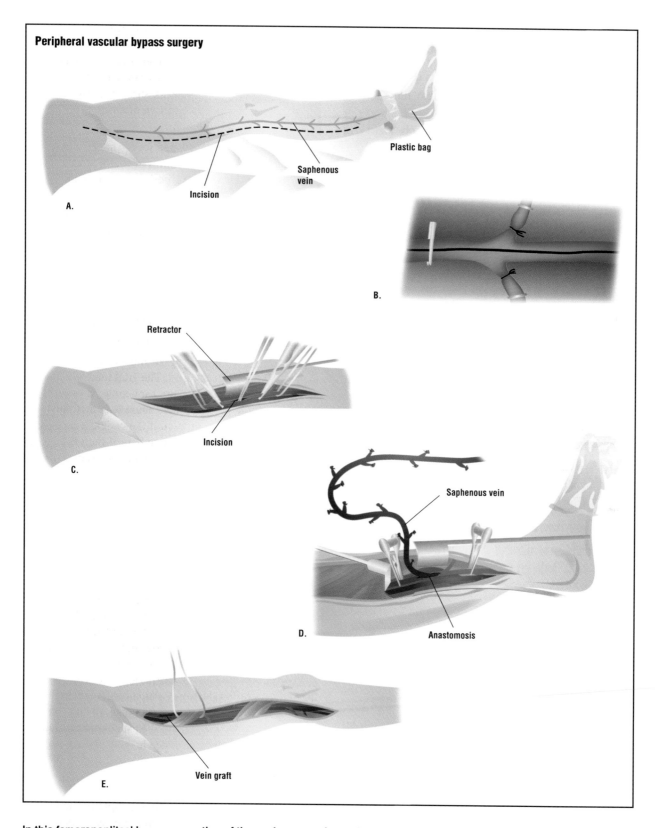

A.

Incision

Saphenous vein

Plastic bag

B.

C.

Retractor

Incision

D.

Saphenous vein

Anastomosis

E.

Vein graft

In this femoropopliteal bypass, a portion of the saphenous vein can be removed and used to bypass a portion of a diseased artery. To accomplish this, an incision is made down the inside of the leg (A). The saphenous vein is tied off from its tributaries and removed (B). An incision is made in the recipient artery (C), and the vein is stitched to it at the top and bottom of the leg (D). *(Illustration by GGS Inc.)*

than age 70. In people younger than age 70, it occurs more often in men than women, particularly in those who have ever smoked or who have diabetes. Women with PAD live longer than men with the same condition, accounting for the equal incidence in older Americans. African-Americans are at greater risk for arterial occlusion than other racial groups in the United States.

Description

The circulatory system delivers blood, oxygen, and vital nutrients to the limbs, organs, and tissues throughout the body. This is accomplished via arteries that deliver oxygen-rich blood from the heart to the tissues and veins that return oxygen-poor blood from organs and tissues back to the heart and lungs for re-oxygenation. In PAD, the gradual accumulation of plaque in the inner lining (endothelium) of the artery walls results in widespread atherosclerosis that can occlude the arteries and reduce or cut off the supply of blood, oxygen, and nutrients to organ systems or limbs.

Peripheral vascular bypass surgery is a treatment option when PAD affects the legs and feet. PAD is similar to coronary artery disease (CAD), which leads to heart attacks and carotid artery disease (CAD), which causes stroke. Atherosclerosis causes each of these diseases. Most often, atherosclerotic blockage or narrowing (stenosis) occurs in the femoral arteries that supply the thighs with blood or in the common iliac arteries, which are branches of the lower abdominal aorta that also supplies the legs. The popliteal arteries (a portion of the femoral arteries near the surface of the legs) or the posterior tibial and peroneal arteries below the knee (portions of the popliteal artery) can be affected.

Just as coronary artery disease can cause a heart attack when plaque blocks the arteries of the heart, or blockage in the carotid artery leading to the brain can cause a stroke, occlusion of the peripheral arteries can create life-threatening conditions. Plaque accumulation in the peripheral arteries blocks the flow of oxygen-carrying blood, causing cells and tissue in the legs and feet to die from lack of oxygen (ischemia) and nutrition. Normal growth

and cell repair cannot take place, which can lead to gangrene in the limbs and subsequent amputation. If pieces of the plaque break off, they can travel from the legs to the heart or brain, causing heart attack, stroke, or death.

The development of atherosclerosis and PAD is influenced by heredity and also by lifestyle factors, such as dietary habits and levels of **exercise**. The risk factors for atherosclerosis include:

• high levels of blood cholesterol and triglycerides.

• high blood pressure (hypertension)

• cigarette smoking or exposure to tobacco smoke

• diabetes, types 1 and 2

• obesity

• inactivity, lack of exercise

• family history of early cardiovascular disease

Sometimes the body will attempt to change the flow of blood when a portion of an artery is narrowed by plaque. Smaller arteries around the blockage begin to take over some of the blood flow. This adaptation of the body (collateral circulation) is one reason for the absence of symptoms in some people who have PAD. Another reason is that plaque develops gradually as people age. Symptoms usually don't occur until a blockage is over 70%, or when a piece of plaque breaks off and blocks an artery completely. Blockage in the legs reduces or cuts off circulation, causing painful cramping during walking, which is relieved on rest (intermittent claudication). The feet may ache even when lying down at night.

When narrowing of an artery occurs gradually, symptoms are not as severe as they are when sudden, complete blockage occurs. Sudden blockage does not allow time for collateral vessels to develop, and symptoms can be severe. Gradual blockage creates muscle aches and pain, cramping, and sensations of fatigue or numbness in the limbs; sudden blockage may cause severe pain, coldness, and numbness. At times, no pulse can be felt, a leg may become blue (cyanotic) from lack of oxygen, or paralysis may occur.

When the lower aorta, femoral artery, and common iliac arteries (all in the lower abdominal and groin areas) are blocked, gradual narrowing may produce cramping pain and numbness in the buttocks and thighs, and men may become impotent. Sudden blockage will cause both legs to become painful, pale, cold, and numb, with no pulse. The feet may become painful, infected, or even gangrenous when gradual or complete blockage limits or cuts off circulation. Feet may become purple or red, a condition called rubor that indicates severe narrowing. Pain in the feet or legs during rest is viewed as an indication for bypass surgery because circulation is reduced to a degree that threatens survival of the limb.

Early treatment for PAD usually includes medical intervention to reduce the causes of atherosclerosis, such as lowering cholesterol and blood pressure, **smoking cessation**, and reducing the likelihood of clot formation. When these measures are not effective, or an artery becomes completely blocked, lower extremity bypass surgery may be performed to restore circulation, reduce foot and leg symptoms, and prevent limb amputation.

Bypass surgery is an open procedure that requires general anesthesia. In femoropopliteal bypass or femorotibial bypass, the surgeon makes an incision in the groin and thigh to expose the affected artery above the blockage, and another incision (behind the knee for the popliteal artery, for example) to expose the artery below the blockage. The arteries are blocked off with vascular clamps. If an autogenous graft is used, the surgeon passes a dissected (cut and removed) segment of the saphenous vein along the artery that is being bypassed. If the saphenous vein is not long enough or is not of good quality, a tubular graft of synthetic (prosthetic) material is used. The surgeon sutures the graft into an opening in the side of one artery and then into the side of the other. In a femoropopliteal bypass, for example, the graft extends from the femoral artery to the popliteal artery. The clamps are then removed and the flow of blood is observed to make sure it bypasses the blocked portion of the affected artery.

Aortobifemoral bypass surgery is conducted in much the same way, although it requires an abdominal incision to access the lower portion of the abdominal aorta and both femoral arteries in the groin. This is generally a longer and more difficult procedure. Synthetic grafts are used because the lower abdominal aorta is a large conduit, and its blood flow cannot be handled by the smaller saphenous vein. Vascular surgeons prefer the saphenous vein graft for femoropopliteal or femorotibial bypass surgery because it has proven to stay open and provide better performance for a longer period of time than synthetic grafts. Bypass surgery patients will be given heparin, a blood thinner, immediately after the surgery to prevent clotting in the new bypass graft.

Diagnosis/Preparation

Diagnosis

After obtaining a detailed history and reviewing symptoms, the physician examines the legs and feet, and orders appropriate tests or procedures to evaluate the vascular system. Diagnostic tests and procedures may include:

• Blood pressure and pulses—pressure measurements are taken in the arms and legs. Pulses are measured in the arms, armpits, wrists, groin, ankles, and behind the

---

knees to determine where blockages may exist, since no pulse is usually felt below a blockage.

• Doppler ultrasonography—direct measurement of blood flow and rates of flow, sometimes performed in conjunction with stress testing (tests that incorporate an exercise component).

• Angiography—an x ray procedure that provides clear images of the affected arteries before surgery is performed.

• Blood tests—routine tests such as cholesterol and glucose, as well as tests to help identify other causes of narrowed arteries, such as inflammation, thoracic outlet syndrome, high homocycteine levels, or arteritis.

• Spiral computed tomography (CT **angiography**) or magnetic resonance angiography (MRA)—less invasive forms of angiography.

Preparation

If not done earlier in the diagnostic process, ultrasonography or angiography procedures may be performed when the patient is admitted to the hospital. These tests help the physician evaluate the amount of plaque and exact location of the narrowing or obstruction. Any underlying medical condition, such as high blood pressure, heart disease, or diabetes is treated prior to bypass surgery to help obtain the best surgical result. Regular medications, such as blood pressure drugs or **diuretics**, may be discontinued in some patients. Routine pre-operative blood and urine tests are performed when the patient is admitted to the hospital.

Aftercare

After bypass surgery, the patient is moved to a recovery area where blood pressure, temperature, and heart rate are monitored for an hour or more. The surgical site is checked regularly. The patient is then transferred to a concentrated care unit to be observed for any signs of complications. The total hospital stay for femoropopliteal bypass or femorotibial bypass surgery may be two to four days. Recovery is slower with aortobifemoral bypass surgery, which involves abdominal incisions, and the hospital stay may extend up to a week. Walking will begin immediately for patients who have had femoropopliteal or femorotibial bypasses, but patients who have had aortobifemoral bypass may be kept in bed for 48 hours. When bypass patients go home, walking more each day, as tolerated, is encouraged to help maintain blood flow and muscle strength. Feet and legs can be elevated on a footstool or pillow when the patient rests. Some swelling of the leg should be expected; it does not indicate a problem and will resolve within a month or two.

During recuperation, the patient may be given pain medication if needed, and clot prevention (anticoagulant) medication. Any redness of the surgical site or other signs of infection will be treated with **antibiotics**. Patients are advised to reduce the risk factors for atherosclerosis in order to avoid repeat narrowing or blockage of the arteries. Repeat stenosis (restenosis) has been shown to occur frequently in people who do not make the necessary lifestyle modifications, such as changes in diet, exercise, and smoking cessation. The benefits of the bypass surgery may only be temporary if underlying disease, such as atherosclerosis, high blood pressure, or diabetes, is not also treated.

Risks

The risks associated with peripheral vascular bypass surgery are related to the progressive atherosclerosis that led to arterial occlusion, including a return of pre-operative symptoms. In patients with advanced PAD, heart attack or heart failure may occur. Build up of plaque has also taken place in the patient's arteries of the heart. Restenosis, the continuing build up of plaque, can occur within months to years after surgery if risk factors are not controlled. Other complications may include:

- clot formation in a saphenous vein graft
- failed grafts or blockages in grafts
- reactions to anesthesia
- breathing difficulties

- embolism (clot from the surgical site traveling to vessels in the heart, lungs, or brain)
- changes in blood pressure
- infection of the surgical wound
- nerve injury (including sexual function impairment after aortobifemoral bypass)
- post-operative bleeding
- failure to heal properly

Normal results

A femoropopliteal or femorotibial bypass with an autogenous graft of good quality saphenous vein has been shown to have a 60–70% chance of staying open and functioning well for five to 10 years. Aortobifemoral bypass grafts have been shown to stay open and reduce symptoms in 80% of patients for up to 10 years. Pain and walking difficulties should be relieved after bypass surgery. Success rates improve when the underlying causes of atherosclerosis are monitored and managed effectively.

Morbidity and mortality rates

The risk of death or heart attack is about 3–5% in all patients undergoing peripheral vascular bypass surgery. Following bypass surgery, amputation is still an outcome in about 40% of all surgeries performed, usually due to progressive atherosclerosis or complications caused by the patient's underlying disease condition.

Alternatives

Peripheral vascular bypass surgery is a mechanical way to reroute blood, and there is no alternative method. Alternative ways to prevent plaque build-up and reduce the risk of narrowing or blocking the peripheral arteries include nutritional supplements and alternative therapies, such as:

- Folic acid can help lower homocysteine levels and increase the oxygen-carrying capacity of red blood cells.
- Vitamins B_6 and B_{12} can help lower homocysteine levels.
- Antioxidant vitamins C and E work together to promote healthy blood vessels and improve circulation.
- Angelica, an herb that contains coumadin, a recognized anticoagulant, which may help prevent clot formation in the blood.
- Essential fatty acids, as found in flax seed and other oils, to help reduce blood pressure and cholesterol, and maintain blood vessel elasticity.
- Chelation therapy, used to break up plaque and improve circulation.

KEY TERMS

Atheroma—An accumulation of plaque blocking a portion of an artery.

Atherosclerosis (arteriosclerosis)—Process of thickening and hardening of large- and medium-sized arteries as a result of fatty deposits on their inner linings.

Intermittent claudication—Pain that occurs on walking and is relieved on rest.

Ischemia—An inadequate blood supply (circulation) in a part of the body where arteries are blocked.

Peripheral arterial disease (PAD)—An occlusive disease of the arteries most often caused by progressive atherosclerosis.

Peripheral arteries—Arteries other than those of the heart and brain, especially those that supply the lower body organs and limbs.

Plaque—A collection of wax-like fatty deposits on the insides of artery walls.

Restenosis—The repeat narrowing of blood vessels that may occur after surgical removal of plaque when preventive measures are not taken.

Revascularization—Restoring normal blood flow (circulation) in the body's vascular (veins and arteries) system.

Stenosis—Narrowing of a blood vessel.

Resources

BOOKS

Cranton, Elmer M.D., ed. *Bypassing Bypass Surgery: Chelation Therapy: A Non-Surgical Treatment for Reversing Arteriosclerosis, Improving Blocked Circulation, and Slowing the Aging Process.* Hampton Roads Pub. Co., 2001.

McDougal, Gene. *Unclog Your Arteries: How I Beat Atherosclerosis.* 1st Books Library, 2001.

ORGANIZATIONS

American Heart Association (AHA). 7272 Greenville Ave., Dallas, TX 75231. (800) 242-8721. <www.americanheart.org>.

Vascular Disease Foundation. 3333 South Wadsworth Blvd. B104-37, Lakewood, CO 80227. (303) 949-8337 or (866)PADINFO (723-4636). <www.vdf.org>.

OTHER

Bypass Surgery for Peripheral Arterial Disease. Patient Information, Vascular Disease Foundation, 2003. <www.vdf.org.>

Hirsch, M.D., Alan T. "Occlusive Peripheral Arterial Disease." *The Merck Manual of Medicine—Home Edition, Heart and Blood Vessel Disorders* 34:3. <www.merck.com/pubs>.

L. Lee Culvert

Peritoneal dialysis *see* **Kidney dialysis**
Peritoneal fluid analysis *see* **Paracentesis**

Peritoneovenous shunt

Definition

A peritoneovenous shunt refers to the surgical insertion of a shunting tube to achieve the continuous emptying of ascitic fluid into the venous system.

Purpose

Ascites is a serious medical disorder characterized by the pathological accumulation of fluid in the peritoneal cavity, the smooth membrane that lines the cavity of the abdomen and surrounds the organs. Ascites is usually related to acute and chronic liver disease (cirrhosis) and to a lesser degree, to malignant tumors arising in the ovary, colon, or breast. Ascites may also be associated with chronic kidney disease and congestive heart failure. The formation of ascitic fluid results from the interplay of three factors: abnormally high pressure within the liver or the veins draining into the liver (portal hypertension); abnormally low amounts of albumin in the blood (hypoalbuminemia); and changes in sodium and water excretion by the kidneys.

When medical therapy fails, peritoneovenous shunts help manage chronic ascites.

Demographics

Cirrhosis is the seventh leading cause of death by disease in the United States, killing over 25,000 people each year. Fifty percent of patients with cirrhosis will develop ascites over a period of 10 years. Cirrhosis—regardless of its cause—greatly increases the risk for liver cancer. Few studies have been conducted on the risk for liver cancer in patients with primary biliary cirrhosis; however, one study reported an incidence of 2.3%. Approximately 4% of patients with cirrhosis caused by hepatitis C develop liver cancer. In Asia, about 15% of people who have chronic hepatitis B develop liver cancer, but this high rate is not seen in other parts of the world. One Italian study that followed a group of hepatitis B patients for 11 years found no liver cancer over that period of time.

Description

A variety of shunts have been designed for peritoneovenous shunting, including the Hyde shunt (1966-1974), LaVeen shunt (1974-1980), and Denver shunt. The latter predates the LaVeen shunt, but is more popular as of 2003. All designs work about equally well.

For the peritoneovenous shunt insertion procedure, the patient only requires a local anesthetic and a sedative. A long needle is inserted into the jugular vein in the neck, and is passed down through the superior vena cava, the large vein that delivers blood from the head, neck, and upper limbs back to the heart. This serves to widen the vein. The surgeon makes an incision and inserts a tube traversing the subcutaneous tissue of the chest wall. The tube connects the peritoneal cavity to the neck, where it enters the widened jugular vein. There the surgeon attaches a pressure-sensitive one-way valve to prevent backflow.

Diagnosis/Preparation

Ascites may go unnoticed for quite some time until the patient notices a slight increase in waistline. Severe ascites with marked abdominal distension becomes very disabling, especially when associated with swelling of the legs, pleural effusions (fluid around the lungs), and shortness of breath.

Diagnosis can be established by examination of the ascitic fluid, which allows the physician to differentiate between cirrhosis and tumor-induced ascites. The fluid is taken from the peritoneal cavity in a procedure called a **paracentesis**. Ascitic fluid analysis includes a total polymorph count, protein and albumin concentrations, and placement of at least 10 ml of ascitic fluid each into blood culture bottles for processing. If a measurement called the serum-ascitic fluid albumin gradient is greater than 11 g/L, cirrhosis, not cancer, is suspected.

Aftercare

After surgery, the patient's **vital signs** are monitored in a **recovery room**. Pain medication and **antibiotics** are administered as needed. Once released from the hospital, the patient is expected to abstain from alcohol, and follow a low-salt diet and medication regime designed to control ascites.

Patients also require training in shunt maintenance. To keep the fluid moving out of the abdomen, the shunt has to be properly pumped on a daily basis. Twice a day—once at bedtime and again prior to rising in the morning—the shunt is pumped about 20 times. This is essential to limit the accumulation of fibrin and other debris within the shunt, and to avoid the formation of an occlusive fibrin sheath at the venous tip.

Risks

Complications following peritoneovenous shunt insertion are common and include infection, leakage of ascitic fluid, accumulation of abnormally large amounts of fluid in the intercellular tissue spaces of the body (edema), deregulation of the blood clotting mechanism (coagulopathy), and shunt blockage. Clogging of the shunt with debris is the most common complication. Some patients develop further complications from the ascitic fluid entering directly into their bloodstream. Often, scar tissue develops, making future liver transplants difficult.

Normal results

In spite of the complications associated with the procedure, many patients obtain useful relief from ascites following peritoneovenous shunt insertion.

Morbidity and mortality rates

The most recent guidelines from the American Association for the Study of Liver Diseases recommend peritoneovenous shunting only under these conditions:

KEY TERMS

Ascites—An effusion and accumulation of serous fluid in the abdominal cavity.

Ascitic fluid—The fluid that accumulates in the peritoneal cavity in ascites.

Coagulopathy—A defect in the blood clotting mechanism.

Edema—The presence of abnormally large amounts of fluid in the intercellular tissue spaces of the body.

Inferior vena cava—Large vein that returns blood from the lower part of the body to the heart.

Jugular vein—Major vein of the neck that returns blood from the head to the heart.

Hypoalbuminemia—An abnormally low concentration of albumin in the blood.

Paracentesis—Surgical puncture of the abdominal cavity for the aspiration of peritoneal fluid.

Peritoneal cavity—The space enclosed by the peritoneum.

Peritoneum—The smooth membrane that lines the cavity of the abdomen, and surrounds the viscera, forming a closed sac.

Portal hypertension—Abnormally high pressure within the veins draining into the liver.

Subcutaneous—Beneath the skin.

Superior vena cava—Large vein that returns blood to the heart from the head, neck, and upper limbs.

Venous system—Circulation system that carries blood that has passed through the capillaries of various tissues, except the lungs, and is found in the veins, the right chambers of the heart, and the pulmonary arteries; it is usually dark red as a result of a lower oxygen content.

• Patient is diuretic-resistant, and is not a transplant candidate.

• Patient is not a candidate for serial therapeutic paracentesis because of multiple abdominal surgical scars.

• A physician is unavailable to perform serial paracentesis.

Cirrhosis is irreversible, but the rate of progression can be very slow depending on its cause and other factors. Five-year survival rates are about 85% in the Unites States and can be lower or higher depending on severity.

Alternatives

Alternative treatments for ascites include:

• **Diuretics**. Diuretics are medications that promote the excretion of urine and help eliminate excess fluids. The treatment of ascites always involves restricting dietary salt and taking diuretic pills to increase the output of salt in the urine. This treatment is effective, at least in the short-term, in 90% of patients.

• Repeated large-volume paracentesis. This approach, also called serial paracentesis, features repeated surgical puncture of the abdominal cavity and aspiration of the ascitic fluid.

• Transjugular portosystemic shunt. A shunting procedure designed to relieve portal hypertension.

• Portocaval shunt. Another shunting procedure designed to relieve portal hypertension.

• **Liver transplantation**. Replacement of the patient's liver by one obtained from a donor. Liver transplantation is the only definitive treatment for ascites, and the only treatment that has been clearly shown to improve survival.

There is no satisfactory treatment for refractory ascites in patients with cirrhosis. Both peritoneovenous shunts and paracentesis have been used, but there is uncertainty about their relative merits.

See also Portal vein bypass.

Resources

BOOKS

Arroyo, V., P. Gines, J. Rodes. and R. W. Schrier, eds. *Ascites and Renal Dysfunction in Liver Disease: Pathogenesis, Diagnosis, and Treatment.* Oxford, UK: Blackwell Science Inc, 1999.

Moore, W. S. ed. *Vascular Surgery: A Comprehensive Review.* Philadelphia: W. B. Saunders Co., 2001.

PERIODICALS

Gines, P., and V. Arroyo. "Hepatorenal Syndrome." *Journal of the American Society of Nephrology* 10 (1999): 1833-9.

Hu, R. H. and P. H. Lee. "Salvaging Procedures for Dysfunctional Peritoneovenous Shunt." *Hepatogastroenterology* 48 (May-June 2001): 794-7.

Koike, T., S. Araki, H. Minakami, S. Ogawa, M. Sayama, H. Shibahara, and I. Sato. "Clinical Efficacy of Peritoneovenous Shunting for the Treatment of Severe Ovarian Hyperstimulation Syndrome." *Human Reproduction* 15 (2000): 113-17.

Orsi, F., R.F. Grasso, G. Bonomo, C. Monti, I. Marinucci and M. Bellomi. "Percutaneous Peritoneovenous Shunt Positioning: Technique and Preliminary Results." *European Radiology* 12 (May 2002): 1188-92.

Wagayama, H., T. Tanaka, M. Shimomura, K. Ogura, and K. Shiraki. "Pancreatic Cancer with Chylous Ascites Demonstrated by Lymphoscintigraphy: Successful Treatment with Peritoneovenous Shunting." *Digestive Disturbance Science* 10 (August 2002): 1836-8.

ORGANIZATIONS

American Gastroenterological Association. 4930 Del Ray Avenue, Bethesda, MD 20814. (301) 654-2055. <www.gastro.org>.

Society for Vascular Surgery. 900 Cummings Center, Beverly, MA 01915-1314. (978) 927-8330. <svs.vasculaweb.org>.

OTHER

"Ascites." *Family Practice Notebook.* <www.fpnotebook.com/GI35.htm>.

Monique Laberge, Ph.D.

Permanent pacemakers *see* **Pacemakers**

PET scan *see* **Positron emission tomography (PET)**

Phacoemulsification for cataracts

Definition

Phacoemulsification cataract surgery is a procedure in which an ultrasonic device is used to break up and then remove a cloudy lens, or cataract, from the eye to improve vision. The insertion of an intraocular lens (IOL) usually immediately follows phacoemulsification.

Purpose

Phacoemulsification, or phaco, as surgeons refer to it, is used to restore vision in patients whose vision has become cloudy from cataracts. In the first stages of a cataract, people may notice only a slight cloudiness as it affects only a small part of the lens, the part of the eye that focuses light on the retina. As the cataract grows, it blocks more light and vision becomes cloudier. As vision worsens, the surgeon will recommend cataract surgery, usually phaco, to restore clear vision. With advancements in cataract surgery such as the IOL patients can sometimes experience dramatic vision improvement.

Demographics

As people age, cataracts are likely to form. The National Eye Institute (NEI) reports in a 2002 study that more than half of all United States residents 65 and older have a cataract. People who smoke are at a higher risk for cataracts. Increased exposure to sunlight without eye protection may also be a cause.

Cataracts also can occur anytime because of injury, exposure to toxins, or diseases such as diabetes. Congenital cataracts are caused by genetic defects or developmental problems, or exposure to some contagious diseases during pregnancy.

However, the most common form of cataract in the United States is age related. According to the NEI, cataracts are more common in women than in men, and Caucasians have cataracts more frequently than other races, especially as people age. People who live close to the equator also are at higher risk for cataracts because of increased sunlight exposure.

More than 1.5 million cataract surgeries are performed in the United States each year. The NEI reports that the federal government, through **Medicare**, spends more than $3.4 billion each year treating cataracts. Cataract surgery is one of the most common surgeries performed, and also one of the safest and most effective. Phaco is currently the most popular version of cataract surgery.

Description

Phacoemulsification is a variation of **extracapsular cataract extraction**, a procedure in which the lens and the front portion of the capsule are removed. Formerly the most popular cataract surgery, the older method of extracapsular extraction involves a longer incision, about 0.4 in (10 mm), or almost half of the eye. Recovery from the larger incision extracapsular extraction also requires almost a week-long hospital stay after surgery, and limited physical activity for weeks or even months.

Charles Kelman created phacoemulsification in the late 1960s. His goal was to remove the cataract with a smaller incision, less pain, and shorter recovery time. He discovered that the cataract could be broken up, or emulsified, into small pieces using an ultrasound tip. At first, phaco was slow to catch on because of its high learning curve. With its success rate and shorter recovery period, surgeons slowly learned the technique. Over the past decades, surgeons have constantly refined phaco to make it even safer and more successful. Innovations in technology such as the foldable IOL also have helped improve outcomes by allowing surgeons to make smaller incisions.

During surgery, the patient will probably breathe through an oxygen tube because it might be difficult to

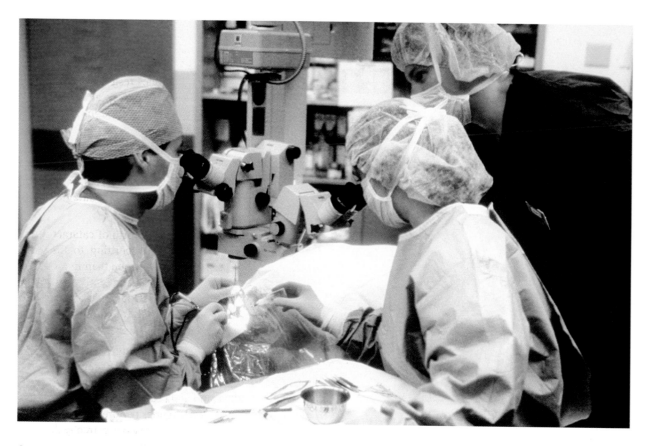

Ophthalmologists treating a patient for cataracts using phacoemulsification. *(Custom Medical Stock Photo. Reproduced by permission.)*

breathe with the draping. The patient's blood pressure and heart rate also are likely to be monitored.

Before making the incision, the surgeon inserts a long needle, usually through the lower eyelid, to anesthetize the area behind the eyeball. The surgeon then puts pressure on the eyeball with his or her hand or a weight to see if there is any bleeding (possibly caused by inserting the anesthetic). The pressure will stop this bleeding. This force also decreases intraocular pressure, which lowers the chances of complications.

After applying the pressure, the surgeon looks through a microscope and makes an incision about 0.1 in (3 mm) on the side of the anesthetized cornea. As of 2003, surgeons are beginning to favor the temporal location for the incision because it has proved to be safer. The incision site also varies depending on the size and denseness of the cataract. Once the incision is made, a viscoelastic fluid is injected to reduce shock to the intraocular tissues. The surgeon then makes a microscopic circular incision in the membrane that surrounds the cataract; this part of the procedure is called capsulorhexis. A water stream then frees the cataract from the cortex. The surgeon inserts a small titanium needle, or phaco tip,

into the cornea. The ultrasound waves from the phaco tip emulsify the cataract so that it can be removed by suction. The surgeon first focuses on the cataract's central nucleus, which is denser.

While the cataract is being emulsified, the machine simultaneously aspirates the cataract through a small hole in the tip of the phaco probe. The surgeon then removes the cortex of the lens, but leaves the posterior capsule, which is used to support the intraocular lens.

The folded IOL is inserted by an injector. The folded IOL means that a larger incision is not required. After the IOL is inserted into the capsular bag, the viscoelastic fluid is removed. No sutures are usually required after the surgery. Some surgeons may recommend that patients wear an eye shield immediately after the surgery.

The entire procedure takes about 20 minutes. The phaco procedure itself takes only minutes.

Most surgeons prefer a certain technique for the procedure, although they might vary due to the cataract's density and size. The variations on the phaco procedure lie mostly on what part of the nucleus the surgeon focuses on first, and how the cataract is emulsified. Some sur-

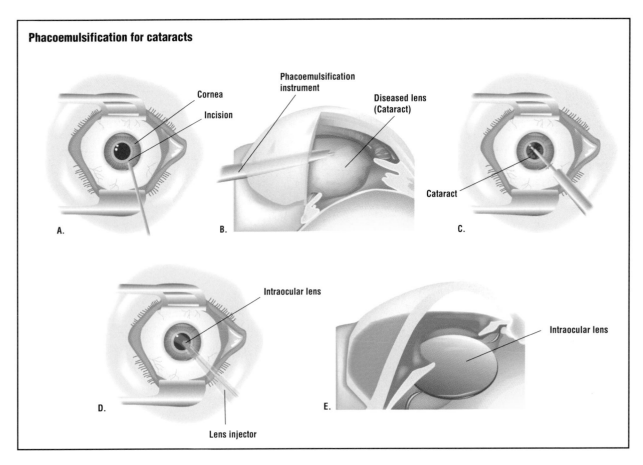

Phacoemulsification for cataracts

In a phacoemulsification procedure, an incision is first made in the cornea, the outer covering of the eye (A). A phacoemulsification instrument uses ultrasonic waves to break up the cataract (B). Pieces of the cataract are then suctioned out (C). To repair the patient's vision, a folded intraocular lens is pushed through the same incision (D) and opened in place (E). *(Illustration by GGS Inc.)*

geons prefer a continuous "chop," while others divide the cataract into quadrants for removal. One procedure, called the "phaco flip," involves the surgeon inverting and then rotating the lens for removal. Advances in technology also may allow for even smaller incisions, some speculate as small as 0.05 in (1.4 mm).

Diagnosis/Preparation

People might have cataracts for years before vision is impaired enough to warrant surgery. Eye doctors may first suggest eyeglasses to temporarily help improve vision. But as the lens grows cloudier, vision deteriorates.

As cataracts develop and worsen, patients may notice these common symptoms:

• gradual (and painless) onset of blurry vision

• poor central vision

• frequent changes in prescription for corrective lenses

• increased glare from lights

• near vision improvement to the point where reading glasses may no longer be needed

• poor vision in sunlight

Cataracts grow faster in younger people or diabetics, so doctors will recommend surgery more quickly in those cases. Surgery may also be recommended sooner if the patient suffers from other eye diseases such as age-related macular degeneration and if the cataract interferes with complete eye examination.

When symptoms worsen to the point that everyday activities become problematic, surgery becomes necessary. A complete ocular exam will determine the severity of the cataract and what type of surgery the patient will receive. For some denser cataracts, the older method of extracapsular extraction is preferred.

The diagnostic exam should include measurement of visual acuity under both low and high illumination, microscopic examination of eye structures and pupil dilation, assessment of visual fields, and measurement of intraocular pressure (IOP).

If cataracts are detected in both eyes, each must be treated separately.

Overall patient health must also be considered, and how it will affect the surgery's outcome. Surgeons may recommend a complete **physical examination** before surgery.

Although preoperative instructions may vary, patients are usually required not to eat or drink anything after midnight the day of the surgery. Patients must disclose all medications to determine if they must be discontinued before surgery. Patients taking **aspirin** for blood thinning usually are asked to stop for two weeks before surgery. Blood-thinning medications may put patients at risk for intraocular bleeding or hemorrhage. Coumadin, the prescription medicine for blood thinning, might still be taken if the risk for stroke is high. People should consult with their eye doctor and internist to decide the best course of action.

An A-scan measurement, which determines the length of the eyeball, will be performed. This helps determine the refractive power of the IOL. Other pre-surgical testing such as a **chest x ray**, blood work, or **urinalysis** may be requested if other medical problems are an issue.

The surgeon may also request patients begin using antibiotic drops before the surgery to limit the chance of infection.

Cataract surgery is done on an outpatient basis, so patients must arrange for someone to take them home after surgery. On the day of the surgery, doctors will review the pre-surgical tests and insert dilating eye drops, antibiotic drops, and a corticosteriod or nonsteroidal anti-inflammatory drop. Anesthetic eye drops will be given in both eyes to keep both eyes comfortable during surgery. A local anesthetic will be administered. Patients are awake for the surgery, but are kept in a relaxed state.

The patient's eye is scrubbed prior to surgery and sterile drapes are placed over the shoulders and head. The patient is required to lie still and focus on the light of the operating microscope. A speculum is inserted to keep the eyelids open.

Aftercare

Immediately following surgery, the patient is monitored in an outpatient recovery area. The patient is advised to rest for at least 24 hours, until he or she returns to the surgeon's office for follow-up. Only light meals are recommended on the day of surgery. The patient may still feel drowsy and may experience some eye pain or discomfort. Usually, over-the-counter medications are advised for pain relief, but patients should check with

WHO PERFORMS THE PROCEDURE AND WHERE IS IT PERFORMED?

Ophthalmologists and optometrists may detect cataracts; however, only an ophthalmologist can perform cataract surgery. An anesthesiologist may be on hand during surgery to administer the local anesthetic. Surgical nurses will assist the ophthalmologist in the **operating room** and assist the patient preoperatively and postoperatively.

The **outpatient surgery** is performed in a hospital or surgery suite designed for ophthalmic surgery.

their doctors to see what is recommended. Other side effects such as severe pain, nausea, or vomiting should be reported to the surgeon immediately.

There will be some changes in the eye during recovery. Patients may see dark spots, which should disappear a few weeks after surgery. There also might be some discharge and itching of the eye. Patients may use a warm, moist cloth for 15 minutes at a time for relief and to loosen the matter. All matter should be gently cleared away with a tissue, not a fingertip. Pain and sensitivity to light are also experienced after surgery. Some patients may also have slight drooping or bruising of the eye which will improve as the eye heals.

Patients have their first postoperative visit the day after surgery. The surgeon will remove the eye shield and prescribe eye drops to prevent infections and control intraocular pressure. These eye drops are used for about a month after surgery.

Patients are advised to wear an eye shield while sleeping, and refrain from rubbing the eye for at least two weeks. During that time, the doctor will give the patient special tinted sunglasses or request that he or she wear current prescription eyeglasses to prevent possible eye trauma from accidental rubbing or bumping. Unlike other types of cataract extraction, patients can resume normal activity almost immediately after phaco.

Subsequent exams are usually at one week, three weeks, and six to eight weeks following surgery. This can change, however, depending on any complications or any unusual postoperative symptoms.

After the healing process, the patient will probably need new corrective lenses, at least for close vision.

QUESTIONS TO ASK THE DOCTOR

- Will Medicare pay for the surgery and my aftercare?

- If I have a cataract in the other eye, how long must I wait to have the other eye treated?

- Will I still need reading glasses after surgery? Will I still need eyeglasses to see far away even if you insert an intraocular lens?

- How many cataract surgeries have you performed? How many of these have been phacoemulsification?

- What precautions should I take to protect my eye after surgery?

- When can I resume my normal activities after surgery? Contact sports?

While IOLs can remove the need for myopic correction, patients will probably need new lenses for close work.

Risks

Complications are unlikely, but can occur. Patients may experience spontaneous bleeding from the wound and recurrent inflammation after surgery. Flashing, floaters, and double vision may also occur a few weeks after surgery. The surgeon should be notified immediately of these symptoms. Some can easily be treated, while others such as floaters may be a sign of a retinal detachment.

Retinal detachment is one possible serious complication. The retina can become detached by the surgery if there is any weakness in the retina at the time of surgery. This complication may not occur for weeks or months.

Infections are another potential complication, the most serious being endophthalmitis, which is an infection in the eyeball. This complication, once widely reported, is much more uncommon today because of newer surgery techniques and **antibiotics**.

Patients may also be concerned that their IOL might become displaced, but newer designs of IOLs also have limited reports of intraocular lens dislocation.

Other possible complications are the onset of glaucoma and, in very rare cases, blindness.

It is possible that a secondary cataract may develop in the remaining back portion of the capsule. This can occur for as long as one to two years after surgery. YAG capsulotomy, using a laser, is most often used for the secondary cataract. This outpatient procedure requires no incision. The laser makes a small opening in the remaining back part of the lens to allow light to penetrate.

Normal results

Most patients have restored visual acuity after surgery, and some will have the best vision of their lives after the insertion of IOLs. Some patients will no longer require the use of eyeglasses or contact lenses after cataract surgery. Patients will also have better color and depth perception and be able to resume normal activities they may have stopped because of impaired vision from the cataract, such as driving, reading, or sports.

Morbidity and mortality rates

Phacoemulsification has taken the previous risks from cataract surgery, making it a much safer procedure. Before phacoemulsification, death after cataract surgery was still rare, but usually stemmed from the possible complications of general anesthesia. Phaco is performed under local anesthesia, limiting the risk of general anesthetic use.

Other serious complications such as blindness also have been reduced with the widespread use of phaco. Better antibiotics have enabled physicians to combat former debilitating infections that previously would have caused blindness.

Alternatives

Some older methods of cataract surgery may have to be used if the cataract is too large to remove with a small incision, including:

- Extracapsular cataract extraction. While phaco is considered a type of extracapsular extraction, the older version of this technique requires a much larger incision and does not use the phaco machine. It is similar in that the lens and the front portion of the capsule are removed and the back part of the capsule remains. The surgeon might consider this technique if the patient has corneal disease or if the pupil becomes too small during the first stages of surgery.

- Intracapsular cataract extraction. This also requires a larger incision than phaco. It differs in that the lens and the entire capsule are removed. While it is the easiest cataract surgery for the surgeon technically, this method carries an increased risk for the patient with increased potential for detachment of the retina and swelling after surgery. Recovery is long and most patients will have to use large "cataract glasses" to see.

See also Extracapsular cataract extraction.

KEY TERMS

Astigmatism—Asymmetric vision defects due to irregularities in the cornea.

Cornea—Clear, bowl-shaped structure at the front of the eye. It is located in front of the colored part of the eye (iris). The cornea lets light into the eye and partially focuses it.

Floaters—Spots in the field of vision.

Glaucoma—Disease of the eye characterized by increased pressure of the fluid inside the eye. Untreated, glaucoma can lead to blindness.

Lens (the crystalline lens)—A transparent structure in the eye that focuses light onto the retina.

Myopia—A refractive error that causes distant objects to appear blurry. Myopia results when light does not focus properly on the retina.

Retina—The inner, light-sensitive layer of the eye containing rods and cones.

Resources

BOOKS

Buettner, Helmut, ed. *Mayo Clinic on Vision and Eye Health.* Rochester, MN: Mayo Clinic Health Information, 2002.

Cassel, Gary H., Michael D. Billig, and Harry G. Randall. *The Eye Book: A Complete Guide to Eye Disorders and Health.* Baltimore, MD: Johns Hopkins University Press, 1998.

Jaffe, Norman S., Mark S. Jaffe, and Gary F. Jaffe. *Cataract Surgery and Its Complications, 6th Edition.* St. Louis: Mosby, 1997.

Massengill, R.K. *Supersight: The Lens Implant Miracle.* Boston, MA: Health Institute Press, 1987.

Slade, Stephen G., Richard N. Baker, and Dorothy Kay Brockman. *The Complete Book of Laser Eye Surgery.* Naperville, IL: Sourcebooks, Inc., 2000.

Spaeth, George L., ed. *Ophthalmic Surgery Principles and Practice.* Philadelphia, PA: W.B. Saunders Company, 1982.

ORGANIZATIONS

American Academy of Ophthalmology. P.O. Box 7424, San Francisco, CA 94120-7424. (415) 561-8500. <http://www.aao.org>.

American Optometric Association. 243 North Lindbergh Blvd., St. Louis, MO 63141. (314) 991-4100. <http://www.aoanet.org>.

American Society of Cataract and Refractive Surgery. 4000 Legato Road, Suite 850, Fairfax, VA 22033-4055. (703) 591-2220. E-mail: <ascrs@ascrs.org>. <http://www.ascrs.org>.

National Eye Institute. 2020 Vision Place Bethesda, MD 20892-3655. (301) 496-5248. <http://www.nei.nih.gov>.

OTHER

"Cataract Surgery." *EyeMdLink.com,* [cited March 28, 2003]. <http://www.eyemdlink.com/EyeProcedure.asp.EyeProcedureID=19>.

Samalonis, Lisa B. "Cataract Surgery Today." *Eye World,* February 2002 [cited March 28, 2003] <http://www.eyeworld.org/feb02/0202p34.html>.

Mary Bekker

Pharyngectomy

Definition

A pharyngectomy is the total or partial surgical removal of the pharynx, the cavity at the back of the mouth that opens into the esophagus at its lower end. The pharynx is cone-shaped, has an average length of about 3 in (76 mm), and is lined with mucous membrane.

Purpose

A pharyngectomy procedure is performed to treat cancers of the pharynx that include:

- Throat cancer. Throat cancer occurs when cells in the pharynx or larynx (voice box) begin to divide abnormally and out of control. A total or partial pharyngectomy is usually performed for cancers of the hypopharynx (last part of the throat), in which all or part of the hypopharynx is removed.

- Hypopharyngeal carcinoma (HPC). A carcinoma is a form of cancerous tumor that may develop in the pharynx or adjacent locations and for which surgery may be indicated.

Description

Whether a pharyngectomy is performed in total or with only partial removal of the pharynx depends on the localized amount of cancer found. The procedure may also involve removal of the larynx, in which case it is called a laryngopharyngectomy. Well-localized, early stage HPC tumors can be amenable to a partial pharyngectomy or a laryngopharyngectomy, but laryngopharyngectomy is more commonly performed for more advanced cancers. It can be total, involving removal of the entire larynx, or partial and may also involve removal of part of the esophagus (esophagectomy). Patients undergoing laryngopharyngectomy will lose some speaking ability and require special techniques or reconstructive procedures to regain the use of their voice.

Pharyngectomy

WHO PERFORMS THE PROCEDURE AND WHERE IS IT PERFORMED?

A pharyngectomy is major surgery performed by a surgeon trained in otolaryngology. An anesthesiologist is responsible for administering anesthesia and the operation is performed in a hospital setting. Otolaryngology is the oldest medical specialty in the United States. Otolaryngologists are physicians trained in the medical and surgical management and treatment of patients with diseases and disorders of the ear, nose, throat (ENT), and related structures of the head and neck. They are commonly referred to as ENT physicians.

With cancer involved in pharyngectomy procedures, the otolaryngologist surgeon usually works with radiation and medical oncologists in a treatment team approach.

Following a total or partial pharyngectomy, the surgeon may also need to reconstruct the throat so that the patient can swallow. A **tracheotomy** is used when the tumor is too large to remove. In this procedure, a hole is made in the neck to bypass the tumor and allow the patient to breathe.

For this type of surgery, patient positioning requires access to the lower part of the neck for the surgeon. This is conveniently achieved by placing the patient on a table fitted with a head holder, allowing the head to be bent back but well supported.

If a laryngopharyngectomy is performed, the surgeon starts with a curved horizontal neck skin incision. The **laryngectomy** incision is usually made from the breastbone to the lower most of the laryngeal cartilages, such that a 1–2 in (2.54–5.08 cm) bridge of skin is preserved. Once the incision is deepened, flaps are elevated until the larynx is exposed. The anterior jugular veins and strap muscles are left undisturbed. The sternocleidomastoid muscle is then identified. The layer of cervical fibrous tissue is cut (incised) longitudinally from the hyoid (the bony arch that supports the tongue) above to the clavicle (collarbone) below. Part of the hyoid is then divided, which allows the surgeon to enter the loose compartment bounded by the sternomastoid muscle and carotid sheath (which covers the carotid artery) and by the pharynx and larynx in the neck. The pharyngectomy incisions and laryngeal removal are performed, and a view of the pharynx is then possible. Using scissors, the surgeon performs bilateral (on both sides), direct cuts, separating the pharynx from the larynx. If a preliminary tracheotomy has not been performed, the oral endotracheal tube is withdrawn from the tracheal stump and a new, cuffed, flexible tube inserted for connection to new anesthesia tubing. The wound is thoroughly irrigated (flushed); all clots are removed; and the wound is closed. The pharyngeal wall is closed in two layers. The muscle layer closure always tightens the opening to some extent and is usually left undone at points where narrowing may be excessive. In fact, studies show that a mucosal (inner layer) closure alone is sufficient for proper healing.

Diagnosis/Preparation

The initial **physical examination** for a pharyngectomy usually includes examination of the neck, mouth, pharynx, and larynx. A neurologic examination is sometimes also performed. Laryngoscopy is the examination of choice, performed with a long-handled mirror, or with a lighted tube called a laryngoscope. A local anesthetic might be used to ease discomfort. A MRI of the oral cavity and neck may also be performed.

If the physician suspects throat cancer, a biopsy will be performed—this involves removing tissue for examination in the laboratory under a microscope. Throat cancer can only be confirmed through a biopsy or using fine needle aspiration (FNA). The physician also may use an imaging test called a computed tomography (CT) scan. This is a special type of x ray that provides images of the body from different angles, allowing a cross-sectional view. A CT-scan can help to find the location of a tumor, to judge whether or not a tumor can be removed surgically, and to determine the cancer's stage of development.

Before surgery, the patient is also examined for nutritional assessment and supplementation, and careful staging of cancer, while surgical airway management is planned with the anesthesiologist such that a common agreement is reached with the surgeon concerning the timing of tracheotomy and intubation. The anesthesiologist may elect to use an orotracheal (through the mouth and trachea) tube with anesthetic, which can be removed if a subsequent tracheotomy is planned.

Aftercare

After undergoing a pharyngectomy, special attention is given to the patient's pulmonary function and fluid/nutritional balance, as well as to local wound conditions in the neck, thorax, and abdomen. Regular postoperative checks of calcium, magnesium, and phospho-

1146

GALE ENCYCLOPEDIA OF SURGERY

rus levels are necessary; supplementation with calcium, magnesium, and 1,25-dihydroxycholecalciferol is usually required. A patient may be unable to take in enough food to maintain adequate nutrition and experience difficulty eating (dysphagia). Sometimes it may be necessary to have a feeding tube placed through the skin and muscle of the abdomen directly into the stomach to provide extra nutrition. This procedure is called a **gastrostomy**.

Reconstructive surgery is also required to rebuild the throat after a pharyngectomy in order to help the patient with swallowing after the operation. Reconstructive surgeries represent a great challenge because of the complex properties of the tissues lining the throat and underlying muscle that are so vital to the proper functioning of this region. The primary goal is to re-establish the conduit connecting the oral cavity to the esophagus and thus retaining the continuity of the alimentary tract. Two main techniques are used:

- Myocutaneous flaps. Sometimes a muscle and area of skin may be rotated from an area close to the throat, such as the chest (pectoralis major flap), to reconstruct the throat.

- Free flaps. With the advances of microvascular surgery (sewing together small blood vessels under a microscope), surgeons have many more options to reconstruct the area of the throat affected by a pharyngectomy. Tissues from other areas of the patient's body such as a piece of intestine or a piece of arm muscle can be used to replace parts of the throat.

Risks

Potential risks associated with a pharyngectomy include those associated with any head and neck surgery, such as excessive bleeding, wound infection, wound slough, fistula (abnormal opening between organs or to the outside of the body), and, in rare cases, blood vessel rupture. Specifically, the surgery is associated with the following risks:

- Drain failure. Drains unable to hold a vacuum represent a serious threat to the surgical wound.

- Hematoma. Although rare, blood clot formation requires prompt intervention to avoid pressure separation of the pharyngeal repair and compression of the upper windpipe.

- Infection. A subcutaneous infection after total pharyngectomy is recognized by increasing redness and swelling of the skin flaps at the third to fifth post-operative day. Associated odor, fever, and elevated white blood cell count will occur.

QUESTIONS TO ASK THE DOCTOR

- How will the surgery affect my ability to swallow and to eat?
- What type of anesthesia will be used?
- How long will it take to recover from the surgery?
- When can I expect to return to work and/or resume normal activities?
- To what extent will my ability to speak be affected?
- What are the risks associated with a pharyngectomy?
- How many pharyngectomies do you perform in a year?

- Pharyngocutaneous fistula. Patients with poor pre-operative nutritional status are at significant risk for fistula development.

- Narrowing. More common at the lower, esophageal end of the pharyngeal reconstruction than in the upper end, where the recipient lumen of the pharynx is wider.

- Functional swallowing problems. Dysphagia is also a risk which depends on the extent of the pharyngectomy.

Normal results

Oral intake is usually started on the seventh postoperative day, depending on whether the patient has had preoperative radiation therapy, in which case it may be delayed. Mechanical voice devices are sometimes useful in the early, post-operative phase, until the pharyngeal wall heals. Results are considered normal if there is no re-occurrence of the cancer at a later stage.

Morbidity and mortality rates

Smokers are at high risk of throat cancer. According to the Harvard Medical School, throat cancer also is associated closely with other cancers: 15% of throat-cancer patients also are diagnosed with cancer of the mouth, esophagus, or lung. Another 10–20% of throat-cancer patients develop these other cancers later. Other people at risk include those who drink a lot of alcohol, especially if they also smoke. Vitamin A deficiency and certain types of human papillomavirus (HPV) infection also have been associated with an increased risk of throat cancer.

KEY TERMS

Anesthesia—A combination of drugs administered by a variety of techniques by trained professionals that provide sedation, amnesia, analgesia, and immobility adequate for the accomplishment of the surgical procedure with minimal discomfort, and without injury, to the patient.

Biopsy—Procedure that involves obtaining a tissue specimen for microscopic analysis to establish a precise diagnosis.

Carcinoma—A malignant growth that arises from epithelium, found in skin or, more commonly, the lining of body organs.

Computed tomography (CT) scan—An imaging technique that creates a series of pictures of areas inside the body, taken from different angles. The pictures are created by a computer linked to an x ray machine.

Dysphagia—Difficulty in eating as a result of disruption in the swallowing process. Dysphagia can be a serious health threat because of the risk of aspiration pneumonia, malnutrition, dehydration, weight loss, and airway obstruction.

Esophagectomy—Surgical removal of the esophagus.

Esophagus—A long hollow muscular tube that connects the pharynx to the stomach.

Fine needle aspiration (FNA)—Technique that allows a biopsy of various bumps and lumps. It allows the otolaryngologist to retrieve enough tissue for microscopic analysis and thus make an accurate diagnosis of a number of problems, such as inflammation or cancer.

Fistula—An abnormal passage or communication, usually between two internal organs or leading from an internal organ to the surface of the body.

Hypopharynx—The last part of the throat or the pharynx.

Laryngopharyngectomy—Surgical removal of both the larynx and the pharynx.

Laryngoscopy—The visualization of the larynx and vocal cords. This may be done directly with a fibre-optic scope (laryngoscope) or indirectly with mirrors.

Laryngectomy—Surgical removal of the larynx.

Larynx—Voice box.

Magnetic resonance imaging (MRI)—A procedure in which a magnet linked to a computer is used to create detailed pictures of areas inside the body.

Pharynx—The cavity at the back of the mouth. It is cone shaped and has an average length of about 3 in (76 mm) and is lined with mucous membrane. The pharynx opens into the esophagus at the lower end.

Tracheotomy—Opening of the trachea (windpipe) to the outside through a hole in the neck.

Surgical treatment for hypopharyngeal carcinomas is difficult as most patients are diagnosed with advanced disease, and five-year disease specific survival is only 30%. Cure rates have been the highest with surgical resection followed by postoperative radiotherapy. Immediate reconstruction can be accomplished with regional and free tissue transfers. These techniques have greatly reduced morbidity, and allow most patients to successfully resume an oral diet.

See also Laryngectomy; Tracheotomy.

Resources

BOOKS

Orlando, R. C., ed. *Esophagus and Pharynx.* London: Churchill Livingstone, 1997.

Pitman, K. T., J. L. Weissman, and J. T. Johnson. *The Parapharyngeal Space: Diagnosis and Management of Commonly Encountered Entities (Continuing Education Program (American Academy of Otolaryngology—Head and Neck Surgery Foundation).)* Alexandria, VA: American Academy of Otolaryngology, 1998.

Shin, L.M., L. M. Ross, and K. Bellenir, eds. *Ear, Nose, and Throat Disorders Sourcebook: Basic Information About Disorders of the Ears, Nose, Sinus Cavities, Pharynx, and Larynx Including Ear Infections, Tinnitus, Vestibular Disorders.* Holmes, PA: Omnigraphics Inc., 1998.

PERIODICALS

Chang, D. W., C. Hussussian, J. S. Lewin, et al. "Analysis of pharyngocutaneous fistula following free jejunal transfer for total laryngopharyngectomy." *Plastic and Reconstructive Surgery* 109 (April 2002): 1522–1527.

Ibrahim, H. Z., M. S. Moir, and W. W. Fee. "Nasopharyngectomy after failure of 2 courses of radiation therapy." *Archives of Otolaryngology - Head & Neck Surgery* 128 (October 2002): 1196–1197.

Iwai, H., H. Tsuji, T. Tachikawa, et al. "Neoglottic formation from posterior pharyngeal wall conserved in surgery for hypopharyngeal cancer." *Auris Nasus Larynx* 29 (April 2002): 153–157.

ORGANIZATIONS

American Academy of Otolaryngology. One Prince Street, Alexandria, VA 22314-3357. (703) 836-4444. <http://www.entnet.org/>

American Cancer Society (ACS). 1599 Clifton Rd. NE, Atlanta, GA 30329-4251. (800) 227-2345. <http://www.cancer.org>

OTHER

"Throat Cancer." Harvard Medical School. [cited May 31,2003] <http://www.intelihealth.com/IH/ihtIH/WSIHW000/8987/29425/211361.html?d=dmtHealthAZ>.

"Treatment of Laryngeal and Hypopharyngeal Cancers." American Cancer Society. [cited May 31, 2003]. <http://www.cancer.org/docroot/CRI/content/CRI_2_2_4X_Treatment_of_laryngeal_and_hypopharyngeal_cancers_23.asp?sitearea=>.

Monique Laberge, Ph.D.

Pharynx removal *see* **Pharyngectomy**

Phenobarbital *see* **Barbiturates**

Phlebectomy *see* **Vein ligation and stripping**

Phlebography

Definition

Phlebography is an x ray test that provides an image of the leg veins after a contrast dye is injected into a vein in the patient's foot.

Purpose

Phlebography is primarily performed to diagnose deep vein thrombosis—a condition in which clots form in the veins of the leg. Pulmonary embolism can occur when those clots break off and travel to the lungs and pulmonary artery. Phlebography can also be used to evaluate congenital vein problems, assess the function of the deep leg vein valves, and identify a vein for arterial bypass grafting. Ultrasound has replaced phlebography in many cases; but phlebography is the "gold standard," or the best test by which others are judged, even though it is not used routinely.

Description

Phlebography (also called venography, ascending contrast phlebography, or contrast phlebography) is an invasive diagnostic test that provides a constant image of leg veins on a fluoroscope screen. Phlebography identifies the location and extent of blood clots, and enables the condition of the deep leg veins to be assessed. It is especially useful when there is a strong suspicion of deep vein thrombosis, after noninvasive tests have failed to identify the disease.

Phlebography is the most accurate test for detecting deep vein thrombosis. It is nearly 100% sensitive and specific in making this diagnosis. (Pulmonary embolism is diagnosed in other ways.) Accuracy is crucial since deep vein thrombosis can lead to pulmonary embolism, a potentially fatal condition.

Phlebography is not used often; however, because it is painful, expensive, time-consuming, exposes the patient to a fairly high dose of radiation, and can cause complications. In about 5% of cases, there are technical problems in conducting the test.

Phlebography takes 30–45 minutes, and can be done in a physician's office, a laboratory, or a hospital. During the procedure, the patient lies on a tilting x ray table. The area where the catheter will be inserted is shaved, if necessary, and cleaned. In some cases, a local anesthetic is injected to numb the skin at the site of the insertion. A small incision may be required to make a point for insertion. The catheter is inserted and the contrast solution (or dye) is slowly injected. Injection of the dye causes a warm, flushing feeling in the leg that may spread through the body. The contrast solution may also cause slight nausea. Approximately 18% of patients experience discomfort from the contrast solution.

In order to fill the deep venous system with dye, a tight band (tourniquet) may be tied around the ankle or below the knee of the side into which the dye is injected, or the lower extremities may be tilted. The patient is asked to keep the leg still. The physician observes the movement of the solution through the vein with a fluoroscope. At the same time, a series of x rays is taken. When the test is finished, fluid is injected to clear the contrast from the veins, the catheter is removed, and a bandage is applied over the injection site.

Preparation

Fasting or drinking only clear liquids is necessary for four hours before the test, although the procedure may be done in an emergency even if the patient has eaten. The contrast solution contains iodine, to which some people are allergic. Patients should tell their physician if they have allergies or hay fever, or if they have had a reaction to a contrast solution.

Aftercare

Patients should drink large amounts of fluids to flush the remaining contrast solution from their bodies. The area around the incision will be sore for a few days. The physician should be notified if there is swelling, redness, pain, or fever. Pain medication is rarely needed. In most cases, the patient can resume normal activities the next day.

Risks

Phlebography can cause complications such as phlebitis, tissue damage, and the formation of deep vein thrombosis in a healthy leg. A rare side effect in up to 8% of cases is a severe allergic reaction to the dye. This usually happens within 30 minutes after injection of the dye, and requires medical attention.

Normal results

Normal phlebography results show proper blood flow through the leg veins.

Abnormal phlebography results show well-defined filling defects in veins. These findings confirm a diagnosis of deep vein thrombosis:

- blood clots
- consistent filling defects
- an abrupt end of a contrast column
- major deep veins that are unfilled
- dye flow that is diverted

Resources

BOOKS

DeBakey, Michael E., and Antonio M. Gotto, Jr. "Invasive Diagnostic Procedures." In *The New Living Heart.* Holbrook, MA: Adams Media Corporation, 1997, 78.

"Phlebography." In *Mayo Clinic Practice of Cardiology,* 3rd ed. St. Louis, MO: Mosby, 1996, 1840-1.

Texas Heart Institute. "Diseases of the Peripheral Arteries and Veins." In *Texas Heart Institute Heart Owner's Handbook.* New York: Wiley & Sons, 1996.

"Venous Imaging." In *Diagnostic Nuclear Medicine,* 3rd ed., Vol. 1. Baltimore, MD: Williams & Wilkins, 1996, 586-7.

PERIODICALS

Barloon T. J., G. R. Bergus, and J. E. Seabold. "Diagnostic Imaging of Lower Limb Deep Venous Thrombosis." *American Family Physician* 56 (September 1, 1997): 791-801.

Tapson, Victor F. "Pulmonary Embolism—New Diagnostic Approaches." *New England Journal of Medicine* 336 (May 15, 1997).

KEY TERMS

Contrast solution—A liquid dye injected into the body that allows structures, including veins, to be seen by x rays. Without the dye, the veins could not be seen on x rays.

Deep vein thrombosis—The development or presence of a blood clot in a vein deep within the leg. Deep vein thrombosis can lead to pulmonary embolism.

Invasive—A diagnostic test that invades healthy tissue; in the case of phlebography, through an incision in a healthy vein.

Pulmonary embolism—An obstruction of a blood vessel in the lungs, usually due to a blood clot that blocks a pulmonary artery. A pulmonary embolism can be very serious and in some cases is fatal.

OTHER

"Lower-Limb Venography." *Test Universe Website.* 11 July 2001. <http://www.testuniverse.com/mdx/MDX-2970.html>.

Springhouse Corporation. "Catching Deep Vein Thrombosis in Time: Diagnostic Tests at a Glance." *SpringNet.* 2001. 11 July 2001. <http://www.springnet.com/ce/p507bs4.htm>.

Lee A. Shratter, M.D.
Lori De Milto
Stéphanie Islane Dionne

Phlebotomy

Definition

Phlebotomy is the act of drawing or removing blood from the circulatory system through a cut (incision) or puncture in order to obtain a sample for analysis and diagnosis. Phlebotomy is also done as part of the patient's treatment for certain blood disorders.

Purpose

Phlebotomy that is part of treatment (therapeutic phlebotomy) is performed to treat polycythemia vera, a condition that causes an elevated red blood cell volume (**hematocrit**). Phlebotomy is also prescribed for patients with disorders that increase the amount of iron in their blood to dangerous levels, such as hemochromatosis, hepatitis B, and hepatitis C. Patients with pulmonary edema may undergo phlebotomy procedures to decrease their total blood volume.

Phlebotomy is also used to remove blood from the body during blood donation and for analysis of the substances contained within it.

Description

Phlebotomy is performed by a nurse or a technician known as a phlebotomist. Blood is usually taken from a vein on the back of the hand or just below the elbow. Some blood tests, however, may require blood from an artery. The skin over the area is wiped with an antiseptic, and an elastic band is tied around the arm. The band acts as a tourniquet, retaining blood within the arm and making the veins more visible. The phlebotomy technician feels the veins in order to select an appropriate one. When a vein is selected, the technician inserts a needle into the vein and releases the elastic band. The appropriate amount of blood is drawn and the needle is withdrawn from the vein. The patient's pulse and blood pressure may be monitored during the procedure.

For some tests requiring very small amounts of blood for analysis, the technician uses a finger stick. A lance, or small needle, makes a small cut in the surface of the fingertip, and a small amount of blood is collected in a narrow glass tube. The fingertip may be squeezed to get additional blood to surface.

The amount of blood drawn depends on the purpose of the phlebotomy. Blood donors usually contribute a unit of blood (500 mL) in a session. The volume of blood needed for laboratory analysis varies widely with the type of test being conducted. Typically one or several small (5–10 mL) tubes are drawn. Therapeutic phlebotomy removes a larger amount of blood than donation and blood analysis require. Phlebotomy for treatment of hemochromatosis typically involves removing a unit of blood—250 mg of iron—once a week. Phlebotomy sessions are required until iron levels return to a consistently normal level, which may take several months to several years. Phlebotomy for polycythemia vera removes enough blood to keep the patient's hematocrit (proportion of red blood cells) below 45%. The frequency and duration of sessions depends on the patient's individual needs.

Diagnosis/Preparation

Patients having their blood drawn for analysis may be asked to discontinue medications or to avoid food (to fast) for a period of time before the blood test. Patients donating blood will be asked for a brief medical history, have their blood pressure taken, and have their hematocrit checked with a finger stick test prior to donation.

Aftercare

After blood is drawn and the needle is removed, pressure is placed on the puncture site with a cotton ball to stop bleeding, and a bandage is applied. It is not uncommon for a patient to feel dizzy or nauseated during or after phlebotomy. The patient may be encouraged to rest for a short period once the procedure is completed. Patients are also instructed to drink plenty of fluids and eat regularly over the next 24 hours to replace lost blood volume. Patients who experience swelling of the puncture site or continued bleeding after phlebotomy should seek immediate medical treatment.

Risks

Most patients will have a small bruise or mild soreness at the puncture site for several days. Therapeutic phlebotomy may cause thrombocytosis and chronic iron deficiency (anemia) in some patients. As with any invasive procedure, infection is also a risk. This risk is minimized by the use of prepackaged sterilized equipment and careful attention to proper technique. There is no risk of HIV infection from phlebotomy, since all needles are disposed of after a single use. Arterial blood collection carries a higher risk than venous collection, and is performed by a physician or other specially trained professional. Patients who are anemic or have a history of cardiovascular disease may not be good candidates for phlebotomy.

Normal results

Normal results include obtaining the needed amount of blood with the minimum of discomfort to the patient.

Morbidity and mortality rates

Properly performed, phlebotomy does not carry the risk of mortality. It may cause temporary pain and bleeding, but these are usually easily managed.

Alternatives

Phlebotomy is a necessary medical procedure, and is required for a wide variety of other procedures.

Resources

PERIODICALS

Messinezy, Maria and T. C. Pearson. "Polycythaemia, Primary (Essential) Thrombocythaemia and Myelofibrosis (ABC of Clinical Haematology)." *British Medical Journal* 314 (22 February 1997): 587–90.

Wolfe, Yun Lee. "Case of the Ceaseless Fatigue." *Prevention Magazine* (July 1997): 88–94.

Paula Anne Ford-Martin
Richard Robinson

Photocoagulation therapy

Definition

Photocoagulation therapy is a method of treating detachments (tears) of the retina (the layer of light-sensitive cells at the back of the eye) with an argon laser. The high-intensity beam of light from the laser is converted into heat, which forces protein molecules in the affected tissue to condense and seal the tear.

Purpose

The purpose of photocoagulation therapy is to reattach a torn or detached portion of the retina and/or prevent further growth of abnormal blood vessels in the retina that can cause a detachment.

Demographics

The incidence of RD in the United States is about 0.3%, or one in 15,000 people.

The most common risk factors associated with RD are extreme nearsightedness (5% risk); cataract removal without lens implantation (2%); and cataract removal with loss of the vitreous body during surgery (10%). It is estimated that 15% of people with RD in one eye will eventually develop it in the other eye.

Males account for 60% and females for 40% of patients with RD below the age of 45. Above age 45, there is no significant gender difference.

With regard to racial or ethnic background, the incidence of RD is higher among Jews in the United States than in the general population; the incidence of RD among African Americans is lower than average.

Description

Structure of the human eye

To fully understand how photocoagulation therapy works, it is helpful to have a basic picture of the structure of the human eye. The retina is the innermost tunica, or covering, of the posterior part of the eyeball. It is made of several layers of cells, one of which contains the rod and cone cells that are sensitive to light. Behind the retina are the other two tunicae of the eye, the choroid and the sclera. The sclera is a tough white layer of tissue that covers the exterior of the eyeball. At the front of the eye, the sclera is continuous with a transparent area of tissue known as the cornea.

At the back of the eye, the retina is continuous with the optic nerve. The macula, which is a yellowish oval-shaped area that is the central point of vision, lies in the center of the retina. In front of the retina is the vitreous body, which is also known as the vitreous humor, or simply the vitreous. The vitreous body is a clear gel that consists primarily of water and collagen fibers.

Types of retinal detachment (RD)

RHEGMATOGENOUS. A rhegmatogenous RD is the most common of the three types of retinal detachment. The word rhegmatogenous comes from a Greek word that means "tear." A rhegmatogenous RD typically occurs in older people. As the vitreous body in the center of the eyeball ages, it shrinks and pulls away from the retina. This separation is called a posterior vitreous detachment (PVD). A PVD is not the same thing as a retinal detachment, although it may slightly increase the risk of an RD. In places where the retina is still attached to the vitreous body, a small hole or tear can develop. Over time, fluid can seep into the area around the hole or tear and thus enlarge the area of detached tissue.

TRACTION. Traction RDs are most often found in adults with diabetic retinopathy or infants with retinopathy of prematurity (ROP). Diabetic retinopathy is a disorder that develops when the patient's diabetes affects the small blood vessels in the eye. Although diabetic retinopathy is more severe in patients with type 1 diabetes (insulin-dependent), it can also occur in patients with type 2. Retinal detachment is most likely to occur in a subtype of the disorder known as proliferative diabetic retinopathy. The term proliferative refers to the abnormal growth of new blood vessels along the surface of the vitreous body. These new blood vessels can bleed into the vitreous body and form scar tissue that pulls on the retina. Eventually, the scar tissue can exert enough pulling force to cause a retinal detachment.

In ROP, a traction RD can develop because premature birth interrupts the normal development of the blood vessels in the baby's eyes. After the baby is born, some of these blood vessels grow along the retina, bleed into the vitreous body, and form scar tissue similar to that found in diabetic retinopathy. Retinal detachment in ROP can be treated with photocoagulation.

EXUDATIVE. Exudative RDs occur when tissue fluid builds up in the space between the retina and the choroid underneath it. If enough fluid leaks into this space, it can push the retina away from the choroid and cause it to detach. Exudative RDs are associated with certain inflammatory disorders of the eye; tumors, including melanoma (cancer) of the choroid; and a congenital disorder known as Coats' disease, which affects the growth of the blood vessels in the retina.

Risk factors for retinal detachment

Retinal detachment is associated with a number of different factors and conditions, including:

- extreme nearsightedness
- genetic factors (retinal detachment tends to run in families)
- premature birth (the risk of ROP is highest in premature infants weighing less than 2.2 lb [1 kg] at birth)
- type 1 or type 2 diabetes

- cataract surgery
- sickle cell disease
- Coats' disease
- Eales' disease
- Marfan's syndrome
- breast cancer or melanoma
- leukemia
- history of previous retinal detachment
- age (Retinal detachment is most common in people between the ages of 40 and 70.)
- traumatic injury to the eye
- laser in situ keratomileusis surgery (**LASIK**, a procedure done to correct vision without the need for glasses or contact lenses)

Photocoagulation therapy for retinal detachment is usually performed with an argon laser. A laser is a device that produces high-intensity, narrowly focused monochromatic light by exciting atoms and causing them to give off their energy in phases. The word laser comes from "light amplification by stimulated emission of radiation." An argon laser uses ionized argon to generate its light, which is in the blue-green portion of the visible light spectrum.

In a laser photocoagulation treatment, the patient is asked to sit in front of the instrument. After applying anesthetic eye drops, the ophthalmologist places a contact lens on the patient's eye and focuses the laser beam through it. He or she operates the laser by foot. The patient may see a brief burst of blue-green light. When the laser beam reaches the retina at the back of the eye, its light is absorbed by the pigment in the cells and converted to heat, which seals the edge of the retinal detachment

QUESTIONS TO ASK THE DOCTOR

- What are my chances of having normal vision after the laser therapy?
- What is the likelihood of my needing another laser treatment?
- Am I likely to develop retinal detachment in my other eye?
- How often should I schedule preventive eye examinations from now on?

against the underlying choroid. The procedure is short, taking about 10–30 minutes.

Diagnosis/Preparation

Diagnosis

The diagnosis of retinal detachment requires direct examination of the eye as well as taking the patient's medical history. The diagnosis may be made in some cases by an optometrist, who is a health professional qualified to examine the eye for diseases and disorders as well as taking measurements for corrective lenses. If the symptoms of RD appear suddenly, however, the patient is more likely to be diagnosed by an ophthalmologist, who is a physician specializing in treating disorders of the eye.

PATIENT HISTORY. Retinal detachment is not usually painful, and the patient's eye will look normal from the outside. In almost all cases, a patient with RD consults a doctor because he or she is having one or more of the following visual disturbances:

- blurring of vision that is not helped by blinking the eye
- a gray or black curtain or shade coming across the field of vision from one direction
- floaters, which appear as moving black spots in front of the eye (The sudden appearance of a large group, or "shower," of floaters is a serious symptom of RD.)
- flashes of light
- objects appearing wavy or distorted in shape
- blind spot in the visual field

The visual symptoms of retinal detachment may develop either gradually or suddenly. In a very small number of cases, a sudden retinal detachment may cause complete loss of vision in the affected eye.

Patients who have gone to a primary care physician or emergency room for these visual symptoms are re-ferred to an ophthalmologist. Many ophthalmologists will give patients a piece of paper with a circle on it and ask them to draw what they are seeing on the circle in the area corresponding to the part of their visual field that is affected. In some cases, the location of the spots, light flashes, or shadows that a patient sees is a clue to the part of the retina that is detached.

The ophthalmologist will take a patient history, asking about a family history of eye disorders; previous diseases or disorders of the eye; other diseases or disorders that the patient may have, particularly diabetes or sickle cell disease; and a history of head trauma, direct blows to the eye, or surgical removal of a foreign body from the eye. If the patient suffered a head or eye injury within the past six months, the ophthalmologist will ask whether the visual disturbances started at the time of the injury or several months later.

EYE EXAMINATION. After taking the history, the ophthalmologist will examine the eye itself. This examination has several parts, including:

- A test of visual clarity or sharpness. This test is the same one used by an optometrist when fitting a patient for glasses or contact lenses.
- An external check for bleeding or any other signs of trauma to the eye.
- A test that measures the response of the pupil of the eye to changes in light intensity. One sign of RD is a difference in the pupillary reaction between the affected eye and the normal one. The pupil will not contract as far as it normally does when the doctor shines a light into the affected eye.
- A test that measures the amount of fluid pressure inside each eyeball. In RD, the affected eye typically has a lower pressure measurement than the other eye.
- Examination of the eye with a slit lamp, which is an instrument with a high-intensity light source that can be focused as a thin sliver of light. The examiner uses the slit lamp together with a binocular ophthalmoscope (an instrument that looks like a microscope with two eyepieces) in order to check first the front and then the back of the eye for any abnormalities. To check the front part, the doctor will touch the side of the eye with a strip of paper containing an orange dye. The dye stains the film of tear fluid on the outer surface of the eye, making it easier to see the structures in the front of the eye. Patients with RD usually have normal results for this part of the slit-lamp examination. In the second part, the doctor puts some drops in the patient's eye to make the pupil dilate. This procedure allows him or her to see the structures in the back of the eye. If the patient has RD, the doctor may see the retina lifted upward or forward, pos-

KEY TERMS

Choroid—The middle of the three tunicae or coats that surround the eyeball; the choroid lies between the retina and the sclera.

Coats' disease—A chronic and progressive disorder of the retina marked by exudative RD. It is named for George Coats (1876-1915), a British ophthalmologist. It occurs most frequently in preadolescent boys and young adults.

Cornea—The transparent front portion of the exterior cover of the eye.

Cryopexy—Reattachment of a detached retina by freezing the tissue behind the tear with nitrous oxide.

Diabetic retinopathy—Degeneration of the retina related to diabetes; both type 1 and type 2 diabetes can lead to diabetic retinopathy.

Eales disease—A disorder marked by recurrent hemorrhages into the retina and vitreous body. It occurs most often in males between the ages of 10 and 25.

Exudative RD—A type of retinal detachment caused by the accumulation of tissue fluid underneath the retina.

Floaters—Spots seen in front of the eyes, caused by clumping of the collagen fibers in the vitreous body.

Laser—A device that produces high-intensity, narrowly focused monochromatic light by exciting atoms and causing them to give off their energy in phase.

Laser in situ keratomileusis (LASIK)—A procedure in which the shape of the cornea is changed with an excimer laser in order to correct the patient's vision.

Macula—A small, yellowish depressed area on the retina that absorbs the shorter wave lengths of visible light and is responsible for fine detailed vision.

Marfan's syndrome—A hereditary disorder that affects the connective tissues of the body, the lens of the eye, and the cardiovascular system.

sibly moving back and forth. The retina will have a grayish color with darker blood vessels visible. It may have a pitted surface resembling an orange peel, and there may also be a line visible at the edge of the detachment.

LABORATORY AND IMAGING STUDIES. Today, there are no laboratory tests for retinal detachment. Ultrasound, however, can be used to diagnose retinal detachment if the doctor cannot see the retina with a slit lamp because of cataracts or blood seeping into the vitreous body. If the RD is exudative, ultrasound can be used to detect a tumor or hemorrhage underneath the retina.

Preparation

Treatment of RD follows as soon as possible after the diagnosis; however, an immediate procedure is not usually necessary since the time frame for treatment of a detached retina is several hours rather than only a few minutes.

If the patient has suffered a traumatic injury to the eye, the eye may be covered with a protective shield prior to treatment.

Preparation for photocoagulation therapy consists of eye drops that dilate the pupil of the eye and numb the eye itself. The laser treatment is painless, although some patients require additional anesthetic for sensitivity to the laser light.

Aftercare

Patients who have had photocoagulation therapy for retinal detachment are asked to have a friend or family member drive them home. The reason for this precaution is that the eye medication used to dilate the pupil of the patient's eye before the procedure takes several hours to wear off. During this period, the eye is unusually sensitive to light. The patient can go to work the next day with no restrictions on activity.

Risks

The most common risks of laser photocoagulation therapy are mild discomfort at the beginning of the procedure and the possibility that a second laser treatment will be needed to reattach the retina securely.

Normal results

Over 90% of retinal detachments can be repaired with prompt treatment, although sometimes a second procedure is needed. About 40% of patients treated for retinal detachment will have good vision within six months of surgery. The results are less favorable if the retina has been detached for a long time or if there is a large growth of fibrous tissue that has caused a traction

Ophthalmology—The branch of medicine that deals with the diagnosis and treatment of eye disorders.

Optometrist—A primary health care provider who examines eyes and diagnoses disorders of the eye as well as prescribing eyeglasses, contact lenses, and other vision aids.

Pneumatic retinopexy—Reattachment of a detached retina using an injected gas bubble to hold the retina against the back of the eye.

Pupil—The opening in the center of the iris of the eye that allows light to enter the eye.

Retina—The innermost of three layers of tissue surrounding the human eyeball. The retina surrounds the vitreous body and joins the optic nerve at the back of the eye.

Retinal detachment (RD)—A condition in which the inner layers of cells in the retina separate from the underlying pigmented layers of cells called the choroid.

Retinopathy of prematurity (ROP)—A disorder that occurs in premature infants in which blood vessels in the eye continue to grow in an abnormal pattern after delivery. It can lead to retinal detachment and blindness. ROP is also known as retrolental fibroplasia.

Sclera—The tough white outer tunica or coat of the eyeball.

Tunica (plural, tunicae)—The medical term for a membrane or piece of tissue that covers or lines a body part. The retina is the innermost of three tunicae that surround the eyeball.

Vitrectomy—Surgical removal of the vitreous body.

Vitreous body—The transparent gel that fills the inner portion of the eyeball between the lens and the retina. It is also called the vitreous humor or crystalline humor.

---

detachment. These patients, however, will still have some degree of reading or traveling vision after the retina has been reattached. In a very small minority of patients, the surgeon cannot reattach the retina because of extensive growths of fibrous scar tissue on it.

Morbidity and mortality rates

The mortality rate for laser photocoagulation treatment of retinal detachment is extremely low; morbidity depends to a large extent on the cause of the RD. A study done in 2001 reported that laser therapy for rhegmatogenous RDs is as effective as pneumatic retinopexy or **scleral buckling**, but has the advantage of fewer complications after the procedure. In the treatment of ROP, laser photocoagulation has been found to be more effective than cryopexy in reducing the infant's risk of nearsightedness in later life.

Alternatives

Alternatives to laser photocoagulation as a treatment for RD depend on the location and size of the retinal detachment. Photocoagulation treatment works best on small tears in the retina. One alternative for the treatment of small areas of detachment is cryopexy, which is performed as an outpatient procedure under local anesthe-sia. In cryopexy, the ophthalmologist uses nitrous oxide to freeze the tissue underneath the retinal tear. This procedure leads to the formation of scar tissue that seals the edges of the tear in place.

Pneumatic retinopexy is a procedure that can be used if the RD is located in the upper part of the eye. After numbing the patient's eye with a local anesthetic, the ophthalmologist injects a small bubble of gas into the vitreous body. The gas bubble rises and presses the torn part of the retina back against the underlying choroid. The bubble is slowly absorbed over the next two weeks. The ophthalmologist then uses either photocoagulation or cryopexy to complete the reattachment of the retina.

If the RD is large, the doctor may decide to perform a scleral buckle treatment or a vitrectomy. These procedures are more invasive than laser photocoagulation or cryopexy; however, they are still usually done as outpatient procedures. In a scleral buckle procedure, the doctor attaches a tiny silicon band to the sclera. The buckle, which remains in the eye permanently, puts pressure on the retina to hold it in place.

In a vitrectomy, the ophthalmologist removes the vitreous body and replaces it with air or a saline solution that puts pressure on the retina to hold it in place. Vitrectomies are usually performed if there is a very large tear in the retina; if the macula is involved; or if blood that has leaked into the vitreous body is interfering with diagnosis or treatment.

See also Retinal cryopexy; Scleral buckling.

Resources

BOOKS

"Retinal Disorders." Section 8, Chapter 99 in *The Merck Manual of Diagnosis and Therapy,* edited by Mark H. Beers, and Robert Berkow. Whitehouse Station, NJ: Merck Research Laboratories, 1999.

"Retinopathy of Prematurity." Section 19, Chapter 260 in *The Merck Manual of Diagnosis and Therapy,* edited by Mark H. Beers, and Robert Berkow. Whitehouse Station, NJ: Merck Research Laboratories, 1999.

PERIODICALS

Arevalo, J. Fernando, et al. "Retinal Detachment in Myopic Eyes after Laser in situ Keratomileusis." *Journal of Refractive Surgery,* 18 (November–December 2002): 708–714.

Dellone-Larkin, Gregory, and Cecilia A. Dellone. "Retinal Detachment." *eMedicine,* August 10, 2001 [March 21, 2003]. <www.emedicine.com/emerg/topic504.htm>.

El-Asrar, A. M., and S. A. Al-Kharashi. "Full Panretinal Photocoagulation and Early Vitrectomy Improve Prognosis of Retinal Vasculitis Associated with Tuberculoprotein Hypersensitivity (Eales' Disease)." *British Journal of Ophthalmology,* 86 (November 2002): 1248–1251.

Foroozan, R., B. P. Conolly, and W. S. Tasman. "Outcomes after Laser Therapy for Threshold Retinopathy of Prematurity." *Ophthalmology,* 108 (September 2001): 1644–1646.

Greenberg, P. B., and C. R. Baumal. "Laser Therapy for Rhegmatogenous Retinal Detachment." *Current Opinion in Ophthalmology,* 12 (June 2001): 171–174.

Lee, E. S., H. J. Koh, O. W. Kwon, and S. C. Lee. "Laser Photocoagulation Repair of Recurrent Macula-Sparing Retinal Detachments." *Yonsei Medical Journal,* 43 (August 2002): 446–450.

Vakili, Roya, Shachar Tauber, and Edward S. Lim. "Successful Management of Retinal Tear Post-Laser in situ Keratomileusis Retreatment." *Yale Journal of Biology and Medicine,* 75 (2002): 55–57.

van Meurs, J. C., et al. "Postoperative Laser Coagulation as Retinopexy in Patients with Rhegmatogenous Retinal Detachment Treated with Scleral Buckling Surgery: A Prospective Clinical Study." *Retina,* 22 (December 2002): 733–739.

Wu, Lihteh, and Carlos Cabezas. "Retinal Detachment, Exudative." *eMedicine,* June 28, 2001 [March 24, 2003]. <www.emedicine.com/OPH/topic407.htm>.

ORGANIZATIONS

American Academy of Ophthalmology. P. O. Box 7424, San Francisco, CA 94120-7424. (415) 561-8500. <www.aao.org>.

American Optometric Association. 243 North Lindbergh Blvd., St. Louis, MO 63141. (314) 991-4100. <www.aoanet.org>.

Canadian Ophthalmological Society (COS). 610-1525 Carling Avenue, Ottawa ON K1Z 8R9 Canada. <www.eyesite.ca>.

Diabetic Retinopathy Foundation. 350 North LaSalle, Suite 800, Chicago, IL 60610. <www.retinopathy.org>.

Wills Eye Hospital. 840 Walnut Street, Philadelphia, PA 19107. (215) 928-3000. <www.willseye.org>.

Rebecca Frey, PhD

Photorefractive keratectomy (PRK)

Definition

Photorefractive keratectomy (PRK) is a noninvasive refractive surgery in which the surgeon uses an excimer laser to reshape the cornea of the eye by removing the epithelium, the gel-like outer layer of the cornea.

Purpose

PRK, one of the first (and once the most popular) refractive surgeries, eliminates or reduces moderate nearsightedness (myopia), hyperopia (farsightedness), and astigmatism; it is most commonly used to treat myopia. Successfully treated PRK patients no longer require corrective lenses, and those who do still require correction, require much less.

PRK is an elective, **outpatient surgery**, and people choose the treatment for different reasons. Some simply no longer want to wear eyeglasses for cosmetic reasons. Sports enthusiasts may find eyeglasses or contact lenses troublesome during physical activities. Others may experience pain or dryness while wearing contact lenses, or have corneal ulcers that make wearing contact lenses painful. Firefighters and police officers may have trouble seeing in emergency situations when their contact lenses get dry or their eyeglasses fog up.

Demographics

There is no such thing as a typical PRK patient. Because it is an **elective surgery**, patients come from every age group and income bracket. PRK candidates, however, must be 18 or older; have myopia, hyperopia, or astigmatism; and have had stable vision for at least two years. While PRK is experiencing a slight resurgence in popularity, it lags behind the newer and less painful **laser in-situ keratomileusis (LASIK)**. The American Acade-

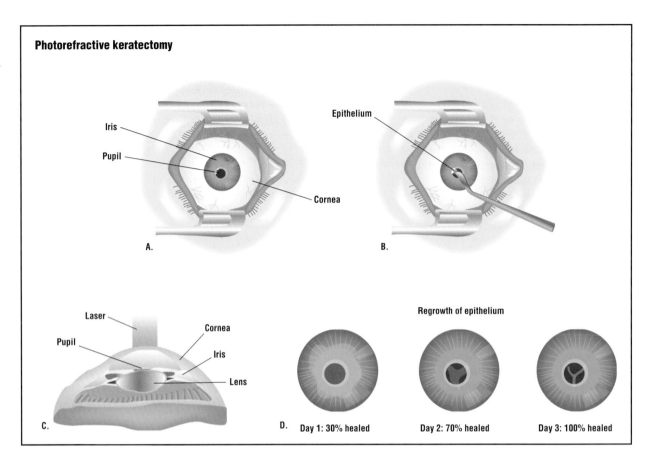

Photorefractive keratectomy

Iris

Pupil

Cornea

A.

Epithelium

B.

Laser

Pupil

Cornea

Iris

Lens

C.

Regrowth of epithelium

D.

Day 1: 30% healed

Day 2: 70% healed

Day 3: 100% healed

In PRK surgery, the eye is held open with a speculum (A). The gel-like coating on the eye, called the epithelium, is scraped away (B). A laser is used to reshape the cornea and improve vision (C). The epithelium repairs itself in a few days (D). *(Illustration by GGS Inc.)*

my of Ophthalmology (AAO) estimates that 95% of all refractive surgeries are LASIK.

The first PRK patients are sometimes referred to as "early adopters." These are people who are always interested in the latest technology and have the financial resources to take advantage of it. In the mid-1990s when PRK was first approved, patients were in their early 30s to mid-40s and financially stable. Prices have now stabilized at about $2,500 per eye for PRK.

While it has lost favor with the general public, PRK is the choice of the United States military. Military doctors prefer PRK over LASIK because the latter involves cutting a flap that doctors fear may loosen and become unhinged during combat.

Description

PRK was first performed in the 1980s and widely used in Europe and Canada in the early 1990s, but was not approved in the United States until 1995. PRK was the most popular refractive procedure until the creation

of LASIK, which has a much shorter recovery time. PRK is still the preferred option for patients with thin corneas, corneal dystrophies, corneal scars, or recurrent corneal erosion.

PRK takes about 10 minutes to perform. Immediately before the procedure, the ophthalmologist may request corneal topography (a corneal map) to compare with previous maps to ensure the treatment plan is still correct. Ophthalmic personnel will perform a refraction to make sure the refractive correction the surgeon will program into the excimer laser is correct.

Patients may be given a sedative such as Valium to relax them before the surgery. Anesthetic drops will be applied to numb the eye and prevent pain during the procedure.

After the eye drops are inserted, the surgeon prepares the treated eye for surgery. If both eyes are being treated on the same day, the non-treated eye is patched. The surgeon inserts a speculum in the first eye to be treated to hold the eyelids apart and prevent movement. The patient stares at the blinking light of a laser microscope and must fixate his or her gaze on that light. The patient must remain still.

The surgeon double-checks the laser settings to make sure they are programmed correctly for the refractive error. With everything in place, the eye surgeon removes the surface corneal cells (epithelium) with a sponge, mechanical blade, or the excimer laser. With the epithelium completely removed, the surgeon will begin reshaping, or ablating, the cornea. This takes 15–45 seconds, and varies for refractive error; the stronger the error, the longer the ablation. Patients may worry that moving could cause irreversible eye damage, but they should know that, at the slightest movement, the doctor immediately stops the laser. When the ablation is completed, the surgeon places a bandage contact lens on the treated eye to protect it and allow the healing process to take place; it also eases some of the pain of the exposed cornea. The surgeon will also dispense anti-inflammatory and antibiotic eye drops to stop infection and reduce pain.

Diagnosis/Preparation

Patients should have a complete eye evaluation and medical history taken before surgery. Soft contact lens wearers should stop wearing their lenses at least one week before the initial exam. Gas-permeable lens wearers should not wear their lenses from three weeks to a month before the exam. Contact lens wear alters the cornea's shape, which should be allowed to return to its natural shape before the exam.

Patients should also disclose current medications. Allergy medications and birth control pills have been known to cause haze after surgery. Physicians will want to examine the potential risks involved with these medications.

Patients who have these conditions/history should not have the procedure, including:

• pregnant women or women who are breastfeeding
• patients with very small or very large refractive errors
• patients with scarred corneas or macular disease
• people with autoimmune diseases
• diabetics
• glaucoma patients
• patients with persistent blepharitis

Physicians will perform a baseline eye evaluation, including a manifest and cycloplegic refraction, measurement of intraocular pressure (to determine if the patient has glaucoma), slit-lamp biomicroscopy, tear film evaluation, corneal topography, evaluation of corneal thickness, dilated fundus examination, and measurement of scotopic pupil size.

WHO PERFORMS THE PROCEDURE AND WHERE IS IT PERFORMED?

An ophthalmologist performs PRK with the aid of ophthalmic technicians and nurses. The surgeon may have received specific refractive surgery training in medical school, but because it is a relatively new procedure, older surgeons may not have completed such training. Instead, these surgeons may have completed continuing medical education courses or may have had training provided by the laser companies.

Preparation and aftercare may be handled by an optometrist who works with the ophthalmologist on these cases. The optometrist usually establishes eligibility for PRK, and may also perform much of the follow-up, with the exception of the first post-PRK visit.

Hospitals are one setting for this surgery, but the most common location is an ambulatory surgery center or surgery suite. Surgeons at surgery centers owned by refractive surgery companies also perform PRK. These businesses hire support staff, optometrists and surgeons in a stand-alone surgery center or in a hospital.

If the patient is an appropriate candidate, he or she must sign an **informed consent** form that states he or she is aware of possible complications and outcomes of the procedure.

Pre-surgery preparations

The patient is advised to discontinue contact lens wear immediately and refrain from using creams, lotions, makeup, or perfume for at least two days before surgery. Patients may also be asked to scrub their eyelashes for a period of time to remove any debris.

Aftercare

Patients usually have follow-up appointments at 24 hours, four days, one week, one month, three months, six months, and then annually following PRK. More frequent visits may be necessary, if there are complications.

Patients should refrain from strenuous activity for at least one month after surgery. Creams, lotions, and makeup must also be avoided for at least two weeks.

The bandage contact lens is removed by the surgeon usually after four days (during the second visit). Patients must be diligent in using antibiotic drops and steroid drops. Because the epithelium is completely removed, there is a greater chance of infection and pain; the eye drops are needed to minimize these possible complications. The eye drops must be used for at least four months for some patients. The slow healing process is imperative to keeping the desired correction.

PRK has a long recovery rate, which is why LASIK gained popularity so quickly. Unlike LASIK, in which patients notice improved vision immediately and are back to normal routines the next day, PRK patients are advised to rest for at least two days. PRK patients also experience moderate pain the first few days of recovery, and may need pain relievers such as Demerol to ease the pain. Vision also fluctuates the first few weeks of recovery as the epithelium grows back. This can cause haze, and patients become concerned that the surgery was unsuccessful. PRK patients need to be aware that vision can fluctuate for as long as up to six months after surgery. Incorrect use of eye drops can cause regression.

Risks

PRK patients may experience glare, vision fluctuation, development of irregular astigmatism, vision distortion (even with corrective lenses), glaucoma, loss of best visual acuity, and, though extremely rare, total vision loss.

A more common side effect is long-term haze. Some patients who have aggressive healing processes can form corneal scars that can cause haze. With proper screening for this condition and with the use of eye drops, this risk can be lessened.

Complications associated with LASIK, such as photophobia, haloes, and dry eye, are not as common with PRK. However, The patient may be under-corrected or overcorrected, and enhancements might be needed to attain the best visual acuity.

Normal results

Most PRK patients achieve 20/40 vision, which means in most states they can legally drive a car without vision correction. Some patients will still need corrective lenses, but the lenses will not need to be as powerful.

There have been reports of regression after the PRK healing process is completed. Sometimes a patient will require an enhancement, and the surgeon must repeat the surgery. Patients should also be aware that with the onset of presbyopia after age 40, they will probably require vision correction for reading or close work.

Morbidity and mortality rates

Information about PRK mortality and morbidity is limited because the procedure is elective. Complications that can lead to more serious conditions, such as infection, are treated with topical **antibiotics**. There is also a chance the patient could have a severe reaction to the antibiotics or steroids used in the healing process.

Alternatives

Because these patients only have mild to moderate myopia, hyperopia, or astigmatism, they can choose from most refractive surgeries and non-surgical procedures.

Surgical alternatives

- Laser in-situ keratomileusis (LASIK). The most popular refractive surgery, it is similar to PRK, but differs in how it reshapes the cornea. Instead of completely removing tissue, LASIK leaves a "flap" of tissue that the surgeon moves back into place after ablation. LASIK is less painful with a shorter recovery time. However, there are more complications associated with LASIK.
- Radial keratotomy (RK). RK was the first widely used surgical correction for mild to moderate myopia. The surgeon alters the shape of the cornea without a laser. This is one of the oldest refractive procedures, and has proved successful on lower and moderate corrections.
- Astigmatic keratotomy (AK). AK is a variation of RK used to treat mild to moderate astigmatism. AK has proved successful if the errors are mild to moderate.

Non-surgical alternatives

Contact lenses and eyeglasses also can correct refractive errors. Improvements in contact lenses have

KEY TERMS

Ablation—The vaporization of eye tissue.

Astigmatism—Asymmetric vision defects due to irregularities in the cornea.

Cornea—The clear, curved tissue layer in front of the eye. It lies in front of the colored part of the eye (iris) and the black hole in the center of the iris (pupil).

Corneal topography—Mapping the cornea's surface with a specialized computer that illustrates corneal elevations.

Dry eye—Corneal dryness due to insufficient tear production.

Enhancement—A secondary refractive procedure performed in an attempt to achieve better visual acuity.

Excimer laser—An instrument that is used to vaporize tissue with a cold, coherent beam of light with a single wavelength in the ultraviolet range.

Hyperopia—The inability to see near objects as clearly as distant objects, and the need for accommodation to see objects clearly.

Myopia—A vision problem in which distant objects appear blurry. People who are myopic or nearsighted can usually see near objects clearly, but not far objects.

Presbyopia—A condition affecting people over the age of 40 in which the focusing of near objects fails to work because of age-related hardening of the lens of the eye.

Caster, Andrew I. *The Eye Laser Miracle: The Complete Guide to Better Vision.* New York, NY: Ballantine Books, 1997.

Slade, Stephen G., Richard N. Baker, and Dorothy Kay Brockman. *The Complete Book of Laser Eye Surgery.* Naperville, IL: Sourcebooks, Inc., 2000.

ORGANIZATION

American Academy of Ophthalmology. P.O. Box 7424, San Francisco, CA 94120-7424. (415) 561-8500. <www.aao.org>.

American Society of Cataract and Refractive Surgery. 4000 Legato Road, Suite 850, Fairfax, VA 22033-4055. (703) 591-2220. E-mail: <ascrs@ascrs.org>. <www.ascrs.org>.

Council for Refractive Surgery Quality Assurance. 8543 Everglade Drive, Sacramento, CA 95826-0769. (916) 381-0769. E-mail: <info@usaeyes.org>. <www.usaeyes.org>.

OTHER

Bethke, Walt. "Surface Procedures: The State of the Art." *Review of Ophthalmology,* February 2003 [cited March 16, 2003]. <;www.revopth.com/index.asp?page=1_283.htm>.

"Identify Allergies Before Performing LASIK, PRK." *Ocular Surgery News.* October 25, 2002 [cited March 16, 2003]. <www.osnsupersite.com/view.asp?ID=3802>.

"PRK: Photorefractive Keratectomy." *EyeMdLink.com.* [cited March 20, 2003]. <www.eyemdlink.com/EyeProcedure.asp?EyeProcedureID=7>.

Sabar, Ariel. "Laser Gives Kids Vision to Fly." *The Baltimore Sun.* February 27, 2003 [cited March 16, 2003]. <www.sunspot.net/features/health/bal-te.ar.laser27feb27,0,3705843.story?coll=bal-home-headlines>.

Segre, Liz. "PRK: The Original Laser Eye Surgery." *All About Vision.* [cited March 16, 2003]. <www.allaboutvision.com/visionsurgery/prk.htm>.

Mary Bekker

made them easier to wear, and continuous-wear contact lenses, which a patient can sleep in for as long as 30 days, can provide a similar effect to PRK. A customized rigid gas-permeable contact lens is used for orthokeratology (Ortho-K), in which a patient wears the lens for a predetermined amount of time to reshape the cornea. After removing the lens, the patient's vision is improved and remains improved until the cornea returns to its natural shape. At that time, the patient repeats the process.

See also Laser in-situ keratomileusis (LASIK).

Resources

BOOKS

Brint, Stephen F., Dennis Kennedy, and Corinne Kuypers-Denlinger. *The Laser Vision Breakthrough.* Roseville, CA: Prima Health, 2000.

Physical examination

Definition

A physical examination is the evaluation of a body to determine its state of health. The techniques of inspection include palpation (feeling with the hands and/or fingers), percussion (tapping with the fingers), auscultation (listening), and smell. A complete health assessment also includes gathering information about a person's medical history and lifestyle, conducting laboratory tests, and screening for disease. These elements constitute the data on which a diagnosis is made and a plan of treatment is developed.

Purpose

The term annual physical examination has been replaced in most health care circles by periodic health examination. The frequency with which it is conducted depends on factors such as the age, gender, and the presence of risk factors for disease in the person being examined. Health-care professionals often use guidelines that have been developed by organizations such as the United States Preventative Services Task Force. Organizations such as the American Cancer Society or American Heart Association, which promote detection and prevention of specific diseases, generally recommend more intensive or frequent examinations, or suggest that examinations be focused on particular organ systems of the body.

Comprehensive physical examinations provide opportunities for health care professionals to obtain baseline information about individuals that may be useful in the future. They also allow health care providers to establish relationships before problems occur. Physical examinations are appropriate times to answer questions and teach good health practices. Detecting and addressing problems in their early stages can have beneficial long-term results.

Every person should have periodic physical examinations. These occur frequently (monthly at first) in infants and gradually reach a frequency of once per year for adolescents and adults.

Description

A complete physical examination usually starts at the head and proceeds all the way to the toes. However, the exact procedure will vary according to the needs of the person being examined and the preferences of the examiner. An average examination takes about 30 minutes. The cost of an examination will depend on the charge for professional time and any tests that are included. Most health plans cover routine physical examinations, including some tests.

The examination

Before examiners question the patient, they will observe a person's overall appearance, general health, and behavior. Measurements of height and weight are made. **Vital signs** such as pulse, breathing rate, body temperature, and blood pressure are recorded.

With the person being examined in a sitting position, the following systems are reviewed:

• Skin. The exposed areas of the skin are observed; the size and shape of any lesions are noted.

• Head. The hair, scalp, skull, and face are examined.

• Eyes. The external structures are observed. The internal structures can be observed using an ophthalmoscope (a lighted instrument) in a darkened room.

• Ears. The external structures are inspected. A lighted instrument called an otoscope may be used to inspect internal structures.

• Nose and sinuses. The external nose is examined. The nasal mucosa and internal structures can be observed with the use of a penlight and a nasal speculum.

• Mouth and pharynx. The lips, gums, teeth, roof of the mouth, tongue, and pharynx are inspected.

• Neck. The lymph nodes on both sides of the neck and the thyroid gland are palpated.

• Back. The spine and muscles of the back are palpated and checked for tenderness. The upper back, where the lungs are located, is palpated on the right and left sides and a **stethoscope** is used to listen for breath sounds.

• Breasts and armpits. A woman's breasts are inspected with the arms relaxed and then raised. In both men and women, the lymph nodes in the armpits are felt with the examiner's hands. While the person is still sitting, movement of the joints in the hands, arms, shoulders, neck, and jaw can be checked.

While the person is lying down on the examining table, the examination includes:

• Breasts. The breasts are palpated and inspected for masses.

• Front of chest and lungs. The area is inspected with the fingers, using palpation and percussion. A stethoscope is used to listen to internal breath sounds.

The head should be slightly raised to examine:

• Heart. A stethoscope is used to listen to the heart's rate and rhythm. The blood vessels in the neck are observed and palpated.

The person being examined should lie flat for an examination of the:

- Abdomen. Light and deep palpation is used on the abdomen to feel the outlines of internal organs, including the liver, spleen, kidneys, and aorta, a large blood vessel.

- Rectum and anus. With the person lying on the left side, the outside areas are observed. An internal digital examination (using a gloved finger), is usually done for persons over 40 years old. In men, the prostate gland is also palpated.

- Reproductive organs. The external sex organs are inspected and the area is examined for hernias. In men, the scrotum and testicles are palpated. In women, a pelvic examination is completed using a speculum and a sample for a Papanicolaou test (Pap test) may be taken.

- Legs. While lying flat, the legs are inspected for swelling, and pulses in the knee, thigh, and foot area are found. The groin area is palpated for the presence of lymph nodes. The joints and muscles are observed.

- Musculoskeletal system. With the person standing, the straightness of the spine and the alignment of the legs and feet is noted.

- Blood vessels. The presence of any abnormally enlarged veins (varicose), usually in the legs, is noted.

In addition to evaluating a person's alertness and mental ability during the initial conversation, inspection of the nervous system may include:

- Neurologic screen. The person's ability to take a few steps, hop, and do deep knee bends is observed. The strength of the handgrip is felt. While sitting in an upright position, the reflexes in the knees and feet can be tested with a small hammer. The sense of touch in the hands and feet can be evaluated by testing reaction to pain and vibration.

- The 12 nerves in the head (cranial) that are connected directly to the brain. They control the senses of smell and taste, strength of muscles in the head, reflexes in the eye, facial movements, gag reflex, vision, hearing, and muscles in the jaw. General muscle tone and coordination, and the reaction of the abdominal area to stimulants like pain, temperature, and touch may also be evaluated.

Diagnosis/Preparation

The individual being examined should be comfortable and treated with respect throughout the examination. As the examination continues, examiners should explain what they are doing and share any relevant findings. Using language appropriate to the person being examined improves the effectiveness of communications and ultimately fosters better relations between examiners and examinees.

QUESTIONS TO ASK THE DOCTOR

- What are my results, both normal and abnormal?

- What has changed since the last physical examination?

- What do you recommend as a result of the findings of this physical examination?

- When do you want to repeat the physical examination?

Before visiting a health care professional, individuals should write down important facts and dates about their own medical history, as well as those of family members. There should be a complete listing of all medications and their dosages. This list should include over-the-counter preparations, vitamins, and herbal supplements. Some people bring their bottles of medications with them. Any questions or concerns about medications should be written down.

Before the physical examination begins, the bladder should be emptied. A urine specimen is usually collected in a small container at this time. The urine is tested for the presence of glucose (sugar), protein, and blood cells. For some blood tests, individuals may be told ahead of time not to eat or drink for 12 hours prior to the test.

Individuals being examined usually remove all clothing and put on a loose-fitting hospital gown. An additional sheet is provided to keep persons covered and comfortable during the examination.

Aftercare

Once a physical examination has been completed, the person being examined and the examiner should review what laboratory tests have been ordered, why they have been selected, and how and with whom the results will be shared. A health professional should discuss any recommendations for treatment and follow-up visits. Special instructions should be put in writing. This is also an opportunity for persons to ask any remaining questions about their own health concerns.

Risks

There are virtually no risks associated with a physical examination. Complications with the process of a physical examination are unusual. Occasionally, a useful piece of information or data may be overlooked. More

KEY TERMS

Auscultation—The process of listening to sounds that are produced in the body. Direct auscultation uses the ear alone, such as when listening to the grating of a moving joint. Indirect auscultation involves the use of a stethoscope to amplify sounds from within the body, such as those coming from the heart or intestines.

Hernia—The bulging of an organ, or part of an organ, through the tissues normally containing it; also called a rupture.

Inspection—The visual examination of the body using the eyes and a lighted instrument if needed. The sense of smell may also be used.

Ophthalmoscope—Lighted device for studying the interior of the eyeball.

Otoscope—An instrument with a light for examining the internal ear.

Palpation—The examination of the body using the sense of touch. There are two types: light and deep.

Percussion—An assessment method in which the surface of the body is struck with the fingertips to obtain sounds that can be heard or vibrations that can be felt. It can determine the position, size, and consistency of an internal organ. It is performed over the chest to determine the presence of normal air content in the lungs, and over the abdomen to evaluate air in the loops of the intestine.

Reflex—An automatic response to a stimulus.

Speculum—An instrument for enlarging the opening of any canal or cavity in order to facilitate inspection of its interior.

Stethoscope—A Y-shaped instrument that amplifies body sounds such as heartbeat, breathing, and air in the intestine. Used in auscultation.

Varicose veins—The permanent enlargement and twisting of veins, usually in the legs. They are most often seen in people working in occupations requiring long periods of standing, and in pregnant women.

commonly, results of associated laboratory tests compel physicians to recheck an individual or reexamine portions of the body already reviewed. In a sense, complications may arise from the findings of a physical examination. These usually trigger further investigations or initiate treatment. They are really more beneficial than negative, as they often begin a process of treatment and recovery.

Normal results

Normal results of a physical examination correspond to the healthy appearance and normal functioning of the body. For example, appropriate reflexes will be present, no suspicious lumps or lesions will be found, and vital signs will be normal.

Abnormal results of a physical examination include any findings that indicate the presence of a disorder, disease, or underlying condition. For example, the presence of lumps or lesions, fever, muscle weakness or lack of tone, poor reflex response, heart arrhythmia, or swelling of lymph nodes will indicate possible health problems.

Resources

BOOKS

Bickley, L. S., P. G. Szilagyi, and J. G. Stackhouse. *Bates' Guide to Physical Examination & History Taking, 8th edition.* Philadelphia: Lippincott Williams & Wilkins, 2002.

Chan, P. D., and P. J. Winkle. *History and Physical Examination in Medicine, 10th edition.* New York: Current Clinical Strategies, 2002.

Seidel, Henry M. *Mosby's Physical Examination Handbook, 4th edition.* St. Louis, MO: Mosby-Year Book, 2003.

Swartz, Mark A., and William Schmitt. *Textbook of Physical Diagnosis: History and Examination, 4th edition.* Philadelphia: Saunders, 2001.

PERIODICALS

Ahmed, A. M. "Deficiencies of Physical Examination Among Medical Students." *Saudi Medical Journal,* 24, no.1 (2003): 108–111.

ORGANIZATIONS

American Academy of Family Physicians. 11400 Tomahawk Creek Parkway, Leawood, KS 66211-2672. (913) 906-6000. E-mail: <fp@aafp.org>. <http://www.aafp.org>.

American Academy of Pediatrics. 141 Northwest Point Boulevard, Elk Grove Village, IL 60007-1098. (847) 434-4000; Fax: (847) 434-8000. E-mail: <kidsdoc@aap.org>. <http://www.aap.org/default.htm>.

American College of Physicians. 190 N Independence Mall West, Philadelphia, PA 19106-1572. (800) 523-1546, x2600, or (215) 351-2600. <http://www.acponline.org>.

American Medical Association. 515 N. State Street, Chicago, IL 60610. (312) 464-5000. <http://www.ama-assn.org>.

OTHER

Karolinska Institute. [cited March 1, 2003]. <http://isp.his. ki.se/text/physical.htm>.

Loyola University Chicago Stritch School of Medicine. [cited March 1, 2003]. <http://www.meddean.luc.edu/lumen/MedEd/MEDICINE/PULMONAR/PD/Pdmenu.htm>.

National Library of Medicine. [cited March 1, 2003]. <http://www.nlm.nih.gov/medlineplus/ency/article/002274.htm>.

Review of Systems School of Medical Transcription. [cited March 1, 2003]. <http://www.mtmonthly.com/student corner/cpe.htm>.

L. Fleming Fallon, Jr. MD, DrPH

Pitocin *see* **Uterine stimulants**

Pituitary gland removal *see* **Hypophysectomy**

Planning a hospital stay

Definition

Planning a hospital stay includes determining what hospitals or facilities are covered by the patient's insurance plan, evaluating the credentials of the health care providers and hospital, gathering information about the hospital, including services offered, scheduling the hospital stay, completing pre-admission testing, receiving and following all of the appropriate pre-admission instructions, registering at the hospital upon arrival, as well as completing an **informed consent** form.

Purpose

Patients are admitted to the hospital for a variety of reasons, including scheduled tests, procedures, or surgery; emergency medical treatment; administration of medication; or to stabilize or monitor an existing medical condition.

Planning a hospital stay helps the patient understand what to expect before **admission to the hospital** and ensures the patient is physically and psychologically ready.

Description

If the hospital stay was planned, some of the steps involved in preparing for the hospital stay will take place one to two weeks before the patient is admitted to the hospital. Many of these steps will not apply if the hospital stay was unexpected or was the result of an emergency.

Determining insurance coverage

Although there are many types of hospitals available to meet the needs of different patients, the patient's choice of hospital may be limited by his or her insurance plan. The patient should find out if the selected hospital is approved by his or her insurance plan. If the patient receives care from a facility that is not approved by the health care plan, the patient may be responsible for paying for most or all of the medical expenses related to the hospital stay.

Managed care insurance plans often require pre-certification before any hospital stay, except for emergency hospital admissions. Usually, the patient's doctor has to authorize the hospital stay, and some types of care provided in the hospital may require insurance clearance.

If the patient has **Medicare** insurance (for patients over age 65), a semiprivate room, meals, general nursing care, and other **hospital services** and supplies are covered services. Those services not covered by Medicare include private duty nursing, a private room (unless medically necessary), and television and telephone fees.

The patient may desire to seek a **second opinion** to confirm the doctor's treatment recommendations. The patient should check with his or her insurance provider to determine if the second opinion consultation is covered.

FOR PATIENTS WITHOUT INSURANCE COVERAGE. For patients who do not have insurance coverage, other payment options and sources of financial aid can be discussed. The patient should ask to speak with the hospital's financial counselor for more information.

Evaluating credentials

The patient should find out if the physicians who will provide care in the hospital are board certified. Even though board certification is not required for an individual physician to practice medicine, most hospitals require that a certain percentage of their staff be board certified. There are 24 certifying boards recognized by the American Board of Member Specialties (ABMS) and the American Medical Association (AMA). Most of the ABMS boards issue time-limited certificates, valid for six to 10 years. This requires physicians to become re-certified to maintain their board certification—a process that includes a credential review, continuing education in the specialty, and additional examinations.

A physician's membership in professional societies is also an important consideration. Professional societies provide an independent forum for medical specialists to discuss issues of national interest and mutual concern. Examples of professional societies include the Society of Thoracic Surgeons (STS) and the American College of Physicians–American Society of Internal Medicine (ACP-ASIM).

To find information about a physician's qualifications, the patient can call a state or county medical association for assistance. A reference book is also available, *The Official ABMS Directory of Board-Certified Medical Specialists,* that lists all physicians who are certified by approved boards. This publication also contains brief information about each physician's medical education and training, and it can be found in many libraries.

Evaluating the health care team

Selecting a hospital that has a multi-disciplinary team of specialists is important. The medical team should include surgeons (as applicable), physicians who specialize in the patient's medical condition (such as cardiologists for heart disease and pulmonologists for lung disease), infectious disease specialists, pharmacologists, and advanced care registered nurses. Other medical team members may include fellows, residents, interns, clinical coordinators, physical therapists, occupational therapists, respiratory therapists, registered dietitians, social workers, and financial counselors.

Evaluating the hospital

The patient should find out if the hospital has been accredited by the Joint Commission on Accreditation of Healthcare Organizations, a professionally sponsored program that stimulates a high quality of patient care in health care facilities. Joint Commission accreditation means the hospital voluntarily sought accreditation and met national health and safety standards.

Here are some questions to consider when evaluating a hospital:

- Does the hospital offer treatment for the patient's specific condition? How experienced is the hospital staff in treating that condition?

- What is the hospital's success record in providing the specific medical treatment or procedure the patient needs?

- Does the hospital have experience treating other patients the same age as the potential patient?

- Does the hospital explain the patient's rights and responsibilities?

- Does the hospital have a written description of its services and fees?

- How much does the patient's type of treatment cost at the hospital?

- Is financial help available?

- Who will be responsible for the patient's specific care plan while he or she is in the hospital?

- If the hospital is far from the patient's home; will accommodations be provided for caregivers?

- What type of services are available during the patient's hospital stay?

- Will a discharge plan be developed before the patient goes home from the hospital?

- Does the hospital provide training to help the patient care for his or her condition at home?

Hospital services

Usually, the patient receives information about the hospital from the admitting office when the hospital stay is scheduled. This information should include directions to the hospital, parking information, lodging information if the patient is from out of town, types of rooms, and services offered.

Hospital services offered may include:

- Ethics consultation: Bioethics professionals are available at most hospitals to provide advice or help the patient identify, analyze, and resolve ethical issues that may arise during the patient's care at the hospital.

- Barber or beautician: These services may incur a fee, in addition to the fees of the patient's hospital stay.

- Complementary techniques such as guided imagery and relaxation tapes, massage therapy, or aromatherapy (to reduce a patient's level of stress and anxiety).

- **Home care**: If home health services will be needed after the patient is discharged, they can be arranged by the social worker or nursing staff.

- Interpreter: An interpreter or other special services may be available to assist patients and family members who do not speak the language or are from out of the country.

- Nutrition therapy: Registered dietitians are available to provide comprehensive nutrition assessment, counseling, and education.

- Ombudsman: Health care personnel available to address concerns and problems about medical services that cannot be resolved by reporting these concerns to the nursing staff.

- Pastoral care: Clergy members are available at most hospitals to provide religious support and services to meet patients' spiritual needs. Many hospitals also have a small chapel that provides a quiet retreat for patients and family members of all religious backgrounds and faiths.

- Patient education: A variety of services are available to teach patients about their medical condition or to help them prepare for their scheduled tests or procedures. Patient education may include one-on-one instruction from a health care provider, educational sessions in a group setting, or self-guided learning videos or modules. Informative and instructional handouts are usually provided to explain specific medications, tests, or procedures.

- Pediatric services: Many hospitals have dedicated services and programs available to help children, teenagers, and their parents feel better prepared to cope more effectively with hospital stays, surgery, procedures, and other health-related events.

- Social work: Social workers are available to help patients manage the changes that may occur as a result of the patient's hospitalization. Socials workers provide referrals to community resources and can help the family make arrangements for care in the home as necessary after the patient is discharged from the hospital.

Patient rights and responsibilities

All hospitals have a list of **patient rights** and responsibilities, established by the American Hospital Association. These rights and responsibilities are usually published and posted throughout the hospital. By law, all patients have certain rights. Some patient rights include the right to:

- considerate and respectful care

- complete information about diagnosis, treatment, and expected recovery in terms the patient can understand

- knowledge of the name and function of any health care professional providing care

- informed consent

- the right to refuse treatment to the extent permitted by law and be informed of the medical consequences of refusing treatment

Each patient should obtain a list of his or her rights and responsibilities prior to a hospital admission.

Hospital environment

Most hospital rooms have a bed, bedside table, chair telephone, television, and bathroom. Some hospitals charge a fee for use of the telephone or television; patients should be notified of these charges prior to their hospital admission. Each patient area has a call signal button so the patient can notify the nursing staff if help is needed. Most hospital rooms are doubles that are shared by two patients, unless a private room was previously requested. Some hospitals also have wards in which four or more patients stay in one room. Three nutritionally balanced meals are provided to the patient daily during a hospital stay; daily menus are usually provided for patients to select their food choices, as applicable. (Some patients have dietary restrictions so their food choices may be limited.)

Hospital caregivers

Sometimes, the patient's personal or family physician is not the attending physician who is in charge of the patient's overall care and treatment in the hospital. The attending physician may be a doctor on the hospital staff or a specialist. Fellows, residents, or interns may also provide care. Fellows are doctors who receive training in a special area of medicine after their residency training; residents are doctors who have recently graduated from medical school and are training in a medical specialty; and interns are first-year residents.

Nurses work closely with doctors to supervise the care provided in the hospital. Nurses take the patient's **vital signs**, administer medications, provide treatments, and teach patients how to care for themselves. The head nurse, also called the clinical nurse manager, coordinates care for each patient on the nursing unit.

Other health care providers include medical technologists, radiographers, and nuclear medicine technicians who perform diagnostic tests; therapists such as physical therapists, occupational therapists, and speech therapists who provide specialized care as needed; and dietitians to provide nutrition counseling and nutrition assessments. There are several other health care providers who may assist patients during their hospital stay; patients should ask for more information about the types of providers they may be in contact with during their hospital stay.

Information for visitors and family members

It may be helpful for the patient to select a spokesperson from the family to communicate with the health care providers. This may improve communication with the health care providers as well as to other family members. The patient should also communicate his or her wishes regarding the spokesperson's telephone communications to other family members.

Educational classes may be available for family members to learn more about the patient's condition and what to expect during the patient's **recovery at home**.

If a family member needs to contact the patient or the patient's other family members, the family member should call the hospital and ask for the nursing unit where the patient is staying. The nursing unit staff can connect the caller to the patient's room, take a message, or connect the caller to the patient's family members who are present. Since every hospital has **patient confidentiality** rules, some information may not be able to be disclosed over the telephone.

Most hospitals prohibit the use of cellular phones in patient care areas, as they interfere with the operation of medical equipment.

Most hospitals are smoke-free environments. There are usually designated outside areas where visitors can smoke.

Most hospitals have designated visiting hours that should be adhered to by family members and friends.

Most hospitals have on-site pharmacies where family members can fill the patient's prescriptions; gift shops; and a cafeteria. Usually a list of on-site and off-site dining options can be obtained from the hospital's information desk or social work department.

Preadmission testing

Preadmission testing includes a review of the patient's medical history, a complete **physical examination**, a variety of tests, patient education, and meetings with the health care team. The review of the patient's medical history includes an evaluation of the patient's previous and current medical conditions, surgeries and procedures, medications, and any other health conditions such as allergies that may impact the patient's hospital stay. Preadmission testing is generally scheduled a few days before the hospital admission.

The patient may find it helpful to bring along a family member or friend to the preadmission testing appointments. This caregiver can help the patient remember important details to prepare for the hospital stay.

Preadmission instructions

Preadmission instructions include information about reserving blood products if necessary, taking or discontinuing medications, eating and drinking, **smoking cessation**, limiting activities, and preparing items to bring to the hospital.

Blood transfusions and blood donation

Blood transfusions may be necessary during surgery. A blood **transfusion** is the delivery of whole blood or blood components to replace blood lost through trauma, surgery, or disease. About one in three hospitalized patients will require a blood transfusion. The surgeon can provide an estimate of how much blood the patient's procedure may require.

To decrease the risk of infection and immunologic complications, some hospitals offer a blood donation program if surgery is scheduled or if it is known that blood products will be needed by the patient during his or her hospital stay. Autologous blood (from the patient) is the safest blood available for transfusion, since there is no risk of disease transmission. Methods of autologous donation or collection include:

• Intraoperative blood collection: The blood lost during surgery is processed, and the red blood cells are re-infused during or immediately after surgery.

• Preoperative donation: The patient donates blood once a week for about one to three weeks before surgery. The blood is separated and the blood components needed are re-infused during surgery.

• Immediate preoperative hemodilution: The patient donates blood immediately before surgery to decrease the loss of red blood cells during surgery. Immediately after donating, the patient receives fluids to compensate for the amount of blood removed. Since the blood is diluted, fewer red blood cells are lost from bleeding during surgery.

• Postoperative blood collection: Blood lost from the surgical site right after surgery is collected and re-infused after the surgical site has been closed.

The physician determines what type of blood collection process, if any, is appropriate.

Medication guidelines

Depending on the reason for the hospital stay, certain medications may be prescribed or restricted. The health care team will provide specific guidelines. If certain medications need to be restricted before the hospital stay, the patient will receive a complete list of the medications (including prescription, over-the-counter, and herbal medications) to avoid taking. The patient should not bring any medications to the hospital; all necessary medications, as ordered by the doctor, will be provided in the hospital.

Eating and drinking guidelines

Before most procedures, the patient is advised not to eat or drink anything after midnight the evening before the surgery. This includes no smoking and no gum chewing. The patient should not drink any alcoholic beverages for at least 24 hours before being hospitalized, unless instructed otherwise.

Smoking cessation

Patients are encouraged to quit smoking and stop using tobacco products prior to their hospital admission and to make a commitment to be a nonsmoker. Quitting smoking will help the patient recover more quickly. There are several smoking cessation programs available in the community. The patient should ask a health care provider for more information if he or she needs help quitting smoking.

Activity

The patient should eat healthy foods, rest, and **exercise** as normal before a hospitalization, unless given other instructions. The patient should try to get enough sleep to build up energy for the surgery.

The patient should make arrangements ahead of time for someone to care for children and take care of any other necessary activities at home such as getting the mail or newspapers. The patient should inform family members about the scheduled hospital stay, so they can provide help and support.

Items to bring to the hospital

The patient should bring a list of current medications, allergies, and appropriate medical records upon admission to the hospital. The patient should also bring a prepared list of questions to ask.

The patient should not bring valuables such as jewelry, credit cards, checkbook, or other such items. A small amount of cash (no more than $20) may be packed to purchase items such as newspapers or magazines. If necessary, patients can secure their personal belongings in the hospital cashier's office, safe, or vault for safekeeping until discharge. Most hospitals state in their policies that they are not responsible for lost or stolen personal items.

The patient should only pack what is needed. Some essential items include a toothbrush, toothpaste, comb or brush, deodorant, razor (not electric), slippers, robe, pajamas, and one change of comfortable clothes to wear when going home. The patient should also pack eyeglasses, hearing aids, and dentures, including their carrying cases, if applicable. These items should be labeled with the patient's name when not in use, should be stored in their carrying cases, and put in the bedside stand so they are not lost.

The patient should bring a list of family members' names and phone numbers to contact in an emergency. The patient may also want to pack a book or other personal item such as a family picture.

Personal electronic devices such as hair dryers, curling irons, electric razors, personal televisions, computers, and other electronic devices are not permitted in the hospital, since these devices may interfere with the hospital's medical equipment.

Transportation

The patient should arrange for transportation home, since the effects of certain medications given in the hospital make it unsafe to drive.

Hospital registration and admission

Upon arriving at the hospital, the patient first reports to the hospital registration or admitting area. The patient

---

QUESTIONS TO ASK THE DOCTOR

- How can I prepare myself for the hospital stay?
- Who are the members of the health care team at this hospital?
- What types of questions should I ask my insurance provider to determine if the medical expenses of my hospital stay will be covered?
- What type of tests or procedures will be performed?
- What types of precautions must I follow before and after my hospital stay?
- Will I have to have blood transfusions during my hospital stay?
- Can I take my medications the day I am admitted to the hospital?
- Should I change my diet or eating habits before my hospital stay?
- How long will I have to stay in the hospital?
- What kind of pain or discomfort will I experience and what can I take to relieve it?
- What types of resources are available to me during my hospital stay, and during my recovery at home?
- After I go home from the hospital, how long will it take me to recover?
- What are the signs of infection, and what types of symptoms should I report to my doctor?
- What types of medications will I have to take? How long will I have to take them?
- When will I be able I resume my normal activities? When will I be able to drive? When will I be able to return to work?
- What lifestyle changes (including diet, **weight management,** exercise, and activity changes) are recommended to improve my condition?
- How often do I need to see my doctor for follow-up visits?

---

will be required to complete paperwork and show an insurance identification card, if insured. Often, a pre-registration process performed prior to the date of hospital admission helps make the registration process run smoothly. An identification bracelet that includes the patient's name and doctor's name will be placed on the patient's wrist.

KEY TERMS

Anesthesiologist—A specially trained physician who administers anesthesia.

Case manager—A health care professional who can provide assistance with a patient's needs beyond the hospital.

Catheter—A small, flexible tube used to deliver fluids or medications or used to drain fluid or urine from the body.

Clinical nurse specialists—Nurses with advanced training as well as a master's degree.

Discharge planner—A health care professional who helps patients arrange for health and home care needs after they go home from the hospital.

Electrocardiogram (ECG, EKG)—A test that records the electrical activity of the heart using small electrode patches attached to the skin on the chest.

General anesthesia—Anesthesia that makes the patient unconscious and not feel pain.

Guided imagery—A form of focused relaxation that coaches the patient to visualize calm, peaceful images.

Infectious disease team—A team of physicians who help control the hospital environment to protect patients against harmful sources of infection.

Informed consent—An educational process between health care providers and patients intended to instruct the patient about the nature and purpose of the procedure or treatment, the risks and benefits of the procedure, and alternatives, including the option of not proceeding with the test or treatment.

Inpatient surgery—Surgery that requires an overnight stay of one or more days in the hospital.

Local anesthesia—Anesthesia that numbs a localized area of the body.

NPO—A term that means "nothing by mouth." NPO refers to the time after which the patient is not allowed to eat or drink prior to a procedure or treatment.

Nurse manager—The nurse responsible for managing the nursing care on the nursing unit and also supervises all of the other personnel who work on the nursing unit.

Nursing unit—The floor or section of the hospital where patient rooms are located.

Outpatient surgery—Also called same-day or ambulatory surgery.

Pharmacologist—Medication specialist who checks patients' blood levels to monitor their response to immunosuppressive medications.

Regional anesthesia—Anesthesia that does not makes the patient unconscious; it works by blocking sensation in a region of the body.

Registered nurses—Specially trained nurses who provide care during the patient's hospital stay. Registered nurses provide medical care, medications, and education, as well as assess the patient's condition.

Social worker—A health care provider who can provide support to patients and families, including assistance with a patient's psychosocial adjustment needs and referrals for community support.

If the patient is not feeling well upon arrival to the hospital, a family member or caregiver can help the patient complete the admitting process. Sometimes, a patient's illness may require that the hospital stay be rescheduled.

Informed consent

The health care provider will review the informed consent form and ask the patient to sign it. Informed consent is an educational process between health care providers and patients. Before any procedure is performed or any form of medical care is provided, the patient is asked to sign a consent form. Before signing the form, the patient should understand the nature and purpose of the procedure or treatment, the risks and benefits of the procedure, and alternatives, including the option of not proceeding with the procedure. Signing the informed consent form indicates that the patient permits the surgery or procedure to be performed. During the discussion about the procedure, the health care providers are available to answer the patient's questions about the consent form or procedure.

Advance directives

As part of the admissions evaluation, the patient will be asked about advance directives. Advance directives are legal documents that increase a patient's control over medical decisions. A patient may decide medical treatment in advance, in the event that he or she becomes physically or mentally unable to communicate his or her wishes. Advance directives either state what kind of treatment the patient wants to receive (**living will**), or authorize another person to make medical decisions for the patient when he or she is unable to do so (durable **power of attorney**).

Advance directives are not required and may be changed or canceled at any time. Any change should be written, signed, and dated in accordance with state law, and copies should be given to the physician and to others who received original copies. Advance directives can be revoked either in writing or by destroying the document.

Advance directives are not do-not-resuscitate (**DNR**) orders. A DNR order indicates that a person—usually with a terminal illness or other serious medical condition—has decided not to have **cardiopulmonary resuscitation** (CPR) performed in the event that his or her heart or breathing stops.

Admission tests

Some routine tests will be performed, including blood pressure, temperature, pulse, and weight checks; blood tests; **urinalysis**; **chest x ray**; and electrocardiogram (ECG). A brief physical exam will be performed. The health care team will ask several questions to evaluate the patient's condition. The patient should inform the health care team if he or she drinks alcohol on a daily basis so precautions can be taken to avoid complications.

Results

Patients who receive proper preparation for their hospital experience, including physical and psychological preparation, are less anxious and are more likely to make a quicker recovery at home, with fewer complications.

See also Managed care plans; Medicaid.

Resources

BOOKS

Deardoff, William, and John Reeves. *Preparing for Surgery: A Mind-Body Approach to Enhance Healing and Recovery.* Oakland, CA: New Harbinger Publications, 1997.

Furlong, Monica Winefryck. *Going Under: Preparing Yourself for Anesthesia: Your Guide to Pain Control and Healing Techniques Before, During and After Surgery.* London: Autonomy Publishing Company, 1993.

Marquis Who's Who Staff, and American Board of Medical Specialties Staff, eds. *The Official ABMS Directory of Board Certified Medical Specialist.* New Providence, NJ: Marquis Who's Who, 1998.

"Preoperative Care." *Mosby's Medical, Nursing and Allied Health Dictionary.* 5th ed. Edited by Kenneth Anderson, Lois E. Anderson, and Walter D. Glanze. B. C. Decker, 1998.

ORGANIZATIONS

Agency for Health Care Policy and Research (AHCPR), Publications Clearinghouse. P.O. Box 8547, Silver Spring, MD, 20907. (800) 358-9295. <http://www/ahcpr.gov>.

American Association of Nurse Anesthetists (AANA). 222 South Prospect Avenue, Park Ridge, IL 60068-4001. (847) 692-7050. <http://www.aana.com/>.

American College of Surgeons. 633 N. Saint Clair Street, Chicago, IL 60611-3211. (312) 202-5000. <http://www.facs.org/>.

American Hospital Association. One North Franklin, Chicago, IL 60606. (312) 422-3000. <http://www.hospitalconnect.com>.

American Society of Anesthesiologists (ASA). 520 North Northwest Highway, Park Ridge, IL 60068-2573. (847) 825-5586. <http://www.asahq.org/>.

Joint Commission on Accreditation of Healthcare Organizations (JCAHO). One Renaissance Boulevard, Oakbrook Terrace, IL 60181. (630) 792-5800. <http://www.jcaho.org>.

National Heart, Lung and Blood Institute. Information Center. P.O. Box 30105, Bethesda, MD 20824-0105. (301) 251-2222. <http://www.nhlbi.nih.gov >.

National Institutes of Health. U.S. Department of Health and Human Services. 9000 Rockville Pike, Bethesda, MD 20892. (301) 496-4000. <http://www.nih.gov>.

OTHER

preSurgery.com. <http://www.presurgery.com>.

SurgeryLinx. MDLinx, Inc. 1025 Vermont Avenue, NW, Suite 810, Washington, DC 20005. (202) 543-6544. <http://sgreports.nlm.nih.gov/NN/>.

Angela M. Costello

Plastic, reconstructive, and cosmetic surgery

Definition

Plastic, reconstructive, and cosmetic surgery refers to a variety of operations performed in order to repair or restore body parts to look normal, or to change a body part to look better. These types of surgery are highly specialized. They are characterized by careful preparation of a person's skin and tissues, by precise cutting and suturing techniques, and by care taken to minimize scarring. Recent advances in the development of miniaturized instruments, new materials for artificial limbs and body parts, and improved surgical techniques have expanded the range of plastic surgery procedures that can be performed.

Purpose

Although these three types of surgery share some common techniques and approaches, they have somewhat different emphases. Plastic surgery is usually performed to treat birth defects and to remove skin blemishes such as warts, acne scars, or birthmarks. Cosmetic surgery procedures are performed to make persons look younger or enhance their appearance in other ways. Reconstructive surgery is used to reattach body parts severed in combat or accidents, to perform skin grafts after severe burns, or to reconstruct parts of person's body that were missing at birth or removed by surgery. Reconstructive surgery is the oldest form of plastic surgery, having developed out of the need to treat wounded soldiers in wartime.

Demographics

The top 10 most commonly performed elective cosmetic surgeries in the United States include the following:

• **liposuction**

• breast augmentation

• eyelid surgery

• face lift

• tummy tuck

• collagen injections

• chemical peel

• laser skin resurfacing

• **rhinoplasty**

• forehead lift

There were approximately 29 million surgical procedures performed in the United States in 2001. Because many plastic and reconstructive surgical procedures are performed in private professional offices or as outpatient procedures, accurate statistics concerning the number of procedures performed are not available.

Description

Plastic surgery

Plastic surgery includes a number of different procedures that usually involve skin. Operations to remove excess fat from the abdomen ("tummy tucks"), **dermabrasion** to remove acne scars or tattoos, and reshaping the cartilage in children's ears (**otoplasty**) are common applications of plastic surgery.

Cosmetic surgery

Most cosmetic surgery is done on the face. It is intended either to correct disfigurement or to enhance a person's features. The most common cosmetic procedure for children is correction of a cleft lip or palate. In adults, the most common procedures are remodeling of the nose (rhinoplasty), removal of baggy skin around the eyelids (**blepharoplasty**), face lifts (rhytidectomy), or changing the size or shape of the breasts (mammoplasty). Although many people still think of cosmetic surgery as only for women, growing numbers of men are choosing to have facelifts and eyelid surgery, as well as hair transplants and "tummy tucks."

Reconstructive surgery

Reconstructive surgery is often performed on burn and accident victims. It may involve the rebuilding of severely fractured bones, as well as **skin grafting**. Reconstructive surgery includes such procedures as the reattachment of an amputated finger or toe, or implanting a prosthesis. Prostheses are artificial structures and materials that are used to replace missing limbs or teeth, or arthritic hip and knee joints.

Diagnosis/Preparation

General preparation

Preparation for nonemergency plastic or reconstructive surgery includes individual education, as well as medical considerations. Some operations, such as nose reshaping or the removal of warts, small birthmarks, and tattoos can be done as outpatient procedures under local anesthesia. Most plastic and reconstructive surgery, however, involves a stay in the hospital and general anesthesia.

Medical preparation

Preparation for plastic surgery includes the surgeon's detailed assessment of the parts of an individual's body that will be involved. Skin grafts require evaluating suitable areas of skin for the right color and texture to match the skin at the graft site. Face lifts and cosmetic surgery in the eye area require very close attention to the texture of the skin and the placement of surgical cuts (incisions).

Persons scheduled for plastic surgery under general anesthesia will be given a **physical examination**, blood and urine tests, and other tests to make sure that they do not have any previously undetected health problems or blood clotting disorders. The surgeon will check the list of prescription medications that the prospective patient may be taking to make sure that none of them will interfere with normal blood clotting or interact with the anesthetic.

Individuals are asked to avoid using **aspirin** or medications containing aspirin for a week to two weeks before surgery, because these drugs lengthen the time of blood clotting. Smokers are asked to stop smoking two weeks before surgery because smoking interferes with the healing process. For some types of plastic surgery, individuals may be asked to donate several units of their own blood before the procedure, in case a **transfusion** is needed during the operation. The prospective patient will be asked to sign a consent form before the operation.

Personal education

The surgeon will meet with the prospective patient before the operation is scheduled, in order to explain the procedure and to be sure that the individual is realistic about the expected results. This consideration is particularly important for people undergoing cosmetic surgery.

Medical considerations

Some people should not have plastic surgery because of certain medical risks. These groups include:

- persons recovering from a heart attack, severe infection (for example, pneumonia), or other serious illnesses

- people with infectious hepatitis or HIV infections

- individuals with cancer whose cancer might spread (metastasize)

- people who are extremely overweight (Individuals who are more than 30% overweight should not have liposuction.)

- persons with blood clotting disorders

Psychological

Plastic, cosmetic, and reconstructive surgeries have an important psychological dimension because of the high value placed on outward appearance in Western society. Many people who are born with visible deformities or disfigured by accidents later in life develop emotional problems related to social rejection. Other people work in fields such as acting, modeling, media journalism, and even politics, where their employment depends on how

> ## QUESTIONS TO ASK THE DOCTOR
>
> - Will insurance cover the surgery?
> - How long will the recovery be?
> - What will be the resulting appearance?
> - Is the surgeon board certified in plastic and reconstructive surgery?
> - How many similar procedures has the surgeon performed?
> - What is the surgeon's complication rate?

they look. Some people have unrealistic expectations of cosmetic surgery and think that it will solve all their life problems. It is important for anyone considering non-emergency plastic or cosmetic surgery to be realistic about its results. One type of psychiatric disorder, called body dysmorphic disorder, is characterized by an excessive preoccupation with imaginary or minor flaws in appearance. Persons with this disorder frequently seek unnecessary plastic surgery.

Aftercare

Medical

Medical aftercare following plastic surgery under general anesthesia includes bringing patients to a **recovery room**, monitoring their **vital signs**, and giving medications to relieve pain as necessary. Persons who have had fat removed from the abdomen may be kept in bed for as long as two weeks. Individuals who have had mammoplasties, **breast reconstruction**, and some types of facial surgery typically remain in the hospital for a week after the operation. Those who have had liposuction or eyelid surgery are usually sent home in a day or two.

People who have had outpatient procedures are usually given **antibiotics** to prevent infection and are sent home as soon as their vital signs are normal.

Psychological

Some individuals may need follow-up psychotherapy or counseling after plastic or reconstructive surgery. These people typically include children whose schooling and social relationships have been affected by birth defects, as well as persons of any age whose deformities or disfigurements were caused by trauma from accidents, war injuries, or violent crimes.

KEY TERMS

Blepharoplasty—Surgical reshaping of the eyelid.

Dermabrasion—A technique for removing the upper layers of skin with planing wheels powered by compressed air.

Face lift—Plastic surgery performed to remove sagging skin and wrinkles from an individual's face.

Liposuction—A surgical technique for removing fat from under the skin by vacuum suctioning.

Mammoplasty—Surgery performed to change the size or shape of breasts.

Rhinoplasty—Surgery performed to change the shape of the nose.

Risks

The risks associated with plastic, cosmetic, and reconstructive surgery include the postoperative complications that can occur with any surgical operation under anesthesia. These complications include wound infection, internal bleeding, pneumonia, and reactions to the anesthesia.

In addition to these general risks, some plastic, cosmetic, and reconstructive surgical procedures carry specific risks:

- formation of undesirable scar tissue

- development of persistent pain, redness, or swelling in the area of the surgery

- infection inside the body related to inserting a prosthesis (These infections can result from contamination at the time of surgery or from bacteria migrating into the area around the prosthesis at a later time.)

- anemia or fat embolisms from liposuction

- rejection of skin grafts or tissue transplants

- loss of normal feeling or function in the area of the operation (For example, it is not unusual for women who have had mammoplasties to lose sensation in their nipples.)

- complications resulting from unforeseen technological problems (The best-known example of this problem was the discovery in the mid-1990s that **breast implants** made with silicone gel could leak into the recipient's body.)

Normal results

Normal results include an individual's recovery from the surgery with satisfactory results and without complications.

Morbidity and mortality rates

Morbidity and mortality rates vary with the complexity and severity of different procedures. Mortality is similar to that associated with all surgical procedures. Morbidity is influenced by personal expectations. From a surgical perspective, most morbidity is due to errors associated with anesthesia, procedure, pain medications, and after care. From an individual's perspective, morbidity involves the degree to which actual results compared to expected outcomes. The latter distinction is very subjective.

Alternatives

Alternatives to plastic, reconstructive, and cosmetic surgical procedures include using various products that may be affixed to articles of clothing or the surface of the body.

See also Cleft lip repair; Face lift.

Resources

BOOKS

Kaminer, Michael S., Jeffrey S. Dover, and Kenneth A. Arndt. *Atlas of Cosmetic Surgery.* Philadelphia: Saunders, 2002.

Loftus, Jean M. *The Smart Woman's Guide to Plastic Surgery: Essential Information from a Female Plastic Surgeon.* New York: McGraw Hill, 2000.

Mason, Aaron C. *Handbook of Plastic Surgery.* St. Louis: Mosby, 2001.

Narins, Rhoda S. *Cosmetic Surgery: An Interdisciplinary Approach.* New York: Marcel Dekker, 2001.

PERIODICALS

Butler, P. E., and M. Khan. "Assessing Technical Skills of Plastic Surgeons." *Plastic and Reconstructive Surgery* 111 (2003): 491–492.

Cockerill, J. W. "Improving Digital Imaging." *Plastic and Reconstructive Surgery* 111 (2003): 503–504.

Goldwyn, R. M. "Get a Life or Two or More!" *Plastic and Reconstructive Surgery* 111 (2003): 934–936.

Melmed, E. P. "Who Decides the Criteria?" *Plastic and Reconstructive Surgery* 111 (2003): 513–514.

ORGANIZATIONS

American Academy of Facial Plastic and Reconstructive Surgery. 310 S. Henry Street, Alexandria, VA 22314. (703) 299-9291. <http://www.facial-plastic-surgery.org/index.asp>.

American Board of Plastic Surgery. Seven Penn Center, Suite 400, 1635 Market Street, Philadelphia, PA 19103-2204. (215) 587-9322. <http://www.abplsurg.org/>.

American College of Plastic and Reconstructive Surgery. <http://www.breast-implant.org>.

American College of Surgeons. 633 North Saint Claire Street, Chicago, IL, 60611. (312) 202-5000. <http://www.facs.org/>.

American Society for Aesthetic Plastic Surgery. 11081 Winners Circle, Los Alamitos, California 90720. (800) 364-2147. (562) 799-2356. <http://www.surgery.org/>.

American Society of Plastic Surgeons. 444 E. Algonquin Rd., Arlington Heights, IL 60005. (888) 475-2784. <http://www.plasticsurgery.org/>.

OTHER

Johns Hopkins University. [cited March 2, 2003]. <http://www.hopkinsmedicine.org/plasticsurgery/>.

National Library of Medicine. [cited March 2, 2003]. <http://www.nlm.nih.gov/medlineplus/plasticcosmeticsurgery.html>.

University of Iowa. [cited March 2, 2003]. <http://aboutplastic.surgery.uiowa.edu/surgery/plastic/>.

L. Fleming Fallon, Jr., MD, DrPH

Platelet count *see* **Complete blood count**

Pneumonectomy

Definition

Pneumonectomy is the medical term for the surgical removal of a lung.

Purpose

A pneumonectomy is most often used to treat lung cancer when less radical surgery cannot achieve satisfactory results. It may also be the most appropriate treatment for a tumor located near the center of the lung that affects the pulmonary artery or veins, which transport blood between the heart and lungs. In addition, pneumonectomy may be the treatment of choice when the patient has a traumatic chest injury that has damaged the main air passage (bronchus) or the lung's major blood vessels so severely that they cannot be repaired.

Demographics

Pneumonectomies are usually performed on patients with lung cancer, as well as patients with such non-cancerous diseases as chronic obstructive pulmonary disease (COPD), which includes emphysema and chronic bronchitis. These diseases cause airway obstruction.

Approximately 361,000 Americans die of lung disease every year. Lung disease is responsible for one in seven deaths in the United States, according to the American Lung Association. More than 25 million Americans are now living with chronic lung disease.

Lung cancer

Lung cancer is the leading cause of cancer-related deaths in the United States. It is expected to claim nearly 157,200 lives in 2003. Lung cancer kills more people than cancers of the breast, prostate, colon, and pancreas combined. Cigarette smoking accounts for nearly 90% of cases of lung cancer in the United States.

Lung cancer is the second most common cancer among both men and women and is the leading cause of death from cancer in both sexes. In addition to the use of tobacco as a major cause of lung cancer among smokers, second-hand smoke contributes to the development of lung cancer among nonsmokers. Exposure to asbestos and other hazardous substances is also known to cause lung cancer. Air pollution is also a probable cause, but makes a relatively small contribution to incidence and mortality rates. Indoor exposure to radon may also make a small contribution to the total incidence of lung cancer in certain geographic areas of the United States.

In each of the major racial/ethnic groups in the United States, the rates of lung cancer among men are about two to three times greater than the rates among women. Among men, age-adjusted lung cancer incidence rates (per 100,000) range from a low of about 14 among Native Americans to a high of 117 among African Americans, an eight-fold difference. For women, the rates range from approximately 15 per 100,000 among Japanese Americans to nearly 51 among Native Alaskans, only a three-fold difference.

Chronic obstructive pulmonary disease

The following are risk factors for COPD:

• current smoking or a long-term history of heavy smoking

• employment that requires working around dust and irritating fumes

• long-term exposure to second-hand smoke at home or in the workplace

• a productive cough (with phlegm or sputum) most of the time

• shortness of breath during vigorous activity

• shortness of breath that grows worse even at lower levels of activity

• a family history of early COPD (before age 45)

Diagnosis/Preparation

Diagnosis

In some cases, the diagnosis of a lung disorder is made when the patient consults a physician about chest pains or other symptoms. The symptoms of lung cancer vary somewhat according to the location of the tumor; they may include persistent coughing, coughing up blood, wheezing, fever, and weight loss. In cases involving direct trauma to the lung, the decision to perform a pneumonectomy may be made in the emergency room. Before scheduling a pneumonectomy, however, the surgeon reviews the patient's medical and surgical history and orders a number of tests to determine how successful the surgery is likely to be.

In the case of lung cancer, blood tests, a bone scan, and computed tomography scans of the head and abdomen indicate whether the cancer has spread beyond the lungs. **Positron emission tomography (PET)** scanning is also used to help stage the disease. Cardiac screening indicates how well the patient's heart will tolerate the procedure, and extensive pulmonary testing (e.g., breathing tests and quantitative ventilation/perfusion scans) predicts whether the remaining lung will be able to make up for the patient's diminished ability to breathe.

Preparation

A patient who smokes must stop as soon as a lung disease is diagnosed. Patients should not take **aspirin** or ibuprofen for seven to 10 days before surgery. Patients should also consult their physician about discontinuing any blood-thinning medications such as coumadin or warfarin. The night before surgery, patients should not eat or drink anything after midnight.

Description

In a conventional pneumonectomy, the surgeon removes only the diseased lung itself. The patient is given general anesthesia. An intravenous line inserted into one arm supplies fluids and medication throughout the operation, which usually lasts one to three hours.

The surgeon begins the operation by cutting a large opening on the same side of the chest as the diseased lung. This posterolateral **thoracotomy** incision extends from a point below the shoulder blade around the side of the patient's body along the curvature of the ribs at the front of the chest. Sometimes the surgeon removes part of the fifth rib in order to have a clearer view of the lung and greater ease in removing the diseased organ.

A surgeon performing a traditional pneumonectomy then:

- deflates (collapses) the diseased lung
- ties off the lung's major blood vessels to prevent bleeding into the chest cavity
- clamps the main bronchus to prevent fluid from entering the air passage
- cuts through the bronchus
- removes the lung
- staples or sutures the end of the bronchus that has been cut
- makes sure that air is not escaping from the bronchus
- inserts a temporary drainage tube between the layers of the pleura (pleural space) to draw air, fluid, and blood out of the surgical cavity
- closes the chest incision

Aftercare

Chest tubes drain fluid from the incision and a respirator helps the patient breathe for at least 24 hours after the operation. The patient may be fed and medicated intravenously. If no complications arise, the patient is transferred from the surgical **intensive care unit** to a regular hospital room within one to two days.

A patient who has had a conventional pneumonectomy will usually leave the hospital within 10 days. Aftercare during hospitalization is focused on:

- relieving pain
- monitoring the patient's blood oxygen levels
- encouraging the patient to walk in order to prevent formation of blood clots
- encouraging the patient to cough productively in order to clear accumulated lung secretions

If the patient cannot cough productively, the doctor uses a flexible tube (bronchoscope) to remove the lung secretions and fluids.

Recovery is usually a slow process, with the remaining lung gradually taking on the work of the lung that has been removed. The patient may gradually resume normal non-strenuous activities. A pneumonectomy patient who does not experience postoperative problems may be well enough within eight weeks to return to a job that is not physically demanding; however, 60% of all pneumonectomy patients continue to struggle with shortness of breath six months after having surgery.

Risks

The risks for any surgical procedure requiring anesthesia include reactions to the medications and breathing problems. The risks for any surgical procedure include bleeding and infection.

Between 40% and 60% of pneumonectomy patients experience such short-term postoperative difficulties as:

• prolonged need for a mechanical respirator

• abnormal heart rhythm (cardiac arrhythmia); heart attack (myocardial infarction); or other heart problem

• pneumonia

• infection at the site of the incision

• a blood clot in the remaining lung (pulmonary embolism)

• an abnormal connection between the stump of the cut bronchus and the pleural space due to a leak in the stump (bronchopleural fistula)

• accumulation of pus in the pleural space (empyema)

• kidney or other organ failure

Over time, the remaining organs in the patient's chest may move into the space left by the surgery. This condition is called postpneumonectomy syndrome; the surgeon can correct it by inserting a fluid-filled prosthesis into the space formerly occupied by the diseased lung.

Normal results

The doctor will probably advise the patient to refrain from strenuous activities for a few weeks after the operation. The patient's rib cage will remain sore for some time.

A patient whose lungs have been weakened by non-cancerous diseases like emphysema or chronic bronchitis may experience long-term shortness of breath as a result of this surgery. On the other hand, a patient who develops a fever, chest pain, persistent cough, or shortness of

QUESTIONS TO ASK THE DOCTOR

• Why is it necessary to remove the whole lung?

• What benefits can I expect from a pneumonectomy?

• What are the risks of this operation?

• What are the normal results?

• How long will my recovery take?

• Are there any alternatives to this surgery?

breath, or whose incision bleeds or becomes inflamed, should notify his or her doctor immediately.

Morbidity and mortality rates

In the United States, the immediate survival rate from surgery for patients who have had the left lung removed is between 96% and 98%. Due to the greater risk of complications involving the stump of the cut bronchus in the right lung, between 88% and 90% of patients survive removal of this organ. Following lung volume reduction surgery, most investigators now report mortality rates of 5–9%.

Alternatives

Lung cancer

The treatment options for lung cancer are surgery, radiation therapy, and chemotherapy, either alone or in combination, depending on the stage of the cancer.

After the cancer is found and staged, the cancer care team discusses the treatment options with the patient. In choosing a treatment plan, the most significant factors to consider are the type of lung cancer (small cell or non-small cell) and the stage of the cancer. It is very important that the doctor order all the tests needed to determine the stage of the cancer. Other factors to consider include the patient's overall physical health; the likely side effects of the treatment; and the probability of curing the disease, extending the patient's life, or relieving his or her symptoms.

Chronic obstructive pulmonary disease

Although surgery is rarely used to treat COPD, it may be considered for people who have severe symptoms that have not improved with medication therapy. A significant number of patients with advanced COPD

KEY TERMS

Bronchodilator—A drug that relaxes bronchial muscles resulting in expansion of the bronchial air passages.

Bronchopleural fistula—An abnormal connection between an air passage and the membrane that covers the lungs.

Corticosteroids—Any of various adrenal-cortex steroids used as anti-inflammatory agents.

Emphysema—A chronic disease characterized by loss of elasticity and abnormal accumulation of air in lung tissue.

Empyema—An accumulation of pus in the lung cavity, usually as a result of infection.

Malignant mesothelioma—A cancer of the pleura (the membrane lining the chest cavity and covering the lungs) that typically is related to asbestos exposure.

Pleural space—The small space between the two layers of the membrane that covers the lungs and lines the inner surface of the chest.

Pulmonary embolism—Blockage of a pulmonary artery by a blood clot or foreign matter.

Pulmonary rehabilitation—A program to treat COPD, which generally includes education and counseling, exercise, nutritional guidance, techniques to improve breathing, and emotional support.

face a miserable existence and are at high risk of death, despite advances in medical technology. This group includes patients who remain symptomatic despite the following:

• smoking cessation

• use of inhaled bronchodilators

• treatment with **antibiotics** for acute bacterial infections, and inhaled or oral corticosteroids

• use of supplemental oxygen with rest or exertion

• pulmonary rehabilitation

After the severity of the patient's airflow obstruction has been evaluated, and the foregoing interventions implemented, a pulmonary disease specialist should examine him or her, with consideration given to surgical treatment.

Surgical options for treating COPD include laser therapy or the following procedures:

• Bullectomy. This procedure removes the part of the lung that has been damaged by the formation of large air-filled sacs called bullae.

• Lung volume reduction surgery. In this procedure, the surgeon removes a portion of one or both lungs, making room for the remaining lung tissue to work more efficiently. Its use is considered experimental, although it has been used in selected patients with severe emphysema.

• Lung transplant. In this procedure a healthy lung from a donor who has recently died is given to a person with COPD.

Resources

BOOKS

Argenziano, Michael, M.D., and Mark E. Ginsburg, M.D., eds. *Lung Volume Reduction Surgery*, 1st ed. Totowa, NJ: Humana Press, 2002.

Devita, Vincent T., Samuel Hellman, and Steven A. Rosenberg, eds. *Cancer: Principles and Practice of Oncology*, 6th ed. Philadelphia, PA: Lippincott Williams & Wilkins Publishers, 2001.

Henschke, Claudia I., Peggy McCarthy, and Sarah Wernick. *Lung Cancer: Myths, Facts, Choices—And Hope*, 1st ed. New York, NY: W. W. Norton & Company, Inc., 2002.

Johnston, Lorraine. *Lung Cancer: Making Sense of Diagnosis, Treatment, and Options*. Sebastopol, CA: O'Reilly & Associates, 2001.

Pass, H., M. D., D. Johnson, M. D., James B. Mitchell, PhD., et al., eds. *Lung Cancer: Principles and Practice*, 2nd ed. Philadelphia, PA: Lippincott Williams & Wilkins, 2000.

PERIODICALS

Crystal, Ronald G. "Research Opportunities and Advances in Lung Disease." *Journal of the American Medical Association* 285 (2001): 612-618.

Grann, Victor R., and Alfred I. Neugut. "Lung Cancer Screening at Any Price?" *Journal of the American Medical Association* 289 (2003): 357-358.

Mahadevia, Parthiv J., Lee A. Fleisher, Kevin D. Frick, et al. "Lung Cancer Screening with Helical Computed Tomography in Older Adult Smokers: A Decision and Cost-Effectiveness Analysis." *Journal of the American Medical Association* 289 (2003): 313-322.

Pope, C. Arden, III, Richard T. Burnett, Michael J. Thun, et al. "Lung Cancer, Cardiopulmonary Mortality, and Long-Term Exposure to Fine Particulate Air pollution." *Journal of the American Medical Association* 287 (2002): 1132-1141.

ORGANIZATIONS

American Cancer Society. 1599 Clifton Road, N.E., Atlanta, GA 30329-4251. (800) 227-2345. <www.cancer.org>.

American Lung Association, National Office. 1740 Broadway, New York, NY 10019. (800) LUNG-USA. <www.lungusa.org>.

National Cancer Institute (NCI), Building 31, Room 10A03, 31 Center Drive, Bethesda, MD 20892-2580. Phone: (800) 4-CANCER. (301) 435-3848. <www.nci.nih.gov>.

National Comprehensive Cancer Network. 50 Huntingdon Pike, Suite 200, Rockledge, PA 19046. (215) 728-4788. Fax: (215) 728-3877. <www.nccn.org/>.

National Heart, Lung and Blood Institute (NHLBI). 6701 Rockledge Drive, P.O. Box 30105, Bethesda, MD 20824-0105. (301) 592-8573. <www.nhlhi.nih.gov/>.

OTHER

Aetna InteliHealth Inc. *Lung Cancer.* [cited May 17, 2003]. <www. intelihealth.com.>.

American Cancer Society (ACS). *Cancer Reference Information.* [cited May 17, 2003].<www3.cancer.org/cancerinfo>.

Maureen Haggerty
Crystal H. Kaczkowski, M Sc

Portacaval shunting *see* **Portal vein bypass**

Portal vein bypass

Definition

Portal vein bypass surgery diverts blood from the portal vein into another vein. It is performed when pressure in the portal vein is so high that it causes internal bleeding from blood vessels in the esophagus.

Purpose

The portal vein carries blood from the stomach and abdominal organs to the liver. It is a major vein that splits into many branches. In people with liver failure and cirrhosis, a chronic degenerative liver disease causing irreversible scarring of the liver, the liver is incapable of processing blood from the bowels. As a result, an abnormally high pressure develops in the veins that drain blood from the bowels as the body tries to form other channels for the blood to empty into the main circulation. These channels consist of fragile veins that surround the esophagus, stomach, or other areas of the digestive tract. Because of the fragility of these veins, they are prone to rupturing, which can result in massive amounts of bleeding. The abnormally high pressure within the veins draining into the liver, called portal hypertension, can also result in the formation of fluid seeping from the surface of the liver and collecting in large quantities in the abdominal cavity, a condition known as ascites.

Massive internal bleeding caused by portal hypertension occurs in about 40% of patients with cirrhosis. It is initially fatal in at least half of these patients. Patients who survive are likely to experience bleeding recurrence.

> ## WHO PERFORMS THE PROCEDURE AND WHERE IS IT PERFORMED?
>
> Portal vein bypass surgery is performed by a surgeon specialized in gastroenterology or hepatology in a hospital setting, very often as an emergency operation.

Portal vein bypass, also called portacaval shunting, is performed on these surviving patients to control bleeding.

The purpose of portal vein bypass surgery is to lower portal hypertension by shunting blood away from the portal venous system and into the main venous system.

Demographics

Cirrhosis of the liver is caused by chronic liver disease. Common causes of chronic liver disease in the United States include hepatitis C infection and long-term alcohol abuse. Men and women are equally affected, but onset is earlier in men.

Description

Different portal vein bypass procedures are available. The surgery is usually performed under general anesthesia. The surgeon makes an abdominal incision and locates the portal vein. In portacaval shunting, blood from the portal vein is diverted into the inferior vena cava (one of the main veins leading back to the heart). This is the most common type of bypass. In splenorenal shunting, the splenic vein (a part of the portal vein) is connected to the renal (kidney) vein. A mesocaval shunt connects the superior mesenteric vein (another part of the portal vein) to the inferior vena cava.

Another procedure, called transvenous intrahepatic portosystemic shunt (TIPS), has become the favored surgical approach. A TIPS is performed through a small nick in the skin, working through specialized instruments that are passed through the body using an x ray camera for guidance. The TIPS procedure creates a shunt within the liver itself, by linking the portal vein with a vein draining away from the liver together with a device called a stent, which acts as a scaffold to support the connection between these two veins inside the liver.

Diagnosis/Preparation

A radiologist assesses patients for bypass surgery based on their medical history, **physical examination**, blood work, and liver imaging studies performed using

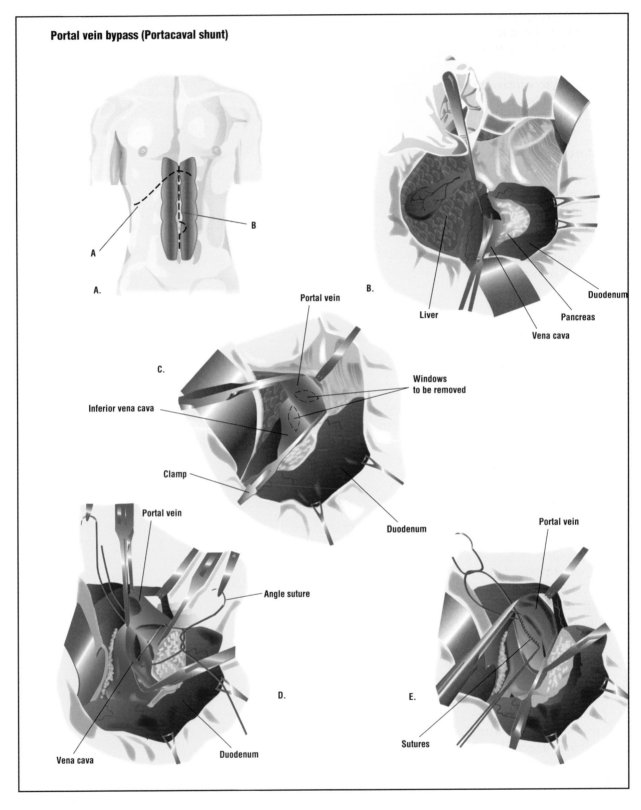

Portal vein bypass (Portacaval shunt)

Portal vein bypass can be achieved through one of two incisions (A). Once the abdomen is entered, the inferior vena cava is exposed (B). Further exposure reveals the portal vein. Both the portal vein and inferior vena cava are clamped (C). Windows are cut in both vessels (D), and the two are connected with sutures (E). *(Illustration by GGS Inc.)*

computed tomagraphy (CT) scans, ultrasounds, or **magnetic resonance imaging** (MRI) scans, and in consultation with the treating gastroenterologist, hepatologist, or surgeon.

Standard preoperative blood and urine tests are also performed. The heart and arterial blood pressure are monitored both during and after the operation.

Aftercare

The patient is connected to a heart monitor and fed through a nasogastric tube. Vital functions are monitored through blood and urine tests. Patients receive pain medication and **antibiotics**. Once released from the hospital, patients are expected to abstain from alcohol and to follow a diet and medication schedule designed to reduce the risks of bleeding.

Risks

Portal vein bypass surgery is high risk because it is performed on patients who are generally in poor health. Only half the patients survive, although the chances of survival are greater with TIPS surgery. The rate of serious complications in TIPS is only 1–2%. Those patients who survive the operation still face the risk of heart failure, brain disease due to a decrease in the liver's conversion of waste products (liver encephalopathy), hemorrhage, lung complications, infection, coma, and death.

Normal results

More than 90% of patients that undergo TIPS to prevent bleeding from varices will have a relief in their symptoms and experience little to no bleeding after surgery. When TIPS is performed for ascites, 60–80% of people will have relief in their ascites. The survival rate is directly related to the amount of liver damage patients have; the less damage, the more likely the patient is to recover. Cooperation with restrictions on alcohol and diet affect long-term survival.

Morbidity and mortality rates

Liver cirrhosis is a major medical problem worldwide and is associated with significant morbidity and mortality from its complications such as liver cell insufficiency and portal hypertension with ascites and gastrointestinal bleeding.

Alternatives

Before resorting to bypass surgery, physicians first attempt to treat portal hypertension with medications known

---

QUESTIONS TO ASK THE DOCTOR

- What are the possible complications involved in portal vein bypass surgery?
- Why is the surgery required?
- Are there any alternatives?
- What type of anesthesia will be used?
- How is the surgery performed?
- How long will I be in the hospital?
- How much portal vein bypass surgery do you perform in a year?

---

as nonselective beta-blockers. These medications need to be taken daily to produce an effect and some patients may not be able to remain on beta-blocker therapy if they develop side effects. Other patients on beta-blocker therapy also remain at risk for bleeding from varices and from ascites.

Another approach is to seal off the veins to prevent rupturing. In sclerotherapy, a camera (endoscope) is passed down through the esophagus to inject the abnormal veins with substances that close them off. This can also be achieved with variceal band ligation, a procedure by which the abnormal veins are tied off with small rubber bands. Although sclerotherapy and variceal band ligation are very effective in targeting the abnormal and fragile veins around the esophagus, they do not lower the pressure of the blood inside the portal venous system. Thus, portal hypertension may still result in fluid accumulation inside the abdominal cavity, or in bleeding.

The best approach to relieve portal hypertension within a patient is by replacing their liver with a new one capable of filtering the blood. However, not many patients are suitable candidates for a liver transplant.

See also Liver transplantation; Sclerotherapy for esophageal varices.

Resources

BOOKS

Current Medical Diagnosis and Treatment, 1998, 37th Edition. Edited by Stephen McPhee, et al. Stamford: Appleton & Lange, 1997.
"Stomach and Duodenum." In *Current Surgical Diagnosis and Treatment,* 10th Edition. Edited by Lawrence W. Way. Stamford: Appleton & Lange, 1994.

PERIODICALS

Bambini, D. A., R. Superina, P. S. Almond, P. F. Whitington, and E. Alonso. "Experience with the Rex Shunt (Mesen-

KEY TERMS

Ascites—Fluid buildup in the abdominal cavity caused by fluid leaks from the surface of the liver and intestine.

Cirrhosis—A chronic degenerative liver disease causing irreversible scarring of the liver.

Inferior vena cava—A large vein that returns blood from the legs, pelvis, and abdomen to the heart.

Portal hypertension—Abnormally high pressure within the veins draining into the liver.

Portal vein—A large vein that carries blood from the stomach and intestines to the liver.

Varices—Uneven, permanent dilation of veins.

terico-left Portal Bypass) in Children with Extrahepatic Portal Hypertension." *Journal of Pediatric Surgery* 35 (January 2000): 13–18.

Fuchs, J., et al. "Mesenterico-left Portal Vein Bypass in Children with Congenital Extrahepatic Portal Vein Thrombosis: A Unique Curative Approach." *Journal of Pediatric Gastroenterology and Nutrition* 36 (February 2003): 213–216.

de Ville de Goyet, J., et al. "Treatment of Extrahepatic Portal Hypertension in Children by Mesenteric-to-left Portal Vein Bypass: A New Physiological Procedure." *European Journal of Surgery* 165 (August 1999): 777–781.

ORGANIZATIONS

American College of Surgeons. 633 N. Saint Clair St., Chicago, IL 60611. (312) 202-5000. <http://www.faacs.org>.

Society for Vascular Surgery. 900 Cummings Center, Beverly, MA 01915-1314. (978) 927-8330. <http://svs.vascula web.org>.

OTHER

"Cirrhosis and Portal Hypertension." *Family Doctor.* <http://familydoctor.org/handouts/188.html>.

Tish Davidson, AM
Monique Laberge, PhD

Positron emission tomography (PET)

Definition

Positron emission tomography (PET) is a non-invasive scanning technique that utilizes small amounts of radioactive positrons (positively charged particles) to visualize body function and metabolism.

Purpose

PET is the fastest growing nuclear medicine tool in terms of increasing acceptance and applications. It is useful in the diagnosis, staging, and treatment of cancer because it provides information that cannot be obtained by other techniques such as computed tomography (CT) and **magnetic resonance imaging** (MRI).

PET scans are performed at medical centers equipped with a small cyclotron. Smaller cyclotrons and increasing availability of certain radiopharmaceuticals are making PET a more widely used imaging modality.

Physicians first used PET to obtain information about brain function, and to study brain activity in various neurological diseases and disorders including stroke, epilepsy, Alzheimer disease, Parkinson disease, and Huntington disease; and in psychiatric disorders such as schizophrenia, depression, obsessive-compulsive disorder, attention deficit hyperactivity disorder (ADHD), and Tourette syndrome. PET is now used to evaluate patients for these cancers: head and neck, lymphoma, melanoma, lung, colorectal, breast, and esophageal. PET also is used to evaluate heart muscle function in patients with coronary artery disease or cardiomyopathy.

Description

PET involves injecting a patient with a radiopharmaceutical similar to glucose. An hour after injection of this tracer, a PET scanner images a specific metabolic function by measuring the concentration and distribution of the tracer throughout the body.

When it enters the body, the tracer courses through the bloodstream to the target organ, where it emits positrons. The positively charged positrons collide with negatively charged electrons, producing gamma rays. The gamma rays are detected by photomultiplier-scintillator combinations positioned on opposite sides of the patient. These signals are processed by the computer and images are generated.

PET provides an advantage over CT and MRI because it can determine if a lesion is malignant. The two other modalities provide images of anatomical structures, but often cannot provide a determination of malignancy. CT and MRI show structure, while PET shows function. PET has been used in combination with CT and MRI to identify abnormalities with more precision and indicate areas of most active metabolism. This additional information allows for more accurate evaluation of cancer treatment and management.

KEY TERMS

Electron—One of the small particles that make up an atom. An electron has the same mass and amount of charge as a positron, but the electron has a negative charge.

Gamma ray—A high-energy photon emitted by radioactive substances.

Half-life—The time required for half of the atoms in a radioactive substance to disintegrate.

Photon—A light particle.

Positron—One of the small particles that make up an atom. A positron has the same mass and amount of charge as an electron, but the positron has a positive charge.

See also CT scans; Magnetic resonance imaging.

Resources

BOOKS

Bares, R., and G. Lucignani. *Clinical PET.* Kluwer Academic Publishers, 1996.

Gulyas, Balazs, and Hans Muller-Gartner. *Positron Emission Tomography: A Critical Assessment of Recent Trends.* Kluwer Academic Publishers, 1996.

Kevles, Bettyann Holtzmann. *Medical Imaging in the Twentieth Century.* Rutgers University Press, 1996.

PERIODICALS

"Brain Imaging and Psychiatry: Part 1." *Harvard Mental Health Letter* 13 (January 1997): 1.

"Brain Imaging and Psychiatry: Part 2." *Harvard Mental Health Letter* 13 (February 1997): 1403.

Goerres, G. "Position Emission Tomography and PET CT of the Head and Neck: FDG Uptake in Normal Anatomy, in Benign Lesions, and Changes Resulting from Treatment." *American Journal of Roentgenology* (November 2002): 1337.

Kostakoglu, L. "Clinical Role of FDG PET in Evaluation of Cancer Patients." *Radiographics* (March-April 2003): 315.

Shreve, P. "Pitfalls in Oncologic Diagnosis with FDG PET Imaging: Physiologic and Benign Variants." *Radiographics* 62 (January/February 1999).

"Studies Argue for Wider Use of PET for Cancer Patients." *Cancer Weekly Plus* 15 (December 1997): 9.

OTHER

Di Carli, M. F. "Positron Emission Tomography (PET)." *1st Virtual Congress of Cardiology.* October 4, 1999. <http://www.fac.org>.

Madden Yee, Kate. "Start-up Enters Breast Imaging Arena with Scintimammography, PET Offerings." *Radiology News.* March 14, 2001. <http://www.auntminnie.com>.

"Nycomed Amersham and the Medical Research Council: Major Collaboration in World Leading Imaging Technology." *Medical Research Center.* 2001. <http://www.mrc.ac.uk/whats_new/press_releases/PR_2001/mrc_02_01.html>.

Dan Harvey
Lee A. Shratter, M D

Post-surgical pain

Definition

Post-surgical pain is a complex response to tissue trauma during surgery that stimulates hypersensitivity of the central nervous system. The result is pain in areas not directly affected by the surgical procedure. Post-operative pain may be experienced by an inpatient or outpatient. It can be felt after any surgical procedure, whether it is minor dental surgery or a triple-bypass heart operation.

Purpose

Post-operative pain increases the possibility of post-surgical complications, raises the cost of medical care, and most importantly, interferes with recovery and return to normal activities of daily living. Management of post-surgical pain is a basic patient right. When pain is controlled or removed, a patient is better able to participate in activities such as walking or eating, which will encourage his or her recovery. Patients will also sleep better, which aids the healing process.

Description

Pain is recognized in two different forms: physiologic pain and clinical pain. Physiologic pain comes and goes, and is the result of experiencing a high-intensity sensation. It often acts as a safety mechanism to warn individuals of danger (e.g., a burn, animal scratch, or broken glass). Clinical pain, in contrast, is marked by hypersensitivity to painful stimuli around a localized site, and also is felt in non-injured areas nearby. When a patient undergoes surgery, tissues and nerve endings are traumatized, resulting in incision pain. This trauma overloads the pain receptors that send messages to the spinal cord, which becomes overstimulated. The resultant central sensitization is a type of posttraumatic stress to the spinal cord, which interprets any stimulation—painful or otherwise—as unpleasant. That is why a patient may feel pain in movement or physical touch in locations far from the surgical site.

Patients handle post-operative pain in high individualized ways. Health care professionals have observed that some patients report that they are in extreme pain after surgery, demanding large doses of pain medications while others seem to do well with much less medication. Several theories have been put forth for this discrepancy. For example, differences in body size seemed to require differing amounts of medication, but this theory did not explain differences in pain perception among patients of the same build. Emotional well-being was considered a better indicator of the ability to tolerate pain. It has been theorized that patients with stronger support systems and better attitudes actually perceive less pain than others. Some health care professionals have even speculated that extreme pain was not real in many cases, but was a way to seek attention.

Clear biological evidence proving that individuals are born with varying thresholds of pain perception was only recently discovered. Psychiatrist and radiologist Jon-Kar Zubieta, from the Mental Health Research Institute at the University of Michigan, found that variations in an amino acid in a newly discovered gene, which codes for an enzyme that accesses neurotransmitters in the brain, produce different levels of pain perception. Only three combinations produce the variation. One individual may be able to fully access and metabolize the opioid neurotransmitters that reduce the sensation of pain. This person would have a higher threshold of pain tolerance and a lower level of pain perception. Another might not be able to do so at all, and that individual would experience more intense pain from the same stimulus. A third person might be able to tolerate a moderate amount of pain.

This variation in genes not only shows that individuals do indeed experience pain at different levels, but it also points to differences in how people behave toward other stressors. Genetic variation may be a factor in the impact of long-term illness and depression that often accompanies chronic pain.

Since pain perception is highly subjective, it is important for the health care team to be aware of pain sensitivity differences in patients, and to value patient self-report as a reliable tool for pain assessment. The most common self-report system in use is the pain intensity scale. The patient is asked to identify where the pain falls on a scale of 0 "no pain at all" to 10 "the worst pain in the world." This scale, however, does have limitations. The Short-Form McGill Questionnaire, which uses sensory words or synonyms, may allow the patient to communicate more accurate, descriptive information about pain and may be a better tool in planning **pain management** strategies.

It is clear that there is a real need for providing different approaches to post-surgical pain management. A variety of interventions may be used before, during, and after surgery. Most of these methods involve medications given orally, intravenously, intramuscularly, or topically (via the skin). Some must be administered by a health care professional; others by the patient.

Pain management methods

Pre-surgery pain management

The goal of post-surgical pain management is to reduce the amount pain a patient experiences after surgery. New research has suggested that preventing the nervous system from being overtaxed by pain from the trauma of surgery may lead to a less painful postoperative experience. Pretreated patients may require less post-surgical medications, and they may recover more quickly, possibly experiencing pain-free days far sooner than patients who have used traditional post-surgical pain methods.

Also, in view of improved, less-invasive surgical techniques and the insurance industry's trend after the turn of the twenty-first century to trim rising medical costs by reducing the length of hospital stays, many patients have no longer been required to remain overnight in a hospital. Recently, outpatient (also called ambulatory) surgery has become a procedure of choice for many complex surgeries, such as **hysterectomy** and prostatectomy. The patient must now be made comfortable enough to return home and manage his or her own pain.

Preemptive analgesia introduces anesthetic drugs near the spinal cord or, sometimes, in nerve blocks in specific regions of the body. An epidural catheter, a thin plastic tube through which pain medication is delivered, is inserted into the patient's back before surgery. The patient may also receive general anesthesia and post-surgical pain medications as needed. Sometimes, the epidural catheter remains in place for several hours or days after surgery, and is attached to a pump so the patient can administer medication on demand.

In other cases, peripheral nerve blocks are used to limit sensation in specific regions of the body. By injecting local anesthetic near a nerve or nerve plexus that supplies the area where the surgery will be performed, all sensation is blunted and the affected area is numbed and feels "asleep." Some patients remain awake, but sedated, during surgery; others are given general anesthesia. Two important advantages to the use of peripheral nerve blocks in patients who are awake during surgery is the avoidance of the side effects of general anesthesia (nausea and vomiting) and complications that could occur during intubation, placing a tube in the patient's airway. The use of peripheral nerve blocks alone may be best suited to surgical procedures involving the arms, legs, and shoulders.

Pain management during surgery

General anesthesia has been the standard for pain management during surgery. Topical local anesthetics are also being used to numb the surgical site before any incisions are made. This has been the method used frequently with laparoscopic procedures. In a **laparoscopy**, the surgeon inserts a laparascope (an instrument that has a tiny video camera attached) through a small incision, often in the abdomen. Other small incisions are made for the surgeon to insert **surgical instruments** into, and to do repairs or remove diseased or damaged tissues. Local anesthetics minimize pain trauma to the surgical site and the central nervous system.

Post-surgery pain management

In most hospitals during the past century, post-surgical pain management consisted only of the administration of **analgesics** and narcotics immediately after surgery. These drugs were usually given by intravenous or intramuscular injection, or by mouth. This is still a viable method for managing post-operative pain.

Management of these drugs, nevertheless, has variant applications. Some hospitals insist on a routine of scheduled medications, rather than giving medications as needed. The health care staff in these instances state that when patients take medications before the pain appears, the body does not over-react to the pain stimulus. Therefore, staying ahead of the pain is critical.

Other hospitals advocate continuous around-the-clock dosing through the use of a pump-type device that immediately delivers medication into the veins (intravenously, the most common method), under the skin (subcutaneously), or between the dura mater and the skull (epidurally). A health care provider programs the device with the specific dosage to deliver at each request made by the patient, as well as the total permitted during the time for which the device is set (commonly eight hours, sometimes 12, especially if the health care providers are working 12-hour shifts). Some of these devices are very sophisticated and even monitor themselves, ringing an alarm bell if there is an indication that they might be malfunctioning. The patient administers the dose by pushing a button, and is encouraged to keep a steady supply of medication within his or her system. This is called **patient-controlled analgesia** (PCA).

PCA provides pain medication at the patient's need. However, because opium-like pain-relievers (opioids) are the medications these pumps deliver, there has been some concern about possible narcotic addiction. The pumps are calibrated to a maximum dosage, and are limited to a maximum dose every eight (or 12) hours. The health care staff checks the equipment regularly, and records the number of times the patient pushes the pump button. If the patient has pushed the button more times than allowed, the pump refuses to administer more medication. The patient should notify the health care staff if a specific medication is ineffective. In some cases, the patient needs encouragement to use the pump more, if necessary.

Nonsteroid anti-inflammatory analgesics (NSAIDs) are best used for continuous around-the-clock pain relief. This prevents the extremes in pain perception that occur with on-demand dosing; sometimes the patient feels no pain and extreme pain at other times. Opioids are best given on a schedule or in a computerized pump, which can prevent overdoses.

Another method used post-surgically is the On-Q or the "pain relief ball." It is a balloon-type device that administers non-narcotic medication to the incision site through a small catheter. When the incision site is closed, the catheter is attached to the surgical site and the balloon or pump is either taped to the patient's skin, carried in a pocket or pouch, or attached to the patient's clothing. The pump numbs the incision site by flooding it with anesthetic. Recent tests show that On-Q reduces narcotic use by 40% in cesarean patients, and eliminates all narcotics in 43% of hysterectomy patients.

Alternative non-medical methods

Some non-medical methods can help reduce post-operative pain. Patient education about the surgical procedure and the aftermath can help reduce stress, which can affect the perception of pain. Education, like visualization, prepares the mind for surgery and recovery. The patient knows what to expect, thereby removing fear of the unknown. Education also enlists the patient's cooperation and may encourage a feeling of control and empowerment, which reduces stress, fear, and helplessness. These factors can contribute to less perceived pain. Therefore, both education and visualization can be helpful in minimizing pain perception and encouraging a positive attitude after surgery, which can promote healing.

Meditation and deep breathing techniques also can reduce stress. These techniques can lower blood pressure and increase oxygen levels, which are critical to a healthy recovery. Hypnosis before and after surgery may calm the mind and emotions, and mute the perception of pain.

Multiple methods

Multimodal analgesia uses more than one method of pain management. Multiple methods can actually reduce the amount of medications necessary to relieve pain, and can minimize uncomfortable side-effects. Using pre-surgical, surgical, and post-surgical techniques allows the patient to arise from surgery with the pain already under con-

- level of sensation after regional anesthesia

- pain status

- nausea/vomiting

The patient is discharged from the PACU when he or she meets established criteria for discharge, as determined by a scale. One example is the Aldrete scale, which scores the patient's mobility, respiratory status, circulation, consciousness, and pulse oximetry. Depending on the type of surgery and the patient's condition, the patient may be admitted to either a general surgical floor or the **intensive care unit**. Since the patient may still be sedated from anesthesia, safety is a primary goal. The patient's call light should be in the hand and side rails up. Patients in a day surgery setting are either discharged from the PACU to the unit, or are directly discharged home after they have urinated, gotten out of bed, and tolerated a small amount of oral intake.

First 24 hours

After the hospitalized patient transfers from the PACU, the nurse taking over his or her care should assess the patient again, using the same previously mentioned categories. If the patient reports "hearing" or feeling pain during surgery (under anesthesia) the observation should not be discounted. The anesthesiologist or nurse anesthetist should discuss the possibility of an episode of awareness under anesthesia with the patient. Vital signs, respiratory status, pain status, the incision, and any drainage tubes should be monitored every one to two hours for at least the first eight hours. Body temperature must be monitored, since patients are often hypothermic after surgery, and may need a warming blanket or warmed IV fluids. Respiratory status should be assessed frequently, including assessment of lung sounds (auscultation) and chest excursion, and presence of an adequate cough. Fluid intake and urine output should be monitored every one to two hours. If the patient does not have a urinary catheter, the bladder should be assessed for distension, and the patient monitored for inability to urinate. The physician should be notified if the patient has not urinated six to eight hours after surgery. If the patient had a vascular or neurological procedure performed, circulatory status or neurological status should be assessed as ordered by the surgeon, usually every one to two hours. The patient may require medication for nausea or vomiting, as well as pain.

Patients with a **patient-controlled analgesia** pump may need to be reminded how to use it. If the patient is too sedated immediately after the surgery, the nurse may push the button to deliver pain medication. The patient should be asked to rate his or her pain level on a pain scale in order to determine his or her acceptable level of pain. Controlling pain is crucial so that the patient may perform coughing, deep breathing exercises, and may be able to turn in bed, sit up, and, eventually, walk.

Effective preoperative teaching has a positive impact on the first 24 hours after surgery. If patients understand that they must perform respiratory exercises to prevent pneumonia; and that movement is imperative for preventing blood clots, encouraging circulation to the extremities, and keeping the lungs clear; they will be much more likely to perform these tasks. Understanding the need for movement and respiratory exercises also underscores the importance of keeping pain under control. Respiratory exercises (coughing, deep breathing, and incentive spirometry) should be done every two hours. The patient should be turned every two hours, and should at least be sitting on the edge of the bed by eight hours after surgery, unless contraindicated (e.g., after **hip replacement**). Patients who are not able to sit up in bed due to their surgery will have sequential compression devices on their legs until they are able to move about. These are stockings that inflate with air in order to simulate the effect of walking on the calf muscles, and return blood to the heart. The patient should be encouraged to splint any chest and abdominal incisions with a pillow to decrease the pain caused by coughing and moving. Patients should be kept NPO (nothing by mouth) if ordered by the surgeon, at least until their cough and gag reflexes have returned. Patients often have a dry mouth following surgery, which can be relieved with oral sponges dipped in ice water or lemon ginger mouth swabs.

Patients who are discharged home after a day surgery procedure are given prescriptions for their pain medications, and are responsible for their own pain control and respiratory exercises. Their families (or caregivers) should be included in preoperative teaching so that they can assist the patient at home. The patient should be reminded to call his or her physician if any complications or uncontrolled pain arise. These patients are often managed at home on a follow-up basis by a hospital-connected visiting nurse or **home care** service.

After 24 hours

After the initial 24 hours, vital signs can be monitored every four to eight hours if the patient is stable. The incision and dressing should be monitored for the amount of drainage and signs of infection. The surgeon may order a dressing change during the first postoperative day; this should be done using sterile technique. For home-care patients this technique must be emphasized.

The hospitalized patient should be sitting up in a chair at the bedside and ambulating with assistance by

KEY TERMS

Ambulate—To move from place to place (walk).

Auscultation—The act of listening to sounds arising within organs as an aid to diagnosis and treatment.

Catheter—A tubular medical device inserted into canals, vessels, passageways, or body cavities to permit injection or withdrawal of fluids, or to keep a passage open.

Deep vein thrombosis—Potentially life-threatening blood clot in one of the deep veins of the body, and often in the legs secondary to immobility after surgery. Symptoms include pain, warmth, swelling, and redness.

Dehiscence—Separation of a surgical incision or rupture of a wound closure.

Ileus—Obstruction in or immobility of the intestines. Symptoms include nausea and vomiting, absent bowel sounds, abdominal pain, and abdominal distension.

Incentive spirometer—Device that is used postoperatively to prevent lung collapse and promote maximum inspiration. The patient inhales until a preset volume is reached, then sustains the volume by holding his or her breath for three to five seconds.

Oximetry—Measuring the degree of oxygen saturation of circulating blood.

PACU—The postanesthesia care unit, where the patient is cared for after surgery.

Patency—The quality or state of being open or unobstructed.

Patient-controlled analgesia pump—A pump that the patient uses to self-administer medication to control pain.

Pulmonary embolism—Potentially life-threatening blockage of a pulmonary artery by fat, air, or a blood clot that originated elsewhere in the body. Symptoms include acute shortness of breath and sudden chest pain.

---

this time. Respiratory exercises are still be performed every two hours, and incentive spirometry values should improve. Bowel sounds are monitored, and the patient's diet gradually increased as tolerated, depending on the type of surgery and the physician's orders.

The patient should be monitored for any evidence of potential complications, such as leg edema, redness, and pain (deep vein thrombosis), shortness of breath (pulmonary embolism), dehiscence (separation) of the incision, or ileus (intestinal obstruction). The surgeon should be notified immediately if any of these occur. If dehiscence occurs, sterile saline-soaked dressing packs should be placed on the wound.

Preparation

Patients receive a great deal of information on postoperative care. They may be offered pain medication in preparation for any procedure that is likely to cause discomfort. Patients may receive educational materials such as handouts and video tapes, so that they will have a clear understanding of what to expect postoperatively.

Aftercare

Aftercare includes ensuring that patients are comfortable, either in bed or chair, and that they have their call lights accessible. After dressing changes, blood-soaked dressings should be properly disposed of in a biohazard container. Pain medication should be offered before any procedure that might cause discomfort. Patients should be given the opportunity to ask questions. In some cases, they may ask the nurse to demonstrate certain techniques so that they can perform them properly once they return home.

Normal results

The goal of postoperative care is to ensure that patients have good outcomes after surgical procedures. A good outcome includes recovery without complications and adequate **pain management**. Another objective of postoperative care is to assist patients in taking responsibility for regaining optimum health.

See also Preoperative care.

Resources

BOOKS

Beauchamp, Daniel R., M.D., Mark B. Evers, M.D., Kenneth L. Mattox, M.D., Courtney M. Townsend, and David C. Sabiston, eds. *Sabiston Textbook of Surgery: The Biological Basis of Modern Surgical Practice.* 16th ed. London: W B Saunders Co., 2001.

Lawrence, Peter F., Richard M. Bell, and Merril T. Dayton, eds. *Essentials of General Surgery.* 3rd ed. Philadelphia: Lippincott, Williams & Wilkins, 2000.

Lubin, Michael F., H. Kenneth Walker, and Robert B. Smith, eds. *Medical Management of the Surgical Patient.* 4th ed. Cambridge, UK: Cambridge University Press, 2003.

Ponsky, Jeffrey, Michael Rosen, Jason Brodsky, M. D., Frederick Brody, M.D., and Jeffrey L. Ponsky. *The Cleveland Clinic Guide to Surgical Patient Management,* 1st ed. Philadelphia: Mosby, 2002.

PERIODICALS

Barone, C. P., M. L. Lightfoot, and G. W. Barone. "The Postanesthesia Care of an Adult Renal Transplant Recipient." *Journal of PeriAnesthesia Nursing* 18, no.1 (February 2003): 32 41.

Smykowski, L., and W. Rodriguez. "The Post Anesthesia Care Unit Experience: A Family-centered Approach." *Journal of Nursing Care Quality* 18, no. 1 (January-March 2003): 5-15.

Wills, L. "Managing Change Through Audit: Post-operative Pain in Ambulatory Care." *Paediatric Nursing* 14, no.9 (November 2002): 35-8.

ORGANIZATIONS

National Institutes of Health. 9000 Rockville Pike, Bethesda, MD 20892. (301) 496-4000. Email: NIHInfo@OD.NIH.GOV. <http://www.nih.gov/>.

Abby Wojahn, RN , BSN, CCRN
Crystal H. Kaczkowski, MSc.

Potassium test *see* **Electrolyte tests**

Power of attorney

Definition

Power of attorney, also known as durable medical power of attorney, is a legal mechanism that empowers a designated person to make medical decisions for a patient should the patient be unable to make the decisions due to incapacitation.

Purpose

Power of attorney assures that a patient's wishes are acknowledged in the medical setting. Along with other legal documents such as a **living will** and a do not resuscitate (**DNR**) order, the power of attorney designates the agent or person who is legally authorized to act for the patient in the medical setting. All three mechanisms are a part of what is know as advanced medical directives.

Description

The patient's agent is the person appointed by the patient to represent him or her in medical situations where decisions must be made. According to the Patient Self-Determination Act of 1991, patient autonomy is represented in the health care agent. This surrogate, through his/her power of attorney authorization, has all of the rights that the patient has with respect to deciding on medical procedure. These include the rights to refuse treatment, to agree to treatment, or to have treatment withdrawn.

Guided by a living will, which is a document developed in advance that reflects the patient's wishes, the agent acts on behalf of the patient with providers, administrators, and other legal agents. In most states, surrogates can act for the patient on any medical procedure, including a decision to refuse life support procedures such as resuscitation. States differ, however, on whether health agents can invoke a DNR order.

In the difficult times that families experience with a seriously ill or terminally ill family member, health agents play a major role in making decisions and stipulating what the patient's wishes are with respect to his or her medical and/or dying needs. Health agents can work with or without a living will. The crucial feature is that the person having power of attorney is empowered to respond to changes in the patient's health and to make flexible decisions. It is the health agent, rather than the patient, who must be apprised of all medical options, weigh the risk and benefits, and make a decision based on the specific situation.

Preparation

The person who has the medical power of attorney for a patient is only as good as his or her level of understanding of the patient and level of respect for the patient's wishes. There are some specific steps that can be taken to prepare the health care agent for power of attorney responsibilities. These steps include:

• The patient must think about medical treatments he or she would or would not like to have in different medical situations such as accidents, acute and life-threatening injuries, nursing home care, etc.

• If possible, the patient should write down his or her medical wishes and have these developed into a living will.

• The patient will want to convey these medical wishes to family and friends, as well as the identity of the person who will have power of attorney.

• Whether a written document is drafted or not, it is important that the patient have discussions with the designated agent so that his or her wishes can be carried out in the concrete situation. Not all elements of the medical decisions required can be known in advance. Hence, it is very important that the health agent knows the patient, knows the patient's wishes and rationale, and understands fully what is of value to the patient. Family and health providers should also be brought into knowledge of the patient's wishes.

Medical decisions likely to be faced in severe health emergencies include options for **cardiopulmonary resuscitation** (CPR), diagnostic tests, dialysis, administration of drugs, surgery, and organ and tissue use. However, there are also other decisions that can come into play at these crucial medical moments and these may involve the power of family members, traditional and non-traditional, having a say in the decision making and issues of children visitation, etc., that the health agent may have to understand and honor.

Once the initial steps for the advanced instructions are in place, an official medical power of attorney form for the state of residence or health care must be filled out. These may be two different states. It is important to have a medical power of attorney for any and all states in which medical care might be provided.

Normal results

All medical directives, whether the living will, power of attorney, or **do not resuscitate order**, are respected by all health personnel in whatever medical setting the chosen state stipulates. Usually these include hospitals, emergency rooms, emergency vehicles, and short- or long-term care facilities such as hospice care. Many states also include the home. The medical directives become a part of the patient's medical record and must be honored by any and all health personnel involved in the patient's treatment or care.

Resources

BOOKS

"Death and Dying." *Merck Manual—Home Edition.* Miami Lakes, FL: Merck, 2003.

PERIODICALS

Kish, S. K. "Advance Directives in Critically Ill Cancer Patients." *Critical Care Nursing Clinics North America* 12, no. 3 (September 1, 2000) 373–83.

Matousek, M. "Start the Conversation: The Modern Maturity Guide to End-of-Life Care," and "The Last Taboo." *Modern Maturity* (September–October, 2000).

ORGANIZATIONS

National Library of Medicine, NIH/MedlinePlus. <www.nlm.nih.gov/medlineplus/deathanddying. html>.

Partnership for Caring. 1620 Eye St., NW, Suite 202, Washington, DC 20006. (202) 296-8071; Fax: (202) 296-8352, Toll-free hotline: (800) 989-9455 <www.partnershipfor caring.org/>.

KEY TERMS

Advanced medical directives—Documents prepared in advance of medical care that reflect the wishes of patients for or against medical procedures should they become incapacitated.

Health care agent—Also known as the surrogate or patient representative, this is the person who has power of attorney to have the patient's wishes carried out if the patient is incapacitated.

Living will—A document that is usually included in advanced medical directives containing explicit medical procedures that patients' wishes to have or to refuse should they become incapacitated.

OTHER

"Choosing a Health Care Agent." *WebMD Health.* <www.Web MD.com>.

"Living Wills And Other Advance Directives." *Aetha Intelitteattibal* <www.intelihealth.com>.

"What You Can Cover in Your Healthcare Directives." *Nolo Law for All.* <www.nololaw.com>.

Nancy McKenzie, PhD

Prednisone *see* **Corticosteroids**

Preoperative autologous blood donation *see* **Autologous blood donation**

Preoperative care

Definition

Preoperative care is the preparation and management of a patient prior to surgery. It includes both physical and psychological preparation.

Purpose

Patients who are physically and psychologically prepared for surgery tend to have better surgical outcomes. Preoperative teaching meets the patient's need for information regarding the surgical experience, which in turn may alleviate most of his or her fears. Patients who are more knowledgeable about what to expect after surgery, and who have an opportunity to express their goals and opinions, often cope better with postoperative pain and decreased mobility. Preoperative care is extremely important prior to any invasive procedure, regardless of whether the procedure is minimally invasive or a form of major surgery.

Preoperative teaching must be individualized for each patient. Some people want as much information as possible, while others prefer only minimal information because too much knowledge may increase their anxiety. Patients have different abilities to comprehend medical procedures; some prefer printed information, while others learn more from oral presentations. It is important for the patient to ask questions during preoperative teaching sessions.

Description

Preoperative care involves many components, and may be done the day before surgery in the hospital, or during the weeks before surgery on an outpatient basis. Many surgical procedures are now performed in a day surgery setting, and the patient is never admitted to the hospital.

Physical preparation

Physical preparation may consist of a complete medical history and physical exam, including the patient's surgical and anesthesia background. The patient should inform the physician and hospital staff if he or she has ever had an adverse reaction to anesthesia (such as anaphylactic shock), or if there is a family history of malignant hyperthermia. Laboratory tests may include **complete blood count**, electrolytes, prothrombin time, activated partial thromboplastin time, and **urinalysis**. The patient will most likely have an electrocardiogram (EKG) if he or she has a history of cardiac disease, or is over 50 years of age. A **chest x ray** is done if the patient has a history of respiratory disease. Part of the preparation includes assessment for risk factors that might impair healing, such as nutritional deficiencies, steroid use, radiation or chemotherapy, drug or alcohol abuse, or metabolic diseases such as diabetes. The patient should also provide a list of all medications, vitamins, and herbal or food supplements that he or she uses. Supplements are often overlooked, but may cause adverse effects when used with general anesthetics (e.g., St. John's wort, valerian root). Some supplements can prolong bleeding time (e.g., garlic, gingko biloba).

Latex allergy has become a public health concern. Latex is found in most sterile surgical gloves, and is a common component in other medical supplies including general anesthesia masks, tubing, and multi-dose medication vials. It is estimated that 1–6% of the general population and 8–17% of health care workers have this allergy. Children with disabilities are particularly susceptible. This includes children with spina bifida, congenital urological abnormalities, cerebral palsy, and Dandy-Walker syndrome. At least 50% of children with spina bifida are latex-sensitive as a result of early, frequent surgical exposure. There is currently no cure available for latex allergy, and research has found that the allergy accounts for up to 19% of all anaphylactic reactions during surgery. The best treatment is prevention, but immediate symptomatic treatment is required if the allergic response occurs. Every patient should be assessed for a potential latex reaction. Patients with latex sensitivity should have their chart flagged with a caution label. Latex-free gloves and supplies must be used for anyone with a documented latex allergy.

Bowel clearance may be ordered if the patient is having surgery of the lower gastrointestinal tract. The patient should start the bowel preparation early the evening before surgery to prevent interrupted sleep during the night. Some patients may benefit from a sleeping pill the night before surgery.

The night before surgery, skin preparation is often ordered, which can take the form of scrubbing with a special soap (i.e., Hibiclens), or possibly hair removal from the surgical area. Shaving hair is no longer recommended because studies show that this practice may increase the chance of infection. Instead, adhesive barrier drapes can contain hair growth on the skin around the incision.

Psychological preparation

Patients are often fearful or anxious about having surgery. It is often helpful for them to express their concerns to health care workers. This can be especially beneficial for patients who are critically ill, or who are having a high-risk procedure. The family needs to be included in psychological preoperative care. Pastoral care is usually offered in the hospital. If the patient has a fear of dying during surgery, this concern should be expressed, and the surgeon notified. In some cases, the procedure may be postponed until the patient feels more secure.

Children may be especially fearful. They should be allowed to have a parent with them as much as possible, as long as the parent is not demonstrably fearful and contributing to the child's apprehension. Children should be encouraged to bring a favorite toy or blanket to the hospital on the day of surgery.

Patients and families who are prepared psychologically tend to cope better with the patient's postoperative course. Preparation leads to superior outcomes since the goals of recovery are known ahead of time, and the patient is able to manage postoperative pain more effectively.

Informed consent

The patient's or guardian's written consent for the surgery is a vital portion of preoperative care. By law, the physician who will perform the procedure must explain the risks and benefits of the surgery, along with other treatment options. However, the nurse is often the person who actually witnesses the patient's signature on the consent form. It is important that the patient understands everything he or she has been told. Sometimes, patients are asked to explain what they were told so that the health care professional can determine how much is understood.

Patients who are mentally impaired, heavily sedated, or critically ill are not considered legally able to give consent. In this situation, the next of kin (spouse, adult child, adult sibling, or person with medical **power of attorney**) may act as a surrogate and sign the consent form. Children under age 18 must have a parent or guardian sign.

Preoperative teaching

Preoperative teaching includes instruction about the preoperative period, the surgery itself, and the postoperative period.

Instruction about the preoperative period deals primarily with the arrival time, where the patient should go on the day of surgery, and how to prepare for surgery. For example, patients should be told how long they should be NPO (nothing by mouth), which medications to take prior to surgery, and the medications that should be brought with them (such as inhalers for patients with asthma).

Instruction about the surgery itself includes informing the patient about what will be done during the surgery, and how long the procedure is expected to take. The patient should be told where the incision will be. Children having surgery should be allowed to "practice" on a doll or stuffed animal. It may be helpful to demonstrate procedures on the doll prior to performing them on the child. It is also important for family members (or other concerned parties) to know where to wait during surgery, when they can expect progress information, and how long it will be before they can see the patient.

Knowledge about what to expect during the postoperative period is one of the best ways to improve the patient's outcome. Instruction about expected activities can also increase compliance and help prevent complications. This includes the opportunity for the patient to practice coughing and deep breathing exercises, use an incentive spirometer, and practice splinting the incision. Additionally, the patient should be informed about early ambulation (getting out of bed). The patient should also

KEY TERMS

Activated partial thromboplastin time (APTT)—A lab test that detects coagulation defects in the intrinsic clotting cascade. Used to regulate heparin dosing.

Ambulate—Move from place to place (walk).

Anaphylactic shock—A systemic reaction that is often severe and occasionally fatal due to a second exposure to a specific antigen (i.e., wasp venom or penicillin) after previous sensitization that results in symptoms (particularly respiratory symptoms, fainting, itching, and hives).

Anesthesia—A safe and effective means of alleviating pain during a medical procedure.

Complete blood count (CBC)—A lab test that determines the number of red and white blood cells per cubic millimeter of blood.

Electrocardiogram (EKG)—A graphic record showing the electrical activity of the heart.

Incentive spirometer—Device that is used postoperatively to prevent lung collapse and promote maximum inspiration. The patient inhales until a preset volume is reached, then sustains the volume by holding the breath for three to five seconds.

Patient-controlled analgesia pump—A pump that the patient uses to self-administer medication to control pain.

Prothrombin time (PT)—A lab test that detects coagulation defects in the extrinsic clotting cascade. Used to regulate coumadin dosing.

be taught that the respiratory interventions decrease the occurrence of pneumonia, and that early leg exercises and ambulation decrease the risk of blood clots.

Patients hospitalized postoperatively should be informed about the tubes and equipment that they will have. These may include multiple intravenous lines, drainage tubes, dressings, and monitoring devices. In addition, they may have sequential compression stockings on their legs to prevent blood clots until they start ambulating.

Pain management is the primary concern for many patients having surgery. Preoperative instruction should include information about the pain management method that they will utilize postoperatively. Patients should be encouraged to ask for or take pain medication before the pain becomes unbearable, and should be taught how to rate their discomfort on a pain scale. This instruction allows the patients, and others who may be assessing them, to evaluate the pain consistently. If they will be using a **patient-controlled analgesia** pump, instruction should take place during the preoperative period. Use of alternative methods of pain control (distraction, imagery, positioning, mindfulness meditation, music therapy) may also be presented.

Finally, the patient should understand long-term goals such as when he or she will be able to eat solid food, go home, drive a car, and return to work.

Preparation

It is important to allow adequate time for preparation prior to surgery. The patient should understand that he or she has the right to add or strike out items on the generic consent form that do not pertain to the specific surgery. For example, a patient who is about to undergo a **tonsillectomy** might choose to strike out (and initial) an item that indicates sterility might be a complication of the operation.

Normal results

The anticipated outcome of preoperative care is a patient who is informed about the surgical course, and copes with it successfully. The goal is to decrease complications and promote recovery.

See also Pediatric concerns; Postoperative care.

Resources

BOOKS

Beauchamp, Daniel R., M.D., Mark B. Evers, M.D., Kenneth L. Mattox, M.D., Courtney M. Townsend, and David C. Sabiston, eds. *Sabiston Textbook of Surgery: The Biological Basis of Modern Surgical Practice.* 16th ed. London: W. B. Saunders Co., 2001.

Lawrence, Peter F., Richard M. Bell, and Merril T. Dayton, eds. *Essentials of General Surgery,* 3rd ed. Philadelphia, PA: Lippincott, Williams & Wilkins, 2000.

Lubin, Michael F., H. Kenneth Walker, and Robert B. Smith, eds. *Medical Management of the Surgical Patient,* 4th ed. Cambridge, UK: Cambridge University Press, 2003.

Ponsky, Jeffrey, Michael Rosen, Jason Brodsky, M.D., Frederick Brody, M.D., and Jeffrey L. Ponsky. *The Cleveland Clinic Guide to Surgical Patient Management,* 1st ed. Philadelphia, PA: Mosby, 2002.

Switzer, Bobbiejean, M.D., ed. *Handbook of Preoperative Assessment and Management.* Philadelphia, PA: Lippincott Williams & Wilkins, 2000.

PERIODICALS

Dean, A., and T. Fawcett. "Nurses' use of evidence in pre-operative fasting." *Nursing Standard* 17, no.12 (December 2002): 33-7.

ORGANIZATIONS

National Institutes of Health. 9000 Rockville Pike, Bethesda, MD 20892. (301) 496-4000. Email: NIHInfo@OD.NIH.GOV. <http://www.nih.gov/>.

Abby Wojahn, RN , BSN , CCRN
Crystal H. Kaczkowski, M Sc

Preparing for surgery

Definition

Preparing for a planned surgery (also called **elective surgery**) includes selecting a surgery center and surgeon to perform the procedure, scheduling the surgery, undergoing pre-surgical testing, meeting with health care professionals and the **surgical team**, receiving education about the procedure, receiving and following all of the appropriate preoperative instructions, and signing a consent form.

Purpose

Preparing for surgery helps the patient understand what to expect before surgery and ensures the patient is physically and psychologically ready for the surgery.

Description

Most patients go to the surgery center or hospital the same day as the scheduled surgery; thus, many of the steps involved in preparing for surgery will take place from one to four weeks before the scheduled surgery. Many surgeries are performed on an outpatient basis, which means that the patient goes home the same day as the surgery.

Selecting a surgeon and surgery center

SURGEON. A surgeon, along with a multi-disciplinary team of surgical specialists, will perform the surgery. The surgeon should be board certified by the American Board of Surgery, as well as certified by the medical specialty board or boards related to the type of surgery performed. Certification from a medical specialty board means that the surgeon has completed an approved educational training program (including three to seven years of full-time training in an accredited residency program). Certification also includes an evaluation, including an examination that assessed the surgeon's knowledge, skills, and experience necessary to perform high-quality patient care in that specialty.

There are 24 certifying boards recognized by the American Board of Member Specialties (ABMS) and the American Medical Association (AMA). Most of the ABMS boards issue time-limited certificates, valid for six to 10 years. This requires physicians to become re-certified to maintain their board certification—a process that includes a credential review, continuing education in the specialty, and additional examinations. Even though board certification is not required for an individual physician to practice medicine, most hospitals require that a certain percentage of their staff be board certified.

The letters FACS (Fellow of the American College of Surgeons) after a surgeon's name are a further indication of a surgeon's qualifications. Those who become Fellows of the American College of Surgeons have passed a comprehensive evaluation of their surgical training and skills; they also have demonstrated their commitment to high standards of ethical conduct. This evaluation is conducted according to national standards that were established to ensure that patients receive the best possible surgical care.

A surgeon's membership in professional societies is also an important consideration. Professional societies provide an independent forum for medical specialists to discuss issues of national interest and mutual concern. Examples of professional societies include the Society of Thoracic Surgeons (STS) and the American College of Physicians–American Society of Internal Medicine (ACP-ASIM).

To find information about a surgeon's qualifications, the patient can call a state or county medical association for assistance. A reference book is also available: *The Official ABMS Directory of Board Certified Medical Specialists* that lists all surgeons who are certified by approved boards. This publication also contains brief information about each surgeon's medical education and training, and it can be found in many libraries.

SURGERY CENTER. The surgeon will arrange for the procedure to be performed in a hospital where he or she has staff privileges. The patient should make sure the hospital has been accredited by the Joint Commission on Accreditation of Healthcare Organizations, a professionally sponsored program that stimulates a high quality of patient care in health care facilities. Joint Commission accreditation means the hospital voluntarily sought accreditation and met national health and safety standards. There is also an accreditation option that is available for **ambulatory surgery centers**.

Selecting a surgery center that has a multi-disciplinary team of specialists is important. The surgery team should include surgeons, infectious disease specialists, pharmacologists, and advanced care registered nurses.

Other surgical team members may include fellows and residents, clinical coordinators, physical therapists, respiratory therapists, registered dietitians, social workers, and financial counselors.

Choosing a surgery center with experience is important. Some questions to consider when choosing a surgery center or hospital include:

• How many surgeries are performed annually and what are the outcomes/survival rates of those surgeries?

• How do the surgery center's outcomes compare with the national average?

• Does the surgery center offer treatment for a patient's specific condition? How experienced is the staff in treating that condition?

• What is the center's success record in providing the specific medical treatment or procedure?

• Does the surgery center have experience treating patients the same age as the inquiring patient?

• Does the surgery center explain the patient's rights and responsibilities?

• Does the surgery center have a written description of its services and fees?

• How much does the patient's type of treatment cost at this surgery center?

• Is financial help available?

• Who will be responsible for the patient's specific care plan while he or she is in the hospital?

• If the center is far from the patient's home, will accommodations be provided for caregivers?

• What type of services are available during the patient's hospital stay?

• Will a discharge plan be developed before the patient goes home from the hospital?

• Does the hospital provide training to help the patient care for his or her condition at home?

Scheduling the surgery

Depending on the nature of the surgery, it may be scheduled within days or weeks after the surgery is determined to be the appropriate treatment option for the patient. The patient's surgery time may not be determined until the business day before the scheduled surgery. The patient may be instructed to call the surgical center to find out the time of the scheduled surgery.

The time the patient is told to report to the surgery center (arrival time) is not the time when the surgery will take place. Patients are told to arrive at the surgery center far enough in advance (usually about two hours prior to the scheduled surgery time) so they can be properly prepared for surgery. In some cases, the patient's surgery may need to be rescheduled if another patient requires **emergency surgery** at the patient's scheduled time.

The patient should ask the health care providers if the scheduled surgery will be performed on an outpatient or inpatient basis. Outpatient means the patient goes home the same day as the surgery; inpatient means a hospital stay is required.

Pre-surgical testing

Pre-surgical testing, also called preoperative testing or surgical consultation, includes a review of the patient's medical history, a complete **physical examination**, a variety of tests, patient education, and meetings with the health care team. The review of the patient's medical history includes an evaluation of the patient's previous and current medical conditions, surgeries and procedures, medications, and any other health conditions such as allergies that may impact the surgery. Pre-surgical testing is generally scheduled within one week before the surgery.

The patient may find it helpful to bring along a family member or friend to the pre-surgical testing appointments. This caregiver can help the patient remember important details to prepare for surgery.

After attending the surgical consultation, the patient may desire to seek a **second opinion** to confirm the first doctor's treatment recommendations. The patient should check with his or her insurance provider to determine if the second opinion consultation is covered.

Meeting with the surgical team

During the surgical consultation, the patient meets with the surgeon or a member of the surgeon's health care team to discuss the surgery and other potential treatment options for the patient's medical condition. At some time before the surgery, the patient will meet with other health care providers, including the anesthesiologist, nurse clinicians, and sometimes a dietitian, social worker, or rehabilitation specialist.

Patient education

The surgical team will ensure that the patient understands the potential benefits and risks of the procedure as well as what to expect before the procedure and during the recovery. Patient education may include one-on-one instruction from a health care provider, educational sessions in a group setting, or self-guided learning videos or modules. Informative and instructional handouts are usually provided to explain specific pre-surgical requirements.

Some surgery centers offer services such as guided imagery and relaxation tapes, massage therapy, aromatherapy, or other complementary techniques to reduce a patient's level of stress and anxiety before a surgical procedure. Guided imagery is a form of focused relaxation that coaches the patient to visualize calm, peaceful images. Several research studies have proven that guided imagery can significantly reduce stress and anxiety before and after surgical and medical procedures and help the patient recover more rapidly. Guided imagery and relaxation tapes are available at many major bookstores and from some surgery centers. The patient may be able to listen to the tapes during the procedure, depending on the type of procedure being performed.

Preoperative instructions

Preoperative instructions include information about reserving blood products for surgery, taking or discontinuing medications before the surgery, eating and drinking before surgery, quitting smoking, limiting activities before surgery, and preparing items to bring to the hospital the day of surgery.

BLOOD TRANSFUSIONS AND BLOOD DONATION. Blood transfusions may be necessary during surgery. A blood **transfusion** is the delivery of whole blood or blood components to replace blood lost through trauma, surgery, or disease. About one in three hospitalized patients will require a blood transfusion. The surgeon can provide an estimate of how much blood the patient's procedure may require.

To decrease the risk of infection and immunologic complications, some surgery centers offer a preoperative blood donation program. Autologous blood (from the patient) is the safest blood available for transfusion, since there is no risk of disease transmission. Methods of autologous donation or collection include:

• Intraoperative blood collection: the blood lost during surgery is processed, and the red blood cells are re-infused during or immediately after surgery.

• Preoperative donation: the patient donates blood once a week for one to three weeks before surgery. The blood is separated and the blood components needed are re-infused during surgery.

• Immediate preoperative hemodilution: the patient donates blood immediately before surgery to decrease the loss of red blood cells during surgery. Immediately after donating, the patient receives fluids to compensate for the amount of blood removed. Since the blood is diluted, fewer red blood cells are lost from bleeding during surgery.

- Postoperative blood collection: blood lost from the surgical site right after surgery is collected and re-infused after the surgical site has been closed.

The surgeon determines what type of blood collection process, if any, is appropriate.

MEDICATION GUIDELINES. Depending on the type of surgery scheduled, certain medications may be prescribed or restricted before the surgery. The health care team will provide specific guidelines. If certain medications need to be restricted before surgery, the patient will receive a complete list of the medications (including prescription, over-the-counter, and herbal medications) to avoid taking before the scheduled surgery.

If the physician advises the patient to take prescribed medication within 12 hours before surgery, it should be taken with small sips of water.

The patient should not bring any medications to the hospital; all necessary medications, as ordered by the doctor, will be provided in the hospital.

EATING AND DRINKING BEFORE SURGERY. Before most surgeries, the patient is advised not to eat or drink anything after midnight the evening before the surgery. This includes no smoking and no gum chewing. The patient should not drink any alcoholic beverages for at least 24 hours before surgery, unless instructed otherwise. If the patient has diabetes or if the surgery is to be performed on a child, the patient should ask the health care team for specific guidelines about eating and drinking before surgery.

Smoking cessation

Patients who will undergo any surgical procedure are encouraged to quit smoking and stop using tobacco products at least two weeks before the procedure, and to make a commitment to be a nonsmoker after the procedure. Ideally, the patient should quit smoking at least eight weeks prior to surgery. Quitting smoking before surgery helps the patient recover more quickly from surgery. There are several **smoking cessation** programs available in the community. The patient should ask a health care provider for more information if he or she needs help quitting smoking.

Activity before surgery

The patient should eat right, rest, and **exercise** as normal before surgery, unless given other instructions. The patient should try to get enough sleep to build up energy for the surgery. The health care team may advise the patient to scrub the planned surgical site with a special disinfecting soap the evening before the surgery.

MAKING PLANS FOR HOME AND WORK. The patient should make arrangements ahead of time for someone to care for children and take care of any other necessary activities at home such as getting the mail or newspapers. The patient should inform family members about the scheduled surgery in advance, so they can provide help and support before, during, and after surgery.

The patient should ask the health care team what supplies may be needed after surgery during **recovery at home** so these items can be purchased or rented ahead of time. Some supplies that may be needed include an adaptive chair for the toilet or bathtub, or supplies for changing the wound dressing at home. Ask the health care providers if **home care** assistance (in which a visiting nurse visits the home to provide medical care) will be needed after surgery.

Items to bring to the hospital

The patient should bring a list of current medications, allergies, and appropriate medical records upon admission to the surgery center. The patient should also bring a prepared list of questions to ask.

The patient should not bring valuables such as jewelry, credit cards or other items. A small amount of cash (no more than $20) may be packed to purchase items such as newspapers or magazines.

Women should not wear nail polish or makeup the day of surgery.

If a hospital stay is expected after surgery, the patient should only pack what is needed. Some essential items include a toothbrush, toothpaste, comb or brush, deodorant, razor, eyeglasses (if applicable), slippers, robe, pajamas, and one change of comfortable clothes to wear when going home. The patient should also bring a list of family members' names and phone numbers to contact in an emergency.

Transportation

The patient should arrange for transportation home, since the effects of anesthesia and other medications given before surgery make it unsafe to drive.

Preoperative preparation

Upon arriving at the hospital or surgery center, the patient will be required to complete paperwork and show an insurance identification card, if insured. An identification bracelet that includes the patient's name and doctor's name will be placed on the patient's wrist.

INFORMED CONSENT. The health care provider will review the **informed consent** form and ask the patient to sign it. Informed consent is an educational process

QUESTIONS TO ASK THE DOCTOR

- Will I have to have blood transfusions during the surgery?

- Do I take my medications the day of the surgery?

- Can I eat or drink the day of the surgery? If not, how long before the surgery should I stop eating and drinking?

- How long does my type of surgery typically last?

- How long will I have to stay in the hospital after surgery?

- What kind of pain or discomfort will I experience after the surgery and what can I take to relieve it? What type of bruising, swelling, scarring, or pain should be expected after surgery?

- What types of resources are available to me during my hospital stay, and during my recovery at home?

- After I go home from the hospital, how long will it take me to recover?

- What are the signs of infection, and what types of symptoms should I report to my doctor?

- How should I care for my incision?

- What types of medications will I have to take after surgery? How long will I have to take them?

- When will I be able I resume my normal activities? When will I be able to drive? When will I be able to return to work?

- What lifestyle changes (including diet, **weight management,** exercise, and activity changes) are recommended after the surgery to improve my condition?

- How often do I need to see my doctor or surgeon for follow-up visits after surgery?

- Can I receive follow-up care from my primary physician, or do I need to have follow-up visits with the surgeon?

between health care providers and patients. Before any procedure is performed, the patient is asked to sign a consent form. Before signing the form, the patient should understand the nature and purpose of the procedure or treatment, the risks and benefits of the procedure, and alternatives, including the option of not proceeding with the procedure. Signing the informed consent form indicates that the patient permits the surgery or procedure to be performed. During the discussion about the procedure, the health care providers are available to answer the patient's questions about the consent form or procedure.

ADVANCED DIRECTIVES. The health care provider will ask the patient if he or she has any advance directives to be included in the patient's file. Advance directives are legal documents that increase a patient's control over medical decisions. A patient may decide medical treatment in advance, in the event that he or she becomes physically or mentally unable to communicate his or her wishes. Advance directives either state what kind of treatment the patient wants to receive (**living will**), or authorize another person to make medical decisions for the patient when he or she is unable to do so (durable **power of attorney**). Advance directives are not required and may be changed or canceled at any time. Any change should be written, signed and dated in accordance with state law, and copies should be given to the physician and to others who received original copies. Advance directives can be revoked either in writing or by destroying the document. Advance directives are not do-not-resuscitate (**DNR**) orders. A DNR order indicates that a person—usually with a terminal illness or other serious medical condition—has decided not to have **cardiopulmonary resuscitation** (CPR) performed in the event that his or her heart or breathing stops.

TESTS AND PREOPERATIVE EVALUATION. Some routine tests will be performed, including blood pressure, temperature, pulse, and weight checks; blood tests; **urinalysis**; **chest x ray**; and electrocardiogram (ECG). A brief physical exam will be performed. In some cases, an enema may be required. The health care team will ask several questions to evaluate the patient's condition and to complete the final preparations for surgery. The patient should inform the health care team if he or she drinks alcohol on a daily basis so precautions can be taken to avoid complications during and after surgery.

FINAL SURGICAL PREPARATION. Preoperative preparation generally includes these steps:

- The patient changes into a hospital gown.

- The patient removes (as applicable) contact lenses and glasses, dentures, hearing aids, nail polish, and jewelry.

- The patient empties his or her bladder.

- The health-care providers clean and possibly shave the area on the body where the surgery will be performed.

- The patient may receive medication to aid relaxation.

- An intravenous catheter will be placed in a vein in the patient's arm to deliver fluids, medications, or blood during surgery.
- In some hospitals, the patient may wait in an area called a holding area until the **operating room** and surgical team are ready. Depending on the hospital's policy, one or two of the patient's family members may wait with the patient.
- The patient is taken to the operating room in a wheelchair or on a bed (also called a gurney) where monitors are placed to evaluate the patient's condition during surgery.
- Anesthesia is administered; the type of anesthesia administered will depend upon the procedure, the patient's general health, and medications.
- A catheter may be placed in the patient's bladder to drain urine.
- The patient's **vital signs**, including the blood oxygen level, electrical activity of the heart, blood pressure, pulse, temperature, breathing, mental status, and level of consciousness, are continuously monitored during and after the surgery.

Information for families

While the patient is in surgery, the family members wait in a designated waiting area. Some hospitals or surgery centers offer a pager to the patient's family so they can be contacted for updates about the progress of the surgery. It may be helpful for the patient to select a spokesperson from the family to communicate with the health care providers. This may improve communication with the health care providers as well as to other family members. The patient should also communicate his or her wishes regarding the spokesperson's telephone communications to other family members.

Educational classes may be available for family members to learn more about the patient's surgery and what to expect during the recovery.

When the surgery is complete, the surgeon usually contacts the family members to provide information about the surgery. If a problem or complication occurs during surgery, the family members are notified immediately.

Normal results

Patients who receive proper preparation for surgery, including physical and psychological preparation, experience less anxiety and are more likely to make a quicker recovery at home, with fewer complications. Patients who perceive their surgical and postoperative experiences as positive report that they had minimal pain and nausea, were relaxed,

KEY TERMS

Case manager—A health care professional who can provide assistance with a patient's needs beyond the hospital.

Discharge planner—A health care professional who helps patients arrange for health and home care needs after they go home from the hospital.

Electrocardiogram (ECG, EKG)—A test that records the electrical activity of the heart using small electrode patches attached to the skin on the chest.

Infectious disease team—A team of physicians who help control the hospital environment to protect patients against harmful sources of infection.

Informed consent—An educational process between health care providers and patients intended to instruct the patient about the nature and purpose of the procedure or treatment, the risks and benefits of the procedure, and alternatives, including the option of not proceeding with the test or treatment.

Inpatient surgery—Surgery that requires an overnight stay of one or more days in the hospital.

NPO—A term that means nothing by mouth. NPO refers to the time after which the patient is not allowed to eat or drink prior to a procedure or treatment.

Outpatient surgery—Also called same-day or ambulatory surgery. The patient arrives for surgery and returns home on the same day.

had confidence in the skills of their health care team, felt they had some control over their care, and returned to their normal activities within the expected timeframe.

See also Finding a surgeon.

Resources

BOOKS

Deardoff, William, and John Reeves. *Preparing for Surgery: A Mind-Body Approach to Enhance Healing and Recovery.* Oakland, CA: New Harbinger Publications, 1997.

Furlong, Monica Winefryck. *Going Under: Preparing Yourself for Anesthesia: Your Guide to Pain Control and Healing Techniques Before, During and After Surgery.* London: Autonomy Publishing Company, November, 1993.

Marquis Who's Who Staff, and American Board of Medical Specialties Staff, eds. *The Official ABMS Directory of Board Certified Medical Specialist.* New Providence, NJ: Marquis Who's Who, 1998.

"Preoperative Care." *Mosby's Medical, Nursing and Allied Health Dictionary* 5th ed. Edited by Kenneth Anderson, Lois E. Anderson, and Walter D. Glanze. B. C. Decker, 1998.

PERIODICALS

"Recommended Practices for Managing the Patient Receiving Anesthesia." *AORN Journal* 75, no. 4 (April 2002): 849.

ORGANIZATIONS

Agency for Health Care Policy and Research (AHCPR), Publications Clearinghouse. P.O. Box 8547, Silver Spring, MD, 20907. (800) 358-9295. <http://www/ahcpr.gov>.

American Board of Surgery. 1617 John F. Kennedy Boulevard, Suite 860, Philadelphia, PA 19103. (215) 568-4000. <http://www.absurgery.org/>.

American Association of Nurse Anesthetists (AANA). 222 South Prospect Avenue, Park Ridge, IL 60068-4001. (847) 692-7050. <http://www.aana.com/>.

American College of Surgeons. 633 N. Saint Clair Street, Chicago, IL 60611-3211. (312) 202-5000. <http://www.facs.org/>.

American Society of Anesthesiologists (ASA). 520 North Northwest Highway, Park Ridge, IL 60068-2573. (847) 825-5586. <http://http://www.asahq.org/>.

National Heart, Lung and Blood Institute. Information Center. P.O. Box 30105, Bethesda, MD 20824-0105. (301) 251-2222. <http://www.nhlbi.nih.gov>.

OTHER

preSurgery.com. <http://www.presurgery.com>.

Reports of the Surgeon General. National Library of Medicine. <http://sgreports.nlm.nih.gov/NN/>.

SurgeryLinx. MDLinx, Inc. 1025 Vermont Avenue, NW, Suite 810, Washington, DC 20005. (202) 543-6544. <http://sgreports.nlm.nih.gov/NN/>.

Surgical Procedures, Operative. <http://www.mic.ki.se/Diseases/e4.html>.

Team Surgery. 3900 Paseo del Sol, #322, Santa Fe, NM 87507. <http://www.teamsurgery.com/>.

Angela M. Costello

Pressure sores *see* **Bedsores**

Presurgical testing

Definition

Presurgical or preoperative testing is the preparation and management of a patient before surgery.

Purpose

Presurgical testing psychologically and physically prepares a patient for surgery.

Demographics

The U.S. Department of Health and Human Services' National Center for Health Statistics reported more than 40 million inpatient surgical procedures (requiring an overnight hospital stay) performed in the United States in 2000. Data from 1996 indicates more than 30 million outpatient surgical procedures (in which the patient goes home the same day of surgery) were performed.

Obstetrical, cardiovascular, digestive, musculoskeletal, and nervous system surgeries were among the majority of the inpatient surgical procedures performed. The majority of outpatient surgeries were performed on the digestive system, eyes, musculoskeletal system, female reproductive organs, and urinary system.

Description

A planned surgery usually involves a surgical consultation, presurgical testing, the surgery itself, and **recovery at home**.

During the surgical consultation, the patient meets with the surgeon or a member of the surgeon's health care team to discuss the surgery and other potential treatment options for the patient's medical condition. A thorough review of the patient's medical history and a complete physical exam are performed at this time. The medical review includes an evaluation of the patient's previous and current medical conditions, surgeries and procedures, medications, and any other health conditions, such as allergies, that may impact the surgery.

The **surgical team** will ensure that the patient understands the potential benefits and risks of the procedure. Patient education may include one-on-one instruction from a health care provider, educational sessions in a group setting, or self-guided learning videos or modules. Informative and instructional handouts are usually provided to explain specific pre-surgical requirements.

After attending the surgical consultation, the patient may desire to seek a **second opinion** to confirm the first doctor's treatment recommendations.

Diagnosis/Preparation

Presurgical testing, also called preoperative testing, includes a variety of tests, patient education, and meetings with the health care team to inform the patient about what to expect before the procedure and during the recovery. Presurgical testing is generally scheduled within one week before the surgery.

Several tests are performed before surgery to provide complete information about the patient's overall health, to prepare the patient for anesthesia (as applicable), and to identify and treat any potential problems ahead of time. Each surgery patient does not have the same presurgery tests. In addition to a check of the patient's temperature, blood pressure, and pulse, more common tests include:

• blood tests

• urine tests

• chest x rays

• pulmonary function tests

• computed tomography scan (CT or CAT scan)

• heart function tests that may include an electrocardiogram or echocardiogram

If the patient recently had these tests performed (within the past six months), he or she can request the test results be forwarded to the surgical center.

Before some surgical procedures, such as valve surgery, a complete dental exam is needed to reduce the risk of infection. Other precautions will be taken before the surgery to reduce the patient's risk of infection.

Informed consent is an educational process between health-care providers and patients. Before any procedure is performed, the patient is asked to sign a consent form. Before signing the form, the patient should understand the nature and purpose of the diagnostic procedure or treatment, the risks and benefits of the procedure, and alternatives, including the option of not proceeding with the test or treatment. During the discussion about the procedure, the health care providers are available to answer the patient's questions about the consent form or procedure.

Advance directives are legal documents that increase a patient's control over medical decisions. A patient may decide medical treatment in advance, in the event that he or she becomes physically or mentally unable to communicate his or her wishes. Advance directives either state what kind of treatment the patient wants to receive (**living will**), or authorize another person to make medical decisions for the patient when he or she is unable to do so (durable **power of attorney**).

Advance directives are not required and may be changed or canceled at any time. Any change should be written, signed, and dated in accordance with state law, and copies should be given to the physician and to others who received original copies. Advance directives can be revoked either in writing or by destroying the document.

Advance directives are not a do-not-resuscitate (**DNR**) order, which indicates that a person—usually with a terminal illness or other serious medical condition—has decided not to have **cardiopulmonary resuscitation** (CPR) performed in the event that his or her heart or breathing stops.

Patients who will undergo any surgical procedure are encouraged to quit smoking and stop using tobacco products at least two weeks before the procedure, and to make a commitment to be a nonsmoker after the procedure. Quitting smoking before surgery helps the patient recover more quickly from surgery. There are several **smoking cessation** programs available in the community. The patient should ask a health care provider for more information if he or she needs help quitting smoking.

The presurgical evaluation may include meetings with the anesthesiologist, surgeon, nurse clinicians, and other health care providers who will manage the patient's care during and after surgery, such as a dietitian, social worker, or rehabilitation specialist.

The patient's surgery time may not be determined until the business day before the scheduled surgery. The patient may be instructed to call the surgical center to find out the time of the scheduled surgery.

Patients are told to come to the surgery center far enough in advance (usually about two hours prior to the scheduled surgery time) so they can be properly prepared for surgery. In some cases, the patient's surgery may need to be rescheduled if another patient requires **emergency surgery** at the patient's scheduled time.

Some surgery centers offer services such as guided imagery and relaxation tapes, massage therapy, or other complementary techniques to reduce a patient's level of stress and anxiety before a surgical procedure.

Guided imagery is a form of focused relaxation that coaches the patient to visualize calm, peaceful images. Several research studies have proven that guided imagery can significantly reduce stress and anxiety before and after surgical and medical procedures and help the patient recover more rapidly. Guided imagery tapes are available at many major bookstores and from some surgery centers. The patient listens to the guided imagery tapes on his or her own CD or tape player before and after the surgery. The patient may even be able to continue listening to the tapes during the procedure, depending on the type of procedure being performed.

Blood transfusions may be necessary during surgery. A blood **transfusion** is the delivery of whole blood or blood components to replace blood lost through trauma, surgery, or disease. About one in three hospitalized patients will require a blood transfusion. The surgeon can provide an estimate of how much blood the patient's procedure may require.

To decrease the risk of infection and immunologic complications, some surgery centers offer a preoperative blood donation program. Autologous blood (from the patient) is the safest blood available for transfusion, since there is no risk of disease transmission. Methods of autologous donation or collection include:

- Intraoperative blood collection: The blood lost during surgery is processed, and the red blood cells are reinfused during or immediately after surgery.

- Preoperative donation: The patient donates blood once a week for about one to three weeks before surgery. The blood is separated, and the blood components needed are reinfused during surgery.

- Immediate preoperative hemodilution: The patient donates blood immediately before surgery to decrease the loss of red blood cells during surgery. After donating, the patient receives fluids to compensate for the amount of blood removed. Since the blood is diluted, fewer red blood cells are lost from bleeding during surgery.

- Postoperative blood collection: Blood lost from the surgical site right after surgery is collected and reinfused after the surgical site has been closed.

The surgeon determines what type of blood collection process, if any, is appropriate.

Depending on the type of surgery scheduled, certain medications may be prescribed or restricted before the surgery. The health-care team will provide specific guidelines. If certain medications need to be restricted before surgery, the patient will receive a complete list of the medications (including prescription, over-the-counter, and herbal medications) to avoid taking before the scheduled surgery.

Prescribed medications that need to be taken within 12 hours before surgery should be swallowed with small sips of water.

Before most surgeries, the patient is advised not to eat or drink anything after midnight the evening before the surgery. This includes no smoking and no gum chewing. The patient should not drink any alcoholic beverages for at least 24 hours before surgery, unless instructed otherwise.

Most patients are admitted to the surgery center or hospital the same day as the scheduled surgery. The patient should bring a list of current medications, allergies, and appropriate medical records upon admission to the surgery center.

The patient should arrange for transportation home, since the effects of anesthesia and other medications given before surgery make it unsafe to drive.

KEY TERMS

Biopsy—The removal of a small sample of tissue for analysis to determine a diagnosis.

Bone densitometry test—A test that quickly and accurately measures the density of bone.

Catheter—A small, flexible tube used to deliver fluids or medications.

Chest x ray—A diagnostic procedure in which a small amount of radiation is used to produce an image of the structures of the chest (heart, lungs, and bones) on film.

Echocardiogram—An imaging procedure used to create a picture of the heart's movement, valves and chambers. The test uses high-frequency sound waves that come from a hand wand placed on the chest. Echocardiogram may be used in combination with Doppler ultrasound to evaluate the blood flow across the heart's valves.

Electrocardiogram (ECG, EKG)—A test that records the electrical activity of the heart using small electrode patches attached to the skin on the chest.

Pulmonary function test—A test that measures the capacity and function of the lungs, as well as the blood's ability to carry oxygen. During the test, patient breathes into a device called a spirometer.

Resources

BOOKS

Anderson, Kenneth, Lois E. Anderson, and Walter D. Glanze, eds. "Preoperative Care." In *Mosby's Medical, Nursing an Allied Heath Dictionary.* 5th ed. B. C. Decker, 1998.

Deardoff, William, and John Reeves. *Preparing for Surgery: A Mind-Body Approach to Enhance Healing and Recovery.* Oakland, CA: New Harbinger Publications, 1997.

Furlong, Monica Winefryck. *Going Under: Preparing Yourself for Anesthesia: Your Guide to Pain Control and Healing Techniques Before, During and After Surgery.* Albuquerque, NM: Autonomy Publishing Company, 1993.

PERIODICALS

"Recommended Practices for Managing the Patient Receiving Anesthesia." *AORN Journal* 75, 4 (April 2002): 849.

ORGANIZATIONS

American Board of Surgery. 1617 John F. Kennedy Boulevard, Suite 860, Philadelphia, PA 19103. (215) 568-4000. <http://www.absurgery.org/>.

American College of Surgeons. 633 N. Saint Clair Street, Chicago, IL 60611-3211. (312) 202-5000. <http://www.facs.org/>.

National Heart, Lung and Blood Institute. Information Center. P.O. Box 30105, Bethesda, MD 20824-0105. (301) 251-2222. <http://www.nhlbi.nih.gov>.

OTHER

preSurgery.com. <http://www.presurgery.com>.

Reports of the Surgeon General. National Library of Medicine. <http://sgreports.nlm.nih.gov/NN/>.

SurgeryLinx. MDLinx, Inc. 1025 Vermont Avenue, NW, Suite 810, Washington, DC 20005. (202) 543-6544. <http://sgreports.nlm.nih.gov/NN/>.

Surgical Procedures, Operative. <http://www.mic.ki.se/Diseases/e4.html>.

Angela M. Costello

Private insurance plans

Definition

Private insurance plans include all forms of health insurance that are not funded by the government.

Purpose

These plans are intended to protect their beneficiaries from the high costs that may be incurred for health care. Most private insurance plans in the United States are employment-based.

Of the nearly 239 million Americans who are covered by private health insurance, approximately nine in 10 (213 million, or 89%) are enrolled in employment-based plans.

Description

Private health insurance plans may be purchased on an individual or group basis. Most group plans are offered by large employers, although some are available through voluntary associations. Individual policies are usually more expensive than group policies. Furthermore, they may have additional coverage restrictions.

There are several major categories of private health insurance in the United States.

Indemnity plans

Indemnity plans are private insurance plans that allow beneficiaries to choose any physician or hospital when they need medical care. Most indemnity plans have a deductible, or amount that the policyholder must pay before the plan will cover any costs. After the deductible has been satisfied, indemnity plans pay a co-insurance percentage, most often 70–90% of the charges. The beneficiary pays the remainder of the bill.

Preferred provider organization (PPO) plans

PPO plans are similar to indemnity plans in that they usually have both a deductible and a co-insurance percentage. Unlike indemnity plans, PPOs offer a list of physicians and hospitals from which enrollees must select in order to receive the plan's maximum benefit. PPOs tend to be less expensive than indemnity plans because health care providers are often willing to reduce their fees in order to participate in these plans. Many large companies have moved their insured employees into PPOs because of their cost effectiveness.

A person enrolled in a PPO can choose to seek care from a non-network provider. This is called going out of network. Some people find this beneficial because it allows continuity of care from an existing provider. Enrollees may also propose their physician for membership in the PPO so that continuity of service may be provided.

Health maintenance organization (HMO) plans

HMOs usually have no deductible. Beneficiaries are charged a small co-payment, typically $5 or $10, per visit, and the plan covers all other charges. The list of preferred providers is generally smaller than that of a PPO. In most HMOs, each beneficiary selects a primary care physician who is responsible for all health care needs. Referrals to specialists must be made through the primary care physician. Like PPOs, HMOs are usually able to charge lower premiums because their participating health care providers agree to accept substantially reduced fees.

Long-term care (LTC) insurance

Long-term care insurance, or LTC, is a type of private health insurance intended to cover the cost of custodial or nursing **home care**. It can be very expensive, and persons considering this form of insurance should not purchase it if the premiums cause financial hardship in the present.

Medigap insurance plans

Medicare does not offer complete health insurance protection. Medigap insurance is a type of plan intended to supplement Medicare coverage. There are 10 standard Medigap benefit packages. These are identified by the letters A through J, and are available in most states, United States territories, and the District of Columbia. Medigap policies pay most or all of the co-insurance amounts charged by Medicare. Some Medigap policies cover Medicare deductibles.

Medical savings accounts (MSAs)

Medical savings accounts are not health insurance plans in the strict sense, but offer a partial alternative to expensive individual private insurance plans. MSAs are similar to Individual Retirement Accounts (IRAs), and have been considered a significant tax break for self-employed individuals. They were created as a four-year pilot project by the Health Insurance Portability and Accountability Act (HIPAA) of 1996. Effective December 31, 2000, the federal government issued an extension on these accounts for two years. The future of MSAs is not clear; however, the government will not revoke these accounts once they have been opened.

An MSA must be combined with a qualified high-deductible private health plan. Without an MSA, a self-employed individual can deduct qualified medical expenses only under the itemized deductions of a 1040 tax form, and the expenses must exceed 7.5% of the adjusted gross income.

The cost of health insurance

The cost of private health insurance has risen steadily over the past two decades, largely because of the rising cost of health care in the United States. Between 1980 and 1995, the total amount spent on health care in the United States each year rose from $247.2 billion to $1.04 trillion, more than a 400% increase. Between 1995 and 2002, the amount almost doubled again, to $2 trillion per year. The reasons for the escalating costs include the following:

- Increased longevity. The life expectancy of most Americans is approximately 76 years. When older people join an insured group, the entire group's health care risks and costs rise.

- Advances in medical technology. New technology is often expensive.

- Increased use of health care. Between 1991 and 1996, the average annual number of physician office visits rose from 2.7–3.4 per person. The average number of visits has continued to rise, and was just under four per person per year in 2003.

The rising costs of health insurance over the past 30 years have caused many employers to curtail or drop health insurance as an employee benefit. The cost of health insurance premiums increased from $16.8 billion in 1970 to $310 billion in 1995. By 2002, it had almost doubled again, to approximately $500 billion. Many employers have increased the amount of money employees are expected to contribute toward their health care. Others, particularly smaller businesses, do not offer health insurance at all. A 1997 study found that only 34% of workers in smaller businesses were covered through their employers, whereas 82% of employees in the largest companies were covered. Experts feel that this trend will continue. Workers in large-employer health insurance plans generally have policies that cover more health services, have lower deductibles, and offer more opportunities to enroll in HMOs.

Uninsured persons

The U.S. Census Bureau reported in 1997 that 43.4 million people in the United States, or 16.1% of the population, had no health insurance coverage. Between 1998 and 1999, both the number and proportion of uninsured Americans declined slightly, to 42.6 million and 15.5% respectively. As of 2000, the Centers for Disease Control and Prevention estimated that 40.5 million people under age 65 were without health insurance.

Some workers do not have health insurance because they cannot afford it. In the 1950s, employer-based health insurance served most American families reasonably well because many workers were employed by large firms and remained with them for life. The trend over the past two decades is employment by small firms that do not offer health insurance as a benefit, and a tendency to change employers every few years. Most uninsured workers are self-employed, work only part-time, or hold low-wage jobs that do not give them access to lower-cost employer-sponsored group plans. Workers in these three categories do not qualify for coverage by government programs for low-income people.

The other major category of uninsured people includes those who cannot purchase private insurance at affordable rates because they are likely to need expensive medical services. Those who have a high risk of developing cancer or are HIV-positive may not be able to obtain coverage from any insurance company. As early as the 1980s, some insurance companies began introducing clauses that excluded or restricted benefits for persons with pre-existing conditions. These clauses denied private insurance to anyone already diagnosed with a serious medical condition. One of the goals of the Health Insurance Portability and Accountability Act (HIPPA) of 1996 was to help workers who could not change jobs because they had family members with serious health problems. In the past, they would have been denied health insurance by the preexisting condition clauses in the new employer's plan. HIPAA requires employer-sponsored insurance plans to accept transfers from other plans without imposing preexisting condition clauses.

An individual private health insurance plan can be expensive and restrictive. It may, however, be the only choice for a consumer who is not employed; self-employed; or is a new hire at a company and must wait several months or more before the company's coverage takes effect.

Tax credit proposals

One approach to the rising costs of private health insurance that is gaining bipartisan political support is to offer tax credits that would allow more Americans to purchase health insurance. The present federal tax code favors workers who already have employer-sponsored health insurance. Supporters of the tax credit approach maintain that it would give workers a wider choice of health plans, create greater portability of health insurance, and encourage groups other than employment-based populations (e.g., church groups, unions, fraternal organizations) to sponsor insurance plans for their members.

See also Managed care plans.

Resources

BOOKS

Institute of Medicine. *Health Insurance Is a Family Matter.* Washington, DC: National Academy Press, 2002.

Miller, I. *American Health Care Blues: Blue Cross, HMOs, and Pragmatic Reform Since 1960.* Somerset, NJ: Transaction Publishers, 2000.

Nyman J.A. *Theory of Demand for Health Insurance.* Palo Alto, CA: Stanford University Press, 2002.

Stevens, W.S. *Health Insurance: Current Issues and Background.* Hauppauge, NY: Nova Science Publishers, 2003.

PERIODICALS

Cohen, M.A. "Private long-term care insurance: a look ahead." *Journal of Aging and Health* 15, no.1 (2003): 74-98.

Longest, Jr., B.B. "Medicare: How You See it Depends on Where You Stand." *Healthcare Financial Management* 57, no.3 (2003): 88-92.

Newton, L.H. "The Turn to the Local: The Possibility of Returning Health Care to the Community." *Business Ethics Quarterly* 12, no.4 (2002): 505-26.

Sturm, R. and R.L. Pacula. "Private Insurance: What Has Parity Brought?" *Behavioral Healthcare Tomorrow* 10, no.2 (2001): SR26-28.

Taylor, P., L. Blewett, M. Brasure, K.T. Call, E. Larson, J. Gale, A. Hagopian, L.G. Hart, D. Hartley, P. House, M.K. James, T. Ricketts. "Small Town Health Care Safety Nets: Report on a Pilot Study." *Journal of Rural Health* 19, no.2 (2003): 125-34.

ORGANIZATIONS

American Association of Retired Persons (AARP). 601 E. Street NW, Washington, DC 20049. (800) 424-3410, <http://www.aarp.org/>.

American College of Healthcare Executives. One North Franklin, Suite 1700, Chicago, IL 60606-4425. (312) 424-2800, Fax: 312-424-0023 <http://www.ache.org/>.

KEY TERMS

Co-insurance—The percentage of health care charges that an insurance company pays after the beneficiary pays the deductible. Most co-insurance percentages are 70–90%.

Deductible—An amount of money that an insured person is required to pay on each claim made on an insurance policy.

Indemnity—Protection, as by insurance, against damage or loss.

Indemnity plans—Private health insurance plans that allow the policyholder to choose any physician or hospital when health care is needed.

Long-term care (LTC) insurance—A type of private health insurance intended to cover the cost of long-term nursing home or home health care.

Medigap—A group of 10 standardized private health insurance policies intended to cover the coinsurance and deductible costs not covered by Medicare.

Portability—A feature that allows employees to transfer health insurance coverage or other benefits from one employer to another when they change jobs.

Preferred provider organizations (PPOs)—Private health insurance plans that require beneficiaries to select their health care providers from a list approved by the insurance company.

Premium—The amount paid by an insurance policyholder for insurance coverage. Most health insurance policy premiums are payable on a monthly basis.

American Medical Association. 515 N. State Street, Chicago, IL 60610. (312) 464-5000. <http://www.ama-assn.org>.

Health Insurance Association of America. 1201 F Street, NW, Suite 500, Washington, DC 20004-1204. (202) 824-1600. Fax: (202) 824-1722. <http://www.hiaa.org/index_flash.cfm>.

United States Department of Health and Human Services. 200 Independence Avenue SW, Washington, DC 20201. <http://www.hhs.gov>.

OTHER

Agency for Healthcare Research and Quality. [cited May 12, 2003]. <http://www.ahcpr.gov/consumer/insuranc.htm>.

Association of Health Insurance Advisors. [cited May 12, 2003]. <http://www.ahia.net/>.

Council for Affordable Health Insurance. [cited May 12, 2003]. <http://cahionline.org/cahi_index.shtml>.

Georgetown University Health Policy Institute. [cited May 15, 2003]. <http://www.healthinsuranceinfo.net/>.

Health Insurance Information, Counseling & Assistance Program of New York State. [cited May 12, 2003]. <http://hiicap.state.ny.us/>.

L. Fleming Fallon, Jr., MD , DrPH

PRK *see* **Photorefractive keratectomy (PRK)**

Proctosigmoidoscopy *see* **Sigmoidoscopy**

Prophylaxis, antibiotic

Definition

A prophylaxis is a measure taken to maintain health and prevent the spread of disease. Antibiotic prophylaxis is the focus of this article and refers to the use of **antibiotics** to prevent infections.

Purpose

Antibiotics are well known for their ability to treat infections. But some antibiotics also are prescribed to prevent infections. This usually is done only in certain situations or for people with particular medical problems. For example, people with abnormal heart valves have a high risk of developing heart valve infections even after only minor surgery. This happens because bacteria from other parts of the body get into the bloodstream during surgery and travel to the heart valves. To prevent these infections, people with heart valve problems often take antibiotics before having any kind of surgery, including dental surgery.

Antibiotics also may be prescribed to prevent infections in people with weakened immune systems such as those with AIDS or people who are having chemotherapy treatments for cancer. But even healthy people with strong immune systems may occasionally be given preventive antibiotics—if they are having certain kinds of surgery that carry a high risk of infection, or if they are traveling to parts of the world where they are likely to get an infection that causes diarrhea, for example.

In all of these situations, a physician should be the one to decide whether antibiotics are necessary. Unless a physician says to do so, it is not a good idea to take antibiotics to prevent ordinary infections.

Because the overuse of antibiotics can lead to resistance, drugs taken to prevent infection should be used only for a short time.

Description

Among the drugs used for antibiotic prophylaxis are amoxicillin (a type of penicillin) and **fluoroquinolones** such as ciprofloxacin (Cipro) and trovafloxacin (Trovan). These drugs are available only with a physician's prescription and come in tablet, capsule, liquid, and injectable forms.

For surgical prophylaxis, the cephalosporin antibiotics are usually preferred. This class includes cefazolin (Ancef, Kefzol), cefamandole (Mandol), cefotaxime (Claforan), and others. The choice of drug depends on its spectrum and the type of bacteria that are most likely to be encountered. For example, surgery on the intestines, which have many anaerobic bacteria, might call for cefoxitin (Mefoxin), while in heart surgery, where there are no anaerobes, cefazolin might be preferred.

Recommended dosage

The recommended dosage depends on the type of antibiotic prescribed and the reason it is being used. For the correct dosage, the patient is advised to check with the physician or dentist who prescribed the medicine or the pharmacist who filled the prescription. The patient is recommended to be sure to take the medicine exactly as prescribed, and not to take more or less than directed, and to take the medicine only for as long as the physician or dentist says to take it.

The recommended dose of prophylactic antibiotic for surgery has varied with studies. At one time, it was common to give a dose of antibiotic when the patient was called to the **operating room**, and to continue the drug for 48 hours after surgery. More recent studies indicate that a single antibiotic dose, given immediately before the start of surgery, may be just as effective in preventing infection, while reducing the risk of drug side effects.

Precautions

The warnings listed below refer primarily to the effects of the drugs when taken in multiple doses. When prophylactic antibiotics are used as a single dose, adverse effects are very unlikely. The only exceptions are for people who are allergic to the antibiotic used. Since **cephalosporins** are closely related to penicillins, people who are allergic to penicillins should avoid cephalosporin antibiotics.

If the medicine causes nausea, vomiting, or diarrhea, the patient is advised to check with the physician or dentist who prescribed it as soon as possible. Patients who are taking antibiotics before surgery should not wait until the day of the surgery to report problems with the medicine. The physician or dentist needs to know right away if problems occur.

KEY TERMS

AIDS—Acquired immunodeficiency syndrome. A disease caused by infection with the human immunodeficiency virus (HIV). In people with this disease, the immune system breaks down, opening the door to other infections and some types of cancer.

Antibiotic—A medicine used to treat infections.

Chemotherapy—Treatment of an illness with chemical agents. The term is typically used to describe the treatment of cancer with drugs.

Immune system—The body's natural defenses against disease and infection.

For other specific precautions, the patient is advised to see the entry on the type of drug prescribed such as penicillins or fluoroquinolones.

Side effects

Antibiotics may cause a number of side effects. For details, the patient is advised to see entries on specific types of antibiotics. Anyone who has unusual or disturbing symptoms after taking antibiotics should get in contact with the prescribing physician.

Interactions

Whether used to treat or to prevent infection, antibiotics may interact with other medicines. When this happens, the effects of one or both of the drugs may change or the risk of side effects may be greater. Anyone who takes antibiotics for any reason should inform the physician about all the other medicines he or she is taking and should ask whether any possible interactions may interfere with drugs' effects. For details of drug interactions, the candidate is advised to see entries on specific types of antibiotics.

Resources

BOOKS

AHFS: Drug Information. Washington DC: American Society Healthsystems Pharmaceuticals, 2002.

Reynolds, J.E.F., ed. *Martindale The Extra Pharmacopoeia,* 31st ed. London: The Pharmaceutical Press, 1993.

Brody, T.M., J. Larner, K.P. Minneman, and H.C. Neu. *Human Pharmacology: Molecular to Clinical,* 2nd ed. St. Louis: Mosby Year-Book.

PERIODICALS

Braffman-Miller, Judith. "Beware the Rise of Antibiotic-Resistant Microbes." *USA Today (Magazine)* 125 (March 1997): 56.

"Consumer Alert: Antibiotic Resistance Is Growing!" *People's Medical Society Newsletter* 16 (August 1997): 1.

Guthrie, P. "Doctors, Patients Must Act Together to Save Antibiotics' Potency, Experts Say." *Atlanta Journal-Constitution* (March 19, 2003).

Nancy Ross-Flanigan
Sam Uretsky, PharmD

Prostaglandins *see* **Uterine stimulants**

Prostate-specific antigen test *see* **Tumor marker tests**

Prostate resection *see* **Transurethral resection of the prostate**

Prostatectomy, open *see* **Open prostatectomy**

Proton pump inhibitors *see* **Gastric acid inhibitors**

PSA test *see* **Tumor marker tests**

Psyllium *see* **Laxatives**

Pubo-vaginal sling *see* **Sling procedure**

Pulmonary embolism *see* **Venous thrombosis prevention**

Pulse oximeter

Definition

The pulse oximeter is a photoelectric instrument for measuring oxygen saturation of blood.

Purpose

A pulse oximeter measures the amount of oxygen present in blood by registering pulsations within an arteriolar bed (an area between arteries and capillaries). It is a noninvasive method widely used in hospitals on newborns, persons with pulmonary disorders, and individuals undergoing pulmonary and cardiac procedures. Oxygen levels can be estimated during **exercise**, surgery, or other medical procedures, or while a person is asleep.

Description

The oximeter consists of a light-emitting diode (LED), a photodetector probe containing a permanent or disposable sensor, alarms for pulse rate and oxygen levels, a display screen, and cables. The device works by

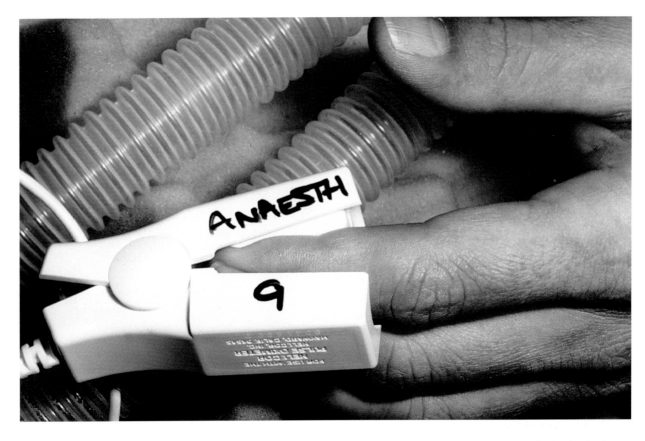

This pulse oximeter on the patient's finger monitors blood oxygen levels while the patient is under general anesthesia during surgery. *(M. English, MD/Custom Medical Stock Photo. Reproduced by permission.)*

emitting beams of red and infrared light that are passed through a pulsating arteriolar bed. Sensors detect the amount of light absorbed by oxyhemoglobin and deoxy-hemoglobin in the red blood cells. The ratio of red to infrared light measured by the photodetector indicates the amount of oxygen present in the blood. The sensor is attached to the body over the arteriolar area in the ear, the fingertip, the big toe, or across the bridge of the nose. Clip sensors can be used on fingers or the earlobe.

The pulse oximeter is widely used in most hospitals and in research laboratories that study pulmonary function. Oximeters are used in hospital settings such as intensive care units, pulmonary units, and in health care centers. Portable hand-held devices are available, and are used to spot check patients and for in-home use under the supervision of a physician.

Usage

Several steps can be taken to enhance accurate readings. If possible, the patient should not smoke 24 hours prior to pulse oximetry. Fingernail polish should be removed if the oximeter will be attached to the finger. For people with poor circulation, hands should be slowly warmed with warm towels before attaching the oximeter. Abnormally high or low temperatures, as well as reduced hemoglobin, can influence the amount of oxygen adhering to the hemoglobin within the red blood cells, altering the reading. The sensor should be wrapped securely around the finger to prevent outside light from interfering with the reading, which could render it invalid. The device must not be used near flammable anesthetics.

Resources

BOOKS

Bartell, Karen H. *Pulmonary Pathophysiology: The Essentials, 6th edition.* Philadelphia: Lippincott Williams & Wilkins, 2003.

Daggett, Sharron. *Handbook of Arterial Blood Gas Interpretation and Ventilator Management.* Bethesda, MD: National Institute of Nurse Education, 1999.

Madama, Vincent C. *Pulmonary Function Testing and Cardiopulmonary Stress Testing, 2nd edition.* Albany, NY: Delmar, 1997.

Moyle, John T. B. *Pulse Oximetry, 2nd edition.* Annapolis Junction, MD: BMJ Books, 2002.

PERIODICALS

Davies, G., A. M. Gibson, M. Swanney, D. Murray, and L. Beckert. "Understanding of Pulse Oximetry among Hos-

KEY TERMS

Arteriolar bed—An area in which arterioles cluster between arteries and capillaries.

Arterioles—The smallest branches of arteries.

Capillaries—Tiny blood vessels with a diameter of a red blood cell through which a single layer of cells flows.

Deoxyhemoglobin—Hemoglobin with oxygen removed.

Oxyhemoglobin—Hemoglobin combined with oxygen.

pital Staff." *New Zealand Medical Journal* 116, no.1168 (2003): 297–299.

Tschupp, A., and S. Fanconi. "A Combined Ear Sensor for Pulse Oximetry and Carbon Dioxide Tension Monitoring: Accuracy in Critically Ill Children." *Anesthesia and Analgesia* 96, no.1 (2003): 82–84.

ORGANIZATIONS

American Academy of Family Physicians. 11400 Tomahawk Creek Parkway, Leawood, KS 66211-2672. (913) 906-6000. fp@aafp.org. <http://www.aafp.org>.

American Academy of Pediatrics. 141 Northwest Point Boulevard, Elk Grove Village, IL 60007-1098. (847) 434-4000; Fax: (847) 434-8000. kidsdoc@aap.org. <http://www.aap.org/default.htm>.

American College of Physicians. 190 N Independence Mall West, Philadelphia, PA 19106-1572. (800) 523-1546, x2600, or (215) 351-2600. <http://www.acponline.org>.

OTHER

Oximeter.Org. [cited March 1, 2003]. <http://www.oximeter.org/pulseox/principles.htm>.

University of Medicine and Dentistry of New Jersey. [cited March 1, 2003] <http://www.umdnj.edu/rspthweb/bibs/pulseox.htm>.

Virtual Hospital. [cited March 1, 2003]. <http://www.vh.org/adult/provider/anesthesia/ProceduralSedation/PulseOximetry.html>.

World Federation of Societies of Anaesthesiologists. [cited March 1, 2003]. <http://www.nda.ox.ac.uk/wfsa/html/u05/u05_003.htm>.

L. Fleming Fallon, Jr. MD, DrPH

Pyloroplasty

Definition

Pyloroplasty is a surgical procedure in which the pylorus valve at the lower portion of the stomach is cut and resutured, relaxing and widening its muscular opening (pyloric sphincter) into the duodenum (first part of the small intestine). Pyloroplasty is a treatment for patients at high risk for gastric or peptic ulcer disease (PUD).

Purpose

Pyloroplasty surgery enlarges the opening through which stomach contents are emptied into the intestine, allowing the stomach to empty more quickly. A pyloroplasty is performed to treat the complications of PUD or when medical treatment has not been able to control PUD in high-risk patients.

Demographics

Nearly four million people in the United States have PUD; about five adults in 100,000 will develop an ulcer. About 1.7% of children being treated in general pediatric practices are diagnosed with PUD. The presence of ulcer-causing *Helicobacter pylori* bacteria occurs in 10% of the population in industrialized countries and is believed to cause 80–90% of primary ulcers. In the United States, *H. pylori* infection occurs more frequently in black and Hispanic populations than in white. The frequency of secondary ulcers (caused by other existing conditions) is not known as it depends on the frequency of other illnesses, chronic diseases, and drug use. Primary and secondary PUD can occur in patients of all ages. Primary PUD is rare in children under age 10, increasing during adolescence. Secondary PUD is more prevalent in children under age six.

Description

Peptic ulcer disease develops when there is an imbalance between normal conditions that protect the lining (mucosa) of the stomach and the intestines and conditions that disrupt normal functioning of the lining. Protective factors include the water-soluble mucosal gel layer, the production of bicarbonate in the lining to balance acidity, the regulation of gastric acid (stomach acid) secretion, and blood flow in the lining. The aggressive factors that work against this protective gastric-wall system are excessive acid production, *H. pylori* bacterial infection, and a reduced blood flow (ischemia) in the mucosal lining. These aggressive factors can cause inflammation and ulcer development. A peptic ulcer is a type of sore or hole (perforation) that forms on the lining of the stomach (gastric ulcer) or intestine (duodenal ulcer), when the lining has been eaten away by stomach acid and digestive juices. Peptic ulcers can be primary, caused by *H. pylori* infection, or secondary, caused by excess acid production, stress, use of medications, and other un-

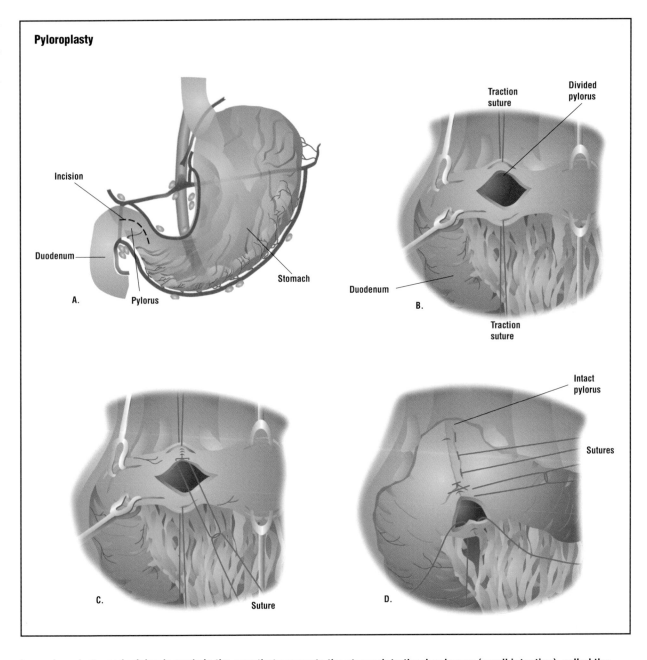

Pyloroplasty

A. — Incision, Duodenum, Pylorus, Stomach

B. — Traction suture, Divided pylorus, Duodenum, Traction suture

C. — Suture

D. — Intact pylorus, Sutures

In a pyloroplasty, an incision is made in the area that connects the stomach to the duodenum (small intestine), called the pylorus (A). The pylorus is divided laterally (B), and then stitched longitudinally (C and D), allowing for a larger connection. *(Illustration by GGS Inc.)*

derlying conditions that disrupt the gastric environment. Although *H. pylori* is believed to cause the majority of all ulcers, not all people infected with it develop ulcers. In high-risk individuals, the bacteria more readily disturb the balance between good factors and destructive factors, upsetting the protective function of the stomach and intestine lining. An ulcer develops when the lining can no longer protect the organs. Secondary ulcers are usually found in the stomach; primary ulcers can be in the stomach or intestine.

Other factors that contribute to mucosal inflammation and ulceration include:

- alcohol and caffeine use
- non-steroidal anti-inflammatory drugs (NSAIDs)
- aspirin
- cigarette smoking
- exposure to certain irritating chemicals
- emotional disturbances and prolonged stress

- traumatic injuries and burns

- respiratory failure

- blood poisoning

- critical illnesses that create imbalances in body chemistry

Symptoms of gastric or peptic ulcer include burning pain, nausea, vomiting, loss of appetite, bloating, burping, and losing weight.

When PUD is diagnosed or high risk established, medical treatment will begin to treat *H. pylori* infection if present and to restore balanced conditions in the mucosal lining. Any underlying condition may be treated simultaneously, including respiratory disorders, fluid imbalance, or stomach and digestive disorders. Medications may be prescribed to help correct gastric disturbances and control gastric acid secretion. Certain drugs that are prescribed for other conditions, especially NSAIDs, may be discontinued if they are known to cause inflammation. Adult patients may be advised to discontinue alcohol and caffeine use and to stop smoking.

When medical treatment alone is not able to improve the conditions that cause PUD, a pyloroplasty procedure may be recommended, particularly for patients with stress ulcers, perforation of the mucosal wall, and gastric outlet obstruction. The surgery involves cutting the pylorus lengthwise and resuturing it at a right angle across the cut to relax the muscle and create a larger opening from the stomach into the intestine. The enlarged opening allows the stomach to empty more quickly. A pyloroplasty is sometimes done in conjunction with a **vagotomy** procedure in which the vagus nerves that stimulate stomach acid production and gastric motility (movement) are cut. This may delay gastric emptying and pyloroplasty will help correct that effect.

Diagnosis

Diagnosis begins with an accurate history of prior illnesses and existing medical conditions as well as a family history of ulcers or other gastrointestinal (stomach and intestines) disorders. A complete history and comprehensive diagnostic testing may include:

- location, frequency, duration, and severity of pain

- vomiting and description of gastric material

- bowel habits and description of stool

- all medications, including over-the-counter products

- appetite, typical diet, and weight changes

- family and social stressors

- alcohol consumption and smoking habits

- heart rate, pulse, and blood pressure

- chest examination and x ray, if necessary

- palpation (touch) of the abdomen

- rectal examination and stool testing

- pelvic examination in sexually active females

- examination of testicles and inguinal (groin) area in males

- testing for the presence of *Helicobacter pylori*

- complete blood count and blood chemistry profile

- urinalysis

- imaging studies of gastrointestinal system (x ray, other types of scans)

- biopsy of stomach lining using a tube-like telescopic instrument (endoscope)

Preparation

Before surgery, standard preoperative blood and urine tests will be performed and various x rays may be ordered. The patient will not be permitted to eat or drink anything after midnight the night before the procedure. When the patient is admitted to the hospital, cleansing enemas may be ordered to empty the intestine. If nausea or vomiting are present, a suction tube may be used to empty the stomach.

Aftercare

The patient will spend several hours in a recovery area after surgery where blood pressure, pulse, respiration, and temperature will be monitored. The patient's breathing may be shallower than normal because of the effect of anesthesia and the patient's reluctance to breathe deeply and experience pain at the site of the surgical incision. The patient will be shown how to support the site while breathing deeply or coughing, and will be given pain medication as needed. Fluid intake and output will be measured. The operative site will be observed for any sign of redness, swelling, or wound drainage. Intravenous fluids are usually given for 24–48 hours until the

Pyloroplasty

QUESTIONS TO ASK THE DOCTOR

- How will this surgery be performed?
- What is your experience with this procedure? How often do you perform this procedure?
- Why must I have the surgery?
- What are my options if I opt not have the surgery?
- How can I expect to feel after surgery?
- What are the risks involved in having this surgery?
- How quickly will I recover? When can I return to school or work?
- What are my chances of getting this condition again?
- What can I do to avoid getting this condition again?

KEY TERMS

Gastric (or peptic) ulcer—An ulcer (sore or hole) in the stomach lining, duodenum, or other part of the gastrointestinal system.

Pyloric sphincter—A broad band of muscle in the pylorus valve at the bottom end of the stomach.

Pylorus—The valve at the bottom end of the stomach that releases food from the stomach into the intestines.

Vagotomy—A surgical procedure in which the nerves that stimulate stomach acid production and gastric motility (movement) are cut.

patient is gradually permitted to eat a special light diet and as bowel activity resumes. About eight hours after surgery, the patient may be allowed to walk a little, increasing movement gradually over the next few days. The average hospital stay, dependent upon the patient's overall recovery status and any underlying conditions, ranges from six to eight days.

Risks

Potential complications of this abdominal surgery include excessive bleeding, surgical wound infection, incisional hernia, recurrence of gastric ulcer, chronic diarrhea, and malnutrition. After the surgery, the surgeon should be informed of an increase in pain, and of any swelling, redness, drainage, or bleeding in the surgical area. The development of headache, muscle aches, dizziness, fever, abdominal pain or swelling, constipation, nausea or vomiting, rectal bleeding, or black stools should also be reported.

Normal results

Complete healing is expected without complications. Recovery and a return to normal activities should take from four to six weeks.

Morbidity and mortality rates

Successful treatment of *Helicobacter pylori* has improved morbidity and mortality rates, and the prognosis for PUD, with proper treatment and avoidance of causative factors, is excellent. Pyloroplasty is rarely performed in primary ulcer disease. Morbidity and mortality are higher in patients with secondary ulcers because of underlying illness that complicates both PUD and surgical treatment.

Resources

BOOKS

Monahan, Frances. *Medical-Surgical Nursing.* Philadelphia: W. B. Saunders Co., 1998.

ORGANIZATIONS

American Gastroenterological Association. 7910 Woodmont Ave., Seventh Floor, Bethesda, MD 20814. (301) 654-2055. <http://www.gastro.org>.

National Institute of Diabetes and Digestive and Kidney Disorders. 31 Center Drive, Bethesda, MD 20892. (301) 496-7422. <http://www.niddk.nih.gov>.

OTHER

"Peptic Ulcer Surgery." *Mayo Clinic Online.* March 5, 1998. <http://www.mayohealth.org>.

"Peptic Ulcer Disease." *Inteli Health.* Harvard Medical School and Aetna Consumer Health Information. March 6, 2001. <http:// www.intelihealth.com>.

Kathleen D. Wright, RN
L. Lee Culvert

Pylorus repair *see* **Pyloroplasty**

Quadrantectomy

Definition

Quadrantectomy is a surgical procedure in which a "quadrant" (approximately one-fourth) of the breast, including tissue surrounding a cancerous tumor, is removed. It is also called a partial or segmental mastectomy.

Purpose

Quadrantectomy is a type of breast-conserving surgery used as a treatment for breast cancer. Prior to the advent of breast-conserving surgeries, total mastectomy (complete removal of the breast) was considered the standard surgical treatment for breast cancer. Procedures such as quadrantectomy and **lumpectomy** (removing the tissue directly surrounding the tumor) have allowed doctors to treat cancer without sacrificing the entire affected breast.

Demographics

The American Cancer Society estimates that approximately 211,300 new cases of breast cancer are diagnosed annually in the United States, and 39,800 women die as a result of the disease. Approximately one in eight women will develop breast cancer at some point in her life. The risk of developing breast cancer increases with age: women ages 30–40 have a one in 252 chance, ages 40–50 a one in 68 chance, ages 50–60 a one in 35 chance, and ages 60–70 a one in 27 chance.

In the 1990s, the incidence of breast cancer was higher among Caucasian women (113.1 cases per 100,000 women) than African American women (100.3 per 100,000). The death rate associated with breast cancer, however, was higher among African American women (29.6 per 100,000) than Caucasian women (22.2 per 100,000). Rates were lower among Hispanic women (14.2 per 100,000), American Indian women (12.0), and Asian women (11.2 per 100,000).

Description

The patient is usually placed under general anesthesia for the duration of the procedure. In some instances, a local anesthetic may be administered with sedation to help the patient relax.

During quadrantectomy, a margin of normal breast tissue, skin, and muscle lining is removed around the periphery of the tumor. This decreases the risk of any abnormal cells being left behind and spreading locally or to other parts of the body (a process called metastasis). The amount removed is generally about one-fourth of the size of the breast (hence, the "quadrant" in quadrantectomy). The remaining tissue is then reconstructed to minimize any cosmetic defects, and then sutured closed. Temporary drains may be placed through the skin to remove excess fluid from the surgical site.

Some patients may have the lymph nodes removed from under the arm (called the axillary lymph nodes) on the same side as the tumor. Lymph nodes are small, oval- or bean-shaped masses found throughout the body that act as filters against foreign materials and cancer cells. If cancer cells break away from their primary site of growth, they can travel to and begin to grow in the lymph nodes first, before traveling to other parts of the body. Removal of the lymph nodes is therefore a method of determining if a cancer has begun to spread. To remove the nodes, a second incision is made in the area of the armpit and the fat pad that contains the lymph nodes is removed. The tissue is then sent to a pathologist, who extracts the lymph nodes from the fatty tissue and examines them for the presence of cancer cells.

Diagnosis/Preparation

Breast tumors may be found during self-examination or an examination by a health care professional. In other cases, they are visualized during a routine mammogram. Symptoms such as breast pain, changes in breast size or shape, redness, dimpling, or irritation may be an indication that medical attention is warranted.

Prior to surgery, the patient is instructed to refrain from eating or drinking after midnight on the night before the operation. The physician will tell the patient what will take place during and after surgery, as well as expected outcomes and potential complications of the procedure.

Aftercare

The patient may return home the same day or remain in the hospital for one to two days after the procedure. Discharge instructions will include how to care for the incision and drains, what activities to restrict (i.e., driving and heavy lifting), and how to manage postoperative pain. Patients are often instructed to wear a well-fitting support bra for at least a week following surgery. A follow-up appointment to remove stitches and drains is usually scheduled 10–14 days after surgery.

If lymph nodes are removed, specific steps should be taken to minimize the risk of developing lymphedema of the arm, a condition in which excess fluid is not properly drained from body tissues, resulting in chronic swelling. This swelling can sometimes become severe enough to interfere with daily activity. Prior to being discharged, the patient will learn how to care for the arm, and how to avoid infection. She will also be told to avoid sunburn, refrain from heavy lifting, and to be careful not to wear tight jewelry and elastic bands.

Most patients undergo radiation therapy as part of their complete treatment plan. The radiation usually begins immediately or soon after quadrantectomy, and involves a schedule of five days of treatment a week for five to six weeks. Other treatments, such as chemotherapy or hormone therapy, may also be prescribed depending on the size and stage of the patient's cancer.

Risks

Risks associated with the surgical removal of breast tissue include bleeding, infection, breast asymmetry, changes in sensation, reaction to the anesthesia, and unexpected scarring.

Some of the risks associated with removal of the lymph nodes include excessive bleeding, infection, pain, excessive swelling, and damage to nerves during surgery. Nerve damage may be temporary or permanent, and may result in weakness, numbness, tingling, and drooping. Lymphedema is also a risk whenever lymph nodes have been removed; it may occur immediately following surgery or months to years later.

Normal results

Most patients will not experience recurrences of the cancer following a treatment plan of quadrantectomy and radiation therapy. One study followed patients for a period of 20 years after breast-conserving surgery, and found that only 9% experienced recurrence of the cancer.

Morbidity and mortality rates

Following removal of the axillary lymph nodes, there is approximately a 10% risk of lymphedema and a 20% risk of abnormal skin sensations. Approximately 17% of women undergoing breast-conserving surgery have a poor cosmetic result (e.g., asymmetry or distortion of shape). The risk of complications associated with general anesthesia is less than 1%.

Alternatives

A full mastectomy, in which the entire affected breast is removed, is one alternative to quadrantectomy. A **simple mastectomy** removes the entire breast, while a

---

KEY TERMS

Mammogram—A set of x rays taken of the front and side of the breast; used to diagnose various abnormalities of the breast.

Pathologist—A medical doctor who specializes in the diagnosis of diseases from the microscopic analyses of cells and tissues.

---

radical mastectomy removes the entire breast plus parts of the chest muscle wall and the lymph nodes. In terms of recurrence and survival rates, breast-conserving surgery has been shown to be equally effective as mastectomy in treating breast cancer.

A new technique that may eliminate the need for removing many axillary lymph nodes is called sentinel node biopsy. When lymph fluid moves out of a region, the "sentinel" lymph node is the first node it reaches. The theory behind **sentinel lymph node biopsy** is that if cancer is not present in the sentinel node, it is unlikely to have spread to other nearby nodes. This procedure may allow individuals with early stage cancers to avoid the complications associated with partial or radical removal of lymph nodes if there is little or no chance that cancer has spread to them.

Resources

BOOKS

Iglehart, J. Dirk, and Carolyn M. Kaelin. "Diseases of the Breast" In *Sabiston Textbook of Surgery.* Philadelphia: W. B. Saunders Company, 2001.

PERIODICALS

Apantaku, Leila. "Breast-Conserving Surgery for Breast Cancer." *American Family Physician* 66, no. 12 (December 15, 2002): 2271-8.

Sainsbury, J. R., T. J. Anderson, and D. A. L. Morgan. "Breast Cancer." *British Medical Journal* 321 (September 23, 2000): 745-50.

Veronesi, U., N. Cascinelli, L. Mariani, et al. "More Long-Term Data for Breast-Conserving Surgery." *New England Journal of Medicine* 347, no. 16 (October 17, 2002): 1227-32.

ORGANIZATIONS

American Cancer Society. 1599 Clifton Rd. NE, Atlanta, GA 30329-4251. (800) 227-2345. <http://www.cancer.org>.

Society of Surgical Oncology. 85 W. Algonquin Rd., Suite 550, Arlington Heights, IL 60005. (847) 427-1400. <http://www.surgonc.org>.

OTHER

"All About Cancer: Detailed Guide." *American Cancer Society.* 2003 [cited April 9, 2003]. <http://www.cancer.org/docroot/CRI/CRI_2_3.asp>.

Stephanie Dionne Sherk

Radical neck dissection

Definition

Radical neck dissection is a surgical operation used to remove cancerous tissue in the head and neck.

Purpose

The purpose of radical neck dissection is to remove lymph nodes and other structures in the head and neck that are likely or known to be malignant. Variations on neck dissections exist, depending on the extent of the cancer. A radical neck dissection removes the most tissue. It is performed when the cancer has spread widely in the neck. A modified neck dissection removes less tissue, and a selective neck dissection even less.

Demographics

Experts estimate that there are approximately 5,000–10,000 radical neck dissections in the United States each year. Men and women undergo radical neck dissections at about the same rate.

Description

Cancers of the head and neck (sometimes inaccurately called throat cancer) often spread to nearby tissues and into the lymph nodes. Removing these structures is one way of controlling the cancer.

Of the 600 lymph nodes in the body, approximately 200 are in the neck. Only a small number of these are removed during a neck dissection. In addition, other structures such as muscles, veins, and nerves may be removed during a radical neck dissection. These include the sternocleidomastoid muscle (one of the muscles that functions to flex the head), internal jugular (neck) vein, submandibular gland (one of the salivary glands), and the spinal accessory nerve (a nerve that helps control speech, swallowing, and certain movements of the head and neck).

The goal is always to remove all the cancer, but to save as many components surrounding the nodes as possible.

An incision is made in the neck, and the skin is pulled back (retracted) to reveal the muscles and lymph nodes. The surgeon is guided in what to remove by tests performed prior to surgery and by examination of the size and texture of the lymph nodes.

Diagnosis/Preparation

This operation should not be performed if cancer has metastasized (spread) beyond the head and neck, or if the cancer has invaded the bones of the cervical vertebrae (the first seven bones of the spinal column) or the skull. In these cases, the surgery will not effectively contain the cancer.

Radical neck dissection is a major operation. Extensive tests are performed before the operation to try to determine where and how far the cancer has spread. These may include lymph node biopsies, computed tomography (CT) scans, **magnetic resonance imaging** (MRI) scans, and barium swallows. In addition, standard preoperative blood and **liver function tests** are performed, and the candidate will meet with an anesthesiologist before the operation. The candidate should tell the anesthesiologist about all drug allergies and all medication (prescription, nonprescription, or herbal) that are presently being taken.

- What tests will be performed to determine if the cancer has spread?
- Which parts of the neck will be removed?
- How will a radical neck dissection affect daily activities after recovery?
- What is the likelihood that all of the cancer can be removed with a radical neck dissection?
- Are the involved lymph nodes on one or both sides of the neck?
- What will be the resulting appearance after surgery?
- How will my speech and breathing be affected?
- Is the surgeon board certified in otolaryngology head and neck surgery?
- How many radical neck procedures has the surgeon performed?
- What is the surgeon's complication rate?

Aftercare

A person who has had a radical neck dissection will stay in the hospital several days after the operation, and sometimes longer if surgery to remove the primary tumor was performed at the same time. Drains are inserted under the skin to remove the fluid that accumulates in the neck area. Once the drains are removed and the incision appears to be healing well, people are usually discharged from the hospital, but will require follow-up doctor visits. Depending on how many structures are removed, a person who has had a radical neck dissection may require physical therapy to regain use of the arm and shoulder.

Risks

The greatest risk in a radical neck dissection is damage to the nerves, muscles, and veins in the neck. Nerve damage can result in numbness (either temporary or permanent) to different regions on the neck and loss of function (temporary or permanent) to parts of the neck, throat, and shoulder. The more extensive the neck dissection, the more function a person is likely to lose. As a result, it is common following radical neck dissection for people to have stooped shoulders, limited ability to lift

one or both arms, and limited head and neck rotation and flexion due to the removal of nerves and muscles. Other risks are the same as for all major surgery: potential bleeding, infection, and allergic reaction to anesthesia.

Normal results

Normal lymph nodes are small and show no cancerous cells under a microscope. Abnormal lymph nodes may be enlarged and show malignant cells when examined under a microscope.

Morbidity and mortality rates

The mortality rate for radical neck dissection can be as high as 14%.

Morbidity rates are somewhat higher and are due to bleeding, post-surgery infection, and medicine errors.

Alternatives

Alternatives to radical neck dissection depend on the reason for the proposed surgery. Most alternatives are far less acceptable. Radiation and chemotherapy may be used instead of a radical neck dissection in the case of cancer. Alternatives for some surgical procedures may reduce scarring, but are not as effective in the removal of all pathological tissue. Chemotherapy and radiation or altered fractionated radiotherapy are reasonable alternatives.

See also Carotid endarterectomy; Parathyroidectomy; Thyroidectomy.

Resources

BOOKS

Bland, K. I., W. G. Cioffi, and M. G. Sarr. *Practice of General Surgery.* Philadelphia: Saunders, 2001.
Braunwald, E., D. L. Longo, and J. L. Jameson. *Harrison's Principles of Internal Medicine, 15th Edition.* New York: McGraw-Hill, 2001.
Goldman, L., and J. C. Bennett. *Cecil Textbook of Medicine, 21st Edition.* Philadelphia: Saunders, 1999.
Schwartz, S. I., J. E. Fischer, F. C. Spencer, G. T. Shires, and J. M. Daly. *Principles of Surgery, 7th edition.* New York: McGraw Hill, 1998.
Townsend, C., K. L. Mattox, R. D. Beauchamp, B. M. Evers, and D. C. Sabiston. *Sabiston's Review of Surgery, 3rd Edition.* Philadelphia: Saunders, 2001.

PERIODICALS

Agrama, M. T., D. Reiter, M. F. Cunnane, A. Topham, and W. M. Keane. "Nodal Yield in Neck Dissection and the Likelihood of Metastases." *Otolaryngology Head and Neck Surgery* 128, no.2 (2003): 185–190.
Cmejrek, R. C., J. M. Coticchia, and J. E. Arnold. "Presentation, Diagnosis, and Management of Deep-neck Abscess-

es in Infants." *Archives of Otolaryngology Head and Neck Surgery* 128, no.12 (2002): 1361–1364.

Ferlito, A., et al. "Is the Standard Radical Neck Dissection No Longer Standard?" *Acta Otolaryngolica* 122, no.7 (2002): 792–795.

Kamasaki, N., H. Ikeda, Z. L. Wang, Y. Narimatsu, and T. Inokuchi. "Bilateral Chylothorax Following Radical Neck Dissection." *International Journal of Oral and Maxillofacial Surgery* 32, no.1 (2003): 91–93.

Myers, E. N., and B. R. Gastman. "Neck Dissection: An Operation in Evolution: Hayes Martin Lecture." *Archives of Otolaryngology Head And Neck Surgery* 129, no.1 (2003): 14–25.

Ohshima, A., et al. "Is a Bilateral Modified Radical Neck Dissection Beneficial for Patients with Papillary Thyroid Cancer?" *Surgery Today* 32, no.12 (2002): 1027–1030.

Wang, L. F., W. R. Kuo, C. S. Lin, K. W. Lee, and K. J. Huang. "Space Infection of the Head and Neck." *Kaohsiung Journal of Medical Sciences* 18, no.8 (2002): 386–392.

ORGANIZATIONS

American College of Surgeons. 633 North St. Clair Street, Chicago, IL 60611-32311. (312) 202-5000, Fax: (312) 202-5001. E-mail: <postmaster@facs.org>. <http://www.facs.org>.

American Academy of Otolaryngology—Head and Neck Surgery. One Prince St., Alexandria, VA 22314-3357. (703) 836-4444. <http://www.entnet.org/index2.cfm>.

American Cancer Society. 1599 Clifton Road NE, Atlanta, GA 30329. (800) 227-2345. <http://www.cancer.org>.

American Osteopathic College of Otolaryngology—Head and Neck Surgery. 405 W. Grand Avenue, Dayton, OH 45405. (937) 222-8820 or (800) 455-9404, Fax: (937) 222-8840. info@aocoohns.org

OTHER

Amersham Health. [cited April 7, 2003] <http://www.amershamhealth.com/medcyclopaedia/Volume%20VI%202/neck%20dissection.asp>.

Baylor College of Medicine. [cited April 7, 2003] <http://www.bcm.tmc.edu/oto/grand/120293.html>.

Eastern Virginia Medical School. [cited April 7, 2003] <http://www.voice-center.com>.

Medical Algorithms Project. [cited April 7, 2003] <http://www.medal.org/docs_ch37/doc_ch37.23.html>.

Thyroid Cancer.Net. [cited April 7, 2003] <http://www.thyroid-cancer.net/topics/what+is+a+neck+dissection?CMS_Session=4ebe4755df4793bda647c0bf21fd977f>.

University of Washington Department of Surgery. [cited April 7, 2003] <http://depts.washington.edu/soar/abstract/ab16.htm>.

L. Fleming Fallon, Jr. MD, DrPH

Radical prostatectomy *see* **Open prostatectomy**

Radioimmunoassay *see* **Immunoassay tests**

Reconstructive surgery *see* **Plastic, reconstructive, and cosmetic surgery**

Recovery at home

Definition

Recovery at home after surgery may require certain dietary and environmental restrictions, recommended rest and limitations to physical activities, and other dos and don'ts as recommended by a physician or surgeon.

Purpose

Post-operative recovery at home should promote physical healing and rest and recovery from the stress of surgery. For patients who undergo orthopedic surgery, the home recovery period will also involve rehabilitation to regain diminished musculoskeletal functioning. Emotional and psychological recovery from life-altering surgeries may also begin during the home recovery period.

Description

When patients are discharged from either an ambulatory surgical facility or a hospital, they will receive written instructions from their physician on restrictions and recommendations for their post-operative recovery at home. A nurse will usually review these instructions verbally with the patient and answer any questions and concerns. They may also call one or up to several days after a surgical discharge to follow up on how the patient is feeling and answer any questions about home recovery.

Restrictions and recommendations outlined in home recovery instructions may include:

• Driving restrictions. A patient may be prohibited from driving for a period of time due to functional limitations or to medication that impairs driving ability.

• Work restrictions. Depending on the nature of a patient's job, they may be required to stay off of work or request alternate duties until recovery is complete.

• Social restrictions. Patients at high risk of complications from infection, such as an organ transplant patient, may be advised to avoid anyone with a cold or flu and to stay away from crowds or social gatherings during the initial recovery period.

• Medication recommendations. Prescription and/or over the counter drugs may be recommended on an as-needed basis for pain and nausea. Other drugs may also be required.

• Dietary limitations. Certain types of gastrointestinal procedures and other surgeries may require a restricted diet during the recovery period. Alcohol may also be prohibited, particularly if pain medication has been prescribed.

• Ambulation recommendations. The doctor will note if the patient should refrain from lifting heavy objects, climbing stairs, having sex, or participating in other potentially strenuous activities.

• **Exercise** recommendations. If movement, stretches, or exercise is encouraged as part of recovery, that fact will also be noted.

• **Incision care**. Patients are instructed on how to care for their incision and educated on signs of infection (i.e., redness, warmth, swelling, fever, odor).

• **Home care** needs. Some patients may require a visiting nurse or live-in health aid for a period of time as they recover from surgery.

• Adaptive equipment. Assistive or adaptive devices such as crutches, a walker, prosthetics, or bed or bathroom hand rails may be necessary.

• Follow-up with physician. A patient may be instructed to call the doctor's office to schedule a follow-up appointment. They should also be given criteria for warning signs and symptoms that may occur with their procedure, and when to call their physician if they do appear.

• Other required medical appointments. If a patient has undergone **orthopedic surgery** or another procedure that requires rehabilitation, he may need to see a physical therapist to regain range of motion, strength, and mobility. Depending on the type of surgery performed, the expertise of other medical professionals may also be required.

The postoperative period is also a time of emotional healing. Patients who face a long recovery and rehabilitation may feel depressed or anxious about their situation. Providing a patient with realistic goals and expectations for recovery both before and after the surgery can help them avoid feelings of failure or let down when things do not progress as quickly as they had hoped. Realistic recovery expectations can also prevent a patient from doing too much too early and potentially hindering the healing process.

Certain life-altering surgeries, such as an **amputation** or a mastectomy, carry their own set of emotional issues. Counseling, therapy, or participation in a patient support group may be an important part of post-operative recovery as a patient adjusts to their new life.

Preparation

Discharge recommendations for home recovery are typically explained to the patient before they are allowed to leave the hospital or ambulatory care facility. In some cases, the patient may be required to sign paperwork indicating that they have both received and understood home care instructions.

Depending on the surgical procedure they undergo, a patient may be taught some home care techniques while still in the hospital. Physical therapy exercises, incision care, and use of assistive devices such as crutches or splints are a few self-care skills that may be demonstrated and practiced in an inpatient environment.

A physical and emotional support system is also a crucial part of a successful home recovery. Faced with restrictions to movement, driving, and possibly more, a patient needs someone at home to assist them with the daily tasks of independent living. If family or friends are not nearby or available, a visiting nurse or home healthcare aid should be hired before the patient is discharged to home recovery.

KEY TERMS

Ambulation—To walk or move.

Ambulatory care—An outpatient facility; designed for patients who do not require inpatient hospital treatment or care.

Prosthetics—A custom-built artificial limb or other body part.

Orthopedic—Related to the musculoskeletal system, including the bones, joints, muscles, ligaments, and tendons.

Normal results

Following home care instructions can help to speed a patient's recovery time and ensure the safe resumption of normal activities. Several studies have indicated that women may have a longer postoperative recovery time than men. In some cases, the familiar, comforting home environment may even speed the healing process or improve the degree of recovery. One study of patients 64 and older undergoing hip surgery found that patients who were allowed to undergo rehabilitation at home had significantly better outcomes than those who underwent rehabilitation as hospital inpatients. On average, the former had better physical capacity and independent living skills when assessed six months after surgery.

Some studies have also indicated that gender may have an impact on the success and speed of post-operative home recovery. A 2001 study in the British Medical Journal found that women recovered from surgery at a 25% slower rate than men. Further research is needed to determine exactly why this gender gap exists, but the authors did hypothesize that both anatomical and physiological differences could be a factor.

Resources

BOOKS

Brubaker, Melinda, et al. *Surgery: A Patient's Guide from Diagnosis to Recovery.* San Francisco: UCFS Nursing Press, 1999.

Klippel, John H., ed. *All You Need to Know About Joint Surgery: Preparing for Surgery, Recovery, and an Active New Lifestyle.* Atlanta: Arthritis Foundation, 2002.

Trehair, RCS. *All About Heart Bypass Surgery.* Philadelphia: Oxford University Press, 2003.

PERIODICALS

Golub, Catherine. "Ready Yourself for Recovery: Tips for Pre- and Post-Op Nutrition." *Environmental Nutrition* 24 (November 2001): 2.

ORGANIZATIONS

National Association for Home Care and Hospice. 228 Seventh Street SE, Washington, DC 20003. (202) 547-7424. <http://www.nahc.org>.

Visiting Nurses Association of America. 99 Summer Street, Suite 1700, Boston, Massachusetts 02110. (617) 737-3200. <http://www.vnaa.org>.

Paula Ford-Martin

Recovery room

Definition

The recovery room, also called a post-anesthesia care unit (PACU), is a space a patient is taken to after surgery to safely regain consciousness from anesthesia and receive appropriate post-operative care.

Description

Patients who have had surgery or diagnostic procedures requiring anesthesia or sedation are taken to the recovery room, where their **vital signs** (e.g., pulse, blood pressure, temperature, blood oxygen levels) are monitored closely as the effects of anesthesia wear off. The patient may be disoriented when he or she regains consciousness, and the recovery room nursing staff will work to ease their anxiety and ensure their physical and emotional comfort.

The recovery room staff will pay particular attention to the patient's respiration, or breathing, as the patient recovers from anesthesia. A **pulse oximeter**, a clamp-like device that attaches to a patient's finger and uses infrared light to measure the oxygen saturation level of the blood, is usually used to assess respiratory stability. If the oxygen saturation level is too low, supplemental oxygen may be administered through a nasal cannula or face mask. Intravenous fluids are also frequently administered in the recovery room.

Because general anesthesia can cause a patient's core body temperature to drop several degrees, retaining body heat to prevent hypothermia and encourage good circulation is also an important part of recovery room care. Patients may be wrapped in blankets warmed in a heater or covered with a forced warm-air blanket system to bring body temperature back up to normal. They may also receive heated intravenous fluids.

The amount of time a patient requires in the recovery room will vary by surgical or diagnostic procedure and the type of anesthesia used. As the patient recovers

Rectal prolapse repair

KEY TERMS

Fast track—A protocol for post-operative patients with projected shorter recovery times. Fast-tracking a patient means that they will either bypass PACU completely, or spend a shorter time there with less intensive staff intervention and monitoring.

Hypothermia—Low core body temperature of 95°F (35°C) or less.

Nasal cannula—A piece of flexible plastic tubing with two small clamps that fit into the nostrils and provide supplemental oxygen flow.

from anesthesia, their post-operative condition is assessed by the recovery room nursing staff. A physician may order analgesic or antiemetic medication for any pain or nausea and vomiting, and the surgeon and/or anesthesiologist may come by to examine the patient.

Both hospitals and ambulatory surgical centers have recovery room facilities, which are generally located in close proximity to the **operating room**. A recovery room may be private, or it may be a large, partitioned space shared by many patients. Each patient bay, or space, is equipped with a variety of medical monitoring equipment. To keep the area sterile and prevent the spread of germs, outside visitors may be required to don a gown and cap or may be prohibited completely. Spouses or partners of women who are recovering after caesarean section and the parents of children recovering from surgery are typically excluded from any visitor prohibitions in the recovery room. In fact, parents are usually encouraged to be with their child in recovery to minimize any emotional trauma.

In some ambulatory surgery facilities, patients may have a different post-operative experience if they receive short-acting anesthetic drugs for their procedure. This protocol, known as "fast tracking," involves either shortening the time spent in the PACU or, if clinically indicated, bypassing the PACU altogether and sending the patient directly to what is known as a phase II step-down unit. A step-down unit is an "in between" transitional care area where patients can rest and recover before discharge with a lesser degree of monitoring and staff attention then in a PACU.

Normal results

After the effects of anesthesia have worn off completely and the patient's condition is considered stable, he or she will either be returned to their hospital room (for inpatient surgery) or discharged (for **outpatient**

surgery). Patients who are discharged will be briefed on post-operative care instructions to follow at home before they are released.

Resources

BOOKS

Hatfield, Anthea, and Michael Tronson. *The Complete Recovery Room Book, 3rd edition.* London: Oxford University Press, 2002.

PERIODICALS

Duncan, Peter, et al. "A Pilot Study of Recovery Room Bypass ("Fast-track Protocol") in a Community Hospital." *Canadian Journal of Anesthesia* 48 (2001): 630.

ORGANIZATIONS

American Society of Anesthesiologists. 520 N. Northwest Highway Park Ridge, IL 60068-2573. (847) 825-5586; Fax: (847) 825-1692. <http://www.asahq.org>.

Paula Ford-Martin

Rectal artificial sphincter *see* **Artificial sphincter insertion**

Rectal prolapse repair

Definition

Rectal prolapse repair surgery treats a condition in which the rectum falls, or prolapses, from its normal anatomical position because of a weakening in the surrounding supporting tissues.

Purpose

A prolapse occurs when an organ falls or sinks out of its normal anatomical place. The pelvic organs normally have tissue (muscle, ligaments, etc.) holding them in place. Certain factors, however, may cause those tissues to weaken, leading to prolapse of the organs. The rectum is the last out of six divisions of the large intestine; the anus is the opening from the rectum through which stool exits the body. A complete rectal prolapse occurs when the rectum protrudes through the anus. If rectal prolapse is present, but the rectum does not protrude through the anus, it is called occult rectal prolapse, or rectal intussusception. In females, a rectocele occurs when the rectum protrudes into the posterior (back) wall of the vagina.

Factors that are linked to the development of rectal prolapse include age, repeated childbirth, constipation, ongoing physical activity, heavy lifting, prolapse of other pelvic organs, and prior **hysterectomy**. Symptoms of rectal prolapse include protrusion of the rectum during and after defecation, fecal incontinence (inadvertent leakage of feces with physical activity), constipation, and rectal bleeding. Women may experience a vaginal bulge, vaginal pressure or pain, painful sexual intercourse, and lower back pain.

Demographics

The overall incidence of rectal prolapse in the United States is approximately 4.2 per 1,000 people. The incidence of the disorder increases to 10 per 1,000 among patients older than 65. Most patients with rectal prolapse are women; the ratio of male-to-female patients is one in six.

Description

Surgery is generally not performed unless the symptoms of the prolapse have begun to interfere with daily life. Because of the numerous defects that can cause rectal prolapse, there are more than 50 operations that may be used to treat the condition. A perineal or abdominal approach may be used. While abdominal surgery is associated with a higher rate of complications and a longer recovery time, the results are generally longer lasting. Perineal surgery is generally used for older patients who are unlikely to tolerate the abdominal procedure well.

Abdominal and laparoscopic approach

Rectopexy and anterior resection are the two most common abdominal surgeries used to treat rectal prolapse. The patient is usually placed under general anesthesia for the duration of surgery. During rectopexy, an incision into the abdomen is made, the rectum isolated from surrounding tissues, and the sides of the rectum lifted and fixed to the sacrum (lower backbone) with stitches or with a non-absorbable mesh. Anterior resection removes the S-shaped sigmoid colon (the portion of the large intestine just before the rectum); the two cut ends are then reattached. This straightens the lower portion of the colon and makes it easier for stool to pass. Rectopexy and anterior resection may also be performed in combination and may lead to a lower rate of prolapse recurrence.

As an alternative to the traditional laparotomy (large incision into the abdomen), laparoscopic surgery may be performed. **Laparoscopy** is a surgical procedure in which a laparoscope (a thin, lighted tube) and various instruments are inserted into the abdomen through small incisions. Rectopexy and anterior resection have been performed laparoscopically with good results. A patient's recovery time following laparoscopic surgery is

shorter and less painful than following traditional abdominal surgery.

Perineal approach

Perineal repair of rectal prolapse involves a surgical approach around the anus and perineum. The patient may be placed under general or regional anesthesia for the duration of surgery.

The most common perineal repair procedures are the Altemeier and Delorme procedures. During the Altemeier procedure (also called a proctosigmoidectomy), the prolapsed portion of the rectum is resected (removed) and the cut ends reattached. The weakened structures supporting the rectum may be stitched into their anatomical position. The Delorme procedure involves the resection of only the mucosa (inner lining) of the prolapsed rectum. The exposed muscular layer is then folded and stitched up and the cut edges of mucosa stitched together.

A rarely used procedure is anal encirclement. Also called the Thiersch procedure, anal encirclement involves the insertion of a thin circular band of non-absorbable material under the skin of the anus. This narrows the anal opening and prevents the protrusion of the rectum through the opening. This procedure, however, does not address the underlying condition and therefore is generally reserved for patients who are not good candidates for more invasive surgery.

Diagnosis/Preparation

Physical examination is most often used to diagnose rectal prolapse. The patient is asked to strain as if defecating; this increase in intra-abdominal pressure will maximize the degree of prolapse and aid in diagnosis. In some instances, imaging studies such as defecography (x rays taken during the process of defecation) may be administered to determine the extent of prolapse.

Before surgery, an intravenous (IV) line is placed so that fluid and/or medications may be easily administered to the patient. A Foley catheter will be placed to drain urine. **Antibiotics** are usually given to help prevent infection. The patient will be given a bowel prep to cleanse the colon and prepare it for surgery.

Aftercare

A Foley catheter may remain for one to two days after surgery. The patient will be given a liquid diet until normal bowel function returns. The recovery time following perineal repair is faster than recovery after abdominal surgery and usually involves a shorter hospital stay (one to three days following perineal surgery, three to seven days following abdominal surgery). The patient will be instructed to avoid activities for several weeks that will cause strain on the surgical site; these include lifting, coughing, long periods of standing, sneezing, straining with bowel movements, and sexual intercourse. High-fiber foods should be gradually added to the diet to avoid constipation and straining that could lead to prolapse recurrence.

Risks

Risks associated with rectal prolapse surgery include potential complications associated with anesthesia, infection, bleeding, injury to other pelvic structures, recurrent prolapse, and failure to correct the defect. Following a resection procedure, a leak may occur at the site where two cut ends of colon are reattached, requiring surgical repair.

Normal results

Most patients undergoing rectal prolapse repair will be able to return to normal activities, including work, within four to six weeks after surgery. The majority of patients will experience a significant improvement in symptoms and have a low chance of prolapse recurrence if heavy lifting and straining is avoided.

Morbidity and mortality rates

The approximate recurrence rates for the most commonly performed surgeries as reported by several studies are as follows:

• Altemeier procedure: 5–54%

• Delorme procedure: 5–26%

• anal encirclement: 25%

• rectopexy: 2–10%

• anterior resection: 7–9%

• rectopexy with anterior resection: 0–4%

• laparoscopic rectopexy

Abdominal surgeries are associated with a higher rate of complications than perineal repairs; rectopexy, for example, has a morbidity rate of 3–29%, and anterior resection a rate of 15–29%. The complication rate for combined rectopexy and anterior resection is slightly lower at 4–23%. Approximately 25% of patients undergoing anal encirclement will eventually require surgery to treat complications associated with the procedure.

Alternatives

There are currently no medical therapies available to treat rectal prolapse. In cases of mild prolapse where the rectum does not protrude through the anus, a high-fiber diet, stool softeners, enemas, or **laxatives** may help to avoid constipation, which may make the prolapse worse.

Resources

BOOKS

Feldman, Mark, et al. *Sleisenger & Fordtran's Gastrointestinal and Liver Disease.* 7th edition. Philadelphia: Elsevier Science, 2002.

Walsh, Patrick C., et al. *Campbell's Urology.* 8th edition. Philadelphia: Elsevier Science, 2002.

PERIODICALS

Felt-Bersma, Richelle J. F., and Miguel A. Cuesta. "Rectal Prolapse, Rectal Intussusception, Rectocele, and Solitary Rectal Ulcer Syndrome." *Gastroenterology Clinics* 30, no. 1 (March 1, 2001): 199–222.

ORGANIZATIONS

American Society of Colon and Rectal Surgeons. 85 W. Algonquin Rd., Suite 550, Arlington Heights, IL 60005. (847) 290-9184. <http://www.fascrs.org>.

OTHER

Flowers, Lynn K. "Rectal Prolapse." *eMedicine,* July 30, 2001. [cited April 9, 2003]. <http://www.emedicine.com/emerg/topic496.htm>.

Poritz, Lisa S. "Rectal Prolapse." *eMedicine,* February 6, 2003. [cited April 9, 2003]. <http://www.emedicine.com/med/topic3533.htm>.

Stephanie Dionne Sherk

Rectal resection

Definition

A rectal resection is the surgical removal of a portion of the rectum.

Purpose

Rectal resections repair damage to the rectum caused by diseases of the lower digestive tract, such as cancer, diverticulitis, and inflammatory bowel disease (ulcerative colitis and Crohn's disease). Injury, obstruction, and ischemia (compromised blood supply) may require rectal resection. Masses and scar tissue can grow within the rectum, causing blockages that prevent normal elimination of feces. Other diseases, such as diverticulitis and ulcerative colitis, can cause perforations in the rectum. Surgical removal of the damaged area can return normal rectal function.

Demographics

Colorectal cancer affects 140,000 people annually, causing 60,000 deaths. Incidence of the disease in 2001 differed among ethnic groups, with Hispanics having 10.2 cases per 100,000 people and African Americans having 22.8 cases per 100,000. Rectal cancer incidence is a portion of the total colorectal incidence rate. Surgery is the optimal treatment for rectal cancer, resulting in cure in 45% of patients. Recurrence due to surgical failure is low, from 4–8%, when the procedure is meticulously performed.

Crohn's disease and ulcerative colitis, both chronic inflammatory diseases of the colon, each affect approximate-

ly 500,000 young adults. Surgery is recommended when medication fails patients with ulcerative colitis. Nearly three-fourths of all Crohn's patients will require surgery to remove a diseased section of the intestine or rectum.

Description

During a rectal resection, the surgeon removes the diseased or perforated portion of the rectum. If the diseased or damaged section is not very large, the separated ends are reattached. Such a procedure is called rectal anastomosis.

Diagnosis/Preparation

Diagnostic tests

A number of tests identify masses and perforations within the intestinal tract.

- A lower GI (gastrointestinal) series is a series of x rays of the colon and rectum that can help identify ulcers, cysts, polyps, diverticuli (pouches in the intestine), and cancer. The patient is given a **barium enema** to coat the intestinal tract, making disease easier to see on the x rays.

- Flexible **sigmoidoscopy** involves insertion of a sigmoidoscope, a flexible tube with a miniature camera, into the rectum to examine the lining of the rectum and the sigmoid colon, the last third of the intestinal tract. The sigmoidoscope can also remove polyps or tissue for biopsy.

- A **colonoscopy** is similar to the flexible sigmoidoscopy, except the flexible tube examines the entire intestinal tract.

- Magnetic resonance imaging (MRI), used both prior to and during surgery, allows physicians to determine the precise margins for the resection, so that all of the diseased tissue can be removed. This also identifies patients who could most benefit from adjuvant therapy such as chemotherapy or radiation.

Preoperative preparation

To cleanse the bowel, the patient may be placed on a restricted diet for several days before surgery, then placed

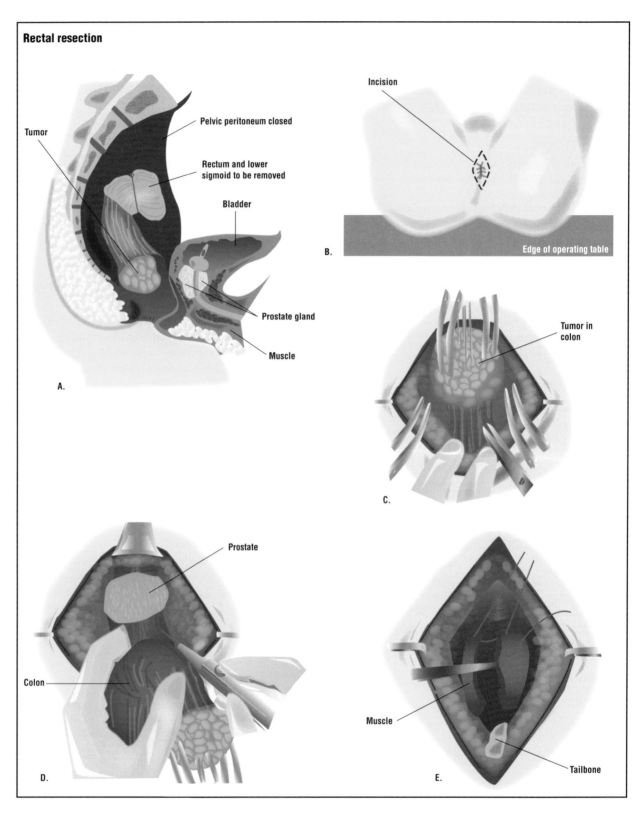

Rectal resection

A tumor in the rectum or lower colon can be removed by a rectal resection (A). An incision is made around the patient's anus (B). The tumor is pulled down through the incision (C). An attached area of the colon is also removed (D). The area is repaired, leaving an opening for bowel elimination (E). *(Illustration by GGS Inc.)*

on a liquid diet the day before, with nothing by mouth after midnight. A series of enemas and/or oral preparations (GoLytely, Colyte, or senna) may be ordered to empty the bowel. Oral anti-infectives (neomycin, erythromycin, or kanamycin sulfate) may be ordered to decrease bacteria in the intestine and help prevent post-operative infection. The operation can be done with an abdominal incision (laparotomy) or using minimally invasive techniques with small tubes to allow insertion of the operating instruments (**laparoscopy**).

Aftercare

Postoperative care involves monitoring blood pressure, pulse, respiration, and temperature. Breathing tends to be shallow because of the effect of the anesthesia and the patient's reluctance to breathe deeply due to discomfort around the surgical incision. The patient is taught how to support the incision during deep breathing and coughing, and given pain medication as necessary. Fluid intake and output is measured, and the wound is observed for color and drainage.

Fluids and electrolytes are given intravenously until the patient's diet can be resumed, starting with liquids, then adding solids. The patient is helped out of bed the evening of the surgery and allowed to sit in a chair. Most patients are discharged in two to four days.

Risks

Rectal resection has potential risks similar those of other major surgeries. Complications usually occur while the patient is in the hospital and the patient's general health prior to surgery will be an indication of the risk potential. Patients with heart problems and stressed immune systems are of special concern. Both during and following the procedure, the physician and nursing staff will monitor the patient for:

- excessive bleeding
- wound infection
- thrombophlebitis (inflammation and blood clot in the veins in the legs)
- pneumonia
- pulmonary embolism (blood clot or air bubble in the lungs' blood supply)
- cardiac stress due to allergic reaction to the general anaesthetic

Symptoms that the patient should report, especially after discharge, include:

- increased pain, swelling, redness, drainage, or bleeding in the surgical area
- flu-like symptoms such as headache, muscle aches, dizziness, or fever

---

QUESTIONS TO ASK THE DOCTOR

- Am I a good candidate for laparoscopic surgery?
- What kinds of preoperative tests will be required?
- What medications will be given for pain relief after the surgery?
- What will I need to do to prepare for surgery?
- What will my recovery time be and what restrictions will I have?

- increased abdominal pain or swelling, constipation, nausea or vomiting, or black, tarry stools

Normal results

Complete healing is expected without complications. The recovery rate varies, depending on the patient's overall health prior to surgery. Typically, full recovery takes six to eight weeks.

Morbidity and mortality rates

Mortality has decreased from nearly 28% to under 6%, through the use of prophylactic **antibiotics** before and after surgery.

Alternatives

If the section of the rectum to be removed is very large, the rectum may not be able to be reattached. Under those circumstances, a **colostomy** would be preformed. The distal end of the rectum would be closed and left to atrophy. The proximal end would be brought through an opening in the abdomen to create an opening, a stoma, for feces to be removed from the body.

Resources

BOOKS

Johnston, Lorraine. *Colon & Rectal Cancer: A Comprehensive Guide for Patients and Families.* Sebastopol, CA: O'Reilly, 2000.

Levin, Bernard. *American Cancer Society Colorectal Cancer.* New York: Villard, 1999.

PERIODICALS

Beets-Tan, R. G. H., et al. "Accuracy of Maganetic Resonance Imaging in Prediction of Tumour-free Resection Margin in Rectal Cancer Surgery." *The Lancet* 357 (February 17, 2001): 497.

KEY TERMS

Adjuvant therapy—Treatment used to increase the effectiveness of surgery, usually chemotherapy or radiation used to kill any cancer cells that might be remaining.

Anastomosis—The surgical connection of two sections of tubes, ducts, or vessels.

Diverticuli—Pouches in the intestinal wall usually created from a diet low in fiber.

Enema—Insertion of a tube into the rectum to infuse fluid into the bowel and encourage a bowel movement. Ordinary enemas contain tap water, mixtures of soap and water, glycerine and water, or other materials.

Intestine—Commonly called the bowels, divided into the small and large intestine. They extend from the stomach to the anus. The small intestine is about 20 ft (6 m) long. The large intestine is about 5 ft (1.5 m) long.

Ischemia—A compromise in blood supply delivered to body tissues that causes tissue damage or death.

Sigmoid colon—The last third of the intestinal tract that is attached to the rectum.

Schwenk, Wolfgang. "Pulmonary Function Following Laparoscopic or Conventional Colorectal Resection: A Randomized Controlled Evaluation." *Journal of the American Medical Association* 281 (April 7, 1999): 1154.

Walling, Anne D. "Follow-up After Resection for Colorectal Cancer Saves Lives. (Tips from Other Journals)." *American Family Physician* 66 (August 1, 2002): 485.

ORGANIZATIONS

American Board of Colon and Rectal Surgery (ABCRS). 20600 Eureka Road, Suite 713, Taylor, MI 48180. (734) 282-9400. <http://www.fascrs.org>.

Mayo Clinic. 200 First St. S.W., Rochester, MN 55905. (507) 284-2511. <http://www.mayoclinic.org>.

Janie Franz

Red blood cell indices

Definition

Red blood cell (RBC) indices are calculations derived from the **complete blood count** that aid in the diagnosis and classification of anemia.

Purpose

Red blood cell indices help classify types of anemia, a decrease in the oxygen carrying capacity of the blood. Healthy people have an adequate number of correctly sized red blood cells containing enough hemoglobin to carry sufficient oxygen to all the body's tissues. Anemia is diagnosed when either the hemoglobin or **hematocrit** of a blood sample is too low.

Description

Measurements needed to calculate RBC indices are the red blood cell count, hemoglobin, and hematocrit. The hematocrit is the percentage of blood by volume that is occupied by the red cells. The three main RBC indices are:

- Mean corpuscular volume (MCV). The average size of the red blood cells expressed in femtoliters (fl). MCV is calculated by dividing the hematocrit (as percent) by the RBC count in millions per microliter of blood, then multiplying by 10.

- Mean corpuscular hemoglobin (MCH). The average amount of hemoglobin inside an RBC expressed in picograms (pg). The MCH is calculated by dividing the hemoglobin concentration in grams per deciliter by the RBC count in millions per microliter, then multiplying by 10.

- Mean corpuscular hemoglobin concentration (MCHC). The average concentration of hemoglobin in the RBCs expressed as a percent. It is calculated by dividing the hemoglobin in grams per deciliter by the hematocrit, then multiplying by 100.

The mechanisms by which anemia occurs will alter the RBC indices in a predictable manner. Therefore, the RBC indices permit the physician to narrow down the possible causes of an anemia. The MCV is an index of the size of the RBCs. When the MCV is below normal, the RBCs will be smaller than normal and are described as microcytic. When the MCV is elevated, the RBCs will be larger than normal and are termed macrocytic. RBCs of normal size are termed normocytic.

Failure to produce hemoglobin results in smaller than normal cells. This occurs in many diseases, including iron deficiency anemia, thalassemia (an inherited disease in which globin chain production is deficient), and anemias associated with chronic infection or disease. Macrocytic cells occur when division of RBC precursor cells in the bone marrow is impaired. The most common causes of macrocytic anemia are vitamin B_{12} deficiency, folate deficiency, and liver disease. Normocytic anemia may be caused by decreased production (e.g., malignancy and other causes of bone marrow failure), increased destruction (hemolytic anemia), or blood loss. The RBC count is low, but the size and amount of hemoglobin in the cells are normal.

A low MCH indicates that cells have too little hemoglobin. This is caused by deficient hemoglobin production. Such cells will be pale when examined under the microscope and are termed hypochromic. Iron deficiency is the most common cause of a hypochromic anemia. The MCH is usually elevated in macrocytic anemias associated with vitamin B_{12} and folate deficiency.

The MCHC is the ratio of hemoglobin mass in the RBC to cell volume. Cells with too little hemoglobin are lighter in color and have a low MCHC. The MCHC is low in microcytic, hypochromic anemias such as iron deficiency, but is usually normal in macrocytic anemias. The MCHC is elevated in hereditary spherocytosis, a condition with decreased RBC survival caused by a structural protein defect in the RBC membrane.

Cell indices are usually calculated from tests performed on an automated electronic cell counter. However, these counters measure the MCV, which is directly proportional to the voltage pulse produced as each cell passes through the counting aperture. Electronic cell counters calculate the MCH, MCHC, hematocrit, and an additional parameter called the red cell distribution width (RDW).

The RDW is a measure of the variance in red blood cell size. It is calculated by dividing the standard deviation (a measure of variation) of RBC volume by the MCV and multiplying by 100. A large RDW indicates abnormal variation in cell size, termed anisocytosis. The RDW aids in differentiating anemias that have similar indices. For example, thalassemia minor and iron deficiency anemia are both microcytic and hypochromic anemias, and overlap in MCV and MCH. However, iron deficiency anemia has an abnormally wide RDW, but thalassemia minor does not.

Diagnosis/Preparation

RBC indices require 3–5 mL of blood collected by vein puncture with a needle. A nurse or phlebotomist usually collects the sample.

Aftercare

Discomfort or bruising may occur at the puncture site. Pressure to the puncture site until the bleeding stops reduces bruising; warm packs relieve discomfort. Some people feel dizzy or faint after blood has been drawn and should be allowed to lie down and relax until they are stable.

Risks

Other than potential bruising at the puncture site, and/or dizziness, there are no complications associated

KEY TERMS

Anemia—A variety of conditions in which a person's blood cannot carry as much oxygen as is needed by the tissues.

Hypochromic—A descriptive term applied to a red blood cell with a decreased concentration of hemoglobin.

Macrocytic—A descriptive term applied to a larger than normal red blood cell.

Mean corpuscular hemoglobin (MCH)—A calculation of the average weight of hemoglobin in a red blood cell.

Mean corpuscular hemoglobin concentration (MCHC)—A calculation of the average concentration of hemoglobin in a red blood cell.

Mean corpuscular volume (MCV)—A measure of the average volume of a red blood cell.

Microcytic—A descriptive term applied to a smaller than normal red blood cell.

Normochromic—A descriptive term applied to a red blood cell with a normal concentration of hemoglobin.

Normocytic—A descriptive term applied to a red blood cell of normal size.

Red cell distribution width (RDW)—A measure of the variation in the size of red blood cells.

with this test. However, certain prescription medications may affect the test results. These drugs include zidovudine (Retrovir), phenytoin (Dilantin), and azathioprine (Imuran). When the hematocrit is determined by centrifugation, the MCV and MCHC may differ from those derived by an electronic cell counter, especially in anemia. Plasma trapped between the RBCs tends to cause an increase in the hematocrit, giving rise to a somewhat higher MCV and lower MCHC.

Normal results

Normal results for red blood cell indices are as follows:

• MCV: 80–96 fl
• MCH: 27–33 pg
• MCHC: 33–36%
• RDW: 12–15%

Resources

BOOKS

Chernecky, Cynthia C., and Barbara J. Berger. *Laboratory Tests and Diagnostic Procedures*. 3rd edition. Philadelphia: W. B. Saunders Company, 2001.

Henry, J.B. *Clinical Diagnosis and Management by Laboratory Methods*. 20th ed. Philadelphia: W. B. Saunders Company, 2001.

Kee, Joyce LeFever. *Handbook of Laboratory and Diagnostic Tests*. 4th edition. Upper Saddle River, NJ: Prentice Hall, 2001.

Wallach, Jacques. *Interpretation of Diagnostic Tests*. 7th edition. Philadelphia: Lippincott Williams & Wilkens, 2000.

OTHER

National Institutes of Health. [cited April 5, 2003]. <http://www.nlm.nih.gov/medlineplus/encyclopedia.html>.

Victoria E. DeMoranville
Robert Harr
Mark A. Best

Red blood cell test *see* **Hemoglobin test**

Regional anesthetic *see* **Anesthesia, local**

Remote surgery *see* **Telesurgery**

Renal transplant *see* **Kidney transplantation**

Reoperation

Definition

Reoperation is a term used by surgeons for the duplication of a surgical procedure. Repeating surgery may involve surgery at the same site, at another site for the same condition, or to repair a feature from a previous surgery.

Purpose

Success for most surgical procedures depends, in large part, upon the lack of a need to repeat the surgery. However, failure of some feature of a procedure may be only one of many reasons that reoperation is necessary. Reasons for repeat surgery depend upon surgical skills, as well as the reason for the primary surgery. Some diseases and conditions necessitate or make probable repeating the operation.

Cancer

Surgeries for cancer are sometimes repeated because a new tumor or more surrounding tissue has been affected by the original malignancy. This is often the case with breast surgery for cancer that involves breast conservation management. Often it is necessary to re-excise the site of the previously bioped primary cancer. In the case of breast cancer, only 50% of re-excision specimens show residual tumors. If cancer cells are found with the re-excision, this may change the treatment protocol. Colon cancer sometimes involves more surgeries to resect newly affected areas beyond the previous primary site.

Coronary artery surgery

Currently, about 10% of coronary artery procedures are reoperations due to the progression of the disease into native vessels between operations, as well as to treat diseased vein grafts. The mortality associated with reoperation is significantly higher than that of the original bypass procedures. In one study, patients undergoing their first coronary artery bypass graft (CABG) had a mortality rate of 1.7% versus 5.2% for elective reoperation.

Orthropedic surgeries

Arthroplasty—the operative restoration of a joint like the elbow, knee, hip, or shoulder, often involve components that need to be repaired. Infections of the joint may also require reoperation with the complete removal of all prostheses and cement. Re-implantation is repeated after a six-week course of **antibiotics**. Other bone surgeries that have a high reoperation rate are back surgeries, including spinal surgeries involving discectomy in which discs are fused together to reduce pain. Due to scaring or infection, there may be a need for reoperation. As the frequency of repeat back surgeries increases, the chance of a satisfactory result drops precipitously.

Gastrointestinal surgeries

Crohn's disease surgeries are often repeated. Operations that cut and stitch only the area of obstruction, called strictureplasty, often have repeat operations if the affected area is the small intestine. Another gastrointestinal surgery that often requires reoperation is fundoplication or flap wrapping of the lower part of the esophagus to prevent the reflux of acid from the stomach back into the esophagus. Folding the loose valve that had prevented reflux in such a way as to tighten its ability to close treats a condition known as gastroesophageal reflux disease (GERD). The surgery has a high failure rate of between 30% after five years and 63% after 10 years. Reoperation may be required because of surgical failure, breakdown of tissue, injury to nearby organs, or an excessively wrapped fundus leading to trouble swallowing.

Vasectomy and penile prostheses

These surgeries often have complications that lead to reoperation, largely due to surgical failure.

Normal results

In general, reoperation, or the repeat of a surgical procedure at the same site, is more difficult and involves more risks that the original procedure. It requires more operative time; more blood is lost; and the incidences of infection and clots are higher. Advancements in design and improvements in cementing techniques for component failure in arthroplasty have improved the results of reoperation.

Resources

OTHER

"Gastroesophageal Reflux Disease and Heartburn." *MD Consult* <http://www.MDConsult.com.>.
"Inflammatory Bowel Disease (Crohn's Disease and Ulcerative Colitis)." *MD Consult* <http://www.MDConsult.com.>.
"Vasectomy and Vasovasotomy: Comprehensive Version." *MD Consult* <http://www.MDConsult.com.>.

Nancy McKenzie, PhD

Replantation of digits *see* **Finger reattachment**

Replantation, tooth *see* **Tooth replantation**

Retinal cryopexy

Definition

Retinal cryopexy, also called retinal **cryotherapy**, is a procedure that uses intense cold to induce a chorioretinal scar and to destroy retinal or choroidal tissue.

Purpose

The retina is the very thin membrane in the back of the eye that acts like the "film" in a camera. It is held against the inside back portion of the eye by pressure from fluid within the eye. In the front part of the eye, the retina is firmly attached at a ring just behind the lens called the pars plana. In the back part of the eye, the retina is continuous with the optic nerve. In between the pars plana and the optic nerve the retina has no fixed attachments. The retina collects information from the images projected on it from the eye lens and sends it along the optic nerve to the brain, where the information is interpreted and experienced as sight.

Several disorders can affect the retina and retinal cryopexy is used to treat the following conditions:

• retinal breaks or detachments

• retinal ischemia (retinal tissue that lacks oxygen)

• neovascularization (proliferation of blood vessels in the retina)

• Coats' disease (abnormal retinal blood vessels that cause loss of vision)

• retinoblastoma (intraocular tumors)

Demographics

Disease and disorders affecting the retina cause the majority of the visual disability and blindness in the United States. Retinal detachment occurs in one in 10,000 Americans each year, with middle-aged and older individuals being at higher risk than the younger population. Coats' disease usually affects children, especially boys, in the first 10 years of life, but it can also affect young adults. The condition affects central vision, typically in only one eye. Severity can range from mild vision loss to total retinal detachment and blindness. No cause has yet been identified for Coats' disease. According to the National Cancer Institute, retinoblastoma accounts for approximately 11% of cancers developing in the first year of life, and for 3% of the cancers developing among children younger than 15 years. In the United States, approximately 300 children and adolecents below the age of 20 are diagnosed with retinoblastoma each year. The majority of cases occur among young children, with 63% of all retinoblastoma occurring before the age of two years.

Description

Usually, retinal cryopexy is administered under local anesthesia. The procedure involves placing a metal probe against the eye. When a foot pedal is depressed, the tip of the cryopexy probe becomes very cold as a result of the rapid expansion of very cold gases (usually nitrous oxide) within the probe tip. When the probe is placed on the eye the formation of water crystals followed by rapid thawing results in tissue destruction. This is followed by healing and scar tissue formation.

In the case of retinal detachment, treatment calls for irritating the tissue around each of the retinal tears. Cryopexy stimulates scar formation, sealing the edges of the tear. This is typically done by looking into the eye using the indirect ophthalmoscope while pushing gently on the outside of the eye using the cryopexy probe, producing a small area of freezing that involves the retina and the tissues immediately underneath it. Using multiple small freezes like this, each of the tears is surrounded. Irritated tissue forms a scar, which brings the retina back into contact with the tissue underneath it.

Diagnosis/Preparation

The earlier the retinal disorder diagnosis is confirmed, the greater the chance of successful outcome. Diagnosis is based on symptoms and a thorough examination of the retina. An ophthalmoscope is used to examine the retina. This is a small, hand-held instrument consisting of a battery-powered light and a series of lenses that is held up to the eye. The ophthalmologist is able to see the retina and check for abnormalities by shining the light into the eye and looking through the lens. Eye drops are placed in the eyes to dilate the pupils and help visualization. Afterwards, an indirect ophthalmoscope is used. This instrument is worn on the specialist's head, and a lens is held in front of the patient's eye. It allows a

better view of the retina. Examination with a slit lamp microscope may also be done. This microscope enables the ophthalmologist to examine the different parts of the eye under magnification. After instilling drops to dilate the pupil, the slit lamp is used to detect retinal tears and detachment. A visual acuity test is also usually performed to assess vision loss. This test involves reading letters from a standard eye chart.

Additional diagnostic procedures are used in the case of Coats' disease and retinoblastoma. Ultrasonography helps in differentiating Coats' disease from retinoblastoma. CT scan may be used to characterize the intraocular features of Coats' disease. MRI is another very useful diagnostic tool used to distinguish retinoblastoma from Coats' disease.

Aftercare

After the procedure, patients are taken to a **recovery room**, and observed for 30–60 minutes. Tylenol or pain medication is usually given. Healing typically takes 10–14 days. Vision may be blurred briefly, and the operated eye is usually red and swollen for some time following cryopexy. Cold compresses applied to the eyelids relieve some of the discomfort. Most patients are able to walk the day after surgery and are discharged from the hospital within a week. After discharge, patients are advised to gently cleanse their eyelids every morning, and as necessary, using warm tap water and cotton balls or tissues. Day surgery patients are usually allowed to go home two hours after the surgery is complete.

Risks

Risks involved in retinal cryopexy include infection, perforation of the eye with the anesthetic needle, bleeding, double vision, and glaucoma. All of these complications however, are quite uncommon.

Normal results

If treated early, the outcome of cryopexy for Coats' disease may be successful in preventing progression and in some cases can improve vision, but this is less effective if the retina has completely detached. For retinal reattachments, the retina can be repaired in about 90% of cases. Early treatment almost always improves the vision of most patients with retinal detachment. Some patients, however, require more than one cryopexy procedure to repair the damage.

Morbidity and mortality rates

Survival rates for children with retinoblastoma are favorable, with more than 93% alive five years after diagnosis. Males and females have similar five-year survival rates for the period 1976–1994, namely 93 and 94% respectively. African American children had slightly lower survival rates (86%) than Caucasian children (94%).

Alternatives

Several alternatives to retinal cryopexy are available, depending on the condition being treated. A few examples include:

- Laser photocoagulation. This type of surgery induces a therapeutic effect by destroying outer retinal tissue, thus reducing the oxygen requirements of the retina, and increasing oxygen delivery to the remaining retina through alterations in oxygen diffusion from the choroid. It is used for repairing retinal tears.

- Pneumatic retinopexy. This procedure is used to reattach retinas. After numbing the eye with a local anesthesia, the surgeon injects a small gas bubble into the inside of the eye. The bubble presses against the retina, flattening it against the back wall of the eye. Since the gas rises, this treatment is most effective for detachments located in the upper portion of the eye.

- Scleral buckle. With this technique, a tiny sponge or silicone band is attached to the outside of the eye, pressing inward and holding the retina in position. After removing the vitreous gel from the eye (vitrectomy), the surgeon seals a few areas of the retina into position with laser or cryotherapy.

- Radiation therapy. For neuroblastomas, this treatment uses high-energy radiation to kill or shrink cancer cells.

- Chemotherapy. Another alternative for neuroblastoma. Chemotherapy uses drugs to kill cancer cells. The drugs are delivered through the bloodstream, and spread throughout the body to the cancer site.

KEY TERMS

Chorioretinal—Relating to the choroid coat of the eye and retina.

Choroid—Middle layer of the eye, between the retina and sclera.

Coats' disease—Also called exudative retinitis, a chronic abnormality characterized by the deposition of cholesterol on the outer retinal layers.

Ophthalmoscope—An instrument for viewing the interior of the eye, particularly the retina. Light is thrown into the eye by a mirror (usually concave), and the interior is then examined with or without the aid of a lens.

Retina—Light-sensitive layer of the eye.

Retinoblastoma—Malignant tumor of the retina.

Sclera—The tough white outer coat of the eyeball.

See also Cryotherapy.

Resources

BOOKS

Packer, A. J., ed. *Manual of Retinal Surgery.* Boston: Butterworth-Heinemann, 2001.

Schepens, C. L., M. E. Hartnett, and T. Hirose, eds. *Schepens's Retinal Detachment and Allied Diseases.* Boston: Butterworth-Heinemann, 2000.

Wong, D. and A. H. Chignell. *Management of Vitreo-Retinal Disease: A Surgical Approach.* New York: Springer Verlag, 1999.

PERIODICALS

Anagnoste, S. R., I. U. Scott, T. G. Murray, D. Kramer, and S. Toledano. "Rhegmatogenous retinal detachment in retinoblastoma patients undergoing chemoreduction and cryotherapy." *American Journal of Ophthalmology* 129 (June 2000): 817–819.

Palner, E. A., et al. "Cryotherapy for Retinopathy of Prematurity Cooperative Group. Multicenter trial of cryotherapy for retinopathy of prematurity: ophthalmological outcomes at 10 years." *Archives of Ophthalmology* 119 (2001): 1110–1118.

Steel, D. H., J. West, and W. G. Campbell. "A randomized controlled study of the use of transscleral diode laser and cryotherapy in the management of rhegmatogenous retinal detachment." *Retina* 20 (2000): 346–357.

Veckeneer, M., K. Van Overdam, D. Bouwens, E. Feron, D. Mertens, et al. "Randomized clinical trial of cryotherapy versus laser photocoagulation for retinopexy in conventional retinal detachment surgery." *American Journal of Ophthalmology* 132 (September 2001): 343–347.

ORGANIZATIONS

American Academy of Ophthalmology. P.O. Box 7424, San Francisco, CA 94120-7424. (415) 561-8500. <http://www.aao.org/index.html>.

New England Ophthalmological Society (NEOS). P.O. Box 9165, Boston, MA 02114. (617) 227-6484. <http://www.neos-eyes.org/>.

OTHER

University Ophthalmology Consultants. "What is cryotherapy?" <http://www.umdnj.edu/eyeweb/faqs/cryo.html>.

Monique Laberge, PhD

Retinal detachment surgery *see* **Scleral buckling**

Retropubic suspension

Definition

Retropubic suspension refers to the surgical procedures used to correct incontinence by supporting and stabilizing the bladder and urethra. The Burch procedure, also known as retropubic urethropexy procedure or Burch colosuspension, and Marshall-Marchetti-Krantz procedure (MMK) are the two primary surgeries for treating stress incontinence. The major difference between these procedures is the method for supporting the bladder. The Burch procedure uses sutures to attach the urethra and bladder to muscle tissue in the pelvic area. MMK uses sutures to attach these organs to the pelvic cartilage. Laparoscopic retropubic surgery can be performed with a video laparoscope through small incisions in the belly button and above the pubic hairline.

Purpose

The urinary system expels a quart and a half of urine per day. The amount of urine produced depends upon diet and medications taken, as well as **exercise** and loss of water due to sweating. The ureters, two tubes connecting the kidneys and the bladder, pass urine almost continually and when the bladder is full the brain sends a signal to the bladder to relax and let urine pass from the bladder to the urethra. People who are continent control the release of urine from the urethra via the sphincter muscles. These two sets of muscles act like rubber bands to keep the bladder closed until a conscious decision is made to urinate. The intrinsic sphincter or urethral sphincter muscles keep the bladder closed and the extrinsic sphincter mus-

cles surround the urethra and prevent leakage. Incontinence is common when either the urethra lacks tautness and stability (genuine stress urine incontinence, SUI) and/or the sphincter muscles are unable to keep the bladder closed (intrinsic sphincter deficiency, ISD).

Incontinence occurs in many forms with four primary types related to anatomic, neurological, dietary, or disease, or injury.

Stress incontinence

The most frequent form of incontinence is stress incontinence. This relates to leakage of the urethra with activity that puts stress on the abdominal muscles. The primary sign of stress incontinence is this leakage at sneezing, coughing, exercise, or other straining activities, which indicates a lack of support for the urethra due to weakened muscles, fascia, or ligaments. Pressure from the abdomen with movement, like exercising, uncompensated by tautness or stability in the urethra, causes the urethra to be displaced or mobile leading to leakage. Essentially, this hypermobility of the urethra is an indication that it is moving down or herniating through weakened pelvic structures.

To diagnose incontinence and determine treatment, three grades of severity for stress incontinence are used.

• Type I: Moderate movement of the urethra, with no hernia or cystocele.

• Type II: Severe or hypermobility in the urethra of more than 0.8 in (2 cm), with or without decent of the urethra into pelvic structures.

• Type III: Hypermobility of the urethra where the primary source of incontinence is the inability of the sphincter muscles to keep the bladder closed. This is due to weakness or deficiency in the intrinsic sphincter muscles.

Urge incontinence

Urge incontinence relates to the frequent need to urinate and may involve going to the bathroom every two hours. Accidents are common when not reaching a bath-

Retropubic suspension

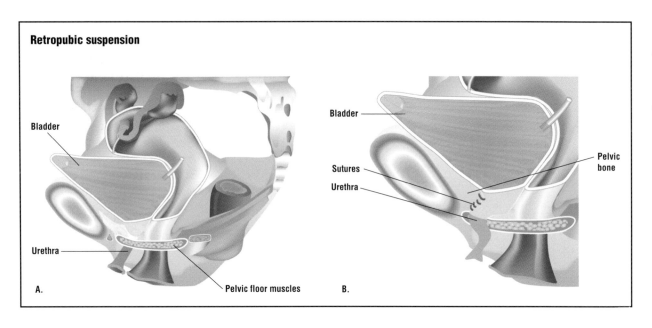

Weak pelvic floor muscles (A) can cause stress incontinence. In a retropubic suspension, the neck of the bladder is elevated and stitched to the pubic bone to hold it in place (B). *(Illustration by GGS Inc.)*

room in time. Urge incontinence is not due to general changes in the urethra or supporting muscles. It is often linked to other disorders that produce muscle spasms in the bladder, such as infections. Urge incontinence can also be due to underlying illnesses like stroke, spinal cord injury, multiple sclerosis and Alzheimer's disease, which cause detrusor hyperflexia—the contracting of the bladder muscle responsible for sending urine from the bladder to the urethra. Urge incontinence is very common in the elderly, especially those in long term care facilities.

Mixed incontinence

Mixed incontinence is a combination of stress incontinence and urge incontinence, especially in older women. Since each form of incontinence pertains to different functions or anatomy, it is very important to distinguish which part of the incontinence is to be treated by surgery.

Overflow incontinence

Overflow incontinence results in leakage from a bladder that never completely empties due to weakened bladder muscles. Overflow incontinence is involuntary and not accompanied by the urge to urinate. Many causes exist for overflow incontinence, including weak bladder muscles due to diabetes, nerve damage, or a blocked urethra. Men are more frequently affected than women.

Demographics

Over 15 million Americans have urinary incontinence and women comprise 85% of all cases. It affects 25% of women of reproductive age and 50% of women past menopause. Due to the female anatomy, women have twice the risk for stress incontinence compared to men. In addition, childbirth places pressure and burden on the pelvic muscles that often weaken with age, thereby weakening urethra stability. Women are more prone to surgeries for urological changes than men and severe urinary incontinence is often associated with these surgeries as well as hysterectomies. The majority of women with incontinence have stress incontinence or mixed incontinence. Male incontinence occurs primarily in response to blockage in the prostate or after prostate surgery. It is usually treated with implants and/or an artificial sphincter insert.

Description

There are a variety of retropubic suspension surgeries available to treat stress incontinence. The variations differ by the types of structures used to support the urethra and bladder. In all procedures, parts of the pelvic anatomy (pubic bone, ligaments) serve as an anchor or wall upon which the urethra is tacked for stability. The surgery is called a suspension surgery because it stabilizes the urethra from tilting by suspending it against a part of the pelvic anatomy. The Burch procedure is often performed when other surgery is needed such as repair of the urethra for cystoceles and urethral reconstruction. However, this procedure is the most difficult of the anti-incontinent surgeries and is more common in mild forms of stress incontinence where intrinsic sphincter deficiency is not present.

The Burch procedure can be done through open abdominal surgery, which requires a long incision at the bikini line, or surgery performed through the vagina. The patient, in stirrups, receives general anesthesia. Within the retropubic area, the anterior vaginal wall is separated from the bladder manually. The bladder neck is identified and old adhesions or fatty tissues are removed. The neck of the bladder is sutured to pubic ligaments where it will form adhesions and thereby gain stability. The surgeon examines for bladder injury and the surgery is completed. Urethral position is tested by placing a cotton-tipped swab in the urethra and measuring the angle. With abdominal surgery or vaginal surgery a catheter may be put in place by the surgeon for postoperative voiding and to decrease the risks of infection. A suction drain may be placed in the retropubic space for bleeding. The drain is removed one to three days after surgery.

Recently, laparoscopic surgery has been used to perform retropubic suspensions. Laparoscopic surgery requires only three or four 0.25-in (0.6-cm) incisions in the belly button, pubic hairline, or groin area and uses small instruments without opening the abdominal cavity. Shorter healing time is involved with this procedure, the hospital stay is usually not more than 24 hours and recovery to normal activities takes about seven to 14 days. However, the Burch procedure performed using laparoscopic techniques requires great skill on the part of the surgeon and research indicates that the results may not be as long lasting as those developed with abdominal or vaginal surgery.

Diagnosis/Preparation

A patient with incontinence may have multiple factors that induce transient or chronic incontinence. It is crucial that the physician obtain a complete history, physical, clinical, neurological, and medication evaluation of the patient, as well as a radiographic assessment before continuing urological tests aimed at a surgical so-

lution. The specific indications for the Burch colosuspension procedure or its variants is the correction of stress urinary incontinence. This can be a patient who also requires abdominal surgery that cannot be performed vaginally, like **hysterectomy** or sigmoid surgery, as well as patients who have SUI without ISD.

A urodynamic study with a point pressure leak test will allow a diagnosis to be made that can distinguish the patient who has a hypermobile urethra from the patient who also has ISD. The point pressure leak test, also known as the Valsalva leak test, measures the amount of abdominal pressure required to induce leakage. The patient is asked to cough or strain in order to encourage leakage. The point at which the patient leaks helps determine if stress incontinence with ISD contribution is present. Obese patients and patients that engage in high impact exercise regimens are not considered good candidates for retropubic suspension.

Aftercare

Patients with open retropubic procedures are given pain medication postoperatively that is tapered down over the next two days. A suprapubic catheter stays in place for approximately five days with voiding difficulties encountered initially in many patients. Patients with laparoscopic suspensions are reported to have less blood loss during surgery, less postoperative narcotic requirements, and shorter hospital stays. Patients are expected to refrain from strenuous activity for three months and to have a follow-up visit within three weeks after surgery.

Risks

As with any major abdominal or pelvic surgical procedures, complications that may occur after a retropubic suspension include bleeding; injury to the bladder, urethra, and ureters; wound infection; and blood clots. Specific to the Burch procedure are complications that involve urethral obstruction because of urethral kinking due to elevation of the vagina or bladder base. Postoperative voiding difficulties are common and depend upon the suture tension of the urethral axis. Corrective surgery and the release of the urethra to a more anatomic position resolves voiding issues with a very high rate of success. Vaginal prolapse is also a risk of this procedure.

Normal results

The patient can expect more than 80–90% cure or great improvement in their incontinence. There is a large body of literature documenting the success of the Burch procedure. Published research shows a cure rate ranging from 63–93%, according to the actual version of colo-suspension used. Laparoscopic surgery has not produced the long term results that open surgery has and there is the possibility that the fibrosis (adhesion) necessary for a successful outcome does not occur as easily with the laparoscopic procedure. Patients not carefully screened out for ISD will not have a high level of success with the Burch procedure since the source of the incontinence will not have been treated. Sling procedures are recommended for patients with ISD instead of colosuspension surgery.

Morbidity and mortality rates

The Burch procedure may aggravate vaginal wall weakness or vaginal prolapse. This incident varies between 3% and 17%. Research on the Marshall-Marchetti-Krantz procedure pertaining to 2,712 patients found a complication rate of 21%, with wound complications and infections making up the majority, 5.5% and 3.9% respectively. Direct wound injury occurred in 1.6% and obstructions in 0.3% overall.

Alternatives

General or simple severe stress incontinence related primarily to weakening of the urethral support can be remedied with changes in diet, weight loss, and certain behavioral and rehabilitative measures. These include:

• Regular, daily exercising of the pelvic muscles called Kegel exercises, requiring 30–200 contractions a day for eight weeks.

• Biofeedback to gain awareness and control of pelvic muscles.

• Vaginal weight training in which small weights are inserted in the vagina to tighten vaginal muscles.

• Mild electrical stimulation to increase contractions in pelvic muscles.

• Bladder retraining in which the patient is taught how to resist the urge to urinate and expand the intervals between urinations.

There are also medications that can facilitate continence for those experiencing stress or urge incontinence. These include some kinds of antidepressants, although the mechanism of action is not quite understood, as well as antispasmodic medication and estrogen therapy. Finally, should behavioral, rehabilitative, and surgical procedures fail, there remain alternatives through the use of vaginal cones and urethral plugs that can be inserted and removed by the patient.

See also Needle neck suspension; Sling procedure.

KEY TERMS

Genuine urinary stress incontinence (USI)— Stress incontinence due to hypermobility of the urethra.

Intrinsic sphincter deficiency (ISD)—A factor in severe stress incontinence due to the inadequacy of the sphincter muscles to keep the bladder closed.

Retropubic urethropexy—A generic term for the Burch procedure and its variants that treat mild stress incontinence by stabilizing the urethra with retropubic surgery.

Stress incontinence—Leakage of urine upon movements that put pressure on the abdominal muscles such as coughing, sneezing, laughing, or exercise. One of four types of incontinence.

Urethra hypermobility—Main factor in stress urinary incontinence, with severity based upon how far the urethra has descended into the pelvic floor through herniation or cystocele.

Resources

BOOKS

Walsh, Patrick. *Campbell's Urology.* 8th ed. Elsevier Science, 2000.

PERIODICALS

Liu, C. Y. "Laparoscopic Treatment of Stress Urinary Incontinence." *Obstetrics and Gynecology Clinics of North America* 26, no. 1 (March 1999): 149-67.

Melton, Lisa. "Targeted Treatment for Incontinence Beckons." *Lancet* 359, no. 9303 (January 2002): 326.

Smoger, S. H., T. L. Felice, and G. H. Kloecker. "Urinary Incontinence Among Male Veterans Receiving Care in Primary Care Clinics." *Annals of Internal Medicine* 132, no. 7 (April 4, 2000): 547-551.

Stoffel, J. T., J. Bresette, and J. J. Smith. "Retropubic Surgery for Stress Urinary Incontinence." *Urologic Clinics of North America* 29, no. 3 (August 2002).

Weber, A. M., and M. D. Walters. "The Burch and Sling Procedures are Similarly Effective for Surgical Treatment of Genuine Stress Urinary Incontinence." *Evidence-based Obstetrics & Gynecology* 4, no. 1 (March 2002).

ORGANIZATIONS

American Foundation for Urologic Diseases. The Bladder Health Council, 1128 North Charles Street, Baltimore, MD 21201. (410) 468-1800. <http://www.afud.org/education/bladder.html>.

National Kidney and Urologic Diseases Information Clearinghouse. 3 Information Way, Bethesda, MD 20892-3580.

---

(800) 891-5390 or (301) 654-4415. <http://www.niddk.
nih.gov>.

The Simon Foundation for Continence, P.O. Box 835, Wilmette, IL 60091. (800) 23-SIMON or (847) 864-3913.
<http://www.simonfoundation.org>.

OTHER

Bladder Control in Women. National Kidney and Urologic Disease Information Clearinghouse. NIH Publication no. 97-
4195. May 2002 [cited May 12, 2003]. < http://www.
niddk.nih.gov/health/urolog/uibcw/bcw/bcw.htm>.

Ginsberg, David. "Trends in Surgical Therapy for Stress Urinary Incontinence." American Urological Association
97th Annual Meeting, WebMD Conference Coverage.
2002 [cited May 12, 2003]. <http://www.medscape.com/
viewarticle/437091>.

Hendrix, Susan L., and S. Gene McNeeley. "Urinary Incontinence and Menopause: Update on Evidence-Based Treatment." *Medscape,* October 28, 2002 [cited May 12, 2003].
<http://www.medscape.com/view program/2052>.

Nancy McKenzie, PhD

Rh typing *see* **Type and screen**

Rhinoplasty

Definition

The term rhinoplasty means "nose molding" or
"nose forming." It refers to a procedure in plastic surgery
in which the structure of the nose is changed. The change
can be made by adding or removing bone or cartilage,
grafting tissue from another part of the body, or implanting synthetic material to alter the shape of the nose.

Purpose

Rhinoplasty is most often performed for cosmetic
reasons. A nose that is too large, crooked, misshapen,
malformed at birth, or deformed by an injury can be
given a more pleasing appearance. If breathing is impaired due to the form of the nose or to an injury, it can
often be improved with rhinoplasty.

Demographics

Rhinoplasty is the third most common cosmetic procedure among both men and women. Total number of
rhinoplasty procedures in the United States in 1999 was
133,058. More than 13,100 of those procedures were
performed on men.

WHO PERFORMS THE PROCEDURE AND WHERE IS IT PERFORMED?

Simple rhinoplasty is usually performed in an
outpatient surgery center or in the surgeon's office. Most procedures take only an hour or two,
and patients go home right away. Complex procedures may be performed in a hospital and require a short stay.

Rhinoplasty is usually performed by a surgeon with advanced training in plastic and reconstructive surgery.

Description

The external nose is composed of a series of interre-
lated parts that include the skin, the bony pyramid, cartilage, and the tip of the nose, which is composed of cartilage and skin. The strip of skin separating the nostrils is
called the columella.

Surgical approaches to nasal reconstruction are varied. Internal rhinoplasty involves making all incisions
from inside the nasal cavity. The external, or "open,"
technique involves a skin incision across the base of the
nasal columella. An external incision allows the surgeon
to expose the bone and cartilage more fully and is most
often used for complicated procedures. During surgery,
the surgeon will separate the skin from the bone and cartilage support. The framework of the nose is then reshaped in the desired form. Shape can be altered by removing or adding bone, cartilage, or skin. The remaining
skin is then replaced over the new framework. If the procedure requires adding to the structure of the nose, the
donated bone, cartilage, or skin can come from another
location on the patient's body or from a synthetic source.

When the operation is completed, the surgeon will
apply a splint to help the bones maintain their new
shape. The nose may also be packed, or stuffed with a
dressing, to help stabilize the septum.

When a local anesthetic is used, light sedation is
usually given first, after which the operative area is
numbed. It will remain insensitive to pain for the length
of the surgery. A general anesthetic is used for lengthy or
complex procedures, or if the doctor and patient agree
that it is the best option.

Diagnosis/Preparation

The quality of the skin plays a major role in the outcome of rhinoplasty. Persons with extremely thick skin

Rhinoplasty

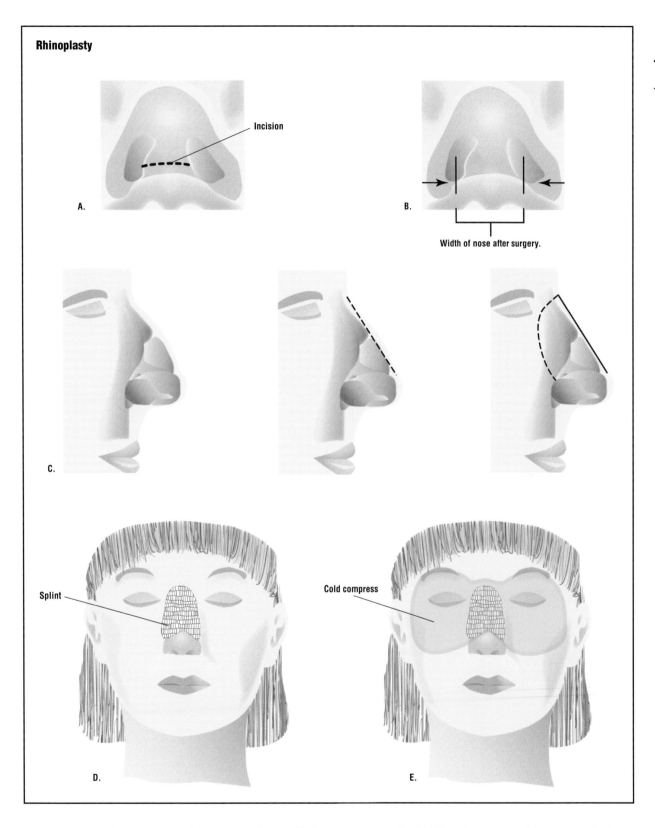

During an open rhinoplasty, an incision is made in the skin between the nostrils (A). Closed rhinoplasty involves only incisions inside the nose. Rhinoplasty may involve a change in nostril width (B) or removal of a hump on the nose (C) using bone sculpting. After surgery, a splint supports the nose (D), and a cold compress reduces swelling (E). *(Illustration by GGS Inc.)*

may not see a significant change in the underlying bone structure after surgery. On the other hand, thin skin provides almost no cushion to hide many minor bone irregularities or imperfections.

Rhinoplasty should not be performed until the pubertal growth spurt is complete, ages 14–15 for girls and older for boys.

During the initial consultation, the candidate and surgeon will determine what changes can be made in the shape of the nose. Most doctors take photographs during that consult. The surgeon will also explain the techniques and anesthesia options available to the candidate.

The candidate and surgeon should also discuss guidelines for eating, drinking, smoking, taking or avoiding certain medications, and washing the face for the weeks immediately following surgery.

Aftercare

Patients usually feel fine immediately after surgery. As a precaution, most surgery centers do not allow patients to drive themselves home after an operation.

The first day after surgery, there will be some swelling of the face. Persons should stay in bed with their heads elevated for at least a day. The nose may hurt and a headache is common. The surgeon will prescribe medication to relieve these conditions. Swelling and bruising around the eyes will increase for a few days, but will begin to diminish after about the third day. Slight bleeding and stuffiness are normal, and vary according to the extent of the surgery performed. Most people are walking in two days, and back to work or school in a week. No strenuous activities are allowed for two to three weeks.

Patients are given a list of postoperative instructions, which include requirements for hygiene, **exercise**, eating, and follow-up visits to the doctor. Patients should not blow their noses for the first week to avoid disruption of healing. It is extremely important to keep the surgical dressing dry. Dressings, splints, and stitches are removed in one to two weeks. Patients should avoid excessive sun or sunburn.

Risks

Any type of surgery carries a degree of risk. There is always the possibility of unexpected events such as an infection or a reaction to the anesthesia.

When the nose is reshaped or repaired from inside, the scars are not visible. If the surgeon needs to make the incision on the outside of the nose, there will be some slight scarring. In addition, tiny blood vessels may burst, leaving small red spots on the skin. These spots are barely visible, but may be permanent.

Normal results

The best candidates for rhinoplasty are those persons with relatively minor deformities. Nasal anatomy and proportions are quite varied and the final look of any rhinoplasty operation depends on a person's anatomy, as well as the surgeon's skill.

A cosmetic change of the nose will change a person's appearance, but it will not change self-image. A person who expects a different lifestyle after rhinoplasty is likely to be disappointed.

The cost of rhinoplasty depends on the difficulty of the work required and on the specialist chosen. If the problem was caused by an injury, insurance will usually cover the cost. A rhinoplasty done only to change a person's appearance is not usually covered by insurance.

Morbidity and mortality rates

Death from a rhinoplasty procedure is exceedingly rare. When it occurs, the cause is often due to an adverse reaction to anesthesia or postoperative medications or to an infection. About 10% of persons receiving rhinoplasty require a second procedure.

Alternatives

The alternative to cosmetic rhinoplasty is to accept oneself, literally, at face value. Persons contemplating rhinoplasty may want to question some of the conventional standards of beauty and work on their body image issues to improve their self-confidence.

See also Blepharoplasty; Forehead lift.

KEY TERMS

Cartilage—Firm supporting tissue that does not contain blood vessels.

Columella—The strip of skin running from the tip of the nose to the upper lip, which separates the nostrils.

Septum—The dividing barrier in the center of the nose.

Resources

BOOKS

Engler, Alan M. *BodySculpture: Plastic Surgery of the Body for Men and Women,* 2nd Edition. Poughkeepsie, NY: Hudson Pub, 2000.

Irwin, Brandith, and Mark McPherson. *Your Best Face: Looking Your Best without Plastic Surgery.* Carlsbad, CA: Hay House, Inc, 2002.

Man, Daniel, and L. C. Faye. *New Art of Man: Faces of Plastic Surgery: Your Guide to the Latest Cosmetic Surgery Procedures, 3rd Edition.* New York: BeautyArt Press, 2003.

Papel, I. D., and S. S. Park. *Facial Plastic and Reconstructive Surgery, 2nd Edition.* New York: Thieme Medical Publishers, 2000.

PERIODICALS

Ahn, M. S., C. S. Maas, and N. Monhian. "A Novel, Conformable, Rapidly Setting Nasal Splint Material: Results of a Prospective Study." *Archives of Facial Plastic Surgery* 5, no.2 (2003): 189–192.

Bagal, A. A., and P. A. Adamson. "Revision Rhinoplasty." *Facial Plastic Surgery* 18, no.4 (2002): 233–244.

Lascaratos, J. G., J. V. Segas, C. C. Trompoukis, and D. A. Assimakopoulos. "From the Roots of Rhinology: The Reconstruction of Nasal Injuries by Hippocrates." *Annals of Otolology Rhinology and Laryngology* 112, no.2 (2003): 159–162.

Rohrich, R. J., and A. R. Muzaffar. "Rhinoplasty in the African-American Patient." *Plastic and Reconstructive Surgery* 111, no.3 (2003): 1322–1339.

Russell, P., and C. Nduka. "Digital Photography for Rhinoplasty." *Plastic and Reconstructive Surgery* 111, no.3 (2003): 1266–1267.

ORGANIZATIONS

American Board of Plastic Surgery. Seven Penn Center, Suite 400, 1635 Market Street, Philadelphia, PA 19103-2204. (215) 587-9322. <http://www.abplsurg.org/>.

American College of Plastic and Reconstructive Surgery. <http://www.breast-implant.org>.

American College of Surgeons. 633 North Saint Claire Street, Chicago, IL 60611. (312) 202-5000. <http://www.facs.org/>.

American Society for Aesthetic Plastic Surgery. 11081 Winners Circle, Los Alamitos, CA 90720. (800) 364-2147 or (562) 799-2356. <http://www.surgery.org/>.

American Society for Dermatologic Surgery. 930 N. Meacham Road, P.O. Box 4014, Schaumburg, IL 60168-4014. (847) 330-9830. <http://www.asds-net.org>.

American Society of Plastic and Reconstructive Surgeons. 44 E. Algonquin Rd., Arlington Heights, IL 60005. (847) 228-9900. <http://www.plasticsurgery.org>.

American Society of Plastic Surgeons. 444 E. Algonquin Rd., Arlington Heights, IL 60005. (888) 475-2784. <http://www.plasticsurgery.org/>.

OTHER

American Academy of Facial and Reconstructive Plastic Surgery. [cited April 9, 2003]. <http://www.facial-plastic-surgery.org/patient/procedures/rhinoplasty.html>.

National Library of Medicine. [cited April 9, 2003]. <http://www.nlm.nih.gov/medlineplus/plasticcosmeticsurgery.html>.

Restoration of Appearance Trust. [cited April 9, 2003]. <http://www.raft.ac.uk/plastics/rhinoplasty.html>.

Revision Rhinoplasty. [cited April 9, 2003]. <http://www.revisionrhinoplasty.net/>.

L. Fleming Fallon, Jr. MD, DrPH

Rhizotomy

Definition

Rhizotomy is the cutting of nerve roots as they enter the spinal cord.

Purpose

Rhizotomy (also called dorsal rhizotomy, selective dorsal rhizotomy, and selective posterior rhizotomy) is a treatment for spasticity that is unresponsive to less invasive procedures.

Demographics

Spasticity (involuntary muscle contraction) affects many thousands of Americans, but very few are affected seriously enough to require surgery for its treatment.

Description

Rhizotomy is performed under general anesthesia. The patient lies face down. An incision is made along the lower spine, exposing the sensory nerve roots at the center the spinal cord. Individual nerve rootlets are electrically stimulated. Since these are sensory nerves, they should not stimulate muscle movement. Those that do (and therefore cause spasticity) are cut. Typically, one-quarter to one-half of nerve rootlets tested are cut.

Diagnosis/Preparation

Rhizotomy is performed on patients with spasticity that is insufficiently responsive to oral medications or injectable therapies (botulinum toxin, phenol, or alcohol). It is most commonly performed for those patients with lower extremity spasticity that interferes with walking or severe spasticity that prevents hygiene or positioning of the legs. It is most commonly performed on children with cerebral palsy.

Patients undergoing rhizotomy receive a large battery of tests before the procedure, in order to document the functional effects of spasticity, and the patient's medical health and likely response to anesthesia and other operative stresses. Rhizotomy is performed as an in-patient procedure, and the patient is likely to require an overnight hospital stay before the operation.

Aftercare

After surgery, the patient will spend one to several days in the hospital. Physical therapy and strength training usually begin the next day, in order to maximize the gains expected from surgery, and to keep the limbs mobile. Medication may be given for pain.

Risks

Rhizotomy carries small but significant risks of nerve damage, permanent loss of sensation or altered sensation, weakness of the lower extremities, bowel and bladder dysfunction, increased likelihood of hip dislocation, and scoliosis progression. Anesthesia carries its own risks.

Normal results

Rhizotomy reduces spasticity, which should allow more normal gait and improve mobility. Patients may require fewer walking aids, such as walkers or crutches.

Morbidity and mortality rates

Other than the risks from anesthesia, rhizotomy does not carry a risk of death during surgery. Morbidity rates vary among centers performing the surgery. Persistent and significant adverse effects may occur in 1–5% of patients, including bowel or bladder changes and low back pain.

Alternatives

Other spasticity treatments include oral medications and an implanted pump delivering baclofen to the space around the spinal cord (intrathecal baclofen). These may be appropriate alternatives for some patients. **Orthopedic surgery** can correct deformities that occur from untreated spasticity. Some controversy exists whether rhizotomy can delay or prevent the need for other spasticity procedures, especially orthopedic surgery such as **tenotomy**, with some evidence suggesting it can, and other evidence suggesting it may not.

Resources

ORGANIZATIONS

United Cerebral Palsy. 1660 L Street, NW, Suite 700, Washington, DC 20036. (800) 872-5827 or (202)776-0406. TTY: (202) 973-7197. Fax: (202) 776-0414. webmaster@ ucp.org. <http://www.UCP.org>.
WE MOVE. <http://www.wemove.org>.

Richard Robinson

Rhytidoplasty *see* **Face lift**

Robot-assisted surgery

Definition

Robot-assisted surgery involves the use of a robot under the direction and guidance of a surgeon.

Purpose

Robot-assisted surgery provides many benefits in the surgical care of patients. Computer-assisted robots provide exact motion and trajectories to minimize the side-effects of surgical intervention. Surgeon-guided robotics allow the surgeon to access patient anatomy with smaller incisions.

Demographics

Patients undergoing surgical procedures classified as **neurosurgery**, **orthopedic surgery**, radio surgery and radiotherapy, prostatectomy, endoscopy, **laparoscopy**, cardiac surgery and craniofacial surgery may experience robot-assisted surgical techniques.

Description

Neurosurgery

A high level of accuracy is required when operating on the brain to avoid damage to the sensitive brain tissue. Biopsies and minor interventions are best assisted by the robotic device. Interventions include drilling into the skull and making an incision through the dura mater to gain brain tissue samples, empty cysts, or eliminate hemorrhage.

Orthopedic surgery

Applications such as cementless hip-replacement, total knee arthroplasties, and pedicle screw placement can benefit for the more accurate cutting and drilling provided by a robot. Femur bone-cutting devices provide improved drilling to carve a cavity in the bone for prosthesis implant. Pins inserted into the bone before surgery are used as landmarks for computerized tomography (CT) imaging. The CT image provides the surgeon with the necessary information for choosing an implant. The surgeon removes the head from the femur bone, eliminating the joint. The leg is secured in position and the robot is brought into po-

sition. A high speed cutter is then applied to create the cavity, and then followed by a smoothing tool. The surgeon manually inserts the implant into the femur and completes the cap implant into the pelvic bone.

Radiosurgery and radiotherapy

Radiation treatment is provided by a robot. The CT image or magnetic resonance image (MRI) is used to determine where the radiation treatment should be delivered. The robot aligns with patient anatomy, delivering specific doses of radiation to the intended location.

Prostatectomy

Removal of all or part of the prostate is another robot-assisted procedure. The robot controls instruments inserted through the urethra to the prostate gland. A diathermic hot wire cutting loop is guided to remove tissue in an appropriate pattern around the urethra. Fastening the guiding frame to the upper legs of the patient secures the device for accurate guidance.

Endoscopy

Endoscopy is used to examine patient cavities for the presence of polyps, tumors, and other disease states. The endoscope can be better passed through cavities such as the colon or trachea. Three-dimensional images of the cavity are obtained and used to dictate the path that will be taken to pass the endoscope. Sedation and heavy analgesia can be avoided.

Laparoscopy

In laparoscopic surgeries, three to four small incisions are made in the abdominal or thoracic cavity to insert the instruments and video equipment. The surgeon performs the operation from a remote console that provides the human machine interface. The console provides video monitoring images that are three dimensional. Joysticks are used to manipulate the tools within the chest cavity to complete the surgical procedure.

Cardiac surgery

Robots are being used in the coronary artery bypass grafting surgeries and cardiac valve replacement and repair surgeries. The harvesting of artery and vein grafts can also be accomplished with the aid of laparoscopic techniques.

Craniofacial surgery

Difficult bone cuts and bone tumor removals are accomplished successfully using robotic instruments. Preplanned trajectories are programmed into the machine. Precision cuts are made in the manner desired to achieve an esthetical and satisfactory result. As the surgeon manipulates the saw, he or she is guided along the path by a predetermined trajectory determined during an initial run on a model of the surgical site.

Aftercare

The patient should expect a faster recovery then that achieved by traditional surgery procedures.

Risks

With some of these procedures, a longer surgical time is required to achieve the same desired outcome as the traditional surgical approach. There is an increased risk of anesthesia related complications as surgical times increase. Additionally, if the robotic procedure is not completed successfully, the surgeon may need to complete the procedure with a traditional technique.

Normal results

Results for each procedure are comparable to or better than the standard surgical procedure.

Morbidity and mortality rates

Complications should be comparable to the standard surgical procedure, and even reduced. Some complications may only be associated with the robot-assisted procedure.

Alternatives

Alternative treatment is to use a traditional surgical approach without the use of robot assistance.

Arthoplastic—Manufactured replacement joint.

Cardiac surgery—Surgery performed on the heart.

Craniofacial surgery—Surgery of the facial tissue and skull.

Endoscopy—Used to visualize internal structures of the body, such as the trachea, esophagus or intestines.

Laparascopy—Surgery on internal structures through small incisions and visualized with the laparoscope.

Neurosurgery—Surgery performed on the brain.

Orthopedic surgery—Surgery performed on the bones. May include joint replacements and surgery of the vertebrae.

Prostatectomy—Performed for the treatment of prostate disease including prostate cancer.

Radio surgery and radiotherapy—Used in the treatment of cancerous growths or kidney stones.

Resources

PERIODICALS

Rembold, Ulrich, and Catherina Burghart. "Surgical Robotics: An Introduction." *Journal of Intelligent Robotic Systems* 30 (2001): 1–28.

Allison Joan Spiwak, MSBME

Root canal treatment

Definition

Root canal treatment, also known as endodontic treatment, is a dental procedure in which the diseased or damaged pulp (central core) of a tooth is removed and the inside areas (the pulp chamber and root canals) are filled and sealed.

Purpose

An inflamed or infected pulp is called pulpitis. It is the most common cause of a toothache. To relieve the pain and prevent further complications, the tooth may be extracted (surgically removed) or saved by root canal treatment.

Demographics

Root canal treatment has become a common dental procedure. According to the American Association of Endodontists, more than 14 million root canal treatments are performed every year, with a 95% success rate.

Description

Inside the tooth, the pulp of a tooth is comprised of soft tissue that contains the blood supply, by which the tooth receives its nutrients; and the nerve, by which the tooth senses hot and cold. This tissue is vulnerable to damage from deep dental decay, accidental injury, tooth fracture, or trauma from repeated dental procedures such as multiple fillings or restorations over time. If a tooth becomes diseased or injured, bacteria may build up inside the pulp, spreading infection from the natural crown of the tooth to the root tips in the jawbone. Pus accumulating at the ends of the roots can form a painful abscess that can damage the bone supporting the teeth. Such an infection may produce pain that is severe, constant, or throbbing. It can also result in prolonged sensitivity to heat or cold, swelling, and tenderness in the surrounding gums, facial swelling, or discoloration of the tooth. In some cases, however, the pulp may die so gradually that there is little noticeable pain.

Root canal treatment is performed under local anesthesia. A thin sheet of rubber, called a rubber dam, is placed in the mouth and around the base of the tooth to isolate the tooth and help to keep the operative field dry. The dentist removes any tooth decay and makes an opening through the natural crown of the tooth into the pulp chamber. Creating this access also relieves the pressure inside the tooth and can dramatically ease pain.

The dentist determines the length of the root canals, usually with a series of x rays. Small wire-like files are then used to clean the entire canal space of diseased pulp tissue and bacteria. The debris is flushed out with large amounts of water (irrigation). The canals are also slightly enlarged and shaped to receive an inert (non-reactive) filling material called gutta percha. However, the tooth is not filled and permanently sealed until it is completely free of active infection. The dentist may place a temporary seal, or leave the tooth open to drain, and prescribe an antibiotic to counter any spread of infection from the tooth. This is why root canal treatment may require several visits to the dentist.

Once the canals are completely clean, they are filled with gutta percha and a sealer cement to prevent bacteria from entering the tooth in the future. A metal post may be placed in the pulp chamber for added structural sup-

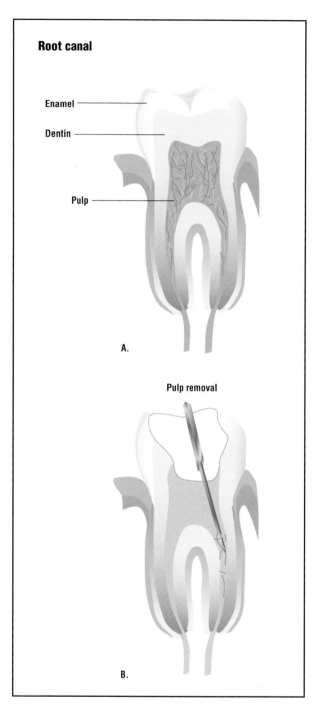

During a root canal, the diseased pulp of a tooth (A), is removed (B). The remaining empty tooth is filled and sealed with a filling or crown. *(Illustration by GGS Inc.)*

port and better retention of the crown restoration. The tooth is protected by a temporary filling or crown until a permanent restoration may be made. This restoration is usually a gold or porcelain crown, although it may be a gold inlay, or an amalgam or composite filling (paste fillings that harden).

Diagnosis/Preparation

Signs that a root canal treatment is necessary include severe pain while chewing, prolonged sensitivity to heat or cold, or a darkening of the tooth. Swelling and tenderness of the gums or pimples appearing on the gums are also common symptoms. However, it is also possible that no symptoms will be noticed. The dentist will take an x ray of the tooth to determine if there is any sign of infection in the surrounding bone.

Aftercare

Once a root canal treatment is performed, the recipient must have a crown placed over the tooth to protect it. The cost of the treatment and the crown may be expensive. However, replacing an extracted tooth with a fixed bridge, a removable partial denture, or an implant to maintain the space and restore the chewing function is typically even more expensive.

During the time when **antibiotics** are being used, care should be taken to avoid using the tooth to chew food. The tooth has been structurally weakened and may break, or there is a possibility of the interior of the tooth becoming reinfected.

If the tooth feels sensitive following the procedure, a standard over-the-counter pain medication such as ibuprofen or naproxen may be taken. This sensitivity will fade after a few days. In most cases the patient can resume regular activity the following day.

Risks

There is a possibility that a root canal treatment will not be successful the first time. If infection and inflammation recur and an x ray indicates a repeat treatment is feasible, the old filling material is removed and the canals are thoroughly cleaned out. The dentist will try to identify and correct problems with the first root canal treatment before filling and sealing the tooth a second time.

In cases where an x ray indicates that another root canal treatment cannot correct the problem, endodontic surgery may be performed. In a procedure called an apicoectomy, or root resectioning, the root end of the tooth is accessed in the bone, and a small amount is shaved away. The area is cleaned of diseased tissue and a filling is placed to reseal the canal.

Normal results

With successful root canal treatment, the tooth will no longer cause pain. However, because it does not contain an internal nerve, it no longer has sensitivity to hot, cold, or sweets. Because these are signs of dental decay, the root canal recipient must receive regular dental check-ups with periodic x rays to avoid further disease in the tooth. The restored tooth may last a lifetime. However, with routine wear, the filling or crown may eventually need to be replaced.

Morbidity and mortality rates

In some cases, despite proper root canal treatment and endodontic surgery, the tooth dies and must be extracted. This is relatively uncommon.

Alternatives

The only alternative to performing a root canal procedure is to extract the diseased tooth. After restoration or extraction, the two main goals are to allow normal chewing and to maintain proper alignment band spacing between teeth. A fixed bridge, a removable partial denture or an implant will accomplish both goals. However, these are usually more expensive than a root canal treatment.

Resources

BOOKS

Peterson, L. J., E. Ellis, J. R. Hupp, and M. R. Tucker. *Contemporary Oral and Maxillofacial Surgery, 4th edition.* Amsterdam: Elsevier, 2002.

KEY TERMS

Abscess—A cavity or space in tooth or gum tissue filled with pus as the result of infection. Its swelling exerts pressure on the surrounding tissues, causing pain.

Apicoectomy—Also called root resectioning. The root tip of a tooth is accessed in the bone and a small amount is shaved away. The diseased tissue is removed and a filling is placed to reseal the canal.

Crown—The natural crown of a tooth is that part of the tooth covered by enamel. Also, a restorative crown is a protective shell that fits over a tooth.

Endodontic—Pertaining to the inside structures of the tooth, including the dental pulp and tooth root, and the periapical tissue surrounding the root.

Endodontist—A dentist who specializes in the diagnosis and treatment of disorders affecting the inside structures of teeth.

Extraction—The surgical removal of a tooth from its socket in a bone.

Gutta percha—An inert, latex-like substance used for filling root canals.

Pulp—The soft innermost layer of a tooth, containing blood vessels and nerves.

Pulp chamber—The area within the natural crown of a tooth occupied by dental pulp.

Pulpitis—Inflammation of the pulp of a tooth involving the blood vessels and nerves.

Root canal—The space within a tooth that runs from the pulp chamber to the tip of the root.

Root canal treatment—The process of removing diseased or damaged pulp from a tooth, then filling and sealing the pulp chamber and root canals.

Tronstad, L. *Clinical Endodontics: A Textbook 2nd edition.* New York: Thieme Medical Publishers, 2003.

Walton, R. E. and M. Torabinejad. *Principles and Practice of Endodontics, 3rd edition.* Philadelphia: Saunders, 2001.

Wray, D. *Textbook of General and Oral Surgery.* Amsterdam: Elsevier, 2003.

PERIODICALS

Bader, H. I. "Treatment Planning for Implants versus Root Canal Therapy: A Contemporary Dilemma." *Implant Dentistry* 11, no. 3 (2002): 217–223.

Buchanan, L. S. "Negotiating Root Canals to their Termini." *Dentistry Today* 19, no. 11(2000): 60–71.

Douglass, A. B., and J. M. Douglass. "Common Dental Emergencies." *American Family Physician* 67, no.3 (2003): 511–516.

Himel, V. T., and M. E. Levitan. "Use of Nickel Titanium Instruments for Cleaning and Shaping Root Canal Systems." *Texas Dental Journal* 120, no. 3 (2003) L 262–268.

ORGANIZATIONS

Academy of General Dentistry, 211 East Chicago Avenue, Chicago, IL 60611. (312) 440-4300. <http://www.agd.org>.

American Academy of Pediatric Dentistry, 211 East Chicago Avenue, #700, Chicago, IL 60611-2663. (312) 337-2169. Fax: (312) 337-6329. <http://www.aapd.org>.

American Association of Endodontists, 211 E. Chicago Ave., Suite 1100, Chicago, IL 60611-2691. (800) 872-3636 or (312) 266-7255. Fax: (866) 451-9020 or (312) 266-9867. info@aae.org. <http://www.aae.org>.

American Dental Association, 211 E. Chicago Avenue, Chicago, IL 60611. (312) 440-2500. Fax: (312) 440-7494. <http://www.ada.org>.

OTHER

Animated-Teeth.com. [cited May 2, 2003]. <http://www.animated-teeth.com/root_canal/t1_root_canal.htm>.

Health Promotion Board of Singapore. [cited May 2, 2003]. <http://www.hpb.gov.sg/hpb/haz/haz03029.asp>.

New Zealand Dental Association. [cited May 2, 2003]. <http://www.nzda.org.nz/public/rootcanals.htm>.

L. Fleming Fallon, Jr., MD, DrPH

Rotator cuff repair

Definition

Rotator cuff surgery is the repair of inflammation or tears of the rotator cuff tendons in the shoulder. There are four tendons in the rotator cuff, and these tendons are attached individually to the following muscles: teres minor, subscapularis, infraspinatus, and the supraspinatus. The tears and inflammation associated with rotator cuff injury occur in the region near where these tendon/muscle complexes attach to the humerus (upper arm) bone.

Purpose

Rotator cuff surgery is necessary when chronic shoulder pain associated with rotator cuff injury does not respond to conservative therapy such as rest, heat/ice application, or the use of non-steroidal anti-inflammatory drugs (NSAIDs). Rotator cuff injuries are often lumped into the category referred to as rotator cuff syndrome. Rotator cuff syndrome describes a range of symptoms from basic sprains and tendon swelling (tendonitis) to total rupture or tearing of the tendon.

Demographics

Approximately 5–10% of the general population is believed to have rotator cuff syndrome at a given time. It is not commonly found in individuals under the age of 20 years, even though many in this population are athletically active. In general, males are more likely than females to develop rotator cuff syndrome and require surgery. Most rotator cuff injuries are associated with athletic activities such as baseball, tennis, weight lifting, and swimming, where the arms are repeatedly lifted over the head. Rotator cuff injuries can also occur in accidents involving falling to the ground or when the humerus is pushed into the shoulder socket. Rotator cuff injuries can also occur in older, active individuals because the rotator cuff tendons begin to deteriorate after age 40. Occupations that have been associated with rotator cuff injuries include nursing, painting, carpentry, tree pruning, fruit picking, and grocery clerking.

Description

For most patients, if the pain begins to subside, they are encouraged to undergo a period of physical therapy. If the pain does not subside after a few weeks, then the physician may suggest the use of cortisone injections into the shoulder region. Rotator cuff repair is then considered if the more conservative methods are not successful.

The primary aim of rotator cuff repair is to repair the connection between the damaged tendon and the bone. Once this bridge is re-established and the connection between the tendon and the bone has thoroughly healed, the corresponding muscles can once again move the arm in a normal fashion. The goal of the surgery is to ensure the smooth movement of the rotator cuff tendons and bursa under the upper part of the shoulder blade. The surgery is also performed to improve the comfort of the patient and to normalize the function of the shoulder and arm. There are a variety of surgical approaches that can be used to accomplish rotator cuff repair. The most common approach is called the anterior acromioplasty approach. This approach allows for excellent access to the most common sites of tears—the biceps groove, anterior cuff, and the undersurface of the joint.

Most rotator cuff repairs are accomplished using incisions that minimize cosmetic changes in the skin following healing. If possible, the surgery is performed with an arthroscope to minimize cosmetic damage to the skin. Typically, the incision made is about the size of a buttonhole. The arthroscope, a pencil-sized instrument, is then inserted into the joint. The surgeon usually accesses the rotator cuff by opening part of the deltoid muscle. If bone spurs, adhesions, and damaged bursa are present in the rotator cuff region, then the surgeon will generally remove these damaged structures to improve function in the joint. In cases where the arthroscopic technique is not advised or when it fails to achieve the desired results, a conversion to open surgery is made. This involves a larger incision and usually requires more extensive anesthesia and a longer recovery period.

The success of the rotator cuff repair is dependent on the following factors:

- age of the patient
- type of surgical technique employed
- degree of damage present
- patient's recovery goals
- patient's ability to follow a physical therapy program following surgery
- smoking status
- number of previous cortisone injections

Diagnosis/Preparation

The diagnosis of rotator cuff injury is based on a combination of clinical signs and symptoms, coupled with diagnostic testing. The most common clinical signs and symptoms include:

- tenderness in the rotator cuff
- pain associated with the movement of the arm above the head

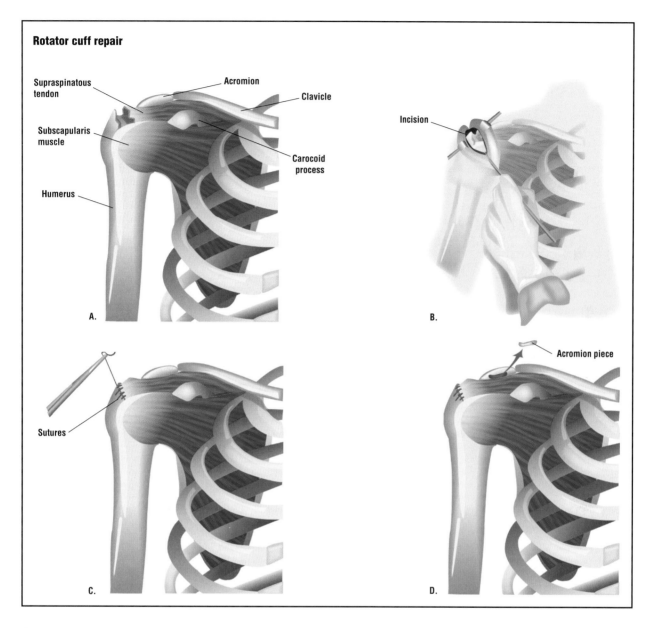

Rotator cuff repair

A.

- Supraspinatous tendon
- Acromion
- Clavicle
- Subscapularis muscle
- Carocoid process
- Humerus

B.

- Incision

C.

- Sutures

D.

- Acromion piece

A rotator cuff injury results in a torn tendon at the top of the shoulder (A). To repair it, an incision is made over the site of the tear (B). The tendon's attachment to the bone is repaired with sutures (C), and a small piece of bone from the acromion may be removed (D) to ensure smoother movement of the tendons. *(Illustration by GGS Inc.)*

- pain that is fairly constant but more intense at night
- weakness or pain with the forward movement of the arm
- muscle atrophy in long-term injuries that involve a complete tendon tear

X rays are used to rule out other types of injuries or abnormalities present in the shoulder region. While x rays are often used to help solidify the diagnosis, **arthrography**, ultrasonography, computed tomography (CT), and **magnetic resonance imaging** (MRI) are the definitive tests in the diagnosis of rotator cuff injury.

Arthography and ultrasonography of the shoulder can help determine whether or not there is a full tear in the rotator cuff. A MRI can help determine whether there is a full tear, partial tear, chronic tendonitis, or other cause of the shoulder pain. The final decision to repair the tear ultimately rests on the amount of pain and restriction suffered by the patient.

Aftercare

Following the procedure, the patient will typically spend several hours in the **recovery room**. Generally, an

cilitate recovery and improve the functioning of the joint in the future.

Risks

Complications following arthroscopic rotator cuff surgery are very rare. Such complications occur in less than 1% of cases. These complications include instrument breakage, blood vessel or nerve damage, blood vessel clots, infection, and inflammation. Complications, though still rare, are more common following open surgery. This is due to the larger incisions and more complicated anesthesia that is often necessary.

Normal results

The prognosis for the long-term relief from rotator cuff syndrome is good, especially when both conservative and surgical therapeutic approaches are used. In those patients who do require surgery, six weeks of physical therapy is typically instituted following surgery. Complete recovery following surgery may take several months. In rare cases, the rotator cuff injury is so severe that the patient may require muscle transfers and tendon grafts. Even more rarely, the injury can be so severe that the tendons are not repairable. This typically occurs when a severe rotator cuff injury is neglected for a long period of time.

Morbidity and mortality rates

Morbidity is rare in both the arthroscopic and open procedures. Mortality is exceedingly rare in patients undergoing rotator cuff repair.

Alternatives

Conservative approaches are typically used before surgery is considered in patients with rotator cuff injury. This is true even in cases where there is evidence of a full tendon tear. Some patients with a full or partial tear do not suffer a significant amount of pain and retain normal or nearly normal range of motion in shoulder movement. A majority of those with rotator cuff syndrome respond to conservative non-surgical approaches. Conservative therapies include the following:

- heat or ice to reduce pain and swelling
- cessation or reduction of activities that involve the movement of the arms overhead
- medication such as non-steroidal anti-inflammatory agents to reduce pain and inflammation
- cortisone injections to reduce pain and inflammation
- rest

ice pack will be applied to the affected shoulder joint for a period up to 48 hours. The patient will usually be given either prescription or non-prescription pain medication. The dressing is usually removed the day after surgery and is replaced by adhesive strips. The patient should contact a physician if there are any significant changes in the affected area once the patient goes home. These changes can include increased swelling, pain, bleeding, drainage in the affected area, nausea, vomiting, or signs of infection. Signs of infection include fever, dizziness, headache, and muscle aches.

It often takes several days for the arthroscopic puncture wounds to heal, and the joint usually takes several weeks to recover. Most patients can resume normal daily activities, with the permission of a physician, within a few days following the procedure. Most patients are advised to undergo a rehabilitation program that includes physical therapy. Such a program can fa-

KEY TERMS

Adhesions—A fibrous band that holds together tissue that are usually separated and that are associated with wound healing.

Arthrography—Visualization of a joint by radiographic means following injection of a contrast dye into the joint space.

Arthroscope—An endoscope, or a tube containing an optical system, that is used to examine the interior of a joint.

Bone spurs—A sharp or pointed calcified projection.

Bursa—A sac found in connective tissue that acts to reduce friction between tendon and bone.

Deltoid muscle—Muscle that covers the prominence of the shoulder.

Once the pain begins to subside, the patient usually is encouraged to begin a program of physical therapy to help re-institute normal motion and function to the shoulder.

Resources

BOOKS

Current Medical Diagnosis & Treatment. New York: McGraw-Hill, 2003.

"Rotator Cuff Tendinitis." In *The Merck Manual,* edited by Keryn A. G. Lane. West Point, PA: Merck & Co., 1999.

"Rotator Cuff Syndrome." In *Ferri's Clinical Advisor,* edited by Fred F. Ferri. St. Louis: Mosby, 2001.

Schwartz, Seymour I., ed. *Principles of Surgery.* New York: McGraw-Hill 1999.

Shannon, Joyce Brennfleck. *Sports Injuries Sourcebook.* Detroit: Omnigraphics, Inc., 2002.

PERIODICALS

Welling, Ken R. "Rotator Cuff Surgery." *Surgical Technologist* 31 (1999): 4.

Mark Mitchell

Routine urinalysis *see* **Urinalysis**

S

Sacral nerve stimulation

Definition

Sacral nerve stimulation, also known as sacral neuromodulation, is a procedure in which the sacral nerve at the base of the spine is stimulated by a mild electrical current from an implanted device. It is done to improve functioning of the urinary tract, to relieve pain related to urination, and to control fecal incontinence.

Purpose

As a proven treatment for urinary incontinence, sacral nerve stimulation (SNS) has recently been found effective in the treatment of interstitial cystitis, a disorder that involves hyperreflexia of the urinary sphincter. SNS is also used to treat pelvic or urinary pain as well as fecal incontinence.

A person's ability to hold urine or feces depends on three body functions:

• a reservoir function represented by the urethra/bladder or colon

• a gatekeeping function represented by the urethral or anal sphincter

• the brain's ability to control urination, defecation, and nerve sensitivity

A dysfunction or deficiency in any of these components can result in incontinence. The most common forms of incontinence are stress urinary incontinence and urge incontinence. Stress incontinence is related to an unstable detrusor muscle that controls the urinary sphincter. When the detrusor muscle is weak, urine can leak out of the bladder from pressure on the abdomen caused by sneezing, coughing, and other movements. Urge incontinence is characterized by a sudden strong need to urinate and inability to hold urine until an appropriate time; it is also associated with hyperactivity of the urinary sphincter. Both conditions can be treated by SNS. SNS requires an

implanted device that sends continuous stimulation to the sacral nerve that controls the urinary sphincter. This treatment has been used with over 1500 patients with a high rate of success. It was approved in Europe in 1994. The Food and Drug Administration (FDA) approved SNS for disturbances that are usually treated by augmentation of the sphincter muscle or implanting an artificial sphincter can benefit from electrical stimulation of the sacral nerve. Although the mechanism of SNS is not completely clear, researchers believe that the patient's control of the pelvic region is restored by the stimulation or activation of afferent fibers in the muscles of the pelvic floor.

Demographics

Urinary incontinence affects between 15% and 30% of American adults living in the community, and as many as 50% of people confined to **nursing homes**. It is a disorder that affects women far more frequently than men; 85% of people suffering from urinary incontinence are women. According to the chief of geriatrics at a Boston hospital, 25 million Americans suffer each year from occasional episodes of urinary or fecal incontinence.

Interstitial cystitis is less common than urinary or fecal incontinence but still affects 700,000 Americans each year. The average age of IC patients is 40; 25% of patients are younger than 30. Although 90% of patients diagnosed with IC are women, it is thought that the disorder may be underdiagnosed in men.

Description

Sacral nerve stimulation (SNS) is conducted through an implanted device that includes a thin insulated wire called a lead and a neurostimulator much like a cardiac pacemaker. The device is inserted in a pocket in the patient's lower abdomen. SNS is first tried on an outpatient basis in the doctor's office with the implantation of a test lead. If the trial treatment is successful, the patient is scheduled for inpatient surgery.

Permanent surgical implantation is done under general anesthesia and requires a one-night stay in the hospital. After the patient has been anesthetized, the surgeon implants the neurostimulator, which is about the size of a pocket stopwatch, under the skin of the patient's abdomen. Thin wires, or leads, running from the stimulator carry electrical pulses from the stimulator to the sacral nerves located in the lower back. After the stimulator and leads have been implanted, the surgeon closes the incision in the abdomen.

Diagnosis/Preparation

Incontinence significantly affects a patient's quality of life; thus patients usually consult a doctor when their urinary problems begin to cause difficulties in the workplace or on social occasions. A family care practitioner will usually refer the patient to a urologist for diagnosis of the cause(s) of the incontinence. Patients with urinary and fecal incontinence are evaluated carefully through the taking of a complete patient history and a **physical examination**. The doctor will use special techniques to assess the capacity of the bladder or rectum as well as the functioning of the urethral or anal sphincter in order to determine the cause or location of the incontinence. **Cystoscopy**, which is the examination of the full bladder with a scope attached to a small tube, allows the physician to rule out certain disorders as well as plan the most effective treatment. These extensive tests are especially important in diagnosing interstitial cystitis because all other causes of urinary urgency, frequency, and pain

must be ruled out before surgery can be suggested. Cystoscopy is done under anesthesia and often works as a treatment for IC. Once the doctor has made the diagnosis of urinary incontinence due to sphincter insufficiency, he or she will explain and discuss the surgical implant with the patient. SNS may be tried out on a temporary basis. The same pattern of diagnosis and treatment is used for patients with IC and fecal incontinence. Temporary implants can help eliminate those patients who will not benefit from a permanent implant.

Aftercare

Following surgery, the patient remains overnight in the hospital. **Antibiotics** may be given to reduce the risk of infection and pain medications to relieve discomfort. The patient will be given instructions on **incision care** and follow-up appointments before he or she leaves the hospital.

Aftercare includes fine-tuning of the SNS stimulator. The doctor can adjust the strength of the electrical impulses in his or her office with a handheld programmer. The stimulator runs for about five to 10 years and can be replaced during an outpatient procedure. About a third of patients require a second operation to adjust or replace various elements of the stimulator device.

Risks

In addition to the risks of bleeding and infection that are common to surgical procedures, implanting an SNS device carries the risks of pain at the insertion site, discomfort when urinating, mild electrical shocks, and displacement or dislocation of the leads.

Normal results

Patients report improvement in the number of urinations, the volume of urine produced, lessened urgency, and higher overall quality of life after treatment with SNS. Twenty-two patients undergoing a three to seven-day test of sacral nerve stimulation on an outpatient basis reported significant reduction in urgency and frequency, according to the American Urological Association. Studies have indicated complete success in about 50% of patients. Sacral nerve stimulation is being used to treat fecal incontinence in the United States and Europe, with promising early reports. As of 2003, SNS is the least invasive of the recognized surgical treatments for fecal incontinence.

Morbidity and mortality rates

Sacral nerve stimulation has been shown to be a safe and effective procedure for the treatment of both urinary and fecal incontinence. Two groups of researchers, in

Spain and the United Kingdom respectively, have reported that "the effects of neuromodulation are long-lasting and associated morbidity is low." The most commonly reported complications of SNS are pain at the site of the implant (15.3% of patients), pain on urination (9%), and displacement of the leads (8.4%).

Alternatives

There are three types of nonsurgical treatments that benefit some patients with IC:

• Behavioral approaches. These include biofeedback, diet modifications, bladder retraining, and pelvic muscle exercises.

• Medications. These include antispasmodic drugs, tricyclic antidepressants, and pentosan polysulfate sodium, which is sold under the trade name Elmiron. Elmiron appears to work by protecting the lining of the bladder from bacteria and other irritating substances in urine.

• Intravesical medications. These are medications that affect the muscular tissues of the bladder. Oxybutynin is a drug that is prescribed for patients who are incontinent because their bladders fail to store urine properly. Capsaicin and resiniferatoxin are used to treat hyperreflexia of the detrusor muscle.

Surgical alternatives to SNS are considered treatments of last resort for IC because they are invasive, irreversible, and benefit only 30–40% of patients. In addition, some studies indicate that these surgeries can lead to long-term kidney damage. They include the following procedures:

• Augmentation cystoplasty. In this procedure, the surgeon removes the patient's bladder and replaces it with a section of the bowel—in effect creating a new bladder. The patient passes urine through the urethra in the normal fashion.

• Urinary diversion. The surgeon creates a tube from a section of the patient's bowel and places the ureters (tubes that carry urine from the kidneys to the bladder) in this tube. The tube is then attached to a stoma, or opening in the abdomen. Urine is carried into an external collection bag that the patient must empty several times daily.

• Internal pouch. The surgeon creates a new bladder from a section of the bowel and attaches it inside the abdomen. The patient empties the pouch by self-catheterization four to six times daily.

Resources

BOOKS

Walsh, Patrick C., MD, et al., eds. *Campbell's Urology*, 8th ed. Philadelphia: W. B. Saunders Company, 2002.

KEY TERMS

Afferent fibers—Nerve fibers that conduct nerve impulses from tissues and organs toward the central nervous system.

Detrusor muscle—The medical name for the layer of muscle tissue covering the urinary bladder. When the detrusor muscle contracts, the bladder expels urine.

Fecal incontinence—Inability to control bowel movements.

Hyperreflexia—A condition in which the detrusor muscle of the bladder contracts too frequently, leading to inability to hold one's urine.

Interstitial cystitis—A condition of unknown origin that causes urinary urgency, pain in the bladder and abdomen, and pain during sexual intercourse.

Neuromodulation—Electrical stimulation of a nerve for relief of pain.

Sacral nerve—The nerve in the lower back region of the spine that controls the need to urinate.

Sphincter—A ringlike band of muscle that tightens or closes the opening to a body organ.

Urgency—A sudden compelling need to urinate.

Urinary incontinence—Inability to control urination.

PERIODICALS

Elliott, Daniel S., MD. "Medical Management of Overactive Bladder." *Mayo Clinic Proceedings* 76 (April 2001): 353-355.

Ganio, E., A. Masin, C. Ratto, et al. "Short-Term Sacral Nerve Stimulation for Functional Anorectal and Urinary Disturbances: Results in 40 Patients: Evaluation of a New Option for Anorectal Functional Disorders." *Disorders of the Colon and Rectum* 44 (September 2001): 1261-1267.

Kenefick, N. J., C. J. Vaisey, R. C. Cohen, et al. "Medium-Term Results of Permanent Sacral Nerve Stimulation for Faecal Incontinence." *British Journal of Surgery* 89 (July 2002); 896-601.

Linares Quevedo, A. I., M. A. Jiminez Cidre, E. Fernandez Fernandez, et al. "Posterior Sacral Root Neuromodulation in the Treatment of Chronic Urinary Dysfunction. [in Spanish] *Actas urologicas espanolas* 26 (April 2002): 250-260.

ORGANIZATIONS

American Urological Association (AUA). 1120 North Charles Street, Baltimore, MD 21201. (410) 727-1100. <www.auanet.org>.

National Association for Continence (NAFC). P. O. Box 1019, Charleston, SC 29402-1019. (843) 377-0900. <www.nafc.org>.

National Kidney Foundation. 30 East 33rd Street, Suite 1100, New York, NY 10016. (800) 622-9010 or (212) 889-2210. <www.kidney.org>.

National Kidney and Urologic Diseases Information Clearinghouse (NKUDIC). 3 Information Way, Bethesda, MD 20892-3580.

OTHER

Interstitial Cystitis Association. *Sacral Nerve Stimulation Can Relieve Interstitial Cystitis, Studies Suggest.* <www.ichelp.com/research/SacralNerveStimulationCanRelieveIC.html>.

Mayo Clinic. *Sacral Nerve Stimulation.* <www.mayoclinic.org/incontinence-jax/sacralstim.html.>

Nancy McKenzie, PhD

Salpingo-oophorectomy

Definition

Unilateral salpingo-oophorectomy is the surgical removal of a fallopian tube and an ovary. If both sets of fallopian tubes and ovaries are removed, the procedure is called a bilateral salpingo-oophorectomy.

Purpose

This surgery is performed to treat ovarian or other gynecological cancers, or infections caused by pelvic inflammatory disease. Occasionally, removal of one or both ovaries may be done to treat endometriosis, a condition in which the lining of the uterus (the endometrium) grows outside of the uterus (usually on and around the pelvic organs). The procedure may also be performed if a woman has been diagnosed with an ectopic pregnancy in a fallopian tube and a **salpingostomy** (an incision into the fallopian tube to remove the pregnancy) cannot be done. If only one fallopian tube and ovary are removed, the woman may still be able to conceive and carry a pregnancy to term. If both are removed, however, the woman is rendered permanently infertile. This procedure is commonly combined with a **hysterectomy** (surgical removal of the uterus); the ovaries and fallopian tubes are removed in about one-third of hysterectomies.

Until the 1980s, women over age 40 having hysterectomies routinely had healthy ovaries and fallopian tubes removed at the same time. Many physicians reasoned that a woman over 40 was approaching menopause and soon her ovaries would stop secreting estrogen and releasing eggs.

Removing the ovaries would eliminate the risk of ovarian cancer and only accelerate menopause by a few years.

In the 1990s, the thinking about routine salpingo-oophorectomy began to change. The risk of ovarian cancer in women who have no family history of the disease is less than 1%. Moreover, removing the ovaries increases the risk of cardiovascular disease and accelerates osteoporosis unless a woman takes prescribed hormone replacements.

Demographics

Overall, ovarian cancer accounts for only 4% of all cancers in women. For women at increased risk, **oophorectomy** may be considered after the age of 35 if childbearing is complete. Factors that increase a woman's risk of developing ovarian cancer include age (most ovarian cancers occur after menopause), the presence of a mutation in the BRCA1 or BRCA2 gene, the number of menstrual periods a woman has had (affected by age of onset, pregnancy, breastfeeding, and oral contraceptive use), history of breast cancer, diet, and family history. The incidence of ovarian cancer is highest among American Indian (17.5 cases per 100,000 population), Caucasian (15.8 per 100,000), Vietnamese (13.8 per 100,000), Caucasian Hispanic (12.1 per 100,000), and Hawaiian (11.8 per 100,000) women; it is lowest among Korean (7.0 per 100,000) and Chinese (9.3 per 100,000) women. African American women have an ovarian cancer incidence of 10.2 per 100,000 population.

Endometriosis, another reason why salpingo-oophorectomy may be performed, has been estimated to affect up to 10% of women. Approximately four out of every 1,000 women are hospitalized as a result of endometriosis each year. Women 25–35 years of age are affected most, with 27 being the average age of diagnosis.

Description

General or regional anesthesia will be given to the patient before the procedure begins. If the procedure is

Salpingo-oophorectomy

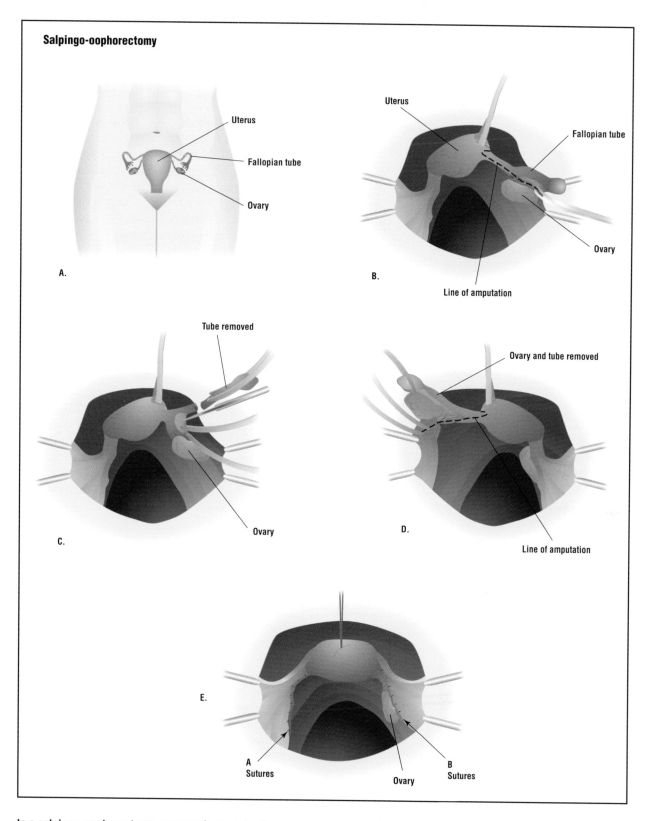

A.

B.

C.

D.

E.

In a salpingo-oophorectomy, a woman's reproductive organs are accessed through an incision in the lower abdomen, or laparoscopically (A). Once the area is visualized, a diseased fallopian tube can be severed from the uterus and removed (B and C). The ovary can also be removed with the tube (D). The remaining structures are stitched (E), and the wound is closed. *(Illustration by GGS Inc.)*

performed through a laparoscope, the surgeon can avoid a large abdominal incision and can shorten recovery. With this technique, the surgeon makes a small cut through the abdominal wall just below the navel. A tube containing a tiny lens and light source (a laparoscope) is then inserted through the incision. A camera can be attached that allows the surgeon to see the abdominal cavity on a video monitor. When the ovaries and fallopian tubes are detached, they are removed though a small incision at the top of the vagina. The organs can also be cut into smaller sections and removed. When the laparoscope is used, the patient can be given either regional or general anesthesia; if there are no complications, the patient can leave the hospital in a day or two.

If a laparoscope is not used, the surgery involves an incision 4–6 in (10–15 cm) long into the abdomen extending either vertically up from the pubic bone toward the navel, or horizontally (the "bikini incision") across the pubic hairline. The scar from a bikini incision is less noticeable, but some surgeons prefer the vertical incision because it provides greater visibility while operating. A disadvantage to abdominal salpingo-oophorectomy is that bleeding is more likely to be a complication of this type of operation. The procedure is more painful than a laparoscopic operation and the recovery period is longer. A woman can expect to be in the hospital two to five days and will need three to six weeks to return to normal activities.

Diagnosis/Preparation

Before surgery, the doctor will order blood and urine tests, and any additional tests such as ultrasound or x rays to help the surgeon visualize the woman's condition. The woman may also meet with the anesthesiologist to evaluate any special conditions that might affect the administration of anesthesia. A colon preparation may be done, if extensive surgery is anticipated.

On the evening before the operation, the woman should eat a light dinner, then take nothing by mouth, including water or other liquids, after midnight.

Aftercare

If performed through an abdominal incision, salpingo-oophorectomy is major surgery that requires three to six weeks for full recovery. However, if performed laparoscopically, the recovery time can be much shorter. There may be some discomfort around the incision for the first few days after surgery, but most women are walking around by the third day. Within a month or so, patients can gradually resume normal activities such as driving, exercising, and working.

Immediately following the operation, the patient should avoid sharply flexing the thighs or the knees. Persistent back pain or bloody or scanty urine indicates that a ureter may have been injured during surgery.

If both ovaries are removed in a premenopausal woman as part of the operation, the sudden loss of estrogen will trigger an abrupt premature menopause that may involve severe symptoms of hot flashes, vaginal dryness, painful intercourse, and loss of sex drive. (This is also called "surgical menopause.") In addition to these symptoms, women who lose both ovaries also lose the protection these hormones provide against heart disease and osteoporosis many years earlier than if they had experienced natural menopause. Women who have had their ovaries removed are seven times more likely to develop coronary heart disease and much more likely to develop bone problems at an early age than are premenopausal women whose ovaries are intact. For these reasons, some form of hormone replacement therapy (HRT) may be prescribed to relieve the symptoms of surgical menopause and to help prevent heart and bone disease.

Reaction to the removal of fallopian tubes and ovaries depends on a wide variety of factors, including the woman's age, the condition that required the surgery, her reproductive history, how much social support she has, and any previous history of depression. Women who have had many gynecological surgeries or chronic pelvic pain seem to have a higher tendency to develop psychological problems after the surgery.

Risks

Major surgery always involves some risk, including infection, reactions to the anesthesia, hemorrhage, and scars at the incision site. Almost all pelvic surgery causes some internal scars, which in some cases can cause discomfort years after surgery.

Potential complications after a salpingo-oophorectomy include changes in sex drive, hot flashes, and other symptoms of menopause if both ovaries are removed. Women who have both ovaries removed and who do not take estrogen replacement therapy run an increased risk for cardiovascular disease and osteoporosis. Women with a history of psychological and emotional problems before an oophorectomy are more likely to experience psychological difficulties after the operation.

Normal results

If the surgery is successful, the fallopian tubes and ovaries will be removed without complication, and the underlying problem resolved. In the case of cancer, all the cancer will be removed. A woman will become infertile following a bilateral salpingo-oophorectomy.

Morbidity and mortality rates

Studies have shown that the complication rate following salpingo-oophorectomy is essentially the same as that following hysterectomy. The rate of complications differs by the type of hysterectomy performed. Abdominal hysterectomy is associated with a higher rate of complications (9.3%), while the overall complication rate for vaginal hysterectomy is 5.3%, and 3.6% for laparoscopic vaginal hysterectomy. The risk of death is about one in every 1,000 (1/1,000) women having a hysterectomy. The rates of some of the more commonly reported complications are:

- excessive bleeding (hemorrhaging): 1.8–3.4%

- fever or infection: 0.8–4.0%

- accidental injury to another organ or structure: 1.5–1.8%

Because of the cessation of hormone production that occurs with a bilateral oophorectomy, women who lose both ovaries also prematurely lose the protection these hormones provide against heart disease and osteoporosis. Women who have undergone bilateral oophorectomy are seven times more likely to develop coronary heart disease and much more likely to develop bone problems at an early age than are premenopausal women whose ovaries are intact.

Alternatives

Depending on the specific condition that warrants an oophorectomy, it may be possible to modify the surgery so at least a portion of one ovary remains, allowing the woman to avoid early menopause. In the case of endometriosis, there are a number of alternative treatments that are usually pursued before a salpingo-oophorectomy (with or without hysterectomy) is performed. These include excising the growths without re-

KEY TERMS

BRCA1 or BRCA2 genetic mutation—A genetic mutation that predisposes otherwise healthy women to breast cancer.

Endometriosis—A painful disease in which cells from the lining of the uterus (endometrium) become attached to other organs in the pelvic cavity. The condition is hard to diagnose and often causes severe pain as well as infertility.

Fallopian tubes—Tubes that extend from either end of the uterus that convey the egg from the ovary to the uterus during each monthly cycle.

Hysterectomy—The surgical removal of the uterus.

Ureter—The tube that carries urine from the bladder to the kidneys.

moving any organs, blocking or destroying the nerves that provide sensation to some of the pelvic structures, or prescribing drugs that decrease estrogen levels.

Resources

PERIODICALS

Kauff, N. D., J. M. Satagopan, M. E. Robson, et al. "Risk-Reducing Salpingo-oophorectomy in Women with a BRC1 or BRC2 Mutation." *New England Journal of Medicine* 346 (May 23, 2002): 1609–15.

ORGANIZATIONS

American Cancer Society. 1599 Clifton Road NE, Atlanta, GA 30329. (800) ACS-2345. <http://www.cancer.org>.
American College of Obstetricians and Gynecologists. 409 12th St., SW, PO Box 96920, Washington, DC 20090-6920. <http://www.acog.org>.
Midlife Women's Network. 5129 Logan Ave. S., Minneapolis, MN 55419. (800) 886-4354.

OTHER

Hernandez, Manuel and Robert McNamara. "Endometriosis." *eMedicine.* December 23, 2002 [cited March 15, 2003]. <http://www.emedicine.com/aaem/topic181.htm>.
Kapoor, Dharmesh. "Endometriosis." *eMedicine.* September 17, 2002 [cited March 15, 2003]. <http://www.emedicine.com/med/topic3419.htm>.
Surveillance, Epidemiology, and End Results. "Racial/Ethnic Patterns of Cancer in the United States: Ovary." *National Cancer Institute.* 1996 [cited March 14, 2003]. <http://seer.cancer.gov/publications/ethnicity/ovary.pdf>.
"What Is Endometriosis?" *Endo-Online.* 2002 [cited March 15, 2003]. <http://www.endometriosisassn.org/endo.html>.

Carol A. Turkington
Stephanie Dionne Sherk

Salpingostomy

Definition

A salpingostomy is a surgical incision into a fallopian tube. This procedure may be done to repair a damaged tube or to remove an ectopic pregnancy (one that occurs outside of the uterus).

Purpose

The fallopian tubes are the structures that carry a mature egg from the ovaries to the uterus. These tubes, which are about 4 in (10 cm) long and 0.2 in (0.5 cm) in diameter, are found on the upper outer sides of the uterus, and open into the uterus through small channels. It is within the fallopian tubes that fertilization, the joining of an egg and a sperm, takes place.

During a normal pregnancy, the fertilized egg passes from the fallopian tubes into the uterus and then implants into the lining of the uterus. If the fertilized egg implants anywhere outside of the uterus, it is called an ectopic (or tubal) pregnancy. The majority of ectopic pregnancies occur in the fallopian tubes (95%); they may also occur in the uterine muscle (1–2%), the abdomen (1–2%), the ovaries (less than 1%), and the cervix (less than 1%).

As an ectopic pregnancy progresses, the fallopian tubes are unable to contain the growing embryo and may rupture. A ruptured ectopic pregnancy is considered a medical emergency as it can cause significant hemorrhaging (excessive bleeding). If an ectopic pregnancy is diagnosed early (i.e., before rupture has occurred), it may be possible to manage medically; the drug methotrexate targets rapidly dividing fetal cells, preventing the fetus from developing further. If medical management is not possible or has failed, surgical intervention may be necessary. A salpingostomy may then be performed to remove the pregnancy.

Salpingostomy may also be performed in an effort to restore fertility to a woman whose fallopian tubes have been damaged, such as by adhesions (bands of scar tissue that may form after surgery or trauma). In the case of hydrosalpinx, a condition in which a tube becomes blocked and filled with fluid, a salpingostomy may be performed to create a new tubal ostium (opening).

Demographics

Ectopic pregnancy occurs in approximately 2% of all pregnancies. Once a woman has an ectopic pregnancy, she has an increased chance (10–25%) of having another. Women between the ages of 25 and 34 have a higher incidence of ectopic pregnancy, although the mor-

tality rate among women over the age of 35 is 2.5–5.9 times higher. Minority women are also at an increased risk of ectopic pregnancy-related death.

Description

Salpingostomy may be performed via laparotomy or **laparoscopy**, under general or regional anesthesia. A laparotomy is an incision made in the abdominal wall through which the fallopian tubes are visualized. If the tube has already ruptured as a result of an ectopic pregnancy, a salpingectomy will be performed to remove the damaged fallopian tube. If rupture has not occurred, a drug called vasopressin is injected into the fallopian tube to minimize the amount of bleeding. An incision (called a linear salpingostomy) is made through the wall of the tube in the area of the ectopic pregnancy. The products of conception are then flushed out of the tube with an instrument called a suction-irrigator. Any bleeding sites are treated by suturing or by applying pressure with forceps. The incision is not sutured but instead left to heal on its own (called closure by secondary intent). The abdominal wall is then closed.

A neosalpingostomy is similar to a linear salpingostomy but is performed to treat a tubal blockage (e.g., hydrosalpinx). An incision is made to create a new opening in the fallopian tube; the tissue is folded over and stitched into place. The new hole, or ostium, replaces the normal opening of the fallopian tube through which the egg released by an ovary each menstrual cycle is collected.

Salpingostomy may also be performed laparoscopically. With this surgery, a tube (called a laparoscope) containing a tiny lens and light source is inserted through a small incision in the navel. A camera can be attached that allows the surgeon to see the abdominal cavity on a video monitor. The salpingostomy is then performed with instruments inserted through trocars, small incisions of 0.2–0.8 in (0.5–2 cm) made through the abdominal wall.

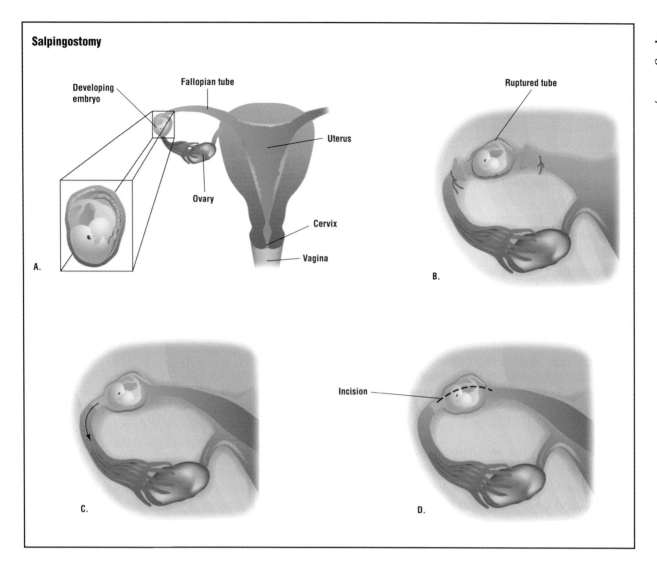

Salpingostomy

A tubal or ectopic pregnancy can be removed in several ways. If the fallopian tube is ruptured (A), the tube is tied off on both sides, and the embryo removed. If the tube is intact, the embryo can be pulled out the end of the tube (C), or tube can be cut open and the contents removed (D). *(Illustration by GGS Inc.)*

An advantage of laparoscopic salpingostomy is that the operation is less invasive, thus recovery time is quicker and less painful as compared to a laparotomy; the average duration of recovery following laparoscopy is 2.4 weeks, compared to 4.6 weeks for laparotomy. An abdominal incision, on the other hand, allows the surgeon a better view of and easier access to the pelvic organs. Several studies have indicated a reduced rate of normal pregnancy after salpingostomy by laparoscopy versus laparotomy.

Diagnosis/Preparation

It has been estimated that 40–50% of ectopic pregnancies are incorrectly diagnosed when first presenting to emergency room medical personnel. Often the symptoms of ectopic pregnancy are confused with other conditions such as miscarriage or pelvic inflammatory disease. Diagnosis is usually based on presentation of symptoms, a positive pregnancy test, and detection of a pregnancy outside of the uterus by means of ultrasonography (using a machine that transmits high frequency sound waves to visualize structures in the body).

Diagnosis of hydrosalpinx or other defects of the fallopian tubes may be done surgically, using a laparoscope to visualize the fallopian tubes. Alternatively, a hysterosalpingogram may be performed, in which the uterus is filled with a dye and an x ray is taken to see if the dye flows through the fallopian tubes.

KEY TERMS

Adhesions—Bands of scar tissue that may form after surgery or trauma.

Hydrosalpinx—A condition in which a fallopian tube becomes blocked and filled with fluid.

Methotrexate—A drug that targets rapidly dividing fetal cells, preventing a fetus from developing further.

Salpingectomy—The surgical removal of a fallopian tube.

Aftercare

If performed through an abdominal incision, a salpingostomy requires three to six weeks for full recovery. If salpingostomy is performed laparoscopically, the recovery time can be much shorter (an average of 2.4 weeks). There may be some discomfort around the incision for the first few days after surgery, but most women are walking by the third day. Within a month or so, patients can gradually resume normal activities such as driving, exercising, and working.

Risks

Complications associated with the surgical procedure include reaction to anesthesia, excessive bleeding, injury to other organs, and infection. With an ectopic pregnancy, there is a chance that not all of the products of conception will be removed and that the persistent tissue will continue growing. If this is the case, further treatment will be necessary.

Normal results

In the case of ectopic pregnancy, the products of conception will be removed without significantly impairing fertility. If salpingostomy is being performed to restore fertility, the procedure will increase a woman's chance of conceiving without resorting to artificial reproductive techniques.

Morbidity and mortality rates

Abdominal pain occurs in 97% of women with an ectopic pregnancy, vaginal bleeding in 79%, abdominal tenderness in 91%, and infertility in 15%. Persistent ectopic pregnancy after surgical treatment occurs in 5–10% of cases. Ectopic pregnancy accounts for 10–15% of all maternal death; the mortality rate for ectopic pregnancy is approximately one in 2,500 cases.

Alternatives

Some ectopic pregnancies may be managed expectantly (allowing the pregnancy to progress to see if it will resolve on its own). This may occur in up to 25% of ectopic pregnancies. There is, of course, a chance that the fallopian tube will rupture during the period of observation. Treatment with methotrexate is gaining popularity and has been shown to have success rates similar to laparoscopic salpingostomy if multiple doses are given and the patient is in stable condition. Salpingectomy is another surgical option and is indicated if a tube has ruptured or is seriously damaged.

Resources

PERIODICALS

Hajenius, P. J., B. Mol, P. Bossuyt, W. Ankum, and F. Van der Veen. "Interventions for Tubal Ectopic Pregnancy (Cochrane Review)." *The Cochrane Library* 1 (January 20, 2003).

Tay, J. I., J. Moore, and J. J. Walker. "Ectopic Pregnancy." *British Medical Journal* 320 (April 1, 2000): 916–19.

Tenore, Josie L. "Ectopic Pregnancy." *American Family Physician* (February 15, 2000): 1073–79.

Watson, A., P. Vandekerckhove, and R. Lilford. "Techniques for Pelvic Surgery in Subfertility (Cochrane Review)." *The Cochrane Library* 1 (January 20, 2003).

ORGANIZATIONS

American College of Obstetricians and Gynecologists. 409 12th St., SW, PO Box 96920, Washington, DC 20090-6920. <http://www.acog.org>.

OTHER

Braun, R. Daniel. "Surgical Management of Ectopic Pregnancy." *eMedicine.* January 13, 2003 [cited March 16, 2003]. <http://www.emedicine.com/med/topic3316.htm>.

Daiter, Eric. "Ectopic Pregnancy." *OBGYN.net.* [cited March 16, 2003]. <http://www.obgyn.net/pb/cotm/9902/9902.htm>.

"Early Diagnosis and Management of Ectopic Pregnancy." *American Society for Reproductive Medicine (Technical*

Bulletin). March 2001 [cited March 16, 2003]. <http://www.asrm.org/Media/Practice/ectopicpregnancy.PDF>.

"Hysterosalpingogram." *The Harvard Medical School Family Health Guide.*" [cited March 16, 2003]. <http://www.health.harvard.edu/fhg/diagnostics/hystero/hystero.shtml>.

"Salpingostomy." *The McGill Gynecology Page.* August 27, 2002 [cited March 16, 2003]. <http://sprojects.mmip.mcgill.ca/gynecology/lapmain.html>.

Stephanie Dionne Sherk

Saphenous vein bypass *see* **Peripheral vascular bypass surgery**

Scar revision surgery

Definition

Scar revision surgery refers to a group of procedures that are done to partially remove scar tissue following surgery or injury, or to make the scar(s) less noticeable. The specific procedure that is performed depends on the type of scar; its cause, location, and size; and the characteristics of the patient's skin.

Purpose

Scar revision surgery is performed to improve the appearance of the patient's face or other body part, but it is also done to restore or improve functioning when the formation of a scar interferes with the movement of muscles and joints. The shortening or tightening of the skin and underlying muscles that may accompany scar formation is known as contracture. Contractures may interfere with range of motion and other aspects of joint functioning, as well as deform the shape of the hand or other body part. Contractures in the face often affect the muscles that control facial expressions.

Scar revision surgery may be considered as either a cosmetic procedure or a reconstructive surgery, depending on whether the patient's concern is primarily related to appearance or whether contractures have also affected functioning. Some insurance companies will cover the cost of scar revision surgery if the scarring resulted from injury. Patients who are considering scar revision surgery should consult their insurance carriers to learn whether their condition may be covered. According to the American Academy of Facial Plastic and Reconstructive Surgery (AAFPRS), the average cost for scar revision surgery on the face is $1,135, compared to $238 for microdermabrasion and $3,260 for **laser skin resurfacing**.

Demographics

The demographics of scar revision are difficult to establish precisely because of the number of different procedures that are grouped under this heading and the different types of scars that they are intended to treat. In addition, although **dermabrasion** and laser resurfacing of the skin are often described as surgical methods of scar treatment to distinguish them from medical modalities, they are usually listed separately in statistical tables. According to the American Society of Plastic Surgeons (ASPS), in 2001 the number of procedures, by type, were as follows: 227,911 for scar revision; 51,065 for dermabrasion; 175,927 for laser resurfacing; and 1,035,769 for microdermabrasion.

The female to male ratio for scar revision surgery is about four to three, whereas women are almost five times as likely as men to have laser skin resurfacing and almost 13 times as likely to have a microdermabrasion procedure. Most patients who have scar revision surgery are between 15 and 39, although a significant number choose to undergo this type of surgery in their 40s and 50s.

It is difficult to compare scar revision surgery with other treatments across ethnic and racial groups because skin color is a factor in the effectiveness of some forms of therapy. In addition, some types of scars—particularly keloids—are more likely to form in darker skin. On the whole, it is estimated that between 4.5% and 16% of the United States population is affected by keloids and hypertrophic scars. These are the most difficult scars to treat, and are discussed in further detail below.

Description

Scar formation

A description of the process of scar formation may be helpful in understanding scar revision surgery and other procedures intended to improve the appearance of scarred skin. There are three phases in the formation of a scar:

• Inflammation. This phase begins right after the injury and lasts until the wound is closed. It is the body's way of preventing infection, because a wound is not sterile until it is covered by a new outer layer of skin.

• Transitional repair. Scar tissue is formed during this phase to hold the wound together. The length of this phase depends on the severity of the injury.

• Maturation. This phase usually begins about seven to 12 weeks after the injury occurs. It is also the phase in which problem scars appear. Under normal conditions, a repair process takes place in which the development of new skin is combined with breaking down the scar tissue that was formed in the second phase of healing.

A problem scar is likely to develop when the repair process is interrupted or disturbed.

Causes and types of problem scars

Problem scars may result from inflammatory diseases—particularly acne; trauma can include cuts and burns, previous surgery, and a genetic predisposition for skin to overreact to injury. Tension on the skin around the wound, foreign material in the wound, infection, or anything that delays closure of the wound may also contribute to scar formation.

The most difficult types of scars to treat are characterized by overproduction of collagen, which is the extracellular protein found in connective tissue that gives it strength and flexibility. The two types of scars that are most often considered for treatment are keloids and hypertrophic scars. Keloids are shiny, smooth benign tumors that arise in areas of damaged skin and look like irregular growths in the wound area. Hypertrophic scars, on the other hand, are thick, ropy-textured scars that are often associated with contractures.

Keloids can be distinguished from hypertrophic scars by the following characteristics:

- Timing. Hypertrophic scars usually begin to form within weeks of the injury, whereas keloids may not appear until a year later.
- Growth pattern. Hypertrophic scars do not continue to grow after they form, and remain within the original area of injury. Keloids continue to grow and spread outward into normal tissue.
- Role of genetic factors. Keloids tend to run in families, whereas hypertrophic scars do not.
- Racial and age distribution. Keloids occur more frequently in persons with darker skin than in fair-skinned persons. They are also more likely to develop during adolescence and pregnancy, which are periods of high hormone production.
- Recurrence. Hypertrophic scars may fade with time and do not recur. Keloids, on the other hand, may recur even after surgical removal.
- Collagen structure. The collagen fibers in a hypertrophic scar are shorter and generally arranged in a wavelike pattern, whereas the collagen fibers in keloids tend to be randomly arranged.

Surgical approaches to scar revision

The treatment of scars is highly individualized. Most plastic surgeons use a variety of nonsurgical and surgical approaches to improve the appearance of scars. In addition, patients might need several different surgical procedures if their scar revisions require a series of operations at different stages of the healing process.

SURGICAL EXCISION. Surgical excision is a procedure in which the surgeon shaves down and cuts out scar tissue to reduce the size of the scar. This technique is most commonly used on large scars that cannot be treated adequately with medications or other nonsurgical means. When excision is done in stages, it is referred to as "serial excision." This is performed if the area of the scar is too large to remove at one time without distorting nearby skin.

FLAPS, GRAFTS, AND ARTIFICIAL SKIN. Flaps, grafts, and artificial skin are used to treat contractures and large areas of scarring resulting from burns and other traumatic injuries. When there is not enough skin at the site of the injury to cover an incision made to remove scar tissue, the surgeon implants a skin graft or flap after cutting out the scar tissue itself. Skin grafts are thin layers of skin that are removed from another part of the patient's body and carefully matched to the color and texture of the face or other area where the graft is to be placed. A skin flap is a full-thickness piece of tissue with its own blood supply that is taken from a site as close as possible to the scarred area.

Dermal regeneration templates, often called "artificial skin," are used to treat people with contracture scars or severe burns. These devices were approved by the Food and Drug Administration (FDA) in April 2002. The templates are made of two layers of material, a bottom layer composed of collagen derived from cows and a top layer made of silicone. To use the artificial skin, the surgeon first removes all the burned skin or scar tissue from the patient's wound. The collagen layer, which is eventually absorbed, allows the patient's body to start growing new skin while the silicone layer closes and protects the wound. After 14–21 days, the silicone layer can be removed and a very thin graft of the patient's own skin is applied to the surface of the wound. The advantages of using a dermal regeneration template are that it lowers the risk of infection and minimizes the amount of tissue that must be removed from the patient's other body sites.

Z-PLASTY AND W-PLASTY. Z-plasty and W-plasty are surgical techniques used to treat contractures and to minimize the visibility of scars by repositioning them along the natural lines and creases in the patient's skin. They are not usually used to treat keloids or hypertrophic scars. In Z-plasty, the surgeon makes a Z-shaped incision with the middle line of the Z running along the scar tissue. The flaps of skin formed by the other lines of the Z are rotated and sewn into a new position that reorients the scar about 90 degrees. In effect, the Z-plasty minimizes the appearance of the scar by breaking up the straight line of the scar into smaller units.

A W-plasty is similar to a Z-plasty in that the goal of the procedure is to minimize the visibility of a scar by turning a straight line into an irregular one. The surgeon makes a series of short incisions to form a zigzag pattern to replace the straight line of the scar. The primary difference between a Z-plasty and a W-plasty is that a W-plasty does not involve the formation and repositioning of skin flaps. A variation on the W-plasty is known as the geometric broken line closure, or GBLC.

LASER SKIN RESURFACING AND DERMABRASION. Skin resurfacing and dermabrasion are techniques used to treat acne scars or to smooth down scars with raised or uneven surfaces. They are known as ablative skin treatments because they remove the top layer of skin, or the epidermis. In dermabrasion, the surgeon moves an instrument with a high-speed rotating wheel over the scar tissue and surrounding skin several times in order to smooth the skin surface down to the lowest level of scarring. Laser skin resurfacing involves the use of a carbon dioxide or Er:YAG laser to evaporate the top layer of skin and tighten the underlying layer. Keloid or hypertrophic scars are treated with a pulsed dye laser. Dermabrasion or laser resurfacing can be used about five weeks after a scar excision to make the remaining scar less noticeable.

Laser skin resurfacing, however, is less popular than it was in the late 1990s because of increasing awareness of its potential complications. The skin of patients who have undergone laser skin resurfacing takes several months to heal, often with considerable discomfort as well as swelling and reddish discoloration of the skin. In

addition, there is a 33–85% chance that changes in the color of the skin will be permanent; the risk of permanent discoloration is higher for patients with darker skin. As of 2003, some plastic surgeons are recommending laser resurfacing only for patients with deep wrinkles or extensive sun damage who are willing to accept the pain and permanent change in skin color.

Diagnosis/Preparation

Preparation for scar revision surgery includes the surgeon's assessment of the patient's psychological stability as well as the type and extent of potential scar tissue. Many patients respond to scarring following trauma with intense anger, particularly if the face is disfigured or their livelihood is related to their appearance. Some people are impatient to have the scars treated as quickly as possible, and may have the idea that revision surgery will restore their skin to its original condition. During the initial interview, the surgeon must explain that scar revision may take months or years to complete; that some techniques essentially replace one scar with another, rather than remove all scar tissue; and that it is difficult to predict the final results in advance. Most plastic surgeons recommend waiting at least six months, preferably a full year, for a new scar to complete the maturation phase of development. Many scars will begin to fade during this period of time, and others may respond to more conservative forms of treatment.

Good candidates for scar revision surgery are people who have a realistic understanding of its risks as well as its benefits, and equally realistic expectations of its potential outcomes. On the other hand, the following are considered psychological warning signs:

- The patient is considering scar revision surgery to please someone else—most often a spouse or partner.
- The patient has a history of multiple cosmetic procedures and/or complaints about previous surgeons.

- The patient has an unrealistic notion of what scar revision surgery will accomplish.
- The patient seems otherwise emotionally unstable.

In addition to discussing the timing and nature of treatments, the surgeon will take a careful medical history, noting whether the patient is a heavy smoker or has a family history of keloids, as well as other disorders that may influence the healing of scar tissue. These disorders include diabetes, lupus, scleroderma, and other disorders that compromise body's immune system.

Aftercare

Aftercare following Z-plasty or surgical removal of a scar is relatively uncomplicated. The patient is given pain medication, told to rest for a day or two at home, and advised to avoid any activities that might put tension or pressure on the new incision(s). Most patients can return to work on the third day after surgery. The most important aspect of long-term aftercare is protecting the affected area from the sun because the surgical scar will take about a year to mature and is only about 80% as strong as undamaged skin. Sunlight can cause burns, permanent redness, loss of pigment in the skin, and breakdown of the collagen that maintains the elasticity of the skin.

Aftercare following the use of skin grafts, flaps, or dermal regeneration templates begins in the hospital with standard postoperative patients care. If sutures have been used, they are usually removed three to four days after surgery on the face and five to seven days after surgery for incisions elsewhere on the body. Patients are usually asked to return to the hospital at regular intervals so that the graft sites can be monitored. If artificial skin has been used, the patients must keep the site absolutely dry, which may require special precautions or restrictions on bathing or showering.

Aftercare for some patients includes going for psychotherapy or joining a support group to deal with emotions related to disfigurement and scar treatment.

Risks

Scar revision surgery carries the same risks as other surgical procedures under anesthesia, such as bleeding, infection at the incision site, and an adverse reaction to the anesthetic. The chief risk specific to this type of surgery is that the scar may grow, change color, or otherwise become more noticeable. Some plastic surgeons use the "90–10 rule," which means that there is a 90% chance that the scar will look better after surgery; a 9% chance that it will look about the same; and a 1% chance that it will look significantly worse.

Normal results

Normal results of scar revision surgery and associated nonsurgical treatments are a less noticeable scar.

Morbidity and mortality rates

Mortality rates for scar revision surgery are very low. Rates of complications depend on the specific technique that was used, the condition of the patient's general health, and genetic factors affecting the condition of the patient's skin.

Alternatives

There are a number of nonsurgical treatments that can be used before, after, or in place of scar revision surgery.

Drugs

Medications may be used during the initial inflammatory phase of scar formation, as well as therapy for such specific skin disorders as acne. Keloids are often treated by direct injections of **corticosteroids** to reduce itching, redness, and burning; steroid treatment may also cause the keloid to shrink. Corticosteroid injections, gels, or tapes impregnated with medication are also used after scar excisions and Z-plasty to prevent recurrence or formation of hypertrophic scars. Acne scars are treated with oral **antibiotics** or isotretinoin.

Massage, wraps, radiation, and nonablative treatments

The most conservative treatments of scar tissue include several techniques that help to minimize scar formation and improve the appearance of scars that existing already. The simplest approach is repeated massage of the scarred area with cocoa butter or vitamin E preparations. Burn scars are treated typically with the application of pressure dressings, which restrict movement of the affected area and provide insulation. Another technique that is often used is silicone gel sheeting. The sheeting is applied to the scarred area, and remains for a minimum of 12 hours a day over a period of three to six months. It is effective in improving the appearance of keloids in about 85% of cases.

Keloids that do not respond to any other form of treatment may be treated with low-dose radiation therapy.

Nonablative treatments, which do not remove the epidermal layer of skin, include microdermabrasion and superficial chemical peels. Microdermabrasion, the use of which has increased widely since 2000, is a technique for smoothing the skin. During this procedure, the physician uses a handheld instrument that buffs the skin with aluminum oxide crystals; skin flakes are removed through a vacuum tube. Microdermabrasion does not remove deep wrinkles or extensive scar tissue, but can make scars somewhat less noticeable without the risk of serious side effects. Mild chemical peels, such as those made with alpha-hydroxy acid (AHA), are used sometimes to treat acne scars or uneven skin pigmentation resulting from other types of scar revision treatment.

Camouflage

Scars on the face and legs can often be covered with specially formulated cosmetics that even out the color of the surrounding skin and help to make the scar less noticeable. Some of these preparations are available in waterproof formulations for use during swimming and other athletic activities during which one perspires.

See also Laser skin resurfacing; Skin grafting.

Resources

BOOKS

"Acne." Section 10, Chapter 116 in *The Merck Manual of Diagnosis and Therapy*, edited by Mark H. Beers, M.D. and Robert Berkow, M.D. Whitehouse Station, NJ: Merck Research Laboratories, 1999.

"Burns." Section 20, Chapter 276 in *The Merck Manual of Diagnosis and Therapy*, edited by Mark H. Beers, M.D., and Robert Berkow, M.D. Whitehouse Station, NJ: Merck Research Laboratories, 1999.

"Keloid." Section 10, Chapter 125 in *The Merck Manual of Diagnosis and Therapy*, edited by Mark H. Beers, M.D., and Robert Berkow, M.D. Whitehouse Station, NJ: Merck Research Laboratories, 1999.

PERIODICALS

Alam, M., N. E. Omura, J. S. Dover, and K. A. Arndt. "Glycolic Acid Peels Compared to Microdermabrasion: A Right-Left Controlled Trial of Efficacy and Patients Satisfaction." *Dermatologic Surgery* 28 (June 2002): 475-479.

Ang, P., and R. J. Barlow. "Nonablative Laser Resurfacing: A Systematic Review of the Literature." *Clinical and Experimental Dermatology* 27 (November 2002): 630-635.

Chang, C. W., and W. R. Ries. "Nonoperative Techniques for Scar Management and Revision." *Facial Plastic Surgery* 17 (November 2001): 283-288.

Chen, J. S., R. B. Shack, L. Reinisch, et al. "A Comparison of Scar Revision with the Free Electron and Carbon Dioxide Resurfacing Lasers." *Plastic and Reconstructive Surgery* 108 (October 2001): 1268-1275.

Clark, J. M., and T. D. Wang. "Local Flaps in Scar Revision." *Facial Plastic Surgery* 17 (November 2001): 295-308.

Fanous, N. "A New Patients PLURAL CORRECT? Classification for Laser Resurfacing and Peels: Predicting Responses, Risks, and Results." *Aesthetic Plastic Surgery* 26 (March-April 2002): 99-104.

Ghadishah, D., and J. Gorchynski. "Airway Compromise After Routine Alpha-Hydroxy Facial Peel Administration." *Journal of Emergency Medicine* 22 (May 2002): 353-355.

Heimbach, D. M., G. D. Warden, A. Luterman, et al. "Multicenter Postapproval Clinical Trial of Integra(R) Dermal Regeneration Template for Burn Treatment." *Journal of Burn Care and Rehabilitation* 24 (January-February 2003): 42-48.

Hutmacher, D. W., and W. Vanscheidt. "Matrices for Tissue-Engineered Skin." *Drugs of Today* 38 (February 2002): 113-133.

Leach, J. "Proper Handling of Soft Tissue in the Acute Phase." *Facial Plastic Surgery* 17 (November 2001): 227-238.

Lupton, J. R., and T. S. Alster. "Laser Scar Revision." *Dermatologic Clinics* 20 (January 2002): 55-65.

Moran, M. L. "Scar Revision." *Otolaryngologic Clinics of North America* 34 (August 2001): 767-780.

Mostafapour, S. P., and C. S. Murakami. "Tissue Expansion and Serial Excision in Scar Revision." *Facial Plastic Surgery* 17 (November 2001): 245-252.

Rodgers, B. J., E. F. Williams, and C. R. Hove. "W-Plasty and Geometric Broken Line Closure." *Facial Plastic Surgery* 17 (November 2001): 239-244.

KEY TERMS

Collagen—A type of protein found in connective tissue that gives it strength and flexibility.

Contracture—A condition in which the skin and underlying muscles shorten and tighten as the result of the formation of scar tissue or a disorder of the muscle fibers.

Dermabrasion—Planing of the skin done by a mechanical device, most commonly fine sandpaper or a wire brush.

Epidermis—The outermost layer of the skin.

Flap—A piece of tissue used for grafting that has kept its own blood supply.

Hypertrophic—A type of thick scar that is raised above the surface of the skin, usually caused by increasing or prolonging the inflammation stage of wound healing.

Keloid—A raised, irregularly shaped scar that gradually increases in size due to the overproduction of collagen during the healing process. The name comes from a Greek word that means "crablike."

Microdermabrasion—A technique for skin resurfacing that uses abrasive crystals passed through a hand piece to even out skin irregularities.

Nonablative—Not requiring removal or destruction of the epidermis. Some techniques for minimizing scars are nonablative.

Sclafani, Anthony P., MD, and Andrew J. Parker, MD. "Z-Plasty." *eMedicine*, July 24, 2001 [April 9, 2003]. <www.emedicine.com/ent/topic652.htm>.

ORGANIZATIONS

American Academy of Facial Plastic and Reconstructive Surgery (AAFPRS). 310 South Henry Street, Alexandria, VA 22314. (703) 299-9291. <www.facemd.org>.

American Burn Association. 625 North Michigan Avenue, Suite 1530, Chicago, IL 60611. (312) 642-9260. <www.ameriburn.org>.

American Society of Plastic Surgeons (ASPS). 444 East Algonquin Road, Arlington Heights, IL 60005. (847) 228-9900. <www.plasticsurgery.org>.

FACES: The National Craniofacial Association. P. O. Box 11082, Chattanooga, TN 37401. (800) 332-2373. <www.faces-cranio.org>.

OTHER

American Academy of Facial Plastic and Reconstructive Surgery. *2001 Membership Survey: Trends in Facial Plastic Surgery*. Alexandria, VA: AAFPRS, 2002.

American Academy of Facial Plastic and Reconstructive Surgery. *Procedures: Understanding Facial Scar Treatment*. [April 8, 2003]. <www.facial-plastic-surgery.org/patients/procedures/facial_scar.html>.

American Society of Plastic Surgeons. *Procedures: Scar Revision*. [April 7, 2003] <www.plasticsurgery.org/public_education/procedures/ScarRevision.cfm>.

Rebecca Frey, Ph.D.

Scleral buckling

Definition

Scleral buckling is a surgical procedure in which a piece of silicone plastic or sponge is sewn onto the sclera at the site of a retinal tear to push the sclera toward the retinal tear. The buckle holds the retina against the sclera until scarring seals the tear. It also prevents fluid leakage which could cause further retinal detachment.

Purpose

Scleral buckling is used to reattach the retina if the break is very large or if the tear is in one location. It is also used to seal breaks in the retina.

Demographics

Retinal detachment occurs in 25,000 Americans each year. Patients suffering from retinal detachments are commonly nearsighted, have had eye surgery, experi-

---

WHO PERFORMS THE PROCEDURE AND WHERE IS IT PERFORMED?

Scleral buckling can be performed by a general ophthalmologist, an M.D. who specializes in treatment of the eye. Even more specialized ophthalmologists, vitreo-retinal surgeons who specialize in diseases of the retina, may be called upon for serious cases.

The surgery is usually performed in hospital settings. Because of the delicacy of the procedure, sometimes an overnight hospital stay is required. Less severe retinal detachments can be treated on an outpatient basis at surgery centers.

---

enced ocular trauma, or have a family history of retinal detachments. Retinal detachments also are common after cataract removal. White males are at a greater risk, as are people who are middle-aged or older. Patients who already have had a retinal detachment also have a greater chance for another detachment.

Some conditions, such as diabetes or Coats' disease in children, make people more susceptible to retinal detachments.

Description

Scleral buckling is performed in an **operating room** under general or local anesthetic. Immediately before the procedure, patients are given eye drops to dilate the pupil to allow better access to the eye. The patient is given a local anesthetic. After the eye is numbed, the surgeon cuts the eye membrane, exposing the sclera. If bleeding or inflammation blocks the surgeon's view of the retinal detachment or hole, he or she may perform a vitrectomy before scleral buckling.

Vitrectomy is necessary only in cases in which the surgeon's view of the damage is hindered. The surgeon makes two incisions into the sclera, one for a light probe and the other for instruments to cut and aspirate. The surgeon uses a tiny, guillotine-like device to remove the vitreous, which he then replaces with saline. After the removal, the surgeon may inject air or gas to hold the retina in place.

After, the surgeon is able to see the retina, he or she will perform one of two companion procedures.

• Laser photocoagulation. The laser is used when the retinal tear is small or the detachment is slight. The surgeon points the laser beam through a contact lens to

---

Scleral buckling

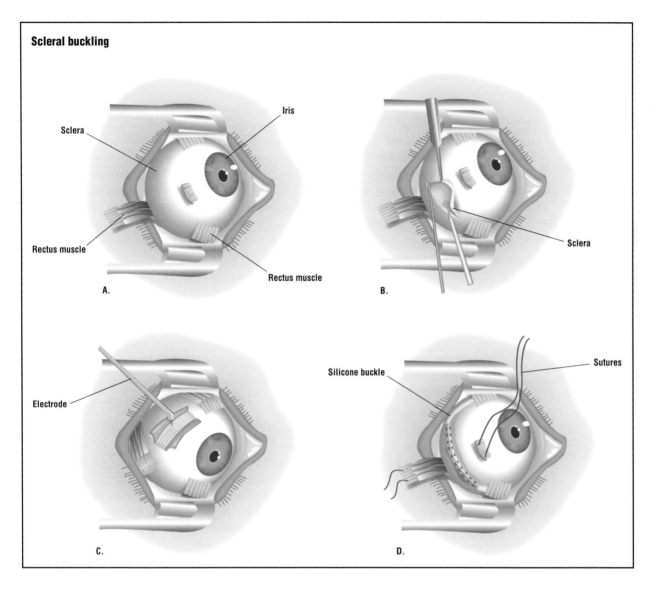

In a scleral buckling procedure, one of the eye's rectus muscles are severed to gain access to the sclera (A). The sclera is cut open (B), and an electrode is applied to the area of retinal detachment (C). A silicone buckle is threaded into place beneath the rectus muscles (D), and the severed muscle is repaired. *(Illustration by GGS Inc.)*

burn the area around the retinal tear. The laser creates scar tissue that will seal the hole and prevent leakage. It requires no incision.

• Cryopexy. Using a freezing probe, the surgeon freezes the outer surface of the eye over the tear or detachment. The inflammation caused by the freezing leads to scar formation that seals the hole and prevents leakage. Cryopexy is used for larger holes or detachments, and for areas that may be hard to reach with a laser.

After the surgeon has performed laser photocoagulation or cryopexy, he or she indents the affected area of the sclera with silicone. The silicone, either in the form of a sponge or buckle, closes the tear and reduces the eyeball's

circumference. This reduction prevents further pulling and separation of the vitreous. Depending on the severity of the detachment or hole, a buckle may be placed around the entire eyeball.

When the buckle is in place, the surgeon may drain subretinal fluid that might interfere with the retina's reattachment. After the fluid is drained, the surgeon will suture the buckle into place and then cover it with the conjunctiva. The surgeon then inserts an antibiotic (drops or ointment) into the affected eye and patches it.

For less severe detachments, the surgeon may choose a temporary buckle that will be removed later. Usually, however, the buckle remains in place for the patient's lifetime. It

QUESTIONS
TO ASK THE DOCTOR

- How many scleral buckling procedures have you performed?
- Could other treatments be an option?
- Will I have to stay in the hospital?
- Will my sight be completely restored?
- What is the probability of having another retinal detachment in the same eye?
- Am I likely to have a retinal detachment in my unaffected eye?

does not interfere with vision. Scleral buckles in infants, however, will need to be removed as the eyeball grows.

Diagnosis/Preparation

Retinal detachment is considered an emergency situation. In the case of an acute onset detachment, the longer it takes to repair the detachment, the less chance of successful reattachment. Usually the patient sees floating spots and experiences peripheral visual field loss. Patients commonly describe the vision loss as having someone pull a shade over their eyes. In extreme cases, patients may lose vision completely.

An ophthalmologist or optometrist will take a complete medical history, including family history of retinal detachment and any recent ocular trauma. In addition to performing a general eye exam, which includes a slit lamp examination, examination of the macula and lens evaluation, physicians may perform the following tests to determine the extent of retinal detachment:

- echography
- 3-mirror contact lens/panfunduscopic
- scleral indentation

Small breaks in the retina will not require surgery, but patients with acute onset detachment require reattachment in 24–48 hours. Chronic retinal detachments should be repaired within one week.

Because scleral buckling is usually an emergency procedure, there is no long-term preparation. Patients are required to fast for at least six hours before surgery.

Aftercare

Immediately following the surgery, patients will need help with meals and walking. Some patients must remain hospitalized for several days. Many scleral buckling procedures however are performed on an outpatient basis.

After release from the hospital, patients should avoid heavy lifting or strenuous **exercise** that could increase intraocular pressure. Rapid eye movements should also be avoided; reading may be prohibited until the surgeon gives permission. Sunglasses should be worn during the day and an eye patch at night. Pain and a scratchy sensation as well as redness in the eye also may occur after surgery. Ice packs may be applied if the conjunctiva swells. Patients may take pain medication, but should check with their physician before taking any over-the-counter medication.

Excessive pain, swelling, bleeding, discharge from the eye or decreased vision is not normal, and should immediately be reported to the physician.

If a vitrectomy was performed in conjunction with the scleral buckling, patients must sleep with their heads elevated. They also must avoid air travel until the air bubble is absorbed.

After scleral buckling, patients will use dilating, antibiotic or corticosteroid eye drops for up to six weeks to decrease inflammation and the chance of infection. Best visual acuity cannot be determined for at least six to eight weeks after surgery. Driving may be prohibited or restricted while vision stabilizes. At the six-to-eight week postoperative visit, physicians determine if the patient needs corrective lenses or stronger prescription lenses. Full vision restoration depends on the location and severity of the detachment.

Risks

Complications are rare but may be severe. In some instances, patients lose sight in the affected eye or lose the entire eye.

Scar tissue, even pre-existing scar tissue, may interfere with the retina's reattachment and the scleral buckling procedure may have to be repeated. Scarring, along with infection, is the most common complication.

Other possible but infrequent complications include:

- bleeding under the retina
- cataract formation
- double vision
- glaucoma
- vitreous hemorrhage

Patients may also become more nearsighted after the procedure. In some instances, although the retina reattaches, vision is not restored.

Normal results

The National Institutes of Health reports that scleral buckling has a success rate of 85–90%. Restored vision depends largely on the location and extent of the detachment, and the length of time before the detachment was repaired. Patients with a peripheral detachment have a quicker recovery then those patients whose detachment was located in the macula. The longer the patient waits to have the detachment repaired, the worse the prognosis.

Morbidity and mortality rates

The danger of mortality and loss of vision depends on the cause of the retinal detachment. Patients with Marfan syndrome, pre-eclampsia and diabetes, for example, are more at risk during the scleral buckling procedure than a patient in relatively good health. The risk of surgery also rises with the use of general anesthesia. Scleral buckling, however, is considered a safe, successful procedure.

Severe infections that are left untreated can cause vision loss, but following the prescribed regimen of eye drops and follow-up treatment by the physician greatly minimizes this risk.

Alternatives

Vitrectomy is sometimes performed alone to treat retinal detachments. Laser photocoagulation and cryopexy also may be used to treat less serious tears. The more common alternative, however, is pneumatic retinopexy, which is used when the tear is located in the upper portion of the eye. The surgeon uses cryopexy to freeze the area around the tear, then removes a small amount of fluid. When the fluid is drained and the eye softened, the surgeon injects a gas bubble into the vitreous cavity. As the gas bubble expands, it seals the retinal tear by pushing the retina against the choroid. Eventually, the bubble will be absorbed.

The patient is required to remain in a certain position for at least a few days after surgery while the bubble helps seal the hole. Pneumatic retinopexy also is not as successful as scleral buckling. Complications include recurrent retinal detachments and the chance of gas getting under the retina.

Resources

BOOKS

Buettner, Helmut, M.D., editor. *Mayo Clinic on Vision and Eye Health.* Rochester, MN: Mayo Clinic Health Information, 2002.

Cassel, Gary H., M.D., Michael D., Billig, O.D., and Harry G. Randall, M.D. *The Eye Book: A Complete Guide to Eye Disorders and Health.* Baltimore, MD: Johns Hopkins University Press, 1998.

Everything You Need to Know About Medical Treatments, edited by Stephen Daly. Springhouse, PA: Springhouse Corp., 1996.

Sardgena, Jill, et al. *The Encyclopedia of Blindness and Vision Impairment,* 2nd Edition. New York, NY: Facts on File, Inc. 2002.

ORGANIZATIONS

American Academy of Ophthalmology. PO Box 7424, San Francisco, CA 94120-7424. (415) 561-8500. <http://www.aao.org>.

American Board of Ophthalmology. 111 Presidential Boulevard, Suite 241, Bala Cynwyd, PA 19004-1075. (610) 664-1175. info@abop.org. <http://www.abop.org>.

National Eye Institute. 2020 Vision Place, Bethesda, MD 20892-3655. (301) 496-5248. <http://www.nei.nih.gov>.

OTHER

Handbook of Ocular Disease Management: Retinal Detachment *Review of Ophthalmology* [cited April 21, 2003]. <http://www.revoptom.com/handbook/SECT5R.HTM>.

"Retinal Detachment." VisionChannel.net [cited April 12, 2003]. <http://www.visionchannel.net/retinaldetachment/treatment.shtml>.

"Retinal Detachment Repair." EyeMdLink.com [cited May 1, 2003]. <http://www.eyemdlink.com/EyeProcedure.asp?EyeProcedureID=52>.

Wu, Lihteh, M.D. "Retinal Detachment, Exudative." emedicine.com. June 28, 2001 [cited May 1, 2003]. <http://www.emedicine.com/oph/topic407htm>.

Mary Bekker

Sclerostomy

Definition

A sclerostomy is a procedure in which the surgeon makes a small opening in the outer covering of the eyeball to reduce intraocular pressure (IOP) in patients with open-angle glaucoma. It is classified as a type of glaucoma filtering surgery. The name of the surgery comes from the Greek word for "hard," which describes the tough white outer coat of the eyeball, and the Greek word for "cutting" or "incision."

Purpose

Sclerostomies are usually performed to reduce IOP in open-angle glaucoma patients who have not been helped by less invasive forms of treatment, specifically medications and **laser surgery**. In some cases—most commonly patients who are rapidly losing their vision or who cannot tolerate glaucoma medications—an ophthalmologist (eye specialist) may recommend a sclerostomy without trying other forms of treatment first.

As of 2003, glaucoma is not considered a single disease but rather a group of diseases characterized by three major characteristics: elevated intraocular pressure (IOP) caused by an overproduction of aqueous humor in the eye or by resistance to the normal outflow of fluid; atrophy of the optic nerve; and a resultant loss of visual field. A sclerostomy works to reduce the IOP by improving the outflow of aqueous humor. Between 80% and 90% of aqueous humor leaves the eye through the trabecular meshwork while the remaining 10–20% passes through the ciliary muscle bundles. A sclerostomy allows the fluid to collect under the conjunctiva, which is the thin membrane lining the eyelids, to form a filtration bleb.

Demographics

In 1995, the World Health Organization (WHO) reported that over five million people around the world have lost their sight due to complications of glaucoma; about 120,000 Americans are blind as a result of glaucoma. According to the National Eye Institute (NEI), nearly three million people in the United States have the disorder; however, nearly half are unaware that they have it. Primary open-angle glaucoma (POAG) accounts for 60–70% of cases. "Primary" means that the glaucoma is not associated with a tumor, injury to the eye, or other eye disorder.

Although glaucoma can occur at any age, it is most common in adults over 35. One major study reported that less than 1% of the United States population between 60 and 64 suffer from POAG. The rate rises to 1.3% for persons between 70 and 74, however, and rises again to 3% for persons between 80 and 84.

With regard to race, African-Americans are four times as likely to develop glaucoma as Caucasians, and six to eight times more likely to lose their sight to the disease. African Americans also develop glaucoma at earlier ages; while everyone over age 60 is at increased risk for POAG, the risk for African Americans rises sharply after age 40. A 2001 study reported that the rate for Mexican Americans lies between the rate of POAG in African Americans and that in Caucasians. Mexican Americans, however, are more likely to suffer from undiagnosed glaucoma—62% as compared to 50% for other races and ethnic groups in the United States. In addition, the rate of POAG in Mexican Americans was found to rise rapidly after age 65; in the older age groups, it approaches the rates reported for African Americans. Among Caucasians, people of Scandinavian, Irish, or Russian ancestry are at higher risk of glaucoma than people from other ethnic groups.

The question of a sex ratio in open-angle glaucoma is debated. Three studies done in the United States between 1991 and 1996 reported that the male:female ratio for open-angle glaucoma is about 1:1. Three other studies carried out in the United States, Barbados, and the Netherlands, however, found that the male:female ratio was almost 2:1. A 2002 study from western Africa reported a male:female ratio of 2.26:1. It appears that further research is needed in this area.

Description

Most sclerostomies are performed as outpatient procedures under local anesthesia. In some cases the patient may be given an intravenous sedative to help him or her relax before the procedure.

Conventional sclerostomy

After the patient has been sedated, the surgeon injects a local anesthetic into the area around the eye as well as a medication to prevent eye movement. Using very small instruments with the help of a microscope, the surgeon makes a tiny hole in the sclera as a passageway for aqueous humor. Some surgeons use an erbium YAG laser to create the hole. Most surgeons apply an antimetabolite drug during the procedure to minimize the risk that the new drainage channel will be closed by tissue regrowth. The most common antimetabolites that are used are mitomycin and 5-fluouracil.

After the surgery, the aqueous humor begins to flow through the sclerostomy hole and forms a small blister-like structure on the upper surface of the eye. This structure is known as a bleb or filtration bleb, and is covered by the eyelid. The bleb allows the aqueous humor to leave the eye in a controlled fashion.

Enzymatic sclerostomy

A newer technique that was first described in 2002 is enzymatic sclerostomy, which was developed at the

Weizmann Institute of Science in Israel. In enzymatic sclerostomy, the surgeon applies an enzyme called collagenase to the eye to increase the release of aqueous humor. The collagenase is applied through an applicator that is attached to the eye with tissue glue for 22–24 hours and then removed. According to the researchers, the procedure reduced the intraocular pressure in all patients immediately following the procedure and in 80% of the subjects at one-year follow-up. None of the patients developed systemic complications. Enzymatic sclerostomy is considered experimental as of mid-2003.

Diagnosis/Preparation

Diagnosis

Open-angle glaucoma is not always diagnosed promptly because it is insidious in onset, which means that it develops slowly and gradually. Unlike closed-angle glaucoma, open-angle glaucoma rarely has early symptoms. It is usually diagnosed either in the course of an eye examination or because the patient has noticed that they are having problems with their peripheral vision—that is, they are having trouble seeing objects at the side or out of the corner of the eye. In some cases the patient notices that he or she is missing words while reading; having trouble seeing stairs or other objects at the bottom of the visual field; or having trouble seeing clearly when driving. Other symptoms of open-angle glaucoma may include headaches, seeing haloes around lights, or difficulty adjusting to darkness. It is important to diagnose open-angle glaucoma as soon as possible because the vision that has been already lost cannot be recovered. Although open-angle glaucoma cannot be cured, it can be stabilized and controlled in almost all patients. Because of the importance of catching open-angle glaucoma as early as possible, adults should have their eyes examined every two years at least.

HIGH-RISK GROUPS. Not everyone is at equal risk for glaucoma. People with any of the risk factors listed below should consult their doctor for advice about the frequency of eye checkups:

• Age over 40 (African Americans) or over 60 (other races and ethnic groups).

• Ocular hypertension. The normal level of IOP is between 11 mm Hg and 21 mm Hg. It is possible for people to have an IOP above 21 mm Hg without signs of damage to the optic nerve or loss of visual field; this condition is referred to as ocular hypertension. Conversely, about one out of six of patients diagnosed with open-angle glaucoma have so-called normal-tension glaucoma, which means that their optic nerve is being damaged even though their IOP is within the "normal"

range. Ocular hypertension does, however, increase a person's risk of developing glaucoma in the future.

• Family history of glaucoma in a first-degree relative. As of 2003, at least six different genes related to glaucoma have been identified.

• An unusually thin cornea (the clear front portion of the outer cover of the eye). A recent National Eye Institute (NEI) study found that patients whose corneas are thinner than 555 microns are three times as likely to develop glaucoma as those whose corneas are thicker than 588 microns.

• Extreme nearsightedness. People who are very nearsighted are two to three times more likely to develop glaucoma than those who are not nearsighted.

• Diabetes.

• History of traumatic injury to the eye or surgery for other eye disorders.

• Use of steroid medications.

• Migraine headaches or sleep-related breathing disorder.

• Male sex.

Some patients should not be treated with filtration surgery. Contraindications for a sclerostomy include cardiovascular disorders and other severe systemic medical problems; eyes that are already blind; or the presence of an intraocular tumor or bleeding in the eye.

DIAGNOSTIC TESTS. Ophthalmologists use the following tests to screen patients for open-angle glaucoma:

• Tonometry. Tonometry is a painless procedure for measuring IOP. One type of tonometer blows a puff of pressurized air toward the patient's eye as the patient sits near a lamp; it measures the changes in the light reflections on the patient's corneas. Another method of tonometry involves the application of a local anesthetic to the outside of the eye and touching the cornea briefly with an instrument that measures the fluid pressure directly.

- Visual field test. This test measures loss of peripheral vision. In the simplest version of this test, the patient sits directly in front of the examiner with one eye covered. The patient looks at the examiner's eye and indicates when he or she can see the examiner's hand. In the automated version, the patient sits in front of a hollow dome and looks at a central target inside the dome. A computer program flashes lights at intervals at different locations inside the dome, and the patient presses a button whenever he or she sees a light. At the end of the test, the computer prints an assessment of the patient's responses.

- Gonioscopy. Gonioscopy measures the size of the angle in the anterior chamber of the eye with the use of a special mirrored contact lens. The examiner numbs the outside of the eye with a local anesthetic and touches the outside of the cornea with the gonioscopic lens. He or she can use a slit lamp to magnify what appears on the lens. Gonioscopy is necessary in order to distinguish between open- and closed-angle glaucoma; it can also distinguish between primary and many secondary glaucomas.

- Ophthalmoscopic examination of the optic nerve. An ophthalmoscope is an instrument that contains a perforated mirror as well as magnifying lenses. It allows the examiner to view the interior of the eye. If the patient has open-angle glaucoma, the examiner can see a cup-shaped depression in the optic disk.

Newer diagnostic devices include a laser-scanning microscope known as the Heidelberg retinal tomograph (HRT) and ultrasound biomicroscopy (UBM). UBM has proved to be a useful method of long-term follow-up of sclerostomies.

Preparation

Preparation for a sclerostomy begins with the patient's decision to undergo incisional surgery rather than continuing to take medications or having repeated laser procedures. Three factors commonly influence the decision: the present extent of the patient's visual loss; the speed of visual deterioration; and the patient's life expectancy.

With regard to the procedure itself, patients may be asked to take oral antibiotic and anti-inflammatory medications for several days prior to surgery.

Aftercare

Patients can use their eyes after filtering surgery, although they should have a friend or relative to drive them home after the procedure. They can go to work the next day, although they will probably notice some blurring of vision in the operated eye for about a month. Patients can carry out their normal activities with the exception of heavy lifting, although they should not drive until their vision has completely cleared. Most ophthalmologists recommend that patients wear their eyeglasses during the day and tape an eye shield over the operated eye at night. They should apply eye drops prescribed by the ophthalmologist to prevent infection, manage pain, and reduce swelling. They should also avoid rubbing, bumping, or getting water into the operated eye. Complete recovery after filtering surgery usually takes about six weeks. Long-term aftercare includes avoiding damage to or infection of the bleb.

It is important for patients recovering from filtering surgery to see their doctor for frequent checkups in the first few weeks following surgery. In most cases the ophthalmologist will check the patient's eye the day after surgery and about once a week for the next several weeks.

Risks

The risks of a sclerostomy include the following:

- Infection. Infections may develop in the bleb (blebitis), but may spread to the interior of the eye (endophthalmitis). The symptoms of an infection include pain and redness in the eye, blurred vision, teariness, and a discharge. Infections must be treated promptly, as they can lead to loss of vision.

- Hyphema. Hyphema refers to the presence of blood inside the anterior chamber of the eye. Hyphemas are most common within the first two to three days after surgery and are usually treated with corticosteroid medications to reduce inflammation.

- Suprachoroidal hemorrhage. A suprachoroidal hemorrhage, or massive bleeding behind the retina, is a serious complication that can occur during as well as after eye surgery.

- Cataract formation.

- Hypotony (low IOP). If hypotony is not corrected, it can lead to failure of the bleb and eventual cataract formation.

- Loss of central vision. This is a very rare complication.

- Bleb leak or failure. Blebs can develop leaks at any time from several days after surgery to years later. Bleb failure usually results from inadequate control of the intraocular pressure and a new obstruction of aqueous humor outflow.

- Closing of the opening in the sclera by new tissue growth. A sclerostomy can be repeated if necessary.

Normal results

According to the National Eye Institute, sclerostomy is 80–90% effective in lowering intraocular pressure. The success rate is highest in patients who have not had previous eye surgery.

Morbidity and mortality rates

Mortality following a sclerostomy is very low because the majority of procedures are performed under local anesthesia. The most common complications of filtering surgery are cataract formation (30% of patients develop cataracts within five years of a sclerostomy) and closure of the drainage opening requiring additional surgery (10–15% of patients). Bleeding or infection occur in less than 1% of patients.

Alternatives

Nonpenetrating deep sclerectomy

There are two surgical alternatives to sclerostomy that are called nonpenetrating deep sclerectomies because they do not involve entering the anterior chamber of the eye. The first alternative, viscocanalostomy, is a procedure that involves creating a window in Descemet's membrane (a layer of tissue in the cornea) to allow aqueous humor to leave the anterior chamber; and injecting a viscoelastic substance into Schlemm's canal, which is the main pathway for aqueous humor to leave the eye. The viscoelastic helps to keep the canal from scarring shut following surgery.

The second type of nonpenetrating surgery involves implanting a device called the Aquaflow® collagen wick about 0.8 in (2 cm) long under the sclera. The wick keeps open a space created by the surgeon to allow drainage of the aqueous humor. The wick is made of a material that is absorbed by the body within six to nine months, but the drainage pathway remains open after the wick is absorbed. The Aquaflow wick was approved by the Food and Drug Administration (FDA) in July 2001.

Both types of nonpenetrating deep sclerectomies allow patients to recover faster, with fewer complications than traditional sclerostomies. Their drawbacks include a lower success rate and the need for additional procedures to control the patient's IOP. Viscocanalostomy in particular is not as effective in reducing IOP levels as traditional filtering surgery.

Complementary and alternative (CAM) approaches

Bilberry (European blueberry) extract has been recommended as improving night vision; it was given to RAF pilots during World War II for this reason. There is evidence that 80–160 mg of bilberry extract taken three times a day does improve night vision temporarily. The plant does not have any serious side effects, but it should not be used in place of regular eye examinations or other treatments for glaucoma.

People who support the medicinal use of marijuana have argued that cannabinoids, the active chemical compounds found in the plant, lower intraocular pressure in patients with glaucoma. According to the Glaucoma Research Foundation, however, very high doses of marijuana are required to produce any significant effect on IOP. A Canadian researcher has concluded that the effects of cannabinoids on IOP "....are not sufficiently strong, long lasting or reliable to provide a valid basis for therapeutic use [of marijuana]."

See also Iridectomy; Laser iridotomy; Trabeculectomy.

Resources

BOOKS

Pelletier, Kenneth R., MD. "CAM Therapies for Specific Conditions: Eye Disorders." In *The Best Alternative Medicine*. New York: Simon & Schuster, 2002.

"Primary Open-Angle Glaucoma." In *The Merck Manual of Diagnosis and Therapy*, edited by Mark H. Beers, MD, and Robert Berkow, MD. Whitehouse Station, NJ: Merck Research Laboratories, 1999.

PERIODICALS

Daboue, A., N. D. Meda, and A. Ahnoux-Zabsonre. "Eye Tension and Open-Angle Glaucoma in a Burkina Faso Hospital." [in French] *Journal français d'ophtalmologie* 25 (January 2002): 39–41.

Dan, J. A., S. G. Honavar, D. A. Belyea, et al. "Enzymatic Sclerostomy: Pilot Human Study." *Archives of Ophthalmology* 120 (May 2002): 548–553.

Kalant, H. "Medicinal Use of Cannabis: History and Current Status." *Pain Research and Management* 6 (Summer 2001): 80–91.

Angle—The open point in the anterior chamber of the eye at which the iris meets the cornea.

Aqueous humor—The watery fluid produced in the eye that ordinarily leaves the eye through the angle of the anterior chamber and Schlemm's canal.

Atrophy—Wasting away or degeneration. Atrophy of the optic nerve is one of the defining characteristics of glaucoma.

Bleb—A thin-walled auxiliary drain created on the outside of the eyeball during filtering surgery for glaucoma. It is sometimes called a filtering bleb.

Conjunctiva—The thin membrane that lines the eyelids and covers the visible surface of the sclera.

Cornea—The transparent front portion of the exterior cover of the eye.

Endophthalmitis—An infection on the inside of the eye, which may result from an infected bleb. Endophthalmitis can result in vision loss.

Glaucoma—A group of eye disorders characterized by increased fluid pressure inside the eye that eventually damages the optic nerve. As the cells in the optic nerve die, the patient gradually loses vision.

Gonioscopy—A technique for examining the angle between the iris and the cornea with the use of a special mirrored lens applied to the cornea.

Hyphema—Blood inside the anterior chamber of the eye. Hyphema is one of the risks associated with sclerostomies.

Hypotony—Intraocular fluid pressure that is too low.

Insidious—Developing in a stealthy and inconspicuous way. Open-angle glaucoma is an insidious disorder.

Ocular hypertension—A condition in which fluid pressure inside the eye is higher than normal but the optic nerve and visual fields are normal.

Open-angle glaucoma—A form of glaucoma in which fluid pressure builds up inside the eye even though the angle of the anterior chamber is open and looks normal when the eye is examined with a gonioscope. Most cases of glaucoma are open-angle.

Ophthalmology—The branch of medicine that deals with the diagnosis and treatment of eye disorders.

Peripheral vision—The outer portion of the visual field.

Schlemm's canal—A circular channel located at the point where the sclera of the eye meets the cornea. Schlemm's canal is the primary pathway for aqueous humor to leave the eye.

Sclera—The tough white fibrous membrane that forms the outermost covering of the eyeball.

Tonometry—Measurement of the fluid pressure inside the eye.

Trabecular meshwork—The main drainage passageway for fluid to leave the anterior chamber of the eye.

Visual field—The total area in which one can see objects in one's peripheral vision while the eyes are focused on a central point.

Kazakova, D., S. Roters, C. C. Schnyder, et al. "Ultrasound Biomicroscopy Images: Long-Term Results After Deep Sclerectomy with Collagen Implant." *Graefe's Archive for Clinical and Experimental Ophthalmology* 240 (November 2002): 918–923.

Lachkar, Y., and P. Hamard. "Nonpenetrating Filtering Surgery." *Current Opinion in Ophthalmology* 13 (April 2002): 110–115.

Luke, C., T. S. Dietlin, P. C. Jacobi, et al. "A Prospective Randomized Trial of Viscocanalostomy Versus Trabeculectomy in Open-Angle Glaucoma: A 1-Year Follow-Up Study." *Journal of Glaucoma* 11 (August 2002): 294–99.

Mizota, A., M. Takasoh, K. Kobayashi, et al. "Internal Sclerostomy with the Er:YAG Laser Using a Gradient-Index (GRIN) Endoscope." *Ophthalmic Surgery and Lasers* 33 (May-June 2002): 214–220.

Mizota, A., M. Takasoh, Y. Tsuyama, et al. "Sclerostomy with an Erbium YAG Laser. The Relationship with Pulse Energy." *Japanese Journal of Ophthalmology* 45 (January 2001): 111.

Pascotto, Antonio, MD, Giorgio Cusati, MD, Elena Soreca, MD, and Sergio Saccà, MD. "Glaucoma, Complications and Management of Glaucoma Filtering." *eMedicine*, November 15, 2002 [cited May 17, 2003]. <http://www.emedicine.com/oph/topic720.htm>.

Rastogi, Shobit, MD, Enrique Garcia-Valenzuela, MD, and Monica Allen, MD. "Hyphema, Postoperative." *eMedicine*, October 26, 2001 [cited May 18, 2003]. <http://www.emedicine.com/oph/topic68.htm>.

Shaarawy, T., C. Nguyen, C. Schnyder, and A. Mermoud. "Five-Year Results of Viscoanalostomy." *British Journal of Ophthalmology* 87 (April 2003): 441–445.

ORGANIZATIONS

American Academy of Ophthalmology. P.O. Box 7424, San Francisco, CA 94120-7424. (415) 561-8500. <http://www.aao.org>.

American Optometric Association. 243 North Lindbergh Blvd., St. Louis, MO 63141. (314) 991-4100.

Canadian Ophthalmological Society (COS). 610-1525 Carling Avenue, Ottawa ON K1Z 8R9. <http://www.eyesite.ca>.

(The) Glaucoma Foundation. 116 John Street, Suite 1605, New York, NY 10038. (212) 285-0080 or (800) 452-8266. <http://www.glaucoma-foundation.org>.

Glaucoma Research Foundation. 490 Post Street, Suite 1427, SanFrancisco, CA 94102. (415) 986-3162 or (800) 826-6693. <http://www.glaucoma.org>.

National Eye Institute. 2020 Vision Place, Bethesda, MD 20892-3655. (301) 496-5248. <http://www.nei.nih.gov>.

Prevent Blindness America. 500 East Remington Road, Schaumburg, IL 60173. (800) 331-2020. <http://www.prevent-blindness.org>.

Wills Eye Hospital. 840 Walnut Street, Philadelphia, PA 19107. (215) 928-3000. <http://www.willseye.org>.

OTHER

Lewis, Thomas L., O. D., Ph.D. *Optometric Clinical Practice Guideline: Care of the Patient with Open Angle Glaucoma.* 2nd ed. St. Louis, MO: American Optometric Association, 2002.

National Eye Institute (NEI). *Facts About Glaucoma.* Bethesda, MD: NEI, 2001. NIH Publication No. 99–651.

NEI Statement. *Prevalence of Glaucoma in Mexican-Americans.* Bethesda, MD: NEI, December 2001 [cited May 18, 2003]. <http://www.nei.nih.gov/news/statements/glauc-mex amer.htm>.

Prevent Blindness America. *Vision Problems in the U.S.: Prevalence of Adult Vision Impairment and Age-Related Eye Disease in America.* Schaumburg, IL: Prevent Blindness America, 2002.

Rebecca Frey, Ph.D.

Sclerotherapy for esophageal varices

Definition

Sclerotherapy for esophageal varices, also called endoscopic sclerotherapy, is a treatment for esophageal bleeding that involves the use of an endoscope and the injection of a sclerosing solution into veins.

Purpose

Esophageal varices are enlarged or swollen veins on the lining of the esophagus which are prone to bleeding.

WHO PERFORMS THE PROCEDURE AND WHERE IS IT PERFORMED?

Sclerotherapy for esophageal varices is performed by a surgeon specialized in gastroenterology or hepatology in a hospital setting, very often as an emergency procedure.

They are life-threatening and can be fatal in up to 50% of patients. Esophageal varices are a complication of portal hypertension, a condition characterized by increased blood pressure in the portal vein resulting from such liver disease, as liver cirrhosis. Increased pressure causes the veins to balloon outward. The vessels may rupture, causing vomiting of blood and bloody stools.

In most hospitals, sclerotherapy for esophageal varices is the treatment of choice to stop esophageal bleeding during acute episodes, and to prevent further incidences of bleeding. Emergency sclerotherapy is often followed by preventive treatments to eradicate distended esophageal veins.

Demographics

Bleeding esophageal varices are a serious complication of liver disease. In the United States, at least 50% of people who survive bleeding esophageal varices are at risk of recurrent bleeding during the next one to two years.

Description

Sclerotherapy for esophageal varices involves injecting a strong and irritating solution (a sclerosant) into the veins and/or the area beside the distended vein. Sclerosant injected directly into the vein causes blood clots to form and stops the bleeding, while sclerosant injected into the area beside the distended vein stops the bleeding by thickening and swelling the vein to compress the blood vessel. Most physicians inject the sclerosant directly into the vein, although injections into the vein and the surrounding area are both effective. Once bleeding has been stopped, the treatment can be used to significantly reduce or destroy the varices.

Sclerotherapy for esophageal varices is performed with the patient awake but sedated. Hyoscine butylbromide (Buscopan) may be administered to freeze the esophagus, making injection of the sclerosant easier. During the procedure, an endoscope is passed through the patient's mouth to the esophagus to allow the surgeon to view the inside. The branches of the blood vessels at or

QUESTIONS TO ASK THE DOCTOR

- What are esophageal varices?
- Are there alternatives to sclerotherapy?
- How do I prepare for surgery?
- What type of anesthesia will be used?
- How is the surgery performed?
- How long will I be in the hospital?
- How many sclerotherapy procedures do you perform in a year?

just above where the stomach and esophagus come together, the usual site of variceal bleeding, are located. After the bleeding vein is identified, a long, flexible sclerotherapy needle is passed through the endoscope. When the tip of the needle's sheath is in place, the needle is advanced, and the sclerosant is injected into the vein or the surrounding area. The most commonly used sclerosants are ethanolamine and sodium tetradecyl sulfate. The needle is withdrawn. The procedure is repeated as many times as necessary to eradicate all distended veins.

Diagnosis/Preparation

A radiologist assesses patients for sclerotherapy based on blood work and liver imaging studies performed using **CT scans**, ultrasound or MRI scans, and in consultation with the treating gastroenterologist, hepatologist, or surgeon. Tests to localize bleeding and detect active bleeding are also performed.

Before a sclerotherapy procedure, the patient's **vital signs** and other pertinent data are recorded, an intravenous line is inserted to administer fluid or blood, and a sedative is prescribed.

Aftercare

After sclerotherapy for esophageal varices, the patient will be observed for signs of blood loss, lung complications, fever, a perforated esophagus, or other complications. Vital signs are monitored, and the intravenous line maintained. Pain medication is usually prescribed. After leaving the hospital, the patient follows a diet prescribed by the physician, and, if appropriate, can take mild pain relievers.

Risks

Risks associated with sclerotherapy include complications that can arise from use of the sclerosant or from the endoscopic procedure. Minor complications, which cause discomfort but do not require active treatment or prolonged hospitalization, include transient chest pain, difficulty swallowing, and fever, which usually go away after a few days. Some patients may have allergic reactions to the sclerosant solution. Infection occurs in up to 50% of cases. In 2-10% of patients, the esophagus tightens, but this complication can usually be treated with dilatation. More serious complications may occur in 10-15% of patients. These include perforation or bleeding of the esophaggus and lung problems, such as aspiration pneumonia. Long-term sclerotherapy can also damage the esophagus and increase the patient's risk of developing cancer.

Patients with advanced liver disease complicated by bleeding are very poor risks for this procedure. The surgery, premedications, and anesthesia may be sufficient to tip the patient into protein intoxication and hepatic coma. The blood in the bowels acts like a high protein meal and may induce protein intoxication.

Normal results

Normal sclerotherapy results include the control of acute bleeding if present and the shrinking of the esophageal varices.

Morbidity and mortality rates

Sclerotherapy for esophageal varices has a 20-40% incidence of complications and a 1–2% mortality rate. The procedure controls acute bleeding in about 90% of patients, but it may have to be repeated within the first 48 hours to achieve this success rate. During the initial hospitalization, sclerotherapy is usually performed two or three times. Preventive treatments are scheduled every few weeks or so, depending on the patient's risk level and healing rate. Several studies have shown that the risk of recurrent bleeding is much lower in patients treated with sclerotherapy: 30-50% as opposed to 70–80% for patients not treated with sclerotherapy.

Alternatives

Pharmacological agents are also used in the treatment of esophageal varices. Such drugs as vasopressin and somatostatin are administered to actively bleeding patients on admission, while propranolol, nadolol or subcutaneous octreotide are used to prevent subsequent bleeding after successful endoscopic variceal eradication. Vasopressin or vasopressin with nitroglycerin has been proven effective in the acute control of variceal hemorrhage. Somatostatin is more effective in the control of active bleeding when compared to vasopressin, glypressin, endoscopic sclerotherapy or balloon tamponade.

KEY TERMS

Cirrhosis—A chronic degenerative liver disease causing irreversible scarring of the liver.

Endoscope—An instrument used to examine the inside of a canal or hollow organ. Endoscopic surgery is less invasive than traditional surgery.

Esophagus—The part of the digestive canal located between the pharynx (part of the digestive tube) and the stomach. Also called the food pipe.

Portal hypertension—Abnormally high pressure within the veins draining into the liver.

Sclerosant—An irritating solution that stops bleeding by hardening the blood or vein it is injected into.

Varices—Swollen or enlarged veins, in this case veins in the lining of the esophagus.

Octreotide has comparable outcomes to vasopressin, terlipressin or endoscopic sclerotherapy. **Liver transplantation** should be considered as an alternative for patients with bleeding varices from liver disease.

Another alternative treatment is provided by Transjugular intrahepatic portal-systemic shunting (TIPS). In TIPS, a catheter fitted with a stent, a wire mesh tube used to prop open a vein or artery, is inserted through a vein in the neck into the liver. Under x ray guidance, the stent is placed in an optimal position within the liver so as to allow blood to flow more easily through the portal vein. This treatment reduces the excess pressure in the esophageal varices, and thus decreases the risk of recurrent bleeding.

See also Portal vein bypass.

Resources

BOOKS

Belcaro, G., and G. Stansby. *The Venous Clinic: Diagnosis, Prevention, Investigations, Conservative and Medical Treatment, Sclerotherapy and Surgery.* River Edge, NJ: World Scientific Pub. Co., 1999.

Green, Frederick L., and Jeffrey L. Ponsky, eds. "Endoscopic Management of Esophageal Varices." In *Endoscopic Surgery.* Philadelphia: W. B. Saunders Co., 1994.

Sadick, N. S. *Manual of Sclerotherapy.* Philadelphia: Lippincott, Williams & Wilkins, 2000.

Shearman, David J. C., et al., eds. "Endoscopy" and "Gastrointestinal Bleeding." In *Diseases of the Gastrointestinal Tract and Liver.* New York: Churchill Livingstone, 1997.

Yamada, Tadataka, et al., eds. "Endoscopic Control of Upper Gastrointestinal Variceal Bleeding." In *Textbook of Gastroenterology.* Philadelphia: J. B. Lippincott Co., 1995.

PERIODICALS

Dhiman, R. K., and Y. K. Chawla. "A new technique of combined endoscopic sclerotherapy and ligation for variceal bleeding." *World Journal of Gastroenterology* 9 (May 2003): 1090–1093.

Mahesh, B., S. Thulkar, G. Joseph, A. Srivastava, and R. K. Khazanchi. "Colour duplex ultrasound-guided sclerotherapy. A new approach to the management of patients with peripheral vascular malformations." *Clinical Imaging* 27 (May-June 2003): 171–179.

Miyazaki, K., T. Nishibe, F. Sata, T. Imai, F. A. Kudo, J. Flores, Y. J. Miyazaki, and K. Yasuda. "Stripping Operation with Sclerotherapy for Primary Varicose Veins Due to Greater Saphenous Vein Reflux: Three-Year Results." *World Journal of Surgery* 27 (May 2003): 551–553.

ORGANIZATIONS

Society of American Gastrointestinal Endoscopic Surgeons (SAGES). 2716 Ocean Park Boulevard, Suite 3000, Santa Monica, CA 90405. (310) 314-2404. <http://www.sages.org>.

OTHER

SAGES: The Role of Endoscopic Sclerotherapy. <http://www.sages.org/sg_asgepub1019.html>.

Lori De Milto
Monique Laberge, Ph.D.

Sclerotherapy for varicose veins

Definition

Sclerotherapy, which takes its name from a Greek word meaning "hardening," is a method of treating enlarged veins by injecting an irritating chemical called a sclerosing agent into the vein. The chemical causes the vein to become inflamed, which leads to the formation of fibrous tissue and closing of the lumen, or central channel of the vein.

Purpose

Sclerotherapy in the legs is performed for several reasons. It is most often done to improve the appearance of the legs, and is accomplished by closing down spider veins—small veins in the legs that have dilated under increased venous blood pressure. A spider vein is one type of telangiectasia, which is the medical term for a reddish-colored lesion produced by the permanent enlargement of the capillaries and other small blood vessels. The word telangiectasia comes from three Greek words that mean "end," "blood vessel," and "stretch out." In a spider vein, also called a "sunburst varicosity" there is a central reddish area that is visible to the eye because it lies close to the surface of the skin; smaller veins spread outward from it in the shape of a spider's legs. Spider veins may also appear in two other common patterns—they may look like tiny tree branches or like extra-fine separate lines.

In addition to the cosmetic purposes sclerotherapy serves, it is also performed to treat the soreness, aching, muscle fatigue, and leg cramps that often accompany small- or middle-sized varicose veins in the legs. It is not, however, used by itself to treat large varicose veins.

Because sclerotherapy is usually considered a cosmetic procedure, it is usually not covered by health insurance. People who are being treated for cramps and discomfort in their legs, however, should ask their insurance companies whether they are covered for sclerotherapy. In 2001, the average cost of the procedure was $227.

Sclerotherapy as a general treatment modality is also performed to treat hemorrhoids (swollen veins) in the esophagus.

Demographics

The American College of Phlebology (ACP), a group of dermatologists, plastic surgeons, gynecologists, and general surgeons with special training in the treatment of venous disorders, comments that more than 80 million people in the United States suffer from spider veins or varicose veins. The American Society of Plastic Surgeons (ASPS) estimates that 50% of women over 21 in the United States have spider veins.

Women are more likely to develop spider veins than men, but the incidence among both sexes increases with age. The results of a recent survey of middle-aged and elderly people in San Diego, California, show that 80% of the women and 50% of the men had spider veins. Men are less likely to seek treatment for spider veins for cosmetic reasons, however, because the discoloration caused by spider veins is often covered by leg hair. On the other hand, men who are bothered by aching, burning sensations or leg cramps, can benefit from sclerotherapy.

According to the ASPS, there were 616,879 sclerotherapy procedures performed in the United States in 2001; 97% were performed on women and 3% were done on men. Most people who are treated with sclerotherapy are between the ages of 30 and 60.

Spider veins are most noticeable and common in Caucasians. Hispanics are less likely than Caucasians but more likely than either African or Asian Americans to develop spider veins.

Description

Causes of spider veins

To understand how sclerotherapy works, it is helpful to begin with a brief description of the venous system in the human body. The venous part of the circulatory system returns blood to the heart to be pumped to the lungs for oxygenation. This is in contrast to the arterial system, which carries oxygenated blood away from the heart to be distributed throughout the body. The smallest parts of the venous system are the capillaries, which feed into larger superficial veins. All superficial veins lie between the skin and a layer of fibrous connective tissue called fascia, which covers and supports the muscles and the internal organs. The deeper veins of the body lie within the muscle fascia. This distinction helps to explain why superficial veins can be treated by sclerotherapy without damage to the larger veins.

Veins contain one-way valves that push blood inward and upward toward the heart when they are functioning normally. The blood pressure in the superficial veins is usually low, but if it rises and remains at a higher level over a period of time, the valves in the veins begin to fail and the veins dilate, or expand. Veins that are not functioning properly are said to be "incompetent." As the veins expand, they become more noticeable because they lie closer to the surface of the skin, forming the typical patterns seen in spider veins.

Some people are at greater risk for developing spider veins. These risk factors include:

- Sex. Females in any age group are more likely than males to develop spider veins.

- Genetic factors. Some people have veins with abnormally weak walls or valves. They may develop spider veins even without a rise in blood pressure in the superficial veins.

- Pregnancy. A woman's total blood volume increases during pregnancy, which increases the blood pressure in the venous system. In addition, the hormonal changes of pregnancy cause the walls and valves in the veins to soften.

- Using birth control pills.

- Obesity. Excess body weight increases pressure on the veins.

- Occupational factors. People whose jobs require standing or sitting for long periods of time without the opportunity to walk or move around are more likely to develop spider veins than people whose jobs allow more movement.

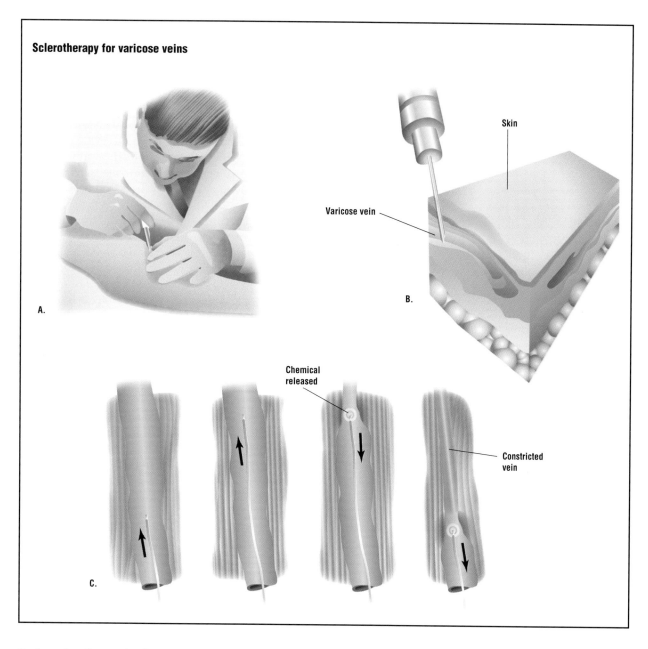

Sclerotherapy for varicose veins

Skin

Varicose vein

B.

A.

Chemical released

Constricted vein

C.

During sclerotherapy for the treatment of varicose veins, the doctor injects a chemical solution directly into the vein (A and B). The needle travels up the vein, and as it is pulled back, the chemical is released, causing the vein to form fibrous tissue that collapses the inside of it (C). *(Illustration by GGS Inc.)*

• Trauma. Falls, deep bruises, cuts, or surgical incisions may lead to the formation of spider veins in or near the affected area.

As of 2003, there is no known method to prevent the formation of spider veins.

Sclerotherapy procedures

In typical outpatient sclerotherapy treatment, the patient changes into a pair of shorts at the doctor's office and lies on an examination table. After cleansing the skin surface with an antiseptic, the doctor injects a sclerosing agent into the veins. This agent is eliminated when the skin is stretched tightly over the area with the other hand. The doctor first injects the larger veins in each area of the leg, then the smaller ones. In most cases, one injection is needed for every inch of spider vein; a typical treatment session will require five to 40 separate injections. No anesthetic is needed for sclerotherapy, although the patient may feel a mild stinging or burning sensation at the injection site.

WHO PERFORMS THE PROCEDURE AND WHERE IS IT PERFORMED?

Sclerotherapy is usually performed by general surgeons, dermatologists, or plastic surgeons, but it can also be done by family physicians or naturopaths who have been trained to do it. The American College of Phlebology holds workshops and intensive practical courses for interested practitioners. The ACP can be contacted for a list of members in each state.

Sclerotherapy is done as an outpatient procedure, most often in the doctor's office or in a plastic surgery clinic.

The liquid sclerosing agents that are used most often to treat spider veins are polidocanol (aethoxysklerol), sodium tetradecyl sulfate, and saline solution at 11.7% concentration. Some practitioners prefer to use saline because it does not cause allergic reactions. The usual practice is to use the lowest concentration of the chemical that is still effective in closing the veins.

A newer type of sclerosing agent is a foam instead of a liquid chemical that is injected into the veins. The foam has several advantages: It makes better contact with the wall of the vein than a liquid sclerosing agent; it allows the use of smaller amounts of chemical; and its movement in the vein can be monitored on an ultrasound screen. Sclerosing foam has been shown to have a high success rate with a lower cost, and causes fewer major complications.

After all the veins in a specific area of the leg have been injected, the doctor covers the area with a cotton ball or pad and compression tape. The patient may be asked to wait in the office for 20–30 minutes after the first treatment session to ensure that there is no hypersensitivity to the sclerosing chemicals. Most sclerotherapy treatment sessions are short, lasting from 15 to 45 minutes.

It is not unusual for patients to need a second treatment to completely eliminate the spider veins; however, it is necessary to wait four to six weeks between procedures.

Diagnosis/Preparation

Diagnosis

The most important aspect of diagnosis prior to undergoing sclerotherapy is distinguishing between telangiectasias and large varicose veins, and telangiectasias and spider nevi. Because sclerotherapy is intended to treat only small superficial veins, the doctor must confirm that the patient does not have a more serious venous disorder.

Spider nevi, which are also called "spider angiomas," are small, benign reddish lesions that consist of a central arteriole, which is a very small branch of an artery with smaller vessels radiating from it. Although the names are similar, spider nevi occur in the part of the circulatory system that carries blood (away) from the heart, whereas spider veins occur in the venous system that returns blood to the heart. To distinguish between the two, the doctor will press gently on the spot in the center of the network. A spider nevus will blanch, or lose its reddish color, when the central arteriole is compressed. When the doctor releases the pressure, the color will return. Spider veins are not affected by compression in this way. In addition, spider nevi occur most frequently in children and pregnant women, rather than in older adults. They are treated by laser therapy or electrodesiccation, rather than by sclerotherapy.

After taking the patient's medical history, the doctor examines the patient from the waist down, both to note the location of spider veins and to palpate (touch with gentle pressure) them for signs of other venous disorders. Ideally, the examiner will have a small raised platform for the patient to stand on during the examination. The doctor will ask the patient to turn slowly while standing, and will be looking for scars or other signs of trauma, bulges in the skin, areas of discolored skin, or other indications of chronic venous insufficiency. While palpating the legs, the doctor will note areas of unusual warmth or soreness, cysts, and edema (swelling of the soft tissues due to fluid retention). Next, the doctor will percuss certain parts of the legs where the larger veins lie closer to the surface. By gently tapping or thumping on the skin over these areas, the doctor can feel fluid waves in the veins and determine whether further testing for venous insufficiency is required. If the patient has problems related to large varicose veins, these must be treated before sclerotherapy can be performed to eliminate spider veins.

Some conditions and disorders are considered contraindications for sclerotherapy:

- Pregnancy and lactation. Pregnant women are advised to postpone sclerotherapy until at least three months after the baby is born, because some spider veins will fade by themselves after delivery. Nursing mothers should postpone sclerotherapy until the baby is weaned because it is not yet known whether the chemicals used in sclerotherapy may affect the mother's milk.

- Diabetes.

- A history of AIDS, hepatitis, syphilis, or other diseases that are carried in the blood.

- Heart conditions.
- High blood pressure, blood clotting disorders, and other disorders of the circulatory system.

Preparation

Patients are asked to discontinue **aspirin** or aspirin-related products for a week before sclerotherapy. Further, they are told not to apply any moisturizers, creams, tanning lotions, or sunblock to the legs on the day of the procedure. Patients should bring a pair of shorts to wear during the procedure, as well as compression stockings and a pair of slacks or a long skirt to cover the legs afterwards.

Most practitioners will take photographs of the patient's legs before sclerotherapy to evaluate the effectiveness of treatment. In addition, some insurance companies request pretreatment photographs for documentation purposes.

Aftercare

Aftercare following sclerotherapy includes wearing medical compression stockings that apply either 20–30 mmHg or 30–40 mmHg of pressure for at least seven to 10 days (preferably four to six weeks) after the procedure. Wearing compression stockings minimizes the risk of edema, discoloration, and pain. Fashion support stockings are a less acceptable alternative because they do not apply enough pressure to the legs.

The surgical tape and cotton balls used during the procedure should be left in place for 48 hours after the patient returns home.

Patients are encouraged to walk, ride a bicycle, or participate in other low-impact forms of **exercise** (examples: yoga and tai chi) to prevent the formation of blood clots in the deep veins of the legs. They should, however, avoid prolonged periods of standing or sitting, and such high-impact activities as jogging.

Risks

Cosmetically, the chief risk of sclerotherapy is that new spider veins may develop after the procedure. New spider veins are dilated blood vessels that can form when some of the venous blood forms new pathways back to the larger veins; they are not the original blood vessels that were sclerosed. Some patients may develop telangiectatic matting, which is a network of new spider veins that surface around the treated area. Telangiectatic matting usually clears up by itself within three to 12 months after sclerotherapy, but it can also be treated with further sclerosing injections.

Other risks of sclerotherapy include:

QUESTIONS TO ASK THE DOCTOR

- How likely am I to develop new spider veins in the treated areas?
- Do you use the newer sclerosing foams when you administer sclerotherapy?
- What technique(s) do you prefer to use for sclerotherapy and why?

- Venous thrombosis. A potentially serious complication, thrombosis refers to the formation of blood clots in the veins.
- Severe inflammation.
- Pain after the procedure lasting several hours or days. This discomfort can be eased by wearing medical compression stockings and by walking briskly.
- Allergic reactions to the sclerosing solution or foam.
- Permanent scarring.
- Loss of feeling resulting from damage to the nerves in the treated area.
- Edema (swelling) of the foot or ankle. This problem is most likely to occur when the foot or ankle is treated for spider veins. The edema usually resolves within a few days or weeks.
- Brownish spots or discoloration in the skin around the treated area. These changes in skin color are caused by deposits of hemosiderin, which is a form of iron that is stored within tissue cells. The spots usually fade after several months.
- Ulceration of the skin. This complication may result from reactive spasms of the blood vessels, the use of overly strong sclerosing solutions, or poor technique in administering sclerotherapy. It can be treated by diluting the sclerosing chemical with normal saline solution.
- Hirsutism. Hirsutism is the abnormal growth of hair on the area treated by sclerotherapy. It usually develops several months after treatment and goes away on its own. It is also known as hypertrichosis.

Normal results

Normal results of sclerotherapy include improvement in the external appearance of the legs and relief of aching or cramping sensations associated with spider veins. It is common for complete elimination of spider veins to require three to four sclerotherapy treatments.

Morbidity and mortality rates

Mortality associated with sclerotherapy for spider veins is almost 0% when the procedure is performed by a competent doctor. The rates of other complications vary somewhat, but have been reported as falling within the following ranges:

- Hemosiderin discoloration: 10%–80% of patients, with fewer than 1% of cases lasting longer than a year.

- Telangiectatic matting: 5%–75% of patients.

- Deep venous thrombosis: Fewer than 1%.

- Mild aching or pain: 35%–55%.

- Skin ulceration: About 4%.

Alternatives

Conservative treatments

Patients who are experiencing some discomfort from spider veins may be helped by any or several of the following approaches:

- Exercise. Walking or other forms of exercise that activate the muscles in the lower legs can relieve aching and cramping because these muscles keep the blood moving through the leg veins. One exercise that is often recommended is repeated flexing of the ankle joint. By flexing the ankles five to 10 times every few minutes and walking around for one to two minutes every half hour throughout the day, the patient can prevent the venous congestion that results from sitting or standing in one position for hours at a time.

- Avoiding high-heeled shoes. Shoes with high heels do not allow the ankle to flex fully when the patient is walking. This limitation of the range of motion of the ankle joint makes it more difficult for the leg muscles to contract and force venous blood upwards toward the heart.

- Elevating the legs for 15–30 minutes once or twice a day. This change of position is frequently recommended for reducing edema of the feet and ankles.

- Wearing compression hosiery. Compression benefits the leg veins by reducing inflammation as well as improving venous outflow. Most manufacturers of medical compression stockings now offer some relatively sheer hosiery that is both attractive and that offers support.

- Medications. Drugs that have been used to treat the discomfort associated with spider veins include **nonsteroidal anti-inflammatory drugs** (NSAIDs) and preparations of vitamins C and E. One prescription medication that is sometimes given to treat circulatory problems in the legs and feet is pentoxifylline, which improves blood flow in the smaller capillaries. Pentoxifylline is sold under the brand name Trendar.

If appearance is the patient's primary concern, spider veins on the legs can often be covered with specially formulated cosmetics that come in a wide variety of skin tones. Some of these preparations are available in waterproof formulations for use during swimming and other athletic activities.

Electrodesiccation, laser therapy, and pulsed light therapy

Electrodesiccation is a treatment modality whereby the doctor seals off the small blood vessels that cause spider veins by passing a weak electric current through a fine needle to the walls of the veins. Electrodesiccation seems to be more effective in treating spider veins in the face than in treating those in the legs; it tends to leave pitted white scars when used to treat spider veins in the legs or feet.

Laser therapy, like electrodesiccation, works better in treating facial spider veins. The sharply focused beam of intense light emitted by the laser heats the blood vessel, causing the blood in it to coagulate and close the vein. Various lasers have been used to treat spider veins, including argon, KTP 532nm, and alexandrite lasers. The choice of light wavelength and pulse duration are based on the size of the vein to be treated. Argon lasers, however, have been found to increase the patient's risk of developing hemosiderin discoloration when used on the legs. The KTP 532nm laser gives better results in treating leg spider veins, but is still not as effective as sclerotherapy.

Intense pulsed light (IPL) systems differ from lasers because the light emitted is noncoherent and not monochromatic. The IPL systems enable doctors to use a wider range of light wavelengths and pulse frequencies when treating spider veins and such other skin problems, as pigmented birthmarks. This flexibility, however, requires considerable skill and experience on the part of the doctor to remove spider veins without damaging the surrounding skin.

Complementary and alternative (CAM) treatments

According to Dr. Kenneth Pelletier, the former director of the program in complementary and alternative treatments at Stanford University School of Medicine, California, horse chestnut extract is as safe and effective as compression stockings when used as a conservative treatment for spider veins. Horse chestnut (*Aesculus hippocastanum*) has been used in Europe for some years to treat circulatory problems in the legs; most recent research has been conducted in Great Britain and Germany. The usual dosage is 75 mg twice a day, at meals.

KEY TERMS

Arteriole—A very small branch of an artery, usually close to a capillary network.

Edema—The presence of abnormally large amounts of fluid in the soft tissues of the body.

Electrodesiccation—A method of treating spider veins or drying up tissue by passing a small electric current through a fine needle into the affected area.

Hemosiderin—A form of iron that is stored inside tissue cells. The brownish discoloration of skin that sometimes occurs after sclerotherapy is caused by hemosiderin.

Hirsutism—Abnormal hair growth on the part of the body treated by sclerotherapy. It is also called hypertrichosis.

Incompetent—In a medical context, insufficient. An incompetent vein is one that is not performing its function of carrying blood back to the heart.

Lumen—The channel or cavity inside a tube or hollow organ of the body.

Palpation—Examining by touch as part of the process of physical diagnosis.

Percussion—Thumping or tapping a part of the body with the fingers for diagnostic purposes.

Phlebology—The study of veins, their disorders, and their treatments. A phlebologist is a doctor who specializes in treating spider veins, varicose veins, and associated disorders.

Sclerose—To harden or undergo hardening. Sclerosing agents are chemicals that are used in sclerotherapy to cause swollen veins to fill with fibrous tissue and close down.

Spider nevus (plural, nevi)—A reddish lesion that consists of a central arteriole with smaller branches radiating outward from it. Spider nevi are also called spider angiomas; they are most common in small children and pregnant women.

Spider veins—Telangiectasias that appear on the surface of the legs, characterized by a reddish central point with smaller veins branching out from it like the legs of a spider.

Telangiectasia—The medical term for the visible discolorations produced by permanently swollen capillaries and smaller veins.

Varicose—Abnormally enlarged and distended.

The most common side effect of oral preparations of horse chestnut is occasional indigestion in some patients.

See also Sclerotherapy for esophageal varices; Vein ligation and stripping.

Resources

BOOKS

Pelletier, Kenneth R., M.D. *The Best Alternative Medicine*, Part II, "CAM Therapies for Specific Conditions: Varicose Veins." New York: Simon & Schuster, 2002.

"Varicose Veins." Section 16, Chapter 212 in *The Merck Manual of Diagnosis and Therapy*, edited by Mark H. Beers, M.D., and Robert Berkow, M.D. Whitehouse Station, NJ: Merck Research Laboratories, 1999.

PERIODICALS

Brunnberg, S., S. Lorenz, M. Landthaler, and U. Hohenleutner. "Evaluation of the Long Pulsed High Fluence Alexandrite Laser Therapy of Leg Telangiectasia." *Lasers in Surgery and Medicine* 31 (2002): 359-362.

Crowe, Mark A., M.D. "Nevus Araneus (Spider Nevus)." *eMedicine*, April 12, 2002 [April 11, 2003]. <www.emedicine.com/derm/topic293.htm>.

Feied, Craig, M.D., Robert Weiss, M.D., and Robert B. Hashemiyoon, M.D. "Varicose Veins and Spider Veins." *eMedicine*, November 20, 2001 [April 10, 2003]. <www.emedicine.com/derm/topic475.htm>.

Frullini, A., and A. Cavezzi. "Sclerosing Foam in the Treatment of Varicose Veins and Telangiectases: History and Analysis of Safety and Complications." *Dermatologic Surgery* 28 (January 2002): 11-15.

Goldman, M. P. "Treatment of Varicose and Telangiectatic Leg Veins: Double-Blind Prospective Comparative Trial Between Aethoxyskerol and Sotradecol." *Dermatologic Surgery* 28 (January 2002): 52-55.

Kern, P. "Sclerotherapy of Varicose Leg Veins. Technique, Indications, and Complications." *International Angiology* 21 (June 2002): 40-45.

Loo, W. J., and S. W. Lanigan. "Recent Advances in Laser Therapy for the Treatment of Cutaneous Vascular Disorders." *Lasers in Medical Science* 17 (2002): 9-12.

MacKay, D. "Hemorrhoids and Varicose Veins: A Review of Treatment Options." *Alternative Medicine Review* 6 (April 2001): 126-140.

Pittler, M. H., and E. Ernst. "Horse-Chestnut Seed Extract for Chronic Venous Insufficiency. A Criteria-Based Systematic Review." *Archives of Dermatology* 134 (November 1998): 1356-1360.

Raulin, C., B. Greve, and H. Grema. "IPL Technology: A Review." *Lasers in Surgery and Medicine* 32 (2003): 78-87.

ORGANIZATIONS

American Academy of Dermatology. 930 East Woodfield Rd., PO Box 4014, Schaumburg, IL 60168. (847) 330-0230. <www.aad.org>.

American Association for Vascular Surgery (AAVS). 900 Cummings Center, #221-U, Beverly, MA 01915. <www.aavs. vascularweb.org>.

American College of Phlebology. 100 Webster Street, Suite 101, Oakland, CA 94607-3724. (510) 834-6500. <www. phlebology.org>.

American Society of Plastic Surgeons (ASPS). 444 East Algonquin Road, Arlington Heights, IL 60005. (847) 228-9900. <www.plasticsurgery.org>.

Peripheral Vascular Surgery Society (PVSS). 824 Munras Avenue, Suite C, Monterey, CA 93940. (831) 373-0508. <www.pvss.org>.

OTHER

American Society of Plastic Surgeons. *Procedures: Sclerotherapy*. [cited April 10, 2003]. <www.plasticsurgery.org/public_education/procedures/Sclerotherapy.cfm>.

Feied, Craig, M.D. *Venous Anatomy and Physiology*. [cited April 10, 2003] <www.phlebology.org/syllabus1.htm>.

Fronek, Helane S., M.D. *Conservative Therapy for Venous Disease*. [cited April 10, 2003] <www.phlebology.org/syllabus4.htm>.

Goldman, M. P., M.D. *Complications of Sclerotherapy*. [cited April 10, 2003] <www.phlebology.org/syllabus9.htm>.

Marley, Wayne, M.D. *Physical Examination of the Phlebology Patient*. [cited April 10, 2003] <www.phlebology.org/syllabus2.htm>.

Sadick, Neil S., M.D. *Technique for Treating Telangiectasias and Reticular Veins*. [cited April 10, 2003] <www.phlebology.org/syllabus6.htm>.

Weiss, Robert A., M.D., and Mitchel P. Goldman, M.D. *Treatment of Leg Telangiectasias with Lasers and High-Intensity Pulsed Light*. [cited April 10, 2003] <www.phlebology.org/syllabus10.htm>.

Rebecca Frey, Ph.D.

Scoliosis surgery, Arthrodesis *see*
Spinal fusion

Scopolamine patch

Definition

A scopolamine patch (Transdermal Scop or Transderm-V) is an adhesive medication patch that is applied to the skin behind the ear. The patch is treated with the belladonna alkaloid scopolamine, an anticholinergic

drug that is a central nervous system depressant and an antiemetic.

Purpose

Scopolamine patches are prescribed to reduce postoperative nausea and vomiting (PONV) associated with anesthesia and surgery. Scopolamine also has a mild analgesic and sedative effect, which adds to its therapeutic value for some surgical patients. In addition to PONV, scopolamine patches are also used for the treatment of motion sickness.

Demographics

Elderly patients may be more sensitive to scopolamine treatment and its use should be prescribed with caution in this group. The safety of scopolamine patches has not been determined in children; therefore the drug's use in pediatric patients is not recommended.

Description

A potent drug derived from an alkaloid of belladonna (*Atropa belladonna*; common name deadly nightshade), scopolamine works by depressing the action of the nerve fibers near the ear and the vomiting center of the brain and central nervous system (CNS). The patch itself is designed with special layered materials that slowly release a small dose of the drug transdermally (through the skin) over a period of several days.

Patients who are instructed to apply their patch at home should wash their hands thoroughly both before and after the procedure. Scopolamine can be spread to the eyes by hand, which can cause blurred vision and pupil dilation. Patches should never be cut into pieces, as cutting destroys the time-release mechanism of the drug. The directions for use for the patch should be read thoroughly before application, and specific physician instructions should also be followed. The drug will start to work approximately four hours after the patch is applied.

Diagnosis/Preparation

The dime-sized scopolamine patch is applied just behind either the left or right ear. The area should be clean and hairless prior to the application, which should occur the evening before a scheduled surgery. For women who are prescribed a scopolamine patch to reduce nausea and vomiting related to a **cesarean section**, the patch should be applied just one hour before the procedure to minimize the baby's exposure to the drug. Scopolamine does cross the placental barrier, but as of early 2003, clinical studies have not shown any negative affects on newborn babies of mothers who used the drug in a caesarean delivery.

Patients with a history of glaucoma, prostate enlargement, kidney or liver problems, bladder obstruction, gastrointestinal obstruction, or contact dermatitis (allergic skin rash) in response to topical drugs may not be suitable candidates for scopolamine patch therapy. A physician or anesthesiologist should take a full medical history before prescribing scopolamine to determine if the medication is appropriate.

Aftercare

Patients who receive a scopolamine patch should not drive or operate heavy machinery until the therapy is complete. Patch therapy generally lasts about three days. Patches should be disposed of according to the manufacturer's directions in a secure place to ensure that small children or pets do not get access to them. If PONV has not resolved after patch therapy has ended, patients should talk to their doctor about their treatment options.

Risks

Possible complications or side effects from transdermal scopolamine include but are not limited to: short-

term memory loss, fatigue, confusion, hallucinations, difficulty urinating, and changes in heart rate. The drug can trigger seizures and psychotic delusions in patients with a history of these problems. Dizziness, nausea, headache, and hypotension (low blood pressure) have also been reported in some patients upon discontinuation of scopolamine patch therapy.

Patients who experience eye pain with redness and possible blurred vision should remove the patch immediately and call their doctor, since these symptoms could be signs of a rare but possible side effect of scopolamine called narrow-angle glaucoma. Blurriness with or without pupil dilation is also a potential but generally harmless side effect of the drug.

Normal results

When scopolamine patch therapy works, it reduces or eliminates post-surgical nausea and vomiting. Patients frequently experience dry mouth as a common side effect of the drug.

Alternatives

Intravenous or intramuscular injection of scopolamine may be used as alternatives to patch therapy for some patients. Other antiemetics that may be prescribed for PONV include anti-droperidol drugs, dopaminergic drugs (i.e., promethazine, droperidol), antihistamines (i.e., diphenhydramine), and the serotonin receptor antagonists (i.e., ondansetron, granisetron, tropisetron, dolasetron). Corticosteroids may also be recommended for PONV in some patients.

Resources

BOOKS

Litwack, Kim, ed. *Core Curriculum for Perianesthesia Nursing Practice,* 4th edition. Philadelphia: W.B. Saunders, 1999.

PERIODICALS

Gan, T. J. "Postoperative nausea and vomiting—can it be eliminated?" *Journal of the American Medical Association* 287 (March 13, 2002): 1233–6.

Paula Ford-Martin

Secobarbital *see* **Barbiturates**

Second-look surgery

Definition

Second-look surgery is performed after a procedure or course of treatment to determine if the patient is free of disease. If disease is found, additional procedures may or may not be performed at the time of second-look surgery.

Purpose

Second-look surgery may be performed under numerous circumstances on patients with various medical conditions.

Cancer

A second-look procedure is sometimes performed to determine if a cancer patient has responded successfully to a particular treatment. Examples of cancers that are assessed during second-look surgery are ovarian cancer and colorectal cancer. In many cases, before a round of chemotherapy and/or radiation therapy is started, a patient will undergo a surgical procedure called cytoreduction to reduce the size of a tumor. This debulking increases the sensitivity of the tumor and decreases the number of necessary treatment cycles. Following cytoreduction and chemotherapy, a second-look procedure may be necessary to determine if the area is cancer-free.

An advantage to second-look surgery following cancer treatment is that if cancer is found, it may be removed during the procedure in some patients. In other cases, if a tumor cannot be entirely removed, the surgeon can debulk the tumor and improve the patient's chances of responding to another cycle of chemotherapy. However, second-look surgery cannot definitively prove that a patient is free of cancer; some microscopic cancer cells can persist and begin to grow in other areas of the body. Even if no cancer is found during second-look surgery, the rate of cancer relapse is approximately 25%.

Pelvic disease

Second-look surgery may benefit patients suffering from a number of different conditions that affect the pelvic organs. Endometriosis is a condition in which the tissue that lines the uterus grows elsewhere in the body, usually in the abdominal cavity, leading to pain and scarring. Endometrial growths may be surgically removed or treated with medications. A second-look procedure may be performed following the initial surgery or course of medication to determine if treatment was successful in reducing the number of growths. Additional growths may be removed at this time.

Second-look surgery may also be performed following the surgical removal of adhesions (bands of scar tissue that form in the abdomen following surgery or injury) or uterine fibroids (noncancerous growths of the uterus). If the results are positive, an additional procedure may be performed to remove the adhesions or growths. Patients undergoing treatment for infertility may benefit from a second-look procedure to determine if the cause of infertility has been cured before ceasing therapy.

Abdominal disease

In patients suffering from bleeding from the gastrointestinal (GI) tract, recurrence of bleeding after attempted treatment remains a significant risk; approximately 10–25% of cases do not respond to initial treatment. Second-look surgery following treatment for GI bleeding may be beneficial in determining if bleeding has recurred and treating the cause of the bleeding before it becomes more extensive.

Patients suffering from a partial or complete blockage of the intestine are at risk of developing bowel ischemia (death of intestinal tissue due to a lack of oxygen). Initial surgery is most often necessary to remove the diseased segment of bowel; a second-look procedure is commonly performed to ensure that only healthy tissue remains and that the new intestinal connection (called an anastomosis) is healing properly.

Other conditions

A variety of other conditions can be assessed with second-look surgery. Patients who have undergone surgical repair of torn muscles in the knee might undergo a procedure called second-look arthroscopy to assess how the repair is healing. A physician may use second-look mastoidoscopy to visualize the middle ear after removal of a cholesteatoma (a benign growth in the middle ear). A second endoscopic procedure may be performed on a patient who underwent endoscopic treatment for sinusitis (chronic infection of the sinuses) to evaluate the surgical site and remove debris.

Description

Second-look surgery may be done within hours, days, weeks, or months of the initial procedure or treatment. This time interval depends on the patient's condition and the type of procedure.

Laparotomy

A laparotomy is a large incision through the abdominal wall to visualize the structures inside the abdominal cavity. After placing the patient under general anesthesia, the surgeon first makes a large incision through the skin, then through each layer under the skin in the region that the surgeon wishes to explore. The area will be assessed for evidence of remaining disease. For example, in the case of second-look laparotomy following treatment for endometriosis, the abdominal organs will be examined for evidence of endometrial growths. In the case of cancer, a "washing" of the abdominal cavity may be performed; sterile fluid is instilled into the abdominal cavity and washed around the organs, then extracted with a syringe. The fluid is then analyzed for the presence of cancerous cells. Biopsies may also be taken of various abdominal tissues and analyzed.

If the surgeon discovers evidence of disease or a failed surgical repair, additional procedures may be performed to remove the disease or repair the dysfunction. For example, if adhesions are encountered during a second-look procedure on an infertile female patient, the surgeon may remove the adhesions at that time. Upon completion of the procedure, the incision is closed.

Laparoscopy

Laparoscopy is a surgical technique that permits a view of the internal abdominal organs without an extensive surgical incision. During laparoscopy, a thin lighted tube called a laparoscope is inserted into the abdominal cavity through a tiny incision. Images taken by the laparoscope are seen on a video monitor connected to the scope. The surgeon may then examine the abdominal cavity, albeit with a more limited operative view than with laparotomy. Such procedures as the removal of growths or repair of deformities can be performed by instruments inserted through other small incisions in the abdominal wall. After the procedure is completed, any incisions are closed with stitches.

Other procedures

Depending on the area of the body in question, other procedures may be used to perform second-look surgery. These include:

> ## KEY TERMS
>
> **Endoscopy**—A surgical technique that uses an endoscope (a thin lighted telescope-like instrument) to visualize structures inside the human body.
>
> **Infertility**—The inability to become pregnant or carry a pregnancy to term.
>
> **Kidney stones**—Small solid masses that form in the kidney.

- Arthroscopy. Arthroscopy uses a thin endoscope to visualize the inner space of a joint such as the knee or elbow. Second-look arthroscopy may be used to determine if previous surgery on the joint is healing properly.
- Percutaneous nephrolithotomy (PNL). This minimally invasive procedure is used to remove kidney stones. Second-look PNL may be used to remove fragments of stones that could not be removed during the initial procedure.
- **Hysteroscopy**. A hysteroscope is an instrument used to visualize and perform procedures on the inner cavity of the uterus. Second-look hysteroscopy may be used after surgery or medical treatment to treat adhesions or benign growths in the uterus to determine if they have been effectively removed.
- Mastoidectomy. This surgical procedure is used to treat cholesteatoma; a second-look procedure is generally performed to ensure that the entire cholesteatoma was removed during the initial procedure.

Resources

BOOKS

Ryan, Kenneth J., Ross S. Berkowitz, Robert L. Barbieri, and Andrea Dunaif, eds. *Kistner's Gynecology and Women's Health,* 7th edition. St. Louis: Mosby, Inc., 1999.

PERIODICALS

Im, Dwight D., William P. McGuire, and Neil B. Rosenshein. "Contemporary Management of Ovarian Cancer." *Obstetrics and Gynecology Clinics* 28, no. 4 (December 2001): 759–73.

Marmo, Riccardo, Gianluca Rotandano, Maria Antonia Bianca, Roberto Piscopo, Antonio Prisco, and Livio Cipolletta. "Outcome of Endoscopic Treatment for Peptic Ulcer Bleeding: Is a Second Look Necessary?" *Gastrointestinal Endoscopy* 57, no. 1 (January 2003): 62–7.

Palter, Steven F. "Office Microlaparoscopy Under Local Anesthesia." *Obstetrics and Gynecology Clinics* 26, no. 1 (1999): 109–20.

ORGANIZATIONS

American College of Surgeons. 633 N. Saint Clair St., Chicago, IL 60611-3211. (312) 202-5000. <http://www.facs.org>.

Society of Surgical Oncology. 85 W. Algonquin Rd., Suite 550, Arlington Heights, IL 60005. (847) 427-1400. <http://www.surgonc.org>.

OTHER

Horlbeck, Drew, and Matthew Ng. "Middle Ear Endoscopy." *eMedicine.* December 13, 2001. [cited May 20, 2003] <http://www.emedicine.com/ENT/topic483.htm>.

Johnson, Darren L., and Jeffrey B. Selby. "Meniscal Transplantation: Indications and Results." *Medscape General Medicine,* August 3, 2001. [cited May 20, 2003] <http://www.medscape.com/viewarticle/408541_1>.

Stephanie Dionne Sherk

Second opinion

Definition

A second opinion is the process of seeking an evaluation by another doctor or surgeon to confirm the diagnosis and treatment plan of a primary physician, or to offer an alternative diagnosis and/or treatment approach.

Purpose

Getting a second surgical opinion can fill an important emotional need as well as establishing medical needs and treatment goals. When a second opinion confirms initial findings, it can provide reassurance and feelings of acceptance for the patient, and may reduce anxiety and uncertainty.

From a cost-effectiveness point of view, second opinions can save health insurance providers money by establishing the certainty of a clinical need (or lack of need) for surgery, particularly when the diagnosis is a life-threatening.

Patients with a diagnosis of cancer may also benefit from a second-opinion pathology review of their biopsy material. A John Hopkins study reported that 1.4% of patients scheduled for cancer-related surgery at their facility were found to have been misdiagnosed when their tissue samples were reevaluated by a second pathologist. Similarly, a study published in the *Annals of Surgical Oncology* in 2002 found that a pathological second opinion of breast cancers changed the initial diagnosis, prognosis, or treatment approach in 80% of the 340 study subjects.

Several clinical research studies, however, have found that patients often seek second opinions not necessarily because they doubt the diagnosis or recommendations of their first provider, but because they were dissatisfied with either the amount of information given to them or the style of communication of their doctor. A 2002 Northwestern University study found that only 46% of patients coming into a breast cancer treatment center for a second opinion had been offered a complete discussion of treatment options during their initial consultation.

Description

Doctors often have differing viewpoints as to how a particular medical problem should be managed, whether through surgery or less invasive treatment means. One surgeon may prefer to take a "watchful waiting" approach before recommending surgery, while another may believe in performing surgery as soon as possible to avoid later complications. In some cases, several surgical techniques may be viable options for a patient. Medicine is not as black-and-white as many patients are led to believe, and physicians are not infallible. For these reasons, and because surgery is a major procedure with associated risks that should not be taken lightly, second opinions are an important part of the process of **informed consent** and decision-making.

Although a physician may strive to be objective, personal views and subjective experiences can influence their treatment recommendations. In addition, both the education and experience of a doctor in a given medical area can also influence the advice they offer a patient. For these reasons, seeking a second opinion from another physician and/or surgeon can be invaluable in making a decision on a course of treatment.

Second opinions are most frequently sought in cases of elective (nonemergency) surgery when the patient has time to consider options and make a more informed choice about his or her course of treatment. While a second surgical opinion may be requested in some cases of **emergency surgery**, they are not as common, simply because of the logistical limitations involved with getting a qualified second opinion if a patient requires immediate care.

In some cases, a doctor or surgeon may encourage seeking a second opinion, particularly when the preferred course of treatment is not clear-cut or another surgeon with advanced training or expertise may provide more insights into surgical options.

Patients should remember that it is their right to seek a second opinion before committing to surgery or another treatment plan. Embarrassment or fear of disapproval from a primary care provider should not be a barrier to getting a second opinion. A competent physician will not consider the decision to seek a second opinion an insult to their ability or experience. Instead, they will consider the patient an informed individual who is proactive and responsible for their own health care.

Patient seeking a second-opinion consultation may ask the provider questions similar to those they asked their primary provider. Questions may include:

- Are there other options besides surgery?

- What are the risks and benefits of each treatment option?

- How might each possible treatment impact quality-of-life for the patient?

- What kind of success rate is associated with surgery and other potential therapies?

- How is the surgery performed?

- Is surgery a permanent, long-term, or temporary solution to the condition?

- What type of anesthesia will be used?

- If surgery is chosen by the patient, how soon must it be done?

- What type of aftercare and recovery time is required once the surgery is complete?

- How much pain is to be expected postoperatively, and how is it typically treated?

- What are the costs involved with surgery and other treatment options, including postoperative care?

Providing the second surgeon with appropriate background information is important, but so is refraining from detailed descriptions of what the first provider did or did not recommend before the consultation begins. Patients should allow the surgeon to draw objective conclusions based on the medical history and diagnostic data before them. If the second opinion differs from the first provider's opinion, and the patient feels comfortable doing so, he or she might then offer information on the first provider's recommendations to get further feedback and input for a final decision.

Preparation

Before seeking a second opinion, patients should contact their health insurance provider to find out if the service is covered. Some insurance companies may request that a second opinion be sought before major **elective surgery**, and may reserve the right to designate a physician or surgeon to provide the patient evaluation. As of mid-2003, **Medicare** Part B covered 80% of costs for surgical second opinions after deductible, and 80% for a third opinion if the first two opinions were contradictory. Other Medicare programs may cover second opinions as well; patients should check with their Medicare carrier for details.

There are several ways to find an appropriate health care professional to provide a second opinion. Patients can:

- Ask friends and family for references.

- Ask their primary care physician or another trusted health care provider for a referral.

- Contact an appropriate specialty medical organization (e.g., American College of Surgeons) for a referral.

- Call their local medical licensing board.

- Check with their insurance provider or Medicare carrier.

When seeking a second surgical opinion, patients should find a surgeon who is board-certified in the appropriate specialty by an organization that is part of the American Board of Medical Specialties (ABMS). For example, surgery of the urinary tract may be performed by a provider who is board certified by the American Board of Urology and/or the American Board of Surgery (ABS), two member organizations of the ABMS. Diplomates of ABMS member boards are surgeons who have passed rigorous written and oral testing on these specialties and have met specific accredited educational and residency requirements. In some cases, surgeons may also be certified in subspecialties within a discipline (for example, a vascular surgeon may be board certified by the **vascular surgery** board of the ABS). The ABMS provides a verification service for patients to check on the certification status of their provider.

In addition, the surgeon may also be a Fellow of the American College of Surgery (ACS), as indicated by the designation F.A.C.S. after their name. This indicates that he or she has met standards of clinical experience, education, ethical conduct, and professional expertise as prescribed by the ACS.

Once a second health care provider is selected, patients should speak with their primary doctor about providing the appropriate medical history, test results, and other pertinent information to the physician who will give the second opinion. The patient may have to sign an information release form to allow the files to be sent. If x rays, **magnetic resonance imaging** (MRI), or other radiological testing was performed, the second physician may request to see the original films, rather than the radiologist's report of the results, in order to interpret them objectively. In some cases, the office of the surgeon giving the second opinion can arrange to have these materials transferred with a patient's written approval. Patients should call ahead to ensure that all needed materials arrive at the second provider's office before the appointment, to give that physician adequate time to review them and to avoid potentially costly repeat testing.

Normal results

Second opinions that agree with the first provider's conclusions may help ease the patient's mind and provide a clearer picture of the necessary course of treatment or surgery. However, if a patient still feels uncomfortable with the treatment plan outlined by the first and second physicians, or strongly disagrees with their conclusions, a third opinion from another provider is an option.

In cases in which the second provider disagrees with the first provider on diagnosis and/or treatment, the patient has harder choices to face. Again, a third evaluation may be in order from yet another physician, and some insurance companies may actually require this step in cases of conflicting opinions. If a patient is very comfortable with and confident in their primary care provider, they may wish to revisit them to review the second opinion.

In all cases, a patient should remember that their personal preferences, beliefs, and lifestyle considerations must also be considered in their final decision on surgery or treatment, as they are the ones who will live with the results.

Resources

BOOKS

Rose, Eric. *Second Opinion: The Columbia Presbyterian Guide to Surgery.* New York: St. Martin's Press, 2000.

PERIODICALS

Staradub, V. L., et al. "Changes in Breast Cancer Therapy Because of Pathology Second Opinions." *Annals of Surgical Oncology* 9, no.10 (December 2002): 982–7.

ORGANIZATIONS

American Board of Medical Specialties (ABMS). 1007 Church St., Suite 404, Evanston, IL 60201. (866) ASK-ABMS. <http://www.abms.org>.
American College of Surgeons (ACS). 63 N. St. Clair Drive, Chicago, IL 60611. (312) 202-5000. E-mail: <postmaster @facs.org>. <http://www.facs.org>.

OTHER

Center for Medicare and Medicaid Services (CMS). *Getting a Second Opinion Before Surgery.* Publication CMS-02173. Revised April 2002. <http://www.medicare.gov/Publications/Pubs/pdf/02173.pdf>.

Paula Ford-Martin

Sedation, conscious

Definition

Conscious sedation, produced by the administration of certain medications, is an altered level of consciousness that still allows a patient to respond to physical stimulation and verbal commands, and to maintain an unassisted airway.

Purpose

The purpose of conscious sedation is to produce a state of relaxation and/or pain relief by using benzodiazepine-type and narcotic medications, to facilitate performing a procedure such as a biopsy, radiologic imaging study, endoscopic procedure, radiation therapy, or bone marrow aspiration.

Description

Sedation is used inside or outside the **operating room**. Outside the operating suite, medical specialists use sedation to calm and relax their patients.

If the patient is to undergo a minor surgical procedure, screening and assessment of medical conditions that may interfere with conscious sedation must be explored. These potential risk factors include advanced age, history of adverse reactions to the proposed medications and a past medical history of severe cardiopulmonary (heart/lung) disease.

Once it has been established that the patient would be a good candidate for conscious sedation, just prior to the surgery or procedure, the patient will receive the sedating drug intravenously. A clip-like apparatus will be placed on the patient's finger to monitor oxygen intake during the sedation. This oxygen monitoring is called pulse oximetry and is a valuable continuous monitor of patient oxygenation.

Dosing of medications that produce conscious sedation is individualized, and the medication is administered slowly to gauge a patient's response to the sedative. The two most common medications used to sedate patients for medical procedures are midazolam and fentanyl.

Fentanyl is a medication classified as an opioid narcotic analgesic (pain reliever) that is 50 to 100 times more potent than morphine. Given intravenously, the onset of action of fentanyl is almost immediate, and peak analgesia occurs with in 10 to 15 minutes. A single dose of fentanyl given intravenously can produce good analgesia for only 20 to 45 minutes for most patients because the drug's distribution shifts from the brain (central nervous system) to peripheral tissues. The key to correct dosage is titration, or giving the medication in small amounts until the desired patient response is achieved.

Midazolam is a medication classified as a short-acting benzodiazepine (sedative) that depresses the central nervous system. Midazolam is ineffective for pain and has no analgesic effect during conscious sedation. The drug is a primary choice for conscious sedation because midazolam causes patients to have no recollection of the medical procedure. In general, midazolam has a fast-acting, short-lived sedative effect when given intravenously, achieving sedation within one to five minutes and peaking within 30 minutes. The effects of midazolam typically last one hour but may persist for six hours (including the amnestic effect). Patients who receive midazolam for conscious sedation should not be allowed to drive home after the procedure.

Monitoring

Patient monitoring during conscious sedation must be performed by a trained and licensed health care professional. This clinician must not be involved in the pro-

cedure, but should have primary responsibility of monitoring and attending to the patient. Equipment must be in place and organized for monitoring the patient's blood pressure, pulse, respiratory rate, level of consciousness, and, most important, the oxygen saturation (the measure of oxygen perfusion inside the body) with a **pulse oximeter** (a machine that provides a continuous real-time recording of oxygenation). The oxygen saturation is the most sensitive parameter affected during increased levels of conscious sedation. **Vital signs** and other pertinent recordings must be monitored before the start of the administration of medications, and then at a minimum of every five minutes thereafter until the procedure is completed. After the procedure has been completed, monitoring should continue every 15 minutes for the first hour after the last dose of medication(s) was administered. After the first hour, monitoring can continue as needed.

Risks and risk management

The American Academy of Pediatrics (AAP) has established safe practice guidelines to manage conscious sedation without an anesthesiologist for minor procedures. These AAP criteria include (1) a full-time licensed clinician (nurse, physician, physician assistant, surgeon assistant, respiratory therapist) who is strictly and exclusively monitoring the patient's breathing, level of consciousness, vital signs, and airway; (2) standard procedures for monitoring vital signs; and (3) immediate availability (on site) of airway equipment, resuscitative medications, suction apparatus, and supplemental oxygen delivery systems.

If adverse reactions occur while using fentanyl, the antidote is a drug called naloxone. It provides rapid reversal of fentanyl's narcotic effect. The incidence of oversedation or decreased respiration is low using fentanyl if the medication is carefully titrated.

See also Pulse oximeter.

Resources

BOOKS

Behrman, R. *Nelson Textbook of Pediatrics,* 16th ed. Philadelphia: W. B. Saunders Company, 2000.

PERIODICALS

"Recommended Practices: Monitoring the Patient Receiving IV Conscious Sedation." *Association of Operating Room Nurses* 57, no. 4 (April 1993).

U. S. Department of Health and Human Services. *Acute Pain Management: Operative or Medical Procedures and Trauma. Clinical Practice Guidelines.* Department of Health and Human Services Pub. No AHCPR 92-0032.

ORGANIZATIONS

American Association of Nurse Anesthetists. 222 South Prospect Avenue Park Ridge, IL 60068-4001. Telephone: (847) 692–7050. Fax: (847) 692–6968. E-mail: info@aana.com.

Laith Farid Gulli, M.D.,M.S.
Alfredo Mori, MBBS

Segmental resection *see* **Segmentectomy**

Segmentectomy

Definition

Segmentectomy is the excision (removal) of a portion of any organ or gland. The procedure has several variations and many names, including segmental resection, wide excision, **lumpectomy**, tumorectomy, **quadrantectomy**, and partial mastectomy.

Purpose

Segmentectomy is the surgical removal of a defined segment or portion of an organ or gland performed as a treatment. In this case, the purpose is the removal of a cancerous tumor. Common organs that have segments are the breasts, lungs, and liver.

Demographics

Segmentectomies are usually performed on patients with lung, liver, or breast cancer.

WHO PERFORMS THE PROCEDURE AND WHERE IS IT PERFORMED?

Segmentectomies are performed in a hospital by a general surgeon, a medical doctor who specializes in surgery. If there are complicating factors, a specialized surgeon may perform the surgery.

Lung cancer is the second most common cancer among both men and women, and is the leading cause of cancer death for both genders. Lung cancer kills more people (approximately 157,000 per year) than cancers of the breast, prostate, colon, and pancreas combined. Almost 90% of all lung cancers are caused by cigarette smoking. Other causes include secondhand smoke and exposure to asbestos and other occupation-related substances.

In each of the racial and ethnic groups, the rates among men are about two to three times greater than the rates among women. Among men, age-adjusted lung cancer incidence rates (per 100,000) range from a low of about 14 among American Indians to a high of 117 among African Americans, an eight-fold difference. For women, the rates range from approximately 15 per 100,000 among Japanese to nearly 51 among Alaska Natives, approximately a three-fold difference.

Excluding cancers of the skin, breast cancer is the most common form of cancer among women in the United States. The increase in incidence is primarily due to increased screening by **physical examination** and **mammography**. Although breast cancer occurs among both women and men, it is quite rare among men. White non-Hispanic women have the highest rates of breast cancer, over twice the rate for Hispanic women. There are a low number of cases for Alaska Native, American Indian, Korean, and Vietnamese women.

Primary cancers of the liver account for approximately 1.5% of all cancer cases in the United States. About two-thirds of liver cancers are most clearly associated with hepatitis B and hepatitis C viral infections and cirrhosis. This type of liver cancer occurs more frequently in men than in women by a ratio of two to one.

Description

When cancer is confined to a segment of an organ, removal of that portion may offer cancer-control results equivalent to those of more extensive operations. This is especially true for breast and liver cancers. For breast and lung cancers, a segmentectomy is often combined with removal of some or all regional lymph nodes.

Treatment options for lung cancer depend on the stage of the cancer (whether it is in the lung only or has spread to other places in the body); tumor size; the type of lung cancer; presence (or lack) of symptoms; and the patient's general health.

A disease in which malignant (cancer) cells form in the tissues of the lung is called non-small cell lung cancer (NSCLC). There are five types of NSCLC; each consists of different types of cancer cells, which grow and spread in different ways. The types of NSCLC are named for the kinds of cells found in the cancer, and how the cells appear when viewed under a microscope.

Segmentectomy may be the treatment of choice for cancerous tumors in the occult, or hidden stage, as well as in stage 0, stage I, or stage II NSCLC. When the site and nature of the primary tumor is defined in occult stage lung cancer, it is generally removed by segmentectomy.

Segmentectomy is the usual treatment for stage 0 cancers of the lung, as they are limited to the layer of tissue that lines air passages, and have not invaded the nearby lung tissue. Chemotherapy or radiation therapy is not normally required.

Segmentectomy is recommended only for treating the smallest stage I cancers and for patients with other medical conditions that make removing part or the entire lobe of the lung (lobectomy) dangerous. If the patient does not have sufficient pulmonary function to tolerate this more extensive operation, a segmentectomy will be performed. Additional chemotherapy after surgery for stage I NSCLC is not routinely recommended. If a patient has serious medical problems, radiation therapy may be the primary treatment.

A cancerous tumor will be surgically removed by segmentectomy or lobectomy in cases of stage II NSCLC. A wedge resection might be done if the patient cannot withstand lobectomy. Sometimes **pneumonectomy** (removal of the entire lung) is needed. Radiation therapy may be used to destroy cancer cells left behind after surgery, especially if malignant cells are present at the edge of the tissue removed by surgery. Some doctors may recommend additional radiation therapy even if the edges of the sample have no detectable cancer cells.

Segmentectomy is under investigation for the treatment of small-cell lung cancers.

Because of the need for radiotherapy after segmentectomy, some patients, such as pregnant women and those with syndromes not compatible with radiation treatment, may not be candidates for segmentectomy. As in any surgery, patients should alert their physician about all allergies and any medications they are taking.

QUESTIONS TO ASK THE DOCTOR

- Is segmentectomy an option for treatment?
- When will it be known whether or not all the cancer has been removed?
- What benefits can be expected from this operation?
- What is the risk of tumor recurrence after undergoing this procedure?
- What should be done to prepare for surgery?
- What happens if this operation does not go as planned?

Diagnosis/Preparation

The following methods may be used to help diagnose breast cancer:

- complete physical exam and family medical history
- clinical breast exam
- mammography
- biopsy (incisional, excisional, or needle)
- ultrasonography
- fine-needle aspiration

Tests help to determine whether cancer cells have spread within the lungs or to other parts of the body after a diagnosis of lung cancer. The following tests and procedures may be used in the staging process to diagnose lung cancer:

- complete physical exam, including personal and family medical history
- chest x ray
- computed tomography (CT) scan
- positron emission tomography (**PET**) scan
- other radiologic exams
- laboratory tests (tissue, blood, urine, or other substances in the body)
- bronchoscopy
- mediastinoscopy
- anterior mediastinotomy
- lymph node biopsy

Treatment is determined when the stage of the tumor is known.

Such routine preoperative preparations, as not eating or drinking after midnight on the night before surgery

KEY TERMS

Angiogram—An examination of a part of the body by injecting dye into an artery so that the blood vessels show up on an x ray.

Anterior mediastinotomy—A surgical procedure to look at the organs and tissues between the lungs and between the breastbone and spine for abnormal areas. An incision (cut) is made next to the breastbone and a thin lighted tube is inserted into the chest. Tissue and lymph node samples may be taken for biopsy.

Biopsy—Removal and examination of tissue, cells, or fluids from the living body

Bronchoscope—A tubular illuminated instrument used for inspecting or passing instruments into the bronchi.

Chemoprevention—The use of drugs, vitamins, or other substances to reduce the risk of developing cancer or of the cancer returning.

Chemotherapy—Cancer treatment that uses drugs to stop the growth of cancer cells, either by killing the cells or by stopping them from dividing.

Clinical breast exam—An examination of the breast and surrounding tissue by a physician who is feeling for lumps and looking for other signs of abnormality.

Computed tomography—An x-ray machine linked to a computer that takes a series of detailed pictures of the organs and blood vessels in the body.

Conservation surgery—Surgery that preserves the aesthetic appearance of the area undergoing an operation.

Excision—To surgically remove.

Excisional biopsy—Procedure in which a surgeon removes all of a lump or suspicious area and an area of healthy tissue around the edges. The tissue is then examined under a microscope to check for cancer cells.

Fine-needle aspiration—A procedure in which a thin needle removes fluid and cells from a breast lump to be examined.

Incisional biopsy—A procedure in which a surgeon cuts out a sample of a lump or suspicious area.

Laser therapy—A cancer treatment that uses a laser beam (a narrow beam of intense light) to kill cancer cells.

Lobectomy—Removal of a section of the lung.

Lymph node biopsy—The removal of all or part of a lymph node to view under a microscope for evidence of cancer cells.

are typically ordered for a segmentectomy. Information about expected outcomes and potential complications is also part of the preparation for this surgery.

Aftercare

After a segmentectomy, patients are usually cautioned against doing moderate lifting for several days. Other activities may be restricted (especially if lymph nodes were removed) according to individual needs. Pain is often enough to limit inappropriate motion, and is generally controlled with medication. If pain medications are ineffective, the patient should contact the physician, as severe pain may be a sign of a complication requiring medical attention. Women who undergo segmentectomy of the breast are often instructed to wear a well-fitting support bra both day and night for approximately one week after surgery.

The length of the hospital stay depends on the specific surgery performed and the extent of organ or tissue removed, as well as other factors.

Radiation therapy usually begins four to six weeks after surgery, and continues for four to five weeks. The timing of additional therapy is specific to each patient.

Risks

The risks for any surgical procedure requiring anesthesia include reactions to the medications and breathing problems. Bleeding and infection are risks for any surgical procedure. Infection in the area affecting a segmentectomy occurs in only 3–4% of patients. Pneumonia is also a risk.

Normal results

Successful removal of the tumor with no major bleeding or infection at the wound site after surgery is considered a normal outcome.

Morbidity and mortality rates

Although the incidence of breast cancer has been rising in the United States for the past two decades, the

Lymph nodes—Small, bean-shaped organs located throughout the lymphatic system. Lymph nodes store special cells that can trap cancer cells and bacteria traveling through the body.

Magnetic resonance imaging (MRI)—A powerful magnet linked to a computer used to make detailed images of areas inside the body. These pictures are viewed on a monitor and can also be printed.

Mammography—An x ray of the breast

Mediastinoscopy—A surgical procedure to look at the organs, tissues, and lymph nodes between the lungs for abnormal areas. An incision (cut) is made at the top of the breastbone and a thin lighted tube is inserted into the chest. Tissue and lymph node samples may be taken for biopsy.

Needle biopsy—The use of a needle to remove tissue from an area that looks suspicious on a mammogram but cannot be felt. Tissue removed in a needle biopsy goes to a lab to be checked for cancer cells.

Photodynamic therapy—A cancer treatment that uses a drug that is activated by exposure to light. When the drug exposed to light, the cancer cells are killed.

Positron emission tomography (PET) scan—A procedure to find malignant tumor cells in the body. A small amount of radionuclide glucose (sugar) is injected into a vein. The PET scanner rotates around the body and makes a picture of where the glucose is being used in the body. Malignant tumor cells show up brighter in the picture because they are more active and take up more glucose than normal cells.

Radiation therapy—A cancer treatment that uses high-energy x rays or other types of radiation to kill cancer cells.

Radiologic exams—The use of radiation or other imaging methods to find signs of cancer.

Radiosurgery—A method of delivering radiation directly to the tumor. This method does not involve surgery and causes little damage to healthy tissue.

Radiotherapy—The treatment of disease with such high-energy radiation, as x rays or gamma rays.

Ultrasonography—A proceduring using high-frequency sound waves to show whether a lump is a fluid-filled cyst (not cancer) or a solid mass (which may or may not be cancer).

Ultrasound test—A device using sound waves that produce a pattern of echoes as they bounce off internal organs. The echoes create a picture of the organs.

mortality rate has remained relatively stable since the 1950s. Mortality rates range from 15% of the incidence rate for Japanese women to 33% of the incidence rate for African American women. The highest age-adjusted mortality occurs among African American women, followed by Caucasian and Hawaiian women.

African American women have the highest mortality rates in the age groups 30–54 years and 55–69 years, followed by Hawaiian, and Caucasian non-Hispanic women. The mortality rate for Caucasian women exceeds that for African American women in the 70-year and older age group.

Five-year survival rates for liver cancer patients are usually less than 10% in the United States. The reported statistics for these cancers often include mortality rates that exceed the incidence rates. The discrepancy occurs when the cause of death is misclassified as "liver cancer" for patients whose cancer originated as a primary tumor in another organ and spread to the liver, becoming a secondary cancer.

For primary liver cancer, non-Hispanic white men and women have the lowest age-adjusted mortality rates in the United States, roughly one-half that of the African American and Hispanic populations.

Liver cancer mortality rates for Asian American groups are several times higher than that of the Caucasian population. The highest age-adjusted mortality rates for all groups are among the Chinese population. Alaskan Native and American Indian populations have a very low incidence of liver cancer.

Factors that affect the prognosis (chance of recovery) for lung cancer include:

• stage of the cancer (whether it is in the lung only or has spread to other places in the body)

• tumor size

• type of lung cancer

• presence of symptoms

• shortness of breath during activities

• shortness of breath with less and less activity

• the patient's general health

Current treatments are not a cure for most patients with non-small cell lung cancer. If it returns after treatment, it is called recurrent non-small cell lung cancer. The cancer may reappear in the brain, lung, or other parts of the body. Further treatment is then required.

Alternatives

Other cancer treatments include:

• chemotherapy

• radiation therapy

• radiosurgery

• laser therapy

• photodynamic therapy

• chemoprevention

Using a segmentectomy to remove breast cancers (as a technique that conserves the aesthetic appearance of a breast) is being investigated for large tumors after several cycles of preoperative chemotherapy.

Cancers in some locations (such as where the windpipe divides into the left and right main bronchi) are difficult to remove completely by surgery without also removing an entire lung.

See also Quadrantectomy.

Resources

BOOKS

Benedet, Rosalind Dolores, and Shannon Abbey (Illustrator). *After Mastectomy: Healing Physically and Emotionally.* Omaha, NE: Addicus Books, 2003.

Clavien, Pierre-Alain, and Nuria Roca, eds. *Malignant Liver Tumors: Current and Emerging Therapies,* 2nd edition. Sudbury, MA: Jones & Bartlett Pub., 2003.

Farrell, Susan. *Mammograms and Mastectomies: Facing Them With Humor and Prayer.* Battle Creek, MI: Acorn Publishing, 2003.

Henschke, Claudia I., Peggy McCarthy, and Sarah Wernick. *Lung Cancer: Myths, Facts, Choices—And Hope.* New York, NY: W.W. Norton & Company, 2002.

Simone, John. *The LCIS & DCIS Breast Cancer Fact Book.* Raleigh, NC: Three Pyramids Publishing, 2002.

PERIODICALS

Mahadevia, Parthiv J., Lee A. Fleisher, Kevin D. Frick, John Eng, Steven N. Goodman, and Neil R. Powe. "Lung Cancer Screening with Helical Computed Tomography in Older Adult Smokers: A Decision and Cost-Effectiveness Analysis." *Journal of the American Medical Association* 289 (2003): 313-22. <http://www.atcs.jp/journal/abstract.php?ac=3&bn=030901&no=10>

Shimizu J. J., Y. Ishida, T. Kinoshita., T. Terada, Y. Tatsuzawa, Y. Kawaura, et al. "Left Upper Division Sleeve Segmentectomy for Early Stage Squamous Cell Carcinoma of the Segmental Bronchus: Report of Two Cases." *Annals of Thoracic Cardiovascular Surgery* 9, no.1 (2003): 62-7.

Vastag, Brian. "Consensus Panel Recommendations for Treatment of Early Breast Cancer." *Journal of the American Medical Association* 284 (2002): 2707-8.

ORGANIZATIONS

American Cancer Society. 1599 Clifton Road, N.E. Atlanta, GA 30329-4251. (800) 227-2345. <http://www.cancer.org>.

National Alliance of Breast Cancer Organizations (NABCO). 9 East 37th Street, 10th Floor, New York, NY 10016. (888) 80-NABCO. <http://www.nabco.org>.

National Comprehensive Cancer Network. 50 Huntingdon Pike, Suite 200, Rockledge, PA 19046. (215) 728-4788. Fax: (215) 728-3877. Email: information@nccn.org. <http://www.nccn.org/ >.

National Institutes of Health (NIH), Department of Health and Human Services. 9000 Rockville Pike. Bethesda, MD 20892. (800) 422-6237.

U.S. Department of Health and Human Services. 200 Independence Avenue, S.W., Washington, D.C. 20201. (877) 696-6775.

Y-ME National Breast Cancer Organization. Suite 500-212 West Van Buren St., Chicago, IL 60607-3908. (800) 986-9505. 312-986-8338. Fax: 312-294-8597. <http://www.y-me.org>.

OTHER

National Cancer Institute. *Types of Cancer.* 2003. [cited April 28, 2003] <http://www.nci.nih.gov/cancerinfo/types/>.

Laura Ruth, Ph.D.
Crystal H. Kaczkowski, M.Sc.

Selective dorsal rhizotomy *see* **Rhizotomy**

Senna *see* **Laxatives**

Sentinel lymph node biopsy

Definition

Sentinel lymph node biopsy (SLNB) is a minimally invasive procedure in which a lymph node near the site of a cancerous tumor is first identified as a sentinel node and then removed for microscopic analysis. SLNB was developed by researchers in several different cancer centers following the discovery that the human lymphatic system can be mapped with radioactive dyes, and that the lymph node(s) closest to a tumor serve to filter and trap cancer cells. These nodes are known as sentinel nodes because they act like sentries to warn doctors that a patient's cancer is spreading.

Sentinel lymph node biopsy

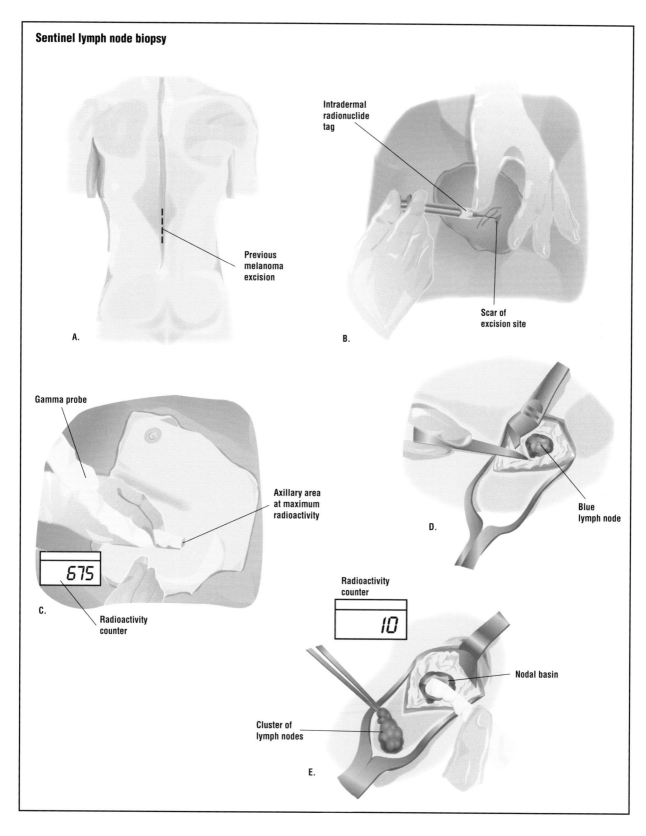

At the site of a previous cancer removal, a radionuclide dye is injected (A and B). The area of maximum radioactivity is traced to a lymph node under the arm (C). The area is cut open, and the lymph node is identified by its blue dye (D). After the lymph node is removed, the area is checked for further radioactivity (E). *(Illustration by GGS Inc.)*

The first descriptions of sentinel nodes come from studies of penile and testicular cancers done in the 1970s. A technique that uses blue dye to map the lymphatic system was developed in the 1980s and applied to the treatment of melanoma in 1989. The extension of sentinel lymph node biopsy to the treatment of breast cancer began at the John Wayne Cancer Institute in Santa Monica, California, in 1991. As of 2003, SLNB is used in the diagnosis and treatment of many other cancers, including cancers of the head and neck, anus, bladder, lung, and male breast.

Purpose

Sentinel lymph node biopsy has several purposes:

• Improving the accuracy of cancer staging. Cancer staging is a system that classifies malignant tumors according to the extent of their spread in the body. It is used to guide decisions about treatment.

• Catching the spread of cancer to nearby lymph nodes as early as possible.

• Defining homogeneous patient populations for clinical trials of new cancer treatments.

Description

A sentinel lymph node biopsy is done in two stages. In the first part of the procedure, which takes one to two hours, the patient goes to the nuclear medicine department of the hospital for an injection of a radioactive tracer known as technetium 99. A doctor who specializes in nuclear medicine first numbs the area around the tumor with a local anesthetic and then injects the radioactive technetium. He or she usually injects a blue dye as well. The doctor will then use a gamma camera to take pictures of the lymph nodes before surgery. This type of imaging study is called lymphoscintigraphy.

After the lymphoscintigraphy, the patient must wait several hours for the dye and the radioactive material to travel from the tissues around the tumor to the sentinel lymph node. He or she is then taken to the **operating room** and put under general anesthesia. Next, the surgeon injects more blue dye into the area around the tumor. The surgeon then uses a hand-held probe connected to a gamma ray counter to scan the area for the radioactive technetium. The sentinel lymph node can be pinpointed by the sound made by the gamma ray counter. The surgeon makes an incision about 0.5 in long to remove the sentinel node. The blue dye that has been injected helps to verify that the surgeon is removing the right node. The incision is then closed and the tissue is sent to the hospital laboratory for examination.

Preparation

Some cancer patients should not be given an SLNB. They include women with cancer in more than one part of the breast; women who have had previous breast surgery, including plastic surgery; women with breast cancer in advanced stages; and women who have had radiation therapy. Melanoma patients who have undergone wide excision (removal of surrounding skin as well as the tumor) of the original skin cancer are also not candidates for an SLNB.

Apart from evaluating the patient's fitness for an SLNB, no additional preparation is necessary.

Aftercare

A sentinel lymph node biopsy does not require extensive aftercare. In most cases, the patient goes home after the procedure or after an overnight stay in the hospital.

The surgeon will discuss the laboratory findings with the patient. If the sentinel node was found to contain cancer cells, the surgeon will usually recommend a full axillary lymph node dissection (ALND). This is a more invasive procedure in which a larger number of lymph nodes—usually 12–15—is surgically removed. A drainage tube is placed for two to three weeks and the patient must undergo physical therapy at home.

Risks

Risks associated with an SLNB include the following:

- Mild discomfort after the procedure.
- Lymphedema (swelling of the arm due to disruption of the lymphatic system after surgery).
- Damage to the nerves in the area of the biopsy.
- Temporary discoloration of the skin in the area of the dye injection.
- False negative laboratory report. A false negative means that there is cancer in other lymph nodes in spite of the absence of cancer in the sentinel node. False negatives usually result from either poor timing of the dye injection, the way in which the pathologist prepared the tissue for examination, or the existence of previously undiscovered sentinel nodes.

Normal results

Sentinel lymph node biopsies have a high degree of accuracy, with relatively few false negatives. A negative laboratory report means that there is a greater than 95% chance that the other nearby lymph nodes are also free of cancer.

Morbidity and mortality rates

Compared to axillary lymph node dissection, sentinel lymph node biopsy has a significantly lower rate of complications. One study found that only 2.6% of patients who had SLNB developed lymphedema, compared to 27% of patients who had ALND. Another study found that 71% of SLNB patients were able to return to normal activity within 4 days of the procedure, compared to 7% of the ALND patients.

Alternatives

Breast cancer patients who should not have a sentinel lymph node biopsy usually undergo an axillary lymph node dissection to determine whether their cancer has spread. Melanoma patients who have already had a wide excision of the original melanoma may have nearby lymph nodes removed to prevent the cancer from spreading. This procedure is called a prophylactic lymph node dissection.

QUESTIONS TO ASK THE DOCTOR

- Am I a candidate for sentinel lymph node biopsy?
- How many SLNBs have you performed?
- Do you perform this procedure on a regular basis?
- What is your false-negative rate?

Resources

PERIODICALS

Burak, W. E., S. T. Hollenbeck, E. E. Zervos, et al. "Sentinel Lymph Node Biopsy Results in Less Postoperative Morbidity Compared with Axillary Lymph Node Dissection for Breast Cancer." *American Journal of Surgery* 183 (January 2002): 23-27.

Burrall, Barbara, and Vijay Khatri. "Still Debating Sentinel Lymph Node Biopsy?" *Dermatology Online Journal* 7 (2):1 [April 22, 2003].

Fukui, Y., T. Yamakawa, T. Taniki, et al. "Sentinel Lymph Node Biopsy in Patients with Papillary Thyroid Carcinoma." *Cancer* 92 (December 1, 2001): 2868-2874.

Golshan, M., W. J. Martin, and K. Dowlatshahi. "Sentinel Lymph Node Biopsy Lowers the Rate of Lymphedema When Compared with Standard Axillary Lymph Node Dissection." *American Surgeon* 69 (March 2003): 209-211.

McMasters, K. M., D. S. Reintgen, M. I. Ross et al. "Sentinel Lymph Node Biopsy for Melanoma: Controversy Despite Widespread Agreement." *Journal of Clinical Oncology* 19 (June 1, 2001): 2851-2855.

Peley, C., E. Farkas, I. Sinkovics, et al. "Inguinal Sentinel Lymph Node Biopsy for Staging Anal Cancer." *Scandinavian Journal of Surgery* 91 (2002): 336-338.

Port, E. R., J. V. Fey, H. S. Cody III, and P. I. Borgen. "Sentinel Lymph Node Biopsy in Patients with Male Breast Carcinoma." *Cancer* 91 (January 15, 2001): 319-323.

Pow-Sang, Julio, MD. "The Spectrum of Genitourinary Malignancies." *Cancer Control* 9 (July-August 2002): 275-276.

Schmalbach, C. E., B. Nussenbaum, R. S. Rees, et al. "Reliability of Sentinel Lymph Node Mapping with Biopsy for Head and Neck Cutaneous Melanoma." *Archives of Otolaryngology—Head and Neck Surgery* 129 (January 2003): 61-65.

Tanis, Pieter J., Omgo E. Nieweg, Renato A. Valdés Olmos, et al. "History of Sentinel Node and Validation of the Technique." *Breast Cancer Research* 3 (2001): 109-112.

Uren, R. F., R. Howman-Giles, and J. F. Thompson. "Patterns of Lymphatic Drainage from the Skin in Patients with Melanoma." *Journal of Nuclear Medicine* 44 (April 2003): 570-582.

ORGANIZATIONS

American Cancer Society (ACS). (800) ACS-2345. <www.cancer.org>.

National Cancer Institute (NCI). NCI Public Inquiries Office, Suite 3036A, 6116 Executive Boulevard, MSC8332, Bethesda, MD 20892-8322. (800) 4-CANCER or (800) 332-8615 (TTY). <www.nci.nih.gov>.

Society of Nuclear Medicine (SNM). 1850 Samuel Morse Drive, Reston, VA 20190. (703) 708-9000. <www.snm.org>.

Rebecca Frey, Ph.D.

Septoplasty

Definition

Septoplasty is a surgical procedure to correct the shape of the septum of the nose. The goal of this procedure is to correct defects or deformities of the septum. The nasal septum is the separation between the two nostrils. In adults, the septum is composed partly of cartilage and partly of bone. Septal deviations are either congenital (present from birth) or develop as a result of an injury. Most people with deviated septa do not develop symptoms. It is typically only the most severely deformed septa that produce significant symptoms and require surgical intervention. However, many septoplasties are performed during **rhinoplasty** procedures, which are most often performed for cosmetic purposes.

Purpose

Septoplasty is performed to correct a crooked (deviated) or dislocated septum, often as part of plastic surgery of the nose (rhinoplasty). The nasal septum has three functions: to support the nose, to regulate air flow, and to support the mucous membranes (mucosa) of the nose. Septoplasty is done to correct the shape of the nose caused by a deformed septum or correct deregulated airflow caused by a deviated septum. Septoplasty is often needed when the patient is having an operation to reduce the size of the nose (reductive rhinoplasty), because this operation usually reduces the amount of breathing space in the nose.

During surgery, the patient's own cartilage that has been removed can be reused to provide support for the nose if needed. External septum supports are not usually needed. Splints may be needed occasionally to support cartilage when extensive cutting has been done. External splints can be used to support the cartilage for the first few days of healing. Tefla gauze is inserted in the nostril to support the flaps and cartilage and to absorb any bleeding or mucus.

Demographics

About one-third of the population may have some degree of nasal obstruction. Among those with nasal obstruction, about one-fourth have deviated septa.

Diagnosis/Preparation

The primary conditions that may suggest a need for septoplasty include:

• nasal air passage obstruction
• nasal septal deformity
• headaches caused by septal spurs
• chronic and uncontrolled nosebleeds
• chronic sinusitis associated with a deviated septum
• obstructive sleep apnea
• polypectomy (polyp removal)
• tumor excision
• turbinate surgery
• ethmoidectomy (removal of all or part of a small bone on the upper part of the nasal cavity)

Septoplasty

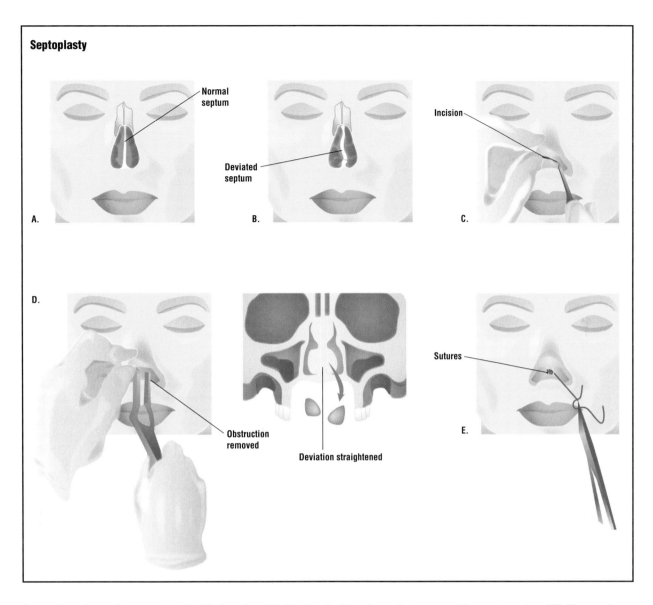

Septoplasty is used to correct a deviated septum (B). First an incision is made to expose the nasal septum (C). Pieces of septum that are obstructing air flow are removed (D), and the incision is then closed (E). *(Illustration by GGS Inc.)*

Septal deformities can cause nasal airway obstruction. Such airway obstruction can lead to mouth breathing, chronic nasal infections, or obstructive sleep apnea. Septal spurs can produce headaches when these growths lead to increased pressure on the nasal septum. Polypectomy, ethmoidectomy, **tumor removal**, and turbinate surgical procedures often include septoplasty. Individuals who have used significant quantities of cocaine over a long period of time often require septoplasty because of alterations in the nasal passage structures.

Septal deviation is usually diagnosed by direct observation of the nasal passages. In addition, a computed tomography (CT) scan of the entire nasal passage is often performed. This scan allows the physician to fully assess the structures and functioning of the area. Additional tests that evaluate the movement of air through the nasal passages may also be performed.

Before performing a septoplasty, the surgeon will evaluate the difference in airflow between the two nostrils. In children, this assessment can be done very simply by asking the child to breathe out slowly on a small mirror held in front of the nose.

As with any other operation under general anesthesia, patients are evaluated for any physical conditions that might complicate surgery and for any medications that might affect blood clotting time. If a general anesthetic is used, then the patient is advised not to drink or eat after midnight the night before the surgery. In many cases, septoplasty can be performed on an outpatient basis using local anesthesia. Conditions that might preclude a patient from receiving a septoplasty include excessive cocaine abuse, Wegener's granulomatosis, malignant lymphomas, and an excessively large septal perforation.

Aftercare

Patients who receive septoplasty are usually sent home from the hospital later the same day or in the morning after the surgery. All dressings inside the nose are usually removed before the patient leaves. Aftercare includes a list of detailed instructions for the patient that focus on preventing trauma to the nose.

The head needs to be elevated while resting during the first 24-48 hours after surgery. Patients will have to breathe through the mouth while the nasal packing is still in place. A small amount of bloody discharge is normal but excessive bleeding should be reported to the physician immediately. **Antibiotics** are usually not prescribed unless the packing is left in place more than 24 hours. Most patients do not suffer significant amounts of pain, but those who do have severe pain are sometimes given narcotic pain relievers. Patients are often advised to place an ice pack on the nose to enhance comfort during the recovery period. Patients who have splint placement usually return seven to 10 days after the surgery for examination and splint removal.

Risks

The risks from septoplasty are similar to those from other operations on the face: postoperative pain with some bleeding, swelling, bruising, or discoloration. A few patients may have allergic reactions to the anesthetics. The operation in itself, however, is relatively low-risk in that it does not involve major blood vessels or vital organs. Infection is unlikely if proper surgical tech-

nique is observed. One of the extremely rare but serious complications of septoplasty is cerebrospinal fluid leak. This complication can be treated with proper nasal packing, bed rest, and antibiotic use. Follow-up surgery may be necessary if the nasal obstruction relapses.

Normal results

Normal results include improved breathing and airflow through the nostrils, and an acceptable outward shape of the nose. Most patients have significant improvements in symptoms following surgery.

Morbidity and mortality rates

Significant morbidity associated with septoplasty is rare and is outlined in the Risks section above. Mortality is extremely rare and associated with the risks involving anesthesia. This procedure can be performed using local

KEY TERMS

Cartilage—A tough, elastic connective tissue found in the joints, outer ear, nose, larynx, and other parts of the body.

Obstructive sleep apnea—A temporary cessation of breathing that occurs during sleep and is associated with poor sleep quality.

Polyp—A tumor commonly found in vascular organs such as the nose that are often benign but can become malignant.

Rhinoplasty—Plastic surgery of the nose.

Septum (plural, septa)—The dividing partition in the nose that separates the two nostrils. It is composed of bone and cartilage.

Sinusitis—Inflammation of the sinuses.

Splint—A thin piece of rigid material that is sometimes used during nasal surgery to hold certain structures in place until healing is underway.

Spurs—A sharp horny outgrowth of the skin.

Wegener's granulomatosis—A rare condition that consists of lesions within the respiratory tract.

anesthesia on an outpatient basis or under general anesthesia during a short hospital stay. General anesthesia is associated with a greater mortality rate, but this risk is minimal.

Alternatives

In cases of sinusitis or allergic rhinitis, nasal airway breathing can be improved by using such nasal sprays, as phenylephrine (Neo-Synephrine). Patients with a history of chronic uncontrolled nasal bleeding should receive conservative therapy that includes nasal packing to identify the source of the bleeding before surgery is contemplated. Those who have been diagnosed with obstructive sleep apnea have a variety of conservative alternatives before surgery is seriously considered. These alternatives include weight loss, changes in sleep posture, and the use of appliances during sleep that enlarge the upper airway.

Resources

BOOKS

Muth, Annemarie S., and Karen Bellenir, eds. *Surgery Sourcebook.* New York: Omnigraphics, 2002.
Schwartz, Seymour I., ed. *Principles of Surgery.* New York: McGraw-Hill, 1999.
"Septal deviation and perforation." In *The Merck Manual,* edited by Keryn A. G. Lane. West Point, PA: Merck & Co., 1999.

OTHER

"Septoplasty." *MEDLINEplus Medical Encyclopedia* [cited July 7, 2003]. <http://www.nlm.nih.gov>.

Mark Mitchell

Serum electrolyte tests *see* **Electrolyte tests**

Seton glaucoma surgery *see* **Tube-shunt surgery**

Sex reassignment surgery

Definition

Also known as sex change or gender reassignment surgery, sex reassignment surgery is a procedure that changes genital organs from one gender to another.

Purpose

There are two main reasons to alter the genital organs from one sex to another.

• Newborns with intersex deformities must early on be assigned to one sex or the other. These deformities represent intermediate stages between the primordial female genitals and the change into male genitals caused by male hormone stimulation.

• Both men and women occasionally believe they are physically a different sex than they are mentally and emotionally. This dissonance is so profound that they are willing to be surgically altered.

In both cases, technical considerations favor successful conversion to a female rather than a male. Newborns with ambiguous organs will almost always be assigned to the female gender unless the penis is at least an inch long. Whatever their chromosomes, they are much more likely to be socially well adjusted as females, even if they cannot have children.

Demographics

Reliable statistics are extremely difficult to obtain. Many sexual reassignment procedures are conducted in private facilities that are not subject to reporting requirements. Sexual reassignment surgery is often conducted outside of the United States. The number of gender reassignment procedures conducted in the United States each year is estimated at between 100 and 500. The number worldwide is estimated to be two to five times larger.

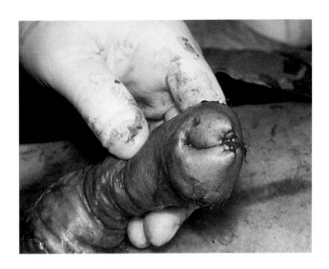

Penis constructed from the patient's previously female genitalia during sex change surgery. *(Custom Medical Stock Photo. Reproduced by permission.)*

Description

Converting male to female anatomy requires removal of the penis, reshaping genital tissue to appear more female, and constructing a vagina. A vagina can be successfully formed from a skin graft or an isolated loop of intestine. Following the surgery, female hormones (estrogen) will reshape the body's contours and stimulate the growth of satisfactory breasts.

Female to male surgery has achieved lesser success due to the difficulty of creating a functioning penis from the much smaller clitoral tissue available in the female genitals. Penis construction is not attempted less than a year after the preliminary surgery to remove the female organs. One study in Singapore found that a third of the persons would not undergo the surgery again. Nevertheless, they were all pleased with the change of sex. Besides the genital organs, the breasts need to be surgically altered for a more male appearance. This can be successfully accomplished.

The capacity to experience an orgasm, or at least "a reasonable degree of erogenous sensitivity," can be expected by almost all persons after gender reassignment surgery.

Diagnosis/Preparation

Gender identity is an extremely important characteristic for human beings. Assigning it must take place immediately after birth, for the mental health of both children and their parents. Changing sexual identity is among the most significant changes that a human can experience. It should therefore be undertaken with extreme care and caution. By the time most adults come

to surgery, they have lived for many years with a dissonant identity. The average in one study was 29 years. Nevertheless, even then they may not be fully aware of the implications of becoming a member of the opposite gender.

In-depth psychological counseling should precede and follow any gender reassignment surgical procedure.

Sex change surgery is expensive. The cost for male to female reassignment is $7,000 to $24,000. The cost for female to male reassignment can exceed $50,000.

WHO PERFORMS THE PROCEDURE AND WHERE IS IT PERFORMED?

Gender reassignment surgery is performed by surgeons with specialized training in urology, gynecology, or plastic and reconstructive surgery. The surgery is performed in a hospital setting, although many procedures are completed in privately owned clinics.

Aftercare

Social support, particularly from one's family, is important for readjustment as a member of the opposite gender. If surgical candidates are socially or emotionally unstable before the operation, over the age of 30, or have an unsuitable body build for the new gender, they tend not to fare well after gender reassignment surgery. However, in no case studied did the gender reassignment procedure diminish their ability to work.

Risks

All surgery carries the risks of infection, bleeding, and a need to return for repairs. Gender reassignment surgery is irreversible, so a candidate must have no doubts about accepting the results and outcome.

Normal results

Persons undergoing gender reassignment surgery can expect to acquire the external genitalia of a member of the opposite gender. Persons having male to female gender reassignment surgery retain a prostate. Individuals undergoing female to male gender reassignment surgery undergo a **hysterectomy** to remove the uterus and **oophorectomy** to remove their ovaries. Developing the habits and mannerisms characteristic of the patient's new gender requires many months or years.

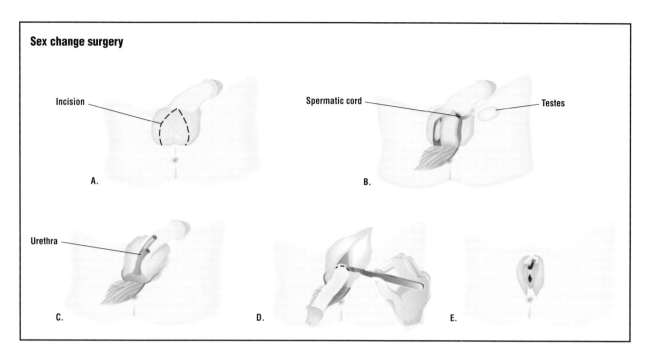

Sex change surgery

Incision — A.

Spermatic cord — Testes — B.

Urethra — C.

D.

E.

To change male genitalia to female genitalia, an incision is made into the scrotum (A). The flap of skin is pulled back, and the testes are removed (B). The skin is stripped from the penis but left attached, and a shorter urethra is cut (C). All but a stump of the penis is removed (D). The excess skin is used to create the labia (external genitalia) and vagina (E). *(Illustration by GGS Inc.)*

Morbidity and mortality rates

The risks that are associated with any surgical procedure are present in gender reassignment surgery. These include infection, postoperative pain, and dissatisfaction with anticipated results. Accurate statistics are extremely difficult to find. Intraoperative death has not been reported.

The most common complication of male to female surgery is narrowing of the new vagina. This can be corrected by dilation or using a portion of colon to form a vagina.

A relatively common complication of female to male surgery is dysfunction of the penis. Implanting a penile prosthesis is technically difficult and does not have uniformly acceptable results.

Psychiatric care may be required for many years after sex-reassignment surgery.

The number of deaths in male-to-female transsexuals was five times the number expected, due to increased numbers of suicide and death from unknown cause.

Alternatives

There is no alternative to surgical reassignment to alter one's external genitalia. The majority of persons who experience gender disorder problems never surgically alter their appearance. They dress as members of the desired gender, rather than gender of birth. Many use creams or pills that contain hormones appropriate to the desired gender to alter their bodily appearance. Estrogens (female hormones) will stimulate breast development, widening of the hips, loss of facial hair and a slight increase in voice pitch. Androgens (male hormones) will stimulate the development of facial and chest hair and cause the voice to deepen. Most individuals who undergo gender reassignment surgery lead happy and productive lives.

See also Breast implants; Penile prostheses.

Resources

BOOKS

Bostwick, John. *Plastic and Reconstructive Breast Surgery,* 2nd edition. St. Louis: Quality Medical Publishers, 1999.

Engler, Alan M. *Body Sculpture: Plastic Surgery of the Body for Men and Women,* 2nd edition. New York: Hudson, 2000.

Tanagho, Emil A. and Jack W. McAninch. *Smith's General Urology,* 15th Edition. New York: McGraw-Hill, 2000.

Walsh, Patrick C. and Alan B. Retik. *Campbell's Urology,* 8th Edition. Philadelphia: Saunders, 2002.

Wilson, Josephine F. *Biological Foundations of Human Behavior.* New York: Harcourt, 2002.

PERIODICALS

Asscheman, H., L. J. Gooren, and P. L. Eklund. "Mortality and Morbidity in Transsexual Patients with Cross-Gender Hormone Treatment." *Metabolism* 38, No. 9 (1989): 869–73.

KEY TERMS

Androgens—A class of chemical compounds (hormones) that stimulates the development of male secondary sexual characteristics.

Chromosomes—The carriers of genes that determine gender and other characteristics.

Estrogens—A class of chemical compounds (hormones) that stimulate the development of female secondary sexual characteristics.

Hysterectomy—Surgical removal of the uterus.

Oophorectomy—Surgical removal of the ovaries.

Docter, R. F. and J. S. Fleming. "Measures of Transgender Behavior." *Archives of Sexual Behavior* 30, No. 3 (2001): 255–71.

Fugate, S. R., C. C. Apodaca, and M. L. Hibbert. "Gender Reassignment Surgery and the Gynecological Patient." *Primary Care Update for Obstetrics and Gynecology* 8, No. 1 (2001): 22–4.

Harish, D., and B. R. Sharma. "Medical Advances in Transsexualism and the Legal Implications." *American Journal of Forensic Medicine and Pathology* 24, No. 1 (2003): 100–05.

Jarolim, L. "Surgical Conversion of Genitalia in Transsexual Patients." *British Journal of Urology International* 85, No. 7 (2000): 851–56.

Monstrey, S., P. Hoebeke, M. Dhont, G. De Cuypere, R. Rubens, M. Moerman, M. Hamdi, K. Van Landuyt, and P. Blondeel. "Surgical Therapy in Transsexual Patients: A Multi-disciplinary Approach." *Annals of Surgery* (Belgium) 101, No. 5 (2001): 200–09.

ORGANIZATIONS

American Medical Association. 515 N. State Street, Chicago, IL 60610, Phone: (312) 464-5000. <http://www.ama-assn.org/>.

American Psychiatric Association. 1400 K Street NW, Washington, DC 20005, (888) 357-7924. Fax: (202) 682-6850. apa@psych.org.

American Psychological Association. 750 First Street NW, Washington, DC, 20002-4242. (800) 374-2721 or (202) 336-5500. <http://www.apa.org/>.

American Urological Association. 1120 North Charles Street, Baltimore, MD 21201-5559. (410) 727-1100. <http://www.auanet.org/index_hi.cfm>.

OTHER

Health A to Z [cited March 24, 2003]. <http://www.healthatoz.com/healthatoz/Atoz/ency/sex_change_surgery.html>.

Hendrick Health System [cited March 24, 2003]. <http://www.hendrickhealth.org/healthy/001240.htm>.

Intersex Society of North America [cited March 24, 2003]. <http://www.isna.org/newsletter/>.

University of Missouri-Kansas City [cited March 24, 2003]. <http://www.umkc.edu/sites/hsw/gendid/srs.html>.

L. Fleming Fallon, Jr., MD, DrPH

Shoulder arthroscopic surgery *see* **Rotator cuff repair; Bankart procedure**

Shoulder joint replacement

Definition

Shoulder joint replacement surgery is performed to replace a shoulder joint with artificial components (prostheses) when the joint is severely damaged by such degenerative joint diseases as arthritis, or in complex cases of upper arm bone fracture.

Purpose

The shoulder is a ball-and-socket joint that allows the arms to be raised, twisted, bent, and moved forward, to the side and backward. The head of the upper arm bone (humerus) is the ball, and a circular cavity (glenoid) in the shoulder blade (scapula) is the socket. A soft-tissue rim (labrum) surrounds and deepens the socket. The head of the humerus is also covered with a smooth, tough tissue (articular cartilage); and the joint, also called the acromioclavicular (AC) joint, has a thin inner lining (synovium) that facilitates movement while surrounding muscles and tendons provide stability and support.

The AC joint can be damaged by the following conditions to such an extent as to require replacement by artificial components:

Shoulder joint replacement

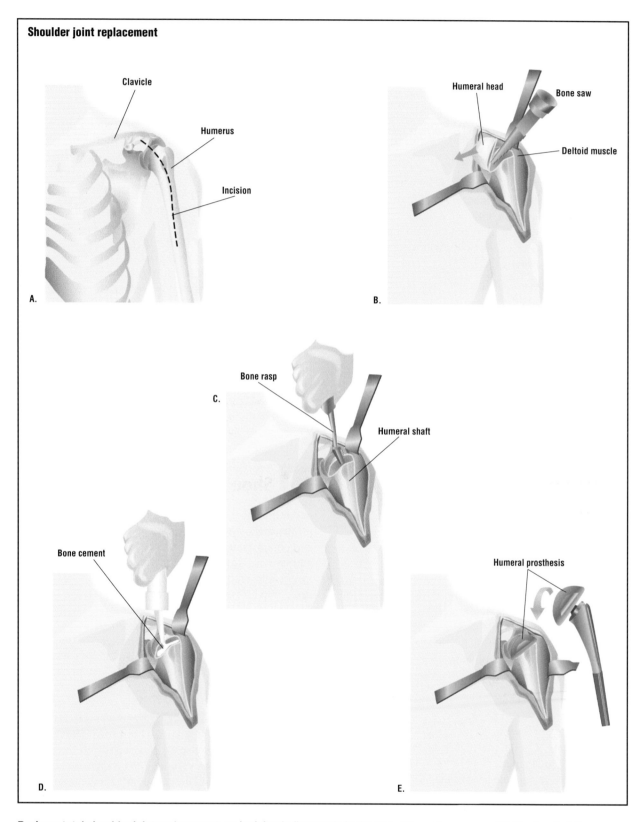

During a total shoulder joint replacement, an incision is first made in the shoulder and upper arm (A). The head of the humerus is removed with a bone saw (B). The shaft of the humerus is reamed with a bone rasp to ready it for the prosthesis (C). After the shoulder joint, or glenoid cavity, is similarly prepared, bone cement is applied to areas to receive prostheses (D). The ball and socket prostheses are put in place, and the incision is closed (E). *(Illustration by GGS Inc.)*

- Osteoarthritis. This is a degenerative joint disease characterized by destruction or thinning of the articular cartilage. When non-surgical treatment is no longer effective and shoulder resection not possible, joint replacement surgery is usually indicated.

- Rheumatoid arthritis. Shoulder replacement surgery is the most commonly performed procedure for the arthritic shoulder with severe inflammatory or rheumatoid arthritis.

- Severe fracture of the humerus. A fracture of the upper arm bone can be so severe as to require replacement of the AC joint.

- Osteonecrosis. This condition usually follows a three- or four-part fracture of the humeral head that disrupts the blood supply, resulting in bone death and disruption of the AC joint.

- Charcot's arthropathy. Also called neuropathic arthropathy or arthritis, Charcot's arthropathy is a condition in which the shoulder joint is destroyed following loss of its nerve supply.

Demographics

Shoulder arthritis is among the most prevalent causes of shoulder pain and loss of function. In the United States, arthritis of the shoulder joint is less common than arthritis of the hip or knee. Individuals with arthritis in one joint are more likely to get it in another joint. Overall, arthritis is quite common in the United States, affecting about 16 million Americans. Osteoarthritis is also the most common joint disorder, extremely common by age 70. Men and women are equally affected, but onset is earlier in men.

Description

Shoulder joint replacement surgery can either replace the entire AC joint, in which case it is referred to as total shoulder joint replacement or total shoulder **arthroplasty**; or replace only the head of the humerus, in which case the procedure is called a hemiarthroplasty.

Implants

The two artificial components that can be implanted in the shoulder during shoulder joint replacment surgery are:

- The humeral component. This part replaces the head of the humerus. It is usually made of cobalt or chromium-based alloys and has a rounded ball attached to a stem that can be inserted into the bone. It comes in various sizes and may consist of a single piece or a modular unit.

- The glenoid component. This component replaces the glenoid cavity. It is made of very high-density polyethelene. Some models feature a metal tray, but the 100% polyethylene type is more common.

Shoulder joint replacement surgery is performed under either regional or general anesthesia, depending on the specifics of the case. The surgeon makes a 3–4 in (7.6–10.2 cm) incision on the front of the shoulder from the collarbone to the point where the shoulder muscle (deltoid) attaches to the humerus. The surgeon also inspects the muscles to see if any are damaged. He or she then proceeds to dislocate the humerus from the socket-like glenoid cavity to expose the head of the humerus. Only the portion of the head covered with articular cartilage is removed. The center cavity of the humerus (humeral shaft) is then cleaned and enlarged with reamers of gradually increasing size to create a cavity matching the shape of the implant stem. The top end of the bone is smoothed so that the stem can be inserted flush with the bone surface.

If the glenoid cavity of the AC joint is not damaged and the surrounding muscles are intact, the surgeon does not replace it, thus performing a simple hemiarthroplasty. However, if the glenoid cavity is damaged or diseased, the surgeon moves the humerus to the back and implants the artificial glenoid component as well. The surgeon prepares the surface by removing the cartilage and equalizes the glenoid bone to match the implant. Protrusions on the polyethylene glenoid implant are then fitted into holes drilled in the bone surface. Once a precise fit is achieved, the implant is cemented into position. The humerus, with its new implanted artificial head, is replaced in the glenoid socket. The surgeon reattaches the supporting tendons and closes the incision.

Diagnosis/Preparation

Damage to the AC joint is usually assessed using x rays of the joint and humerus. They provide information on the state of the joint space, the position of the humeral head in relation to the glenoid, the presence of bony defects or deformity, and the quality of the bone. If glenoid wear is observed, a computed tomography (CT) scan is usually performed to evaluate the degree of bone loss.

The treating physician usually performs a general medical evaluation several weeks before shoulder joint replacement surgery to assess the patient's general health

1310

condition and risk for anesthesia. The results of this examination are forwarded to the orthopedic surgeon, along with a surgical clearance. Patients are advised to eat properly and take a daily iron supplement some weeks before surgery. Several types of tests are usually required, including blood tests, a cardiogram, a urine sample, and a **chest x ray**. Patients may be required to stop taking certain medications until surgery is over.

Aftercare

Following surgery, the operated arm is placed in a sling, and a support pillow is placed under the elbow to protect the repair. A drainage tube is used to remove excess fluid and is usually removed on the day after surgery.

A careful and well-planned rehabilitation program is very important for the successful outcome of a shoulder joint replacement. It should start no later than the first postoperative day. A physical therapist usually starts the patient with gentle, passive-assisted range of motion exercises. Before the patient leaves the hospital (usually two or three days after surgery), the therapist provides instruction on the use of a pulley device to help bend and extend the operated arm.

Risks

Complications after shoulder replacement surgery occur less frequently than with other joint replacement surgeries. However, there are risks associated with the surgery such as infection; intra-operative fracture of the humerus or postoperative fractures; biceps tendon rupture; and postoperative instability and loosening of the glenoid implant. Advances in surgical techniques and prosthetic innovations are helping to significantly lower the occurrence of complications.

Normal results

Pain relief is expected after shoulder joint replacement because the diseased joint surfaces have been replaced with smooth gliding surfaces. Improved motion, however, is variable and depends on the following:

• The surgeon's ability to reconstruct the shoulder's supporting tissues, namely the shoulder ligaments, capsule, and muscle attachments.

• The patient's preoperative muscle strength.

• The patient's motivation and compliance in participating in postoperative rehabilitation therapy.

Morbidity and mortality rates

Good to excellent outcomes usually follow shoulder joint replacement surgery, including pain relief and a

---

QUESTIONS TO ASK THE DOCTOR

• What type of joint replacement surgery does my shoulder require?

• What are the risks associated with the surgery?

• How long will it take for my shoulder to recover from the surgery?

• How long will the artificial components last?

• Is there a risk of implant infection?

• How many shoulder joint replacement surgeries do you perform in a year?

---

functional range of motion that provides the ability to dress and perform the normal activities of daily living. In the hands of experienced orthopedic surgeons, such outcomes occur 90% of the time. Shoulders with artificial joints are reported to function well for more than 20 years. No death has ever been reported for shoulder joint replacement procedures.

Alternatives

Arthritis treatment is very complex, as it depends on the type of arthritis and the severity of symptoms. Alternatives to joint replacement may include medications and therapy. It is known that arthritis is characterized by an increased rate of cartilage degradation and a decreased rate of cartilage production. An experimental therapy featuring the use of such joint supplements as glucosamine and chondroitin is being investigated for its effectiveness to repair cartilage. The pain and inflammation resulting from arthritis are also commonly treated with nonsteroidal anti-inflammatory pain medication (NSAIDs) or cortisone injections (steroidal).

See also Shoulder resection arthroplasty.

Resources

BOOKS

Wallace, W. A., ed. *Joint Replacement in the Shoulder and Elbow.* London: Edward Arnold Pub., 1998.

PERIODICALS

Godeneche, A., et al. "Prosthetic Replacement in the Treatment of Osteoarthritis of the Shoulder: Early Results of 268 Cases." *Journal of Shoulder and Elbow Surgery* 11 (January–February 2002): 11–18.

Miller, S. L., Y. Hazrati, S. Klepps, A. Chiang, and E. L. Flatow. "Loss of Subscapularis Function after Total Shoulder Replacement: A Seldom Recognized Problem." *Journal of*

KEY TERMS

Acromioclavicular (AC) joint—The shoulder joint. Articulation and ligaments between the collarbone and the acromion of the shoulder blade.

Acromion—The triangular projection of the spine of the shoulder blade that forms the point of the shoulder and articulates with the collarbone.

Arthroplasty—The surgical repair of a joint.

Charcot's arthropathy—Also called neuropathic arthropathy, a condition in which the shoulder joint is destroyed following loss of its nerve supply.

Glenoid cavity—The hollow cavity in the head of the shoulder blade that receives the head of the humerus to make the glenohumeral or shoulder joint.

Humerus—The bone of the upper part of the arm.

Inflammatory arthritis—An inflammatory condition that affects joints.

Osteoarthritis—Non-inflammatory degenerative joint disease occurring chiefly in older persons, characterized by degeneration of the articular cartilage.

Osteonecrosis—Condition resulting from poor blood supply to an area of a bone and causing bone death.

Rheumatoid arthritis—Chronic inflammatory disease that destroys joints.

Shoulder resection arthroplasty—Surgery performed to repair a shoulder acromioclavicular (AC) joint. The procedure is most commonly recommended for AC joint problems resulting from osteoarthritis or injury.

Shoulder and Elbow Surgery 12 (January–February 2003): 517–521.

Roos, E. M. "Effectiveness and Practice Variation of Rehabilitation after Joint Replacement." *Current Opinions in Rheumatology* 15 (March 2003): 160–162.

Steinmann, S. P., and R. H. Cofield. "Bone Grafting for Glenoid Deficiency in Total Shoulder Replacement." *Journal of Shoulder and Elbow Surgery,* 9 (September–October 2000): 361–367.

Vitale, M. G., et al. "Geographic Variations in the Rates of Operative Procedures Involving the Shoulder, Including Total Shoulder Replacement, Humeral Head Replacement, and Rotator Cuff Repair." *Journal of Bone and Joint Surgery,* 81 (June 1999): 763–772.

ORGANIZATIONS

American Academy of Orthopaedic Surgeons (AAOS). 6300 North River Road, Rosemont, Illinois 60018-4262. (847) 823-7186. <http://www.aaos.org>.

American Shoulder and Elbow Surgeons (ASES). 6300 North River Road, Suite 727, Rosemont, IL, 60018-4226. (847) 698-1629. <http://www.ases-assn.org>.

OTHER

Getting a Shoulder Replacement. <http://www.jointreplacement.com/xq/ASP.default/mn.local/pg.cat/joint_id.1/cat_id.6/newFont.2/joint_nm.Shoulder/local_id.8/qx/default.htm>.

"A Patient's Guide to Artificial Shoulder Replacement." *Medical MultiMedia.* <http://www.medicalmultimediagroup.com/pated/joints/shoulder/shoulder_replacement.html>.

Monique Laberge, PhD

Shoulder resection arthroplasty

Definition

Shoulder resection **arthroplasty** is surgery performed to repair a shoulder acromioclavicular (AC) joint. The procedure is most commonly recommended for AC joint problems resulting from osteoarthritis or injury.

Purpose

The shoulder consists of three bones: the shoulder blade, the upper arm bone (humerus), and the collarbone (clavicle). The part of the shoulder blade that makes up the roof of the shoulder is called the acromion and the joint where the acromion and the collarbone join is called the acromioclavicular (AC) joint.

Some joints in the body are more likely to develop problems due to normal wear and tear, or deterioration resulting from osteoarthritis, a progressive and degenerative joint disease. The AC joint is a common target for developing osteoarthritis in middle age. This condition can lead to pain and difficulty using the shoulder for everyday activities. Besides osteoarthritis, AC joint disease (arthrosis) may develop from an old injury to the joint such as an acromioclavicular dislocation, which is the disruption of the normal articulation between the acromion and the collarbone. This type of injury is quite common in competitive sports, but can also result from a simple fall on the shoulder.

The goal of shoulder resection arthroplasty is to restore function to an impaired shoulder, with its required motion range, stability, strength, and smoothness.

Demographics

According to the National Ambulatory Medical Care Survey, osteoarthritis is one of the most common confirmed diagnoses in individuals over the age of 65, with the condition starting to develop in middle age.

As for AC joint injuries, they are seen especially in such professional athletes as football or hockey players, and occur most frequently in the second decade of life. Males are more commonly affected than females, with a male-to-female ratio of approximately five to one.

Description

A resection arthroplasty involves the surgical removal of the last 0.5 in (1.3 cm) of the collarbone. This removal leaves a space between the acromion and the cut end of the collarbone where the AC joint used to be. The joint is replaced by scar tissue, which allows movement to occur, but prevents the rubbing of the bone ends. The end result of the surgery is that the flexible connection between the acromion and the collarbone is restored. The procedure is usually performed by making a small 2 in (5 cm) incision in the skin over the AC joint. In some cases, the surgery can be done arthroscopically. In this approach, the surgeon uses an endoscope to look through a small hole into the shoulder joint. The endoscope is an instrument of the size of a pen, consisting of a tube fitted with a light and a miniature video camera, which transmits an image of the joint interior to a television monitor. The surgeon proceeds to remove the segment of collarbone through a small incision with little disruption of the other shoulder structures.

Diagnosis/Preparation

The diagnosis is made by physical exam. Tenderness over the AC joint is usually present, with pain upon compression of the joint. X rays of the AC joint may show narrowing of the joint and bone spurs around the joint. A **magnetic resonance imaging** (MRI) scan may also be performed. An MRI scan is a special imaging test that uses magnetic waves to create pictures that show the tissues of the shoulder in slices and has the advantage of showing tendons as well as bones. In some cases, an ultrasound test may be also be performed to inspect the soft tissues of the joint.

Prior to arthroplasty surgery, all the standard preoperative blood and urine tests are performed. The patient also meets with the anesthesiologist to discuss any special conditions that may affect the administration of anesthesia.

Aftercare

The rehabilitation following surgery for a simple resection arthroplasty is usually fairly rapid. Patients

should expect the soreness to last for three to six weeks. Postoperatively, patients usually have the affected arm in a sling for two weeks. Thereafter, a progressive passive range of shoulder motion **exercise** is started, usually with range-of-motion exercises that gradually evolve into active stretching and strengthening. The patient's arm remains in the sling between sessions. At six weeks, healing is sufficient to encourage progressive functional use. Physiotherapy usually continues until range of motion and strength are maximized. The therapist may also use massage and other types of hands-on treatments to ease muscle spasm and pain. Heavy physical use of the shoulder is prohibited for an additional six weeks.

Risks

Patients who undergo shoulder resection arthroplasty are susceptible to the same complications associated with any such surgery. These include wound infection, osteomyelitis, soft tissue ossification, and failure of fixation (remaining in place), with recurrent deformity. Symptomatic AC joint arthritis may develop in patients who undergo the surgery as a result of injury.

Specific risks associated with shoulder resection arthroplasty include:

- Fractures. Fractures of the humerus may occur after surgery, although the risk is considered low.

- Shoulder instability. Early shoulder dislocations may occur during the early postoperative period due to soft tissue imbalance or to inadequate postoperative protection; late dislocation may result from glenoid cavity wear.

- Degenerative changes. Progressive degeneration of the AC joint is a common late complication.

Normal results

Shoulder resection arthroplasty is generally very effective in reducing pain and restoring motion of the shoulder.

QUESTIONS TO ASK THE DOCTOR

- How can I regain the use of my shoulder?
- What will it take to make my shoulder healthy again?
- Why do I have problems with my shoulder?
- What surgical procedures do you follow?
- How many shoulder resection arthroplasties do you perform each year?
- Will surgery on my shoulder allow me to resume my activities?

Morbidity and mortality rates

In a recent four-year follow-up study on shoulder arthroplasty patients, all patients experienced relief from pain. Functional improvement was good in 77% of patients. Average shoulder abduction improved from 37–79° and forward flexion from 52–93°. No deaths resulting from shoulder resection arthroplasty have ever been reported.

Alternatives

Non-surgical treatments

Doctors commonly attempt to treat AC joint problems using conservative treatments. Patients may be prescribed such anti-inflammatory medications as **aspirin** or ibuprofen. Treatment also may include such disease-modifying drugs as methotrexate, sulfasalazine and gold injections. Researchers are also working on biologic agents that can interrupt the progress of osteoarthritis. These agents target specific chemicals in the body to prevent them from acting on the joints. Resting the sore joint and applying ice to it can also ease pain and inflammation. Injections of cortisone into the joint may also be prescribed. Cortisone is a strong steroidal medication that decreases inflammation and reduces pain. The effects of the drug are temporary, but it provides effective relief in the short term. Physicians may also prescribe sessions with a physical or occupational therapist, who may use various treatments to relieve inflammation of the AC joint, including heat and ice.

Surgical alternatives

Alternative surgical approaches include replacing the entire shoulder joint with a prosthesis (total shoulder arthroplasty) or replacing the head of the humerus (hemiarthroplasty).

KEY TERMS

Acromioclavicular dislocation—Disruption of the normal articulation between the acromion and the collarbone. The acromioclavicular joint (AC joint) is normally stabilized by several ligaments that can be torn in the process of dislocating the AC joint.

Acromioclavicular (AC) joint—Articulation and ligaments between the collarbone and the acromion of the shoulder blade.

Acromion—The triangular projection of the spine of the shoulder blade that forms the point of the shoulder and articulates with the collarbone.

Arthroplasty—The surgical repair of a joint.

Arthrosis—A disease of a joint.

Glenoid cavity—The hollow cavity in the head of the shoulder blade that receives the head of the humerus to make the glenohumeral or shoulder joint.

Osteoarthritis—Non-inflammatory degenerative joint disease occurring chiefly in older persons, characterized by deterioration of the articular cartilage.

See also Arthroplasty; Shoulder joint replacement.

Resources

BOOKS

Friedman, R. J. *Arthroplasty of the Shoulder.* New York: Thieme Medical Pub., 1994.

Lajtai, G., S. J. Snyder, G. Applegate, G. Aitzetmuller, and C. Gerber, eds. *Shoulder Arthroscopy and MRI-Techniques.* New York: Springer Verlag, 2003.

Walch, G., and P. Boileau., eds. *Shoulder Arthroplasty.* New York: Springer Verlag, 1999.

Wallace, W. A., ed. *Joint Replacement in the Shoulder and Elbow.* London: Edward Arnold Pub., 1998.

PERIODICALS

Iannotti, J. P., and T. R. Norris. "Influence of Preoperative Factors on Outcome of Shoulder Arthroplasty for Glenohumeral Osteoarthritis." *Journal of Bone and Joint Surgery* 85 (February 2003): 251–258.

Mileti, J., J. W. Sperling, and R. H. Cofield. "Shoulder Arthroplasty for the Treatment of Postinfectious Glenohumeral Arthritis." *Journal of Bone and Joint Surgery* 85 (April 2003): 619–614.

Nagels, J., M. Stokdijk, and P. M. Rozing. "Stress Shielding and Bone Resorption in Shoulder Arthroplasty." *Journal of Shoulder and Elbow Surgery* 12 (January–February 2003): 35–39.

Sanchez-Sotelo, J., J. W. Sperling, C. M. Rowland, and R. H. Cofield. "Instability after Shoulder Arthroplasty: Results of Surgical Treatment." *Journal of Bone and Joint Surgery* 85 (April 2003): 622–631.

Sofka, C. M., and R. S. Adler. "Sonographic Evaluation of Shoulder Arthroplasty." *American Journal of Roentgenology* 180 (April 2003): 1117–1120.

Woodruff, J., P. Cohen, and G. Bradley. "Arthroplasty of the Shoulder in Rheumatoid Arthritis with Rotator Cuff Dysfunction." *International Orthopaedics* 27 (2003): 7–10.

ORGANIZATIONS

American Academy of Orthopaedic Surgeons. 6300 North River Road, Rosemont, Illinois 60018-4262. (847) 823-7186. <http://www.aaos.org>.

American Shoulder and Elbow Surgeons (ASES). 6300 North River Road, Suite 727, Rosemont, IL, 60018-4226. (847) 698-1629. <http://www.ases-assn.org>.

OTHER

"Arthroplasty of the Shoulder." *Wheeless' Textbook of Orthopaedics.* <http://www.ortho-u.net/orthoo/44.htm>.

"Rehabilitation After Shoulder Arthroplasty." *University of Washington Orthopaedics and Sports Medicine.* <http://www.orthop.washington.edu/shoulder_elbow/roughness/management/rehab/01>.

Monique Laberge, PhD

Sigmoidoscopy

Definition

Sigmoidoscopy is a diagnostic and screening procedure in which a rigid or flexible tube with a camera on the end (a sigmoidoscope) is inserted into the anus to examine the rectum and lower colon (bowel) for bowel disease, cancer, precancerous conditions, or causes of bleeding or pain.

Purpose

Sigmoidoscopy is used most often in screening for colorectal cancer or to determine the cause of rectal bleeding. It is also used in diagnosis of inflammatory bowel disease, microscopic and ulcerative colitis, and Crohn's disease.

Cancer of the rectum and colon is the second most common cancer in the United States. About 155,000 cases are diagnosed annually. Between 55,000 and 60,000 Americans die each year of cancer in the colon or rectum.

After reviewing a number of studies, experts recommend that people over 50 be screened for colorectal can-

> ### WHO PERFORMS THE PROCEDURE AND WHERE IS IT PERFORMED?
>
> A colonoscopy procedure is usually performed by a gastroenterologist, a physician with specialized training in diseases of the colon. Alternatively, general surgeons or experienced family physicians perform sigmoidoscopic examinations. In the United States, the procedure is usually performed in an outpatient facility of a hospital or in a physician's professional office.
>
> Persons with rectal bleeding may need a full colonoscopy in a hospital setting. Individuals whose blood does not clot well (possibly as a result of blood-thinning medications) may require the procedure to be performed in a hospital setting.

cer using sigmoidoscopy every three to five years. Individuals with such inflammatory bowel conditions as Crohn's disease or ulcerative colitis, and thus are at increased risk for colorectal cancer, may begin their screenings at a younger age, depending on when their disease was diagnosed. Many physicians screen such persons more often than every three to five years. Screening should also be performed in people who have a family history of colon or rectal cancer, or small growths in the colon (polyps).

Some physicians do this screening with a colonoscope, which allows them to see the entire colon. However, most physicians prefer sigmoidoscopy, which is less time-consuming, less uncomfortable, and less costly.

Studies have shown that one-quarter to one-third of all precancerous or small cancerous growths can be seen with a sigmoidoscope. About one-half are found with a 1 ft (30 cm) scope, and two-thirds to three-quarters can be seen using a 2 ft (60 cm) scope.

In some cases, the sigmoidoscope can be used therapeutically in conjunction with such other equipment as electrosurgical devices to remove polyps and other lesions found during the sigmoidoscopy.

Demographics

Experts estimate that in excess of 500,000 sigmoidoscopy procedures are performed each year. This number includes most of the persons who are diagnosed with colon cancer each year, a greater number who are screened and receive negative results, persons who have been treated for colon conditions and receive a sigmoidoscopy as a follow-up procedure, and individuals who are diagnosed with other diseases of the large colon.

Description

Sigmoidoscopy may be performed using either a rigid or flexible sigmoidoscope. A sigmoidoscope is a thin tube with fiberoptics, electronics, a light source, and camera. A physician inserts the sigmoidoscope into the anus to examine the rectum (the first 1 ft [30 cm] of the colon) and its interior walls. If a 2 ft (60 cm) scope is used, the next portion of the colon can also be examined for any irregularities. The camera of the sigmoidoscope is connected to a viewing monitor, allowing the interior of the rectum and colon to be enlarged and viewed on the monitor. Images can then be recorded as still pictures or the entire procedure can be videotaped. The still pictures are useful for comparison purposes with the results of future sigmoidoscopic examinations.

If polyps, lesions, or other suspicious areas are found, the physician biopsies them for analysis. During the sigmoidoscopy, the physician may also use forceps, graspers, snares, or electrosurgical devices to remove polyps, lesions, or tumors.

The sigmoidoscopy procedure requires five to 20 minutes to perform. Preparation begins one day before the procedure. There is some discomfort when the scope is inserted and throughout the procedure, similar to that experienced when a physician performs a rectal exam using a finger to test for occult blood in the stool (another important screening test for colorectal cancer). Individuals may also feel some minor cramping pain. There is rarely severe pain, except for persons with active inflammatory bowel disease.

Private insurance plans almost always cover the cost of sigmoidoscopy examinations for screening in healthy individuals over 50, or for diagnostic purposes. **Medicare** covers the cost for diagnostic exams, and may cover the costs for screening exams. **Medicaid** benefits vary by state, but sigmoidoscopy is not a covered procedure in many states. Some community health clinics offer the procedure at reduced cost, but this can only be done if a local gastroenterologist (a physician who specializes in treating stomach and intestinal disorders) is willing to donate personal time to perform the procedure.

Diagnosis/Preparation

The purpose of preparation for sigmoidoscopy is to cleanse the lower bowel of fecal material or stool so the physician can see the lining. Preparation begins 24 hours before the procedure, when an individual must begin a clear liquid diet. Preparation kits are available in drug stores. In normal preparation, about 20 hours before the exam, a person begins taking a series of **laxatives**, which may be oral tablets or liquid. The individual must stop drinking any liquid four hours before the exam. An hour or two prior to the examination, the person uses an enema or laxative suppository to finish cleansing the lower bowel.

Individuals need to be careful about medications before having sigmoidoscopy. They should not take **aspirin**, products containing aspirin, or products containing ibuprofen for one week prior to the exam, because these medications can exacerbate bleeding during the procedure. They should not take any iron or vitamins with iron for one week prior to the exam, since iron can cause color changes in the bowel lining that interfere with the examination. They should take any routine prescription medications, but may need to stop certain medications. Prescribing physicians should be consulted regarding routine prescriptions and their possible effect(s) on sigmoidoscopy.

Individuals with renal insufficiency or congestive heart failure need to be prepared in an alternative way, and must be carefully monitored during the procedure.

Aftercare

There is no specific aftercare necessary following sigmoidoscopy. If a biopsy was taken, a small amount of blood may appear in the next stool. Persons should be encouraged to pass gas following the procedure to relieve any bloating or cramping that may occur after the procedure. In addition, an infection may develop following sigmoidoscopy. Persons should be instructed to call their physician if a fever or pain in the abdomen develops over the few days after the procedure.

Risks

There is a slight risk of bleeding from the procedure. This risk is heightened in individuals whose blood does not clot well, either due to disease or medication, and in those with active inflammatory bowel disease. Rarely, trauma to the bowel or other organs can occur, resulting in an injury (perforation) that must be repaired, or peritonitis, which must be treated with medication.

Sigmoidoscopy may be contraindicated in persons with severe active colitis or toxic megacolon (an extremely dilated colon). In general, people experiencing continuous ambulatory peritoneal dialysis are not candidates due to a high risk of developing intraperitoneal bleeding.

Normal results

The results of a normal examination reveal a smooth colon wall, with sufficient blood vessels for good blood flow.

Morbidity and mortality rates

For a cancer screening sigmoidoscopy, an abnormal result is one or more noncancerous or precancerous polyps, or clearly cancerous polyps. People with polyps have an increased risk of developing colorectal cancer in the future and may be required to undergo additional procedures such as **colonoscopy** or more frequent sigmoidoscopic examinations.

Small polyps can be completely removed. Larger polyps may require the physician to remove a portion of the growth for laboratory biopsy. Depending on the laboratory results, a person is then scheduled to have the polyp removed surgically, either as an urgent matter if it is cancerous, or as an elective procedure within a few months if it is non-cancerous.

In a diagnostic sigmoidoscopy, an abnormal result shows signs of active inflammatory bowel disease, either a thickening of the intestinal lining consistent with ulcerative colitis, or ulcerations or fissures consistent with Crohn's disease.

Mortality from a sigmoidoscopy examination is rare and is usually due to uncontrolled bleeding or perforation of the colon.

Alternatives

A screening examination for colorectal cancer is a test for fecal occult blood. A dab of fecal material from toilet tissue is smeared onto a card. The card is treated in a laboratory to reveal the presence of bleeding. This test is normally performed prior to a sigmoidoscopic examination.

A less invasive alternative to a sigmoidoscopic examination is an x ray of the colon and rectum. Barium is used to coat the inner walls of the colon. This lower GI (gastrointestinal) x ray may reveal the outlines of suspicious or abnormal structures. It has the disadvantage of not allowing direct visualization of the colon. It is less costly than a sigmoidoscopic examination.

A more invasive procedure is direct visualization of the colon during surgery. This procesdure is rarely performed in the United States.

See also Colonoscopy; Cystoscopy.

Resources

BOOKS

Bland, K. I., W. G. Cioffi, and M. G. Sarr. *Practice of General Surgery.* Philadelphia: Saunders, 2001.

Grace, P. A., A. Cuschieri, D. Rowley, N. Borley, and A. Darzi. *Clinical Surgery,* 2nd Edition. London: Blackwell Publishers, 2003.

Miller, B. E. *Atlas of Sigmoidoscopy and Cytoscopy.* Boca Raton, FL: CRC Press, 2001.

Schwartz, S. I., J. E. Fischer, F. C. Spencer, G. T. Shires, and J. M. Daly. *Principles of Surgery,* 7th Edition. New York: McGraw Hill, 1998.

Townsend, C., K. L. Mattox, R. D. Beauchamp, B. M. Evers, and D. C. Sabiston. *Sabiston's Review of Surgery,* 3rd Edition. Philadelphia: Saunders, 2001.

Wigton, R. S. *Flexible Sigmoidoscopy and Other Gastrointestinal Procedures.* St. Louis: Mosby-Year Book, 2000.

PERIODICALS

Mandel, J. S. "Sigmoidoscopy Screening Probably Works, But How Well Is Still Unknown." *Journal of the National Cancer Institute* 95, no.8 (2003): 571–573.

Nelson, D. E., J. Bolen, S. Marcus, H. E. Wells, and H. Meissner. "Cancer Screening Estimates for U.S. Metropolitan Areas." *American Journal of Preventive Medicine* 24, no.4 (2003): 301–309.

Newcomb, P. A., B. E. Storer, L. M. Morimoto, A. Templeton, and J. D. Potter. "Long-term Efficacy of Sigmoidoscopy in the Reduction of Colorectal Cancer Incidence." *Journal of the National Cancer Institute* 95, no.8 (2003): 622–625.

Walsh, J. M., and J. P. Terdiman. "Colorectal Cancer Screening: Clinical Applications." *Journal of the American Medical Association* 289, no.10 (2003): 1297–1302.

Walsh, J. M., and J. P. Terdiman. "Colorectal Cancer Screening: Scientific Review." *Journal of the American Medical Association* 289, no.10 (2003): 1288–1296.

ORGANIZATIONS

American Academy of Family Physicians. 11400 Tomahawk Creek Parkway, Leawood, KS 66211-2672. (913) 906-6000. E-mail: <fp@aafp.org>. <http://www.aafp.org>.

American College of Surgeons. 633 North St. Clair Street, Chicago, IL 60611-32311. (312) 202-5000, Fax: (312) 202-5001. E-mail: <postmaster@facs.org>. <http://www.facs.org>.

American Society for Gastrointestinal Endoscopy. 1520 Kensington Road, Suite 202, Oak Brook, IL 60523. (630) 573-0600, Fax: (630) 573-0691. E-mail: <info@asgeoffice.org>. <http://www.asge.org>.

Society of American Gastrointestinal Endoscopic Surgeons. 2716 Ocean Park Blvd., Suite 3000, Santa Monica, CA 90405. (310) 314-2404, Fax: (310) 314-2585. E-Mail: <sagesweb@sages.org>. <http://www.sages.org>.

OTHER

American Academy of Family Physicians [cited May 5, 2003] <http://www.aafp.org/afp/990115ap/313.html>.

American Cancer Society. [cited May 5, 2003] <http://www. cancer.org/docroot/SPC/content/SPC_1_Colonoscopy_and _Sigmoidoscopy_FAQ.asp>.

American Society for Gastrointestinal Endoscopy. [cited May 5, 2003] <http://www.asge.org/gui/patient/flex.asp>.

Colonoscope.org. [cited May 5, 2003] <http://www.colon scope.org/Hbw/your_colon.asp>.

National Institute of Diabetes and Digestive and Kidney Diseases. [cited May 5, 2003] <http://www.niddk.nih.gov/ health/digest/pubs/diagtest/sigmo.htm>.

National Library of Medicine. [cited May 5, 2003] <http:// www.nlm.nih.gov/medlineplus/ency/article/003885.htm>.

Society of American Gastrointestinal and Endoscopic Surgeons. [cited May 5, 2003] <http://www.sages.org/pi_ flexible_sigmoidoscopy.html>.

L. Fleming Fallon, Jr, MD, DrPH

Simple mastectomy

Definition

Simple mastectomy is the surgical removal of one or both breasts. The adjacent lymph nodes and chest muscles are left intact. If a few lymph nodes are removed, the procedure is called an extended simple mastectomy. Breast-sparing techniques may be used to preserve the patient's breast skin and nipple, which is helpful in cosmetic **breast reconstruction**.

Purpose

Removal of a patient's breast is usually recommended when cancer is present in the breast or as a prophylactic when the patient has severe fibrocystic disease and a family history of breast cancer. The choice of a simple mastectomy may be determined by evaluating the size of the breast, the size of the cancerous mass, where the cancer is located, and whether any cancer cells have spread to adjacent lymph nodes or other parts of the body. If the cancer has not been contained within the breast, it calls for a **modified radical mastectomy**, which removes the entire breast and all of the adjacent lymph nodes. Only in extreme circumstances is a radical mastectomy, which also removes part of the chest wall, indicated.

A larger tumor usually is an indication of more advanced disease and will require more extensive surgery such as a simple mastectomy. In addition, if a woman has small breasts, the tumor may occupy more area within the contours of the breast, necessitating a simple mastectomy in order to remove all of the cancer.

Very rapidlygrowing tumors usually require the removal of all breast tissue. Cancers that have spread to such adjacent tissues as the chest wall or skin make simple mastectomy a good choice. Similarly, multiple sites of cancer within a breast require that the entire breast be removed. In addition, simple mastectomy is also recommended when cancer recurs in a breast that has already undergone a **lumpectomy**, which is a less invasive procedure that just removes the tumor and some surrounding tissue without removing the entire breast.

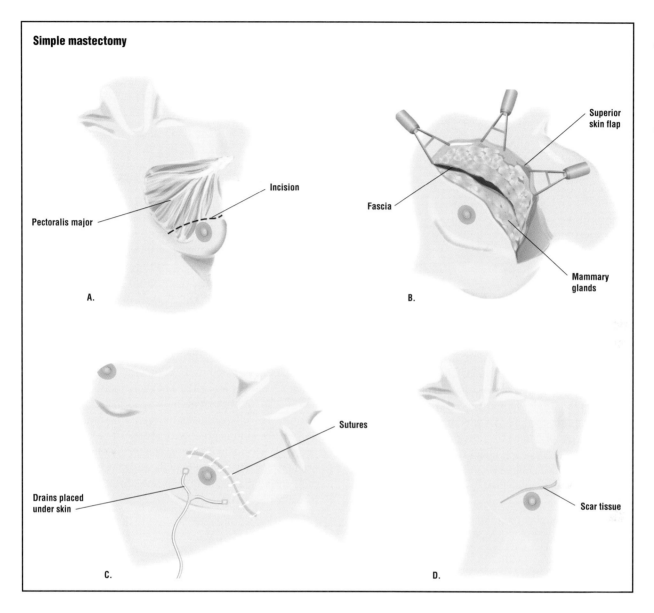

Simple mastectomy

A.
Pectoralis major
Incision

B.
Superior skin flap
Fascia
Mammary glands

C.
Drains placed under skin
Sutures

D.
Scar tissue

In a simple mastectomy, the skin over the tumor is cut open (A). The tumor and tissue surrounding it are removed (B), and the wound is closed (C). *(Illustration by GGS Inc.)*

Sometimes, surgeons recommend simple mastectomy for women who are unable to undergo the adjuvant radiation therapy required after a lumpectomy. Radiation treatment is not indicated for pregnant women, those who have had previous therapeutic radiation in the chest area, and patients with collagen vascular diseases such as scleroderma or lupus. In these cases, simple mastectomy is the treatment of choice.

Finally, some women, with family histories of breast cancer and who test positive for a cancer-causing gene, choose to have one or both of their breasts removed as a preventative for future breast cancer. This procedure is highly controversial. Though prophylactic mastectomy reduces the occurrence of breast cancer by 90% in high-risk patients, it is not a foolproof method. There has been some incidence of cancer occurring after both breasts were removed.

Demographics

According to the American Cancer Society in 2003, it was estimated that more than 260,000 new cases of breast cancer in women would occur that year. New cases of breast cancer in men were expected to reach 1,300. Rates of incidence have increased since 1980, due in part to the aging of the population. During the 1990s, breast cancer incidence increased only in women age 50 and over.

Simple mastectomy is performed by a general surgeon or a gynecological surgeon. If reconstructive breast surgery is to be done, a cosmetic surgeon performs it. Patients undergo simple mastectomies under general anesthesia as an inpatient in a hospital. There is a growing trend, due to reductions in insurance coverage and patient preference, to perform simple mastectomies without reconstructive breast surgery as outpatient procedures.

For approximately 80% of women, the first indication of cancer is the discovery of a lump in the breast, found either by themselves in a monthly self-exam or by a partner or by a mammogram, a special x ray of the breast that looks for anomalies in the breast. Early detection of breast cancer means that smaller tumors are found that require lessintensive surgery and better treatment outcomes. Simple mastectomy has been the standard treatment of choice for breast cancer for the past 60 years. Newer breast-conserving surgery techniques have been gaining in acceptance since the mid-1980s. For larger hospitals, facilities in urban areas, and health care institutions with a cancer center or high cancer patient volume, these newer techniques are being utilized at a more rapid rate, especially on the East Coast.

Interestingly, though, the National Cancer Institute found in 2003 that American women were 21% more likely to have a mastectomy than their counterparts in the United Kingdom. Though breast-conserving procedures are available and have proven to be viable options, some physicians and women still think breast removal will also remove all of their risk of cancer recurrence. It is clear that treatment options for cancer are highly individual and often emotionally charged.

Description

Simple mastectomy is one of several types of surgical treatments for breast cancer. Some techniques are rarely used; others are quite common. These common surgical procedures include:

• Radical mastectomy is rarely used, and then only in cases where cancer cells have invaded the chest wall and the tumor is very large. The breast, muscles under the breast, and all of the lymph nodes are removed.

This produces a large scar and severe disability to the arm nearest the removed breast.

• Modified radical mastectomy was the most common form of mastectomy until the 1980s. The breast is removed along with the lining over the chest muscle and all of the lymph nodes.

• Simple, sometimes called total, mastectomy has been the treatment of choice in the late 1980s and 1990s. Generally, only the breast is removed; though, sometimes, one or two lymph nodes may be removed as well.

• Partial mastectomy is used to remove the tumor, the lining over the chest muscle underneath the tumor, and a good portion of breast tissue, but not the entire breast. This is a good treatment choice for early stage cancers.

• Lumpectomy just removes the tumor and a small amount of tissue surrounding it. Some lymph nodes may be removed as well. This procedure is gaining acceptance among surgeons and patients alike.

Two other surgical procedures are variations on the simple mastectomy. The skin-sparing mastectomy is a new surgical procedure in which the surgeon makes an incision, sometimes called a keyhole incision, around the areola. The tumor and all breast tissue are removed, but the incision is smaller and scarring is minimal. About 90% of the skin is preserved and allows a cosmetic surgeon to perform breast reconstruction at the same time as the mastectomy. The subcutaneous mastectomy, or nipple-sparing mastectomy, preserves the skin and the nipple over the breast.

During a simple mastectomy, the surgeon makes a curved incision along one side of the breast and removes the tumor and all of the breast tissue. A few lymph nodes may be removed. The tumor, breast tissue, and any lymph nodes will be sent to the pathology lab for analysis. If the skin is cancer-free, it is sutured in place or used immediately for breast reconstruction. One or two drains will be put in place to remove fluid from the surgical area. Surgery takes from two to five hours; it is longer with breast reconstruction.

Breast reconstruction

Breast reconstruction, especially if it is begun at the same time as the simple mastectomy, can minimize the sense of loss that women feel when having a breast removed. Although there may be other smaller surgeries later to complete the breast reconstruction, there will not be a second major operation nor an additional scar.

If there is not enough skin left after the mastectomy, a balloon-type expander is put in place. In subsequent weeks, the expander is filled with larger amounts of saline (salt water) solution. When it has reached the appropriate size, the expander is removed and a permanent breast implant is installed.

If there is enough skin, an implant is installed immediately. In other instances, skin, fat, and muscle are removed from the patient's back or abdomen and repositioned on the chest wall to form a breast.

None of these reconstructions have nipples at first. Later, nipples are reconstructed in a separate surgery. Finally, the areola is tattooed in to make the reconstructed breast look natural.

Breast reconstruction does not prevent a potential recurrence of breast cancer.

Diagnosis/Preparation

If a mammogram has not been performed, it is usually ordered to verify the size of the lump the patient has reported. A biopsy of the suspicious lump and/or lymph nodes is usually ordered and sent to the pathology lab before surgery is discussed.

When a simple mastectomy has been determined, such preoperative tests as blood work, a **chest x ray**, and an electrocardiogram may be ordered. Blood-thinning medications such as **aspirin** should be stopped several days before the surgery date. The patient is also asked to refrain from eating or drinking the night before the operation.

At the hospital, the patient will sign a consent form, verifying that the surgeon has explained what the surgery is and what it is for. The patient will also meet with the anesthesiologist to discuss the patient's medical history and determine the choice of anesthesia.

Aftercare

If the procedure is performed as an **outpatient surgery**, the patient may go home the same day of the surgery. The length of the hospital stay for inpatient mastectomies ranges from one to two days. If breast reconstruction has taken place, the hospital stay may be longer.

The surgical drains will remain in place for five to seven days. Sponge baths will be necessary until the stitches are removed, usually in a week to 10 days. It is important to avoid overhead lifting, strenuous sports, and sexual intercourse for three to six weeks. After the surgical drains are removed, stretching exercises may be begun, though some physical therapists may start a patient on shoulder and arm mobility exercises while in the hospital.

Since breast removal is often emotionally traumatic for women, seeking out a support group is often helpful. Women in these groups offer practical advice about such matters as finding well-fitting bras and swimwear, and emotional support because they have been through the same experience.

QUESTIONS TO ASK THE DOCTOR

- Why is this procedure necessary?
- How big is my tumor?
- Are there other breast-saving or less-invasive procedures for which I might be a candidate?
- What can I expect after surgery?
- Do you work with a cosmetic surgeon?
- Will I have to undergo radiation or chemotherapy after surgery?

Finally, for women who chose not to have breast reconstruction, it will be necessary to find the proper fitting breast prosthesis. Some are made of cloth, and others are made of silicone, which are created from a mold from the patient's other breast.

In some case, the patient may be required to undergo additional treatments such as radiation, chemotheraphy, or hormone therapy.

Risks

The risks involved with simple mastectomy are the same for any major surgery. There may, however, be a need for more extensive surgery once the surgeon examines the tumor, the tissues surrounding it, and the lymph nodes nearby. A biopsy of the lymph nodes is usually performed during surgery and a determination is made whether to remove them. Simple mastectomy usually has limited impact on range of motion of the arm nearest the breast that is removed, but physical therapy may still be necessary to restore complete movement.

There is also the risk of infection around the incision. When the lymph nodes are removed, lymphedema may also occur. This condition is a result of damage to the lymph system. The arm on the side nearest the affected breast may become swollen. It can either resolve itself or worsen.

As in any surgery, the risk of developing a blood clot after a mastectomy is a serious matter. All hospitals use a variety of techniques to prevent blood clots from forming. It is important for the patient to walk daily when at home.

Finally, there is the risk that not all cancer cells were removed. Further treatment may be necessary.

Normal results

The breast area will fully heal in three to four weeks. If the patient had breast reconstruction, it may

---

take up to six weeks to recover fully. The patient should be able to participate in all of the activities she has engaged in before surgery. If breast reconstruction is done, the patient should realize that the new breast will not have the sensitivity of a normal breast. In addition, dealing with cancer emotionally may take time, especially if additional treatment is necessary.

Morbidity and mortality rates

Deaths due to breast cancer have declined by 1.4% each year between 1989 and 1995, and by 3.2% each year thereafter. The largest decreases have been among younger women, as a result of cancer education campaigns and early screening, which encourages more women to go to their physicians to be checked.

The five-year survival rate for cancers that were confined to the breast was 97% in 2003. For cancers that had spread to areas within the chest region, the rate was 78%, and it is only 23% for cancers occurring in other parts of the body after breast cancer treatment. The best survival rates were for early-stage tumors.

Two 20-year longitudinal studies concluded in 2002 indicated that the survival rate for patients with modified radical mastectomy (the removal of the entire breast and all lymph nodes) was no different from that of breast-conserving lumpectomy (the removal of the tumor alone). Implications of these studies suggest that the removal of the entire breast may not afford greater protection against future cancer than breast-conserving techniques. However, it should be noted that the majority of cancer recurrences occurred within the first five years for both those with mastectomies and those with lumpectomies.

Alternatives

Skin-sparing mastectomy, also called nipple-sparing mastectomy, is becoming a treatment of choice for women undergoing simple mastectomy. In this procedure, the skin of the breast, the areola, and the nipple are peeled back to remove the breast and its inherent tumor. Biopsies of the skin and nipple areas are performed immediately to assure that they do not have cancer cells in them. Then, a cosmetic surgeon performs a breast reconstruction at the same time as the mastectomy. The breast regains its normal contours once prostheses are inserted. Unfortunately, the nipple will lose its sensitivity and, of course, its function, since all underlying tissue has been removed. If cancer is found near the nipple, this procedure cannot be done.

See also Lumpectomy; Modified radical mastectomy.

Resources

BOOKS

A Breast Cancer Journey. Atlanta: American Cancer Society, 2001.

PERIODICALS

"American Women Still Having Too Many Mastectomies." *Women's Health Weekly* (February 6, 2003): 20.

Jancin, Bruce. "High U.S. Mastectomy Rate Is Cause for Concern." *Family Practice News* 33, no.2 (January 15, 2003): 31–32.

"Procedure Preserves Natural Appearance after Mastectomy." *AORN Journal* 77, no.1 (January 2003): 213–1.

Zepf, Bill. "Mastectomy vs. Less Invasive Surgery for Breast Cancer." *American Family Physician* 67, no.3 (February 1, 2003): 587.

ORGANIZATIONS

American Cancer Society. (800) ACS-2345. <http://www.cancer.org>.

American Society of Plastic Surgeons. 444 E. Algonquin Rd., Arlington Heights, IL 60005. (888) 475-2784. <http://www.plasticsurgery.org>.

National Cancer Institute. 6116 Executive Boulevard, MSC8322, Suite 3036A, Bethesda, MD 20892-8322. (800) 422-6237. <http://www.cancer.gov>.

Janie Franz

Sinus x ray *see* **Skull x rays**

Skeletal traction *see* **Traction**

Skin grafting

Definition

Skin grafting is a surgical procedure in which skin or a skin substitute is placed over a burn or non-healing wound.

Purpose

A skin graft is used to permanently replace damaged or missing skin or to provide a temporary wound covering. This covering is necessary because the skin protects the body from fluid loss, aids in temperature regulation, and helps prevent disease-causing bacteria or viruses from entering the body. Skin that is damaged extensively by burns or non-healing wounds can compromise the health and well-being of the patient.

Demographics

Although anyone can be involved in a fire and need a skin graft, the population groups with a higher risk of fire-related injuries and deaths include:

• children four years old and younger

• adults 65 years and older

• African Americans and Native Americans

• low-income Americans

• persons living in rural areas

• persons living in manufactured homes (trailers) or substandard housing

Description

The skin is the largest organ of the human body. It is also known as the integument or integumentary system because it covers the entire outside of the body. The skin consists of two main layers: the outer layer, or epidermis, which lies on and is nourished by the thicker dermis. These two layers are approximately 0.04–0.08 in (1–2 mm) thick. The epidermis consists of an outer layer of dead cells called keratinocytes, which provide a tough protective coating, and several layers of rapidly dividing cells just beneath the keratinocytes. The dermis contains the blood vessels, nerves, sweat glands, hair follicles, and oil glands. The dermis consists mainly of connective tissue, which is largely made up of a protein called collagen. Collagen gives the skin its flexibility and provides structural support. The fibroblasts that make collagen are the main type of cell in the dermis.

Skin varies in thickness in different parts of the body; it is thickest on the palms and soles of the feet, and thinnest on the eyelids. In general, men have thicker skin than women, and adults have thicker skin than children. After age 50, however, the skin begins to grow thinner again as it loses its elastic fibers and some of its fluid content.

Injuries treated with skin grafts

Skin grafting is sometimes done as part of elective plastic surgery procedures, but its most extensive use is in

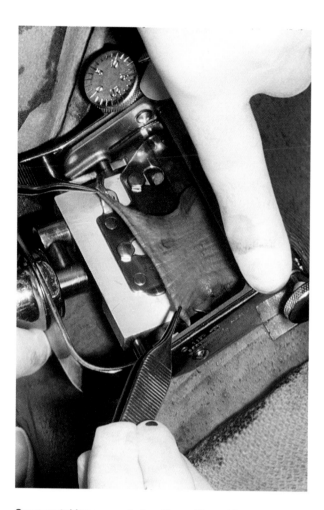

Surgeon taking a sample for skin grafting. *(Custom Medical Stock Photo. Reproduced by permission.)*

the treatment of burns. For first or second-degree burns, skin grafting is generally not required, as these burns usually heal with little or no scarring. With third-degree burns, however, the skin is destroyed to its full depth, in addition to damage done to underlying tissues. People who suffer third-degree burns often require skin grafting.

Wounds such as third-degree burns must be covered as quickly as possible to prevent infection or loss of fluid. Wounds that are left to heal on their own can contract, often resulting in serious scarring; if the wound is large enough, the scar can actually prevent movement of limbs. Non-healing wounds, such as diabetic ulcers, venous ulcers, or pressure sores, can be treated with skin grafts to prevent infection and further progression of the wounded area.

Types of skin grafts

The term "graft" by itself commonly refers to either an allograft or an autograft. An autograft is a type of graft

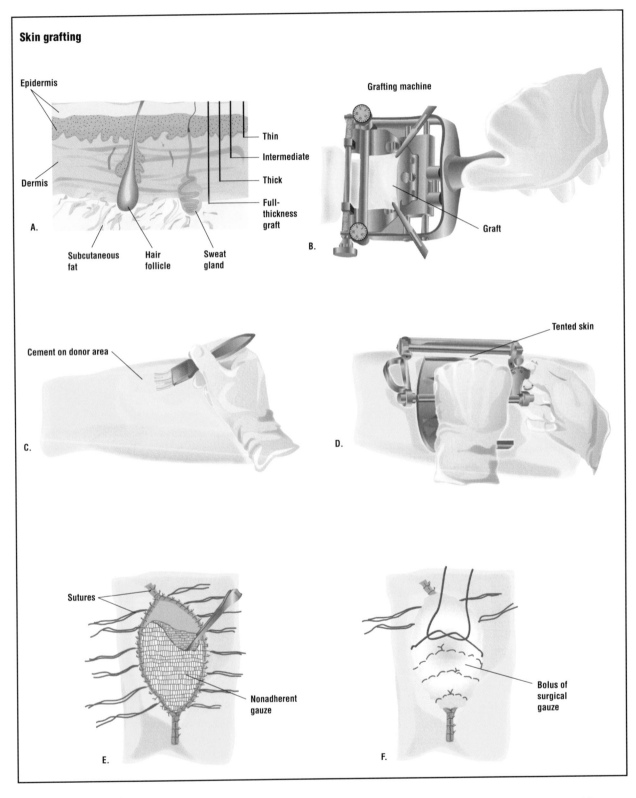

Skin grafting

Epidermis

Dermis

A.

Subcutaneous fat

Hair follicle

Sweat gland

Thin

Intermediate

Thick

Full-thickness graft

Grafting machine

B.

Graft

Cement on donor area

C.

Tented skin

D.

Sutures

Nonadherent gauze

E.

Bolus of surgical gauze

F.

Skin grafts may be used in several thicknesses (A). To begin the procedure, a special cement is used on the donor skin area (C). The grafting machine is applied to the area, and a sample taken (D). After the graft is stitched to the recipient area, it is covered with nonadherent gauze (E) and a layer of fluffy surgical gauze held in place with suture (F). *(Illustration by GGS Inc.)*

that uses skin from another area of the patient's own body if there is enough undamaged skin available, and if the patient is healthy enough to undergo the additional surgery required. An allograft uses skin obtained from another human being, Donor skin from cadavers is frozen, stored, and available for use as allografts. Skin taken from an animal (usually a pig) is called a xenograft because it comes from a nonhuman species. Allografts and xenografts provide only temporary covering because they are rejected by the patient's immune system within seven days. They must then be replaced with an autograft.

SPLIT-THICKNESS GRAFTS. The most important part of any skin graft procedure is proper preparation of the wound. Skin grafts will not survive on tissue with a limited blood supply (cartilage or tendons) or tissue that has been damaged by radiation treatment. The patient's wound must be free of any dead tissue, foreign matter, or bacterial contamination. After the patient has been anesthetized, the surgeon prepares the wound by rinsing it with saline solution or a diluted antiseptic (Betadine) and removes any dead tissue by débridement. In addition, the surgeon stops the flow of blood into the wound by applying pressure, tying off blood vessels, or administering a medication (epinephrine) that causes the blood vessels to constrict.

Following preparation of the wound, the surgeon then harvests the tissue for grafting. A split-thickness skin graft involves the epidermis and a little of the underlying dermis; the donor site usually heals within several days. The surgeon first marks the outline of the wound on the skin of the donor site, enlarging it by 3–5% to allow for tissue shrinkage. The surgeon uses a dermatome (a special instrument for cutting thin slices of tissue) to remove a split-thickness graft from the donor site. The wound must not be too deep if a split-thickness graft is going to be successful, since the blood vessels that will nourish the grafted tissue must come from the dermis of the wound itself. The graft is usually taken from an area that is ordinarily hidden by clothes, such as the buttock or inner thigh, and spread on the bare area to be covered. Gentle pressure from a well-padded dressing is then applied, or a few small sutures used to hold the graft in place. A sterile nonadherent dressing is then applied to the raw donor area for approximately three to five days to protect it from infection.

FULL-THICKNESS GRAFTS. Full-thickness skin grafts may be necessary for more severe burn injuries. These grafts involve both layers of the skin. Full-thickness autografts are more complicated than partial-thickness grafts, but provide better contour, more natural color, and less contraction at the grafted site. A flap of skin with underlying muscle and blood supply is transplanted to the area to be grafted. This procedure is used when tissue loss is

extensive, such as after open fractures of the lower leg, with significant skin loss and underlying infection. The back and the abdomen are common donor sites for full-thickness grafts. The main disadvantage of full-thickness skin grafts is that the wound at the donor site is larger and requires more careful management. Often, a split-thickness graft must be used to cover the donor site.

A composite skin graft is sometimes used, which consists of combinations of skin and fat, skin and cartilage, or dermis and fat. Composite grafts are used in patients whose injuries require three-dimensional reconstruction. For example, a wedge of ear containing skin and cartilage can be used to repair the nose.

A full-thickness graft is removed from the donor site with a scalpel rather than a dermatome. After the surgeon has cut around the edges of the pattern used to determine the size of the graft, he or she lifts the skin with a special hook and trims off any fatty tissue. The graft is then placed on the wound and secured in place with absorbable sutures.

Aftercare

Once a skin graft has been put in place, it must be maintained carefully even after it has healed. Patients who have grafts on their legs should remain in bed for seven to 10 days with their legs elevated. For several months, the patient should support the graft with an Ace bandage or Jobst stocking. Grafts on other areas of the body should be similarly supported after healing to decrease the amount of contracture.

Grafted skin does not contain sweat or oil glands, and should be lubricated daily for two to three months with mineral oil or another bland oil to prevent drying and cracking.

Aftercare of patients with severe burns typically includes psychological or psychiatric counseling as well as **wound care** and physical rehabilitation, particularly if the patient's face has been disfigured. The severe pain and lengthy period of recovery involved in burn treatment are often accompanied by anxiety and depression. If the patient's burns occurred in combat, a transportation disaster, terrorist attack, or other fire involving large numbers of people, he or she is at high risk of developing post-traumatic stress disorder (PTSD). Doctors treating the survivors of a nightclub fire in Rhode Island in February 2003 gave them anti-anxiety medications within a few days of the tragedy in order to reduce the risk of PTSD.

Risks

The risks of skin grafting include those inherent in any surgical procedure that involves anesthesia. These include reactions to the medications, breathing problems, bleeding, and infection. In addition, the risks of an allograft procedure include transmission of an infectious disease from the donor.

The tissue for grafting and the recipient site must be as sterile as possible to prevent later infection that could result in failure of the graft. Failure of a graft can result from inadequate preparation of the wound, poor blood flow to the injured area, swelling, or infection. The most common reason for graft failure is the formation of a hematoma, or collection of blood in the injured tissues.

Normal results

A skin graft should provide significant improvement in the quality of the wound site, and may prevent the serious complications associated with burns or non-healing wounds. Normally, new blood vessels begin growing from the donor area into the transplanted skin within 36 hours. Occasionally, skin grafts are unsuccessful or don't heal well. In these cases, repeat grafting is necessary. Even though the skin graft must be protected from trauma or significant stretching for two to three weeks following split-thickness skin grafting, recovery from surgery is usually rapid. A dressing may be necessary for one to two weeks, depending on the location of the graft. Any **exercise** or activity that stretches the graft or puts it at risk for trauma should be avoided for three to four weeks. A one to two-week hospital stay is most often required in cases of full-thickness grafts, as the recovery period is longer.

Morbidity and mortality rates

According to the American Burn Association, there are more than 1 million burn injuries in the United States each year that require medical attention. Approximately one-half of these require hospitalization, and roughly 25,000 of those burn patients are admitted to a specialized burn unit. About 4,500 people die from burns each year in the United States.

In the United States, someone dies in a fire nearly every two hours, on average, and another person is injured every 23 minutes. Approximately half the deaths occur in homes without smoke alarms. In addition to deaths resulting directly from burns, as many as 10,000 Americans die every year of burn-related infections, pneumonia being the most common infectious complication among hospitalized burn patients.

The average size of a burn injury in a patient admitted to a burn center is approximately 14% of the total body surface area. Smaller burns covering 10% of the total body area or less account for 54% of burn center admissions, while larger burns covering 60% or more account for 4% of admissions. About 6% of patients admitted to burn centers do not survive, mostly as a result of having suffered severe inhalation injuries in a fire.

Treatment for severe burns has improved dramatically in the past 20 years. Today, patients can survive with burns covering up to about 90% of the body, although they often face permanent physical impairment.

Alternatives

There has been great progress in the development of artificial skin replacement products in recent years. Although nothing works as well as the patient's own skin, artificial skin products are important due to the limitation of available skin for allografting in severely burned patients. Unlike allographs and xenographs, artificial skin replacements are not rejected by the patient's body and actually encourage the generation of new tissue. Artificial skin usually consists of a synthetic epidermis and a collagen-based dermis. The artificial dermis consists of fibers arranged in a lattice that act as a template for the formation of new tissue. Fibroblasts, blood vessels, nerve fibers, and lymph vessels from surrounding healthy tissue grow into the collagen lattice, which eventually dissolves as these cells and structures build a new dermis. The synthetic epidermis, which acts as a temporary barrier during this process, is eventually replaced with a split-thickness autograft or with an epidermis cultured in the laboratory from the patient's own epithelial cells.

Several artificial skin products are available for burns or non-healing wounds, including Integra®, Dermal Re-

KEY TERMS

Allograft—Tissue that is taken from one person's body and grafted to another person.

Autograft—Tissue that is taken from one part of a person's body and transplanted to a different part of the same person.

Collagen—A protein that provides structural support for the skin. Collagen is the main component of connective tissue.

Contracture—An abnormal persistent shortening of a muscle or the overlying skin at a joint, usually caused by the formation of scar tissue following an injury.

Débridement—The removal of foreign matter and dead or damaged tissue from a traumatic or infected wound until healthy tissue is reached.

Dermatome—A surgical instrument used to cut thin slices of skin for grafts.

Dermis—The underlayer of skin, containing blood vessels, nerves, hair follicles, and oil and sweat glands.

Epidermis—The outer layer of skin, consisting of a layer of dead cells that perform a protective function and a second layer of dividing cells.

Fibroblasts—A type of cell found in connective tissue; produces collagen.

Hematoma—A localized collection of blood in an organ or tissue due to broken blood vessels.

Integument—A covering; in medicine, the skin as a covering for the body. The skin is also called the integumentary system.

Keratinocytes—Dead cells at the outer surface of the epidermis that form a tough protective layer for the skin. The cells underneath divide to replenish the supply.

Xenograft—Tissue that is transplanted from one species to another (e.g., pigs to humans).

generation Template® (from Integra Life Sciences Technology), Apligraft® (Novartis), Transcyte® (Advance Tissue Science), and Dermagraft®. Researchers have also obtained promising results growing or cultivating the patient's own skin cells in the laboratory. These cultured skin substitutes reduce the need for autografts and can reduce the complications of burn injuries. Laboratory cultivation of skin cells may improve the prognosis for severely burned patients with third-degree burns over 50% of their body. The recovery of these patients has been hindered by the limited availability of uninjured skin from their own bodies for grafting. Skin substitutes may also reduce treatment costs and the length of hospital stays. In addition, other research has demonstrated the possibility of using stem cells collected from bone marrow or blood for use in growing skin grafts.

Patients with less severe burns are usually treated in a doctor's office or a hospital emergency room. Patients with any of the following conditions, however, are usually transferred to hospitals with specialized burn units: third-degree burns; partial-thickness burns over 10% of their total body area; electrical or chemical burns; smoke inhalation injuries; or preexisting medical disorders that could complicate management, prolong recovery, or affect mortality. In addition, burned children in hospitals without qualified personnel should be admitted to a hospital with a burn unit. A **surgical team** that specializes in burn treatment and skin grafts will perform the necessary procedures. The team may include neurosurgeons, ophthalmologists, oral surgeons, thoracic surgeons, psychiatrists, and trauma specialists as well as plastic surgeons and dermatologists.

Resources

BOOKS

Beauchamp, Daniel R., M.D., Mark B. Evers, M.D., Kenneth L. Mattox, M.D., et al., eds. *Sabiston Textbook of Surgery: The Biological Basis of Modern Surgical Practice*, 16th ed. London, UK: W. B. Saunders Co., 2001.

Dipietro, Luisa A., and Aime L. Burns, eds. *Wound Healing: Methods and Protocols.* Totowa, NJ: Humana Press, 2003.

Herndon, David, ed. *Total Burn Care*, 2nd ed. London, UK: W. B. Saunders Co., 2001.

Tura, A., ed. *Vascular Grafts: Experiment and Modelling*, 1st ed. Billerica, MA: WIT Press/Computational Mechanics, 2003.

PERIODICALS

Duenwald, Mary. "Tales from a Burn Unit: Agony, Friendship, Healing." *New York Times*, March 18, 2003 [June 25, 2003].

Eto, M., H. Hackstein, K. Kaneko, et al. "Promotion of Skin Graft Tolerance Across MHC Barriers by Mobilization of Dendritic Cells in Donor Hemopoietic Cell Infusions." *Journal of Immunology* 69 (September 1, 2002): 2390-2396.

Latenser, B. A. and Vern A. Kowal. "Paediatric Burn Rehabilitation." *Pediatric Rehabilitation* 5 (January-March 2002): 3-10.

Losada, F., M.D., Pedro P. Garcia-Luna, M.D., T. Gomez-Cia, M.D., et al. "Effects of Human Recombinant Growth Hormone on Donor-Site Healing in Burned Adults." *World Journal of Surgery* 26 (January 2002): 2-8.

Revis, Don R., Jr., MD, and Michael B. Seagal, MD. "Skin Grafts, Full-Thickness." *eMedicine*, May 17, 2002 [cited June 25, 2003]. <www.emedicine.com/ent/topic48.htm>.

Revis, Don R., Jr., MD, and Michael B. Seagal, MD. "Skin Grafts, Split-Thickness." *eMedicine*, July 20, 2001 [cited June 25, 2003]. <www.emedicine.com/ent/topic47.htm>.

Snyder, R. J., H. Doyle, and T. Delbridge. "Applying Split-Thickness Skin Grafts: A Step-by-Step Clinical Guide and Nursing Implications." *Ostomy Wound Management* 47 (November 2002): 990-996.

ORGANIZATIONS

American Burn Association. 625 N. Michigan Ave., Suite 1530, Chicago, IL 60611. (800) 548-2876. Fax: (312) 642.9130. E-mail: info@ameriburn.org. <www.ameriburn.org>.

American Diabetes Association. 1701 North Beauregard Street, Alexandria, VA 22311. (800) 342-2383. E-Mail: AskADA @diabetes.org. <www.diabetes.org>.

American Society of Plastic Surgeons (ASPS). 444 East Algonquin Road, Arlington Heights, IL 60005. (847) 228-9900. <www.plasticsurgery.org>.

National Institutes of Health, 9000 Rockville Pike, Bethesda, MD 20892. (301) 496-4000. Email: NIHInfo@OD.NIH. GOV. <www.nih.gov>.

Lisa Christenson, PhD
Crystal H. Kaczkowski, M.Sc.

Skin smoothing *see* **Dermabrasion**

Skull x rays

Definition

Skull x rays are performed to examine the nose, sinuses, and facial bones. These studies may also be referred to as sinus x rays. x ray studies produce films, also known as radiographs, by aiming x rays at soft bones and tissues of the body. x ray beams are similar to light waves, except their shorter wavelength allows them to penetrate dense substances, producing images and shadows on film.

Purpose

Doctors may order skull x rays to aid in the diagnosis of a variety of diseases or injuries.

Sinusitis

Sinus x rays may be ordered to confirm a diagnosis of sinusitis, or sinus infection.

Fractures

A skull x ray may detect bone fractures resulting from injury or disease. The skull x ray should clearly show the entire skull, jaw bones, and facial bones.

Tumors

Skull radiographs may indicate tumors in facial bones, tissues, or sinuses. Tumors may be benign (not cancerous) or malignant (cancerous).

Other

Birth defects (referred to as congenital anomalies) may be detected on a skull x ray by changes in bone structure. Abnormal tissues or glands resulting from various conditions or diseases may also be shown on a skull radiograph.

Description

Skull or sinus x rays may be performed in a doctor's office that has x ray equipment and a technologist available. The exam may also be performed in an outpatient radiology facility or a hospital radiology department.

In many instances, particularly for sinus views, the patient will sit upright in a chair, perhaps with the head held stable by a foam vise. A film cassette is located behind the patient. The x ray tube is in front of the patient and may be moved to allow for different positions and views. A patient may also be asked to move his or her head at various angles and positions.

In some cases, technologists will ask the patient to lie on a table and will place the head and neck at various angles. In routine skull x rays, as many as five different views may be taken to allow a clear picture of various bones and tissues. The length of the test will vary depending on the number of views taken, but in general, it should last about 10 minutes. The technologist will usually ask a patient to wait while the films are being developed to ensure that they are adequate before going to the radiologist.

Preparation

There is no preparation for the patient prior to arriving at the radiology facility. Patients will be asked to remove jewelry, dentures, or other metal objects that may produce artifacts on the film. The referring doctor or x ray technologist can answer any questions regarding the procedure. Any woman who is or may be pregnant should tell the technologist.

Aftercare

There is no aftercare required following skull or sinus x ray procedures.

Risks

There are no common side effects from skull or sinus x ray. The patient may feel some discomfort in the positioning of the head and neck, but will have no complications. Any x ray procedure carries minimal radiation risk; children and pregnant women should be protected from radiation exposure to the abdominal or genital areas.

Normal results

Normal results should indicate sinuses, bones, tissues, and other observed areas are of normal size, shape, and thickness for the patient's age and medical history. Results, whether normal or abnormal, will be provided to the referring doctor in a written report.

Abnormal results

Abnormal results may include:

Sinusitis

Air in sinuses will show up on a radiograph as black, but fluid will be cloudy or white (opaque). This helps the radiologist to identify fluid in the sinuses. In chronic sinusitis, the radiologist may also note thickening or destruction of the bony wall of an infected sinus.

Fractures

Radiologists may recognize even tiny facial bone fractures as a line of defect.

Tumors

Tumors may be visible if the bony sinus wall is distorted or destroyed. Abnormal findings may result in follow-up imaging studies.

Other

Skull x rays may also detect disorders that show up as changes in bone structure, such as Paget's disease of the bone or acromegaly (a disorder associated with ex- cess growth hormones from the pituitary gland). Areas of calcification, or gathering of calcium deposits, or destruction may indicate a condition such as an infection of bone or bone marrow (osteomyelitis).

Resources

ORGANIZATIONS

National Cancer Institute. Building 31, Room 10A31, 31 Center Drive, MSC 2580, Bethesda, MD 20892-2580. (800) 422-6237. <http://www.nci.nih.gov>.
National Head Injury Foundation, Inc. (888) 222-5287. <http://www.nhif.org/home.html>.
Radiological Society of North America. 820 Jorie Boulevard, Oak Brook, IL 60523-2251. (630) 571-2670. <http://www.rsna.org>.

Teresa Norris, RN
Lee A. Shratter, MD

Sling procedure

Definition

The sling procedure, or suburethral sling procedure, refers to a particular kind of surgery using ancillary material to aid in closure of the urethral sphincter function of the bladder. It is performed as a treatment of severe urinary incontinence. The sling procedure, also known as the suburethral fascial sling or the pubovaginal sling, has many forms due to advances in the types of material used for the sling. Some popular types of sling material are Teflon (polytetrafluoroethylene), Gore-Tex®, and rectus fascia (fibrous tissue of the rectum). The surgery can be done through the vagina or the abdomen and some clinicians perform the procedure using a laparoscope—a small instrument that allows surgery through very small incisions in the belly button and above the pubic hairline. The long-term efficacy and durability of the laparoscopic suburethral sling procedure for management of stress incontinence are undetermined. A new technique, the Tension-Free Vaginal Tape Sling Procedure (TVT), has gained popularity in recent years and early research indicates high success rates and few postoperative complications. This procedure is done under local anesthetic and offers new opportunities for treatment of stress incontinence. However, TVT has not been researched for its long-term effects. Finally, there are many surgeons who use the sling procedure for all forms of incontinence.

Purpose

Incontinence is very common and not fully understood. Generally defined as the involuntary loss of urine, incontinence comes in many forms and has many etiologies. Four established types of incontinence, according to the Agency for Health Care Policy and Research, affect approximately 13 million adults—most of them older women. Actual prevalence may be higher because incontinence is widely underreported and underdiagnosed. The four types of incontinence are: stress incontinence, urge incontinence (detrusor overactivity or instability), mixed incontinence, and overflow incontinence. There are also other types of incontinence tied to specific conditions, such as neurogenic bladder in which neurological signals to the bladder are impaired.

Stress incontinence is the most frequently diagnosed form of incontinence and occurs largely with physical activity, laughter and coughing, and sneezing. The inability to hold urine can be due to weakness in the internal and external urinary sphincter or due to a weakened urethra. These two conditions, intrinsic sphincter deficiency (ISD) and urethral hypermobility or genuine stress incontinence (GSI), pertain to the inability of the "gatekeeper" sphincter muscles to stay taut and/or the urethra failing to hold urine under pressure from the abdomen. In women, as the pelvic structures relax due to age, injury, or illness, the uterus prolapses and the urethra becomes hypermobile. This allows the urethra to descend at an angle that permits loss of urine and puts pressure upon the sphincter muscles, both internal and external, allowing the mouth of the bladder to stay open.

Urge incontinence, the other frequent type of incontinence, pertains to overactivity of the sphincter in which the muscle contracts frequently, causing the need to urinate. Stress incontinence is often allied with sphincter overactivity and is often accompanied by urge incontinence.

Severe stress incontinence occurs most frequently in women younger than 60 years old. It is thought to be due to the relaxation of the supporting structures of the pelvis that results from childbirth, obesity, or lack of **exercise**. Some researchers believe that aging, perhaps due to estrogen deficiency, is a major cause of severe urinary incontinence in women, but no link has been found between incontinence and estrogen deficiency. Surgery for stress or mixed incontinence is primarily offered to patients who have failed, are not satisfied with, or are unable to comply with more conservative approaches. It is often performed during such other surgeries as urethra prolapse, cystocele surgery, urethral reconstruction, and **hysterectomy**.

The sling procedure gets its name from the tissue attached under the mid- or proximal urethra and sutured at its ends onto a solid structure like the rectus sheath, pubic bone, or pelvic side walls. The procedure is used in the severest cases of stress incontinence, particularly those that have a concomitant sphincter inadequacy (ISD). The sling supports the urethra as it receives pressure from the abdomen and helps the internal sphincter muscles to keep the urethral opening closed. The procedure is the most popular because it has the highest success rate of all surgical remedies for severe stress incontinence related to sphincter inadequacies in both men and women.

Demographics

Urinary incontinence (UI) plagues 10–35% of adults and at least half of the million nursing home residents in the United States. Other studies indicate that between 10% and 30% of women experience incontinence during their lifetimes, compared to about 5% of men. One reason that more women than men have incontinent episodes is the relatively shorter urethras of women. Women have urethras of about 2 in (5 cm) and men have urethras of 10 in (25.4 cm). Studies have documented that about 50% of all women have occasional urinary incontinence, and as many as 10% have regular incontinence. Nearly 20% of women over age 75 experience daily urinary incontinence. Incontinence is a major factor in individuals entering long term care facilities. Women at highest risk are those who have given birth to more than three children and women who were given oxytocin to induce labor. Oxytocin puts more pressure on the pelvic muscles than does ordinary labor. Women who smoke have twice the rate of incontinence, according to one study of 600 women. Those women who do high-impact exercises are at much higher risk for incontinence. According to the medical literature, those at highest risk for urinary leakage are gymnasts, followed by softball, volleyball, and basketball players. Finally, women who have diabetes or are obese have higher rates of incontinence. Women who require sling procedures have often had other surgeries for incontinence, necessitating sling procedure to treat intrinsic sphincter deficiency caused by operative trauma. A rarer cause of stress incontinence in older women is urethral instability. In men, stress incontinence is usually caused by sphincter damage after surgery on the prostate.

Description

Anti-incontinence surgery is used to address the failure of two parts of female urinary continence: loss of support to the bladder neck or central urethra and intrinsic sphincter deficiency (ISD). The surgery does not restore function to the urethra or to the ability for closure to the sphincter. It replaces the mechanism for continence with supporting and compressive aids. Stabilizing the supporting elements of the urethra (ligaments, fascia, and muscles) was thought for many years to be the most important factor in curing incontinence. Called anatomic or genuine stress urinary incontinence (SUI), retropublic procedures, like the Burch procedure, sought only to restore the urethra to a fixed position. However, it became clear with the high failure rate of these procedures that ISD was present and unless surgery could confer some added compressive ability to the closure of the bladder, SUI would persist.

The urethral sling procedure is effective in the treatment of the severest types of incontinence (Types II and III) by re-establishing the "hammock effect" of the proximal or central point of the urethra during abdominal straining. The surgery involves the placement of a piece of material under the urethra at its arterial or vesical juncture and anchoring it on either side of the pubic bone or to the abdominal wall or vaginal wall. This technique involves the creation of a sling from a strip of tissue from the patient's own abdominal fascia (fibrous tissue) or from a cadaver. Synthetic slings also are used, but some are prone to break down over time.

The urethral sling procedure is most often performed as open surgery, which involves entering the pelvic area from the abdomen or from the vagina while the patient is under general or regional anesthesia. Broad-spectrum **antibiotics** are offered intravenously. If the patient is fitted with a urethral catheter, ampicillin and gentamicin are administered instead. The patient is placed in stirrups. Surgery takes place as a 6-to-9-cm by 1.5-cm sling is harvested from rectal tissue and sutured under the urethra at each end within the retropubic space (the area that undergirds the urethra). Synthetic tissue or fascia from a donor may also be used.

The goal of the surgery is to create a compression aid to the urethra. This involves an individualized approach to the tension needed on the sling. While the sling procedure is relatively easy to complete, the issue of tension on the sling is hard to determine and involves the use of tests during surgery for determining the compression effect of the sling on the urethra. Some manual tests are performed or a more sophisticated urodynamic test, like cystourethrography, may determine tension. It is important for the surgeon to test tension during

QUESTIONS TO ASK THE DOCTOR

- Do I have a urethral closure problem as a part of my incontinence?
- How many sling procedures have you performed?
- How soon will I be able to tell if I am going to have urine retention difficulties?
- If this surgery does not work, are there other procedures that will allow me a better quality of life?
- Is patient satisfaction a formal part of your evaluation of the success of the procedure you use?
- What type of material do you use for the sling and why do you choose this material?

surgery because of the high rate of retention of urine (inability to void) after surgery associated with this procedure and the miscalculation of the required tension.

Diagnosis/Preparation

Candidates for surgical treatment of incontinence must undergo a full clinical, neurological, and radiographic evaluation before there can be direct analysis of the condition to be treated and the desired outcome. Both urethral and bladder functions are evaluated and there is an attempt to determine the conditions associated with stress incontinence. In many women, incontinence may be due to vaginal prolapse. Stress incontinence can be identified by observation of urine during pelvic examination or by a sitting or standing **stress test** where patients are asked to cough or strain and evidence of leakage is obtained. Gynecologists often use a Q-tip test to determine the angle and change in the position of the urethra during straining. Other tests include subtracted cystometry to measure how much the bladder can hold, how much pressure builds up inside the bladder as it stores urine, and how full it is when the patients feels the urge to urinate.

The frequency of stress incontinence as measured by typical symptoms ranges between 33% and 65%. The frequency of stress incontinence is around 12% when measured or defined by cystometric findings. The ability to distinguish SUI as the cause of incontinence, as opposed to ISD, becomes more complicated; but it is a very important factor in the decision to have surgery. A combination of pelvic examination for urethral hypermoblity and leak point pressure as measured by coughing or other abdominal straining has been shown to be very effective in distinguishing ISD, and identifying the patient who needs surgery.

Aftercare

IV ketorolac and oral and intravenous pain medication are administered, as are postoperative antibiotics. A general diet is available usually on the evening of surgery. When the patient is able to walk, usually the same day, the urethral catheter is removed. The patient must perform self-catheterization to check urine volume every four hours to protect the urethral wall. If the patient is unwilling to perform catheterization, a tube can be placed suprapubically (in the back of the pubis) for voiding. Catheterization lasts about eight days, with about 98% of patients able to void at three months. Patients are discharged on the second day postoperatively, unless they have had other procedures and need additional recovery time. Patients may not lift heavy objects or engage in strenuous activity for approximately six weeks. Sexual intercourse may be resumed in the fourth week following surgery. Follow-up visits are scheduled for three to four weeks after surgery

Risks

Although the sling treatment has a very high success rate, it is also associated with a prolonged period of voiding difficulties, intraoperative bladder or urethra injury, infections associated with screw or staple points, and rejection of sling material from a donor or erosion of synthetic sling material. Patients should not be encouraged to undergo a sling procedure unless the risk of long-term voiding difficulty and the need for intermittent self-catheterization are understood. Fascial slings seem to be associated with the fewest complications for sling procedure treatment. Synthetic slings have a greater risk of having to be removed due to erosion and inflammation.

Normal results

Regardless of the procedure used, a proportion of patients will remain incontinent. Results vary according to the type of sling procedure used, the type of attachment used for the sling, and the type of material used for the sling. Normal results for the sling procedure overall are recurrent stress incontinence of 3–12% after bladder sling procedures. In general, reported cure rates are lower for second and subsequent surgical procedures. A recent qualitative study published in the *American Journal of Obstetrics and Gynecology* of 57 patients who underwent patient-contributed fascial sling procedures indicates good success with fascial sling procedures. At a median of 42 months after the procedure, the postoperative objective cure rate for stress urinary incontinence was 97%, with 88% of patients indicating that the sling had improved the quality of their lives. Eighty-four percent of patients indicated that the sling relieved their incontinence long term, and 82% of patients stated that they would undergo the surgery again. The study also found that voiding function was a common side effect in 41% of the patients.

Morbidity and mortality rates

The most common complications of sling procedures are voiding problems (10.4%), new detrusor instability (7–27%), and lower urinary tract damage (3%). Some of the complications depend upon tension issues as well as on the materials used for the sling. There are recent and well-designed studies of patient fascia and donor fascia used for slings in five centers with follow-up from 30 to 51 months that report no erosions or vaginal wall complications in any patients. Prolonged retention or voiding issues occurred in 2.3% of patients and de novo or spontaneous urge incontinence developed in 6%. These figures relate only to a large study utilizing patient or donor fascia and one that did not control for other factors like techniques of anchoring. In general, studies of the sling procedure are small and have many variables. There are no long term studies (over five years) of this most popular procedure.

Alternatives

Alternatives to anti-incontinent sling procedure surgery depend upon the severity of the incontinence and the type. Severe stress incontinence with intrinsic sphincter deficiency can benefit from bulking agents for the urethra to increase compression, as well as external devices like a pessary that is placed in the vagina and holds up the bladder to prevent leakage. Urethral inserts can be placed in the urethra until it is time to use the bathroom. The patient learns to put the insertion in and take it out as needed. There are also urine seals that are small foam pads inserted in garments. Milder forms of incontinence can benefit from an assessment of medication usage, pelvic muscle exercises, bladder retraining, weight loss, and certain devices that stimulate the muscles around the urethra to strengthen them. For mild urethral mobility, procedures for tacking or stabilizing the urethra at the neck called Needle Neck Suspension, as well as procedures to hold the urethra in place with sutures, like the Burch method, are alternative forms of surgery.

KEY TERMS

Intrinsic sphincter deficiency (ISD)—One of the major factors in stress incontinence. Loss of support of the urethra causes the internal sphincter muscles to be unable to keep the bladder neck closed due to lack of contractive ability.

Pubovaginal sling—A general term for a procedure that places a sling around the urethra without the use of tension between the sling and the urethra. The is often referred to as the Tension-Free Vaginal Tape (TVT) procedure.

Stress incontinence—Incontinence that occurs when abdominal pressure is placed upon the urethra from such movements as coughing, sneezing, laughter, and exercise.

Urethral fascial sling—A support and compression aid to urethral function using auxillary material made of patient or donor tissue to undergird the urethra.

Resources

BOOKS

"Urologic Surgery." In *Campbell's Urology,* edited by M. F. Campbell, et al., 8th ed. Philadelphia: W. B. Saunders, 2002.

PERIODICALS

Lobel, B., A. Manunta, and A. Rodriguez. "The Management of Female Stress Urinary Incontinence Using the Sling Procedure." *British International Journal of Urology* 88, no. 8 (November 2001): 832.

Melton, Lisa. *"Targeted Treatment for Incontinence Beckons."* Lancet 359, no. 9303, (January 2002): 326.

Richter, H. R. "Effects of Pubovaginal Sling Procedure on Patients with Urethral Hypermobility and Intrinsic Sphincteric Deficiency: Would They Do it Again?" *American Journal of Obstetrics and Gynecology* 184, no. 2 (January 2001): 14–19.

ORGANIZATIONS

American Foundation for Urologic Disease/The Bladder Health Council. 1128 North Charles St., Baltimore, MD 21201. (410) 468-1800. Fax: (410) 468-1808. admin@afud.org. <http://www.afud.org>.

The Simon Foundation for Continence. P.O. Box 835, Wilmette, IL 60091. (800) 23-simon or (847) 864-3913. <http://www.simonfoundation.org/html/>.

OTHER

National Kidney and Urological Diseases Information Clearinghouse. *Bladder Control in Women.* Intellihealth. April 17, 2003 [cited June 25, 2003]. <http://www.intelihealth.

com/IH/ihtIH/WSIHW000/9103/24149/35872.html?d=dmtContent>.

"Urinary Incontinence." MD Consult Patient Handout. [cited June 25, 2003]. <www.MDConsult.com>.

Nancy McKenzie, Ph.D.

Small bowel follow-through (SBFT): Small intestine radiography and fluoroscopy *see* **Upper GI exam**

Small bowel resection

Definition

A small **bowel resection** is the surgical removal of one or more segments of the small intestine.

Purpose

The small intestine is the part of the digestive system that absorbs much of the liquid and nutrients from food. It consists of three segments: the duodenum, jejunum, and ileum; and is followed by the large intestine (colon). A small bowel resection may be performed to treat the following conditions:

• Crohn's disease. This condition is characterized by a chronic inflammatory condition that affects the digestive tract. If other treatment does not effectively control symptoms, the physician may recommend surgery to close fistulas or remove part of the intestine where the inflammation is worst.

• Cancer. Cancer of the small intestine is a rare cancer in which malignant cells are found in the tissues of the small intestine. Adenocarcinoma, lymphoma, sarcoma, and carcinoid tumors account for the majority of small intestine cancers. Surgery to remove the cancer is the most common treatment. When the tumor is large, removal of the small intestine segment containing the cancer is usually indicated.

• Ulcers. Ulcers are crater-like lesions on the mucous membrane of the small bowel caused by an inflammatory, infectious, or malignant condition that often requires surgery and in some cases, bowel resection.

• Intestinal obstruction. This condition involves a partial or complete blockage of the bowel that results in the failure of the intestinal contents to pass through. Intestinal obstruction is usually treated by decompressing the intestine with suction, using a nasogastric

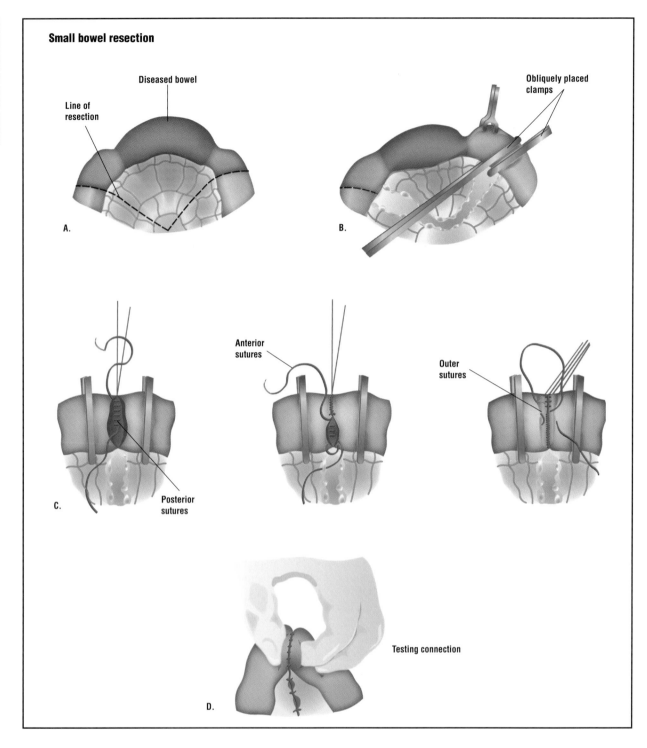

Small bowel resection

Diseased bowel

Line of
resection

Obliquely placed
clamps

A.

B.

Anterior
sutures

Outer
sutures

Posterior
sutures

C.

Testing connection

D.

To remove a diseased portion of the small intestine, an incision is made into the abdomen, and the area to be treated is pulled out (A). Clamps are placed around the area to be removed and the section is cut (B). Three layers of sutures repair the remaining bowel (C). *(Illustration by GGS Inc.)*

tube inserted into the stomach or intestine. In cases where decompression does not relieve the symptoms, or if tissue death is suspected, bowel resection may be considered.

- Injuries. Accidents may result in bowel injuries that require resection.
- Precancerous polyps. A polyp is a growth that projects from the lining of the intestine. Polyps are usually be-

nign and produce no symptoms, but they may cause rectal bleeding and develop into malignancies over time. When polyps have a high chance of becoming cancerous, bowel resection is usually indicated.

Demographics

According to the National Cancer Institute, adenocarcinoma, lymphoma, sarcoma, and carcinoid tumors account for the majority of small intestine cancers which, as a whole, account for only 1–2% of all gastrointestinal cancers diagnosed in the United States.

Crohn's disease occurs worldwide with a prevalence of 10–100 cases per 100,000 people. The disorder occurs most frequently among people of European origin; is three to eight times more common among Jews than among non-Jews; and is more common among whites than nonwhites. Although the disorder can start at any age, it is most often diagnosed between 15 and 30 years of age. Some 20–30% of patients with Crohn's disease have a family history of inflammatory bowel disease.

The occurrence of polyps increases with age; the risk of cancer developing in an unremoved polyp is 2.5% at five years, 8% at 10 years, and 24% at 20 years after the diagnosis. The risk of developing bowel cancer after removal of polyps is 2.3%, compared to 8.0% for patients who do not have them removed.

Description

The resection procedure can be performed using an open surgical approach or laparoscopically. There are three types of surgical small bowel resection procedures:

• Duodenectomy. Excision of all or part of the duodenum.

• Ileectomy. Excision of all or part of the ileum.

• Jejunectomy. Excision of all or a part of the jejunum.

Open resection

Following adequate bowel preparation, the patient is placed under general anesthesia and positioned for the operation. The surgeon starts the procedure by making a midline incision in the abdomen. The diseased part of the small intestine (ileum or duodenum or jejunum) is removed. The two healthy ends are either stapled or sewn back together, and the incision is closed. If it is necessary to spare the intestine from its normal digestive work while it heals, a temporary opening (stoma) of the intestine into the abdomen (**ileostomy**, duodenostomy, or jejunostomy) is made. The ostomy is later closed and repaired.

Laparoscopic bowel resection

Laparoscopic small bowel resection features insertion of a thin telescope-like instrument called a laparo-

---

WHO PERFORMS THE PROCEDURE AND WHERE IS IT PERFORMED?

Bowel resection surgery is performed by a colorectal surgeon, who is a physician fully trained in **general surgery** as evidenced by certification by the American Board of Surgery (ABS). Colorectal surgeons also are certified by the American Society of Colon and Rectal Surgeons (ASCRS), the leading professional society representing more than 1,000 board-certified colon and rectal surgeons and other surgeons dedicated to advancing and promoting the science and practice of the treatment of patients with diseases and disorders affecting the colon, rectum, and anus.

Bowel resection surgery is performed in a hospital setting.

---

scope through a small incision made at the umbilicus (belly button). The laparoscope is connected to a small video camera unit that shows the operative site on video monitors located in the **operating room**. The abdomen is inflated with carbon dioxide gas to allow the surgeon a clear view of the operative area. Four to five additional small incisions are made in the abdomen for insertion of specialized **surgical instruments** that the surgeon uses to perform the surgery. The small bowel is clamped above and below the diseased section and this section is removed. The small bowel ends are reattached using staples or sutures. Following the procedure, the small incisions are closed with sutures or surgical tape.

Diagnosis/Preparation

As with any surgery, the patient is required to sign a consent form. Details of the procedure are discussed with the patient, including goals, technique, and risks. Blood and urine tests, along with various imaging tests and an electrocardiogram (EKG), may be ordered as required. To prepare for the procedure, the patient is asked to completely clean the bowel and is placed on a low residue diet for several days prior to surgery. A liquid diet may be ordered for at least the day before surgery, with nothing taken by mouth after midnight. Preoperative bowel preparation involving mechanical cleansing and administration of **antibiotics** before surgery is the standard practice. This involves the prescription of oral antibiotics (neomycin, erythromycin, or kanamycin sulfate) to decrease bacteria in the intestine and help pre-

QUESTIONS TO ASK THE DOCTOR

- What do I need to do before surgery?
- What happens on the day of surgery?
- What type of anesthesia will be used?
- What happens during surgery, and how is the surgery performed?
- What happens after the surgery?
- What are the risks associated with a small bowel resection?
- How long will I be in the hospital?
- When can I expect to return to work and/or normal activities?
- Will there be a scar?

vent postoperative infection. A nasogastric tube is inserted through the nose into the stomach on the day of surgery or during surgery. This removes the gastric secretions and prevents nausea and vomiting. A urinary catheter (thin tube inserted into the bladder) may also be inserted to keep the bladder empty during surgery, giving more space in the surgical field and decreasing chances of accidental injury.

Aftercare

Once the surgery is completed, the patient is taken to a postoperative or recovery unit where a nurse monitors recovery and ensures that bandages are kept clean and dry. Mild pain at the incision site is commonly experienced and the treating physician usually prescribes pain medication. Postoperative care also involves monitoring of blood pressure, pulse, respiration, and temperature. Breathing tends to be shallow because of the effect of anesthesia and the patient's reluctance to breathe deeply and experience pain that is caused by the abdominal incision. The patient is given instruction on the way to support the operative site during deep breathing and coughing. Fluid intake and output is measured, and the operative site is observed for color and amount of wound drainage. The nasogastric tube remains in place, attached to low intermittent suction until bowel activity resumes. Fluids and electrolytes are infused intravenously until the patient's diet can gradually be resumed, beginning with liquids and progressing to a regular diet as tolerated. The patient is generally out of bed approximately eight to 24 hours after surgery. Patients are usually scheduled for a follow-up examination within two weeks after surgery. During the first few days after surgery, physical activity is restricted.

Risks

Risks include all the risks associated with general anesthesia, namely, adverse reactions to medications and breathing problems. They also include the risks associated with any surgery, such as bleeding or infection. Additional risks associated specifically with bowel resection include:

- bulging through the incision (incisional hernia)
- narrowing (stricture) of the opening (stoma)
- blockage (obstruction) of the intestine from scar tissue.

Normal results

Complete healing is expected without complications after bowel resection, but the period of time required for recovery from the surgery varies depending on the condition requiring the procedure, the patient's overall health status prior to surgery, and the length of bowel removed.

Morbidity and mortality rates

According to the National Cancer Institute, the predominant treatment for small intestine cancers is surgery when bowel resection is possible, and cure depends on the ability to completely remove the cancer. The overall five-year survival rate for resectable adenocarcinoma is 20%. The five-year survival rate for resectable leiomyosarcoma, the most common primary sarcoma of the small intestine, is approximately 50%.

Crohn's disease is a chronic incurable disease characterized by periods of progression and remission with 99% of patients suffering at least one relapse. Physicians are presently unable to predict the extent and severity of the disease over time; thus, while morbidity is very high for Crohn's disease, mortality is essentially zero.

Alternatives

Alternatives to bowel resection depend on the specific medical condition being treated. For most conditions where bowel resection is advised, the only alternative is treatment with drugs.

Resources

BOOKS

Michelassi, F. and J. W. Milsom, eds. *Operative Strategies in Inflammatory Bowel Disease.* New York: Springer Verlag, 1999.

Peppercorn, Mark, ed. *Therapy of Inflammatory Bowel Disease: New Medical and Surgical Approaches.* New York: Marcel Dekker, 1989.

Ratnaike, R. N., ed. *Small Bowel Disorders.* London: Edward Arnold, 2000.

KEY TERMS

Adenocarcinoma—Adenocarcinoma starts in the lining of the small intestine and is the most common type of cancer of the small intestine. These tumors occur most often in the part of the small intestine nearest the stomach and often grow and block the bowel.

Anesthesia—A combination of drugs administered by a variety of techniques by trained professionals that provide sedation, amnesia, analgesia, and immobility adequate for the accomplishment of the surgical procedure with minimal discomfort and without injury to the patient.

Cancer—The uncontrolled growth of abnormal cells which have mutated from normal tissues.

Colon—Also called the large intestine, the colon has six major segments: caecum, ascending colon, transverse colon, descending colon, sigmoid colon, and rectum. Its length is approximately 5 ft (1.5 m) in the adult and it is responsible for forming, storing, and expelling waste matter.

Crohn's disease—Chronic inflammatory process, primarily involving the intestinal tract, that most commonly affects the last part of the small intestine (ileum) and/or the large intestine (colon and rectum).

Duodenectomy—Excision of the duodenum.

Ileectomy—Excision of the ileum.

Jejunectomy—Excision of all or a part of the jejunum.

Leiomyosarcoma—Leiomyosarcomas are cancers that start growing in the smooth muscle lining of the small intestine.

Lymphoma—A lymphoma starts from lymph tissue in the small intestine. Lymph tissue is part of the body's immune system, which helps the body fight infections. Most of these tumors are a type of lymphoma called non-Hodgkin's lymphomas.

Ostomy—An operation to create an opening from an area inside the body to the outside.

Polyp—Growth, usually benign, protruding from a mucous membrane, such as that lining the walls of the intestines.

Resection—Removal of a portion or all of an organ or other structure.

Small intestine—The small intestine consists of three sections: duodenum, jejunum and ileum, all of which are involved in the absorption of nutrients. The total length of the small intestine is approximately 22 ft (6.5 m).

Thompson, J. C., and L. Rose. *Atlas of Surgery of the Stomach, Duodenum, and Small Bowel.* St. Louis: Mosby, 1992.

PERIODICALS

Bines, J. E., R. G. Taylor, F. Justice, et al. "Influence of Diet Complexity on Intestinal Adaptation Following Massive Small Bowel Resection in a Preclinical Model." *Journal of Gastroenterology and Hepatology* 17 (November 2002): 1170–1179.

Dahly, E. M., M. B. Gillingham, Z. Guo, et al. "Role of Luminal Nutrients and Endogenous GLP-2 in Intestinal Adaptation to Mid-Small Bowel Resection." *American Journal of Physiology and Gastrointestinal Liver Physiology* 284 (March 2003): G670–G682.

Libsch, K. D., N. J. Zyromski, T. Tanaka, et al. "Role of Extrinsic Innervation in Jejunal Absorptive Adaptation to Subtotal Small Bowel Resection: A Model of Segmental Small Bowel Transplantation." *Journal of Gastrointestinal Surgery* 6 (March-April 2002): 240–247.

O'Brien, D. P., L. A. Nelson, J. L. Williams, et al. "Selective Inhibition of the Epidermal Growth Factor Receptor Impairs Intestinal Adaptation After Small Bowel Resection." *Journal of Surgical Research* 105 (June 2002): 25–30.

ORGANIZATIONS

American Board of Colorectal Surgeons (ABCRS). 20600 Eureka Rd., Ste. 600, Taylor, MI 48180. (734) 282-9400. <www.abcrs.org>.

American Society of Colorectal Surgeons (ASCRS). 85 West Algonquin, Suite 550, Arlington Heights, IL 60005. (847) 290 9184. <www.fascrs.org>.

United Ostomy Association, Inc. (UOA). 19772 MacArthur Blvd., Suite 200, Irvine, CA 92612-2405. (800) 826-0826. <www.uoa.org>.

OTHER

"Bowel Resection; Patient Discharge Instructions." *Northwest Memorial Hospital Patient Education Brochure.* March 2001 [cited June 25, 2003]. <http://www.nmh.org/patient_ed_pdfs/pt_ed_bowel_resection_discharge.pdf.>.

"Crohn's Disease." American Society of Colon and Rectal Surgeons Patient Brochure. 1996 [cited June 25, 2003]. <http://www.fascrs.org>.

Monique Laberge, Ph.D.

Smoking cessation

Definition

Smoking cessation means "to quit smoking," or "withdrawal from nicotine." Because smoking is highly addictive, quitting the habit often involves irritability, headache, mood swings, and cravings associated with the sudden cessation or reduction of tobacco use by a nicotine-dependent individual.

Purpose

There are many good reasons to stop smoking; not the least is that smoking cessation may speed post-surgery recovery. Smoking cessation helps a person heal and recover faster, especially in the incision area, or if the surgery involved any bones. Research shows that patients who underwent hip and knee replacements, or surgery on other bone joints, healed better and recovered more quickly if they had quit or cut down their tobacco intake several weeks before the operation. Smoking weakens the bone mineral that keeps the skeleton strong and undermines tissue and vessel health. One study suggested that even quitting tobacco for a few days could improve tissue blood flow and oxygenation, and might have a positive effect on wound healing. If a patient has had a history of heart problems, his chances of having a second heart attack will be lowered. Quitting may also reduce wound complications, and lower the risk of cardiovascular trouble after surgery. If surgery was performed to remove cancerous tumors, quitting will reduce the risk of a second tumor, especially if cancer in the lung, head, or neck has been successfully treated.

Description

Quitting smoking is one of the best things a person can do to increase their life expectancy. On average, male smokers who quit at 35 years old can be expected to live to be 76 years old instead of 69 years if they were still smoking. Women who quit would live to be 80 years old instead of 74 years.

Effects of smoking on the body

Nicotine acts as both a stimulant and a depressant on the body. Saliva and bronchial secretions increase along with bowel tone. Some inexperienced smokers may experience tremors or even convulsions with high doses of nicotine because of the stimulation of the central nervous system. The respiratory muscles are then depressed following stimulation.

Nicotine causes arousal as well as relaxation from stressful situations. Tobacco use increases the heart rate about 10–20 beats per minute; and because it constricts the blood vessels, it increases the blood pressure reading by 5–10 mm Hg.

Sweating, nausea, and diarrhea may also increase because of the effects of nicotine upon the central nervous system. Hormonal activities of the body are also affected. Nicotine elevates the blood glucose levels and increases insulin production; it can also lead to blood clots. Smoking does have some positive effects on the body by stimulating memory and alertness, and enhancing cognitive skills that require speed, reaction time, vigilance, and work performance. Smoking tends to alleviate boredom and reduce stress as well as reduce aggressive responses to stressful events because of its mood-altering ability. It also acts as an appetite suppressant, specifically decreasing the appetite for simple carbohydrates (sweets) and inhibiting the efficiency with which food is metabolized. The fear of weight gain prevents some people from quitting smoking. The addictive effects of tobacco have been well documented. It is considered mood-and behavior-altering, psychoactive, and abusable. Tobacco's addictive potential is believed to be comparable to alcohol, cocaine, and morphine.

Health problems associated with smoking

In general, chronic use of nicotine may cause an acceleration of coronary artery disease, hypertension, reproductive disturbances, esophageal reflux, peptic ulcer disease, fetal illnesses and death, and delayed wound healing. The smoker is at greater risk of developing cancer (especially in the lung, mouth, larynx, esophagus, bladder, kidney, pancreas, and cervix); heart attacks and strokes; and chronic lung disease. Using tobacco during pregnancy increases the risk of miscarriage, intrauterine growth retardation (resulting in the birth of an infant small for gestational age), and the infant's risk for sudden infant death syndrome.

The specific health risks of tobacco use include: nicotine addiction, lung disease, lung cancer, emphysema, chronic bronchitis, coronary artery disease and angina, heart attack, atherosclerotic and peripheral vascular disease, aneurysms, hypertension, blood clots, strokes, oral/tooth/gum diseases including oral cancer, and cancer in the kidney, bladder, and pancreas. Nicotine is also associated with decreased senses of taste and smell. During pregnancy, nicotine may cause increased fetal death, premature labor, low birth weight infants, and sudden infant death syndrome.

Nonsmokers who are regularly exposed to second hand smoke also may experience specific health risks including:

- Increased risk of lung cancer.

- An increased frequency of respiratory infections in infants and children (e.g. bronchitis and pneumonia), asthma, and decreases in lung function as the lungs mature.

- Acute, sudden, and occasionally severe reactions including eye, nose, throat, and lower respiratory tract symptoms.

The specific health risks for smokeless tobacco users include many of the diseases of smokers, as well as a 50-fold greater risk for oral cancer with long-term or regular use.

In diabetics taking medication for high blood pressure, it has been reported that smoking may increase the risk of kidney disease and/or kidney failure.

Making a plan to quit

Long lead times for elective procedures like joint operations offer a good opportunity for doctors to encourage their patients to quit smoking, but only the smoker has the power to stop smoking. Before a smoker decides to quit, he should make sure he wants to quit smoking for himself, and not for other people. The following are some questions as well as some suggestions the smoker may want to consider:

- When is the best time to quit smoking? The answer may be different for women and men. Women should set their quit date to begin at the end of their period for best results. The first step is to set a quit date.

- Make a written list of why you want to quit smoking.

- Will you use an aid to help you quit? Will it be the patch, nicotine gum, Zyban, nicotine spray, soft laser therapy, nasal inhaler, or some other method? If you plan to use Zyban, set your quit date for one week after you begin to use it.

- smoke only in certain places, preferably outdoors

- switch to a brand of cigarettes that you don't like

- do not buy cigarettes by the carton

- cut coffee consumption in half (You will not need to give it up.)

- practice putting off lighting up when the urge strikes

- go for a walk every day or begin an **exercise** program

- stock up on non-fattening safe snacks to help with weight control after quitting

- enlist the support of family and friends

- clean and put away all ashtrays the day before quitting

Smokers who are trying to quit should remind themselves that they are doing the smartest thing they have ever done. Because of the preparation for smoking cessation, the smoker won't be surprised or fearful about quitting. The quitter will be willing to do what's necessary, even though it won't be easy. Remember, this will likely add years to the lifespan. The quitting smoker should be prepared to spend more time with nonsmoking friends, if other smokers don't support the attempt to quit.

Since hospitals are smoke-free environments, if a smoking patient is in the hospital for **elective surgery**, it may be a good opportunity to quit smoking. It might be best to set the quit date around the time of the surgery and let the attending doctor know. As the smoker takes the first step, professional hospital staff will be there to give the support and help needed. Medical staff can start the patient on nicotine replacement therapy to help control the cravings and increase the chances of quitting permanently.

Methods of quitting

Cold turkey, or an abrupt cessation of nicotine, is one way to stop smoking. Cold turkey can provide cost savings because paraphernalia and smoking cessation aids are not required; however, not everyone can stop this way as tremendous willpower is needed.

Laser therapy is an entirely safe and pain-free form of acupuncture that has been in use since the 1980s. Using a painless soft laser beam instead of needles the laser beam is applied to specific energy points on the body, stimulating production of endorphins. These natural body chemicals produce a calming, relaxing effect. It is the sudden drop in endorphin levels that leads to withdrawal symptoms and physical cravings when a person stops smoking. Laser treatment not only helps relieve these cravings, but helps with stress reduction and lung detoxification. Some studies indicate that laser therapy is the most effective method of smoking cessation, with an extraordinarily high success rate.

Acupuncture—small needles or springs are inserted into the skin—is another aid in smoking cessation. The needles or springs are sometimes left in the ears and touched lightly by the patient between visits.

Some smokers find hypnosis particularly useful, especially if there is any kind of mental conflict, such as phobias, panic attacks, or weight control. As a smoker struggles to stop smoking, the conscious mind, deciding to quit, battles the inner mind, which is governed by habit and body chemistry. Hypnosis, by talking directly to the inner mind, can help to resolve that inner battle.

Aversion techniques attempt to make smoking seem unpleasant. This technique reminds the person of the distasteful aspects of smoking, such as the smell, dirty ashtrays, coughing, the high cost, and health issues. The most common technique prescribed by psychologists for "thought stopping"—stopping unwanted thoughts—is to wear a rubber band around the wrist. Every time there is an unwanted thought (a craving to smoke) the band is supposed to be pulled so that it hurts. The thought then becomes associated with pain and gradually neutralized.

Rapid smoking is a technique in which smoking times are strictly scheduled once a day for the first three days after quitting. Phrases are repeated such as "smoking irritates my throat" or "smoking burns my lips and tongue." This causes over-smoking in a way that makes the taste and sensations very unpleasant.

There are special mouthwashes available, which, when used before smoking, alter the taste, making cigarettes taste awful. The aim is for smoking to eventually become associated with this very unpleasant taste.

Smoking cessation aids wean a person off nicotine slowly, and the nicotine can be delivered where it does the least bodily harm. Unlike cigarettes, they do not introduce other harmful poisons to the body. They can be used for a short period of time. However, it should be noted that nicotine from any source (smoking, nicotine gum, or the nicotine patch) can make some health problems worse. These include heart or circulation problems, irregular heartbeat, chest pain, high blood pressure, overactive thyroid, stomach ulcers, or diabetes.

The four main brands of the patch are Nicotrol, Nicoderm, Prostep, and Habitrol. All four transmit low doses of nicotine to the body throughout the day. The patch comes in varying strengths ranging from 7 mg to 21 mg. The patch must be prescribed and used under a physician's care. Package instructions must be followed carefully. Other smoking cessation programs or materials should be used while using the patch.

Nicorette gum allows the nicotine to be absorbed through the membrane of the mouth between the cheek and gums. Past smoking habits determine the right strength to choose. The gum should be chewed slowly.

The nicotine nasal spray reduces cravings and withdrawal symptoms, allowing smokers to cut back slowly. The nasal spray acts quickly to stop the cravings, as it is rapidly absorbed through the nasal membranes. One of the drawbacks is a risk of addiction to the spray.

The nicotine inhaler uses a plastic mouthpiece with a nicotine plug, delivering nicotine to the mucous membranes of the mouth. It provides nicotine at about one-third the nicotine level of cigarettes.

Zyban is an oral medication that is making an impact in the fight to help smokers quit. It is a treatment for nicotine dependence.

The nicotine lozenge is another smoking cessation aid recently added to the growing list of tools to combat nicotine withdrawal.

Withdrawal symptoms

Generally, the longer one has smoked and the greater the number of cigarettes (and nicotine) consumed, the more likely it is that withdrawal symptoms will occur and the more severe they are likely to be. When a smoker switches from regular to low-nicotine cigarettes or significantly cuts back smoking, a milder form of nicotine withdrawal involving some or all of these symptoms can occur.

These are some of the withdrawal symptoms that most ex-smokers experience in the beginning of their new smoke-free life:

• dry mouth
• mood swings
• irritability
• feelings of depression
• gas
• tension
• sleeplessness or sleeping too much
• difficulty in concentration
• intense cravings for a cigarette
• increased appetite and weight gain
• headaches

These side effects are all temporary conditions that will probably subside in a short time for most people. These symptoms can last from one to three weeks and are strongest during the first week after quitting. Drinking plenty of water during the first week can help detoxify the body and shorten the duration of the withdrawal symptoms. A positive attitude, drive, commitment, and a willingness to get help from health care professionals and support groups will help a smoker kick the habit.

Researchers from the University of California San Diego strongly suggest that any of the above cessation aids should be used in combination with other types of smoking cessation help, such as behavioral counseling and/or support programs. These products are not designed to help with the behavioral aspects of smoking, but only the cravings associated with them. Counseling and support groups can offer tips on coping with difficult situations that can trigger the urge to smoke.

Even a new heart can't break a bad habit

Why do some people who have heart transplants continue to smoke? In a three-year study at the University of Pittsburgh of 202 heart transplant recipients, 71% of the recipients were smokers before surgery. The overall rate of post-transplant smoking was 27%. All but one of the smokers resumed the smoking habit they had before the trans-

KEY TERMS

Addiction—Compulsive, overwhelming involvement with a specific activity. The activity may be smoking, gambling, alcohol, or may involve the use of almost any substance, such as a drug.

Appetite suppressant—To decrease the appetite.

Constrict—To squeeze tightly, compress, draw together.

Convulsion—To shake or effect with spasms; to agitate or disturb violently.

Depressant—A drug or other substance that soothes or lessens tension of the muscles or nerves.

Detoxification—To remove a poison or toxin or the effect of such a harmful substance; to free from an intoxicating or addictive substance in the body or from dependence on or addiction to a harmful substance.

Endorphins—Any of a group of proteins with analgesic properties that occur naturally in the brain.

Gestational age—The length of time of growth and development of the young in the mother's womb.

Metabolism—The sum of all the chemical processes that occur in living organisms; the rate at which the body consumes energy.

Nicotine—A poisonous, oily alkaloid in tobacco.

Oxygenation—To supply with oxygen.

Paraphernalia—Articles of equipment or accessory items.

Premature—Happening early or occurring before the usual time.

Psychoactive—Affecting the mind or behavior.

Respiratory infections—Infections that relate to or affect respiration or breathing.

Smoking cessation—To quit smoking or withdrawal from nicotine.

Stimulant—A drug or other substance that increases the rate of activity of a body system.

Tremor—A trembling, quivering, or shaking.

Withdrawal—Stopping of administration or use of a drug; the syndrome of sometimes painful physical and psychological symptoms that follow the discontinuance.

---

plant. The biggest reason for resuming smoking was addiction to nicotine. Smoking is a complex behavior, involving social interactions, visual cues, and other factors. Those who smoked until less than six months before the transplant were much more likely to resume smoking early and to smoke more. One of the major causes of early relapse was because of depression and anxiety within two months after the transplant. Another strong predictor of relapse was having a caretaker who smoked. The knowledge of these risk factors could help develop strategies for identifying those in greatest need of early intervention. According to European studies, the five-year survival rate for post-transplant smokers is 37%, compared to 80% for nonsmoking recipients. Smokers can develop inoperable lung cancers within five years after a transplant, thus resulting in a shorter survival rate. There is an alarming incidence of head and neck cancers in transplant recipients who resume smoking.

Overall, there is a 90% relapse rate in the general population but, the more times a smoker tries to quit, the greater the chance of success with each new try.

Resources

BOOKS

Dodds, Bill. *1440 Reasons to Quit Smoking: 1 For Every Minute of the Day.* Minnetonka, MN: Meadowbrook Press, 2000.

Jones, David C. and Derick D. Schermerhorn, eds. *Yes You Can Stop Smoking: Even if You Don't Want To.* Dolphin Pub., 2001.

Kleinman, Lowell, Deborah Messina-Kleinman, and Mitchell Nides. *Complete Idiot's Guide to Quitting Smoking.* London, UK: Alpha Books, 2000.

Mannoia, Richard J. *NBAC Program: Never Buy Another Cigarette: A Cigarette Smoking Cessation Program.* Paradise Publications, 2003.

Shipley, Robert H. *Quit Smart: Stop Smoking Guide With the Quitsmart System, It's Easier Than You Think!* Quitsmart, 2002.

PERIODICALS

Landman, Anne, Pamela M. Ling, and Stanton A. Glantz. "Tobacco Industry Youth Smoking Prevention Programs: Protecting the Industry and Hurting Tobacco Control." *American Journal of Public Health* 92, no. 6 (June 2002): 917–30.

Ling, Pamela M. and Stanton A. Glantz, "Forum on Youth Smoking, Why and How the Tobacco Industry Sells Cigarettes to Young Adults: Evidence From Industry Documents." *American Journal of Public Health* 92, no. 6 (June 2002): 908–16.

Taylor, Donald H., Jr., Vic Hasselblad, S. Jane Henley, Michael J. Thun, and Frank A. Sloan. "Research and Practice, Benefits of Smoking Cessation for Longevity." *American Journal of Public Health* 92, no. 6 (June 2002): 990–6.

OTHER

Illig, David. *Stop Smoking.* Audio CD. Seattle: WA: Success-world, 2001.

Mesmer. *Stop Smoking With America's Foremost Hypnotist.* Audio CD. Victoria, BC: Ace Mirage Entertainment, 2000.

ORGANIZATIONS

Action on Smoking and Health. 2013 H Street, NW, Washington, DC 20006. (202) 659-4310. <http://ash.org>.

American Lung Association. 61 Broadway, 6th Floor, New York, NY. 10006. (800) 586-4872. <www.lungusa.org>.

Crystal H. Kaczkowski, M.Sc.

Snoring surgery

Definition

Snoring is defined as noisy or rough breathing during sleep, caused by vibration of loose tissue in the upper airway. Surgical treatments for snoring include several different techniques for removing tissue from the back of the patient's throat, reshaping the nasal passages or jaw, or preventing the tongue from blocking the airway during sleep.

Purpose

The purpose of snoring surgery is to improve or eliminate the medical and social consequences of heavy snoring. Most insurance companies, however, regard surgical treatment of snoring as essentially a cosmetic procedure—which means that patients must cover its expenses themselves. The major exception is surgery to correct a deviated septum or other obstruction in the nose, on the grounds that nasal surgery generally improves the patient's breathing during the day as well as at night.

Snoring as a medical problem

The connection between heavy snoring, breathing disorders, and other health problems is a relatively recent discovery. Obstructive sleep apnea (OSA) is a breathing disorder that was first identified in 1965. OSA is marked by brief stoppages in breathing during sleep resulting from partial blockage of the airway. A person with OSA may stop breathing temporarily as often as 20–30 times per hour. He or she usually snores or makes choking and gasping sounds between these episodes. The person is not refreshed by nighttime sleep and may suffer from morning headaches as well as daytime sleepiness. He or she may be misdiagnosed as suffering from clinical de-pression when the real problem is physical tiredness. In addition, the high levels of carbon dioxide that build up in the blood when a person is not breathing normally may eventually lead to high blood pressure, irregular heartbeat, heart attacks, and stroke. In children, heavy snoring appears to be a major risk factor for attention-deficit/hyperactivity disorder.

Although people with OSA snore, not everyone who snores has OSA. It is thought that OSA affects about 4% of middle-aged males and 2% of middle-aged females. Most adults who snore have what is called primary snoring, which means that the loud sounds produced in the upper airway during sleep are *not* interrupted by episodes of breathing cessation. Other terms for primary snoring are simple snoring, benign snoring, rhythmical snoring, continuous snoring, and socially unacceptable snoring (SUS). Although primary snoring is not associated with severe disorders to the same extent as OSA, it has been shown to have some negative consequences for health. A study published in April 2003 reported that habitual primary snoring is a risk factor for chronic daily headaches.

Snoring as a social problem

As the term SUS suggests, primary snoring can cause the same social problems for a person as does snoring associated with OSA. People who snore heavily often keep other family members, roommates, or even neighbors from getting a good night's sleep, which leads to considerable anger and resentment. Recent studies have found that the nonsnoring partner or roommate loses an average of an hour's sleep each night. According to Dr. Kingman Strohl, head of a sleep disorders program in a Veterans Administration hospital, even the average volume of snoring (60 decibels or dB) is as loud as normal speech. Some people, however, snore around 80–82 dB, the sound level of a loud yell; a few have been recorded as reaching 90 dB, the sound level of loud rock music. One study found that 80% of people married to heavy snorers end up sleeping in separate rooms. A group of Swedish researchers reported that heavy snoring has the same level of negative effects on quality of life among adult males as high blood pressure, chronic obstructive pulmonary disease, heart disease, and similar chronic medical conditions.

Risk factors for snoring

Some people are at higher risk of developing problem snoring than others. Risk factors in addition to sex and age include:

• Genetic factors. The size and shape of the uvula, soft palate, tonsils, and other parts of the airway are largely determined by heredity.

• Family history of heavy snoring.

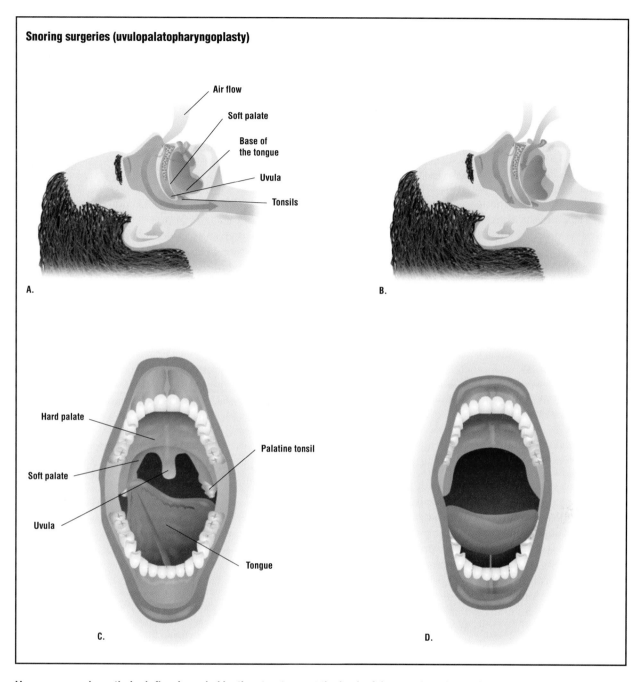

Snoring surgeries (uvulopalatopharyngoplasty)

Air flow

Soft palate

Base of
the tongue

Uvula

Tonsils

A.

B.

Hard palate

Palatine tonsil

Soft palate

Uvula

Tongue

C.

D.

Heavy snorers have their air flow impeded by the structures at the back of the mouth and nose (A and B), which can be alleviated by surgery. In uvulopalatopharyngoplasty, the patient's uvula, soft palate, and tonsils are removed (C and D). *(Illustration by GGS Inc.)*

• Obesity. Severe overweight increases a person's risk of developing OSA.

• Lack of **exercise**. Physical activity helps to keep the muscles of the throat firm and strong as well as the larger muscles of the body.

• Heavy consumption of alcohol and tobacco.

• A history of frequent upper respiratory infections or allergies.

• Trauma to the nose, face, or throat.

Demographics

Snoring is a commonplace problem in the general population in North America. About 12% of children over the age of five are reported to snore frequently and loudly. Among adults, 45% snore occasionally, while 25% snore almost every night. The problem usually grows worse as people age; 50% of people over age 65 are habitual snorers.

Problem snoring is worse among males than among females in all age brackets. With regard to racial and ethnic differences, a sleep research study published in 2003 reported that frequent snoring is more common (in the United States) among African American women, Hispanic women, and Hispanic men than their Caucasian counterparts, even after adjusting for weight and body mass index (BMI). African American, Native American, and Asian American males have the same rates of snoring as Caucasian males. Further research is needed to determine whether these differences are related to variations in the rates and types of health problems in these respective groups.

According to international researchers, heavy snoring appears to be more common in persons of Asian origin than in persons of Middle Eastern, European, or African origin.

Description

With the exception of UPPP, all of the surgical treatments for snoring described in this section are outpatient or office-based procedures.

Uvulopalatopharyngoplasty (UPPP)

Uvulopalatopharyngoplasty, or UPPP, is the oldest and most invasive surgical treatment for snoring. It was first performed in 1982 by a Japanese surgeon named S. Fujita. UPPP requires general anesthesia, one to two nights of inpatient care in a hospital, and a minimum of two weeks of recovery afterward. In a uvulopalatopharyngoplasty, the surgeon resects (removes) the patient's tonsils, part of the soft palate, and the uvula. The procedure works by enlarging the airway and removing some of the soft tissue that vibrates when the patient snores. It is not effective in treating snoring caused by obstructions at the base of the tongue.

UPPP has several drawbacks in addition to its cost and lengthy recovery period. It can result in major complications, including severe bleeding due to removal of the tonsils as well as airway obstruction. In addition, the results may not be permanent; between 50% and 70% of patients who have been treated with UPPP report that short-term improvements in snoring do not last longer than a year.

Laser-assisted uvulopalatoplasty

Laser-assisted uvulopalatoplasty, or LAUP, is an outpatient surgical treatment for snoring in which a carbon dioxide laser is used to vaporize part of the uvula, a small triangular piece of tissue that hangs from the soft palate above the back of the tongue. The patient is seated upright in a comfortable chair in the doctor's office. The doctor first sprays a local anesthetic—usually lidocaine—over the back of the patient's throat, covering the patient's soft palate, tonsils, and uvula. The second step is the injection of more anesthetic into the muscle tissue in the uvula. After waiting for the anesthetic to take effect, the surgeon uses a carbon dioxide laser to make two vertical incisions in the soft palate on either side of the uvula. A third incision is used to remove the tip of the uvula. The surgeon also usually removes part of the soft palate itself. The total procedure takes about half an hour.

LAUP is typically performed as a series of three to five separate treatments. Additional treatment sessions, if needed, are spaced four to eight weeks apart.

LAUP was developed in the late 1980s by Dr. Yves-Victor Kamami, a French surgeon whose first article on the technique was published in 1990. Kamami claimed a high rate of success for LAUP in treating a condition known as obstructive sleep apnea (OSA) as well as snoring. The procedure has become controversial because other surgeons found it less effective than the first reports indicated, and also because most patients suffer considerable pain for about two weeks after surgery. Although some surgeons report a success rate as high as 85% in treating snoring with LAUP, the effectiveness of the procedure is highly dependent on the surgeon's experience and ability.

Somnoplasty

Somnoplasty, or radiofrequency volumetric tissue reduction (RFVTR) is a newer technique in which the surgeon uses a thin needle connected to a source of radiofrequency signals to shrink the tissues in the soft palate, throat, or tongue. It was approved by the Food and Drug Administration (FDA) for the treatment of snoring in 1997. The needle is inserted beneath the surface layer of cells and heated to a temperature between 158°F (70°C) and 176°F (80°C). The upper layer of cells is unaffected, but the heated tissue is destroyed and gradually reabsorbed by the body over the next four to six weeks. Somnoplasty stiffens the remaining layers of tissue as well as reducing the total volume of tissue. Some patients require a second treatment, but most find that their snoring is significantly improved after only one. The procedure takes about 30 minutes and is performed under local anesthesia.

Somnoplasty appears to have a higher success rate (about 85%) than LAUP and is considerably less painful. Most patients report two to three days of mild swelling after somnoplasty compared to two weeks of considerable discomfort for LAUP.

Tongue suspension procedure

The tongue suspension procedure, which is also known as the Repose™ system, is a minimally invasive surgical treatment for snoring that stabilizes the base of the tongue during sleep, preventing it from falling backward and obstructing the airway. The Repose system was approved by the FDA in 1998. It consists of a titanium screw inserted into the lower jaw on the floor of the mouth and a suture passed through the base of the tongue that is then attached to the screw. The attachment holds the tongue forward during sleep.

The Repose system is done as an outpatient procedure under total anesthesia. It takes about 15–20 minutes to complete. The advantages of the tongue suspension procedure include the fact that it is reversible, since no incision is made; and that it can be combined with UPPP, LAUP, or a **tonsillectomy**. Its disadvantages include its relatively long healing time (one to two weeks) and the fact that it appears to be more effective in treating OSA than primary snoring. One team of American and Israeli researchers who conducted a multicenter trial concluded that the tongue suspension procedure requires further evaluation.

Injection snoreplasty

Injection snoreplasty was developed by a team of Army physicians at Walter Reed Hospital and introduced to other ear, nose and throat specialists at a professional conference in 2000. In injection snoreplasty, the surgeon gives the patient a local anesthetic and then injects a hardening agent known as sodium tetradecyl sulfate underneath the skin of the roof of the mouth just in front of the uvula. The chemical, which is also used in sclerotherapy, creates a blister that hardens into scar tissue. The scar tissue pulls the uvula forward, reducing the vibration or flutter that causes snoring.

Preliminary research indicates that injection snoreplasty is safe, has a higher rate of success than LAUP (about 92%), and is also less painful. Most patients need only one treatment, and can manage the discomfort the next day with a mild **aspirin** substitute and throat spray. The primary drawback of injection snoreplasty is that it treats only tissues in the area of the uvula. Snoring caused by tissue vibrations elsewhere in the throat requires another form of treatment. Injection snoreplasty costs about $500 per treatment.

Diagnosis/Preparation

Diagnosis

The most important task in diagnosing a patient's snoring is to distinguish between primary snoring and obstructive sleep apnea. The reason for care in the diagnosis is that surgical treatment without the recommended tests for OSA can complicate later diagnosis of the disorder.

The sounds made when a person snores have a number of different physical causes. Snoring noises may result from one or more of the following:

• An unusually long soft palate and uvula. These structures narrow the airway between the nose and the throat. They act like noisy flutter valves when the person breathes in and out during sleep.

• Too much tissue in the throat. Large tonsils and adenoids can cause snoring, which is one reason why tonsillectomies are sometimes recommended to treat heavy snoring in children.

• Nasal congestion. When a person's nose is stuffy, their attempts to breathe create a partial vacuum in the throat that pulls the softer tissues of the throat together. This suction can also produce a snoring noise. Nasal congestion helps to explain why some people snore only when they have a cold or during pollen season.

• Anatomical deformations of the nose. People who have had their noses or cheekbones fractured or who have a deviated septum are more likely to snore, because their nasal passages develop a twisted or crooked shape and vibrate as air passes through them.

• Sleeping position. People are more likely to snore when they are lying on the back because the force of gravity draws the tongue and soft tissues in the throat backward and downward, blocking the airway.

• Obesity. Obesity adds to the weight of the tissues in the neck, which can cause partial blockage of the airway during sleep.

• Use of alcohol, sleeping medications, or tranquilizers. These substances relax the throat muscles, which may become soft or limp enough to partially close the airway.

Because snoring may be related to lifestyle factors, upper respiratory infections, seasonal allergies, and sleeping habits as well as the anatomy of the person's airway, a complete medical history is the first step in determining suitable treatments. In some cases the patient may have been referred by his or her dentist on the basis of findings during a dental procedure. A primary care doctor can take a history and perform a basic examination of the patient's nose and throat. In addition, the primary care doctor may give the patient one or more short questionnaires to evaluate the severity of daytime sleepiness and other problems related to snoring. The test most commonly used is the Epworth Sleepiness Scale (ESS), which was developed by an Australian physician, Dr. Murray Johns, in 1991. The ESS lists eight situations (reading, watching TV, etc.) and asks the patient to rate his or her chances of dozing off in each situation on a

WHO PERFORMS THE PROCEDURE AND WHERE IS IT PERFORMED?

Snoring surgery is done by a head and neck surgeon, a plastic surgeon, or an otolaryngologist, who is a doctor with special training in treating disorders of the ear, nose, and throat. UPPP is performed under general anesthesia and requires an overnight hospital stay. LAUP, somnoplasty, the tongue suspension procedure, and injection snoreplasty are performed as **outpatient surgery**, usually in a doctor's office or other outpatient facility.

Prosthetic devices to alter the position of the jaw or restrain the tongue during sleep are prescribed and fitted by general dentists or orthodontists.

Polysomnography as a part of a diagnostic workup is done in a special sleep laboratory by experts who are trained in the use of the equipment and interpretation of the results. Recent advances in technology, however, may allow patients to be monitored at home with portable polysomnographs and a computer with an Internet connection.

four-point scale (0–3, with 3 representing a high chance of falling asleep). A score of 6 or lower indicates that the person is getting enough sleep; a score higher than 9 is a danger sign. The ESS is often used to measure the effectiveness of various treatments for snoring as well as to evaluate patients prior to surgery.

The next stage in the differential diagnosis of snoring problems is a detailed examination of the patient's airway by an otolaryngologist, who is a physician who specializes in diagnosing and treating disorders involving the nose and throat. The American Sleep Apnea Association (ASAA) maintains that no one should consider surgery for snoring until their airway has been examined by a specialist. The otolaryngologist will be able to determine whether the size and shape of the patient's uvula, soft palate, tonsils and adenoids, nasal cartilage, and throat muscles are contributing factors, and to advise the patient on specific procedures. It may be necessary for the patient to undergo more than one type of treatment for snoring, as some surgical procedures correct only one or two structures in the nose or throat.

A complete airway examination consists of an external examination of the patient's face and neck; an endoscopic examination of the nasal passages and throat; the use of a laryngeal mirror or magnifying laryngoscope to study the lower portions of the throat; and various imaging studies. The otolaryngologist may use a nasopharyngoscope, which allows for evaluation of obstructions below the palate and the tongue, and may be performed with the patient either awake or asleep. The nasopharyngoscope is a flexible fiberoptic device that is introduced into the airway through the patient's nose. Other imaging studies that may be done include acoustic reflection, computed tomography (CT) scans, or **magnetic resonance imaging** (MRI).

In addition to the airway examination, patients considering surgical treatment for snoring must make an appointment for sleep testing in a specialized laboratory. The American Academy of Sleep Medicine recommends this step in order to exclude the possibility that the patient has obstructive sleep apnea. Sleep testing consists of an overnight stay in a special sleep laboratory. Before the patient goes to sleep, he or she will be connected to a polysomnograph, which is an instrument that monitors the patient's breathing, heart rate, temperature, muscle movements, airflow, body position, and other measurements that are needed to evaluate the cause(s) of sleep disorders. A technician records the data in a separate room. As of 2003, some companies are developing portable polysomnographs that allow patients to connect the device to a computer in their home and transmit the data to the sleep center over an Internet connection.

Preparation

Apart from the extensive diagnostic testing that is recommended, preparation for outpatient snoring surgery is usually limited to taking a mild sedative before the procedure. Preparation for UPPP requires a **physical examination**, EKG, blood tests, and a preoperation interview with the anesthesiologist to evaluate the patient's fitness for general anesthesia.

Aftercare

Aftercare following outpatient snoring surgery consists primarily of medication for throat discomfort, particularly when swallowing. The patient can resume normal work and other activities the same day as the procedure, and speaking is usually not affected.

Risks

In addition to the risk of an allergic reaction to the local anesthetic, snoring surgery is associated with the following risks:

- Severe pain following the procedure that lasts longer than two to three days. This complication occurs more frequently with LAUP than with somnoplasty or injection snoreplasty.

- Causation or worsening of obstructive sleep apnea. LAUP has been reported to cause OSA in patients who had only primary snoring before the operation.

- Nasal regurgitation. This complication refers to food shooting or leaking through the nose when the patient swallows.

- Dehydration. This complication has been reported with the tongue suspension procedure.

- Permanent change in the quality of the patient's voice.

- Recurrence of primary snoring.

Normal results

In general, surgical treatment for snoring appears to be most effective in patients whose primary problem is nasal obstruction. The results of snoring surgery depend to a large degree on a good "fit" between the anatomy of a specific patient's airway and the specific procedure performed, as well as on the individual surgeon's skills.

Morbidity and mortality rates

Mortality rates for UPPP are related to complications of OSA rather than to the procedure itself. With regard to the outpatient procedures for snoring, mortality rates are very close to zero because these surgeries are performed under local anesthesia. Complication rates, however, are high with both UPPP and LAUP. According to one European study, as many as 42% of patients have complications following UPPP, with 14% reporting general dissatisfaction with the results of surgery. Specific complication rates for UPPP are 15% for recurrence of snoring; 13% for nasal regurgitation; 10% for excessive throat secretions; 9% for swallowing problems; and 7% for speech disturbances. Complications for LAUP have been estimated to be 30–40% for recurrence of snoring; 30% for causing or worsening of OSA; 5%–10% for persistent nasal regurgitation; 1% for permanent change in vocal quality.

As of early 2003, no morbidity figures have been published for somnoplasty or injection snoreplasty.

Alternatives

Oral devices and appliances

Oral appliances are intended to reduce snoring by changing the shape of the oral cavity or preventing the tongue from blocking the airway. There are three basic

types of mouthpieces: those that push the lower jaw forward; those that raise the soft palate; and those that restrain the tongue from falling backward during sleep. To work properly, oral appliances should be fitted by an experienced dentist or orthodontist and checked periodically for proper fit. Their major drawback is a low rate of patient compliance; one German study found that only 30% of patients fitted with these devices were still using them after four years. In addition, oral appliances cannot be used by patients with gum disease, **dental implants**, or teeth that are otherwise in poor condition.

Continuous positive airway pressure (CPAP) devices

CPAP devices are masks that fit over the nose during sleep and deliver air into the airway under enough pressure to keep the airway open. If used correctly, CPAP devices can be an effective alternative to surgery. Their main drawback is a relatively low rate of patient compliance; the mask must be used every night, and some people feel mildly claustrophobic when using it. In addition, patients are often asked to lose weight or stop smoking while using CPAP, which are lifestyle adjustments that some would rather not make.

Lifestyle changes

Patients who snore only occasionally or who are light snorers may be helped by one or more of the following changes without undergoing surgery:

- Losing weight and getting adequate physical exercise.

- Avoiding tranquilizers, sleeping pills, antihistamines, or alcoholic beverages before bedtime.

- Quitting smoking.

- Sleeping on the side rather than the back. One do-it-yourself device that is sometimes recommended to keep the patient turned on his or her side is a tennis ball placed inside a sock and attached to the back of the pajamas or nightgown. This approach seems to work for some patients with simple snoring.

• Tilting the head of the bed upward about 4 in (10 cm).

Complementary and alternative (CAM) approaches

There are three forms of alternative treatment that have been shown to be helpful in reducing primary snoring in patients with histories of nasal congestion or swollen tissues in the throat. The first is acupuncture. Treatments for snoring usually focus on acupuncture points on the stomach, arms, and legs associated with the production of excess mucus. Insertion of the acupuncture needles at these points is thought to stimulate the body to release the excess moisture or phlegm.

Homeopathy and aromatherapy also appear to benefit some patients whose snoring is related to colds, allergies, or sore throats. Homeopathic remedies for snoring are available as nose drops and throat sprays as well as the traditional pill formulations. Aromatherapy formulas for snoring typically contain marjoram oil, which may be used alone or combined with lavender and other herbs that clear the nasal passages. Some people find aromatherapy preparations helpful alongside mainstream treatments because their fragrance is pleasant and relaxing.

See also Tonsillectomy; Weight management.

Resources

BOOKS

American Psychiatric Association. *Diagnostic and Statistical Manual of Mental Disorders*, 4th edition, text revision, "Sleep Disorders.". Washington, DC: American Psychiatric Association, 2000.

"Disorders of the Oral Region." Section 9, Chapter 105 in *The Merck Manual of Diagnosis and Therapy*, edited by Mark H. Beers, M.D., and Robert Berkow, M.D. Whitehouse Station, NJ: Merck Research Laboratories, 1999.

Pelletier, Kenneth R., M.D. *The Best Alternative Medicine*, Part I, Chapter 5, "Acupuncture," and Chapter 8, "Homeopathy." New York: Simon & Schuster, 2002.

Price, Shirley. *Practical Aromatherapy*, 3rd ed. London, UK: Thorsons, 1994.

"Sleep Disorders." Section 14, Chapter 173 in *The Merck Manual of Diagnosis and Therapy*, edited by Mark H. Beers, M.D., and Robert Berkow, M.D. Whitehouse Station, NJ: Merck Research Laboratories, 1999.

PERIODICALS

Back, L. J., P. O. Tervahartiala, A. K. Piilonen, et al. "Bipolar Radiofrequency Thermal Ablation of the Soft Palate in Habitual Snorers Without Significant Desaturations Assessed by Magnetic Resonance Imaging." *American Jour-

nal of Respiratory and Critical Care Medicine* 166 (September 15, 2002): 865-871.

Blumen, M. B., S. Dahan, B. Fleury, et al. "Radiofrequency Ablation for the Treatment of Mild to Moderate Obstructive Sleep Apnea." *Laryngoscope* 112 (November 2002): 2086–2092.

Brietzke, S. E., and E. A. Mair. "Injection Snoreplasty: How to Treat Snoring Without All the Pain and Expense." *Otolaryngology and Head and Neck Surgery* 124 (May 2001): 503–510.

Cartwright, R., T. K. Venkatesan, D. Caldarelli, and F. Diaz. "Treatments for Snoring: A Comparison of Somnoplasty and an Oral Appliance." *Laryngoscope* 110 (October 2000): 1680–1683.

Fischer, Y., B. Hafner, and W. J. Mann. "Radiofrequency Ablation of the Soft Palate (Somnoplasty). A New Method in the Treatment of Habitual and Obstructive Snoring." [in German] *HNO* 48 (January 2000): 33–40.

Grontved, A. M., and P. Karup. "Complaints and Satisfaction After Uvulopalatopharyngoplasty." *Acta Otolaryngologica Supplementum* 543 (2000): 190–192.

Hessel, N. S., and N. de Vries. "Diagnostic Workup of Socially Unacceptable Snoring. II. Sleep Endoscopy." *European Archives of Oto-Rhino-Laryngology* 259 (March 2002): 158–161.

Kamami, Y. V. "Laser CO_2 for Snoring. Preliminary Results." *Acta Oto-Rhino-Laryngologica Belgica* 44 (1990): 451–456.

Kyrmizakis, D. E., C. E. Papadakis, J. G. Bizakis, et al. "Sucralfate Alleviating Post-Laser-Assisted Uvulopalatoplasty Pain." *American Journal of Otolaryngology* 22 (January-February 2001): 55–58.

Littner, Michael, M.D., Clete A. Kushida, M.D., Ph.D., Kristyna Hartse, Ph.D., et al. "Practice Parameters for the Use of Laser-Assisted Uvulopalatoplasty: An Update for 2000." *Sleep* 24 (May 2001): 603–609.

Loth, S., B. Petruson, L. Wiren, and L. Wilhelmsen. "Evaluation of the Quality of Life of Male Snorers Using the Nottingham Health Profile." *Acta Oto-Laryngologica* 118 (September 1998): 723–727.

Morgan, Charles E., M.D., and Kenneth Johnson, M.D. "Snoring and Obstructive Sleep Apnea, Surgery." *eMedicine*, May 20, 2002 [cited May 10, 2003]. <http://www.emedicine.com/ent/topic370.htm>.

Nuñez-Fernandez, David, M.D., and Manuel Fernandez-Muradas, M.D. "Snoring and Obstructive Sleep Apnea, Upper Airway Evaluation." *eMedicine*, June 6, 2002 [cited May 10, 2003]. <http://www.emedicine.com/ent/topic410.htm>.

O'Brien, L. M., C. R. Holbrook, C. B. Mervis, et al. "Sleep and Neurobehavioral Characteristics of 5- to 7-Year-Old Children with Parentally Reported Symptoms of Attention-Deficit/Hyperactivity Disorder." *Pediatrics* 111 (March 2003): 554–563.

O'Connor, G. T., B. K. Lind, E. T. Lee, et al. "Variation in Symptoms of Sleep-Disordered Breathing with Race and Ethnicity: The Sleep Heart Health Study." *Sleep* 26 (February 1, 2003): 74–79.

KEY TERMS

Continuous positive airway pressure (CPAP)—A ventilation device that blows a gentle stream of air into the nose during sleep to keep the airway open.

Deviated septum—An abnormal configuration of the cartilage that divides the two sides of the nose. It can cause breathing problems if left uncorrected.

Injection snoreplasty—A technique for reducing snoring by injecting a chemical that forms scar tissue near the base of the uvula, helping to anchor it and reduce its fluttering or vibrating during sleep.

Obstructive sleep apnea (OSA)—A potentially life-threatening condition characterized by episodes of breathing cessation during sleep alternating with snoring or disordered breathing. The low levels of oxygen in the blood of patients with OSA may eventually cause heart problems or stroke.

Palate—The roof of the mouth.

Polysomnography—A test administered in a sleep laboratory to analyze heart rate, blood circulation, muscle movement, brain waves, and breathing patterns during sleep.

Primary snoring—Simple snoring; snoring that is not interrupted by episodes of breathing cessation.

Somnoplasty—A technique that uses radiofrequency signals to heat a thin needle inserted into the tissues of the soft palate. The heat from the needle shrinks the tissues, thus enlarging the patient's airway. Somnoplasty is also known as radiofrequency volumetric tissue reduction (RFVTR).

Uvula—A triangular piece of tissue that hangs from the roof of the mouth above the back of the tongue. Primary snoring is often associated with fluttering or vibrating of the uvula during sleep.

Uvulopalatopharyngoplasty (UPPP)—An operation to remove the tonsils and other excess tissue at the back of the throat to prevent it from closing the airway during sleep.

Raphaelson, M., and T. S. Hakim. "Diagnosing Sleep Apnea in Dental Patients." *Dental Clinics of North America 45 (October 2001): 797–816.*

Rose, E., R. Staats, J. Schulte-Monting, et al. "Long-Term Compliance with an Oral Protrusive Appliance in Patients with Obstructive Sleep Apnoea." [in German] *Deutsche medizinische Wochenschrift* 127 (June 7, 2002): 1245– 1249.

Ryan, C. F., and L. L. Love. "Unpredictable Results of Laser Assisted Uvulopalatoplasty in the Treatment of Obstructive Sleep Apnoea." *Thorax* 55 (May 2000): 399–404.

Scher, A. I., R. B. Lipton, and W. F. Stewart. "Habitual Snoring as a Risk Factor for Chronic Daily Headache." *Neurology* 60 (April 22, 2003): 1366–1368.

Seemann, R. P., J. C. DiToppa, M. A. Holm, and J. Hanson. "Does Laser-Assisted Uvulopalatoplasty Work? An Objective Analysis Using Pre- and Postoperative Polysomnographic Studies." *Journal of Otolaryngology* 30 (August 2001): 212–215.

Truelson, John M., MD, and D. Heath Roberts, DDS. "Snoring and Obstructive Sleep Apnea, Prosthetic Management." *eMedicine*, April 15, 2002 [cited May 10, 2003]. <http://www.emedicine.com/ent/topic498.htm>.

Woodson, B. T., A. Derowe, M. Hawke, et al. "Pharyngeal Suspension Suture with Repose Bone Screw for Obstructive Sleep Apnea." *Otolaryngology and Head and Neck Surgery* 122 (March 2000): 395–401.

ORGANIZATIONS

American Academy of Medical Acupuncture (AAMA). 4929 Wilshire Boulevard, Suite 428, Los Angeles, CA 90010. (323) 937-5514. <http://www.medicalacupuncture.org>.

American Academy of Otolaryngology, Head and Neck Surgery, Inc. One Prince Street, Alexandria, VA 22314-3357. (703) 836-4444. <http://www.entnet.org>.

American Academy of Sleep Medicine (AASM). One Westbrook Corporate Center, Suite 920, Westchester, IL 60154. (708) 492-0930. <http://www.aasmnet.org>.

American Dental Association. 211 East Chicago Avenue, Chicago, IL 60611. (312) 440-2500. <http://www.ada.org>.

American Sleep Apnea Association (ASAA). 1424 K Street NW, Suite 302, Washington, DC 20005. (202) 293-3650. <http://www.sleepapnea.org>.

National Center on Sleep Disorders Research (NCSDR). Two Rockledge Centre, Suite 10038, 6701 Rockledge Drive, MSC 7920, Bethesda, MD 20892-7920. (301) 435-0199. <http://www.nhlbi.nih.gov/about/ncsdr/index.htm>.

OTHER

American Sleep Apnea Association (ASAA). *Considering Surgery for Snoring?* [May 10, 2003]. <http://www.sleepapnea.org/snoring.html>.

National Heart, Lung, and Blood Institute (NHLBI). *Facts About Sleep Apnea.* NIH Publication No. 95-3798 [cited April 13, 2003]. <http://www.nhlbi.nih.gov/health/public/sleep/sleepapn.htm>.

Rebecca Frey, Ph.D.

Sodium test *see* **Electrolyte tests**

Somnoplasty *see* **Snoring surgery**

Sphygmomanometer

Definition

A sphygmomanometer is a device for measuring blood pressure.

Purpose

The sphygmomanometer is designed to monitor blood pressure by measuring the force of the blood in the heart where the pressure is greatest. This occurs during the contraction of the ventricles, when blood is pumped from the heart to the rest of the body (systolic pressure). The minimal force is also measured. This occurs during the period when the heart is relaxed between beats and pressure is lowest (diastolic pressure).

A sphygmomanometer is used to establish a baseline at a healthcare encounter and on admission to a hospital. Checking blood pressure is also performed to monitor the effectiveness of medication and other methods to control hypertension, and as a diagnostic aid to detect various diseases and abnormalities.

Description

A sphygmomanometer consists of a hand bulb pump, a unit that displays the blood pressure reading, and an inflatable cuff that is usually wrapped around a person's upper arm. Care should be taken to ensure that the cuff size is appropriate for the person whose blood pressure is being taken. This improves the accuracy of the reading. Children and adults with smaller or larger than average-sized arms require special sized cuffs appropriate for their needs. A **stethoscope** is also used in conjunction with the sphygmomanometer to hear the blood pressure sounds. Some devices have the stethoscope already built in.

A sphygmomanometer can be used or encountered in a variety of settings:

• home

• hospital

• primary care clinic or professional office

• ambulance

• dental office

• pharmacy and other retail establishment

There are three types of equipment in common use for monitoring blood pressure.

• A mercury-based unit has a manually inflatable cuff attached by tubing to the unit that is calibrated in millimeters of mercury. During **blood pressure measurement**, the unit must be kept upright on a flat surface and the gauge read at eye level. Breakage of the unit may cause dangerous mercury contamination and would require specialist removal for disposal. Due to the hazards of mercury, the use of mercury-based sphygmomanometers has declined sharply since 2000.

• An aneroid unit is mercury free and consists of a cuff that can be applied with one hand for self-testing; a stethoscope that is built in or attached; and a valve that inflates and deflates automatically with the data displayed on an easy-to-read gauge that will function in any position. The unit is sensitive and if dropped may require recalibration.

• An automatic unit is also mercury-free and is typically battery-operated. It has a cuff that can be applied with one hand for self-testing, and a valve that automatically inflates and deflates. Units with manual inflation are also available. The reading is displayed digitally and a stethoscope is not required. This is useful for persons who are hearing-impaired, for emergency situations when staff is limited, and for automatic input into instruments for storage or graphical display. A wrist monitor is also available for home testing. Some more expensive models also remember and print out recordings. The automatic units tend to be more portable than bulkier mercury devices.

Operation

The flow, resistance, quality, and quantity of blood circulating through the heart and the condition of the arterial walls are all factors that influence blood pressure. If blood flow in the arteries is restricted, the reading will be higher.

Blood pressure should be routinely checked every one to two years. It can be checked at any time but is best measured when a person has been resting for at least five minutes, so that exertion prior to the test will not unduly influence the outcome of the reading.

To record blood pressure, the person should be seated with one arm bent slightly, and the arm bare or with the sleeve loosely rolled up. With an aneroid or automatic unit, the cuff is placed level with the heart and wrapped around the upper arm, one inch above the elbow. Following the manufacturer's guidelines, the cuff is inflated and then deflated while an attendant records the reading.

If the blood pressure is monitored manually, a cuff is placed level with the heart and wrapped firmly but not tightly around the arm one inch above the elbow over the brachial artery. Wrinkles in the cuff should be smoothed out. Positioning a stethoscope over the brachial artery in front of the elbow with one hand and listening through the earpieces, the health professional inflates the cuff well above normal levels (to about 200 mm Hg), or until no sound is heard. Alternatively, the cuff should be inflated 10 mm Hg above the last sound heard. The valve in the pump is slowly opened. Air is allowed to escape no faster than 5 mm Hg per second to deflate the pressure in the cuff to the point where a clicking sound is heard over the brachial artery. The reading of the gauge at this point is recorded as the systolic pressure. The sounds continue as the pressure in the cuff is released and the flow of blood through the artery is no longer blocked. At this point, the noises are no longer heard. The reading of the gauge at this point is noted as the diastolic pressure. "Lub-dub" is the sound produced by the normal heart as it beats. Every time this sound is detected, it means that the heart is contracting once. The sounds are created when the heart valves click to close. When one hears "lub," the atrioventricular valves are closing. The "dub" sound is produced by the pulmonic and aortic valves.

With children, the clicking sound does not disappear but changes to a soft muffled sound. Because sounds continue to be heard as the cuff deflates to zero, the reading of the gauge at the point where the sounds change is recorded as the diastolic pressure.

Blood pressure readings are recorded with the systolic pressure first, then the diastolic pressure (e.g. 120/70).

Interpretation

Blood pressure readings must be interpreted in relation to a person's age, physical condition, medical history, and medications being used.

Maintenance

Devices should be checked and calibrated annually by a qualified technician to ensure accurate readings. This is especially important for automatic sphygmomanometers.

Normal results

One elevated reading does not mean that hypertension is present. Repeated measurements may be required if hypertension is suspected. The blood pressure measurement is recorded and compared with normal ranges for an individual's age and medical condition, and a decision is made on whether any further medical intervention is required.

Resources

BOOKS

Bickley, L. S., P. G. Szilagyi, and J. G. Stackhouse. *Bates' Guide to Physical Examination & History Taking.* 8th ed. Philadelphia: Lippincott Williams & Wilkins, 2002.

Chan, P. D., and P. J. Winkle. *History and Physical Examination in Medicine.* 10th ed. New York: Current Clinical Strategies, 2002.
Seidel, Henry M. *Mosby's Physical Examination Handbook.* 4th ed. St. Louis: Mosby-Year Book, 2003.
Swartz, Mark A., and William Schmitt. *Textbook of Physical Diagnosis: History and Examination.* 4th ed. Philadelphia: Saunders, 2001.

PERIODICALS

Doyle, L. W., B. Faber, C. Callanan, and R. Morley. "Blood Pressure in Late Adolescence and Very Low Birth Weight." *Pediatrics* 111, no. 2 (2003): 252–257.
Jones, D. W., L. J. Appel, S. G. Sheps, E. J. Roccella, and C. Lenfant. "Measuring Blood Pressure Accurately: New and Persistent Challenges." *Journal of the American Medical Association* 289, no. 8 (2003): 1027–1030.
O'Brien, E. "Demise of the Mercury Sphygmomanometer and the Dawning of a New Era in Blood Pressure Measurement." *Blood Pressure Monitoring* 8, no. 1 (2003): 19–21.
Pickering, T. G. "What Will Replace the Mercury Sphygmomanometer?" *Blood Pressure Monitoring* 8, no. 1 (2003): 23–25.

ORGANIZATIONS

American Academy of Family Physicians. 11400 Tomahawk Creek Parkway, Leawood, KS 66211-2672. (913) 906-6000. <fp@aafp.org>. <http://www.aafp.org>.
American Academy of Pediatrics. 141 Northwest Point Boulevard, Elk Grove Village, IL 60007-1098. (847) 434-4000. Fax: (847) 434-8000. <kidsdoc@aap.org>. <http://www.aap.org/default.htm>.
American College of Physicians. 190 N. Independence Mall West, Philadelphia, PA 19106-1572. (800) 523-1546, x 2600 or (215) 351-2600. <http://www.acponline.org>.
American Medical Association. 515 N. State Street, Chicago, IL 60610. (312) 464-5000. <http://www.ama-assn.org>.

OTHER

"High Blood Pressure." Medline Plus Health Information. [cited March 12, 2003]. <http://www.nlm.nih.gov/medlineplus/highbloodpressure.html>.

"Hypertension." The Franklin Institute Online. [cited March 12, 2003]. <http://sln.fi.edu/biosci/healthy/pressure.html>.
"Your Guide to Lowering High Blood Pressure." National Heart, Lung and Blood Institute (National Institutes of Health). [cited March 12, 2003]. <http://www.nhlbi.nih.gov/hbp>

L. Fleming Fallon, Jr., MD, DrPH

Sphygmomanometry *see* **Blood pressure measurement**

Spina bifida surgery *see* **Meningocele repair**

Spinal fluid analysis *see* **Cerebrospinal fluid (CSF) analysis**

Spinal fusion

Definition

Spinal fusion is a procedure that promotes the fusing, or growing together, of two or more vertebrae in the spine.

Purpose

Spinal fusion is performed to:

• Straighten a spine deformed by scoliosis, neuromuscular disease, cerebral palsy, or other disorder.

• Prevent further deformation.

• Support a spine weakened by infection or tumor.

• Reduce or prevent pain from pinched or injured nerves.

• Compensate for injured vertebrae or disks.

The goal of spinal fusion is to unite two or more vertebrae to prevent them from moving independently of each other. This may be done to improve posture, increase ability to ventilate the lungs, prevent pain, or treat spinal instability and reduce the risk of nerve damage.

Demographics

According to the American Academy of Orthopaedic Surgeons, approximately a quarter-million spinal fusions are performed each year, half on the upper and half on the lower spine.

Description

Spinal anatomy

The spine is a series of individual bones called vertebrae, separated by cartilaginous disks. The spine is

composed of seven cervical (neck) vertebrae, 12 thoracic (chest) vertebrae, five lumbar (lower back) vertebrae, and the fused vertebrae in the sacrum and coccyx that help to form the hip region.

While the shapes of individual vertebrae differ among these regions, each is essentially a short hollow tube containing the bundle of nerves known as the spinal cord. Individual nerves, such as those carrying messages to the arms or legs, enter and exit the spinal cord through gaps between vertebrae.

The spinal disks act as shock absorbers, cushioning the spine, and preventing individual bones from contacting each other. Disks also help to hold the vertebrae together.

The weight of the upper body is transferred through the spine to the hips and the legs. The spine is held upright through the work of the back muscles, which are attached to the vertebrae.

While the normal spine has no side-to-side curve, it does have a series of front-to-back curves, giving it a gentle "S" shape. The spine curves in at the lumbar region, back out at the thoracic region, and back in at the cervical region.

Surgery for scoliosis, neuromuscular disease, and cerebral palsy

Abnormal side-to-side curvature of the spine is termed scoliosis. An excessive lumbar curve is termed lordosis, and an excessive thoracic curve is kyphosis. "Idiopathic" scoliosis is the most common form of scoliosis; it has no known cause.

Scoliosis and other curves can be caused by neuromuscular disease, including Duchenne muscular dystrophy. Progressive and perhaps uneven weakening of the spinal muscles leads to gradual inability to support the spine in an upright position. The weight of the upper body then begins to collapse the spine, inducing a curve. In addition to pain and disfigurement, severe scoliosis prevents adequate movement of air into and out of the lungs. Scoliosis also occurs in cerebral palsy, due to excess and imbalanced muscle activity pulling on the spine unevenly.

Spinal fusion

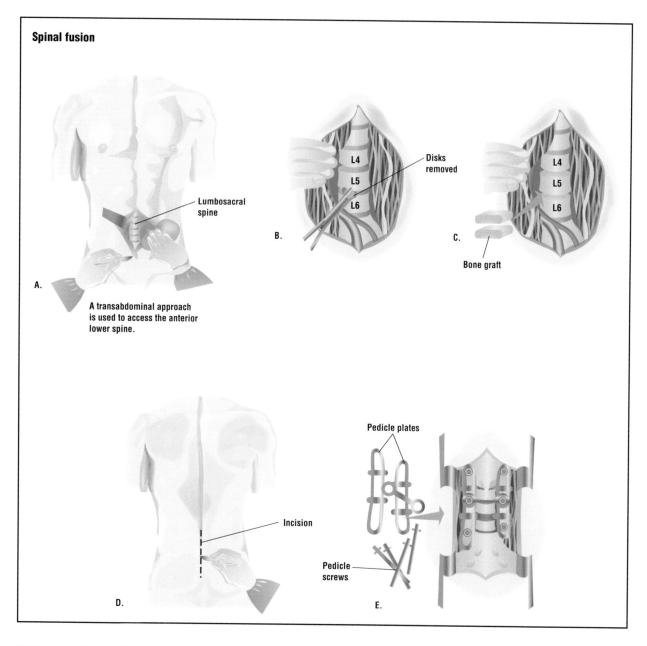

In this spinal fusion, the surgeon makes an incision in the lower abdomen to access the lumbosacral spine (A). The disks between the vertebrae are removed (B), and bone grafts are inserted into the spaces (C). Then another incision is made in the patient's back (D), and the vertebrae are exposed and fixed to the pedicle plates and screws (E) *(Illustration by GGS Inc.)*

Idiopathic scoliosis, which occurs most often in adolescent girls, is usually managed with a brace that wraps the abdomen and chest, allowing the spine to develop straight. Spinal fusion is indicated in patients whose curves are more severe or are progressing rapidly. The indication for surgery in cerebral palsy is similar to that for idiopathic scoliosis.

Spinal fusion in Duchenne muscular dystrophy is usually indicated earlier than in otherwise healthy adolescents. This is because these patients lose ventilatory function rapidly through adolescence, making the surgery more dangerous as time passes. Surgery should occur before excess ventilatory function is lost.

Surgery for herniated disks, disk degeneration, and pain

As people age, their disks become less supple and more prone to damage. A herniated disk is one that has developed a bulge. The bulge can press against nerves located in the spinal cord or exiting from it, causing pain.

QUESTIONS TO ASK THE DOCTOR

- How long will hospitalization be necessary?
- Will patient-controlled analgesia (PCA) be used for pain?
- How soon can the normal regime of school or work be resumed?
- What outcome is expected?
- Is there an alternative to surgery?

Disks can also degenerate, losing mass and thickness, allowing vertebrae to contact each other. This can pinch nerves and cause pain. Disk-related pain is very common in the neck, which is subject to constant twisting forces, and the lower back, which experiences large compressive forces. In these cases, spinal fusion is employed to prevent the nerves from being damaged. The offending disk is removed at the same time. A fractured vertebra may also be treated with fusion to prevent it from causing future problems.

Sometimes, spinal fusion is used to treat back pain even when the anatomical source of the problem cannot be located. This is usually viewed as a last resort for intractable and disabling pain.

The spinal fusion operation

Spinal fusion is performed under general anesthesia. During the procedure, the target vertebrae are exposed. Protective tissue layers next to the bone are removed, and small chips of bone are placed next to the vertebrae. These bone chips can either be from the patient's hip or from a bone bank. The chips increase the rate of fusion. Using bone from the patient's hip (an autograft) is more successful than banked bone (an allograft), but it increases the stresses of surgery and loss of blood.

Fusion of the lumbar and thoracic vertebrae is done by approaching from the rear, with the patient lying face down. Cervical fusion is typically performed from the front, with the patient lying on his or her back.

Many spinal fusion patients also receive **spinal instrumentation**. During the fusion operation, a set of rods, wires, or screws will be attached to the spine. This instrumentation allows the spine to be held in place while the bones fuse. The alternative is an external brace applied after the operation.

An experimental treatment, called human recombinant bone morphogenetic protein-2, has shown promise for its ability to accelerate fusion rates without bone chips and instrumentation. This technique is only available through clinical trials at a few medical centers.

Spinal fusion surgery takes approximately four hours. The patient is intubated (tube placed in the trachea), and has an IV line and Foley (urinary) catheter in place. At the end of the operation, a drain is placed in the incision site to help withdraw fluids over the next several days. The fusion process is gradual and may not be completed for months after the operation.

Diagnosis/Preparation

A potential candidate for spinal fusion undergoes a long series of medical tests. In patients with scoliosis, x rays are taken over many months or years to track progress of the curve. Patients with disk herniation or degeneration may receive x rays, MRI studies, or other tests to determine the location and extent of injury.

Patients in good health may donate several units of their own blood in preparation for surgery. This may be done between six weeks and one week prior to the operation. The patient will probably be advised to take iron supplements to help replace lost iron in the donated blood. Sunburn or sores on the back should be avoided prior to surgery because they increase the risk of infection.

A variety of medical tests will be done shortly before surgery to ensure that the patient is in good health and prepared for the rigors of surgery. Blood and urine tests, x rays, and possibly photographs documenting the curvature will be done. An electroencephalogram (EEG) may be performed to test nerve function along the spine.

The patient will be admitted to the hospital the evening before surgery. No food is allowed after midnight, in order to clear the gastrointestinal tract, which will be immobilized by anesthesia.

Aftercare

The patient will stay in the hospital for four to six days after the operation.

Post-operative pain is managed by intravenous pain medication. Many centers use **patient-controlled analgesia** (PCA) pumps, which allow patients to control the timing of pain medication.

For several days after the operation, the patient is unable to eat or drink because of the lasting effects of the anesthesia on the bowels. Fluids and nutrition are delivered via the IV line.

The nurse helps the patient sit up several times per day, and assists with other needs as well. Physical therapy begins several days after the operation.

Most activities are restricted for several weeks. Strenuous activities such as bike riding or running are usually resumed after six to eight months. The surgical incision should be protected from sunburn for approximately one year to promote healing of the scar.

Risks

Spinal fusion carries a risk of nerve damage. Rarely, delayed paralysis can occur, probably from loss of oxygen to the spine during surgery. Infection may occur. Bone from the bone bank carries a small risk of infection with transmissible diseases from the bone donor. Anesthesia also poses risks. Unsuccessful fusion (pseudoarthrosis) may occur, leaving the patient with the same problem after the operation.

Normal results

Spinal fusion for scoliosis is usually very successful in partially or completely correcting the deformity. Spinal fusion for pain is less uniformly successful because the cause of the pain cannot always be completely identified.

Morbidity and mortality rates

Unsuccessful fusion may occur in 5–25% of patients. Neurologic injury occurs in less than 1–5% of patients. Infection occurs in 1–8%. Death occurs in less than 1% of patients.

Alternatives

Bracing and "watchful waiting" is the alternative to scoliosis surgery. Disk surgery without fusion is possible for some patients. Strengthening exercises and physical therapy may help some back pain patients avoid back surgery.

See also Bone grafting; Disk removal.

Resources

BOOKS

Neuwirth, M.D., Michael. *The Scoliosis Sourcebook.* New York: McGraw-Hill, 2001.

PERIODICALS

Robinson, Richard. "Setting the Record Straight." *Quest Magazine* 4, no.1 (1997). <http://www.mdausa.org/publications/Quest/q41scoliosis.html>

ORGANIZATIONS

National Scoliosis Foundation. (800) NSF-MYBACK (673-6922). <http://www.scoliosis.org>.

Richard Robinson

Spinal instrumentation

Definition

Spinal instrumentation is a method of keeping the spine rigid after **spinal fusion** surgery by surgically attaching hooks, rods, and wire to the spine in a way that redistributes the stresses on the bones and keeps them in proper alignment while the bones of the spine fuse.

Purpose

Spinal instrumentation is used to treat instability and deformity of the spine. Instability occurs when the spine no longer maintains its normal shape during movement. Such instability results in nerve damage, spinal deformities, and disabling pain. Scoliosis (scoliosis) is a side-to-side spinal curvature. Kyphosis is a front-to-back curvature of the upper spine, while lordosis is an excessive curve of the lower spine. More than one type of curve may be present.

Demographics

Spinal deformities may be caused by:

- birth defects
- fractures

• Marfan syndrome

• neurofibromatosis

• neuromuscular diseases

• severe injuries

• tumors

• idiopathic scoliosis (Idiopathic scoliosis is scoliosis of unknown origin. About 85% of cases occur in girls between the ages of 12 and 15 who are experiencing adolescent growth spurt.)

Description

Spinal instrumentation provides a stable, rigid column that encourages bones to fuse after spinal fusion surgery. Its purpose is to aid fusion. Without fusion, the metal will eventually fatigue and break, and so instrumentation is not itself a treatment for spine deformity.

Different types of spinal instrumentation are used to treat different spinal problems. Although the details of the insertion of rods, wires, screws, and hooks vary, the purpose of all spinal instrumentation is the same—to correct and stabilize the backbone while the bones of the spine fuse. The various instruments are all made of stainless steel, titanium, or titanium alloy.

The oldest form of spinal instrumentation is the Harrington rod. While it was simple in design, it required a long period of brace wearing after the operation, and did not allow segmental adjustment of correction. The Luque rod was developed to avoid the long postoperative bracing period. This system threads wires into the space within each vertebra. The risk of injury to the nerves and spinal cord is higher than with some other forms of instrumentation. Cotrel-Dubousset instrumentation uses hooks and rods in a cross-linked pattern to realign the spine and redistribute the biomechanical stress. The main advantage of Cotrel-Dubousset instrumentation is that because of the extensive cross-linking, the patient may not have to wear a cast or brace after surgery.

The disadvantage is the complexity of the operation and the number of hooks and cross-links that may fail.

Several newer systems use screws that are embedded into the portion of the vertebra called the pedicle. Pedicle screws avoid the need for threading wires, but carry the risk of migrating out of the bone and contacting the spinal cord or the aorta (the major blood vessel exiting the heart). During the late 1990s, pedicle screws were the subject of several high-profile lawsuits. The controversies have since subsided, and pedicle screws remain an indispensible part of the spinal instrumentation. Many operations today are performed with a mix of techniques, such as Luque rods in the lower back and hooks and screws up higher. A physician chooses the proper type of instrumentation based on the type of disorder, the age and health of the patient, and the physician's experience.

The surgeon strips the tissue away from the area to be fused. The surface of the bone is peeled away. A piece of bone is removed from the hip and placed along side the area to be fused. The stripping of the bone helps the bone graft to fuse.

After the fusion site is prepared, the rods, hooks, screws, and wires are inserted. There is much variation in how this is done based on the spinal instrumentation chosen. Once the rods are in place, the incision is closed.

Diagnosis/Preparation

Spinal fusion with spinal instrumentation is major surgery. The patient will undergo many tests to determine the nature and exact location of the back problem. These tests are likely to include

• x rays

• magnetic resonance imaging (MRI)

• computed tomography scans (CT scans)

• myleograms

In addition, the patient will undergo a battery of blood and urine tests, and possibly an electrocardiogram to provide the surgeon and anesthesiologist with information that will allow the operation to be performed safely. In Harrington rod instrumentation, the patient may be placed in **traction** or an upper body cast to stretch contracted muscles before surgery.

Aftercare

After surgery, the patient will be confined to bed. A catheter is inserted so that the patient can urinate without getting up. **Vital signs** are monitored, and the patient's position is changed frequently so that **bedsores** do not develop.

Recovery from spinal instrumentation can be a long arduous process. Movement is severely limited for a period of time. In certain types of instrumentation, the patient is put in a cast to allow the realigned bones to stay in position until healing takes place. This can be as long as six to eight months. Many patients will need to wear a brace after the cast is removed.

During the recovery period, the patient is taught respiratory exercises to help maintain respiratory function during the time of limited mobility. Physical therapists assist the patient in learning self-care and in performing strengthening and range-of-motion exercises. Length of hospital stay depends on the age and health of the patient, as well as the specific problem that was corrected. The patient can expect to remain under a physician's care for many months.

Risks

Spinal instrumentation carries a significant risk of nerve damage and paralysis. The skill of the surgeon can affect the outcome of the operation, so patients should look for a hospital and **surgical team** that has a lot of experience doing spinal procedures.

Since the hooks and rods of spinal instrumentation are anchored in the bones of the back, spinal instrumentation should not be performed on people with serious osteoporosis. To overcome this limitation, techniques are being explored that help anchor instrumentation in fragile bones.

After surgery there is a risk of infection or an inflammatory reaction due to the presence of the foreign material in the body. Serious infection of the membranes covering the spinal cord and brain can occur. In the long term, the instrumentation may move or break, causing nerve damage and requiring a second surgery. Some bone grafts do not heal well, lengthening the time the patient must spend in a cast or brace or necessitating additional surgery. Casting and wearing a brace may take an

emotional toll, especially on young people. Patients who have had spinal instrumentation must avoid contact sports, and, for the rest of their lives, eliminate situations that will abnormally put stress on their spines.

Normal results

Many young people with scoliosis heal with significantly improved alignment of the spine. Results of spinal instrumentation done for other conditions vary widely.

Morbidity and mortality rates

Mortality rate for spinal fusion surgery is less than 1%. Neurologic injury may occur in 1–5% of cases. Delayed paralysis is possible but rare.

Alternatives

Not all patients require instrumentation with their spinal fusion. For some patients, a rigid external brace can provide the required rigidity to allow the bones to fuse.

Resources

BOOKS

"Cotrel-Dubousset Spinal Instrumentation." In *Everything You Need to Know About Medical Treatments*. Springhouse, PA: Springhouse Corp., 1996.

"Harrington Rod." In *Everything You Need to Know About Medical Treatments*. Springhouse, PA: Springhouse Corp., 1996.

ORGANIZATIONS

National Scoliosis Foundation. 5 Cabot Place, Stoughton, MA 020724. (800) 673-6922. <http://www.scoliosis.org>

OTHER

Orthogate [cited July 1, 2003]. <http://owl.orthogate.org/>.

Tish Davidson, A.M.
Richard Robinson

Spinal tap *see* **Cerebrospinal fluid (CSF) analysis**

Spirometry tests

Definition

Spirometry is the measurement of air flow into and out of the lungs.

Description

Spirometry requires that the nose is pinched off as the patient breathes through a mouthpiece attached to the spirometer. The patient is instructed on how to breathe during the procedure. Three breathing maneuvers are practiced before recording the procedure, and the highest of three trials is used for evaluation of breathing. This procedure measures air flow by electronic or mechanical displacement principles, and uses a microprocessor and recorder to calculate and plot air flow.

The test produces a recording of the patient's ventilation under conditions involving both normal and maximal effort. The recording, called a spirogram, shows the volume of air moved and the rate at which it travels into and out of the lungs. Spirometry measures several lung capacities. Accurate measurement is dependent upon the patient's performing the appropriate maneuver properly. The most common measurements are:

• Vital capacity (VC). This is the amount of air (in liters) moved out of the lung during normal breathing. The patient is instructed to breathe in and out normally to attain full expiration. Vital capacity is usually about 80% of the total lung capacity. Because of the elastic nature of the lungs and surrounding thorax, a small volume of air will remain in the lungs after full exhalation. This volume is called the residual volume (RV).

• Forced vital capacity (FVC). After breathing out normally to full expiration, the patient is instructed to breathe in with a maximal effort and then exhale as forcefully and rapidly as possible. The FVC is the volume of air that is expelled into the spirometer following a maximum inhalation effort.

• Forced expiratory volume (FEV). At the start of the FVC maneuver, the spirometer measures the volume of air delivered through the mouthpiece at timed intervals of 0.5, 1.0, 2.0, and 3.0 seconds. The sum of these measurements normally constitutes about 97% of the FVC measurement. The most commonly used FEV measurement is FEV-1, which is the volume of air exhaled into the mouthpiece in one second. The FEV-1 should be at least 70% of the FVC.

• Forced expiratory flow 25–75% (FEF 25–75). This is a calculation of the average flow rate over the center portion of the forced expiratory volume recording. It is determined from the time in seconds at which 25% and 75% of the vital capacity is reached. The volume of air exhaled in liters per second between these two times is the FEF 25–75. This value reflects the status of the medium and small sized airways.

• Maximal voluntary ventilation (MVV). This maneuver involves the patient breathing as deeply and as rapidly as possible for 15 seconds. The average air flow (liters per second) indicates the strength and endurance of the respiratory muscles.

Normal values for FVC, FEV, FEF, and MVV are dependent on the patient's age, gender, and height.

Purpose

Spirometry is the most commonly performed pulmonary function test (PFT). The test can be performed at the bedside, in a physician's office, or in a pulmonary laboratory. It is often the first test performed when a problem with lung function is suspected. Spirometry may also be suggested by an abnormal x ray, arterial blood gas analysis, or other diagnostic pulmonary test result. The National Lung Health Education Program recommends that regular spirometry tests be performed on persons over 45 years old who have a history of smoking. Spirometry tests are also recommended for persons with a family history of lung disease, chronic respiratory ailments, and advanced age.

Spirometry measures ventilation, the movement of air into and out of the lungs. The spirogram will identify two different types of abnormal ventilation patterns, obstructive and restrictive.

Common causes of an obstructive pattern are cystic fibrosis, asthma, bronchiectasis, bronchitis, and emphysema. These conditions may be collectively referred to by using the acronym CABBE. Chronic bronchitis, emphysema, and asthma result in dyspnea (difficulty breathing) and ventilation deficiency, a condition known as chronic obstructive pulmonary disease (COPD). COPD is the fourth leading cause of death among Americans.

Common causes of a restrictive pattern are pneumonia, heart disease, pregnancy, lung fibrosis, pneumothorax (collapsed lung), and pleural effusion (compression caused by chest fluid).

Obstructive and restrictive patterns can be identified on spirographs using both a "y" and "x" axis. Volume (liters) is plotted on the y-axis versus time (seconds) on the x-axis. A restrictive pattern is characterized by a normal shape showing reduced volumes for all parameters. The reduction in volumes indicates the severity of the disease. An obstructive pattern produces a spirogram with an abnormal shape. Inspiration volume is reduced. The volume of air expelled is normal but the air flow rate is slower, causing an elongated tail to the FVC.

A flow-volume loop spirogram is another way of displaying spirometry measurements. This requires the FVC maneuver followed by a forced inspiratory volume (FIV). Flow rate in liters per second is plotted on the y-axis and volume (liters) is plotted on the x-axis. The expiration phase is shown on top and the inspiration phase on the bottom. The flow-volume loop spirogram is helpful in diagnosing upper airway obstruction, and can differentiate some types of restrictive patterns.

Some conditions produce specific signs on the spirogram. Irregular inspirations with rapid frequency are caused by hyperventilation associated with stress. Diffuse fibrosis of the lung causes rapid breathing of reduced volume, which produces a repetitive pattern known as the penmanship sign. Serial reduction in the FVC peaks indicates air trapped inside the lung. A notch and reduced volume in the early segments of the FVC is consistent with airway collapse. A rise at the end of expiration is associated with airway resistance.

Spirometry is used to assess lung function over time, and often to evaluate the efficacy of bronchodilator inhalers such as albuterol. It is important for the patient to refrain from using a bronchodilator prior to the evaluation. Spirometry is performed before and after inhaling the bronchodilator. In general, a 12% or greater improvement in both FVC and FEV-1, or an increase in FVC by 0.2 liters, is considered a significant improvement for an adult patient.

Precautions

The patient should inform the physician of any medications he or she is taking, or of any medical conditions that are present; these factors may affect the validity of the test. The patient's smoking habits and history should be thoroughly documented. The patient must be able to understand and respond to instructions for the breathing maneuvers. Therefore, the test may not be appropriate

---

> ## QUESTIONS
> ## TO ASK THE DOCTOR
>
> - What preparation is needed before the test?
> - What results are expected?
> - When will the results be available?
> - What are the risks of the test in this particular case?

---

for very young, unresponsive, or physically impaired persons.

Spirometry is contraindicated in patients whose condition will be aggravated by forced breathing, including:

- hemoptysis (spitting up blood from the lungs or bronchial tubes)
- pneumothorax (free air or gas in the pleural cavity)
- recent heart attack
- unstable angina
- aneurysm (cranial, thoracic, or abdominal)
- thrombotic condition (such as clotting within a blood vessel)
- recent thoracic or abdominal surgery
- nausea or vomiting

The test should be terminated if the patient shows signs of significant head, chest, or abdominal pain while the procedure is in progress.

Spirometry is dependent upon the patient's full compliance with breathing instructions, especially his or her willingness to extend a maximal effort at forced breathing. Therefore, the patient's emotional state must be considered.

Preparation

The patient's age, gender, and race are recorded, and height and weight are measured before the procedure begins. The patient should not have eaten heavily within three hours of the test. He or she should be instructed to wear loose-fitting clothing over the chest and abdominal area. The respiratory therapist or other testing personnel should explain and demonstrate the breathing maneuvers to the patient. The patient should practice breathing into the mouthpiece until he or she is able to duplicate the maneuvers successfully on two consecutive attempts.

Aftercare

In most cases, special care is not required following spirometry. Occasionally, a patient may become light-

KEY TERMS

Bronchodilator—A drug, usually self-administered by inhalation, that dilates the airways.

Forced expiratory volume (FEV)—The volume of air exhaled from the beginning of expiration to a set time (usually 0.5, 1, 2, and 3 seconds).

Forced vital capacity (FVC)—The volume of air that can be exhaled forceably after a maximal inspiration.

Hemoptysis—Spitting up of blood derived from the lungs or bronchial tubes as a result of pulmonary or bronchial hemorrhage.

Thrombosis—Formation or presence of a thrombus; clotting within a blood vessel that may cause infarction of tissues supplied by the vessel.

Thrombotic—Relating to, caused by, or characterized by thrombosis.

Vital capacity (VC)—The volume of air that can be exhaled following a full inspiration.

headed or dizzy. Such patients should be asked to rest or lie down, and should not be discharged until after the symptoms subside. In rare cases, the patient may experience pneumothorax, intracranial hypertension, chest pain, or uncontrolled coughing. In such cases, additional care directed by a physician may be required.

Normal results

The results of spirometry tests are compared to predicted values based on the patient's age, gender, and height. For example, a young adult in good health is expected to have the following FEV values:

- FEV-0.5—50-60% of FVC
- FEV-1—75-85% of FVC
- FEV-2—95% of FVC
- FEV-3—97% of FVC

In general, a normal result is 80–100% of the predicted value. Abnormal values are:

- mild lung dysfunction—60–79%
- moderate lung dysfunction—40–59%
- severe lung dysfunction—below 40%

Resources

BOOKS

Braunwald, Eugene et al., editors. *Harrison's Principles of Internal Medicine.* Philadelphia: McGraw-Hill, 2001.

PERIODICALS

Blonshine, S. and J.B. Fink. "Spirometry: Asthma and COPD Guidelines Creating Opportunities for RTs." *AARC Times* (January 2000): 43-7.

ORGANIZATIONS

National Lung Health Education Program (NLHEP). 1850 High Street, Denver, CO 80218. <http://www.nlhep.org>.

OTHER

Gary, T., et al. "Office Spirometry for Lung Health Assessment in Adults: A Consensus Statement for the National Lung Health Education Program." (March 2000): 1146-61.

National Institutes of Health. [cited April 4, 2003] <http://www.nlm.nih.gov/medlineplus/encyclopedia.html>.

"Spirometry—AARC Clinical Practice Guide." American Association for Respiratory Care. 1130 Ables Lane, Dallas, TX 75229. [cited April 4, 2003] <http://www.muhealth.org/~shrp/rtwww/rcweb/aarc/spirocpg.html>.

Robert Harr
Paul Johnson
Mark A. Best

Spleen removal *see* **Splenectomy**

Splenectomy

Definition

A splenectomy is the total or partial surgical removal of the spleen, an organ that is part of the lymphatic system.

Purpose

The human spleen is a dark purple bean-shaped organ located in the upper left side of the abdomen just behind the bottom of the rib cage. In adults, the spleen is about 4.8 X 2.8 X 1.6 in (12 X 7 X 4 cm) in size, and weighs about 4–5 oz (113–14 g). The spleen plays a role in the immune system of the body. It also filters foreign substances from the blood and removes worn-out blood cells. The spleen regulates blood flow to the liver and sometimes stores blood cells— a function known as sequestration. In healthy adults, about 30% of blood platelets are sequestered in the spleen.

Splenectomies are performed for a variety of different reasons and with different degrees of urgency. Most splenectomies are done after a patient has been diagnosed with hypersplenism. Hypersplenism is not a specific disease but a syndrome (group or cluster of symp-

Splenectomy

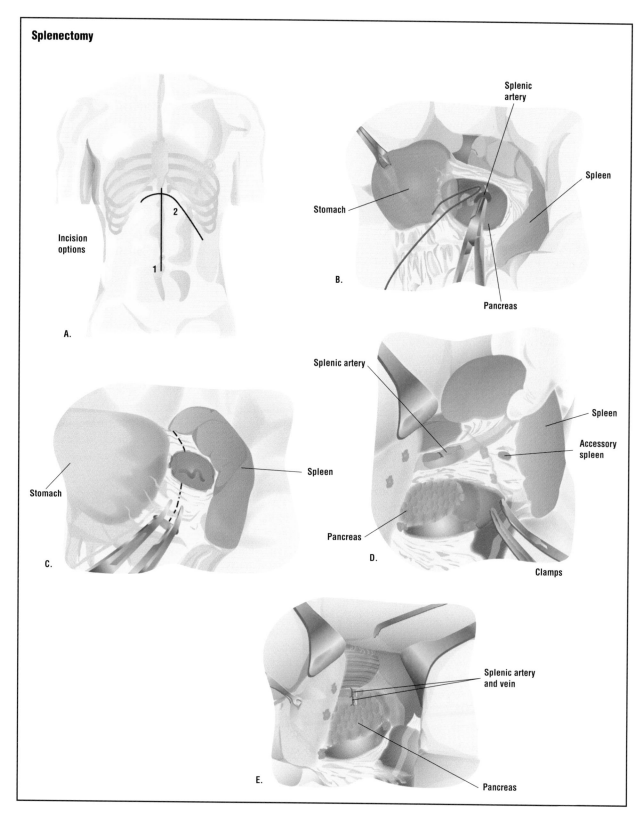

A.

Incision options

1
2

B.

Stomach

Splenic artery

Spleen

Pancreas

C.

Stomach

Spleen

D.

Splenic artery

Spleen

Accessory spleen

Pancreas

Clamps

E.

Splenic artery and vein

Pancreas

There are two options for accessing the spleen for a splenectomy (A, 1 and 2). After the abdomen is entered, the spleen is located, and the artery leading to it is tied off (B). The ligament connecting the stomach and spleen is cut (C), as is the ligament connecting the spleen and colon (D). This frees the spleen for removal (E). *(Illustration by GGS Inc.)*

toms) that may be associated with different disorders. Hypersplenism is characterized by enlargement of the spleen (splenomegaly), defects in the blood cells, and an abnormally high turnover of blood cells. It is almost always associated with such specific disorders as cirrhosis of the liver or certain cancers. The decision to perform a splenectomy depends on the severity and prognosis of the disease that is causing the hypersplenism.

Splenectomy always required

There are two diseases for which a splenectomy is the only treatment—primary cancers of the spleen and a blood disorder called hereditary spherocytosis (HS). In HS, the absence of a specific protein in the red blood cell membrane leads to the formation of relatively fragile cells that are easily damaged when they pass through the spleen. The cell destruction does not occur elsewhere in the body and ends when the spleen is removed. HS can appear at any age, even in newborns, although doctors prefer to put off removing the spleen until the child is five to six years old.

Splenectomy usually required

There are some disorders for which a splenectomy is usually recommended. They include:

• Immune (idiopathic) thrombocytopenic purpura (ITP). ITP is a disease in which platelets are destroyed by antibodies in the body's immune system. A splenectomy is the definitive treatment for this disease and is effective in about 70% of cases of chronic ITP.

• Trauma. The spleen can be ruptured by blunt as well as penetrating injuries to the chest or abdomen. Car accidents are the most common cause of blunt traumatic injury to the spleen.

• Abscesses. Abscesses of the spleen are relatively uncommon but have a high mortality rate.

• Rupture of the splenic artery. This artery sometimes ruptures as a complication of pregnancy.

• Hereditary elliptocytosis. This is a relatively rare disorder. It is similar to HS in that it is characterized by red blood cells with defective membranes that are destroyed by the spleen.

Splenectomy sometimes required

Other disorders may or may not necessitate a splenectomy. These include:

• Hodgkin's disease, a serious form of cancer that causes the lymph nodes to enlarge. A splenectomy is often performed in order to find out how far the disease has progressed.

• Autoimmune hemolytic disorders. These disorders may appear in patients of any age but are most common in adults over 50. The red blood cells are destroyed by antibodies produced by the patient's own body (autoantibodies).

• Myelofibrosis. Myelofibrosis is a disorder in which bone marrow is replaced by fibrous tissue. It produces severe and painful splenomegaly. A splenectomy does not cure myelofibrosis but may be performed to relieve pain caused by the swelling of the spleen.

• Thalassemia. Thalassemia is a hereditary form of anemia that is most common in people of Mediterranean origin. A splenectomy is sometimes performed if the patient's spleen has become painfully enlarged.

Demographics

In the United States, splenomegaly affects as many as 30% of full-term newborns and about 10% of healthy children. Approximately 3% of healthy first-year college students also have spleens that are large enough to be felt when a doctor palpates the abdomen. Some specific causes of splenomegaly are more common in certain racial or ethnic groups. For example, splenomegaly is a common complication of sickle cell disease in patients of African or Mediterranean ancestry. In other parts of the world, splenomegaly is frequently caused by malaria, schistosomiasis, and other infections in areas where these diseases are endemic.

Hereditary spherocytosis (HS) is a disorder is most common in people of northern European descent but has been found in all races. A family history of HS increases the risk of developing this disorder.

Immune thrombocytopenic purpura (ITP) is much more common in children, with male and female children being equally afflicted. Female predominance begins at puberty and continues in adult patients. Overall, 70% of patients with ITP are female; 72% of women diagnosed with ITP are over 40 years old.

Description

Complete splenectomy

REMOVAL OF ENLARGED SPLEEN. A splenectomy is performed under general anesthesia. The most common technique is used to remove greatly enlarged spleens. After the surgeon makes a cut (incision) in the abdomen, the artery to the spleen is tied to prevent blood loss and reduce the size of the spleen. Tying the splenic artery also keeps the spleen from further sequestration of blood cells. The surgeon detaches the ligaments holding the spleen in place and removes the organ. In many cases, tissue samples will be sent to a laboratory for analysis.

REMOVAL OF RUPTURED SPLEEN. When the spleen has been ruptured by trauma, the surgeon approaches the organ from its underside and ties the splenic artery before removing the ruptured organ.

Partial splenectomy

In some cases, the surgeon removes only part of the spleen. This procedure is considered by some to be a useful compromise that reduces pain caused by an enlarged spleen while leaving the patient less vulnerable to infection.

Laparoscopic splenectomy

Laparoscopic splenectomy, or removal of the spleen through several small incisions, has been performed more frequently in recent years. Laparoscopic surgery, which is sometimes called keyhole surgery, is done with smaller **surgical instruments** inserted through very short incisions, with the assistance of a tiny camera and video monitor. Laparoscopic procedures reduce the length of hospital stay, the level of postoperative pain, and the risk of infection. They also leave smaller scars.

As of 2003, however, a laparoscopic procedure is contraindicated if the patient's spleen is greatly enlarged. Most surgeons will not remove a spleen longer than 20 cm (as measured by a CT scan) by this method.

Diagnosis/Preparation

The most important part of a medical assessment in disorders of the spleen is the measurement of spleno-megaly. The normal spleen cannot be felt when the doctor palpates the patient's abdomen. A spleen that is large enough to be felt indicates splenomegaly. In some cases, the doctor will hear a dull sound when he or she thumps (percusses) the patient's abdomen near the ribs on the left side. Imaging studies that can be used to confirm splenomegaly include ultrasound tests, technetium-99m sulfur colloid imaging, and **CT scans**. The rate of

platelet or red blood cell destruction by the spleen can also be measured by tagging blood cells with radioactive chromium or platelets with radioactive indium.

Preoperative preparation for a splenectomy procedure usually includes:

- Correction of abnormalities of blood clotting and the number of red blood cells.
- Treatment of any infections.
- Control of immune reactions. Patients are usually given protective vaccinations about a month before surgery. The most common vaccines used are Pneumovax or Pnu-Imune 23 (against pneumococcal infections) and Meno-mune-A/C/Y/W-135 (against meningococcal infections).

Aftercare

Immediately following surgery, patients are given instructions for **incision care** and medications intended to prevent infection. Blood transfusions may be indicated for some patients to replace defective blood cells. The most important part of aftercare, however, is long-term caution regarding vulnerability to infection. Patients are asked to see their doctor at once if they have a fever or any other sign of infection, and to avoid travel to areas where exposure to malaria or similar diseases is likely. Children with splenectomies may be kept on antibiotic therapy until they are 16 years old. All patients can be given a booster dose of pneumococcal vaccine five to 10 years after undergoing a splenectomy.

Risks

The main risk of a splenectomy procedure is overwhelming bacterial infection, or postsplenectomy sepsis.

KEY TERMS

Computed tomography (CT) scan—An imaging technique that creates a series of pictures of areas inside the body, taken from different angles. The pictures are created by a computer linked to an x ray machine.

Embolization—A treatment in which foam, silicone, or other substance is injected into a blood vessel in order to close it off.

Endemic—Present in a specific population or geographical area at all times. Some diseases that may affect the spleen are endemic to certain parts of Africa or Asia.

Hereditary spherocytosis—A hereditary disorder that leads to a chronic form of anemia (too few red blood cells) due to an abnormality in the red blood cell membrane.

Idiopathic thrombocytopenia purpura (ITP)—A rare autoimmune disorder characterized by an acute shortage of platelets with resultant bruising and spontaneous bleeding.

Laparoscopy—A procedure in which a laparoscope (a thin lighted tube) is inserted through an incision in the abdominal wall to evaluate the presence or spread of disease. Tissue samples may be removed for biopsy.

Lymphatic system—The tissues and organs that produce and store cells that fight infection, together with the network of vessels that carry lymph. The organs and tissues in the lymphatic system include the bone marrow, spleen, thymus gland, and lymph nodes.

Palpate—To examine by means of touch.

Platelet—A disk-shaped structure found in blood that binds to fibrinogen at the site of a wound to begin the clotting process.

Sequestration—A process in which the spleen withdraws blood cells from the circulation and stores them.

Spleen—An organ that produces lymphocytes, filters the blood, stores blood cells and destroys those that are aging. It is located on the left side of the abdomen near the stomach.

Splenomegaly—Enlargement of the spleen.

This condition results from the body's decreased ability to clear bacteria from the blood, and lowered levels of a protein in blood plasma that helps to fight viruses (immunoglobulin M). The risk of dying from infection after undergoing a splenectomy is highest in children, especially in the first two years after surgery. The risk of postsplenectomy sepsis can be reduced by vaccinations before the operation. Some doctors also recommend a two-year course of penicillin following splenectomy, or long-term treatment with ampicillin.

Other risks associated with the procedure include inflammation of the pancreas and collapse of the lungs. In some cases, a splenectomy does not address the underlying causes of splenomegaly or other conditions. Excessive bleeding after the operation is an additional possible complication, particularly for patients with ITP. Infection of the incision immediately following surgery may also occur.

Normal results

Results depend on the reason for the operation. In blood disorders, the splenectomy will remove the cause of the blood cell destruction. Normal results for patients with an enlarged spleen are relief of pain and the complications of splenomegaly. It is not always possible, however, to predict which patients will respond well or to what degree.

Recovery from the operation itself is fairly rapid. Hospitalization is usually less than a week (one to two days for laparoscopic splenectomy), and complete healing usually occurs within four to six weeks. Patients are encouraged to return to such normal activities as showering, driving, climbing stairs, light lifting and work as soon as they feel comfortable. Some patients may return to work in a few days while others prefer to rest at home a little longer.

Morbidity and mortality rates

The outcome of the procedure varies with the underlying disease or the extent of other injuries. Rates of complete recovery from the surgery itself are excellent, in the absence of other severe injuries or medical problems.

Splenectomy for HS patients is usually delayed in children until the age of five to prevent unnecessary infections; reported outcomes are very good.

Studies of patients with ITP show that 80%–90% of children achieve spontaneous and complete remission in two to eight weeks. A small percentage develop chronic or persistent ITP, but 61% show complete remission by

15 years. No deaths in patients older than 15 have been attributed to ITP.

Alternatives

As of 2003 there are no medical alternatives to removing the spleen.

Splenic embolization is a surgical alternative to splenectomy that is used in some patients who are poor candidates for surgery. Embolization involves plugging or blocking the splenic artery with synthetic substances to shrink the size of the spleen. The substances that are injected during this procedure include polyvinyl alcohol foam, polystyrene, and silicone.

See also Gastroduodenostomy; Pancreatectomy.

Resources

BOOKS

Hiatt, J. R., Phillips, E. H., and L. Morgenstern, eds. *Surgical Diseases of the Spleen*. New York: Springer Verlag, 1997.

Wilkins, B. S., and D. H. Wright. *Illustrated Pathology of the Spleen*. Cambridge, UK: Cambridge University Press, 2000.

PERIODICALS

Al-Salem A. H., and Z. Nasserulla. "Splenectomy for Children with Thalassemia." *Internal Surgery* 87 (October-December 2002): 269-273.

Duperier, T., J. Felsherm, and F. Brody. "Laparoscopic Splenectomy for Evans Syndrome." *Surgical Laparoscopy, Endoscopy & Percutaneous Techniques* 13 (February 2003): 45-47.

Schwartz, J., M. D. Leber, S. Gillis, et al. "Long-Term Follow-Up After Splenectomy Performed for Immune Thrombocytopenic Purpura (ITP)." *American Journal of Hematology* 72 (February 2003): 94-98.

Svarch, E., I. Nordet, J. Valdes, et al. "Partial Splenectomy in Children with Sickle Cell Disease." *Haematologica* 88 (February 2003): 281-287.

ORGANIZATIONS

American College of Gastroenterology. 4900 B South 31st St., Arlington, VA 22206. (703) 820-7400. <www.acg.gi.org>

American Gastroenterological Association (AGA). 4930 Del Ray Avenue, Bethesda, MD 20814. (301) 654-2055. <www.gastro.org>

National Cancer Institute (NCI). NCI Public Inquiries Office, Suite 3036A, 6116 Executive Boulevard, MSC8322 Bethesda, MD 20892-8322. (800) 422-6237. <www.cancer.gov>

OTHER

The Body Homepage. *Spleen Cancer.* <www.thebody.com/Forums/AIDS/Cancer/Archive/othertypes/Q141422.html>.

Your surgery.com. *Splenectomy.* <www.yoursurgery.com/ProcedureDetails.cfm?BR=1&Proc=46>.

Teresa Norris, RN
Monique Laberge, Ph. D.

Stapedectomy

Definition

Stapedectomy is a surgical procedure in which the innermost bone (stapes) of the three bones (the stapes, the incus, and the malleus) of the middle ear is removed, and replaced with a small plastic tube surrounding a short length of stainless steel wire (a prosthesis). The operation was first performed in the United States in 1956.

Purpose

A stapedectomy is performed to improve the movement of sound to the inner ear. It is done to treat progressive hearing loss caused by otosclerosis, a condition in which spongy bone hardens around the base of the stapes. This condition fixes the stapes to the opening of the inner ear, so that the stapes no longer vibrates properly. Otosclerosis can also affect the malleus, the incus, and the bone that surrounds the inner ear. As a result, the transmission of sound to the inner ear is disrupted. Untreated otosclerosis eventually results in total deafness, usually in both ears.

Demographics

Otosclerosis affects about 10% of the United States population. It is an autosomal dominant disorder with variable penetrance. These terms mean that a child having one parent with otosclerosis has a 50% chance of inheriting the gene for the disorder, but that not everyone who has the gene will develop otosclerosis. In addition, some researchers think that the onset of the disorder is triggered when a person who has the gene for otosclerosis is infected with the measles virus. This hypothesis is supported by the finding that the incidence of otosclerosis has been steadily declining in countries with widespread measles vaccination.

Otosclerosis develops most frequently in people between the ages of 10 and 30. In most cases, both ears are affected; however, about 10–15% of patients diagnosed with otosclerosis have loss of hearing in only one ear. The disorder affects women more frequently than men by a ratio of 2:1. Pregnancy is a risk factor for onset or worsening of otosclerosis.

With regard to race, Caucasian and Asian Americans are more likely to develop otosclerosis than African Americans.

Description

A stapedectomy does not require any incisions on the outside of the body, as the entire procedure is performed through the ear canal. With the patient under local or general anesthesia, the surgeon opens the ear canal and folds the eardrum forward. Using an operating microscope, the surgeon is able to see the structures in detail, and evaluates the bones of hearing (ossicles) to confirm the diagnosis of otosclerosis.

Next, the surgeon separates the stapes from the incus; freed from the stapes, the incus and malleus bones can now move when pressed. A laser or small drill may be used to cut through the tendon and arch of the stapes bone, which is then removed from the middle ear.

The surgeon then opens the window that joins the middle ear to the inner ear and acts as the platform for the stapes bone. The surgeon directs the laser's beam at the window to make a tiny opening, and gently clips the prosthesis to the incus bone. A piece of tissue is taken from a small incision behind the ear lobe and used to help seal the hole in the window and around the prosthesis. The eardrum is then gently replaced and repaired, and held there by absorbable packing ointment or a gelatin sponge. The procedure usually takes about an hour and a half.

Good candidates for the surgery are those who have a fixed stapes from otosclerosis and a conductive hearing loss of at least 20 dB. Patients with a severe hearing loss might still benefit from a stapedectomy, if only to improve their hearing to the point where a hearing aid can be of help. The procedure can improve hearing in more than 90% of cases.

Diagnosis/Preparation

Diagnosis

Diagnosis of otosclerosis is based on a combination of the patient's family history, the patient's symptoms, and the results of hearing tests. Some patients notice only a gradual loss of hearing, but others experience dizziness, tinnitus (a sensation of buzzing, ringing, or hissing in the ears), or balance problems. The hearing tests should be administered by an ear specialist (audiologist or otologist) rather than the patient's family doctor. The examiner will need to determine whether the patient's hearing loss is conductive (caused by a lesion or disorder in the ear canal or middle ear) or sensorineural (caused by a disorder of the inner ear or the 8th cranial nerve).

Two tests that are commonly used to distinguish conductive hearing loss from sensorineural are Rinne's test and Weber's test. In Rinne's test, the examiner holds the stem of a vibrating tuning fork first against the mastoid bone and then outside the ear canal. A person with normal hearing will hear the sound as louder when it is held near the outer ear; a person with conductive hearing loss will hear the tone as louder when the fork is touching the bone.

In Weber's test, the vibrating tuning fork is held on the midline of the forehead and the patient is asked to indicate the ear in which the sound seems louder. A person with conductive hearing loss on one side will hear the sound louder in the affected ear.

A computed tomography (CT) scan or x ray study of the head may also be done to determine whether the patient's hearing loss is conductive or sensorineural.

Preparation

Patients are asked to notify the surgeon if they develop a cold or sore throat within a week of the scheduled surgery. The procedure should be postponed in order to minimize the risk of infection being carried from the upper respiratory tract to the ear.

Some surgeons prefer to use general anesthesia when performing a stapedectomy, although an increasing number are using local anesthesia. A sedative injection is given to the patient before surgery.

Aftercare

The patient is asked to have a friend or relative drive them home after the procedure. **Antibiotics** are given up to five days after surgery to prevent infection; packing and sutures are removed about a week after surgery.

It is important that the patient not put pressure on the ear for a few days after surgery. Blowing one's nose, lifting heavy objects, swimming underwater, descending rapidly in high-rise elevators, or taking an airplane flight should be avoided.

Right after surgery, the ear is usually quite sensitive, so the patient should avoid loud noises until the ear retrains itself to hear sounds properly.

It is extremely important that the patient avoid getting the ear wet until it has completely healed. Water in the ear could cause an infection; most seriously, water could enter the middle ear and cause an infection within the inner ear, which could then lead to a complete hearing loss. When taking a shower, and washing the hair, the patient should plug the ear with a cotton ball or lamb's wool ball, soaked in Vaseline. The surgeon should give specific instructions about when and how this can be done.

Usually, the patient may return to work and normal activities about a week after leaving the hospital, although if the patient's job involves heavy lifting, three weeks of home rest is recommend. Three days after surgery, the patient may fly in pressurized aircraft.

Risks

The most serious risk is an increased hearing loss, which occurs in about 1% of patients. Because of this risk, a stapedectomy is usually performed on only one ear at a time.

Less common complications include:

- temporary change in taste (due to nerve damage) or lack of taste
- perforated eardrum
- vertigo that may persist and require surgery
- damage to the chain of three small bones attached to the eardrum
- partial facial nerve paralysis
- ringing in the ears

Severe dizziness or vertigo may be a signal that there has been an incomplete seal between the fluids of the middle and inner ear. If this is the case, the patient needs immediate bed rest, an examination by the ear surgeon, and (rarely) an operation to reopen the eardrum to check the prosthesis.

Normal results

Most patients are slightly dizzy for the first day or two after surgery, and may have a slight headache. Hearing improves once the swelling subsides, the slight bleeding behind the ear drum dries up, and the packing is absorbed or removed, usually within two weeks. Hearing continues to get better over the next three months.

About 90% of patients will have markedly improved hearing following the procedure, while 8% experience only minor improvement. About half the patients who had tinnitus before surgery will experience significant relief within 6 weeks after the procedure.

QUESTIONS TO ASK THE DOCTOR

- What is your opinion of medication treatments for otosclerosis?
- Am I a candidate for a stapedotomy without prosthesis?
- What are the chances of my hearing getting worse if I postpone surgery?
- How many stapedectomies have you performed?
- What are the possible complications I could expect following a stapedectomy?

Morbidity and mortality rates

Stapedectomy is a very safe procedure with a relatively low rate of complications. With regard to hearing, about 2% of patients may have additional hearing loss in the operated ear following a stapedectomy; fewer than 1% lose hearing completely in the operated ear. About 9% of patients experience disturbances in their sense of taste. Infection, damage to the eardrum, and facial nerve palsy are rare complications that occur in fewer than 0.1% of patients.

Alternatives

Alternatives to a stapedectomy include:

- Watchful waiting. Some patients with only a mild degree of hearing loss may prefer to postpone surgery.
- Medications. Although there is no drug that can cure otosclerosis, some compounds containing fluoride or calcium are reported to be effective in preventing further hearing loss by slowing down abnormal bone growth. The medication most commonly recommended for the purpose is a combination of sodium fluoride and calcium carbonate sold under the trade name Florical. The medication is taken twice a day over a two-year period, after which the patient's hearing is reevaluated. Florical should not be used during pregnancy, however.
- Hearing aids.
- Stapedotomy. A stapedotomy is a surgical procedure similar to a stapedectomy except that the surgeon uses the laser to cut a hole in the stapes in order to insert the prosthesis rather than removing the stapes. In addition, some ear surgeons use the laser to free the stapes bone without inserting a prosthesis. This variation, however, works best in patients with only mild otosclerosis.

KEY TERMS

Audiologist—A health care professional who performs diagnostic testing of impaired hearing.

Cochlea—The hearing part of the inner ear. This snail-shaped structure contains fluid and thousands of microscopic hair cells tuned to various frequencies, in addition to the organ of Corti (the receptor for hearing).

Conductive hearing loss—A type of medically treatable hearing loss in which the inner ear is usually normal, but there are specific problems in the middle or outer ears that prevent sound from getting to the inner ear in a normal way.

Footplate—A flat oval plate of bone that fits into the oval window on the wall of the inner ear; the base of the stapes.

Incus—The middle of the three bones of the middle ear. It is also known as the "anvil."

Malleus—One of the three bones of the middle ear. It is also known as the "hammer."

Ossicles—The three small bones of the middle ear: the malleus (hammer), the incus (anvil) and the stapes (stirrup). These bones help carry sound from the eardrum to the inner ear.

Otology—The branch of medicine that deals with the diagnosis and treatment of ear disorders.

Otosclerosis—Formation of spongy bone around the footplate of the stapes, resulting in conductive hearing loss.

Stapedotomy—A procedure in which a small hole is cut in the footplate of the stapes.

Tinnitus—A sensation of noise in the ears, usually a buzzing, ringing, clicking, or roaring sound.

Vertigo—A feeling of dizziness together with a sensation of movement and a feeling of rotating in space.

Resources

BOOKS

"Approach to the Patient with Ear Problems." In *The Merck Manual of Diagnosis and Therapy*, edited by Mark H. Beers, M.D., and Robert Berkow, M.D. Whitehouse Station, NJ: Merck Research Laboratories, 2001.

"Congenital Anomalies." In *The Merck Manual of Diagnosis and Therapy*, edited by Mark H. Beers, M.D., and Robert Berkow, M.D. Whitehouse Station, NJ: Merck Research Laboratories, 2001.

"Otosclerosis." In *The Merck Manual of Diagnosis and Therapy*, edited by Mark H. Beers, M.D., and Robert Berkow, M.D. Whitehouse Station, NJ: Merck Research Laboratories, 2001.

PERIODICALS

Brown, D. J., T. B. Kim, E. M. Petty, et al. "Characterization of a Stapes Ankylosis Family with an NOG Mutation." *Otology and Neurotology* 24 (March 2003): 210–215.

House, H. P., M. R. Hansen, A. A. Al Dakhail, and J. W. House. "Stapedectomy Versus Stapedotomy: Comparison of Results with Long-Term Follow-Up." *Laryngoscope* 112 (November 2002): 2046–2050.

Nadol, J. B., Jr. "Histopathology of Residual and Recurrent Conductive Hearing Loss After Stapedectomy." *Otology and Neurotology* 22 (March 2001): 162–169.

Shea, J. J. Jr., and X Ge. "Delayed Facial Palsy After Stapedectomy." *Otology and Neurotology* 22 (July 2001): 465–470.

Shohet, Jack A., M.D., and Frank Sutton, Jr., M.D. "Middle Ear, Otosclerosis." *eMedicine*, July 17, 2001 [cited May 3, 2003]. <http://www.emedicine.com/ent/topic218.htm>.

Vincent, R., J. Oates, and N. M. Sperling. "Stapedotomy for Tympanosclerotic Stapes Fixation: Is It Safe and Efficient? A Review of 68 Cases." *Otology and Neurotology* 23 (November 2002): 866–872.

ORGANIZATIONS

American Academy of Audiology. 11730 Plaza America Drive, Suite 300, Reston, VA 20190. (703) 790-8466. <http://www.audiology.org>.

American Academy of Otolaryngology-Head and Neck Surgery, Inc. One Prince St., Alexandria VA 22314-3357. (703) 836-4444. <http://www.entnet.org>

Better Hearing Institute. 515 King Street, Suite 420, Alexandria, VA 22314. (703) 684-3391.

National Institute on Deafness and Other Communication Disorders (NIDCD), National Institutes of Health. 31 Center Drive, MSC 2320. Bethesda, MD 20892-2320. <http://www.nidcd.nih.gov>.

OTHER

National Institute on Deafness and Other Communication Disorders (NIDCD). *Otosclerosis*, August 1999 [May 2, 2003]. NIH Publication No. 99-4234. <http://www.nidcd.nih.gov/health/hearing/otosclerosis/otosclerosis.htm>.

Carol A. Turkington
Rebecca J. Frey, Ph.D.

Staples *see* **Stitches and staples**

Stem cell transplant *see* **Bone marrow transplantation**

Stents, biliary *see* **Biliary stenting**

Stents, coronary *see* **Coronary stenting**

Stents, ureteral *see* **Ureteral stenting**

Stereotactic radiosurgery

Definition

Stereotactic radiosurgery is the use of a precise beam of radiation to destroy tissue in the brain.

Purpose

This procedure is used to treat brain tumors, arteriovenous malformations in the brain, and in some cases, benign eye tumors or other disorders within the brain.

Demographics

Stereotactic radiosurgery is used to treat a variety of disorders with widely differing demographic profiles.

Description

"Radiosurgery" refers to the use of a high-energy beam of radiation. "Stereotactic" refers to the three-dimensional targeting system used to deliver the beam to the precise location desired. Stereotactic radiosurgery is primarily confined to the head and neck, because the patient must be kept completely still during the delivery of the radiation in order to prevent damage to surrounding tissue. The motion of the patient's head and neck are restricted by a stereotactic frame that holds them in place. It is difficult to immobilize other body regions in this way.

The high energy of the radiation beam disrupts the DNA of the targeted cells, killing them. Multiple weak beams are focused on the target area, delivering maximum energy to it while keeping surrounding tissue safe. Since the radiation passes through the skull to its target, there is no need to cut open the skull to perform the surgery. The beam can be focused on any structure in the brain, allowing access to tumors or malformed blood vessels that cannot be reached by open-skull surgery.

Two major forms of stereotactic radiosurgery are in use as of 2003. The Gamma Knife® is a stationary machine that is most useful for small tumors, blood vessels,

or similar targets. Because it does not move, it can deliver a small, highly localized and precise beam of radiation. Gamma knife treatment is done all at once in a single hospital stay. The second type of radiosurgery uses a movable linear accelerator-based machine that is preferred for larger tumors. This treatment is delivered in several small doses given over several weeks. Radiosurgery that is performed with divided doses is known as fractionated radiosurgery. The total dose of radiation is higher with a linear accelerator-based machine than with gamma knife treatment.

Disorders treated by stereotactic radiosurgery include:

- benign brain tumors, including acoustic neuromas and meningiomas
- malignant brain tumors, including gliomas and astrocytomas
- metastatic brain tumors
- trigeminal neuralgia
- Parkinson's disease
- essential tremor
- arteriovenous malformations
- pituitary tumors

Diagnosis/Preparation

A patient requiring radiosurgery has already been diagnosed with a specific disorder that affects the brain. As preparation for radiosurgery, he or she will undergo neuroimaging studies to determine the precise location of the target area in the brain. These studies may include **CT scans**, MRI scans, and others. Imaging of the blood vessels (**angiography**) or the brain's ventricles (ventriculography) may be done as well. These require the injection of either a harmless radioactive substance or a contrast dye.

the heart. The sounds from each area will be different. "Lub-dub" is the sound produced by the normal heart as it beats. Every time this sound is detected, it means that the heart is contracting once. The noises are created when the heart valves click to close. When one hears "lub," the atrioventricular valves are closing. The "dub" sound is produced by the pulmonic and aortic valves. Other heart sounds, such as a quiet "whoosh," are produced by "murmurs." These sounds are produced when there are irregularities in the path of blood flow through the heart. The sounds reflect turbulence in normal blood flow. If a valve remains closed rather than opening completely, turbulence is created and a murmur is produced. Murmurs are not uncommon; many people have them and are unaffected. They are frequently too faint to be heard and remain undetected.

The lungs and airways require different listening skills from those used to detect heart sounds. The stethoscope must be placed over the chest, and the person being examined must breathe in and out deeply and slowly. Using the bell, the listener should note different sounds in various areas of the chest. Then, the diaphragm should be used in the same way. There will be no wheezes or crackles in normal lung sounds.

Crackles or wheezes are abnormal lung sounds. When the lung rubs against the chest wall, it creates friction and a rubbing sound. When there is fluid in the lungs, crackles are heard. A high-pitched whistling sound called a wheeze is often heard when the airways are constricted.

When the stethoscope is placed over the upper left portion of the abdomen, gurgling sounds produced by the stomach and small intestines can usually be heard just below the ribs. The large intestines in the lower part of the abdomen can also be heard. The noises they make are called borborygmi and are entirely normal. Borborygmi are produced by the movement of food, gas or fecal material.

Operation

Some stethoscopes must be placed directly on the skin, while others can work effectively through clothing.

For the stethoscopes with a two-part sound detecting device in the bell, listeners press the rim against the skin, using the bowl-shaped side, to hear low-pitched sounds. The other flat side, called the diaphragm, detects high-pitched sounds.

A stethoscope is used in conjunction with a device to measure blood pressure (**sphygmomanometer**). The stethoscope detects sounds of blood passing though an artery.

Examination with a stethoscope is noninvasive but very useful. It can assist members of the health care team in localizing problems related to the patient's complaints.

Maintenance

Stethoscopes should be cleaned after each use in order to avoid the spread of infection. This precaution is especially important when they are placed directly onto bare skin.

Aftercare

A stethoscope is a sensitive instrument. It should be handled with some care to avoid damage. It requires periodic cleaning.

Risks

There are no risks to persons being examined with a stethoscope. Users of a stethoscope may be exposed to loud noise if the bell is accidentally dropped or struck against a hard surface while the earpieces are in the user's ears.

Normal results

Stethoscopes produce important diagnostic information when used by a person with training and experience.

Morbidity and mortality rates

Normal use of a stethoscope is not associated with injury to either an examiner or a person being examined.

Alternatives

A tube formed by a roll of paper will function in the same manner as a stethoscope. This improvised instrument was the first form of the modern stethoscope invented by René Laënnec (1781-1826), a French physician. An inverted glass will also function as a stethoscope by placing the open portion on the surface to be listened to and the ear of the examiner on the bottom of the glass. Due to their shape, wine glasses with stems are more effective than flat-bottomed tumblers.

See also Physical examination.

Resources

BOOKS

Bickley, L. S., P. G. Szilagyi, and J. G. Stackhouse, eds. *Bates' Guide to Physical Examination & History Taking*, 8th ed. Philadelphia, PA: Lippincott Williams & Wilkins, 2002.

Blaufox, MD. *An Ear to the Chest: An Illustrated History of the Evolution of the Stethoscope*. Boca Raton, FL: CRC Press-Parthenon Publishers, 2001.

Duffin, J. *To See with a Better Eye*. Princeton, NJ: Princeton University Press, 1998.

Duke, M. *Tales My Stethoscope Told Me*. Santa Barbara, CA: Fithian Press, 1998.

PERIODICALS

Conti, C. R. "The Ultrasonic Stethoscope: The New Instrument in Cardiology?" *Clinical Cardiology* 25 (December 2002): 547-548.

Guinto, C. H., E. J. Bottone, J. T. Raffalli, et al. "Evaluation of Dedicated Stethoscopes as a Potential Source of Nosocomial Pathogens." *American Journal of Infection Control* 30 (December 2002): 499-502.

Hanna, I. R., and M. E. Silverman. "A History of Cardiac Auscultation and Some of its Contributors." *American Journal of Cardiology* 90 (August 1, 2002): 259-267.

Savage, G. J. "On the Stethoscope." *Delaware Medical Journal* 74 (October 2002): 415-416.

ORGANIZATIONS

American Academy of Family Physicians. 11400 Tomahawk Creek Parkway, Leawood, KS 66211-2672. (913) 906-6000. <www.aafp.org>. E-mail: fp@aafp.org

American Academy of Pediatrics. 141 Northwest Point Boulevard, Elk Grove Village, IL 60007-1098. (847) 434-4000; FAX: (847) 434-8000. <www.aap.org>. E-mail: kidsdoc@aap.org

American College of Physicians. 190 N. Independence Mall West, Philadelphia, PA 19106-1572. (800) 523-1546, x2600 or (215) 351-2600. <www.acponline.org>.

American College of Surgeons. 633 North St. Clair Street, Chicago, IL 60611-3231. (312) 202-5000; FAX: (312) 202-5001. <www.facs.org>. E-mail: postmaster@facs.org

OTHER

British Broadcasting Company. <www.bbc.co.uk/radio4/science/guessingtubes.shtml>. (March 1, 2003)

KEY TERMS

Atrioventricular—Referring to the valves regulating blood flow from the upper chambers of the heart (atria) to the lower chambers (ventricles). There are two such valves, one connecting the right atrium and ventricle and one connecting the left atrium and ventricle.

Auscultation—The act of listening to sounds produced by the body.

Bell—The cup-shaped portion of the head of a stethoscope, useful for detecting low-pitched sounds.

Borborygmi—Sounds created by the passage of food, gas or fecal material in the stomach or intestines.

Diaphragm—The flat-shaped portion of the head of a stethoscope, useful for detecting high-pitched sounds.

Murmur—The sound made as blood moves through the heart when there is turbulence in the flow of blood through a blood vessel, or if a valve does not completely close.

Institution of Electrical Engineers. <www.iee.org/News/Press Rel/z18oct2002.cfm>. (March 1, 2003)

McGill University Virtual Stethoscope. <www.music.mcgill.ca/auscultation/auscultation.html>. (March 1, 2003)

University of Minnesota Academic Health Center. <www.ahc.umn.edu/rar/MNAALAS/Steth.html>. (March 1, 2003)

L. Fleming Fallon, Jr., MD, DrPH

Stitches and staples

Definition

Stitches and staples are two methods by which a wound may be closed. Stitches use specialized needles and thread to "sew" a wound closed. Staples are thin pieces of metal that are placed with a stapling device through the edges of a wound to hold it closed.

Description

Wounds to the skin, fat, muscle, blood vessels, and other structures in the body may occur accidentally (as in a cut) or purposefully (as in a surgical incision). A number of different methods exist to close a wound; the method selected depends on the type of injury, the type of tissue injured, the location and depth of the injury, and the patient's health. Stitches and staples are two commonly used wound closure methods.

Stitches

Sutures, as stitches are often called, are the way that most wounds are closed. Suture materials have various characteristics that determine their use. The two main components of suture materials are the needle and thread.

MATERIALS. Suture thread is often characterized by how long it retains its strength in tissue. Absorbable stitches lose their strength in a matter of days or weeks and are eventually absorbed by the tissue. This characteristic is useful for the suturing of subcutaneous tissues. Nonabsorbable stitches retain their strength for months to years and may never be absorbed by the tissue. They are generally used for skin and removed once the wound has sufficiently healed. Suture thread is made of various natural or synthetic components and comes in different diameters for use in different types of tissues. Very fine suture threads are used to close cuts on the face, while threads with a larger diameter are required for subcutaneous tissues.

Suture needles may resemble a conventional sewing needle with an eye through which suture material is threaded, or they come with suture thread attached at one end; this connection is called a swage. Needles may be straight or curved; the most commonly used shape is the semicircle, which permits easier manipulation through tissues by the clinician. Needles vary in length from less than 0.1 in (2 mm) to 2.4 in (60 mm). The point of a needle may be cutting (for such tougher tissues as the skin), rounded (for such easily penetrable tissues as the subcutaneous layers), or blunt (for such easily damaged tissues as the liver).

TECHNIQUE. While various stitching techniques may be used depending on the location of the wound and type of tissue to be sutured, basic suturing technique remains the same. Several instruments are necessary for proper wound closure, including dissecting scissors (for cleaning the wound); suture scissors (for cutting suture thread); a needle holder (for manipulating the needle); and forceps (for manipulating tissue). Wounds resulting from an injury must be cleaned before closure; dead tissue and foreign bodies are removed and the area is cleansed with an antiseptic. Sutures may be interrupted (each stitch is separately placed, tied, and cut) or continuous (one continuous piece of thread composes all the stitches); they may be placed at different angles and depths.

Nonabsorbable stitches should be removed several days to weeks after their placement, depending on their location. For instance, sutures on the face should be removed in approximately 5 days; sutures on the legs and abdomen, in 7 to 10 days; and sutures on the back, in 10 to 14 days. Strips of adhesive tape may be placed over the wound to help support the tissue while it is healing.

Staples

A distinct advantage that staples have over sutures is their quick placement—stapling is approximately three to four times faster than suturing. Staples are also associated with a lower risk of infection and tissue reaction than sutures. It is, however, more difficult to correctly align the edges of a wound for stapling, and staples generally cost more than sutures. Common locations of wounds that may be stapled are the arms, legs, abdomen, back, or scalp; wounds on the hands, feet, neck, or face should not be stapled. Additionally, staples may be used to connect cut ends of larger blood vessels or segments of the bowel.

MATERIALS. Individual staples are composed of stainless steel and have a crossbar that lies parallel to the skin, two legs that enter each edge of the wound, and tips that hold the staple in place. Staples are placed with the aid of a stapling device that generally holds between 5 and 25 staples. Forceps are also necessary to help align the edges of the wound together and hold them in place until staples can be placed.

TECHNIQUE. The wound is first cleaned of dead tissue and foreign bodies and washed with an antiseptic. The edges of the wound are aligned and held together with forceps or the clinician's fingers. The stapling device is held against the wound at the point at which the staple is to be placed. By squeezing the trigger on the stapling device, the staple is automatically placed into the skin; the depth of placement is controlled by how hard the stapling device is held against the skin. The staples should be removed in approximately the same time as sutures; this is done with a specialized staple remover.

Resources

BOOKS

Lammers, Richard L., and Alexander T. Trott. "Methods of Wound Closure." In *Clinical Procedures in Emergency Medicine.* Philadelphia: W. B. Saunders Company, 1998.

Polk, Hiram C., William G. Cheadle, and Glen A. Franklin. "Principles of Operative Surgery." In *Sabiston Textbook of Surgery.* Philadelphia: W. B. Saunders Company, 2001.

OTHER

Doud Galli, Suzanne K. and Minas Constantinides. "Wound Closure." *eMedicine.* January 29, 2002 [cited April 29, 2003]. <http://www.emedicine.com/ent/topic35.htm>.

KEY TERMS

Antiseptic—A substance that inhibits the growth of harmful bacteria and other organisms.

Subcutaneous—Under the skin.

Lai, Stephen Y. "Sutures and Needles." *eMedicine.* September 10, 2001 [cited April 29, 2003]. <http://www.emedicine.com/ent/topic38.htm>.

Terhune, Margaret. "Materials for Wound Closure." *eMedicine.* March 13, 2002 [cited April 29, 2003]. <http://www.emedicine.com/derm/topic825.htm>.

Stephanie Dionne Sherk

Stomach resection *see* **Gastrectomy**

Stomach stapling *see* **Vertical banded gastroplasty**

Stomach tube insertion *see* **Gastrostomy**

Strabismus repair *see* **Eye muscle surgery**

Stress test

Definition

A stress test is primarily used to identify coronary artery disease. It requires patients to **exercise** on a treadmill or exercise bicycle while their heart rate, blood pressure, electrocardiogram (ECG), and symptoms are monitored.

Purpose

The body requires more oxygen during exercise than at rest. To deliver more oxygen during exercise, the heart has to pump more oxygen-rich blood. Because of the increased stress on the heart, exercise can reveal coronary problems that are not apparent when the body is at rest. This is why the stress test, though not perfect, remains the best initial noninvasive practical coronary test.

The stress test is particularly useful for detecting ischemia (inadequate supply of blood to the heart muscle) caused by blocked coronary arteries. Less commonly, it is used to determine safe levels of exercise in people with existing coronary artery disease.

Description

A technician affixes electrodes to the patient's chest, using adhesive patches with a special gel that conducts electrical impulses. Typically, electrodes are placed under each collarbone and each bottom rib, and six electrodes are placed across the chest in a rough outline of the heart. Wires from the electrodes are connected to an ECG, which records the electrical activity picked up by the electrodes.

The technician runs resting ECG tests while the patient is lying down, then standing up, and then breathing heavily for half a minute. These baseline tests can later be compared with the ECG tests performed while the patient is exercising. The patient's blood pressure is taken and the blood pressure cuff is left in place so that blood pressure can be measured periodically throughout the test.

The patient begins riding a stationary bicycle or walking on a treadmill. Gradually the intensity of the exercise is increased. For example, if the patient is walking on a treadmill, then the speed of the treadmill increases and the treadmill is tilted upward to simulate an incline. If the patient is on an exercise bicycle, then the resistance or "drag" is gradually increased. The patient continues exercising at increasing intensity until reaching the target heart rate (generally set at a minimum of 85% of the maximal predicted heart rate based on the patient's age) or experiences severe fatigue, dizziness, or chest pain. During the test, the patient's heart rate, ECG, and blood pressure are monitored.

Sometimes such other tests, as **echocardiography** or thallium scanning, are used in conjunction with the exercise stress test. For instance, recent studies suggest that women have a high rate of false negatives (results showing no problem when one exists) and false positives (results showing a problem when one does not exist) with the stress test. They may benefit from another test, such as exercise echocardiography. People who are unable to exercise may be injected with such drugs, as adenosine, which mimic the effects of exercise on the heart, and then given a thallium scan. The thallium scan or echocardiogram are particularly useful when the patient's resting ECG is abnormal. In such cases, interpretation of exercise-induced ECG abnormalities is difficult.

Preparation

Patients are usually instructed not to eat or smoke for several hours before the test. They should be advised to inform the physician about any medications they are taking, and to wear comfortable sneakers and exercise clothing.

Aftercare

After the test, the patient should rest until blood pressure and heart rate return to normal. If all goes well,

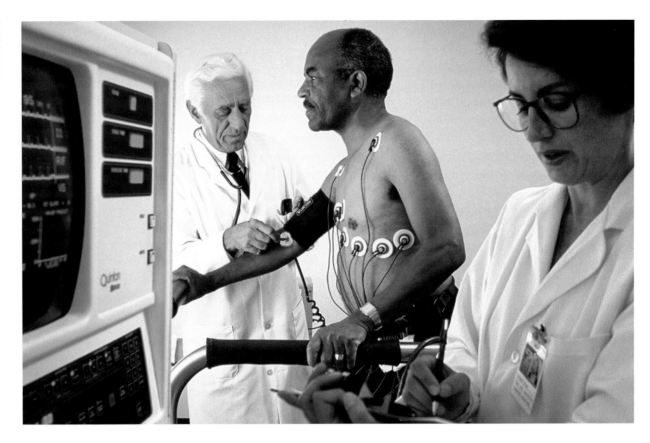

Doctors monitor a patient's vital signs during a stress test. *(Photograph by Mug Shots. The Stock Market. Reproduced by permission.)*

and there are no signs of distress, the patient may return to his or her normal daily activities.

Risks

There is a very slight risk of myocardial infarction (a heart attack) from the exercise, as well as cardiac arrhythmia (irregular heart beats), angina, or cardiac arrest (about one in 100,000). The exercise stress test carries a very slight risk (one in 100,000) of causing a heart attack. For this reason, exercise stress tests should be attended by health care professionals with immediate access to defibrillators and other emergency equipment.

Patients are cautioned to stop the test should they develop any of the following symptoms:

• unsteady gait

• confusion

• skin that is grayish or cold and clammy

• dizziness or fainting

• a drop in blood pressure

• angina (chest pain)

• cardiac arrhythmias (irregular heart beat)

Normal results

A normal result of an exercise stress test shows normal electrocardiogram tracings and heart rate, blood pressure within the normal range, and no angina, unusual dizziness, or shortness of breath.

A number of abnormalities may appear on an exercise stress test. Examples of exercise-induced ECG abnormalities are ST segment depression or heart rhythm disturbances. These ECG abnormalities may indicate deprivation of blood to the heart muscle (ischemia) caused by narrowed or blocked coronary arteries. Stress test abnormalities generally require further diagnostic evaluation and therapy.

Patient education

Patients must be well prepared for a stress test. They should not only know the purpose of the test, but also signs and symptoms that indicate the test should be stopped. Physicians, nurses, and ECG technicians can ensure patient safety by encouraging them to immediately communicate discomfort at any time during the stress test.

KEY TERMS

Angina—Chest pain from a poor blood supply to the heart muscle due to stenosis (narrowing) of the coronary arteries.

Cardiac arrhythmia—An irregular heart rate (frequency of heartbeats) or rhythm (the pattern of heartbeats).

Defibrillator—A device that delivers an electric shock to the heart muscle through the chest wall in order to restore a normal heart rate.

False negative—Test results showing no problem when one exists.

False positive—Test results showing a problem when one does not exist.

Hypertrophy—The overgrowth of muscle.

Ischemia—Dimished supply of oxygen-rich blood to an organ or area of the body.

Resources

BOOKS

Ahya, Shubhada N., Kellie Flood, and Subramanian Paranjothi. *The Washington Manual of Medical Therapeutics,* 30th edition. Philadelphia: Lippincott Williams & Wilkins, 2001, pp. 96–100.

ORGANIZATIONS

American Heart Association. 7272 Greenville Avenue, Dallas, TX 75231. (214) 373-6300. <http://www.amhrt.org>.
National Heart, Lung, and Blood Institute. Information Center. PO Box 30105, Bethesda, MD 20824-0105. (301) 951-3260. <http://www.nhlbi.nih.gov>.

Barbara Wexler
Lee A. Shratter, M.D.

Sulfonamides

Definition

Sulfonamides are a group of anti-infective drugs that prevent the growth of bacteria in the body by interfering with their metabolism. Bacteria are one-celled disease-causing microorganisms that commonly multiply by cell division.

Purpose

Sulfonamides are used to treat many kinds of infections caused by bacteria and certain other microorgan-isms. Physicians may prescribe these drugs to treat urinary tract infections, ear infections, frequent or long-lasting bronchitis, bacterial meningitis, certain eye infections, *Pneumocystis carinii* pneumonia (PCP), traveler's diarrhea, and a number of other infections. These drugs will, however, *not* work for colds, flu, and other infections caused by viruses.

Description

Sulfonamides, which are also called sulfa medicines, are available only with a physician's prescription. They are sold in tablet and liquid forms. Some commonly used sulfonamides are sulfisoxazole (Gantrisin) and the combination drug sulfamethoxazole and trimethoprim (Bactrim, Cotrim, Septra).

Although the sulfonamides have been largely replaced by **antibiotics** for treatment of infections, some bacteria have developed resistance to antibiotics but can still be treated with sulfonamides because the bacteria have not been exposed to these drugs in the past.

Silver sulfadiazine, an ointment containing a sulfonamide, is valuable for the treatment of infections associated with severe burns. The combination drug trimethoprim/sulfamethoxazole (TMP-SMZ) remains in use for many infections, including those associated with HIV infection (AIDS). TMP-SMZ is particularly useful for prevention and treatment of *Pneumocystis carinii* pneumonia, which has been the most dangerous of the infections associated with HIV infection.

Recommended dosage

The recommended dosage depends on the type of sulfonamide, the strength of the medication, and the medical problem for which it is being taken. Patients should check the correct dosage with the physician who prescribed the drug or the pharmacist who filled the prescription.

Patients should always take sulfonamides exactly as directed. To make sure the infection clears up completely, the full course of the medicine must be taken. Patients should not stop taking the drug just because their symptoms begin to improve, because the symptoms may return if the drug is stopped too soon.

Sulfonamides work best when they are at constant levels in the blood. To help keep blood levels constant, patients should take the medicine in doses spaced evenly through the day and night without missing any doses. For best results, sulfa medicines should be taken with a full glass of water, and the patient should drink several more glasses of water every day. This precaution is necessary because sulfa drugs do not dissolve in tissue fluids as easily as some other anti-infective medications. Drinking plenty of water will help prevent some of the medicine's side effects.

Precautions

Symptoms should begin to improve within a few days of beginning to take a sulfa drug. If they do not, or if they get worse, the patient should consult the physician who prescribed the medicine.

Although major side effects are rare, some people have had severe and life-threatening reactions to sulfonamides. These include sudden and severe liver damage; serious blood problems; breakdown of the outer layer of the skin; and a condition called Stevens-Johnson syndrome (erythema multiforme), in which people get blisters around the mouth, eyes, or anus. The patient may be unable to eat and may develop ulcerated areas in the eyes or be unable to open the eyes. It is important to consult a dermatologist and an ophthalmologist as quickly as possible if a patient develops Stevens-Johnson syndrome, to prevent lasting damage to the patient's eyesight. In addition, the syndrome is sometimes fatal.

A physician should be called immediately if any of these signs of a dangerous reaction occur:

- skin rash or reddish or purplish spots on the skin
- such other skin problems as blistering or peeling
- fever
- sore throat
- cough
- shortness of breath
- joint pain
- pale skin
- yellow skin or eyes

Sulfa drugs may also cause dizziness. Anyone who takes sulfonamides should not drive, use machines or do anything else that might be dangerous until they have found out how these drugs affect them.

Sulfonamides may cause blood problems that can interfere with healing and lead to additional infections. Patients should try to avoid minor injuries while taking these medicines, and be especially careful not to injure the mouth when brushing or flossing the teeth or using a toothpick. They should not have dental work done until their blood is back to normal.

Sulfa medications may increase the skin's sensitivity to sunlight. Even brief exposure to sun can cause a severe sunburn or a rash. During treatment with these drugs, patients should avoid exposure to direct sunlight, especially high sun between 10 A.M. and 3 P.M.; wear a hat and tightly woven clothing that covers the arms and legs; use a sunscreen with a skin protection factor (SPF) of at least 15; protect the lips with a lip balm containing sun block; and avoid the use of tanning beds, tanning booths, or sunlamps.

Babies under two months should not be given sulfonamides unless their physician has specifically ordered these drugs.

Older people may be especially sensitive to the effects of sulfonamides, increasing the chance of such unwanted side effects as severe skin problems and blood disorders. Patients who are taking water pills (**diuretics**) at the same time as sulfonamides may also be more likely to have these problems.

Special conditions

People with certain medical conditions or who are taking other medicines may have problems if they take sulfonamides. Before taking these drugs, the patient must inform the doctor about any of these conditions:

ALLERGIES. Anyone who has had unusual reactions to sulfonamides, diuretics, diabetes medicines, or glaucoma medications in the past should let his or her physician know before taking sulfonamides. The physician should also be told about any allergies to foods, dyes, preservatives, or other substances.

PREGNANCY. Some sulfonamides have been found to cause birth defects in studies of laboratory animals. The drugs' effects on human fetuses have not been studied. Pregnant women are advised, however, not to use sulfa drugs around the time of labor and delivery, because they can cause side effects in the baby. Women who are pregnant or who may become pregnant should check with their physicians about the safety of using sulfonamides during pregnancy.

LACTATION. Sulfonamides pass into breast milk and may cause liver problems, anemia, and other problems in nursing babies whose mothers take the medicine. Because of those problems, women should not breastfeed their babies when they are under treatment with sulfa drugs. Women who are breastfeeding but require treatment with sulfonamides should check with their physicians to find out how long they should stop breastfeeding.

OTHER MEDICAL CONDITIONS. People with any of the following medical problems should make sure their physicians are aware of their conditions before they take sulfonamides:

- anemia or other blood problems

KEY TERMS

Anemia—A deficiency of hemoglobin in the blood. Hemoglobin is the compound in blood that carries oxygen from the lungs throughout the body.

Anticoagulant—A type of medication given to prevent blood from clotting. Anticoagulants are also known as blood thinners.

Bronchitis—Inflammation of the air passages of the lungs.

Diuretic—A type of medication given to increase urinary output.

HIV infection—An infectious disease that impairs the immune system. It is also known as acquired immune deficiency syndrome or AIDS.

Inflammation—A condition in which pain, redness, swelling, and warmth develop in a tissue or organ in response to injury or illness.

Meningitis—Inflammation of tissues that surround the brain and spinal cord.

Pneumocystis carinii **pneumonia (PCP)**—A lung infection that affects people with weakened immune systems, such as patients with AIDS or people taking medicines that weaken the immune system.

Porphyria—A disorder in which porphyrins build up in the blood and urine.

Porphyrin—A dark red pigment, sensitive to light, that is found in chlorophyll as well as in a substance in hemoglobin known as heme.

Stevens-Johnson syndrome—A severe inflammatory reaction that is sometimes triggered by sulfa medications. It is characterized by blisters and eroded areas in the mouth, nose, eyes, and anus; it may also involve the lungs, heart, and digestive tract. Stevens-Johnson syndrome is also known as erythema multiforme.

Urinary tract—The passage through which urine flows from the kidneys out of the body.

- kidney disease
- liver disease
- asthma or severe allergies
- alcohol abuse
- poor nutrition
- abnormal intestinal absorption
- porphyria
- folic acid deficiency
- deficiency of an enzyme known as glucose-6-phosphate dehydrogenase (G6PD)

Side effects

The most common side effects are mild diarrhea, nausea, vomiting, dizziness, headache, loss of appetite, and tiredness. These problems usually go away as the body adjusts to the drug and do not require medical treatment.

More serious side effects are not common, but may occur. If any of the following side effects occur, the patient should check with a physician immediately:

- itching or skin rash
- reddish or purplish spots on the skin
- such other skin problems as redness, blistering, or peeling
- severe, watery or bloody diarrhea

- muscle or joint aches
- fever
- sore throat
- cough
- shortness of breath
- unusual tiredness or weakness
- unusual bleeding or bruising
- pale skin
- yellow eyes or skin
- swallowing problems

Other rare side effects may occur. Anyone who has unusual symptoms while taking sulfonamides should get in touch with his or her physician.

Interactions

Sulfonamides may interact with a large number of other medicines. When an interaction occurs, the effects of one or both of the drugs may change or the risk of side effects may be greater. Anyone who takes sulfonamides should give the physician a list of all other medicines that he or she is taking. Among the drugs that may interact with sulfonamides are:

- acetaminophen (Tylenol)
- medicines to treat an overactive thyroid gland

- male hormones (androgens)

- female hormones (estrogens)

- other medicines used to treat infections

- birth control pills

- such medicines for diabetes as glyburide (Micronase)

- warfarin (Coumadin) and other anticoagulants

- disulfiram (Antabuse), a drug used to treat alcohol abuse

- amantadine (Symmetrel), used to treat influenza and also Parkinson's disease

- hydrochlorothiazide (HCTZ, HydroDIURIL) and other diuretics

- the anticancer drug methotrexate (Rheumatrex)

- valproic acid (Depakote, Depakene) and other anti-seizure medications

The list above does not include every drug that may interact with sulfonamides. Patients should be careful to check with a physician or pharmacist before combining sulfonamides with any other prescription or nonprescription (over-the-counter) medicine. This precaution includes herbal preparations. Some herbs, such as bearberry, parsley, dandelion leaf, and sarsaparilla, have a diuretic effect and should not be used while taking sulfa drugs. Basil, which is commonly used in cooking to flavor salad dressings, stews, and tomato recipes, is reported to affect the absorption of sulfonamides.

Resources

BOOKS

"Antibacterial Drugs: Sulfonamides." Section 13, Chapter 153 in *The Merck Manual of Diagnosis and Therapy*, edited by Mark H. Beers, MD, and Robert Berkow, MD. Whitehouse Station, NJ: Merck Research Laboratories, 1999.

Brody, T. M., J. Larner, K. P. Minneman, and H. C. Neu. *Human Pharmacology: Molecular to Clinical*, 2nd ed. St. Louis: Mosby Year-Book, 1995.

"Inflammatory Reactions: Erythema Multiforme." Section 10, Chapter 118 in *The Merck Manual of Diagnosis and Therapy*, edited by Mark H. Beers, MD, and Robert Berkow, MD. Whitehouse Station, NJ: Merck Research Laboratories, 1999.

Karch, A. M. "Lippincott's Nursing Drug Guide." Springhouse, PA: Lippincott Williams & Wilkins, 2003.

Pelletier, Kenneth R., MD. *The Best Alternative Medicine*, Part I, Chapter 6, "Western Herbal Medicine." New York: Simon & Schuster, 2002.

Reynolds, J. E. F., ed. *Martindale: The Extra Pharmacopoeia*, 31st ed. London, UK: The Pharmaceutical Press, 1996.

ORGANIZATIONS

American Society of Health-System Pharmacists (ASHP). 7272 Wisconsin Avenue, Bethesda, MD 20814. (301) 657-3000. <www.ashp.org>.

United States Food and Drug Administration (FDA). 5600 Fishers Lane, Rockville, MD 20857-0001. (888) INFO-FDA. <www.fda.gov>.

OTHER

<http://www.nlm.nih.gov/medlineplus/druginfo/uspdi/202540. html>.

Nancy Ross-Flanigan
Sam Uretsky, PharmD

Surgical debridement *see* **Debridement**

Surgical instruments

Definition

Surgical instruments are tools or devices that perform such functions as cutting, dissecting, grasping, holding, retracting, or suturing. Most surgical instruments are made from stainless steel. Other metals, such as titanium, chromium, vanadium, and molybdenum, are also used.

Purpose

Surgical instruments facilitate a variety of procedures and operations. Specialized surgical packs contain the most common instruments needed for particular surgeries.

In the United States, surgical instruments are used in all hospitals, outpatient facilities, and most professional offices. Instrument users include surgeons, dentists, physicians, and many other health care providers. Millions of new and replacement instruments are sold each year. Many surgical instruments now have electronic or computerized components.

Description

Basic categories of surgical instruments include specialized implements for the following functions:

- cutting, grinding, and dissecting

- clamping

- grasping and holding

- probing

- dilating or enlarging

- retracting

- suctioning

Scissors are an example of cutting instruments. Dissecting instruments are used to cut or separate tissue. Dissectors may be sharp or blunt. One example of a sharp dissector is a scalpel. Examples of blunt dissectors include the back of a knife handle, curettes, and elevators. Clamps, tenacula, and forceps are grasping and holding instruments. Probing instruments are used to enter natural openings, such as the common bile duct, or fistulas. Dilating instruments expand the size of an opening, such as the urethra or cervical os. Retractors assist in the visualization of the operative field while preventing trauma to other tissues. Suction devices remove blood and other fluids from a surgical or dental operative field.

Sharps and related items should be counted four times: prior to the start of the procedure; before closure of a cavity within a cavity; before wound closure begins; and at skin closure or the end of the procedure. In addition, a count should be taken any time surgical personnel are replaced before, during, or after a procedure. Instruments, sharps, and sponges should be counted during all procedures in which there is a possibility of leaving an item inside a patient.

The misuse of surgical instruments frequently causes alignment problems. Instruments should always be inspected before, during, and after surgical or dental procedures. Inspection is an ongoing process that must be carried out by all members of a **surgical team**.

Scissors must be sharp and smooth, and must cut easily. Their edges must be inspected for chips, nicks, or dents.

After a procedure, staff members responsible for cleaning and disinfecting the instruments should also inspect them. The instruments should be inspected again after cleaning and during packaging. Any instrument that is not in good working order should be sent for repair. Depending on use, surgical instruments can last for up to 10 years given proper care.

Preparation

Instruction in the use and care of surgical instruments may range from the medical training required by physicians and dentists to on-the-job training for orderlies and aides.

Surgical instruments are prepared for use according to strict institutional and professional protocols. Instruments are maintained and sterilized prior to use.

Surgical instruments must be kept clean during a procedure. This is accomplished by carefully wiping them with a moist sponge and rinsing them frequently in sterile water. Periodic cleaning during the procedure prevents blood and other tissues from hardening and becoming trapped on the surface of an instrument.

Instruments must be promptly rinsed and thoroughly cleaned and sterilized after a procedure. Ultrasonic cleaning and automatic washing often follow the manual cleaning of instruments. Instruments may also be placed in an autoclave after manual cleaning. The manufacturer's instructions must be followed for each type of machine. Staff members responsible for cleaning instruments should wear protective gloves, waterproof aprons, and face shields to protect themselves and maintain instrument sterility.

Aftercare

Observation of the patient after surgical or dental procedures provides the best indication that correct instrument handling and **aseptic technique** was followed during surgery. After an operation or dental procedure, individuals should show no evidence of the following:

• retained instruments or sponges

• infection at the site of the incision or operation

Risks

Risks associated with surgical instruments include improper use or technique by an operator, leaving an instrument inside a person after an operation, and transmitting infection or disease due to improper cleaning and sterilization techniques. Improperly cleaned or sterilized instruments may contribute to postoperative infections or mortality. Improper use of surgical instruments may contribute to postoperative complications.

See also General surgery

Resources

BOOKS

Bland, K.I., W.G. Cioffi, and M.G. Sarr. *Practice of General Surgery.* Philadelphia: Saunders, 2001.

Burke, K.M., P. Lemone and E. Mohen-Brown. *Understanding Medical Surgical Nursing.* Upper Saddle River, NJ: Prentice Hall, 2002.

Caruthers, B.L., and P. Price. *Surgical Technology for the Surgical Technologist.* Albany, NY: Delmar, 2001.

Grace, P.A., A. Cuschieri, D. Rowley, N. Borley, and A. Darzi. *Clinical Surgery,* 2nd ed. Londin, 2003.

Schwartz, S.I., J.E. Fischer, F. C. Spencer, G.T. Shires, and J.M. Daly. *Principles of Surgery,* 7th ed. New York: McGraw-Hill, 1998.

Townsend, C., K.L. Mattox, R.D. Beauchamp, B.M. Evers, and D.C. Sabiston. *Sabiston's Review of Surgery,* 3rd ed. Philadelphia: Saunders, 2001.

PERIODICALS

Beesley, J. "Creutzfeldt-Jakob Disease—The Perioperative Connection." *British Journal of Perioperative Nursing* 13, no.1 (2003): 21-3.

Guyton, S.W. "Robotic Surgery: The Computer-Enhanced Control of Surgical Instruments." *Otolaryngology Clinics of North America* 35, no.6 (2002): 1303-16.

Pisal, N., M. Sindos, and G. Henson. Risk Factors for Retained Instruments and Sponges after Surgery." *New England Journal of Medicine* 348, no.7 (2003): 1724-5.

Vrancich, A. "Instrumental Care. Creating Longevity through Proper Maintenance." *Materials Management in Health Care* 12, no.3 (2003): 22-5.

Williams, D. "Public Confidence in Medical Technology." *Medical Device Technology* 13, no.10 (2002): 11-13.

ORGANIZATIONS

American Board of Surgery. 1617 John F. Kennedy Boulevard, Suite 860, Philadelphia, PA 19103. (215)568-4000, fax: (215) 563-5718. <http://www.absurgery.org>

American College of Surgeons. 633 North St. Clair Street, Chicago, IL 60611-32311. (312) 202-5000. Fax: (312) 202-5001. E-mail: <postmaster@facs.org>. <http://www.facs.org>.

Association of Perioperative Registered Nurses, Inc. 2170 South Parker Road, Suite 300, Denver, CO 80231-5711. (800) 755-2676. <http://www.aorn.org>

Association of Surgical Technologists. 7108-C South Alton Way, Suite 100, Englewood, CO 80112-2106. (800) 637-7433.

OTHER

Surgical 911. [cited May 6, 2003] <http://www.surgical 911.com>.

United States Bureau of Labor. [cited May 6, 2003] <http://www.bls.gov/oco/ocos106.htm>

University of California-Irvine. [cited May 6, 2003] <http://www.ucihealth.com/News/Releases/DaVinci2.htm>.

University of Indiana. [cited May 6, 2003] <http://www.indiana.edu/~ancmed/instr1.html>.

University of Virginia. [cited May 6, 2003] <http://hsc.virginia.edu/hs-library/historical/antiqua/instru.html>.

L. Fleming Fallon, Jr., M.D., Dr.PH.

Surgical oncology

Definition

Surgical oncology is a specialized area of oncology that engages surgeons in the cure and management of cancer.

Purpose

Cancer has become a medical specialty warranting its own surgical area because of advances in the biology, pathophysiology, diagnostics, and staging of malignant tumors. Surgeons have traditionally treated cancer patients with resection and radical surgeries of tumors, and left the management of the cancer and the patient to other specialists. Advances in the early diagnosis of cancer, the staging of tumors, microscopic analyses of cells, and increased understanding of cancer biology have broadened the range of nonsurgical cancer treatments. These treatments include systematic chemotherapy, hormonal therapy, and radiotherapy as alternatives or adjunctive therapy for patients with cancer.

Not all cancer tumors are manageable by surgery, nor does the removal of some tumors or metastases necessarily lead to a cure or longer life. The oncological surgeon looks for the relationship between tumor excision and the risk presented by the primary tumor. He or she is knowledgeable about patient management with more conservative procedures than the traditional excision or resection.

Demographics

According to the American Association of Cancer Registries, the most commonly diagnosed cancers for males in the United States during 1995–1999, with total of over 1.7 million cases for all races, were:

- prostate–28.6%
- lung–16.3%
- colon and rectum–11.7%
- bladder–6.6%
- non-Hodgkin's lymphoma 4.2%

White males make up more than 1.4 million of the total prostate cancer cases, with African Americans and Hispanic Americans accounting for 160,356 and 75,237 cases respectively. Each of the latter groups had higher stomach cancer incidence in the top five list, replacing non-Hodgkin's lymphoma. For women, the total cases for all races was over 1.6 million, and white women made up more than 1.4 million of this number. There were 140,888 female African American cases and 76,810 Hispanic American female cases.

Leading cancers for all groups were:

- breast–30.7%
- lung–12.5%
- colon & rectum–12.2%
- corpus & uterus–5.9%
- ovary–3.9%

African American women had higher rates of cervical cancer, replacing ovarian cancer in the top five list.

Description

Surgical oncology is guided by principles that govern the routine procedures related to the cancer patient's cure, palliative care, and quality of life. Surgical oncology performs its most efficacious work by local tumor excision, regional lymph node removal, the handling of cancer recurrence (local or widespread), and in rare cases, with surgical resection of metastases from the primary tumor. Each of these areas plays a different role in cancer management.

Excision

Local excision has been the hallmark of surgical oncology. Excision refers to the removal of the cancer and its effects. Resection of a tumor in the colon can end the effects of obstruction, for instance, or removal of a breast carcinoma can stop the cancer. Resection of a primary tumor also stops the tumor from spreading throughout the body. The cancer's spread into other body systems, however, usually occurs before a local removal, giving resection little bearing upon cells that have already escaped the primary tumor. Advances in oncology through patho-

physiology, staging, and biopsy offer a new diagnostic role to the surgeon using excision. These advances provide simple diagnostic information about size, grade, and extent of the tumor, as well as more sophisticated evaluations of the cancer's biochemical and hormonal features.

Regional lymph node removal

Lymph node involvement provides surgical oncologists with major diagnostic information. The sentinel node biopsy is superior to any biological test in terms of prediction of cancer mortality rates. Nodal biopsy offers very precise information about the extent and type of invasive effects of the primary tumor. The removal of nodes, however, may present pain and other morbid conditions for the patient.

Local and regional recurrence

Radical procedures in surgical oncology for local and regional occurrences of a primary tumor provide crucial information on the spread of cancer and prognostic outcomes. However, they do not contribute substantially to the outcome of the cancer. According to most surgical oncology literature, the ability to remove a local recurrence must be balanced by the patient's goals related to aesthetic and pain control concerns. Historically, more radical procedures have not improved the chances for survival.

Surgery for distant metastases

In general, a cancer tumor that spreads further from its primary site is less likely to be controlled by surgery. According to research, except for a few instances where a metastasis is confined, surgical removal of a distant metastasis is not warranted. Since the rapidity of discovering a distant metastasis has little bearing upon cancer survival, the usefulness of surgery is not time-dependent. In the case of liver metastasis, for example, a cure is related to the pathophysiology of the original cancer and level of cancer antigen in the liver rather than the size or time of discovery. While surgery of metastatic cancer may not increase life, there may be indications for it such as pain relief, obstruction removal, control of bleeding, and resolution of infection.

Diagnosis/Preparation

Surgery removes cancer cells and surrounding tissues. It is often combined with radiation therapy and chemotherapy. It is important for the patient to meet with the surgical oncologist to talk about the procedure and begin preparations for surgery. Oncological surgery may be performed to biopsy a suspicious site for malignant cells or tumor. It is also used for **tumor removal** from such organs as the tongue, throat, lung, stomach, intestines, colon, bladder, ovary, and prostate. Tumors of limbs, ligaments, and tendons may also be treated with surgery. In many cases, the biopsy and surgery to remove the cancer cells or tissues are done at the same time as the biopsy.

The impact of a surgical procedure depends upon the diagnosis and the area of the body that is to be treated by surgery. Many cancer surgeries involve major organs and require open abdominal surgery, which is the most extensive type of surgical procedure. This surgery requires medical tests and work-ups to judge the health of the patient prior to surgery, and to make decisions about adjunctive procedures like radiation or chemotherapy. Preparation for cancer surgery requires psychological readiness for a hospital stay, postoperative pain, sometimes slow recovery, and anticipation of complications from tumor excision or resection. It also may require consultation with stomal therapists if a section of the urinary tract or bowel is to be removed and replaced with an outside reservoir or conduit called an ostomy.

Aftercare

After surgery, the type and duration of side effects and the elements of recovery depend on where in the body the surgery was performed and the patient's general health. Some surgeries may alter basic functions in the urinary or gastrointestinal systems. Recovering full use of function takes time and patience. Surgeries that remove such conduits as the colon, intestines, or urinary tract require appliances for urine and fecal waste and the help of a stomal therapist. Breast or prostate surgeries yield concerns about cosmetic appearance and intimate activities. For most cancer surgeries, basic functions like tasting, eating, drinking, breathing, moving, urinating, defecating, or neurological ability may be changed in the short-term. Resources to attend to deficits in daily activities need to be set up before surgery.

Risks

The type of risks that cancer surgery presents depends almost entirely upon the part of the body being biopsied or excised. Risks of surgery can be great when major organs are involved, such as the gastrointestinal system or the brain. These risks are usually discussed explicitly when surgerical decisions are made.

Normal results

Most cancers are staged; that is, they are described by their likelihood of being contained, spreading at the original site, or recurring or invading other bodily systems. The prognosis after surgery depends upon the stage of the disease, and the pathology results on the type of cancer cell involved. General results of cancer surgery depend in large part on norms of success based upon the study of groups of patients with the same diagnosis. The results are often stated in percentages of the chance of cancer recurrence or its spread after surgery. After five disease-free years, patients are usually considered cured. This is because the recurrence rates decline drastically after five years. The benchmark is based upon the percentage of people known to reach the fifth year after surgery with no recurrence or spread of the primary tumor.

Morbidity and mortality rates

Morbidity and mortality of oncological surgery are high if there is organ involvement or extensive excision of major parts of the body. Because there is an ongoing disease process and many patients may be very ill at the time of surgery, the complications of surgery may be quite complex. Each procedure is understood by the surgeon for its likely complications or risks, and these are discussed during the initial surgical consultations.

There are comprehensive surgical procedures for many cancers, and complications may be extensive due to the use of general anesthetic and the opening of body cavities. Open surgery has general risks associated with it that are not related to the type of procedure. These risks include possibility of blood clots and cardiac events.

There is an extensive body of literature about the complication and morbidity rates of surgery performed by high-volume treatment centers. Data show that in

KEY TERMS

Biopsy—The surgical excision of tissue to diagnose the size, type, and extent of a cancerous growth.

Cancer surgery—Surgery in which the goal is to excise a tumor and its surrounding tissue found to be malignant.

Resection—Cutting out tissue to eliminate a cancerous tumor; usually refers to a section of the organ, (e.g., colon, intestine, lung, stomach) that must be cut to remove the tumor and its surrounding tissue.

Tumor staging—The method used by oncologists to determine the risk from a cancerous tumor. A number—ranging from 1A–4B— is assigned to predict the level of invasion by a tumor, and offer a prognosis for morbidity and mortality.

general, large volumes of surgery affect the quality outcomes of surgery, with smaller hospitals having lower rates of procedural success and higher operative and postoperative complications than larger facilities. It is not known whether the surgeon's experience or the advantages of institutional resources in operative or **postoperative care** contributes to these statistics.

Alternatives

Alternatives to cancer surgery exist for almost every cancer now treated in the United States. Research has been very successful for some—but not all—cancers. There are many alternatives to surgery, and chemotherapy and radiation after surgery. Most organizations dealing with cancer patients suggest alternative treatments. Physicians and surgeons expect to be asked about alternatives to surgery, and are usually quite knowledgeable about their use as cancer treatments or as adjuncts to surgery.

Resources

BOOKS

Abeloff, M.D., Martin D. "Surgical Therapy." In *Clinical Oncology.* 2nd ed. Churchill Livingstone, Inc., 2000.

PERIODICALS

Blake, C. "Multidisciplinary Approach to Cancer: The Changing Role of the Surgical Oncologist." *Surgical Clinics of North America* 80, no. 2 (April 2000).

Jemal, A., et.al. "Cancer Statistics, 2002." *CA: A Cancer Journal for Clinicians* 52, no. 1 (2002): 23–47.

Kemeny, M.M. "Cancer Surgery in the Elderly." *Hematology/Oncology Clinics of North America* 14, no.1 (February 1, 2000): 169–93.

ORGANIZATIONS

American Cancer Society. (800) ACS-2345. <www.cancer.org/docroot/home/index.asp.>.

National Cancer Institute's Office of Alternative Medicine. 6120 Executive Boulevard, Suite 450, Bethesda, Maryland, 20892. (800) 4- CANCER, (800) 422-6237.

National Alliance of Breast Cancer Organizations. 9 East 37th Street, Tenth Floor, New York, NY 10016. (212) 719-0154. Fax: 212-689-1213. <http://www.nabco.org.>

OTHER

2001 Cancer Progress Report. National Cancer Institute. <http://www.progressreport.cancer.gov/>.

Nancy McKenzie, Ph.D.

Surgical team

Definition

The surgical team is a unit providing the continuum of care beginning with **preoperative care**, and extending through perioperative (during the surgery) procedures, and postoperative recovery. Each specialist on the team, whether surgeon, anesthesiologist or nurse, has advanced training for his or her role before, during, and after surgery.

Purpose

Surgery, whether elective, required or emergency, is done for a variety of conditions that include:

• cosmetic procedures

• diagnostic and exploratory procedures

• treatment of acute, chronic, and infectious diseases of tissue or organs

• transplantation of organs

• resposition and enhancement of bone, ligaments, tendons, or organ conduits

• replacement or implantation of artificial or electronic devices

The crucial elements of surgery—surgical and operative procedures, pain control, patient safety, and blood and wound control—require individual expertise and high levels of concentration and coordination. Through a team effort, the patient is treated and monitored as he or she undergoes significant acts of bodily invasion and pain control that make up the surgical experience. These surgical acts are true for the most benign and superficial operations, as well as the most intense.

Demographics

According to the Centers for Disease Control and Prevention and the National Center for Health Statistics, 40 million inpatient surgical procedures were performed in the United States in 2000, followed closely by 31.5 million outpatient surgeries. Leading surgeries included:

• digestive system surgeries: 12 million

• musculoskeletal system surgeries: 7.4 million

• cardiovascular system surgeries: 6.8 million

• eye surgeries: 5.4 million

Description

The makeup of the surgical team depends upon the type of surgery, the precise procedures, and the location and the type of anesthesia utilized. The team may include surgeons, anesthesiologists, and nursing and technical staff who are trained in **general surgery** or in a particular surgical specialty. Intense surgeries require larger teams and more comprehensive recovery care. Even though minimally invasive procedures (e.g., **laparoscopy** or endoscopy) are conducted with small instruments and a video camera probe, they require specialized expertise and high technology knowledge. These procedures utilize smaller teams, create less extensive wounds, and yield quicker healing, but often require more operating time and may result in operative injuries.

Types of surgery

Many surgeries are categorized as general surgery, and are associated primarily with accidents, emergencies, and trauma care. Hospitals have general surgeons that staff their emergency rooms or trauma centers. As surgical technology and knowledge have advanced, other surgical specialties have developed for each function and organ of the body. They involve special surgical techniques and anesthesiology requirements, and sometimes require subspecialtists with in-depth knowledge of organ function, operative techniques, complex anesthesiology procedures, and specialized nursing care.

The basic surgical specialties include:

• General surgery—General surgeons manage a broad spectrum of surgical conditions that involve almost any part of the body. They confirm the diagnoses provided by primary care or emergency physicians and radiologists, and perform procedures necessary to correct or alleviate the problem.

• Cardiothoracic surgery—A major surgical specialty with very high demands. The cardiothoracic surgical team oversees the preoperative, operative, and critical care of patients with pathologic conditions within the chest, including the heart and its valves, cancers of the lung, esophagus, and chest wall, and chest vessels.

• Neurosurgery—Neurosurgical teams specialize in surgery of the nervous system, including the brain, spine, and peripheral nervous system, and their supporting structures.

• Oral and maxillofacial surgery—Head and neck surgical teams provide treatment for problems of the ears, sinuses, mouth, pharynx, jaw, and other structures of the head and neck.

• Reconstructive and plastic surgery—Reconstructive surgery is performed on abnormal structures of the body due to injury, birth defects, infection, tumors, or disease. Cosmetic surgery is performed to improve a patient's appearance.

• Transplantation—Transplant surgical teams specialize in specific organ transplant techniques, such as heart and heart-lung transplants, liver transplants, and kidney/pancreas transplants. These highly intricate surgeries require very advanced training and technological support.

• Urology and renal transplantation—Also known as gastrointestinal surgery. The team specializes in problems of the digestive tract (stomach, bowels, liver, and gallbladder) with intensive use of or coordination with transplant team members.

• Vascular surgery—Vascular surgery offers diagnosis and treatment of such arterial and venous disorders as aneurysms, lower extremity revascularization, and other problems.

• Pediatric surgery—Pediatric surgical teams are specially trained to treat a broad range of conditions affecting infants and children. They work closely with specially trained anesthesiologists, and are experts in childhood diseases of the head, neck, chest, and abdomen, with training in birth defects and injuries. Many pediatric surgeons work to increase the use of minimally invasive techniques with children.

Surgical techniques

Open surgeries requiring invasive procedures within the abdominal cavity, brain or extensive limb areas require a hospital stay overnight or up to two weeks. Hospitalization allows the clinical staff to monitor patient recovery (and provide medical attention in the case of a complication), while allowing patients to regain organ functions.

Surgery has been revolutionized by new technology. Ambulatory or outpatient surgeries account for an increasing percentage of surgeries in the United States. Imagery with miniature videoscopes that pass into the patient via tiny incisions is an example of how minimally invasive procedures are replacing open surgeries. Minimally invasive surgeries reduce recovery time and increase the speed of healing. Outpatient or ambulatory surgery environments often allow patients to recover and go home the same day. In such specialty surgery centers, as those designed for ophthalmology, surgery is performed as part of a physician's office practice. These centers contain their own operating rooms and recovery areas.

Minimally invasive procedures that involve the use of a video scope as an exploratory as well as viewing instrument, include the following:

- Arthroscopy—allows viewing of the interior of joints, especially the knee joint.
- Cystoscopy—used to examine the urethra and bladder.
- Endoscopy—much like the laparascope, the endoscope is used in gastrointestinal surgeries of the esophagus, stomach, and colon.
- Laparoscopy—an illuminated tube with a video camera inserted in small incisions in the abdomen.
- Sigmoidoscopy—used for examining the rectum and sigmoid colon.

Types of anesthesia

Surgical procedures and the surgical setting may be associated with different types of anesthesia:

- General anesthesia renders the patient unconscious during surgery. The anesthesia is either inhaled or given intravenously. A breathing tube may be inserted into the windpipe (trachea) to facilitate breathing. The patient is carefully monitored and wakes up in the **recovery room**.
- Regional anesthesia numbs the surgical section of the body. This is usually accomplished via injection through the spinal canal (spinal anesthesia) or through a catheter to the lower part of the back (epidural). Regional anesthetics numb the area of the nerves that provide feeling to the designated part of the body.
- Local anesthesia medicates only the direct operative site, and is administered through injection. The patient remains conscious during the operation.

Surgical team

The basic surgical team consists of experts in operative procedure, **pain management**, and overall or specific patient care. Team members include the surgeon, anesthesiologist, and **operating room** nurse. In teaching hospitals attached to medical schools, the team may be enlarged by those in training, such as interns, residents, and nursing students.

SURGEON. The surgeon performs the operation, and leads the surgical team. Surgeons have medical degrees, specialized surgical training of up to seven years, and in most cases have passed national board certification exams. Board certification means that the surgeon has passed written and oral examinations of academic competence. The American Board of Surgery, a professional organization that strives to improve the quality of care by surgeons, is the certifying board for surgeons. As a peer review organization, the College has advanced standards to certify surgical competence by allowing examined surgeons to become a fellow of the organization. Fellows of the American College of Surgeons (FACS) are the elite members of the profession. An FACS designation after a physician's name and degree denotes attainment of the profession's highest training and expertise. Surgeons' credentials may be explored through the Official American Board of Medical Specialties, available at libraries or online.

ANESTHESIOLOGIST. Anesthesiologists are physicians with at least four years of advanced training in anesthesia. They may attain further specialization in surgical procedures, such as **neurosurgery** or **pediatric surgery**. They are directly or indirectly involved in all three stages of surgery (preoperative, operative, and postoperative) due to their focus on pain management and patient safety.

CERTIFIED REGISTERED NURSE ANESTHETIST (CRNA). The certified nurse anesthetist supports the anesthesiologists, and in an increasing number of hospitals, takes full control of the anesthesia for the operation. Registered nurses must graduate from an approved nursing program and pass a licensing examination. They may be licensed in more than one state. While states determine the training and certification requirements of nurses, the work setting determines their daily responsibilities. Certified registered nurse anesthetists must have advance education and clinical practice experience in anesthesiology.

OPERATING NURSE. The general nursing staff is a critical feature of the surgical team. The nursing staff performs comprehensive care, assistance, and pain management during each surgical phase. He or she is usually the team member providing the most continuity between the stages of care. The operating nurse is the general assistant to the surgeon during the actual operation phase, and usually has advanced training.

Preparation

The surgical team admits the patient to the hospital or surgery center. Many surgeons and anesthesiologists have privileges at more than one hospital and may admit the patient to a center of the patient's choosing. Surgical preparation is the preoperative phase of surgery, and involves special team activities that include monitoring **vital signs**, and administering medications and tests needed immediately before the procedure. In preparation for surgery, the patient meets with the surgeon, anesthesiologist, and surgical nurse. Each team member discusses his or her role in the surgery, and obtains from the patient pertinent information.

Aftercare

After the surgical procedure has been performed, the patient is brought to a recovery room where post-anesthesia staff take over from the surgical team under the guidance of the surgeon and anesthesiologist. The staff carefully monitors the patient by checking vital signs, the surgical wound and its dressings, IV medications, swallowing ability, level of consciousness, and any tubes or drains. Clinical staff also manage the patient's pain and body positioning.

Risks

Because of its risks, surgery should be the option chosen when the benefit includes the removal of life-threatening conditions or improvement in quality of daily life. Radical surgeries for some types of cancer may offer less than a 20% chance of cure, and the operation may pose the same percentage of mortality risk. A failed operation may shorten time with loved ones and friends, or a successful operation may lead to major positive changes in daily life.

Surgery often brings quicker relief from many conditions than other medical treatment. The risks of surgery depend upon a number of factors, including the experience of the surgical team. A recent *New England Journal of Medicine* article reported the findings of a national **Medicare** study that examined 25 million procedures performed between 1994 and 1999 in the United States. Seeking to determine the mortality associated with a number of cardiovascular and cancer surgeries, the researchers found that mortality decreased as patient volume in a surgical setting increased. The variance was dramatic for both pancreatic and esophageal surgeries. The study's messages were that Medicare patients should choose surgical centers where a large number of the type of surgery they need is performed, and that physicians working in low-volume hospitals should find ways to increase volume and reduce their morbidity and mortality rates.

Mortality rates are lower and the care more extensive in teaching hospitals with a "house staff" made up of interns and residents in training.

Health care facilities keep records of the procedures they perform. By contacting the Joint Commission on Accreditation of Healthcare Organizations (JCAHO), a center's success with surgical care, mortality and morbidity rates, and surgical complications can be determined.

The Institute of Medicine estimates that today's anesthesia care is nearly 50 times safer than it was 20 years ago, with one anesthesia-related death per 200,000–300,000 cases. Despite this record of progress, many questions remain about anesthetic safety. Certified registered nurse anesthetists administer over 65 percent of anesthesia in the United States, and are often the primary anesthetists for rural communities and delivery rooms.

Independent of surgical team expertise and experience, patient status, and the level of technological advancement in surgical procedures, cardiac events, blood clots, and infection pose surgical risks. These risks accompany all surgeries and, while great progress has been achieved, they remain factors that are part of any surgical invasion and any use of anesthesia.

Alternatives

Alternatives to surgery should be investigated with the referring physician or primary care physician. Many medical conditions benefit from changes in lifestyle, such as losing weight, increasing **exercise**, and undergoing physical rehabilitation. This is especially true for chronic conditions of the gastrointestinal tract, cardiovascular system, urologic system, and bone and joint issues. Research and other resources offer alternatives to surgery including pharmaceutical and medical remedies.

Patients should obtain a **second opinion** before undergoing most major surgeries. It is very important that patients understand that a second opinion offers them the ability to obtain a confirming or differing diagnosis as well as new treatment options. A study of New York City employees and retirees who sought second opinions found that 30% of the second opinions differed from the first. Many health plans have mandatory second opinion clauses. Second opinions should involve physicians in other facilities or even other cities. A change in surgeon will mean a change in the surgical team.

Resources

BOOKS

McLanahan, S.A., and D.J. McLanahan. *Surgery and Its Alternatives: How to Make the Right Choices for Your Health.* Twin Streams: Kensington Books, 2002.

PERIODICALS

Birkmeyer, J.D., E.V. Finlayson, and C.M. Birkmeyer. "Volume Standards for High-risk Surgical Procedures: Potential Benefits of the Leapfrog Initiative." *Surgery* (130) (September 2001): 415-22.

Finlayson, E.V., and J.D. Birkmeyer. "Operative Mortality with Elective Surgery in Older Adults." *Effective Clinical Practice* 4 (July 2001): 172-7.

KEY TERMS

Anesthesiologist—A physician with advanced training in anesthesia (and sometimes other medical specialties) who administers or oversees the administration of anesthesia to the patient and monitors care after surgery.

Anesthetist—A nurse trained in anesthesiology who, working as an assistant to a anesthesiologist, administers the anesthesia in surgery and monitors the patient after surgery.

Minimally invasive surgery—Surgical techniques, especially the use of small instruments and tiny video cameras, that allow surgery to take place without a full operative wound.

Operative nurse—A nurse specially trained to assist the surgeon and work in all areas of the surgical event to care for the patient.

ORGANIZATIONS

American Board of Medical Specialties. 1007 Church Street, Suite 404, Evanston, IL 60201. (847) 491-9091.

American Board of Surgery. 1617 John F. Kennedy Boulevard, Suite 860, Philadelphia, PA 19103. (215) 568-4000. Fax: 215-563-5718.

American College of Surgeons. 633 North St. Clair Street, Chicago, IL 60611-32311. (312) 202-5000. Fax: (312) 02-5001. <http://www.facs.org/>.

American Society of Anesthesiologists. 520 N. Northwest Highway Park Ridge, IL 60068-2573. (847) 825-5586. Fax: (847) 825-1692. <www.asahq.org>.

OTHER

Joint Commission on Accreditation of Healthcare Organizations. One Renaissance Blvd., Oakbrook Terrace, IL 60181. (630) 792-5000. <www.jcaho.org/>,

Nancy McKenzie, Ph.D.

Sweat test *see* **Electrolyte tests**

Sympathectomy

Definition

Sympathectomy is a surgical procedure that destroys nerves in the sympathetic nervous system. The procedure is performed to increase blood flow and decrease long-term pain in certain diseases that cause narrowed blood vessels. It can also be used to decrease excessive sweating. This surgical procedure cuts or destroys the sympathetic ganglia, which are collections of nerve cell bodies in clusters along the thoracic or lumbar spinal cord.

Purpose

The autonomic nervous system controls such involuntary body functions as breathing, sweating, and blood pressure. It is subdivided into two components, the sympathetic and the parasympathetic nervous systems.

The sympathetic nervous system speeds the heart rate, narrows (constricts) blood vessels, and raises blood pressure. Blood pressure is controlled by means of nerve cells that run through sheaths around the arteries. The sympathetic nervous system can be described as the "fight or flight" system because it allows humans to respond to danger by fighting off an attacker or running away. When danger threatens, the sympathetic nervous system increases heart and respiratory rates and blood flow to muscles, and decreases blood flow to such other areas as skin, digestive tract, and limb veins. The net effect is an increase in blood pressure.

Sympathectomy is performed to relieve intermittent constricting of blood vessels (ischemia) when the fingers, toes, ears, or nose are exposed to cold (Raynaud's phenomenon). In Raynaud's phenomenon, the affected extremities turn white, then blue, and red as the blood supply is cut off. The color changes are accompanied by numbness, tingling, burning, and pain. Normal color and feeling are restored when heat is applied. The condition sometimes occurs without direct cause but is more often caused by an underlying medical condition, such as rheumatoid arthritis. Sympathectomy is usually less effective when Raynaud's syndrome is caused by an underlying medical condition. Narrowed blood vessels in the legs that cause painful cramping (claudication) are also treated with sympathectomy.

Sympathectomy may be helpful in treating reflex sympathetic dystrophy (RSD), a condition that sometimes develops after injury. In RSD, the affected limb is painful (causalgia) and swollen. The color, temperature, and texture of the skin changes. These symptoms are related to prolonged and excessive sympathetic nervous system activity.

Sympathectomy is also effective in treating excessive sweating (hyperhidrosis) of the palms, armpits, or face.

Demographics

Experts estimate that 10,000–20,0000 sympathectomy procedures are performed each year in the united States.

Description

Sympathectomy for hyperhidrosis is accomplished by making a small incision under the armpit and introducing air into the chest cavity. The surgeon inserts a fiberoptic tube (endoscope) that projects an image of the operation on a video screen. The ganglia are cut with fine scissors attached to the endoscope. Laser beams may also be used to destroy the ganglia.

If only one arm or leg is affected, it may be treated with a percutaneous radiofrequency technique. In this technique, the surgeon locates the ganglia by a combination of x ray and electrical stimulation. The ganglia are destroyed by applying radio waves through electrodes on the skin.

Diagnosis/Preparation

A reversible block of the affected nerve cell (ganglion) determines if sympathectomy is needed. This procedure interrupts nerve impulses by injecting the ganglion with a steroid and anesthetic. If the block has a positive effect on pain and blood flow in the affected area, the sympathectomy will probably be helpful. The surgical procedure should be performed only if conservative treatment has not been effective. Conservative treatment includes avoiding exposure to stress and cold, and the use of physical therapy and medications.

Sympathectomy is most likely to be effective in relieving reflex sympathetic dystrophy if it is performed soon after the injury occurs. The increased benefit of early surgery must be balanced against the time needed to promote spontaneous recovery and responses to more conservative treatments.

Patients should discuss expected results and possible risks with their surgeons. They should inform their surgeons of all medications they are taking, and provide a complete medical history. Candidates for surgery should have good general health. To improve general health, a surgical candidate may be asked to lose weight, give up smoking or alcohol, and get the proper amount of sleep and **exercise**. Immediately before the surgery, patients will not be permitted to eat or drink, and the surgical site will be cleaned and scrubbed.

Aftercare

The surgeon informs the patient about specific aftercare needed for the technique used. Doppler ultrasonography, a test using sound waves to measure blood flow, can help to determine whether sympathectomy has had a positive result.

The operative site must be kept clean until the incision closes.

Risks

Side effects of sympathectomy may include decreased blood pressure while standing, which may cause fainting. After sympathectomy in men, semen is sometimes ejaculated into the bladder, possibly impairing fertility. After a sympathectomy is performed by inserting an endoscope in the chest cavity, some persons may experience chest pain with deep breathing. This problem usually disappears within two weeks. They may also experience pneumothorax (air in the chest cavity).

Normal results

Studies show that sympathectomy relieves hyperhidrosis in more than 90% of cases and causalgia in up to 75% of cases. The less invasive procedures cause very little scarring. Most persons stay in the hospital for less than one day and return to work within a week.

Morbidity and mortality rates

In 30% of cases, surgery for hyperhidrosis may cause increased sweating on the chest. In 2% of cases, the surgery may cause increased sweating in other areas, including increased facial sweating while eating. Less frequent complications include Horner's syndrome, a condition of the nervous system that causes the pupil of the eye to close, the eyelid to droop, and sweating to decrease on one side of the face. Other rare complications are nasal blockage and pain to the nerves supplying the skin between the ribs. Mortality is extremely rare, and usually attributable to low blood pressure.

Alternatives

Nonsurgical treatments include physical therapy, medications, and avoidance of stress and cold. These measures reduce or remove the likelihood of triggering a problem mediated by the sympathetic nervous system.

See also Neurosurgery.

Resources

BOOKS

Bland, K.I., W.G. Cioffi, and M.G. Sarr. *Practice of General Surgery.* Philadelphia: Saunders, 2001.

Grace, P.A., A. Cuschieri D. Rowley, N. Borley, and A. Darzi. *Clinical Surgery,* 2nd ed. Londin, 2003.

Schwartz, S.I., J.E. Fischer, F.C. Spencer, G.T. Shires, and J.M. Daly. *Principles of Surgery,* 7th ed. New York: McGraw-Hill, 1998.

Townsend, C., K.L. Mattox, R.D. Beauchamp, B.M. Evers, and D.C. Sabiston. *Sabiston's Review of Surgery,* 3rd Edition. Philadelphia: Saunders, 2001.

PERIODICALS

Atkinson, J.L., and R.D. Fealey. "Sympathotomy Instead of Sympathectomy for Palmar Hyperhidrosis: Minimizing Postoperative Compensatory Hyperhidrosis." *Mayo Clinic Proceedings* 78, no. 2 (2003): 167-72.

Gossot, D., D. Galetta, A. Pascal, D. Debrosse, R. Caliandro, P. Girard, J.B. Stern, and D. Grunenwald. "Long-Term Results of Endoscopic Thoracic Sympathectomy for Upper Limb Hyperhidrosis." *Annals of Thoracic Surgery* 75, no.4 (2003): 1075-9.

Matthews, B.D., H.T. Bui, K.L.Harold, K.W.Kercher, M.A. Cowan, C.A. Van der Veer, and B.T. Heniford. "Thoracoscopic Sympathectomy for Palmaris Hyperhidrosis." *Southern Medical Journal* 96, no.3 (2003): 254-8.

Singh, B., J. Moodley, A.S. Shaik, and J.V. Robbs. "Sympathectomy for Complex Regional Pain Syndrome." *Journal of Vascular Surgery* 37, no. 3 (2003): 508-11.

KEY TERMS

Causalgia—A severe burning sensation sometimes accompanied by redness and inflammation of the skin. Causalgia is caused by injury to a nerve outside the spinal cord.

Claudication—Cramping or pain in a leg caused by poor blood circulation, frequently caused by hardening of the arteries (atherosclerosis). Intermittent claudication occurs only at certain times, usually after exercise, and is relieved by rest.

Fiberoptics—In medicine, fiberoptics uses glass or plastic fibers to transmit light through a specially designed tube inserted into organs or body cavities where it transmits a magnified image of the internal body structures.

Hyperhidrosis—Excessive sweating. Hyperhidrosis can be caused by heat, overactive thyroid glands, strong emotion, menopause, or infection.

Parasympathetic nervous system—The division of the autonomic (involuntary) nervous system that slows heart rate, increases digestive and glandular activity, and relaxes the sphincter muscles that close off body organs.

Percutaneous—Performed through the skin. It is derived from two Latin words, *per* (through) and *cutis* (skin).

Pneumothorax—A collection of air or gas in the chest cavity that causes a lung to collapse. Pneumothorax may be caused by an open chest wound that admits air.

Urschel, H.C., and A. Patel. "Thoracic Outlet Syndromes." *Current Treatment Options in Cardiovascular Medicine* 5, no.2 (2003): 163-8.

ORGANIZATIONS

American Academy of Neurology. 1080 Montreal Avenue, St. Paul, Minnesota 55116. (651) 695-1940. Fax: (651) 695-2791. E-mail: info@aan.org. <http://www.aan.com/>.

American Board of Surgery. 1617 John F. Kennedy Boulevard, Suite 860, Philadelphia, PA 19103. (215) 568-4000. Fax: 215-563-5718. <http://www.absurgery.org/>.

American College of Surgeons. 633 North St. Clair Street, Chicago, IL 60611-32311. (312) 02-5000. Fax: (312) 202-5001. E-mail: postmaster@facs.org. <http://www.facs.org/>.

OTHER

Columbia University College of Physicians and Surgeons. [cited May 15, 2003] <http://www.columbiasurgery.org/divisions/cardiothoracic/dd_hydrosis_endoscopic.html>.

"Excessive Sweating." [cited May 15, 2003] <http://www.excessive-sweating.net/sympathectomy_history.html>.

New York Presbyterian Hospital. [cited May 15, 2003] <http://www.masc.cc/sympathectomy.htm>.

University of Maryland School of Medicine. [cited May 15, 2003] <http://www.umm.edu/thoracic/thoracic5a.html>.

University of Southern California School of Medicine. [cited May 15, 2003] <http://uscneurosurgery.com/glossary/s/sympathectomy.htm>.

L. Fleming Fallon, Jr., M.D., Dr.PH.

Syndactyly surgery *see* **Webbed finger or toe repair**

Syringe and needle

Definition

Syringes and needles are sterile devices used to inject solutions into or withdraw secretions from the body. A syringe is a calibrated glass or plastic cylinder with a plunger at one and an opening that attaches to a needle. The needle is a hollow metal tube with a pointed tip.

Purpose

A syringe and needle assembly is used to administer drugs when a small amount of fluid is to be injected; when a person cannot take the drug by mouth; or when the drug would be destroyed by digestive secretions. A syringe and needle may also be used to withdraw various types of body fluids, most commonly tissue fluid from swollen joints or blood from veins.

Description

The modern hypodermic needle was invented in 1853 by Alexander Wood, a Scottish physician, and independently in the same year by Charles Pravaz, a French surgeon. As of 2003, there are many different types and sizes of syringes used for a variety of purposes. Syringe sizes may vary from 0.25 mL to 450 mL, and can be made from glass or assorted plastics. Latex-free syringes eliminate the exposure of health care professionals and patients to allergens to which they may be sensitive. The most common type of syringe is the piston syringe. Pen, cartridge, and dispensing syringes are also extensively used.

One common type of syringe consists of a hollow barrel with a piston at one end and a nozzle at the other end that connects to a needle. Other syringes have a needle already attached. These devices are often used for subcutaneous injections of insulin and are single-use (i.e., disposable). Syringes have markings etched or printed on their sides, showing the graduations (i.e., in milliliters) for accurate dispensing of drugs or removal of body fluids. Cartridge syringes are intended for multiple uses, and are often sold in kits containing a pre-filled drug cartridge with a needle inserted into the piston syringe. Syringes may also have anti-needlestick features, as well as positive stops that prevent accidental pullouts.

There are three types of nozzles:

- Luer-lock, which locks the needle onto the nozzle of the syringe.
- Slip tip, which secures the needle by compressing the slightly tapered hub onto the syringe nozzle.
- Eccentric, which secures with a connection that is almost flush with the side of the syringe.

A hypodermic needle is a hollow metal tube, usually made of stainless steel and sharpened at one end. It has a female connection at one end that fits into the male connection of a syringe or intravascular administration set. The size of the diameter of the needle ranges from the largest gauge (13) to the smallest (27). The length of the needle ranges from 3.5 inches (8 cm) for the 13-gauge to 0.25 inch (0.6 cm) for the 27-gauge. The needle consists of a hub with a female connection at one end that attaches to the syringe. The bevel, which is a slanted opening on one side of the needle tip, is located at the other end.

Needles are almost always disposable. Reusable needle assemblies are available for home use.

Operation

Syringes and needles are used for injecting or withdrawing fluids from a person. The most common procedure for removing fluids is venipuncture or drawing blood from a vein. In this procedure, the syringe and a needle of the proper size are used with a vacutainer. A vacutainer is a tube with a rubber top from which air has been removed. Fluids enter the container without pressure applied by the person withdrawing the blood. A vacutainer is used to collect blood as it is drawn. The syringe and needle can be left in place while the health care provider changes the vacutainer, allowing for multiple samples to be drawn during a single procedure.

Fluids can be injected by intradermal injection, subcutaneous injection, intramuscular injection, or Z-track injection. For all types of injections, the size of syringe should be chosen based on the amount of fluid being delivered; the gauge and length of needle should be chosen based on the size of the patient and type of medication. A

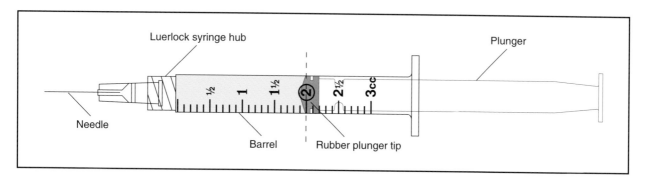

Parts of a syringe. *(From Fundamentals of Nursing, Standards & Practice, 1st edition by DELAUNE. (c) 1998. Reprinted with permission of Delmar Learning, a division of Thomson Learning: www.thomsonrights.com. Fax: 800-730-2215.)*

needle with a larger gauge may be chosen for drawing up the medication into the syringe, and a smaller-gauge needle used to replace the larger one for administering the injection. Proper procedures for infection control should be strictly followed for all injections.

Maintenance

Syringes and needles are normally sterile products and should be stored in appropriate containers. Care should be taken prior to using them. The care provider should ensure that the needles have not been blunted and that the packaging is not torn, as poor handling or storage exposes the contents to air and allows contamination by microorganisms.

Safety

All health care personnel must be offered vaccines against such bloodborne infections as hepatitis B and C.

Used syringes and needles should be discarded quickly in appropriate containers. If a needlestick injury occurs, it must be reported immediately and proper treatment administered to the injured person.

Training

Health care instructors should ensure that staff members are skilled in up-to-date methods of **aseptic technique** as well as the correct handling and use of syringes and needles. All persons administering injections should be aware of current methods of infection prevention.

Teaching the correct use of syringes and needles, as well as their disposal, is important to protect medical staff and people receiving injections from needlestick injuries and contamination from bloodborne infections. As of 2003, some of the more serious infections are human immunodeficiency virus (HIV), hepatitis B (HBV), and hepatitis C (HCV).

Needles are defined as "sharps" for purposes of public health regulation, and must be broken or otherwise "rendered unrecognizable" before being placed in a puncture-proof container labeled with the universal biohazard symbol. This precaution is intended to prevent drug addicts from reusing the needles as well as to protect the hospital environment from contamination by medical waste.

Resources

BOOKS

Basford, Lynn, and Oliver Slevin. *Theory and Practice of Nursing: An Integrated Approach*, 2nd ed. London, UK: Stanley Thornes, 2003.

Ferri, Fred F. *Practical Guide to the Care of the Medical Patient*, 5th ed. St. Louis, MO: Mosby, 2001.

Nettina, Sandra M. *The Lippincott Manual of Nursing Practice*, 7th ed. Philaadelphia, PA: Lippincott Williams & Wilkins, 2001.

Perry, Anne G., and Patricia A. Potter. *Clinical Nursing Skills & Techniques*, 5th ed. St. Louis, MO: Mosby, 2001.

PERIODICALS

Clarke, S. P., D. M. Sloane, and L. H. Aiken. "Needlestick Injuries to Nurses, in Context." *Leonard Davis Institute of Health Economics Issue Brief* 8 (September 2002): 1-4.

Metules, T. "What If You're Stuck by a Needle?" *Registered Nurse* 65 (November 2002): 34-37.

Perry, J., and J. Jagger. "Safer Needles: Not Optional." *Nursing* 32 (October 2002): 20-22.

Ratzlaff, J. I. "Needle Safety Technology." *Spinal Cord Injury Nursing* 19 (Spring 2002): 17-20.

ORGANIZATIONS

American Academy of Family Physicians. 11400 Tomahawk Creek Parkway, Leawood, KS 66211-2672. (913) 906-6000. <www.aafp.org>. E-mail: fp@aafp.org.

American Academy of Pediatrics. 141 Northwest Point Boulevard, Elk Grove Village, IL 60007-1098. (847) 434-4000; FAX: (847) 434-8000. <www.aap.org>. E-mail: kidsdoc@aap.org .

KEY TERMS

Aseptic—Free from infection or diseased material; sterile.

Bevel—The slanted opening on one side of the tip of a needle.

Hypodermic—Applied or administered beneath the skin. The modern hypodermic needle was invented to deliver medications below the skin surface.

Piston—The plunger that slides up and down inside the barrel of a syringe.

Sharps—A general term for needles, lancets, scalpel blades, and other medical devices with points or sharp edges requiring special disposal precautions.

Sterile—Free from living microorganisms.

Subcutaneous—Beneath the skin.

Vacutainer—A tube with a rubber top from which air has been removed.

Z-track injection—A special technique for injecting a drug into muscle tissue so that the drug does not leak (track) into the layers of tissue just beneath the skin.

American College of Physicians. 190 N. Independence Mall West, Philadelphia, PA 19106-1572. (800) 523-1546, x2600 or (215) 351-2600. <www.acponline.org>.

American College of Surgeons. 633 North St. Clair Street, Chicago, IL 60611-3231. (312) 202-5000; FAX: (312) 202-5001. <www.facs.org>. E-mail: postmaster@facs.org.

American Medical Association. 515 N. State Street, Chicago, IL 60610. (312) 464-5000. <www.ama-assn.org>.

American Nurses Association. 600 Maryland Avenue, SW, Suite 100 West, Washington, DC 20024. (202) 651-7000 or (800) 274-4262. <www.nursingworld.org>.

OTHER

American College of Allergy, Asthma, and Immunology, [cited March 13, 2003]. <www.allergy.mcg.edu/advice/latex.html>

American Nurses Association, [cited March 13, 2003]. <www.nursingworld.org/readroom/fsneedle.htm>.

National Institute of Occupational Safety and Health (NIOSH). [cited March 13, 2003]. <www.cdc.gov/niosh/2000-135.html>.

Occupational Safety and Health Administration (OSHA). [cited March 13, 2003]. <www.osha-slc.gov/SLTC/needlestick>.

L. Fleming Fallon, Jr., MD, DrPH

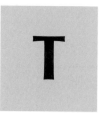

T-PA *see* **Thrombolytic therapy**

Talking to the doctor

Definition

Talking to the doctor is a fundamental requirement for an accurate exchange of information between patient and health care provider. It includes communicating private or potentially sensitive information, and requires a climate of trust. Without trust and accurate information, treatment and healing is difficult at best and impossible at worst.

Purpose

The purpose of talking to a doctor is to exchange information and obtain a cure or relief from pain and suffering. This outcome can only occur in an atmosphere of openness and mutual confidence.

Description

Talking is a basic human mode of communication. Talking to a doctor should be easy, but for many people, this is not the case. Barriers to straightforward communication include inhibition (shyness), fear and guilt. These barriers may be present whether the patient is an adult who can speak for him- or herself or a child or elderly person whose history and symptoms must be described by another family member.

Inhibition

People often hold physicians in high regard. The stated reason for this feeling is a difference in educational level. Doctors have more educational credentials than most people in the general population. This differential tends to make patients self-conscious and hesitant to offer information.

Inhibition is further fueled by the sense of hurry and urgency that many health professionals project. Patients feel uncomfortable when they sense that they are being rushed by their doctor. As a result, they are reluctant to speak freely.

Fear

Apart from vaccinations or routine physical checkups, people in the United States do not ordinarily visit a doctor when they are well. The norm is to make an appointment when something hurts or does not function or feel right. It is natural for people to feel anxious in these circumstances—they are afraid of receiving bad news.

Guilt

Many patients' health complaints are often the direct consequences of their own behavior. Obesity often results from a combination of overeating and inadequate **exercise**. The leading cause of lung cancer is smoking tobacco. Casual sex can lead to unwanted pregnancies and sexually transmitted diseases. Having to accept responsibility for choices that lead to undesirable consequences is painful. Having to tell a person who is an authority figure as well as a trusted confidant often arouses guilt feelings.

Establishing trust

Trust requires time to develop, but it is also a two-way interaction. People seeking the advice of a doctor may reveal only a portion of their symptoms at first. While it is the doctor's task to elicit relevant information, the patient who is answering the questions must be open.

Doctors often assume that patients do not give completely honest answers. Women typically understate their body weight while men overstate their strength. Smokers rarely admit to the true number of cigarettes that they smoke per day. Drinkers underestimate the amount of alcohol that they consume.

Preparation

An important element of any doctor-patient conversation is honesty and openness. Some people may have to make a conscious decision to be open with their doctors. To avoid wasting time and feeling pressured, people should decide to be completely frank before they enter a doctor's office. In addition, inaccurate or incomplete information may lead the doctor to make an incorrect diagnosis or treatment decision.

Bringing records from visits to other health care providers is very useful to a doctor. People who have known their doctors for long periods of time are a steadily shrinking minority. Providing a new doctor with copies of one's medical history saves time and usually improves diagnostic accuracy. For example, old photographs are especially invaluable when evaluating skin problems.

Results

The passage of time, repeated positive interactions, and good outcomes from the information provided by the patient help to establish mutual trust. Trust then enhances the therapeutic interaction. The result may well be better health for the patient.

Preventive care should be part of the interaction between doctor and patient. A frank exchange of information is one form of prevention. If a conversation with one's doctor accomplishes nothing else, it will reduce inhibition, fear and guilt.

See also Health history; Physical examination.

Resources

BOOKS

Bickley, L. S., P. G. Szilagyi, and J. G. Stackhouse, eds. *Bates' Guide to Physical Examination & History Taking*, 8th ed. Philadelphia, PA: Lippincott Williams & Wilkins, 2002.

Chan, P. D., and P. J. Winkle. *History and Physical Examination in Medicine*, 10th ed. New York, NY: Current Clinical Strategies, 2002.

Seidel, Henry M. *Mosby's Physical Examination Handbook*, 4th ed. St. Louis, MO: Mosby-Year Book, 2003.

Swartz, Mark A., and William Schmitt. *Textbook of Physical Diagnosis: History and Examination*, 4th ed. Philadelphia, PA: Saunders, 2001.

PERIODICALS

Lee, S. J., A. L. Back, S. D. Block, and S. K. Stewart. "Enhancing Physician-Patient Communication." *Hematology* (2002): 464-483.

Nadelson, C., and M. T. Notman. "Boundaries in the Doctor-Patient Relationship." *Theoretical Medicine and Bioethics* 23 (March 2002): 191-201.

Nebel, E. J. "Malpractice: Love Thy Patient." *Clinical Orthopedics* 407 (February 2003): 19-24.

Thakur, N. M., and R. L. Perkel. "Prevention in Adulthood: Forging a Doctor-Patient Partnership." *Primary Care* 29 (September 2002): 571-582.

ORGANIZATIONS

American Academy of Family Physicians. 11400 Tomahawk Creek Parkway, Leawood, KS 66211-2672. (913) 906-6000. <www.aafp.org>. E-mail: fp@aafp.org.

American Academy of Pediatrics. 141 Northwest Point Boulevard, Elk Grove Village, IL 60007-1098. (847) 434-4000; FAX: (847) 434-8000. <www.aap.org>. E-mail: kidsdoc@aap.org.

American College of Physicians. 190 N. Independence Mall West, Philadelphia, PA 19106-1572. (800) 523-1546, x2600 or (215) 351-2600. <www.acponline.org>.

American College of Surgeons. 633 North St. Clair Street, Chicago, IL 60611-3231. (312) 202-5000; FAX: (312) 202-5001. <www.facs.org>. E-mail: postmaster@facs.org.

American Hospital Association. One North Franklin, Chicago, IL 60606-3421. (312) 422-3000. <www.aha.org/index.asp>.

American Medical Association. 515 N. State Street, Chicago, IL 60610. (312) 464-5000. <www.ama-assn.org>.

OTHER

Cable News Network (CNN). [cited March 2, 2003]. <www.cnn.com/HEALTH/9906/ 30/internet.house.calls>.

Emory University. [cited March 2, 2003]. <www.emory.edu/WHSC/HSNEWS/releases /jun98/061898kaleidoscope.html>.

University of North Carolina at Chapel Hill. [cited March 2, 2003]. <www.med.unc.edu/wrkunits/2depts/medicine/fgidc/improving_relation ships.htm>.

YourDoctorintheFamily.Com. [cited March 2, 2003]. <www.yourdoctorinthefamily.com/grandtheory/section11.htm>.

L. Fleming Fallon, Jr., MD, DrPH

Tarsorrhaphy

Definition

Tarsorrhaphy is a rare procedure in which the eyelids are partially sewn together to narrow the opening.

Purpose

The eye needs the lid for protection. It also needs tears and periodic blinking to cleanse it and keep it moist. There are many conditions that impair these functions and threaten the eye, specifically the cornea, with drying. Sewing the eyelids partially together helps protect the eye until the underlying condition can be corrected.

A partial list of the conditions that can require tarsorrhaphy includes:

WHO PERFORMS THE PROCEDURE AND WHERE IS IT PERFORMED?

Ophthalmologists perform the procedure on an outpatient basis in a hospital, or sometimes in their offices.

QUESTIONS TO ASK THE DOCTOR

- How long will will the eyes be closed with sutures?
- Will it be painful?
- Will the condition be remedied after the procedure?

- Paralysis or weakness of the eyelids so that they cannot close or blink adequately. Bell's palsy is a nerve condition that weakens the muscles of the face, including the eyelids. It is usually temporary. Myasthenia gravis also weakens facial muscles, but it is usually treatable. A stroke can also weaken eyelids so that they do not close.

- Exophthalmos (eyes bulging out of their sockets) occurs with Graves' disease of the thyroid, and with tumors behind the eyes. If the eyes bulge out too far, the lids cannot close over them.

- Enophthalmos is a condition in which the eye falls back into the socket, making the eyelid ineffective.

- Several eye and corneal diseases cause swelling of the cornea, and require temporary added protection until the condition resolves.

- Sjögren's syndrome reduces tear flow to the point where it can endanger the cornea.

- Dendritic ulcers of the cornea caused by viruses may need to be covered with the eyelid while they heal.

Demographics

People of all ages can suffer from paralysis or corneal diseases that may benefit from tarsorrhaphy. For that reason, physicians can perform tarsorrhaphy on patients of any age. However, it is viewed as a last alternative for many patients, and is not indicated until after other treatments (e.g., patching and eye ointments) have been attempted.

Description

Stitches are carefully placed at the corners of the eyelid opening (palpebral fissure) to narrow it. This provides the eye with improved lubrication and less air exposure. Eyeball motion can help bathe the cornea in tears when it rolls up under the lid. The outpatient procedure is done under local anesthetic.

Diagnosis/Preparation

The use of eye drops and contact lenses to moisten and protect the eyes must be considered before tarsorrha-phy is performed. Tarsorrhaphy is a minor procedure done under local anesthesia. Special preparation is not necessary.

Aftercare

Patients should avoid rubbing the eye and refrain from wearing make-up until given permission from the physician. Driving should be restricted until approval from the ophthalmologist.

Pathways in the home should be cleared of obstacles, and patients should be aware of peripheral vision loss. They will need to compensate by turning their head fully when looking at an object.

An analgesic may be used to ease pain, but severe pain is not normal, and the physician must be alerted. Sutures will be removed in two weeks.

Eye drops or ointment may still be needed to preserve the cornea or treat accompanying disease.

Risks

Tarsorrhaphy carries few risks. Complications may include minor eyelid swelling and superficial infection.

Normal results

The procedure succeeds in protecting the eye and returning moisture to dry eyes.

Morbidity and mortality rates

This is a safe procedure. Only superficial infections have been reported.

Alternatives

Eye drops and contact lenses are widely used to treat conditions that once warranted tarsorrhaphy. The procedure is now considered a last option for treatment.

Resources

BOOKS

Cassel, M.D., H. Gary, Michael D. Billig, O.D.,and Harry G. Randall, M.D. *The Eye Book: A Complete Guide to Eye Disorders and Health.* Baltimore, MD: Johns Hopkins University Press, 1998.

Daly, Stephen, ed. *Everything You Need to Know About Medical Treatments.* Springhouse, PA: Springhouse Corp., 1996.

Sardegna, Jill Otis, et al. *The Encyclopedia of Blindness and Vision Impairment,* 2nd ed. New York: Facts on File Inc., 2002.

J. Ricker Polsdorfer, M.D.
Mary Bekker

Telesurgery

Definition

Telesurgery, also called remote surgery, is performed by a surgeon at a site removed from the patient. Surgical tasks are directly performed by a robotic system controlled by the surgeon at the remote site. The word "telesurgery" is derived from the Greek words *tele*, meaning "far off," and *cheirourgia*, meaning "working by hand."

Description

In the early 2000s, several projects investigating the possibility and practicality of telesurgery were successful in performing complete surgical procedures on human patients from remote locations.

Preceding technologies

Telesurgery became a possibility with the advent of laparoscopic surgery in the late 1980s. **Laparoscopy** (also called minimally invasive surgery) is a surgical procedure in which a laparoscope (a thin lighted tube) and other instruments are inserted into the abdomen through small incisions. The internal operating field may then be visualized on a video monitor connected to the scope. In certain cases, the technique may be used in place of more invasive surgical procedures that require more extensive incisions and longer recovery times.

Computer-assisted surgery premiered in the mid-1990s; it was the next step toward the goal of remote surgery. The ZEUS Surgical System, developed in 1995 by Computer Motion, Inc., was approved by the Federal Drug Administration (FDA) in 2002 for use in general and laparoscopic surgeries with the patient and surgeon in the same room. ZEUS comprises three table-mounted robotic arms—one holding the AESOP endoscope positioner, which provides a view of the internal operating field, the others holding **surgical instruments**. The robotic arms are controlled by the surgeon, who sits at a console several meters away. Visualization of the operating field is controlled by voice activation, while the robotic arms are controlled by movements of the surgeon's hands and wrists.

Computer-assisted surgery has a number of advantages over traditional laparoscopic surgery. The computer interface provides a method for filtering out the normal hand tremors of the surgeon. Two- and three-dimensional visualization of the operating field is possible. The surgeon can perform a maneuver on the console, review it to be sure of its safety and efficacy, then instruct the remote device to perform the task. The surgeon is also seated in an ergonomic position with arms supported by arm rests for the duration of the operation.

Operation Lindbergh

While the concept of telesurgery seems like a logical technological progression—if a surgeon can perform a procedure from several meters away, why not from several thousand meters?—there is a major constraint that could lead to disastrous results during surgery, namely time delay. In the case of computer-assisted surgery, the computer console and remote surgical device are directly connected by several meters of cable; there is therefore virtually no delay in the transmission of data from the console to the surgical device back to the console. The surgeon therefore views his or her movements on the computer interface as they are happening. If the surgical system were removed to a more distant site, however, it would introduce a time delay. Visualization of the operating field could be milliseconds or even seconds behind the real-time manipulations of the surgeon. Studies showed that a delay of more than 150–200 milliseconds would be dangerous; satellite transmission, for example, would introduce a delay of more than 600 milliseconds.

In order to make telesurgery a reality, expert surgeons would need to work with the telecommunication industry to develop secure, reliable, high-speed transmission of data over large distances with imperceptible delays. In January 2000, such a project, labeled "Operation Lindbergh," began under the direction of Dr. Jacques Marescaux, director of the European Institute of Telesurgery; Moji Ghodoussi, project manager at Computer Motions, Inc.; and communication experts from France Télécom. Testing began on a prototype remote system (a modified version of the ZEUS Surgical System called ZEUS TS) in September 2000, with data being relayed between Paris and Strasbourg, France—a distance of approximately 625 mi (1000 km). Once an acceptable length of time delay was established, trials began in July 2001 between New York City and Strasbourg.

On September 7, 2001, Operation Lindbergh culminated in the first complete remote surgery on a human patient (a 68-year-old female), performed over a distance of 4300 mi (7000 km). The patient and surgical system were located in an **operating room** in Strasbourg, while the surgeon and remote console were situated in a high-rise building in downtown New York. A team of surgeons remained at the patient's side to step in if need arose. The procedure performed was a laparoscopic **cholecystectomy** (gall bladder removal), considered the standard of care in minimally invasive surgery. The established time delay during the surgery was 135 ms—remarkable considering that the data traveled a distance of more than 8600 mi (14,000 km) from the surgeon's console to the surgical system and back to the console. The patient left the hospital within 48 hours—a typical stay following laparoscopic cholecystectomy—and had an uneventful recovery.

Applications

Operation Lindbergh has paved the way for wide-ranging applications of telesurgery technology. On February 28, 2003, the first hospital-to-hospital telerobotic-assisted surgery took place in Ontario, Canada, over a distance of 250 mi (400 km). Two surgeons worked together to perform a Nissen fundoplication (surgery to treat chronic acid reflux), with one situated at the patient's side and the other controlling a robotic surgical system from a remote hospital site. Such a scenario may eventually allow surgeons in rural areas to receive expert assistance during minimally invasive procedures.

Other potential applications of telesurgery include:

- training new surgeons
- assisting and training surgeons in developing countries
- treating injured soldiers on or near the battlefield
- performing surgical procedures in space
- collaborating and mentoring during surgery by surgeons around the globe

Resources

PERIODICALS

Marescaux, J., et al. "Transatlantic Robotic Assisted Remote Telesurgery." *Nature* 413, no. 6854 (September 27, 2001): 379-80.

ORGANIZATIONS

Computer Motion, Inc. 130-B Cremona Dr., Goleta, CA 93117. (805) 968-9600. <www.computermotion.com>.
European Institute of Telesurgery. 1, Place de l'Hôpital, F 67091 STRASBOURG Cedex. +33(0)388119000. <www. eits.org>.

OTHER

Ghodoussi, Moji. "Project Lindbergh: World's First Transatlantic Telesurgery." Computer Motion, Inc., 2002 [cited April 13, 2003]. <www.computermotion.com/about/news room/features/projectlindbergh>.
"Operation Lindbergh: First Transatlantic Robot-Assisted Operation." WebSurg, 2003 [cited April 13, 2003]. <www. websurg.com/lindbergh>.
Rola, Monika. "Telerobotics Bridges Rural Health Care Divide." itbusiness.ca, March 4, 2003 [cited April 13, 2003]. <www.itbusiness.ca/index.asp?theaction=61&lid=1&sid= 51570>.
"ZEUS Surgical System." Computer Motion, Inc., 2002 [cited April 13, 2003]. <www.computermotion.com/products andsolutions/products/zeus>.

Stephanie Dionne Sherk

Tendon repair

Definition

Tendon repair refers to the surgical repair of damaged or torn tendons, which are cord-like structures made of strong fibrous connective tissue that connect muscles to bones. The shoulder, elbow, knee, and ankle joints are the most commonly affected by tendon injuries.

Purpose

The goal of tendon repair is to restore the normal function of joints or their surrounding tissues following a tendon laceration.

Demographics

Tendon injuries are widespread in the general adult population. They are more common among people whose occupations or recreational athletic activities require repetitive motion of the shoulder, knee, elbow, or ankle joints. Injuries to the tendons in the shoulder often occur among baseball players, window washers, violinists, dancers, carpenters, and some assembly line workers. Rowers are at increased risk for injuries to the forearm tendons. The repetitive stresses of classical ballet, running, and jogging may damage the Achilles tendon at the back of the heel. So-called tennis elbow, which occurs in many construction workers, highway crews, maintenance workers, and baggage handlers as well as professional golfers and tennis players, is thought to affect 5% of American adults over the age of 30.

Women in all age brackets are at greater risk than men for injuries to the tendons in the elbow and knee joints. It is thought that injuries in these areas are related to the slightly greater looseness of women's joints compared to those in men.

Description

Local, regional or general anesthesia is administered to the patient depending on the extent and location of tendon damage. With a general anesthetic, the patient is asleep during surgery. With a regional anesthetic, a specific region of nerves is anesthetized; with a local anesthetic, the patient remains alert during the surgery, and only the incision location is anesthetized.

After the overlying skin has been cleansed with an antiseptic solution and covered with a sterile drape, the surgeon makes an incision over the injured tendon. When the tendon has been located and identified, the surgeon sutures the damaged or torn ends of the tendon together. If the tendon has been severely injured, a tendon graft may be required. This is a procedure in which a piece of tendon is taken from the foot or other part of the body and used to repair the damaged tendon. If required, tendons are reattached to the surrounding connective tissue. The surgeon inspects the area for injuries to nerves and blood vessels, and closes the incision.

Diagnosis/Preparation

Diagnosis of a tendon injury is usually made when the patient consults a doctor about pain in the injured area. The doctor will usually order radiographs and other imaging studies of the affected joint as well as taking a history and performing an external **physical examination** in the office. In some cases fluid will be aspirated (withdrawn through a needle) from the joint to check for signs of infection, bleeding, or arthritis.

Prior to surgery, the patient is asked not to eat or drink anything, even water. A few days before the operation, patients are also instructed to stop taking such over-the-counter pain medications as **aspirin** or ibuprofen. If the patient has a splint or cast, it is removed before surgery.

To prepare for surgery, the patient typically reports to a preoperative nursing unit, where he or she changes into a hospital gown. Next, the patient is taken to a preoperative holding area, where an anesthesiologist administers an intravenous sedative. The patient is then taken to the **operating room**.

Aftercare

Patients are asked to have someone drive them home after tendon repair surgery. Healing may take as long as 6 weeks, during which the injured part may be immobilized in a splint or cast. Patients are asked not to use the injured tendon until the physician gives permission. The physician will decide how long to rest the tendon. It should not be used for lifting heavy objects or walking. Patients are also asked to avoid driving until the physician gives the go-ahead. To reduce swelling and pain, they should keep the injured limb lifted above the level of the heart as much as possible for the first few days after surgery.

Splints or bandages should be left in place until the next checkup. Patients are advised to keep bandages clean and dry. If patients have a cast, they are asked not to get it wet, to cover it with plastic while bathing, and to avoid exposing the cast to water. Fiberglass casts that get wet may be dried with a hair dryer. Patients are also instructed not to push or lean on the cast to avoid breaking it. If patients have a splint that is held in place with an Ace bandage, they are instructed to ensure that the bandage is not too tight. They are also asked to ensure that

Tendon repair

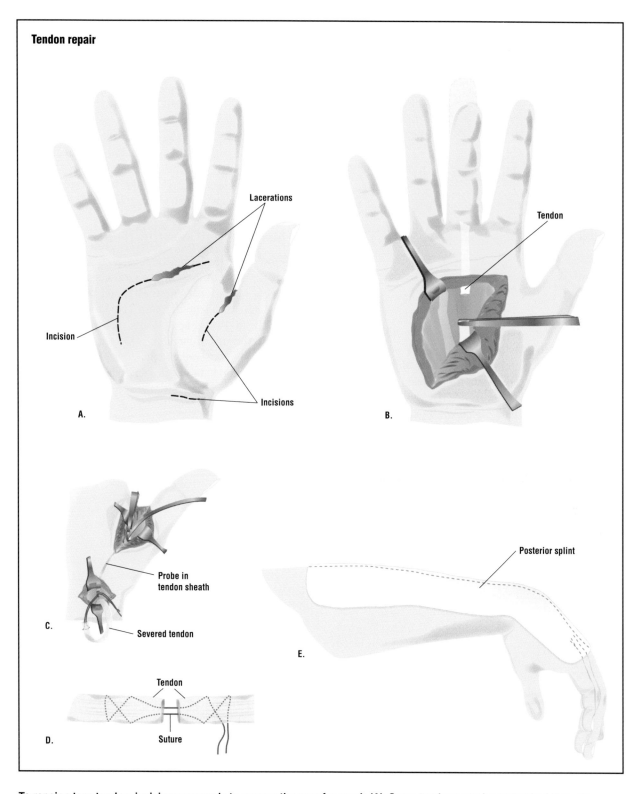

Lacerations

Incision

Incisions

A.

Tendon

B.

Probe in tendon sheath

Severed tendon

C.

Tendon

Suture

D.

Posterior splint

E.

To repair a torn tendon, incisions are made to expose the area for repair (A). Some tendons can be reattached through one incision (B), while others require two to access the severed point and the remaining tendon (C). A special splint that minimizes stretching the tendons may be worn after surgery (E). *(Illustration by GGS Inc.)*

QUESTIONS TO ASK THE DOCTOR

- What happens on the day of surgery?
- What type of anesthesia will be used?
- How long will it take to recover from the surgery?
- Can I expect normal flexibility in the affected area?
- What are the risks associated with tendon repair surgery?
- How many tendon repair procedures do you perform in a year?
- Will there be a scar?

splints remain in exactly the same place. Medications prescribed by the doctor should be taken exactly as directed. Patients who have been given **antibiotics** should take the complete course even if they feel well; this precaution is needed to minimize the risk of drug resistance developing in the disease organism. If patients are taking medicine that makes them feel drowsy, they are advised against driving or using heavy equipment.

Aftercare may also include physical therapy for the affected joint. There are a variety of exercises, wraps, splints, braces, bandages, ice packs, massages, and other treatments that physical therapists may recommend or use in helping a patient recover from tendon surgery.

Risks

Tendon repair surgery includes the risks associated with any procedure requiring anesthesia, such as reactions to medications and breathing difficulties. Risks associated with any surgery are also present, such as bleeding and infection. Additional risks specific to tendon repair include: formation of scar tissue that may prevent smooth movements (adequate tendon gliding); nerve damage; and partial loss of function in the involved joint.

Normal results

Tendon injuries represent a difficult and frustrating problem. Conservative treatment has little if any chance of restoring optimal range of motion in the injured area. Even after surgical repair, a full range of motion is usually not achieved. Permanent loss of motion, joint contractures, weakness and stiffness may be unavoidable. Scar tissue tends to form between the moving surfaces within joints, resulting in adhesions that hamper motion. The surgical repair may also split apart or loosen. Revision surgery may be required to remove scar tissue, insert tendon grafts or other reconstructive procedures. Thus, successful tendon repair depends on many factors. Recovery of the full range of motion is less likely if there is a nerve injury or a broken bone next to the tendon injury; if a long period of time has elapsed between the injury and surgery; if the patient's tissues tend to form thick scars; and if the damage was caused by a crush injury. The location of the injury is also an important factor in determining how well a patient will recover after surgery.

Morbidity and mortality rates

Mortality rates for tendon repairs are very low, partly because some of these procedures can be performed with local or regional anesthesia, and partly because most patients with tendon injuries are young or middle-aged adults in good general health. Morbidity varies according to the specific tendon involved; ruptures of the Achilles tendon or shoulder tendons are more difficult to repair than injuries to smaller tendons elsewhere in the body. In addition, some postoperative complications result from patient noncompliance; in one study, two out of 50 patients in the study sample had new injuries within three weeks after surgery because they did not follow the surgeon's recommendations. In general, tendon repairs performed in the United States are reported as having an infection rate of about 1.9%, with other complications ranging between 5.8% and 9.5%.

Alternatives

There are no alternatives to surgery for tendon repair as of 2003; however, research is providing encouraging findings. Although there is no presently approved drug that targets this notoriously slow and often incomplete healing process, a cellular substance recently discovered at the Lawrence Berkeley National Laboratory may lead to a new drug that would improve the speed and durability of healing for injuries to tendons and ligaments. The substance, called Cell Density Signal-1, or CDS-1, by its discoverer, cell biologist Richard Schwarz, acts as part of a chemical switch that turns on procollagen production. Procollagen is a protein manufactured in large amounts by embryonic tendon cells. It is transformed outside the cell into collagen, the basic component of such connective tissues as tendons, ligaments or bones. Amgen Inc. is planning to use genetic engineering to bring CDS-1 into mass production.

Prolotherapy represents a less invasive alternative to surgery. It is a form of treatment that stimulates the repair of injured or damaged structures. It involves the injection

KEY TERMS

Anesthesia—Loss of normal sensation or feeling induced by anesthetic drugs.

Collagen—Any of a group of about 14 proteins found outside cells. Collagens are a major component of connective tissue, providing its characteristic strength and flexibility.

Contracture—A condition of high resistance to the passive stretching of a muscle, resulting from the formation of fibrous tissue in a joint or from a disorder of the muscle tissue itself.

Fibroblast—A type of cell found in connective tissue involved in collagen production as well as tendon formation and healing.

Laceration—A physical injury that results in a jagged tearing or mangling of the skin.

Meniscus (plural, menisci)—One of two crescent-shaped pieces of cartilage attached to the upper surface of the tibia. The menisci act as shock absorbers within the knee joint.

Prolotherapy—A technique for stimulating collagen growth in injured tissues by the injection of glycerin or dextrose.

Tendon—A fibrous cord of strong connective tissue that connects muscle to bone.

of dextrose or natural glycerin at the exact site of an injury to stimulate the immune system to repair the area. Thus, prolotherapy causes an inflammatory reaction at the exact site of injuries to such structures as ligaments, tendons, menisci, muscles, growth plates, joint capsules, and cartilage to stimulate these structures to heal. Specifically, prolotherapy causes fibroblasts to multiply rapidly. Fibroblasts are the cells that actually make up ligaments and tendons. The rapid production of new fibroblasts means that strong, fresh collagen tissue is formed, which is what is needed to repair injuries to ligaments or tendons.

See also Orthopedic surgery.

Resources

BOOKS

Canale, S. T. *Campbell's Operative Orthopaedics*, 10th ed. St. Louis, MO: Mosby, 2003.

Walsh, W. R., ed. *Repair and Regeneration of Ligament, Tendon, and Capsule*. Totowa, NJ: Humana Press, 2003.

PERIODICALS

Assal, M., M. Jung, R. Stern, et al. "Limited Open Repair of Achilles Tendon Ruptures: A Technique with a New Instrument and Findings of a Prospective Multicenter Study." *Journal of Bone and Joint Surgery, American Volume* 84-A (February 2002): 161-170.

Beredjiklian, P. K. "Biologic Aspects of Flexor Tendon Laceration and Repair." *Journal of Bone and Joint Surgery, American Volume* 85 (March 2003): 539-550.

Forslund, C. "BMP Treatment for Improving Tendon Repair. Studies on Rat and Rabbit Achilles Tendons." *Acta Orthopedica Scandinavica Supplement* 74 (February 2003): 1-30.

Harrell, R. M., Tong, J., Weinhold, P. S., and L. E. Dahners. "Comparison of the Mechanical Properties of Different Tension Band Materials and Suture Techniques." *Journal of Orthopedic Trauma* 17 (February 2003): 119-122.

Herrera, M. F., G. Bauer, F. Reynolds, et al. "Infection After Mini-Open Rotator Cuff Repair." *Journal of Shoulder and Elbow Surgery* 11 (November-December 2002): 605-608.

Joseph, T. A., Defranco, M. J., and G. G. Weiker. "Delayed Repair of a Pectoralis Major Tendon Rupture with Allograft: A Case Report." *Journal of Shoulder and Elbow Surgery* 12 (January-February 2003): 101-104.

Weber, S. C., J. S. Abrams, and W. M. Nottage. "Complications Associated with Arthroscopic Shoulder Surgery." *Arthroscopy* 18 (February 2002) (2 Suppl 1): 88-95.

ORGANIZATIONS

Academic Orthopaedic Society (AOS). 6300 N. River Rd., Suite 505, Rosemont, IL 60018. (847) 318-7330.

American Academy of Orthopaedic Surgeons (AAOS). 6300 North River Road, Rosemont, Illinois 60018-4262. (847) 823-7186; (800) 346-AAOS. <www.aaos.org>

American Physical Therapy Association (APTA). 1111 North Fairfax Street, Alexandria, VA 22314. (703)684-APTA or (800) 999-2782. <www.apta.org>.

OTHER

MedlinePlus. "Tendon Repair." <www.nlm.nih.gov/medlineplus/ency/article/002970.htm>.

Tendon Homepage. <www.eatonhand.com/ten/ten000.htm>.

Monique Laberge, Ph.D.

Tenotomy

Definition

Tenotomy is the cutting of a tendon. This and related procedures are also called tendon release, tendon lengthening, and heel-cord release (for tenotomy of the Achilles tendon).

Purpose

Tenotomy is performed in order to lengthen a muscle that has developed improperly, or become shortened and is resistant to stretch.

Club foot is a common developmental deformity in which the foot is turned inward, with shortening of one or more of the muscles controlling the foot and possibly some bone deformity as well.

A muscle can become shortened and resistant to stretch when it remains in a shortened position for many months. When this occurs, the tendon that attaches muscle to bone can shorten, and the muscle itself can develop fibrous tissue within it, preventing it from stretching to its full range of motion. This combination of changes is called contracture.

Contracture commonly occurs in upper motor neuron syndrome following spinal cord injury; traumatic brain injury; stroke; multiple sclerosis; or cerebral palsy. Damage to the nerves controlling muscles lead to an imbalance of opposing muscle forces across a joint, which may allow one muscle to pull harder than another. For instance, excess pull from the biceps, unless opposed by the triceps, can bend the elbow joint. If the shortened bicep remains in this position, it will develop contracture, becoming resistant to stretching. Tenotomy is performed to lengthen the tendon, allowing the muscle to return to its normal length and allowing the joint to straighten.

When one muscle pulls much more strongly than its opposing muscle, it may cause the joint to become partially dislocated, which is called subluxation. Tenotomy is also performed to prevent or correct subluxation, especially of the hip joint in cerebral palsy.

Chronic pain or bone deformity may prevent a person from moving a joint through its full range of motion, leading to contracture.

Contracture also occurs in a variety of neuromuscular diseases, including muscular dystrophies and polio. Degeneration of one muscle can allow the opposing muscle to pull too hard across the joint, shortening the muscle.

Demographics

Tenotomy is performed in infants with clubfoot, and in older patients who develop contractures or subluxations from neuromuscular disease, the upper motor neuron syndrome, or other disorders.

Description

During a tenotomy, the tendon is cut entirely or partway through, allowing the muscle to be stretched. Tenotomy may be performed through the skin (percutaneous tenotomy) or by surgically exposing the tendon (open tenotomy). The details of the operation differ for each tendon.

During a percutaneous lengthening of the Achilles tendon, a thin blade is inserted through the skin to partially sever the tendon in two or more places. This procedure is called a Z-plasty, and is very rapid, requiring only a few minutes. It may be performed under local anesthesia.

More severe contracture may be treated with an open procedure. In this case, the tendon may be cut lengthwise, and the two pieces joined lengthwise to form a single longer tendon. This procedure takes approximately half an hour. This type of tenotomy is usually performed under general anesthesia.

If multiple joints are to be treated (for example, ankle, knee, and hip), these are often performed at the same time.

Diagnosis/Preparation

Patients requiring tenotomy are those with contracture or developmental deformity leading to muscle shortening that has not responded sufficiently to treatment with casts, splints, stretching exercises, or medication. Tests performed before surgery include determining the range of motion of the joint involved, and possibly x rays to determine if there is a bone deformity impeding movement or subluxation.

Patients undergoing general anesthesia will probably be instructed not to eat anything for up to 12 hours before the procedure.

Aftercare

After tenotomy, the patient may receive pain medication. This may range from over-the-counter **aspirin** to intravenous morphine, depending on the severity of the pain. Ice packs may also be applied. The patient will usually spend the night in the hospital, especially children with swallowing or seizure disorders, who need to be monitored closely after anesthesia.

Casts are applied to the limb receiving the surgery. Before the cast is applied, the contracted muscle is stretched to its normal or near-normal extension. The cast then holds it in that position while the tendon regrows at its extended length. Braces or splints may also be applied.

After the casts come off (typically two to three weeks), intensive physical therapy is prescribed to strengthen the muscle and keep it stretched out.

Risks

Tenotomy carries a small risk of excess bleeding and infection. Tenotomy performed under general anesthesia carries additional risks associated with the anesthesia itself.

Normal results

Tenotomy allows the muscle to stretch out, proving more complete range of motion to the affected joint. This promotes better posture and movement; and may improve the ability to walk, stand, reach, or perform other activities, depending on the location of the procedure. Pain may be reduced as well. Club foot is usually completely fixed by proper treatment. Contracture and subluxation may be only partially remedied, depending on the degree of muscle shortening and fibrotic changes within the muscle before the procedure.

Morbidity and mortality rates

Properly performed, tenotomy does not carry the risk of mortality. It may cause temporary pain and bleeding, but these are usually easily managed.

Alternatives

Tenotomy is usually recommended only after other treatments have failed, or when the rate and severity of contracture or subluxation progression indicates no other more conservative treatment is likely to be effective. Aggressive stretching programs can sometimes prevent or delay development of contracture.

See also Rhizotomy.

Resources

PERIODICALS

Robinson, R. "Fight Against Contractures." *Quest Magazine* (1996). <http://www.mdausa.org/publications/Quest/q34 contrc.html>.

ORGANIZATIONS

Muscular Dystrophy Association. 3300 E. Sunrise Dr. Tucson, AZ 85718. (800) 572-1717. <http://www.mdausa.org>.

Richard Robinson

Testicular cancer surgery *see* **Orchiectomy**

Testicular torsion repair *see* **Orchiopexy**

Tetracyclines

Definition

Tetracyclines are medicines that kill bacteria, which are one-celled disease-causing microorganisms that commonly multiply by cell division. Tetracyclines are also used to treat infections caused by such subcategories of bacteria as rickettsiae and spirochetes.

Tetracyclines are classified as **antibiotics**, which are chemical substances produced by a microorganism that are able to kill other microorganisms without being toxic to the person, animal, or plant being treated. Some tetracyclines are derived directly from a bacterium known as *Streptomyces coelicolor*; others are made in the laboratory from chlortetracycline or oxytetracycline.

Purpose

Tetracyclines are called "broad-spectrum" antibiotics, because they can be used to treat a wide variety of infections. Physicians may prescribe these drugs to treat eye infections, pneumonia, gonorrhea, Rocky Mountain spotted fever, urinary tract infections, Lyme disease, and other infections caused by bacteria. These drugs are also used to treat acne. The tetracyclines will *not* work, however, for colds, flu, and other infections caused by viruses.

Description

Tetracyclines are available only with a physician's prescription. They are sold in capsule, tablet, liquid, and injectable forms. Some commonly used medicines in this group are tetracycline (Achromycin V, Sumycin), demeclocycline (Declomycin), minocycline (Minocin), oxytetracycline (Terramycin), and doxycycline (Doryx, Vibramycin, Vivox).

Tetracyclines have been used for treatment of gum infections in dental surgery. In **orthopedic surgery** they have been used as markers to identify living bone. The patient is given a tetracycline antibiotic for several weeks prior to surgery. Some of the tetracycline is absorbed into the bone during this period. Since tetracyclines glow under ultraviolet light, this absorption helps the surgeon distinguish the living bone from the dead tissue that must be removed.

Tetracycline may also be mixed with bone cement for prevention of infection in bone surgery. In nasal surgery, tetracycline ointments are used to help prevent postsurgical infections.

Recommended dosage

The recommended dosage depends on the specific tetracycline, its strength, and the disease agent and severity of infection for which it is being taken. Patients should check with the physician who prescribed the drug or the pharmacist who filled the prescription for the correct dosage.

To make sure an infection clears up completely, patients should take the full course of antibiotic medication. It is important to not stop taking the drug just because symptoms begin to improve.

Tetracyclines are most effective at constant levels in the blood. To keep blood levels constant, the medicine should be taken in doses spaced evenly throughout the day and night. It is important to not miss any doses.

These medicines work best when taken on an empty stomach with a full glass of water. The water will help prevent irritation of the stomach and esophagus (the tube-like structure that runs from the throat to the stomach). If the medicine still causes stomach upset, the patient may take it with food. Tetracyclines should *never* be taken with milk or milk products, however, as these may prevent the drugs from working properly. Patients should not drink or eat milk or dairy products within one to two hours of taking tetracyclines (except doxycycline and minocycline).

Precautions

The following warnings apply to tetracycline preparations taken by mouth to treat infections; they do not apply to topical ointments or tetracyclines mixed with bone cement. Also, these warnings apply primarily to tetracycline itself. Some members of the tetracycline family, particularly doxycycline and minocycline, have different adverse effects and precautions. Patients should consult their physician or pharmacist about these specific drugs.

Taking outdated tetracyclines can cause serious side effects. Patients should not take these medicines if:

• the color, appearance, or taste have changed

• the drug has been stored in a warm or damp area

• the expiration date on the label has passed

Outdated tetracyclines should be thrown out. Patients should check with their physician or pharmacist if they have any doubts about the effectiveness of their drugs.

Patients should not take antacids, calcium supplements, such salicylates as Magan or Trilisate, magnesium-containing **laxatives**, or sodium bicarbonate (baking soda) within one to two hours of taking tetracyclines. Patients should also not take any medicines that contain iron (including multivitamin and mineral supplements) within two to three hours of taking tetracyclines.

Some people feel dizzy when taking these drugs. Tetracyclines may also cause blurred vision. Because of these possible side effects, anyone who takes these drugs should not drive, use machines or do anything else that might be dangerous until they have found out how the drugs affect them.

Birth control pills may not work properly while tetracyclines are being taken. To prevent pregnancy, women should use alternative methods of birth control while taking tetracyclines.

Tetracyclines may increase the skin's sensitivity to sunlight. Even brief exposure to sun can cause a severe sunburn or a rash. During treatment with these drugs, patients should avoid exposure to direct sunlight, especially high sun between 10 A.M. and 3 P.M.; wear a hat and tightly woven clothing that covers the arms and legs; use a sunscreen with a skin protection factor (SPF) of at least 15; protect the lips with a lip balm containing sun block; and avoid the use of tanning beds, tanning booths, or sunlamps. Sensitivity to sunlight and sunlamps may continue for two weeks to several months after stopping the medicine, so patients must continue to be careful about sun exposure.

Tetracyclines may permanently discolor the teeth of people who took the medicine in childhood. The drugs may also slow down the growth of children's bones. Tetracyclines should not be given to infants or children under eight years of age unless directed by the child's physician.

Special conditions

People with certain medical conditions or who are taking other medicines may have problems if they take tetracyclines. Before taking these drugs, the patient must inform the doctor about any of these conditions:

FOOD OR MEDICATION ALLERGIES. Anyone who has had unusual reactions to tetracyclines in the past should inform his or her physician before taking the drugs again. The physician should also be told about any allergies to foods, dyes, preservatives, or other substances.

PREGNANCY AND LACTATION. Pregnant women should not take tetracyclines during the last four months of pregnancy. These drugs can prevent the baby's bones and teeth from developing properly and may cause the

KEY TERMS

Antibiotic—A chemical substance produced by a microorganism that is able to kill other microorganisms without being toxic to the host. Antibiotics are used to treat diseases in humans, other animals, and plants.

Bacterium (plural, bacteria)—A one-celled microorganism that typically multiplies by cell division and whose nucleus is contained within a cell wall. Most diseases treated with tetracyclines are caused by bacteria.

Gonorrhea—A sexually transmitted disease (STD) that causes infection in the genital organs and may cause disease in other parts of the body.

Microorganism—An organism that is too small to be seen with the naked eye.

Orthopedics—The medical specialty concerned with treatment of diseases of bone.

Rickettsia (plural, rickettsiae)—A microorganism belonging to a subtype of gram-negative bacteria that multiply only within the cells of a living host. Rickettsiae are usually transmitted to humans and other animals through the bites of ticks, fleas, and lice. They are named for Howard Ricketts (1871-1910), an American doctor.

Rocky Mountain spotted fever—An infectious disease that is caused by a rickettsia and spread by ticks. Its symptoms include high fever, muscle pain, and spots on the skin.

Salicylates—A group of drugs that includes aspirin and related compounds. Salicylates are used to relieve pain and reduce inflammation or fever.

Spirochete—A spiral-shaped bacterium. Spirochetes cause such diseases as syphilis and Lyme disease.

---

baby's adult teeth to be permanently discolored. Tetracyclines can also cause liver problems in pregnant women.

Women who are breastfeeding should also not take tetracyclines. The drugs pass into breast milk and can affect the nursing baby's teeth and bones. They may also make the baby more sensitive to sunlight and may increase its risk of contracting fungal infections.

OTHER CONDITIONS. Before using tetracyclines, people with any of these medical problems should make sure their physicians have been informed:

• diabetes

• liver disease

• kidney disease

Side effects

The most common side effects of tetracyclines are stomach cramps or a burning sensation in the stomach, mild diarrhea, nausea, or vomiting. These problems usually go away as the body adjusts to the drug and do not require medical treatment. Less common side effects, such as a sore mouth or tongue and itching of the rectal or genital areas may occur. These reactions do not need medical attention, however, unless they do not go away or are bothersome.

Other rare side effects have been reported, including inflammation of the pancreas, impairment of the kidneys, skin peeling, headache, intracranial hypertension, and ulceration of the esophagus. Anyone who has unusual symptoms during or after treatment with tetracyclines should consult his or her physician.

Drug interactions

Tetracyclines may interact with other medicines. When an interaction occurs, the effects of one or both of the drugs may change or the risk of side effects may be greater. Anyone who takes tetracyclines should give the doctor a list of all other medications that they take on a regular basis, *including over-the-counter drugs, herbal preparations, and traditional Chinese or other alternative medicines.* Standard medications that may interact with tetracyclines include:

• antacids

• calcium supplements

• medicines that contain iron (including multivitamin and mineral supplements)

• laxatives containing magnesium

• cholesterol-lowering drugs, including cholestyramine (Questran) and colestipol (Colestid)

• salicylates

• penicillin compounds

• birth control pills

Herbal preparations containing St. John's wort have been reported to increase sensitivity to sunlight in patients taking tetracyclines. People who have been using St. John's wort to relieve mild depression should discontinue it while they are taking tetracyclines.

Resources

BOOKS

"Antibacterial Drugs: Tetracyclines." Section 13, Chapter 153 in *The Merck Manual of Diagnosis and Therapy*, edited by Mark H. Beers, MD, and Robert Berkow, MD. Whitehouse Station, NJ: Merck Research Laboratories, 1999.

Pelletier, Kenneth R., MD. *The Best Alternative Medicine*, Part I, Chapter 6, "Western Herbal Medicine." New York: Simon & Schuster, 2002.

Wilson, Billie Ann, RN, PhD, Carolyn L. Stang, PharmD, and Margaret T. Shannon, RN, PhD. *Nurses Drug Guide 2000*. Stamford, CT: Appleton and Lange, 1999.

PERIODICALS

Al-Mofarreh, M. A., and I. A. Al Mofleh. "Esophageal Ulceration Complicating Doxycycline Therapy." *World Journal of Gastroenterology* 9 (March 2003): 609-611.

Gottehrer, N. R. "Managing Risk Factors in Successful Nonsurgical Treatment of Periodontal Disease." *Dentistry Today* 22 (January 2003): 64-69.

Grasset, L., C. Guy, and M. Ollagnier. "Cyclines and Acne: Pay Attention to Adverse Drug Reactions! A Recent Literature Review." [in French] *Revue de médecine interne* 24 (May 2003): 305-316.

Lochhead, J., and J. S. Elston. "Doxycycline Induced Intracranial Hypertension." *British Medical Journal* 326 (March 22, 2003): 641-642.

Moore, D. E. "Drug-Induced Cutaneous Photosensitivity: Incidence, Mechanism, Prevention and Management." *Drug Safety* 25 (2002): 345-372.

Wormser, G. P., R. Ramanathan, J. Nowakowski, et al. "Duration of Antibiotic Therapy for Early Lyme Disease. A Randomized, Double-Blind, Placebo-Controlled Trial." *Annals of Internal Medicine* 138 (May 6, 2003): 697-704.

ORGANIZATIONS

American Society of Health-System Pharmacists (ASHP). 7272 Wisconsin Avenue, Bethesda, MD 20814. (301) 657-3000. <www.ashp.org>.

United States Food and Drug Administration (FDA). 5600 Fishers Lane, Rockville, MD 20857-0001. (888) INFO-FDA. <www.fda.gov>.

Nancy Ross-Flanigan
Sam Uretsky, PharmD

Tetralogy of Fallot *see* **Heart surgery for congenital defects**

Therapeutic abortion *see* **Abortion, induced**

Thermometer

Definition

A thermometer is a device used to measure temperature.

Purpose

A thermometer is used in health care to measure and monitor body temperature. In an office, hospital or other health care facility, it allows a caregiver to record a baseline temperature when a patient is admitted. Repeated measurements of temperature are useful to detect deviations from normal levels. Repeated measurements are also useful in monitoring the effectiveness of current medications or other treatments.

The patient's temperature is recorded to check for pyrexia or monitor the degree of hypothermia present in the body.

Demographics

All health care professionals use thermometers. All health care facilities have thermometers. Most homes also have thermometers.

Description

A thermometer can use any of several methods to register temperature. These include mercury; liquid-in-glass; electronic with digital display; infrared or tympanic; and disposable dot matrix. A thermometer can be used in a clinical or emergency setting or at home. Thermometers can record body temperatures in the mouth (oral), armpit (axillary), eardrum (tympanic membrane), or anus (rectal).

A mercury thermometer consists of a narrow glass stem approximately 5 in (12.7 cm) in length with markings along one or both sides indicating the temperature scale in degrees Fahrenheit, Centigrade or both. Liquid mercury is held in a reservoir bulb at one end and rises through a capillary tube when the glass chamber is placed in contact with the body. Mercury thermometers are not used in modern clinical settings.

Electronic thermometers can record a wide range of temperatures between 94°F and 105°F, (35°C and 42°C) and can record oral, axillary, or rectal temperatures. They have temperature sensors inside round-tipped probes that can be covered with disposable guards to prevent the spread of infection. The sensor is connected to a container housing the central processing unit. The information gathered by the sensor is then shown on a display screen. Some electronic models have such other features as memory recall of the last recording or a large display screen for easy reading. To use an electronic thermometer, the caregiver places the probe under the patient's arm or tongue, or in the patient's rectum. The probe is left in place for a period of time that depends on the model used. The device will beep when the peak temperature is reached. The time required to obtain a reading varies from 3–30 seconds.

A tympanic thermometer has a round-tipped probe containing a sensor that can be covered with a disposable guard to protect against the spread of ear infections. It is placed in the ear canal for 1 sec while an infrared sensor records the body heat radiated by the eardrum. The reading then appears on the unit's screen.

Digital and tympanic thermometers should be used in accordance with the manufacturer's guidelines.

Disposable thermometers are plastic strips with dots on the surface that have been impregnated with temperature-sensitive chemicals. The strips are sticky on one side to adhere to the skin under the armpit and prevent slippage. The dots change color at different temperatures as the chemicals in them respond to body heat. The temperature is readable after two to three minutes, depending on the instrument's guidelines. These products vary in length of use; they may be disposable, reusable, or used continuously for up to 48 hours. Disposable thermometers are useful for children, as they can record temperatures while children are asleep.

Diagnosis/Preparation

Training

Caregivers should be given training appropriate for the type of device used in their specific clinical setting.

Operation

The patient should sit or lie in a comfortable position to ensure that temperature readings are taken in similar locations each time and to minimize the effects of stress or excitement on the reading.

The manufacturer's guidelines should be followed when taking a patient's temperature with a digital, tympanic, or disposable thermometer. Dot-matrix thermometers are placed next to the skin and usually held in place by an adhesive strip. With the tympanic thermometer, caregivers should ensure that the probe is properly inserted into the ear to allow an optimal reading. The reading will be less accurate if the sensor cannot accurately touch the tympanic membrane or if the ear canal is clogged by wax or debris.

WHO PERFORMS THE PROCEDURE AND WHERE IS IT PERFORMED?

Most health professionals are trained in the proper operation of thermometers used in clinical settings. Most families have and use thermometers in the home.

A mercury thermometer can be used to monitor a temperature in three body locations:

• Axillary.

• Oral or sublingual. This placement is never used with infants.

• Rectal. This method is used with infants. The tip of a rectal mercury thermometer is usually colored blue to distinguish it from the silver tip of an oral/axillary thermometer.

Before recording a temperature using a mercury thermometer, the caregiver shakes the mercury down by holding the thermometer firmly at the clear end and flicking it quickly a few times with a downward wrist motion toward the silver end. The mercury should be shaken down below 96°F (35.5°C) before the patient's temperature is taken.

In axillary placement, the silver tip of the thermometer is placed under the patient's right armpit, with the patient's arm pressing the instrument against the chest. The thermometer should stay in place for six to seven minutes. The caregiver can record the patient's other **vital signs** during this waiting period. After the waiting period has elapsed, the caregiver removes the thermometer and holds it at eye level to read it. The mercury will have risen to a level indicating the patient's temperature.

The procedure for taking a patient's temperature by mouth with a mercury thermometer is similar to the axillary method except that the silver tip of the thermometer is placed beneath the tongue for four to five minutes before being read. In both cases, the thermometer is wiped clean and stored in an appropriate container to prevent breakage.

To record the patient's rectal temperature with a mercury thermometer, a rectal thermometer is shaken down as described earlier. A small amount of water-based lubricant is placed on the colored tip of the thermometer to make it easier to insert. Infants must be positioned lying on their stomachs and held securely by the caregiver. The tip of the thermometer is inserted into the rectum no more than 0.5 in (1.3 cm) and held there for two to three minutes. The thermometer is removed, read as before, and cleansed with an antibacterial wipe. It is then stored in an appropriate container to prevent breakage. This precaution is important as mercury is poisonous when swallowed.

Liquid-in-glass thermometers contain alternatives to mercury (such as colored alcohol), but are used and stored in the same manner as mercury thermometers.

Maintenance

Many digital and infrared thermometers are self-calibrating and need relatively little care. To ensure accuracy, mercury thermometers should be shaken down prior to every use and left in place for at least three minutes. They require careful storage to prevent breakage and thorough cleaning after each use to prevent cross-infection.

As of early 2003, there is a nationwide initiative to ban the sale of thermometers and blood pressure monitors containing mercury. Health activists are concerned about mercury from broken or unwanted instruments contaminating the environment. A mercury thermometer contains 0.7g (0.025 oz) of mercury; 1 g of the substance is enough to contaminate a 20-acre lake. Several states have banned the use of products containing mercury. Most retail stores have stopped selling mercury thermometers. In October 1999, the Environmental Protection Agency (EPA) advised using alternative products to avoid the need for increased regulations in years to come and to protect human health and wildlife by reducing unnecessary exposure to mercury. According to a 2001 study by the Mayo Clinic, mercury-free devices can monitor information without compromising accuracy.

Aftercare

A thermometer should be cleaned, disinfected and placed in an appropriate container for storage.

Risks

Breakage of a glass thermometer creates a risk of cuts from broken glass and possible mercury poisoning.

Improper operation of a tympanic thermometer can cause injury to the middle ear. As digital devices have replaced glass thermometers, however, the number of injuries has declined.

An additional risk is that old or broken thermometers may give inaccurate results.

Normal results

A normal body temperature is defined as approximately 98.6°F (37°C). Body temperature is not constant throughout a 24-hour period. Some variation (0.3°F) is normal. Individuals also vary in their basal temperatures (0.3°F). A fever is defined as a temperature of 101°F or higher in an infant younger than three months or above 102°F for older children and adults. Hypothermia is recognized as a temperature below 96°F (35.5°C).

Morbidity and mortality rates

Injuries caused by properly inserted and normally functioning thermometers are extremely rare.

Alternatives

There are no convenient alternatives to using a thermometer to measure body temperature.

See also Health history; Physical examination; Vital signs.

Resources

BOOKS

Bickley, L. S., P. G. Szilagyi, and J. G. Stackhouse, eds. *Bates' Guide to Physical Examination & History Taking*, 8th ed. Philadelphia, PA: Lippincott Williams & Wilkins, 2002.

Chan, P. D., and P. J. Winkle. *History and Physical Examination in Medicine*, 10th ed. New York, NY: Current Clinical Strategies, 2002.

Seidel, Henry M. *Mosby's Physical Examination Handbook*, 4th ed. St. Louis, MO: Mosby-Year Book, 2003.

Swartz, Mark A., and William Schmitt. *Textbook of Physical Diagnosis: History and Examination*, 4th ed. Philadelphia, PA: Saunders, 2001.

PERIODICALS

Dowding, D., S. Freeman, S. Nimmo, et al. "An Investigation Into the Accuracy of Different Types of Thermometers." *Professional Nurse* 18 (November 2002): 166-168.

Drake-Lee, A., I. Mantella, and A. Bridle. "Infrared Ear Thermometers Versus Rectal Thermometers." *Lancet* 360 (December 7, 2002): 1883-1886.

Moran, D. S., and L. Mendal. "Core Temperature Measurement: Methods and Current Insights." *Sports Medicine* 32 (2002): 879-885.

Pompei, F. "Insufficiency in Thermometer Data." *Anesthesia and Analgesia* 96 (March 2003): 908-909.

KEY TERMS

Axillary—Pertaining to the armpit.

Hypothermia—Body temperature below 96°F (35.5°C).

Oral—Pertaining to the mouth.

Pyrexia—A temperature of 101°F (38.3°C) or higher in an infant younger than three months or above 102°F (38.9°C) for older children and adults.

Rectal—Pertaining to the rectum.

Sublingual—Under the tongue.

ORGANIZATIONS

American Academy of Family Physicians. 11400 Tomahawk Creek Parkway, Leawood, KS 66211-2672. (913) 906-6000. <www.aafp.org>. E-mail: fp@aafp.org.

American Academy of Pediatrics. 141 Northwest Point Boulevard, Elk Grove Village, IL 60007-1098. (847) 434-4000; FAX: (847) 434-8000. <www.aap.org>. E-mail: kidsdoc @aap.org .

American College of Physicians. 190 N. Independence Mall West, Philadelphia, PA 19106-1572. (800) 523-1546, x2600 or (215) 351-2600. <www.acponline.org>.

American Medical Association. 515 N. State Street, Chicago, IL 60610. (312) 464-5000. <www.ama-assn.org>.

American Nurses Association. 600 Maryland Avenue, SW, Suite 100 West, Washington, DC 20024. (202) 651-7000 or (800) 274-4262. <www.nursingworld.org>.

OTHER

About.com. [cited March 1, 2003]. <www.inventors.about.com/library/inventors/blthermo meter.htm>.

AskLynnRN. [cited March 1, 2003]. <www.asklynnrn.com/html/healthmon_bbt_thermometer.htm>.

How Stuff Works. [cited March 1, 2003]. <www.howstuff works.com/therm.htm>.

Rice University. [cited March 1, 2003]. <www.es.rice.edu/ES/humsoc/Galileo/Things/ thermometer.html>.

L. Fleming Fallon, Jr., MD, DrPH

▌ Thoracic surgery

Definition

Thoracic surgery is any surgery performed in the chest (thorax).

Purpose

The purpose of thoracic surgery is to treat diseased or injured organs in the thorax, including the esophagus (muscular tube that passes food to the stomach), trachea (windpipe that branches to form the right bronchus and the left bronchus), pleura (membranes that cover and protect the lung), mediastinum (area separating the left and right lungs), chest wall, diaphragm, heart, and lungs.

General thoracic surgery is a field that specializes in diseases of the lungs and esophagus. The field also encompasses accidents and injuries to the chest, esophageal disorders (esophageal cancer or esophagitis), lung cancer, **lung transplantation**, and surgery for emphysema.

Description

The most common diseases requiring thoracic surgery include lung cancer, chest trauma, esophageal cancer, emphysema, and lung transplantation.

Lung cancer

Lung cancer is one of the most significant public health problems in the United States and the world. Approximately 171,600 new cases of lung cancer occurred in 1999. It accounts for 28% of cancer deaths, 14% of all cancer diagnoses, and is the leading cause of cancer deaths among women and second most common cause of male cancer deaths. The five-year survival rate in localized disease can approach 50% (stages I and II).

Lung cancer develops primarily by exposure to toxic chemicals. Cigarette smoking is the most important risk factor responsible for the disease. Other environmental factors that may predispose a person to lung cancer include such industrial substances as arsenic, nickel, chromium, asbestos, radon, organic chemicals, air pollution, and radiation.

Most cases of lung cancer develop in the right lung because it contains the majority (55%) of lung tissue. Additionally, lung cancer occurs more frequently in the upper lobes of the lung than in the lower lobes. The tumor receives blood from the bronchial artery (a major artery in the pulmonary system).

Adenocarcinoma of the lung is the most frequent type of lung cancer, accounting for 45% of all cases. This type of cancer can spread (metastasize) earlier than another type of lung cancer called squamous cell carcinoma (which occurs in approximately 30% of lung cancer patients). Approximately 66% of squamous cell carcinoma cases are centrally located. They expand against the bronchus, causing compression. Small-cell carcinoma accounts for 20% of all lung cancers; and the majority (80%) are centrally located. Small-cell carcinoma is a highly aggressive lung cancer, with early metastasis to such distant sites as the brain and bone marrow (the central portion of certain bones, which produce formed elements that are part of blood).

Most lung tumors are not treated with thoracic surgery since patients seek medical care later in the disease process. Chemotherapy increases the rate of survival in patients with limited (not advanced) disease. Surgery may be useful for staging or diagnosis. Pulmonary resection (removal of the tumor and neighboring lymph nodes) can be curative if the tumor is less than or equal to 3 cm, and presents as a solitary nodule. Lung tumors spread to other areas through neighboring lymphatic channels. Even if thoracic surgery is performed, postoperative chemotherapy may also be indicated to provide comprehensive treatment (i.e., to kill any tumor cells that may have spread via the lymphatic system).

Genetic engineering has provided insights related to the growth of tumors. A genetic mutation called a k-ras mutation frequently occurs, and is implicated in 90% of genetic mutations for adenocarcinoma of the lung. Mutations in the cancer cells make them resistant to chemotherapy, necessitating the use of multiple chemotherapeutic agents.

Chest trauma

Chest trauma is a medical/surgical emergency. Initially, the chest should be examined after an airway is maintained. The mortality (death) rate for trauma patients with respiratory distress is approximately 50%. This figure rises to 75% if symptoms include both respiratory distress and shock. Patients with respiratory distress require **endotracheal intubation** (passing a plastic tube from the mouth to the windpipe) and mechanically assisted ventilator support. Invasive thoracic procedures are necessary in emergency situations.

Trauma requiring urgent thoracic surgery may include any of the following problems: a large clotted hemothorax, massive air leak, esophageal injury, valvular cardiac (heart) injury, proven damage to blood vessels in the heart, or chest wall defect.

Esophageal cancer

The number of new cases of esophageal cancer is slowly rising (approximately 3.2 per 100,000 persons under age 80) in the United States, United Kingdom, and Western Europe. The cause of esophageal cancer is not precisely known. The types of esophageal cancers include lymphomas, epithelial tumors, metastatic tumors, and sarcomas. Chronic irritation of the esophagus from a broad range of chemicals may be partially implicated in development of esophageal cancer.

Difficulty swallowing (dysphagia) is the cardinal symptom of esophageal cancer. Radiography, endoscopy, computerized axial tomography (CT scan), and ultrasonography are part of a comprehensive diagnostic evaluation. The standard operation for patients with resectable esophageal carcinoma includes removal of the tumor from the esophagus, a portion of the stomach, and the lymph nodes (within the cancerous region).

Smoking and alcohol consumption are implicated in the development of squamous cell carcinoma. Adenocarcinomas can develop from continued acid reflux (gastroesophageal reflux). Over 90% of patients with esophageal squamous cell carcinoma develop the tumor in the upper and middle thoracic esophagus.

Emphysema

Lung volume reduction surgery (LVRS) is the term used to desribe surgery for patients with emphysema. LVRS is intended to help persons whose disabling dyspnea (difficulty breathing) is related to emphysema and does not respond to medical management. Breathlessness is a result of the structural and functional pulmonary and thoracic abnormalities associated with emphysema. Surgery will assist the patient, but the primary pathogenic process that caused the emphysema is permanent because lung tissues lose the capability of elastic recoil during normal breathing (inspiration and expiration).

Patients are usually transferred out of the **intensive care unit** within one day of surgery. Physical therapy and rehabilitation (coughing and breathing exercises) begin soon after surgery, and the patient is discharged when deemed clinically stable.

Lung transplantation

There are various types of lung transplantations: unilateral (one lung; most common type); bilateral (both lungs); heart-lung; and living donor lobe transplantation.

The long-term survival for persons receiving lung transplantation has not improved over time, and is approximately 3.5 years. A successful outcome is dependent on the patient's general medical condition. Those who have symptomatic osteoporosis (severe disease of the musculoskeletal system) or are users of **corticosteroids** may not have favorable outcomes.

The death rate is due to infections (pulmonary infections) or chronic rejection (bronchiolitis obliterans) if the donor lung was not a perfect genetic match. Patients are given postoperative **antibiotics** to prevent bacterial infections during the early period following surgery.

Bacterial pneumonia is usually severe. A bacterial genus known as *Pseudomonas* accounts for 75% of post-transplant pneumonia cases. Patients can also acquire viral and fungal infections, and an infection caused by a cell parasite known as *Pneumocystis carinii*. Infections are treated with specific medications intended to destroy the invading microorganism. Viral infections require treatment of symptoms.

Acute (quick onset) rejection is common within the first weeks after lung transplantation. Acute rejection is treated with steroids (bolus given intravenously), and is effective in 80% of cases. Chronic rejection is the most common problem, and typically begins with symptoms of fatigue and a vague feeling of illness. Treatment is difficult, and the results are unrewarding. There are several immunosuppressive protocols currently utilized for cases of chronic rejection. The goal of immunosuppressive therapy is to prevent the host's immune reaction from destroying the genetically foreign organ.

Diagnosis/Preparation

The surgeon may use two common incisional approaches: sternotomy (incision through and down the breastbone) or via the side of the chest (**thoracotomy**).

An operative procedure known as video assisted thoracoscopic surgery (VATS) is minimally invasive. During VATS, a lung is collapsed and the thoracoscope and **surgical instruments** are inserted into the thorax through any of three to four small incisions in the chest wall.

Another approach involves the use of a mediastinoscope or bronchoscope to visualize the internal anatomical structures during thoracic surgery or diagnostic procedures.

Preoperative evaluation for most patients (except emergency cases) must include cardiac tests, blood chemistry analysis, and **physical examination**. Like most operative procedures, the patient should not eat or drink food 10–12 hours prior to surgery. Patients who undergo thoracic surgery with the video-assisted approach tend to have shorter inpatient hospital stays.

Aftercare

Patients typically experience severe pain after surgery, and are given appropriate medications. In uncomplicated cases, chest and urine (Foley catheter) tubes

are usually removed within 24–48 hours. A highly trained and comprehensive team of respiratory therapists and nurses is vital for **postoperative care** that results in improved lung function via deep breathing and coughing exercises.

Risks

Precautions for thoracic surgery include coagulation blood disorders (disorders that prevent normal blood clotting) and previous thoracic surgery. Risks include hemorrhage, myocardial infarction (heart attack), stroke, nerve injury, embolism (blood clot or air bubble that obstructs an artery), and infection. Total lung collapse can occur from fluid or air accumulation, as a result of chest tubes that are routinely placed after surgery for drainage.

Resources

BOOKS

Abeloff, M. *Clinical Oncology,* 2nd ed. Churchill Livingstone, Inc., 2000.

Feldman, M. Sleisenger. *Fordtran's Gastrointestinal and Liver Disease,* 7th ed. W. B. Saunders, 2002.

Murray, J. and J. Nadel. *Textbook of Respiratory Medicine,* 3rd ed. W. B. Saunders Company, 2000.

PERIODICALS

Brenner, M. "Lung Volume Reduction Surgery for Emphysema." *Chest* 110, no.1 (July 1996).

Hamacher, J., E. Russi, and Walter Weder. "Lung Volume Reduction Surgery: A Survey on the European Experience." *Chest* 117, no. 6 (June 2000).

ORGANIZATIONS

American Association for Thoracic Surgery. 900 Cummings Center, Suite 221-U, Beverly, Massachusetts 01915. (978) 927-8330. Fax: (978) 524-8890. E-mail: aats@prri.com.

Laith Farid Gulli, M.D., M.S.
Abraham F. Ettaher, M.D.
Nicole Mallory, M.S., PA-C

Thoracotomy

Definition

Thoracotomy is the process of making of an incision (cut) into the chest wall.

Purpose

A physician gains access to the chest cavity (called the thorax) by cutting through the chest wall. Reasons for the entry are varied. Thoracotomy allows for study of the condition of the lungs; removal of a lung or part of a lung; removal of a rib; and examination, treatment, or removal of any organs in the chest cavity. Thoracotomy also provides access to the heart, esophagus, diaphragm, and the portion of the aorta that passes through the chest cavity.

Lung cancer is the most common cancer requiring a thoracotomy. Tumors and metastatic growths can be removed through the incision (a procedure called resection). A biopsy, or tissue sample, can also be taken through the incision, and examined under a microscope for evidence of abnormal cells.

A resuscitative or emergency thoracotomy may be performed to resuscitate a patient who is near death as a result of a chest injury. An emergency thoracotomy provides access to the chest cavity to control injury-related bleeding from the heart, cardiac compressions to restore a normal heart rhythm, or to relieve pressure on the heart caused by cardiac tamponade (accumulation of fluid in the space between the heart's muscle and outer lining).

Demographics

Thoracotomy may be performed to diagnose or treat a variety of conditions; therefore, no data exist as to the overall incidence of the procedure. Lung cancer, a common reason for thoracotomy, is diagnosed in approximately 172,000 people each year and affects more men than women (91,800 diagnoses in men compared to 80,100 in women).

Description

The thoracotomy incision may be made on the side, under the arm (axillary thoracotomy); on the front, through the breastbone (median sternotomy); slanting from the back to the side (posterolateral thoracotomy); or under the breast (anterolateral thoracotomy). The exact location of the cut depends on the reason for the surgery. In some cases, the physician is able to make the incision between ribs (called an intercostal approach) to minimize cuts through bone, nerves, and muscle. The incision may range from just under 5 in (12.7 cm) to 10 in (25 cm).

During the surgery, a tube is passed through the trachea. It usually has a branch to each lung. One lung is deflated for examination and surgery, while the other one is inflated with the assistance of a mechanical device (a ventilator).

A number of different procedures may be commenced at this point. A lobectomy removes an entire lobe or section of a lung (the right lung has three lobes and the left lung has two). It may be done to remove cancer that is contained by a lobe. A **segmentectomy**, or wedge resection, removes a wedge-shaped piece of lung smaller than a lobe. Alternatively, the entire lung may be removed during a **pneumonectomy**.

In the case of an emergency thoracotomy, the procedure performed depends on the type and extent of injury. The heart may be exposed so that direct cardiac compressions can be performed; the physician may use one hand or both hands to manually pump blood through the heart. Internal paddles of a defibrillating machine may be applied directly to the heart to restore normal cardiac rhythms. Injuries to the heart causing excessive bleeding (hemorrhaging) may be closed with staples or stitches.

Once the procedure that required the incision is completed, the chest wall is closed. The layers of skin, muscle, and other tissues are closed with stitches or staples. If the breastbone was cut (as in the case of a median sternotomy), it is stitched back together with wire.

Diagnosis/Preparation

Patients are told not to eat after midnight the night before surgery. The advice is important because vomiting during surgery can cause serious complications or death. For surgery in which a general anesthetic is used, the gag reflex is often lost for several hours or longer, making it much more likely that food will enter the lungs if vomiting occurs.

Thoracotomy

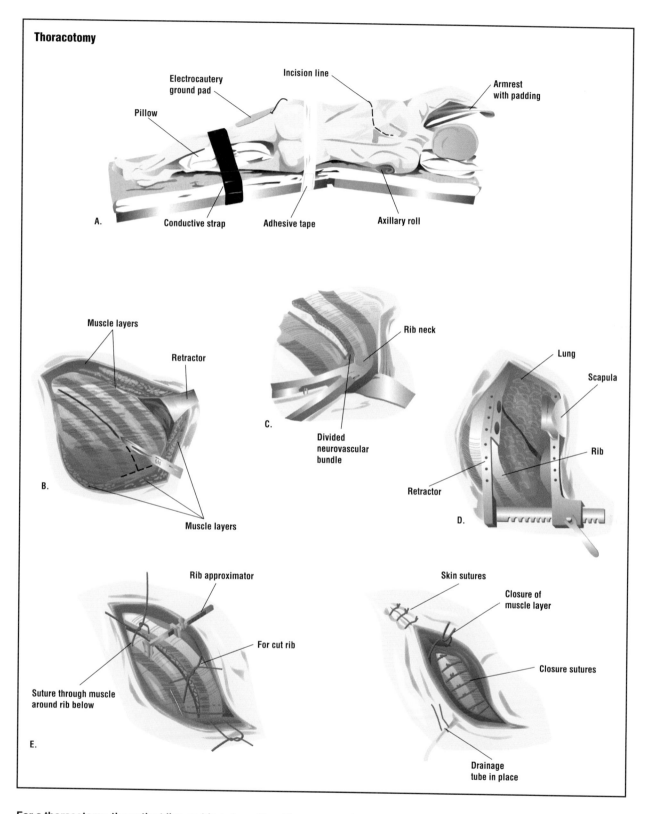

For a thoracotomy, the patient lies on his or her side with one arm raised (A). An incision is cut into the skin of the ribcage (B). Muscle layers are cut, and a rib may be removed to gain access to the cavity. (C). Retractors hold the ribs apart, exposing the lung (D). After any repairs are made, the cut rib is replaced and held in place with special materials (E). Layers of muscle and skin are stitched. *(Illustration by GGS Inc.)*

QUESTIONS TO ASK THE DOCTOR

- Why is thoracotomy being recommended?
- What diagnostic tests will be performed to determine if thoracotomy is necessary?
- What type of incision will be used and where will it be located?
- What type of procedure will be performed?
- How long will is the recovery time and what is expected during this period?
- If a biopsy is the only reason for the procedure, is a thoracoscopy or a guided needle biopsy an option (instead of thoracotomy)?

Patients must tell their physicians about all known allergies so that the safest anesthetics can be selected. Older patients must be evaluated for heart ailments before surgery because of the additional strain on that organ.

Aftercare

Opening the chest cavity means cutting through skin, muscle, nerves, and sometimes bone. It is a major procedure that often involves a hospital stay of five to seven days. The skin around the drainage tube to the thoracic cavity must be kept clean, and the tube must be kept unblocked.

The pressure differences that are set up in the thoracic cavity by the movement of the diaphragm (the large muscle at the base of the thorax) make it possible for the lungs to expand and contract. If the pressure in the chest cavity changes abruptly, the lungs can collapse. Any fluid that collects in the cavity puts a patient at risk for infection and reduced lung function, or even collapse (called a pneumothorax). Thus, any entry to the chest usually requires that a chest tube remain in place for several days after the incision is closed.

The first two days after surgery may be spent in the **intensive care unit** (ICU) of the hospital. A variety of tubes, catheters, and monitors may be required after surgery.

Risks

The rich supply of blood vessels to the lungs makes hemorrhage a risk; a blood **transfusion** may become necessary during surgery. General anesthesia carries such risks as nausea, vomiting, headache, blood pressure issues, or allergic reaction. After a thoracotomy, there may be drainage from the incision. There is also the risk of infection; the patient must learn how to keep the incision clean and dry as it heals.

After the chest tube is removed, the patient is vulnerable to pneumothorax. Physicians strive to reduce the risk of collapse by timing the removal of the tube. Doing so at the end of inspiration (breathing in) or the end of expiration (breathing out) poses less risk. Deep breathing exercises and coughing should be emphasized as an important way that patients can improve healing and prevent pneumonia.

Normal results

The results following thoracotomy depend on the reasons why it was performed. If a biopsy was taken during the surgery, a normal result would indicate that no cancerous cells are present in the tissue sample. The procedure may indicate that further treatment is necessary; for example, if cancer was detected, chemotherapy, radiation therapy, or more surgery may be recommended.

Morbidity and mortality

One study following lung cancer patients undergoing thoracotomy found that 10–15% of patients experienced heartbeat irregularities, readmittance to the ICU, or partial or full lung collapse; 5–10% experienced pneumonia or extended use of the ventilator (greater than 48 hours); and up to 5% experienced wound infection, accumulation of pus in the chest cavity, or blood clots in the lung. The mortality rate in the study was 5.8%, with patients dying as a result of the cancer itself or of postoperative complications.

Alternatives

Video-assisted **thoracic surgery** (VATS) is a less invasive alternative to thoracotomy. Also called thoracoscopy, VATS involves the insertion of a thoracoscope (a thin, lighted tube) into a small incision through the chest wall. The surgeon can visualize the structures inside the chest cavity on a video screen. Such instruments as a stapler or grasper may inserted through other small incisions. Although initially used as a diagnostic tool (to visualize the lungs or to remove a sample of lung tissue for further examination), VATS may be used to remove some lung tumors.

An alternative to emergency thoracotomy is a tube thoracostomy, a tube placed through chest wall to drain excess fluid. Over 80% of patients with a penetrating chest wound can be successfully managed with a thoracostomy.

See also CT-guided biopsy; Thoracoscopy.

KEY TERMS

Aorta—The major artery carrying blood away from the heart.

Catheter—A tube inserted into a body cavity to drain fluid. An example would be a urinary catheter used to drain urine from the urethra.

Diaphragm—The large flat muscle that runs horizontally across the bottom of the chest cavity.

Esophagus—The muscular tube that connects the mouth and the stomach.

Trachea—The tube made of cartilage that carries air from the nose and mouth to the lungs.

Urethra—The tube that carries urine from the bladder to the outside of the body.

Resources

BOOKS

Bartlett, Robert L. "Resuscitative Thoracotomy." (Chapter 17). In *Clinical Procedures in Emergency Medicine.* Philadelphia: W. B. Saunders Company, 1998.

Townsend, Courtney M., et al. "Thoracic Incisions." (Chapter 55). In *Sabiston Textbook of Surgery.* Philadelphia: W. B. Saunders Company, 2001.

PERIODICALS

Blewett, C.J. et al. "Open Lung Biopsy as an Outpatient Procedure." *Annals of Thoracic Surgery* (April 2001): 1113-5.

Handy, John R., et al. "What Happens to Patients Undergoing Lung Cancer Surgery? Outcomes and Quality of Life Before and After Surgery." *Chest* 122, no.1 (August 14, 2002): 21-30.

Swanson, Scott J. and Hasan F. Batirel. "Video-Assisted Thoracic Surgery (VATS) Resection for Lung Cancer." *Surgical Clinics of North America* 82, no.3 (June 1, 2002): 541-9.

ORGANIZATIONS

American Cancer Society. 1599 Clifton Rd. NE, Atlanta, GA 30329-4251. (800) 227-2345. <http://www.cancer.org>.

Society of Thoracic Surgeons. 663 N. Saint Clair St., Suite 2320, Chicago, IL 60611-3658. (312) 202-5800. <http://www.sts.org>.

OTHER

"Detailed Guide: Lung Cancer." *American Cancer Society.* [cited April 28, 2003]. <http://www.cancer.org/docroot/CRI/CRI_2_3x.asp?dt=26>.

Diane M. Calabrese
Stephanie Dionne Sherk

Thrombocyte count *see* **Complete blood count**

Thrombolytic therapy

Definition

Thrombolytic therapy is the use of drugs that dissolve blood clots. The name "thrombolytic" comes from two Greek words that mean "clot" and "loosening."

Purpose

When a blood clot forms in a blood vessel, it may cut off or severely reduce blood flow to parts of the body that are served by that blood vessel. This event can cause serious damage to those parts of the body. If the clot forms in an artery that supplies blood to the heart, for example, it can cause a heart attack. A clot that cuts off blood to the brain can cause a stroke. Thrombolytic therapy is used to dissolve blood clots that could cause serious, and possibly life-threatening, damage if they are not removed. Research suggests that when used to treat stroke, thrombolytic therapy can prevent or reverse paralysis and other problems that otherwise might result.

In heart attacks, thrombolytic therapy is an alternative to stenting, a procedure in which a spring-like device is inserted into a blocked blood vessel. In general, stenting is the preferred treatment, since it both removes the clot and opens the blood vessel, which may have internal cholesterol deposits. Thrombolytic therapy only removes the clot, but it can be administered in hospitals with fewer resources than are required for insertion of a stent.

Thrombolytic therapy is also used to dissolve blood clots that form in catheters or tubes put into people's bodies for medical treatments, such as dialysis or chemotherapy.

Description

Thrombolytic therapy uses drugs called thrombolytic agents, such as alteplase (Activase), anistreplase (Eminase), streptokinase (Streptase, Kabikinase), urokinase (Abbokinase), and tissue plasminogen activator (TPA) to dissolve clots. These drugs are given as injections, and given only under a physician's supervision.

Recommended dosage

The physician supervising thrombolytic therapy decides on the proper dose for each patient. He or she will take into account the type of drug, the purpose for which it is being used, and in some cases, the patient's weight.

Precautions

For thrombolytic therapy to be effective in treating stroke or heart attack, prompt medical attention is very important. The drugs must be given within a few hours of the beginning of a stroke or heart attack. This type of treatment is not right, however, for every patient who has a heart attack or a stroke. Only a qualified medical professional can decide whether a thrombolytic agent should be used. To increase the chance of survival and reduce the risk of serious permanent damage, anyone who has signs of a heart attack or stroke should get immediate medical help.

Thrombolytic therapy may cause bleeding in other parts of the body. This side effect is usually not serious, but severe bleeding does occur in some patients, especially older people. Some people have had minor hemorrhagic strokes in which there has been a small amount of bleeding into the brain. These hemorrhagic strokes have been blocked by clots that would be broken up by use of a thrombolytic agent, so that removal of the harmful clot would cause equally dangerous bleeding. To lower the risk of serious bleeding, people who are given thrombolytic medications should move around as little as possible and should not try to get up on their own unless told to do so by a health care professional. Following all the instructions of the health care providers in charge is very important.

Thrombolytic therapy may be more likely to cause serious bleeding in people who have certain medical conditions or have recently had certain procedures. Before being given a thrombolytic agent, anyone with any of these problems or conditions should tell the physician in charge:

• blood disease or current or past bleeding problems in any part of the body
• heart or blood vessel disease
• stroke (recent or in the past)
• high blood pressure
• brain tumor or other brain disease
• stomach ulcer or colitis
• severe liver disease
• active tuberculosis
• recent falls, injuries, or blows to the body or head
• recent injections into a blood vessel
• recent surgery, including dental surgery
• tubes recently placed in the body for any reason
• recent delivery of a baby

In addition, anyone who has had a recent streptococcal (strep) infection should tell the physician in charge. Some thrombolytic agents may not work properly in people who have just had a strep infection, so the physician may want to use a different drug.

People who take certain medicines may be at greater risk for severe bleeding when they are given a thrombolytic agent.

Women who are pregnant should tell the physician in charge before being given a thrombolytic agent. There is a slight chance that a woman who is given thrombolytic therapy during the first five months of pregnancy will have a miscarriage. Streptokinase and urokinase, however, have both been used without problems in pregnant women.

After being treated with thrombolytic therapy, women who are breastfeeding should check with their physicians before starting to breastfeed again.

Side effects

Anyone who has fever or who notices bleeding or oozing from their gums, from cuts, or from the site where the thrombolytic agent was injected should immediately tell their health care provider.

People who are given thrombolytic therapy should also be alert to the signs of bleeding inside the body and should check with a physician immediately if any of the following symptoms occur:

• blood in the urine
• blood in the stool, or black, tarry stools
• constipation
• coughing up blood
• vomiting blood or material that looks like coffee grounds
• nosebleeds
• unexpected or unusually heavy vaginal bleeding
• dizziness
• sudden, severe, or constant headaches
• pain or swelling in the abdomen or stomach
• back pain or backache
• severe or constant muscle pain or stiffness
• stiff, swollen, or painful joints

Other side effects of thrombolytic agents are possible. Anyone who has unusual symptoms during or after thrombolytic therapy should tell a health care professional.

Interactions

People who take certain medicines may be at greater risk for severe bleeding when they receive a thrombolytic agent. Anyone who is given a thrombolytic agent should tell the physician in charge about all other prescription or nonprescription (over-the-counter) medicines he or she is taking. Among the medicines that may increase the chance of bleeding are:

- aspirin and other medicines for pain and inflammation
- blood thinners (anticoagulants)
- antiseizure medicines, including divalproex (Depakote) and valproic acid (Depakene)
- cephalosporins, including cefamandole (Mandol), cefoperazone (Cefobid), and cefotetan (Cefotan)

In addition, anyone who has been treated with anistreplase or streptokinase within the past year should tell the physician in charge. These drugs may not work properly if they are given again, so the physician may want to use a different thrombolytic agent.

Patients who are taking thrombolytic medications should not take vitamin E supplements or certain herbal preparations without consulting their doctor. High doses of vitamin E can increase the risk of hemorrhagic stroke. Ginger, borage, angelica, dong quai, feverfew, and other herbs can intensify the anticlotting effect of thrombolytic medications and increase the risk of bleeding.

Resources

BOOKS

Brody, T. M., J. Larner, K. P. Minneman, and H. C. Neu. *Human Pharmacology: Molecular to Clinical*, 2nd ed. St. Louis: Mosby Year-Book, 1995.

Karch, A. M. *Lippincott's Nursing Drug Guide*. Springhouse, PA: Lippincott Williams & Wilkins, 2003.

Pelletier, Kenneth R., MD. *The Best Alternative Medicine*, Part I, Chapter 6, "Western Herbal Medicine." New York: Simon & Schuster, 2002.

Reynolds, J. E. F., ed. *Martindale: The Extra Pharmacopoeia*, 31st ed. London, UK: The Pharmaceutical Press, 1996.

Townsend, C. M., ed. *Sabiston Textbook of Surgery*, 16th ed. Philadelphia, PA: W. B. Saunders, 2001.

PERIODICALS

"Acute Myocardial Infarction: Clot-Busting Therapy May Reduce Death in Elderly Heart Attack Patients." *Heart Disease Weekly* May 18, 2003.

Dundar, Y., R. Hill, R. Dickson, and T. Walley. "Comparative Efficacy of Thrombolytics in Acute Myocardial Infarction: A Systematic Review." *QJM* 96 (February 2003): 103-113.

Marsh, P. "Clot-Bust' Drug Right On Target." *Birmingham Post and Mail Ltd*, February 6, 2003.

ORGANIZATIONS

American Society of Health-System Pharmacists (ASHP). 7272 Wisconsin Avenue, Bethesda, MD 20814. (301) 657-3000. <www.ashp.org>.

United States Food and Drug Administration (FDA). 5600 Fishers Lane, Rockville, MD 20857-0001. (888) INFO-FDA. <www.fda.gov>.

OTHER

Harvard Medical School. <www.hms.harvard.edu/news/releases/0302soumerai.html>.

University of Iowa. <www.medicine.uiowa.edu/pharmacology/Lectures/Lecturenotes/111/RJH-Anticoagulants%20(Word).pdf>.

Nancy Ross-Flanigan
Sam Uretsky, PharmD

Thyroid gland removal *see* **Thyroidectomy**

Thyroidectomy

Definition

Thyroidectomy is a surgical procedure in which all or part of the thyroid gland is removed. The thyroid gland is located in the forward (anterior) part of the neck just under the skin and in front of the Adam's apple. The thyroid is one of the body's endocrine glands, which means that it secretes its products inside the body, into the blood or lymph. The thyroid produces several hormones that have two primary functions: they increase the synthesis of proteins in most of the body's tissues, and they raise the level of the body's oxygen consumption.

> **KEY TERMS**
>
> **Arteries**—Blood vessels that carry blood away from the heart to the cells, tissues, and organs of the body.
>
> **Chemotherapy**—Treatment of an illness with chemical agents. The term is usually used to describe the treatment of cancer with drugs that kill cancer cells.
>
> **Dialysis**—A process used to separate waste products from the blood in people whose kidneys are not working well.
>
> **Hemorrhagic stroke**—A disruption of the blood supply to the brain caused by bleeding into the brain.
>
> **Stent**—A thin rodlike or tubelike device, inserted into a vein or artery to keep the vessel open.
>
> **Stroke**—A serious medical event in which blood flow to the brain is stopped by a blood clot in an artery or because an artery has burst. Strokes may cause paralysis and changes in a person's speech, memory, and behavior.

Thyroidectomy

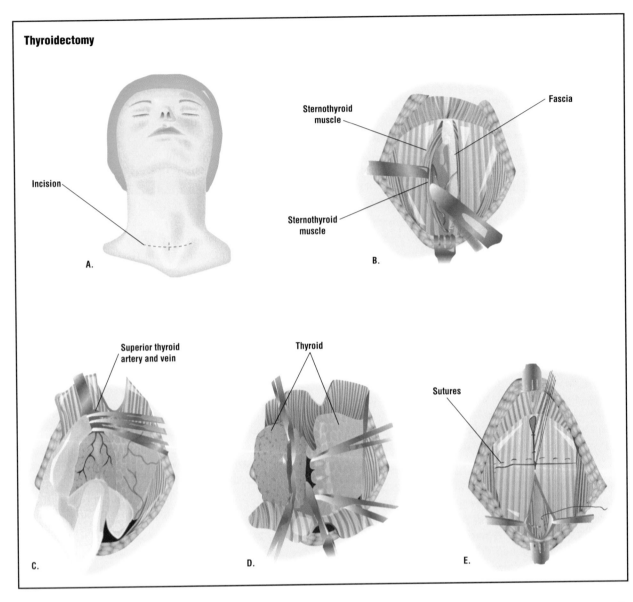

To remove the thyroid gland, an incision is made at the front of the neck (A). Muscles and connecting tissue, or fascia, are divided (B). The veins and arteries above and below the thyroid are severed (C), and the gland is removed in two parts (D). The tissues and muscles are repaired before the skin incision is closed (E). *(Illustration by GGS Inc.)*

Purpose

All or part of the thyroid gland may be removed to correct a variety of abnormalities. If a person has a goiter, which is an enlargement of the thyroid gland that causes swelling in the front of the neck, the swollen gland may cause difficulties with swallowing or breathing. Hyperthyroidism (overactivity of the thyroid gland) produces hypermetabolism, a condition in which the body uses abnormal amounts of oxygen, nutrients, and other materials. A thyroidectomy may be performed if the hypermetabolism cannot be adequately controlled by medication, or if the condition occurs in a child or pregnant woman. Both cancerous and noncancerous tumors (frequently called nodules) may develop in the thyroid gland. These growths must be removed, in addition to some or all of the gland itself.

Demographics

Screening tests indicate that about 6% of the United States population has some disturbance of thyroid function, but many people with mildly abnormal levels of thyroid hormone do not have any disease symptoms. It is estimated that between 12 and 15 million people in the

United States and Canada are receiving treatment for thyroid disorders as of 2002. In 2001, there were approximately 34,500 thyroidectomies performed in the United States. Females are somewhat more likely than males to require a thyroidectomy.

Description

A thyroidectomy begins with general anesthesia administered by an anesthesiologist. The anesthesiologist injects drugs into the patient's veins and then places an airway tube in the windpipe to ventilate (provide air for) the person during the operation. After the patient has been anesthetized, the surgeon makes an incision in the front of the neck at the level where a tight-fitting necklace would rest. The surgeon locates and takes care not to injure the parathyroid glands and the recurrent laryngeal nerves, while freeing the thyroid gland from these surrounding structures. The next step is clamping off the blood supply to the portion of the thyroid gland that is to be removed. Next, the surgeon removes all or part of the gland. If cancer has been diagnosed, all or most of the gland is removed. If other diseases or nodules are present, the surgeon may remove only part of the gland. The total amount of glandular tissue removed depends on the condition being treated. The surgeon may place a drain, which is a soft plastic tube that allows tissue fluids to flow out of an area, before closing the incision. The incision is closed with either sutures (stitches) or metal clips. A dressing is placed over the incision and the drain, if one has been placed.

People generally stay in the hospital one to four days after a thyroidectomy.

Diagnosis/Preparation

Thyroid disorders do not always develop rapidly; in some cases, the patient's symptoms may be subtle or difficult to distinguish from the symptoms of other disorders. Patients suffering from hypothyroidism are sometimes misdiagnosed as having a psychiatric depression. Before a thyroidectomy is performed, a variety of tests and studies are usually required to determine the nature of the thyroid disease. Laboratory analysis of blood determines the levels of active thyroid hormones circulating in the body. The most common test is a blood test that measures the level of thyroid-stimulating hormone (TSH) in the bloodstream. Sonograms and computed tomography scans (**CT scans**) help to determine the size of the thyroid gland and location of abnormalities. A nuclear medicine scan may be used to assess thyroid function or to evaluate the condition of a thyroid nodule, but it is not considered a routine test. A needle biopsy of an abnormality or aspiration (removal by suction) of fluid

from the thyroid gland may also be performed to help determine the diagnosis.

If the diagnosis is hyperthyroidism, a person may be asked to take antithyroid medication or iodides before the operation. Continued treatment with antithyroid drugs may be the treatment of choice. Otherwise, no other special procedure must be followed prior to the operation.

Aftercare

A thyroidectomy incision requires little to no care after the dressing is removed. The area may be bathed gently with a mild soap. The sutures or the metal clips are removed three to seven days after the operation.

Risks

There are definite risks associated with the procedure. The thyroid gland should be removed only if there is a pressing reason or medical condition that requires it.

As with all operations, people who are obese, smoke, or have poor nutrition are at greater risk for developing complications related to the general anesthetic itself.

Hoarseness or voice loss may develop if the recurrent laryngeal nerve is injured or destroyed during the operation. Nerve damage is more apt to occur in people who have large goiters or cancerous tumors.

Hypoparathyroidism (underfunctioning of the parathyroid glands) can occur if the parathyroid glands are injured or removed at the time of the thyroidectomy. Hypoparathyroidism is characterized by a drop in blood calcium levels resulting in muscle cramps and twitching.

Hypothyroidism (underfunctioning of the thyroid gland) can occur if all or nearly all of the thyroid gland is removed. Complete removal, however, may be intentional when the patient is diagnosed with cancer. If a person's thyroid levels remain low, thyroid replacement medications may be required for the rest of his or her life.

A hematoma is a collection of blood in an organ or tissue, caused by a break in the wall of a blood vessel. The neck and the area surrounding the thyroid gland have a rich supply of blood vessels. Bleeding in the area of the operation may occur and be difficult to control or stop. If a hematoma occurs in this part of the body, it may be life-threatening. As the hematoma enlarges, it may obstruct the airway and cause a person to stop breathing. If a hematoma does develop in the neck, the surgeon may need to perform drainage to clear the airway.

Wound infections can occur. If they do, the incision is drained, and there are usually no serious consequences.

Normal results

Most patients are discharged from the hospital one to four days after a thyroidectomy. Most resume their normal activities two weeks after the operation. People who have cancer may require subsequent treatment by an oncologist or endocrinologist.

Morbidity and mortality rates

The mortality of thyroidectomy is essentially zero. Hypothyroidism is thought to occur in 12–50% of persons in the first year after a thyroidectomy. Late-onset hypothyroidism develops among an additional 1–3% of persons each year. Although hypothyroidism may recur many years after a partial thyroidectomy, 43% of recurrences occur within five years.

Mortality from thyroid storm, an uncommon complication of thyroidectomy, is in the range of 20–30%. Thyroid storm is characterized by fever, weakness and wasting of the muscles, enlargement of the liver, restlessness, mood swings, change in mental status, and in some cases, coma. *Thyroid storm is a medical emergency requiring immediate treatment.* After a partial thyroidectomy, thyroid function returns to normal in 90–98% of persons.

Alternatives

Injections of radioactive iodine were used to destroy thyroid tissue in the past. This alternative is rarely performed in 2003.

See also Parathyroidectomy.

Resources

BOOKS

Bland, K. I., W. G. Cioffi, and M. G. Sarr. *Practice of General Surgery.* Philadelphia, PA: Saunders, 2001.

Ruggieri, P. *A Simple Guide to Thyroid Disorders: From Diagnosis to Treatment.* Omaha, NE: Addicus Books, 2003.

Saheen, O. H. *Thyroid Surgery.* Boca Raton, FL: CRC Press, 2002.

Schwartz, S. I., J. E. Fischer, F. C. Spencer, et al. *Principles of Surgery,* 7th ed. New York: McGraw-Hill, 1998.

Townsend, C., K. L. Mattox, R. D. Beauchamp, et al. *Sabiston's Review of Surgery,* 3rd ed. Philadelphia, PA: Saunders, 2001.

PERIODICALS

Bellantone, R., C. P. Lombardi, M. Raffaelli, et al. "Is Routine Supplementation Therapy (Calcium and Vitamin D) Useful After Total Thyroidectomy?" *Surgery* 132 (December 2002): 1109-1113.

Dror, A., M. Salim, and R. Yoseph. "Sutureless Thyroidectomy Using Electrothermal System: A New Technique." *Journal of Laryngology and Otology* 117 (March 2003):198-201.

Ikeda, Y., H. Takami, Y. Sasaki. "Clinical Benefits in Endoscopic Thyroidectomy by the Axillary Approach." *Journal of the American College of Surgery* 196 (February 2003): 189-195.

Oey, I. F., B. D. Richardson, and D. A. Waller. "Video-Assisted Thoracoscopic Thyroidectomy for Obstructive Sleep Apnoea." *Respiratory Medicine* 97 (February 2003): 192-193.

ORGANIZATIONS

American Academy of Otolaryngology-Head and Neck Surgery. One Prince St., Alexandria, VA 22314-3357. (703) 836-4444. <www.entnet.org/index2.cfm>.

American College of Surgeons. 633 North St. Clair Street, Chicago, IL 60611-3231. (312) 202-5000; FAX: (312) 202-5001. <www.facs.org>.

American Medical Association. 515 N. State Street, Chicago, IL 60610. (312) 464-5000. <www.ama-assn.org>.

American Osteopathic College of Otolaryngology-Head and Neck Surgery. 405 W. Grand Avenue, Dayton, OH 45405. (937) 222-8820 or (800) 455-9404; FAX (937) 222-8840. Email: info@aocoohns.org.

Association of Thyroid Surgeons. 717 Buena Vista St., Ventura, CA 93001, FAX: (509) 479-8678. <www.thyroidsurgery.org>.

OTHER

Beth Israel Deaconess Medical Center/Harvard University. <www.bidmc.harvard.edu/thyroidcenter/edu-thysur.asp>. (April 3, 2003).

KEY TERMS

Endocrine—A type of organ or gland that secretes hormones or other products inside the body, into the bloodstream or the lymphatic system. The thyroid is an endocrine gland.

Endocrinologist—A physician who specializes in treating persons with diseases of the thyroid, parathyroid, adrenal glands, and the pancreas.

Goiter—An enlargement of the thyroid gland due to insufficient iodine in the diet.

Hyperthyroidism—Abnormal overactivity of the thyroid gland. People with hyperthyroidism are hypermetabolic, lose weight, exhibit nervousness, have muscular weakness and fatigue, sweat heavily, and have increased urination and bowel movements. This condition is also called thyrotoxicosis.

Hypothyroidism—Abnormal underfunctioning of the thyroid gland. People with hypothyroidism have a lowered body metabolism, gain weight, and are sluggish.

Parathyroid glands—Two pairs of smaller glands that lie close to the lower surface of the thyroid gland. They secrete parathyroid hormone, which regulates the body's use of calcium and phosphorus.

Recurrent laryngeal nerve—A nerve which lies very near the parathyroid glands and serves the larynx or voice box.

Thyroid storm—An unusual complication of thyroid function that is sometimes triggered by the stress of thyroid surgery. It is a medical emergency.

Columbia University School of Medicine. <www.cpmcnet.columbia.edu/dept/thyroid/surgeryHP.html>. (April 3, 2003).

Cornell University Medical College. <www.med.cornell.edu/surgery/endocrine/thyroid.html>. (April 3, 2003).

University of California-San Diego School of Medicine. <www-surgery.ucsd.edu/ent/PatientInfo/th_thyroid.html>. (April 3, 2003).

L. Fleming Fallon, Jr., MD, DrPH

Tissue plasminogen activator *see* **Thrombolytic therapy**

Tissue typing *see* **Human leukocyte antigen test**

Tongue removal *see* **Glossectomy**

Tonsil removal *see* **Tonsillectomy**

Tonsillectomy

Definition

Tonsillectomy is a surgical procedure to remove the tonsils. The tonsils are part of the lymphatic system, which is responsible for fighting infection.

Purpose

Tonsils are removed when a person, most often a child, has any of the following conditions:

• obstruction

• sleep apnea (a condition in which an individual snores loudly and stops breathing temporarily at intervals during sleep)

• inability to swallow properly because of enlarged tonsils

• a breathy voice or other speech abnormality due to enlarged tonsils

• recurrent or persistent abscesses or throat infections

Physicians are not in complete agreement on the number of sore throats that necessitate a tonsillectomy. Most would agree that four cases of strep throat in any one year; six or more episodes of tonsillitis in one year; or five or more episodes of tonsillitis per year for two years indicate that the tonsils should be removed.

Demographics

A tonsillectomy is one of the most common surgical procedures among children. It is uncommon among adults. More than 400,000 tonsillectomies are performed

WHO PERFORMS THE PROCEDURE AND WHERE IS IT PERFORMED?

A tonsillectomy is performed in an outpatient facility associated with a hospital by a general surgeon or otolaryngologist (physician who specializes in treating disorders of the ear, nose, and throat).

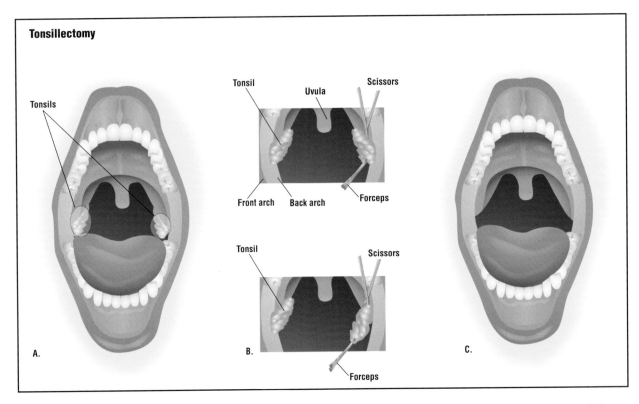

Tonsillectomy

Tonsil | Uvula | Scissors

Front arch | Back arch | Forceps

Tonsil | Scissors

Forceps

A.

B.

C.

Tonsils are removed through the mouth (A). The surgeon uses a scissors to cut away the tonsils, and a forceps to pull them away (B). *(Illustration by GGS Inc.)*

each year in the United States. Approximately 70% of surgical candidates are under age 18.

Description

A tonsillectomy is usually performed under general anesthesia, although adults may occasionally receive a local anesthetic. The surgeon depresses the tongue in order to see the throat, and removes the tonsils with an instrument resembling a scoop.

Alternate methods for removing tonsils are being investigated, including lasers and other electronic devices.

Diagnosis/Preparation

Tonsillectomy procedures are not performed as frequently today as they once were. One reason for a more conservative approach is the risk involved when a person is put under general anesthesia.

In some cases, a tonsillectomy may need to be modified or postponed:

• Bleeding disorders must be adequately controlled prior to surgery.

• Acute tonsillitis should be successfully treated prior to surgery. Treatment may postpone the surgery three to four weeks.

Aftercare

Persons are turned on their side after the operation to prevent the possibility of blood being drawn into the lungs (aspirated). **Vital signs** are monitored. Patients can drink water and other non-irritating liquids when they are fully awake.

Adults are usually warned to expect a very sore throat and some bleeding after the operation. They are given **antibiotics** to prevent infection, and some receive pain-relieving medications. For at least the first 24 hours, individuals are instructed to drink fluids and eat soft, pureed foods.

People are usually sent home the day of surgery. They are given instructions to call their surgeon if there is bleeding or earache, or fever that lasts longer than three days. They are told to expect a white scab to form in the throat between five and 10 days after surgery.

Risks

There is a chance that children with previously normal speech will develop a nasal-sounding voice. In addition, children younger than five years may be emotionally upset by the hospital experience. There are risks associated with any surgical procedure, including post-operative infection and bleeding.

QUESTIONS TO ASK THE DOCTOR

- What will be the resulting functional status of the body after the operation?
- Is the surgeon board certified in head and neck surgery?
- How many tonsillectomy procedures has the surgeon performed?
- What is the surgeon's complication rate?
- Has the surgeon operated on children?

KEY TERMS

Abscess—A localized area of tissue destruction and pus formation.

Sleep apnea—A condition marked by loud snoring during sleep and periodic episodes of suspended breathing.

Tonsils—Oval masses of lymphoid tissue on each side of the throat.

Normal results

Normal results include the correction of the condition for which the surgery was performed.

Morbidity and mortality rates

Morbidity other than minor post-surgical infection is uncommon. About one in every 15,000 tonsillectomies ends in death, either from the anesthesia or bleeding five to seven days after the operation.

Alternatives

There are no alternatives to surgical removal of the tonsils. Drug therapy may be used for recurrent infections involving the tonsils.

See also Adenoidectomy.

Resources

BOOKS

Bland, K.I., W.G. Cioffi, M.G. Sarr. *Practice of General Surgery.* Philadelphia: Saunders, 2001.

Braunwald, E., D.L. Longo, J.L. Jameson. *Harrison's Principles of Internal Medicine,* 15th ed. New York: McGraw-Hill, 2001.

Goldman, L. & J.C. Bennett. *Cecil Textbook of Medicine,* 21st ed. Philadelphia: Saunders, 1999.

Schwartz, S.I., J.E. Fischer, F.C. Spencer, G.T. Shires, J.M. Daly. *Principles of Surgery,* 7th ed. New York: McGraw Hill, 1998.

Townsend, C., K.L. Mattox, R.D. Beauchamp, B.M. Evers, D.C. Sabiston. *Sabiston's Review of Surgery,* 3rd ed. Philadelphia: Saunders, 2001.

PERIODICALS

Remacle, M., J. Keghian, G. Lawson, J. Jamart. "Carbon-dioxide Laser-assisted Tonsil Ablation for Adults with Chronic Tonsillitis: A 6-month Follow-up Study." *European Archives of Otorhinolaryngology* 260, no.4 (2003): 243-6.

Silveira, H., J.S. Soares, H.A. Lima. "Tonsillectomy: Cold Dissection Versus Bipolar Electrodissection." *International Journal of Pediatric Otorhinolaryngology* 67, no.4 (2003): 345-51.

Werle, A.H., P.J. Nicklaus, D.J. Kirse, D.E. Bruegger. "A Retrospective Study of Tonsillectomy in the Under 2-Year-Old Child: Indications, Perioperative Management, and Complications." *International Journal of Pediatric Otorhinolaryngology* 67, no.5 (2003): 453-60.

Yaremchuk, K. "Tonsillectomy by Plasma-Mediated Ablation." *Archives of Otolaryngology Head and Neck Surgery* 129, no.4 (2003): 498-9.

ORGANIZATIONS

American College of Surgeons. 633 North St. Clair Street, Chicago, IL 60611-32311. (312) 202-5000. Fax: (312) 202-5001. E-mail: <postmaster@facs.org>. <http://www.facs.org>.

American Academy of Otolaryngology-Head and Neck Surgery. One Prince St., Alexandria, VA 22314-3357. (703) 836-4444. <http://www.entnet.org/index2.cfm>.

American Cancer Society. 1599 Clifton Road NE, Atlanta, GA 30329. (800) 227-2345. <http://www.cancer.org>.

American Osteopathic College of Otolaryngology-Head and Neck Surgery. 405 W. Grand Avenue, Dayton, OH 45405. (937) 222-8820 or (800) 455-9404, fax (937) 222-8840. Email: <info@aocoohns.org>.

OTHER

Columbia University School of Medicine. [cited May 5, 2003] <http://www.entcolumbia.org/t-aproc.htm>.

Eastern Virginia Medical School. [cited May 5, 2003] <http://www.evmsent.org/ped_ops/tonsillectomy.html>.

National Library of Medicine. [cited May 5, 2003] <http://www.nlm.nih.gov/medlineplus/ency/article/003013.htm>.

University of California-San Diego. [cited May 5, 2003] <http://www-surgery.ucsd.edu/ent/PatientInfo/instructions_tonsillectomy.html>.

University of Florida. [cited May 5, 2003] <http://www.ent.health.ufl.edu/patient%20info/T&A.htm>.

L. Fleming Fallon, Jr., MD, Dr.PH.

Tooth extraction

Definition

Tooth extraction is the removal of a tooth from its socket in the bone.

Purpose

Extraction is performed for positional, structural, or economic reasons. Teeth are often removed because they are impacted. Teeth become impacted when they are prevented from growing into their normal position in the mouth by gum tissue, bone, or other teeth. Impaction is a common reason for the extraction of wisdom teeth. Extraction is the only known method that will prevent further problems with impaction.

Teeth may also be extracted to make more room in the mouth prior to straightening the remaining teeth (orthodontic treatment), or because they are so badly positioned that straightening is impossible. Extraction may be used to remove teeth that are so badly decayed or broken that they cannot be restored. In addition, some patients choose extraction as a less expensive alternative to filling or placing a crown on a severely decayed tooth.

Demographics

Exact statistics concerning tooth extraction are not available. Experts estimate that over 20 million teeth are extracted each year in the United States. Many of these are performed in conjunction with orthodontic procedures. Some extractions are due to tooth decay.

Description

Tooth extraction can be performed with local anesthesia if the tooth is exposed and appears to be easily removable in one piece. The dentist or oral surgeon uses an instrument called an elevator to luxate, or loosen, the tooth; widen the space in the underlying bone; and break the tiny elastic fibers that attach the tooth to the bone. Once the tooth is dislocated from the bone, it can be lifted and removed with forceps.

If the extraction is likely to be difficult, a general dentist may refer the patient to an oral surgeon. Oral surgeons are specialists who are trained to administer nitrous oxide (laughing gas), an intravenous sedative, or a general anesthetic to relieve pain. Extracting an impacted tooth or a tooth with curved roots typically requires cutting through gum tissue to expose the tooth. It may also require removing portions of bone to free the tooth. Some teeth must be cut and removed in sections. The extraction site may or may not require one or more stitches (sutures) to close the incision.

WHO PERFORMS THE PROCEDURE AND WHERE IS IT PERFORMED?

In 2003, teeth are most often extracted by maxillofacial or oral surgeons. Occasionally, a general dentist will extract a tooth. Teeth are most commonly removed in an outpatient facility adjacent to a hospital under general anesthesia.

Diagnosis/Preparation

In some situations, tooth extractions may be temporarily postponed. These situations include:

- Infection that has progressed from the tooth into the bone. Infections may complicate administering anesthesia. They can be treated with **antibiotics** before the tooth is extracted.

- Use of drugs that thin the blood (anticoagulants). These medications include warfarin (Coumadin) and **aspirin**. The patient should stop using these medications for three days prior to extraction.

- People who have had any of the following procedures in the previous six months: heart valve replacement, open heart surgery, prosthetic joint replacement, or placement of a medical shunt. These patients may be given antibiotics to reduce the risk of bacterial infection spreading from the mouth to other parts of the body.

Before extracting a tooth, the dentist will take the patient's medical history, noting allergies and other prescription medications that the patient is taking. A dental history is also recorded. Particular attention is given to previous extractions and reactions to anesthetics. The dentist may then prescribe antibiotics or recommend stopping certain medications prior to the extraction. The tooth is x rayed to determine its full shape and position, especially if it is impacted.

Patients scheduled for deep anesthesia should wear loose clothing with sleeves that are easily rolled up to allow the dentist to place an intravenous line. They should not eat or drink anything for at least six hours before the procedure. Arrangements should be made for a friend or relative to drive them home after the surgery.

Aftercare

An important aspect of aftercare is encouraging a clot to form at the extraction site. The patient should put pressure on the area by biting gently on a roll or wad of gauze for several hours after surgery. Once the clot is

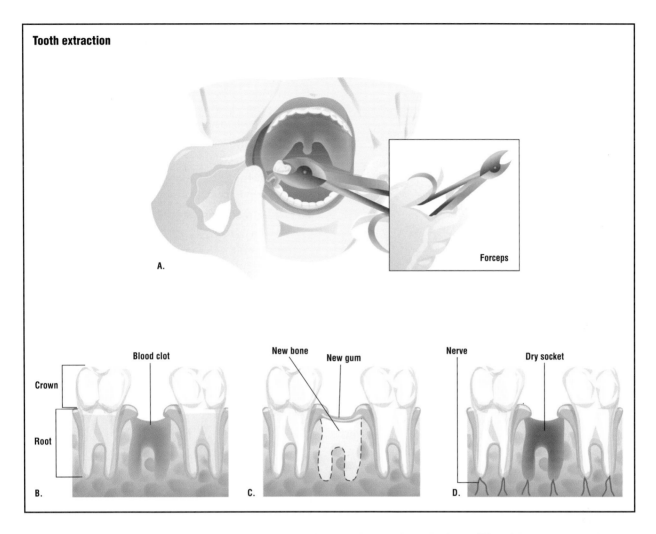

A.

Forceps

Blood clot

New bone   New gum

Nerve   Dry socket

Crown

Root

B.   C.   D.

A dental surgeon uses special forceps to pull out a tooth (A). In its place, a blood clot forms (B), which becomes new bone with gum tissue over the top (C). If the blood clot does not form or falls out, a dry socket occurs (D). No new bone forms, and the nerves are exposed, causing pain. *(Illustration by GGS Inc.)*

formed, it should not be disturbed. The patient should not rinse, spit, drink with a straw, or smoke for at least 24 hours after the extraction and preferably longer. He or she should also avoid vigorous **exercise** for the first three to five days after the extraction.

For the first two days after the procedure, the patient should drink liquids without using a straw and eat soft foods. Any chewing must be done on the side away from the extraction site. Hard or sticky foods should be avoided. The mouth may be gently cleaned with a toothbrush, but the extraction area should not be scrubbed.

Wrapped ice packs can be applied to reduce facial swelling. Swelling is a normal part of the healing process; it is most noticeable in the first 48–72 hours after surgery. As the swelling subsides, the patient's jaw muscles may feel stiff. Moist heat and gentle exercise will restore normal jaw movement. The dentist or oral

surgeon may prescribe medications to relieve postoperative pain.

Risks

Potential complications of tooth extraction include postoperative infection, temporary numbness from nerve irritation, jaw fracture, and jaw joint pain. An additional complication is called dry socket. When a blood clot does not properly form in the empty tooth socket, the bone beneath the socket is exposed to air and contamination by food particles; as a result, the extraction site heals more slowly than is normal or desirable.

Normal results

The wound usually closes in about two weeks after a tooth extraction, but it takes three to six months for the bone and soft tissue to be restructured. Such complications as infection or dry socket may prolong the healing process.

Morbidity and mortality rates

Mortality from tooth extraction is very rare. Complications include a brief period of pain and swelling; post-extraction infections; and migration of adjacent teeth into the empty space created by an extraction. Most people experience some pain and swelling after having a tooth extracted. With the exception of removing wisdom teeth, migration into the empty space is common. Braces or orthodontic appliances usually control this problem.

Alternatives

Alternatives to tooth extraction depend on the reason for the extraction. Postponing or canceling an extraction to correct tooth crowding will cause malocclusion and an undesirable appearance. Not removing an impacted wisdom tooth may cause eventual misalignment, although it may have no impact. Not removing a decayed or abscessed tooth may lead to septicemia and other complications.

See also Wound care.

Resources

BOOKS

Harris, N. O., and F. Garcia-Godoy. *Primary Preventative Dentistry*, 6th ed. Englewood Cliffs, NJ: Prentice Hall, 2003.

Peterson, L. J. *Contemporary Oral and Maxillofacial Surgery*, 4th ed. Amsterdam: Elsevier Science, 2002.

Scully, C. *Oral and Maxillofacial Medicine: A Practical Guide.* London, UK: Butterworth-Heinemann, 2003.

Tronstad, L. *Clinical Endodontics.* New York: Thieme Medical Publishers, 2003.

PERIODICALS

Devlin, H., and P. Sloan. "Early Bone Healing Events in the Human Extraction Socket." *International Journal of Oral and Maxillofacial Surgery* 31 (December 2002): 641-645.

Magheri, P., S. Cambi, and R. Grandini. "Restorative Alternatives for the Treatment of an Impacted Canine: Surgical and Prosthetic Considerations." *Practical Procedures and Aesthetic Dentistry* 14 (October 2002): 659-664.

Moscovich, H. "Fitting Restorations from Extracted Teeth." *Journal of the South African Dental Association* 55 (August 2000): 411-412.

Rosted, P., and V. Jorgensen. "Acupuncture Treatment of Pain Dysfunction Syndrome After Dental Extraction." *Acupuncture in Medicine* 20 (December 2002): 191-192.

ORGANIZATIONS

American Association of Oral and Maxillofacial Surgeons. 9700 West Bryn Mawr Ave., Rosemont, IL 60018-5701. (847) 678-6200. <www.aaoms.org>.

American Board of Oral and Maxillofacial Surgery. 625 North Michigan Avenue, Suite 1820, Chicago, IL 60611. (312) 642-0070; FAX: (312) 642-8584. <www.aboms.org>.

American Dental Association. 211 E. Chicago Avenue, Chicago, IL 60611. (312) 440-2500. <www.ada.org>.

British Association of Oral and Maxillofacial Surgeons, Royal College of Surgeons. 35–43 Lincoln's Inn Fields, London, UK WC2A 3PN. <www.baoms.org.uk>.

OTHER

American Dental Association. [cited April 3, 2003]. <www.ada.org/public/topics/extractions.html>.

Bristol Biomed. [cited April 3, 2003]. <www.brisbio.ac.uk/ROADS/subject-listing/ toothextraction.html>.

Dental Review Online. [cited April 3, 2003]. <www.dentalre-view.com/Tooth_Extraction.htm>.

Emory University. [cited April 3, 2003]. <www.emory.edu/COLLEGE/CULPEPER/RAVINA/PROJECT/Ancient_pages/Tooth_extraction.html>.

L. Fleming Fallon, Jr., MD, DrPH

Tooth replantation

Definition

Tooth replantation is the reinsertion and splinting of a tooth that has been avulsed (knocked or torn out) of its socket.

Purpose

Teeth are replanted to prevent permanent loss of the tooth, and to restore the landscape of the mouth so that the patient can eat and speak normally.

Demographics

According to the National Center for Health Statistics, about 5 million teeth are accidentally avulsed in the United States each year. Most teeth that are replanted are lost through trauma, usually falls and other types of accidents. The most common traumata resulting in tooth avulsion are sports accidents that result in falls or blows to the head. The mandatory use of mouthguards, which are plastic devices that protect the upper teeth, has prevented approximately 200,000 oral injuries each year in football alone. The American Dental Association recommends the use of mouthguards for any sport that involves speed, contact, or the potential for falls. These categories include not only contact sports like football, wrestling, and boxing, but also gymnastics, baseball, hockey, bicycling, skateboarding, and skiing. Without a mouthguard, a person is 60 times more likely to experience dental trauma if he or she participates in these sports.

Other common causes of trauma to the mouth resulting in avulsed teeth include motor vehicle accidents, criminal assaults, and fist fights. Domestic violence is the most common cause of avulsed teeth in women over the age of 21.

Description

In most cases, only permanent teeth are replanted. Primary teeth (baby teeth) do not usually have long enough roots for successful replantation. The only ex-

ception may be the canine teeth, which have longer roots and therefore a better chance of staying in place. In some cases, however, the dentist may choose to replant a child's primary tooth because there is risk to the permanent tooth that has not yet emerged.

To replant a tooth, the dentist or oral surgeon will first administer a local anesthetic to numb the patient's gums. He or she will then reinsert the avulsed tooth in its socket and anchor it within the mouth by installing a splint made of wire and composite resin. Some dentists remove the root canal nerve of the tooth and replace it with a plastic material before reinserting the tooth. The splint holds the tooth in place for two to six weeks. At that time, the splint can be removed and the tooth examined for stability.

Diagnosis/Preparation

When a tooth is dislodged, it is critical to recover the tooth, preserve it under proper conditions, and get the patient to a dentist immediately. The tooth should be handled carefully; it should be picked up or touched by its crown (the top part of the tooth), not by its root. The tooth should be rinsed and kept moist, but not cleaned or brushed. The use of toothpaste, soap, mouthwash, or other chemicals can remove the fibroblasts clinging to the root of the tooth. Fibroblasts are connective tissue cells that act as a glue between teeth and the underlying bone.

The avulsed tooth can be placed in milk or a Save-a-Tooth (R) kit, which is a tooth-preserving cup that contains a medium for preserving the fibroblasts around the tooth. The tooth and the patient should go to the dentist within 30 minutes of the accident since fibroblasts begin to die within that time. Rapid treatment improves the chances for successful replantation. In some cases, artificial fibroblasts can be substituted for the patient's own connective tissue cells.

If the tooth is a primary tooth, it should be rinsed and kept moist also. The dentist should be consulted to determine whether the tooth should be replanted by examining the gums and the emergent tooth. The dentist

QUESTIONS TO ASK THE DOCTOR

- How should I take care of the replanted tooth?
- How long will it take to assess the results of treatment?
- What can be done if the tooth cannot be replanted?
- Where can I be fitted for a mouthguard?

will take a set of x rays to determine how soon the permanent tooth is likely to emerge. Sometimes an artificial spacer is placed where the primary tooth was lost until the permanent tooth comes in.

Any injury to the gum is treated before the tooth is replanted. The dentist may give the patient an antibiotic medication to reduce the risk of infection. Cold compresses can reduce swelling. Stitches may be necessary if the gum is lacerated. The dentist may also take x rays of the mouth to see if there are other injuries to the jawbone or nearby teeth.

Aftercare

The patient may take **aspirin** or **acetaminophen** for pain. **Antibiotics** may also be given for infection. The patient should avoid rinsing the mouth, spitting, or smoking for the first 24 hours after surgery. He or she should limit food to a soft diet for the next few days.

Beginning 24 hours after surgery, the patient should rinse the mouth gently with a solution of salt and lukewarm water every one to two hours. The salt helps to reduce swelling in the tissues around the tooth.

Any kind of traumatic injury always carries the risk of infection. Patients with heart disease or disorders of the immune system should be monitored following tooth replantation. Dentists recommend consulting a physician within 48 hours of the dental surgery to determine the risk of tetanus, particularly if the patient has not received a tetanus booster within the past five years.

Adults with replanted teeth should have periodic checkups. According to the American Association of Endodontists, it takes about two to three years after replantation before the dentist can fully evaluate the outcome of treatment.

Risks

In addition to infection, tooth replantation carries the risks of excessive bleeding and rejection of the tooth.

Rejection is a rare complication. An additional risk is that the root of the tooth may become fused to the underlying bone.

Normal results

Most permanent tooth replantations are successful when the patient acts quickly (within 2 hours). If the tooth is rejected, the dentist may attach the tooth to the bone with tissue glue.

Morbidity and mortality rates

Mortality following tooth replantation is almost unheard of. The rate of complications varies according to the circumstances of the injury, the patient's age, and his or her general health. A history of smoking increases the risk of rejection of the tooth as well as infection.

Alternatives

There are no effective medical alternatives to oral surgery for replanting an avulsed tooth. Over-the-counter **analgesics** (pain relievers), prescription antibiotics, and some herbal preparations may be useful in relieving pain, reducing swelling, or preventing infection.

Herbal preparations that have been found useful as mouthwashes following oral surgery include calendula *Calendula officinalis* and clove (*Eugenia caryophyllata*).

Resources

BOOKS

"Dental Emergencies: Fractured and Avulsed Teeth." Section 9, Chapter 107 in *The Merck Manual of Diagnosis and Therapy*, edited by Mark H. Beers, MD, and Robert Berkow, MD. Whitehouse Station, NJ: Merck Research Laboratories, 1999.

PERIODICALS

Douglass, Alan B., MD, and Joanna M. Douglass, DDS. "Common Dental Emergencies." *American Family Physician* 67 (February 1, 2003): 511-516.

Franklin, Deeanna. "How to Save a Tooth, Save a Smile." *Pediatric News* 36 (February 2002): 1-2.

Pavek, D. I., and P. K. Radtke. "Postreplantation Management of Avulsed Teeth: An Endodontic Literature Review." *General Dentistry* 48 (March-April 2000): 176-181.

"Pedia Trick: Handle with Care." *Pediatrics for Parents* 20 (February 2002): 12.

ORGANIZATIONS

American Academy of Pediatric Dentistry. 211 East Chicago Avenue, Ste. 700, Chicago, IL 60611-2616. (312) 337-2169. <www.aapd.org>.

American Association of Endodontists. 211 East Chicago Avenues, Ste. 1100, Chicago, IL 60611-2691. (312) 266-7255. <www.aae.org>.

Avulsion—A ripping out or tearing away of a tooth or other body part.

Canine tooth—In humans, the tooth located in the mouth next to the second incisor. The canine tooth has a pointed crown and the longest root of all the teeth.

Crown—The top part of the tooth.

Endodontist—A dentist who specializes in the diagnosis and treatment of disorders affecting the pulp of a tooth, the root of the tooth, or the tissues surrounding the root. Some patients with avulsed teeth may be treated by an endodontist.

Eruption—The emergence of a tooth through the gum tissue.

Fibroblasts—Connective tissue cells that help to hold the teeth in their sockets in the jawbone.

Mouthguard—A plastic device that protects the upper teeth from injury during athletic events.

Primary teeth—A child's first set of teeth, sometimes called baby teeth.

American Association of Oral and Maxillofacial Surgeons. 9700 West Bryn Mawr Avenue, Rosemont, IL 60018-5701. (847) 678-6200. <www.aaoms.org>.
American Dental Association. 211 East Chicago Avenue, Chicago, IL 60611. (312) 440-2500. <www.ada.org>.

Janie Franz

Topical antibiotics *see* **Antibiotics, topical**

Total hip replacement *see* **Hip replacement**

Total knee replacement *see* **Knee replacement**

Total shoulder replacement *see* **Shoulder joint replacement**

Total wrist replacement *see* **Wrist replacement**

Trabeculectomy

Definition

Trabeculectomy is a surgical procedure that removes part of the trabeculum in the eye to relieve pressure caused by glaucoma.

Purpose

Glaucoma is a disease that injures the optic nerve, causing progressive vision loss. Glaucoma is a major cause of blindness in the United States. If caught early, glaucoma-related blindness is easily prevented. However, because it does not produce symptoms until late in its cycle, periodic tests for the disease are necessary.

Glaucoma is usually associated with an increase in the pressure inside the eye, called intraocular pressure (IOP). This increase occurs in front of the iris in a fluid called the aqueous humor. Aqueous humor exits through tiny channels between the iris and the cornea, in an area called the trabeculum. When the trabeculum is blocked, pressure from the build up of aqueous humor either increases rapidly with pain and redness, or builds slowly with no symptoms until there is a significant loss of vision. Trabeculectomy is the last treatment employed for either type of glaucoma. It is used only after medications and laser trabeculoplasty have failed to alleviate IOP.

Demographics

Glaucoma can develop at any age, but people over 45 are at higher risk. African Americans are more likely to develop glaucoma, especially primary open-angle glaucoma. Other factors, such as a family history of glaucoma, greatly increase the risk of contracting the disease. Diabetes and previous eye injury also increase chances of developing glaucoma.

Description

The procedure is performed in an **operating room**, usually under local anesthetic. However, some ophthalmologists give patients only a topical anesthetic. A trabeculectomy involves removing a tiny piece of the eye-

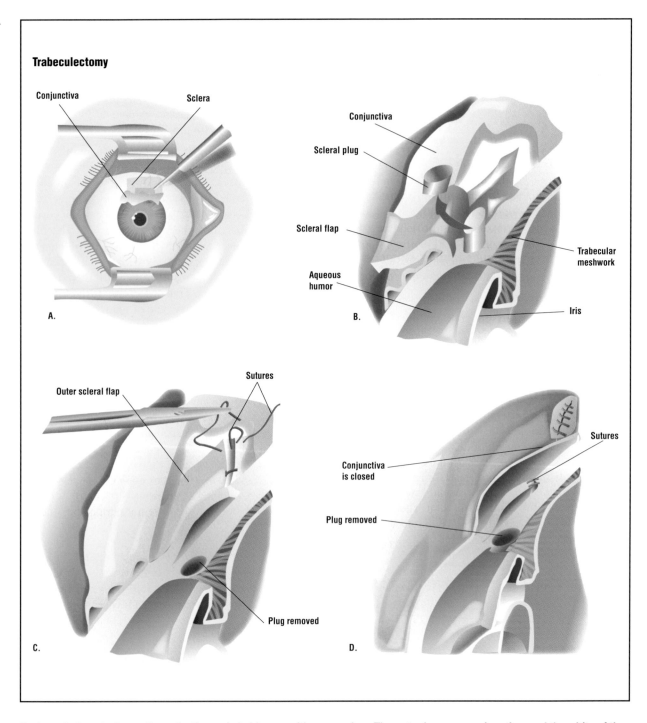

Trabeculectomy

During a trabeculectomy, the patient's eye is held open with a speculum. The outer layer, or conjunctiva, and the white of the eye, or sclera, are cut open (A). A superficial scleral flap is created and a plug of sclera and underlying trabecular network is removed (B). This allows the fluid in the eye to circulate, relieving pressure. The scleral flap is closed and sutured (C). The conjunctiva is closed (D). *(Illustration by GGS Inc.)*

ball, where the cornea connects to the sclera, to create a flap that allows fluid to escape the anterior chamber without deflating the eye. The area is called the trabeculum. After the procedure, fluid can flow out onto the eye's surface, where it is absorbed by the conjuncti-

va, the transparent membrane that lines the sclera and the eyelids.

Sometimes, an additional piece is taken from the iris so that anterior chamber fluid can also flow backward into the vitreous. This procedure is called an **iridectomy**.

Diagnosis/Preparation

The procedure is fully explained and any alternative methods to control intraocular pressure are discussed. Antiglaucoma drugs are prescribed before surgery. Added pressure on the eye caused from coughing or sneezing should be avoided.

Several eye drops are applied immediately before surgery. The eye is sterilized, and the patient draped. A speculum is inserted to keep the eyelids apart during surgery.

Aftercare

Eye drops, and perhaps patching, will be needed until the eye is healed. Driving should be restricted until the ophthalmologist grants permission. The patient may experience blurred vision. Severe eye pain, light sensitivity, and vision loss should be reported to the physician.

Antibiotic and anti-inflammatory eye drops must be used for at least six weeks after surgery. Additional medicines may be prescribed to reduce scarring.

Risks

Infection and bleeding are risks of any surgery. Scarring can cause the drainage to stop. One-third of trabeculectomy patients will develop cataracts.

Normal results

Trabeculectomy will delay the progression of glaucoma. In many cases, people still require medication to lower IOP.

Morbidity and mortality rates

Trabeculectomy is considered a safe procedure. Infection is a complication that could lead to more serious medical problems; however, it is controllable with eye drops.

Alternatives

Physicians will first try to lower IOP with glaucoma medications. Several types of eye drops are effective for this use. Sometimes a patient must instill more than one eye drop, several times a day. Compliance is very important when using these eye drops; missed dosages will raise IOPs.

Lasers are now used to treat both closed-angle and open-angle glaucoma. Peripheral iridectomy is used for people with acute angle-closure glaucoma attacks and chronic closed-angle glaucoma. The procedure creates a hole to improve the flow of aqueous humor.

Laser trabeculoplasty uses an argon laser to create tiny burns on the trabecular meshwork, which lowers IOP. The effects, however, are not permanent, and the patient must be retreated.

Transscleral cyclophotocoagulation treats the ciliary body with a laser to decrease production of aqueous humor, which reduces IOP.

A tube shunt might be implanted to create a drainage pathway in patients who are not candidates for trabeculectomy.

Resources

BOOKS

Cassel, Gary H., M.D., Michael D. Billig, O.D., and Harry G. Randall, M.D. *The Eye Book: A Complete Guide to Eye Disorders and Health.* Baltimore, MD: Johns Hopkins University Press, 1998.

Daly, Stephen, ed. *Everything You Need to Know About Medical Treatments.* Springhouse, PA: Springhouse Corp., 1996.

Sardegna, Jill, et. al. *The Encyclopedia of Blindness and Vision Impairment,* 2nd ed. New York: Facts on File, Inc., 2002.

Vaughan, Daniel, Ed. *General Ophthalmology,* 13th ed. Stamford, CT: Appleton & Lange, 1993.

ORGANIZATIONS

The Glaucoma Foundation. 116 John Street, Suite 1605 New York, NY 10038. (212) 285-0080. info@glaucomafoundation.org. <www.glaucomafoundation.org>

OTHER

"Glaucoma Filtration Procedure." *EyeMdLink.com.* [cited May 18, 2003] <www.eyemdlink.com/EyeProcedure.asp>EyeProcedureID=44>.

J. Ricker Polsdorfer, M.D.
Mary Bekker

Tracheoesophageal fistula repair *see*
Esophageal atresia repair

Tracheostomy *see* **Tracheotomy**

Tracheotomy

Definition

A tracheotomy is a surgical procedure that opens up the windpipe (trachea). It is performed in emergency situations, in the **operating room**, or at bedside of critically ill patients. The term tracheostomy is sometimes used interchangeably with tracheotomy. Strictly speaking, however, tracheostomy usually refers to the opening itself while a tracheotomy is the actual operation.

Purpose

A tracheotomy is performed if enough air is not getting to the lungs, if the person cannot breathe without help, or is having problems with mucus and other secretions getting into the windpipe because of difficulty swallowing. There are many reasons why air cannot get to the lungs. The windpipe may be blocked by a swelling; by a severe injury to the neck, nose, or mouth; by a large foreign object; by paralysis of the throat muscles; or by a tumor. The patient may be in a coma, or need a ventilator to pump air into the lungs for a long period of time.

Demographics

Emergency tracheotomies are performed as needed in any person requiring one.

Description

Emergency tracheotomy

There are two different procedures that are called tracheotomies. The first is done only in emergency situations

and can be performed quite rapidly. The emergency room physician or surgeon makes a cut in a thin part of the voice box (larynx) called the cricothyroid membrane. A tube is inserted and connected to an oxygen bag. This emergency procedure is sometimes called a **cricothyroidotomy**.

Surgical tracheotomy

The second type of tracheotomy takes more time and is usually done in an operating room. The surgeon first makes a cut (incision) in the skin of the neck that lies over the trachea. This incision is in the lower part of the neck between the Adam's apple and top of the breastbone. The neck muscles are separated and the thyroid gland, which overlies the trachea, is usually cut down the middle. The surgeon identifies the rings of cartilage that make up the trachea and cuts into the tough walls. A metal or plastic tube, called a tracheotomy tube, is inserted through the opening. This tube acts like a windpipe and allows the person to breathe. Oxygen or a mechanical ventilator may be hooked up to the tube to bring oxygen to the lungs. A dressing is placed around the opening. Tape or stitches (sutures) are used to hold the tube in place.

After a nonemergency tracheotomy, the patient usually stays in the hospital for three to five days, unless there is a complicating condition. It takes about two weeks to recover fully from the surgery.

Diagnosis/Preparation

Emergency tracheotomy

In the emergency tracheotomy, there is no time to explain the procedure or the need for it to the patient. The patient is placed on his or her back with face upward (supine), with a rolled-up towel between the shoulders. This positioning of the patient makes it easier for the doctor to feel and see the structures in the throat. A local anesthetic is injected across the cricothyroid membrane.

Nonemergency tracheotomy

In a nonemergency tracheotomy, there is time for the doctor to discuss the surgery with the patient, to explain what will happen and why it is needed. The patient

Tracheotomy

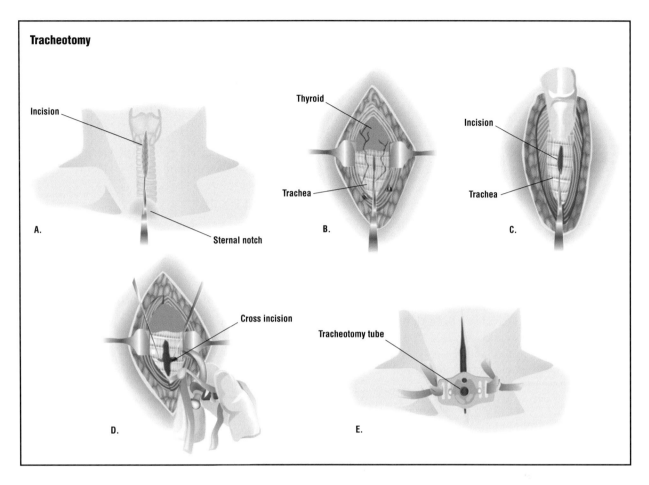

For a tracheotomy, an incision is made in the skin just above the sternal notch (A). Just below the thyroid, the membrane covering the trachea is divided (B), and the trachea itself is cut (C). A cross incision is made to enlarge the opening (D), and a tracheostomy tube may be put in place (E). *(Illustration by GGS Inc.)*

is then put under general anesthesia. The neck area and chest are then disinfected and surgical drapes are placed over the area, setting up a sterile surgical field.

Aftercare

Postoperative care

A **chest x ray** is often taken, especially in children, to check whether the tube has become displaced or if complications have occurred. The doctor may prescribe **antibiotics** to reduce the risk of infection. If the patient can breathe without a ventilator, the room is humidified; otherwise, if the tracheotomy tube is to remain in place, the air entering the tube from a ventilator is humidified. During the hospital stay, the patient and his or her family members will learn how to care for the tracheotomy tube, including suctioning and clearing it. Secretions are removed by passing a smaller tube (catheter) into the tracheotomy tube.

It takes most patients several days to adjust to breathing through the tracheotomy tube. At first, it will be hard even to make sounds. If the tube allows some air to escape and pass over the vocal cords, then the patient may be able to speak by holding a finger over the tube. Special tracheostomy tubes are also available that facilitate speech.

The tube will be removed if the tracheotomy is temporary. Then the wound will heal quickly and only a small scar may remain. If the tracheotomy is permanent, the hole stays open and, if it is no longer needed, it will be surgically closed.

Home care

After the patient is discharged, he or she will need help at home to manage the tracheotomy tube. Warm compresses can be used to relieve pain at the incision site. The patient is advised to keep the area dry. It is recommended that the patient wear a loose scarf over the opening when going outside. He or she should also avoid contact with water, food particles, and powdery substances that could enter the opening and cause serious breathing problems. The doctor may prescribe pain medication and antibiotics to minimize the risk of infections. If the tube is to be kept in place permanently, the patient can be referred to a speech therapist in order to learn to speak with the tube in place. The tracheotomy tube may be replaced four to 10 days after surgery.

Patients are encouraged to go about most of their normal activities once they leave the hospital. Vigorous activity is restricted for about six weeks. If the tracheotomy is permanent, further surgery may be needed to widen the opening, which narrows with time.

Risks

Immediate risks

There are several short-term risks associated with tracheotomies. Severe bleeding is one possible complication. The voice box or esophagus may be damaged during surgery. Air may become trapped in the surrounding tissues or the lung may collapse. The tracheotomy tube can be blocked by blood clots, mucus, or the pressure of the airway walls. Blockages can be prevented by suctioning, humidifying the air, and selecting the appropriate tracheotomy tube. Serious infections are rare.

Long-term risks

Over time, other complications may develop following a tracheotomy. The windpipe itself may become damaged for a number of reasons, including pressure from the tube, infectious bacteria that forms scar tissue, or friction from a tube that moves too much. Sometimes the opening does not close on its own after the tube is removed. This risk is higher in tracheotomies with tubes remaining in place for 16 weeks or longer. In these cases, the wound is surgically closed. Increased secretions may occur in patients with tracheostomies, which require more frequent suctioning.

High-risk groups

The risks associated with tracheotomies are higher in the following groups of patients:

- children, especially newborns and infants
- smokers
- alcoholics
- obese adults
- persons over 60
- persons with chronic diseases or respiratory infections
- persons taking **muscle relaxants**, sleeping medications, tranquilizers, or cortisone

Normal results

Normal results include uncomplicated healing of the incision and successful maintenance of long-term tube placement.

Morbidity and mortality rates

The overall risk of death from a tracheotomy is less than 5%.

Alternatives

For most patients, there is no alternative to emergency tracheotomy. Some patients with pre-existing neuromuscular disease (such as ALS or muscular dystrophy) can be sucessfully managed with emergency noninvasive ventilation via a face mask, rather than with tracheotomy. Patients who receive nonemergency tracheotomy in preparation for **mechanical ventilation** may often be managed instead with noninvasive ventilation, with proper planning and education on the part of the patient, caregiver, and medical staff.

Resources
BOOKS
Bach, John R. *Noninvasive Mechanical Ventilation.* NJ: Hanley and Belfus, 2002.
Fagan, Johannes J., et al. *Tracheotomy.* Alexandria, VA: American Academy of Otolaryngology-Head and Neck Surgery Foundation, Inc., 1997.
"Neck Surgery." In *The Surgery Book: An Illustrated Guide to 73 of the Most Common Operations*, ed. Robert M. Younson, et al. New York: St. Martin's Press, 1993.
Schantz, Nancy V. "Emergency Cricothyroidotomy and Tracheostomy." In *Procedures for the Primary Care Physician*, ed. John Pfenninger and Grant Fowler. New York: Mosby, 1994.
OTHER
"Answers to Common Otolaryngology Health Care Questions." Department of Otolaryngology–Head and Neck Surgery Page. University of Washington School of Medicine [cited July 1, 2003]. <http://weber.u.washington.edu/~otoweb/trach.html>.

Cartilage—A tough, fibrous connective tissue that forms various parts of the body, including the trachea and larynx.

Cricothyroidotomy—An emergency tracheotomy that consists of a cut through the cricothyroid membrane to open the patient's airway as fast as possible.

Larynx—A structure made of cartilage and muscle that connects the back of the throat with the trachea. The larynx contains the vocal cords.

Trachea—The tube that leads from the larynx or voice box to two major air passages that bring oxygen to each lung. The trachea is sometimes called the windpipe.

Ventilator—A machine that helps patients to breathe. It is sometimes called a respirator.

Sicard, Michael W. "Complications of Tracheotomy." The Bobby R. Alford Department of Otorhinolaryngology and Communicative Sciences. December 1, 1994 [cited July 1, 2003]. <http:www.bcm.tmc.edu/oto/grand/12194.html>.

Jeanine Barone, Physiologist
Richard Robinson

Traction

Definition

Traction is force applied by weights or other devices to treat bone or muscle disorders or injuries.

Purpose

Traction treats fractures, dislocations, or muscle spasms in an effort to correct deformities and promote healing.

Description

Traction is referred to as a pulling force to treat muscle or skeletal disorders. There are two major types of traction: skin and skeletal traction, within which there are a number of treatments.

Skin traction

Skin traction includes weight traction, which uses lighter weights or counterweights to apply force to fractures or dislocated joints. Weight traction may be employed short-term, (e.g., at the scene of an accident) or on a temporary basis (e.g., when weights are connected to a pulley located above the patient's bed). The weights, typically weighing five to seven pounds, attach to the skin using tape, straps, or boots. They bring together the fractured bone or dislocated joint so that it may heal correctly.

In obstetrics, weights pull along the pelvic axis of a pregnant woman to facilitate delivery. In elastic traction, an elastic device exerts force on an injured limb.

Skin traction also refers to specialized practices, such as Dunlop's traction, used on children when a fractured arm must maintain a flexed position to avoid circulatory and neurological problems. Buck's skin traction stabilizes the knee, and reduces muscle spasm for knee injuries not involving fractures. In addition, splints, surgical collars, and corsets also may be used.

Skeletal traction

Skeletal traction requires an invasive procedure in which pins, screws, or wires are surgically installed for use in longer term traction requiring heavier weights. This is the case when the force exerted is more than skin traction can bear, or when skin traction is not appropriate for the body part needing treatment. Weights used in skeletal traction generally range from 25–40 lbs (11–18 kg). It is important to place the pins correctly because they may stay in place for several months, and are the hardware to which weights and pulleys are attached. The pins must be clean to avoid infection. Damage may result if the alignment and weights are not carefully calibrated.

Other forms of skeletal traction are tibia pin traction, for fractures of the pelvis, hip, or femur; and overhead arm traction, used in certain upper arm fractures. Cervical traction is used when the neck vertebrae are fractured.

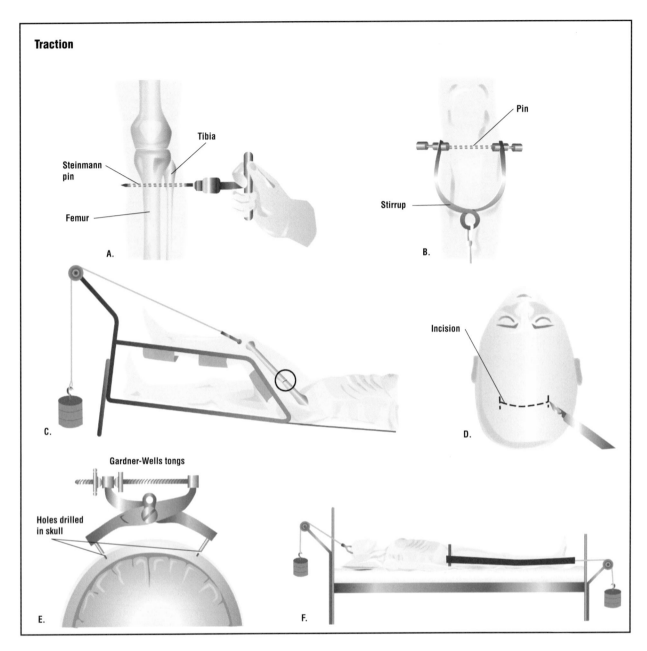

Traction

For tibial traction, a pin is surgically placed in the lower leg (A). The pin is attached to a stirrup (B), and weighted (C). In cervical traction, an incision is made into the head (D). Holes are drilled into the skull, and a halo or tongs are applied (E). Weights are added to pull the spine into place (F). *(Illustration by GGS Inc.)*

Proper care is important for patients in traction. Prolonged immobility should be avoided because it may cause **bedsores** and possible respiratory, urinary, or circulatory problems. Mobile patients may use a trapeze bar, giving them the option of controlling their movements. An **exercise** program instituted by caregivers will maintain the patient's muscle and joint mobility. Traction equipment should be checked regularly to ensure proper position and exertion of force. With skeletal traction, it is important to check for inflammation of the bone, a sign of foreign matter introduction (potential source of infection at the screw or pin site).

Preparation

Both skin and skeletal traction require x rays prior to application. If skeletal traction is required, standard pre-op surgical tests are conducted, such as blood and urine studies. X rays may be repeated over the course of treatment to insure that alignment remains correct, and that healing is proceeding.

KEY TERMS

Skeletal traction—Traction in which pins, screws, or wires are surgically connected to bone to which weights or pulleys are attached to exert force.

Skin traction—Traction in which weights or other devices are attached to the skin.

Weight traction—Sometimes used interchangeably with skin traction.

Normal results

There have been few scientific studies on the effects of traction. Criteria (such as randomized controlled trials and monitored compliance) do exist, but an outcome study incorporating all of them has not yet been done. Some randomized controlled trials emphasize that traction does not significantly influence long-term outcomes of neck pain or lower back pain.

Resources

BOOKS

"Cervical Spine Traction." In *Noble: Textbook of Primary Care Medicine,* 3rd ed.Mosby, Inc., (2001): 1132.

PERIODICALS

Glick, J.M. "Hip Arthroscopy. The Lateral Approach." *Clinics in Sports Medicine* 20, no.4 (October 1, 2001): 733-41.

Overly, M.D., Frank and Dale W. Steele, M.D. "Common Pediatric Fractures and Dislocations." *Clinical Pediatric Emergency Medicine* 3, no.2 (June 2002).

Nancy McKenzie, Ph.D.

Tranquilizers *see* **Antianxiety drugs**

Transfusion

Definition

Transfusion is the process of transferring whole blood or blood components from a donor to a recipient.

Purpose

Transfusions are given to restore lost blood, to improve clotting time, and to improve the ability of the blood to deliver oxygen to the body's tissues. About 32,000 pints of donated blood are transfused each day in the United States.

In the United States, blood collection is strictly regulated by the Food and Drug Administration (FDA). The FDA has rules for the collection, processing, storage, and transportation of blood and blood products. In addition, the American Red Cross, the American Association of Blood Banks (AABB), and most states have specific rules for the collection and processing of blood. The main purpose of regulation is to ensure the quality of transfused blood and to prevent the transmission of infectious diseases through donated blood. Before blood and blood products are used, they are extensively tested for such infectious agents as hepatitis and human immunodeficiency virus (HIV).

Blood and its components

Either whole blood or its components can be used for transfusion. Most blood collected from donors is broken down (fractionated) into components that are used to treat specific problems or diseases. Treating patients with fractionated blood is the most efficient way to use the blood supply.

WHOLE BLOOD. Whole blood is used exactly as received from the donor. Blood components are parts of whole blood, such as red blood cells (RBCs), white blood cells (WBCs), plasma, platelets, clotting factors, and immunoglobulins. Whole blood is used only when needed or when fractionated components are not available, because too much whole blood can raise the recipient's blood pressure. Use of blood components is a more efficient way to use the blood supply, because blood that has been fractionated can be used to treat more than one person.

Whole blood is generally used when a person has lost a large amount of blood. Such blood loss can be caused by injury or surgical procedures. Whole blood is given to help restore the blood volume, which is essential for maintaining blood pressure. It is also given to ensure that the body's tissues are receiving enough oxygen. Whole blood is occasionally given when a required blood fraction is unavailable in isolated form.

RED BLOOD CELLS. Red blood cells (RBCs) carry oxygen throughout the body. They pick up oxygen as they pass through the lungs and give up oxygen to the other tissues of the body as they are pumped through the arteries and veins. When patients do not have enough RBCs to properly oxygenate their bodies, they can be given a transfusion with RBCs obtained from donors. This type of transfusion will increase the amount of oxygen carried to the tissues of the body. RBCs are recovered from whole blood after donation. They are then typed, removed from the watery blood plasma to minimize their volume (packed), and stored. RBCs are given to people with anemia (including thalassemia), whose bone marrow does not make enough RBCs, or who have other conditions that decrease the number of RBCs in the blood. Occasionally, red blood cells from rare blood types are frozen. Once frozen, RBCs can survive for as long as ten years. Packed RBCs are given in the same manner as whole blood.

WHITE BLOOD CELLS. White blood cells (WBCs) are another infection-fighting blood component. On rare occasions, white blood cells are given by transfusion to treat life-threatening infections. Such transfusions are given when the WBC count is very low or when the patient's WBCs are not functioning normally. Most of the time, however, **antibiotics** are used in these cases.

PLASMA. Plasma is the clear yellowish liquid portion of blood. It contains many useful proteins, especially clotting factors and immunoglobulins. After plasma or plasma factors are processed, they are usually frozen. Some plasma fractions are freeze-dried. These fractions include clotting factors I through XIII. Some people have an inherited disorder in which the body produces too little of the clotting factors VIII (hemophilia A) or IX (hemophilia B). Transfusions of these clotting factors help to stop bleeding in people with hemophilia. Frozen plasma must be thawed before it is used; freeze-dried plasma must be mixed with liquid (reconstituted). In both cases, these blood fractions are usually small in volume and can be injected with a **syringe and needle**.

PLATELETS. Platelets are small disk-shaped structures in the blood that are essential for clotting. People who do not have enough platelets (a condition called thrombocytopenia) have bleeding problems. People who have lymphoma or leukemia and people who are receiving cancer therapy do not make enough platelets. Platelets have a very short shelf life; they must be used within 5 days of blood donation. After a unit of blood has been donated and processed, the platelets in it are packed into bags. A platelet transfusion is given in the same manner as whole blood.

IMMUNOGLOBULINS. Immunoglobulins are the infection-fighting fractions in blood plasma. They are also known as gamma globulin, antibodies, and immune sera. Immunoglobulins are given to people who have difficulty fighting infections, especially people whose immune systems have been depressed by such diseases as AIDS. Immunoglobulins are also used to prevent tetanus after a cut has been contaminated; to treat animal bites when rabies is suspected; or to treat severe childhood diseases. Generally, the volume of immunoglobulins used is small, and it can be injected.

Demographics

In order to donate blood, an individual must be at least 17 years old, weigh at least 110 lb (50 kg), and be in generally good health. The average blood donor is a white, married, college-educated male between the ages of 30 and 50. Twenty-five percent of people receiving blood transfusions are over the age of 65, although the elderly constitute only 13% of the population. Fewer than 5% of Americans donate blood each year.

Description

Blood is collected from the donor by inserting a large needle into a vein in the arm, usually one of the larger veins near the inside of the elbow. A tourniquet is placed on the upper arm to increase the pressure in the arm veins, which makes them swell and become more accessible. Once the nurse or technician has identified a suitable vein, she or he sterilizes the area where the needle will be inserted by scrubbing the skin with a soap solution or an antiseptic that contains iodine. Sometimes both solutions are used. The donor lies on a bed or cot during the procedure, which usually takes between 10 and 20 minutes. Generally, an 18-gauge needle is used. This size of needle fits easily into the veins and yet is large enough to allow blood to flow easily. Human blood will sometimes clot in a smaller needle and stop flowing. The donor's blood is collected in a sterile plastic bag that holds one pint (450 ml). The bags contain an anticoagulant to prevent clotting and preservatives to keep the blood cells alive. A sample of the donor's blood is collected at the time of donation and tested for infectious diseases. The blood is not used until the test results confirm that it is safe. Properly handled and refrigerated, whole blood can last for 42 days.

The recipient of a transfusion is prepared in much the same way as the blood donor. The site for the needle insertion is carefully washed with a soap-based solution followed by an antiseptic containing iodine. The skin is then dried and the transfusion needle inserted into the vein. During the early stages of a transfusion, the recipient is monitored closely to detect any adverse reactions. If no signs of adverse reaction are evident, the patient is monitored occasionally for the duration of the transfusion period. Upon completion of the transfusion, a compress is placed over the needle insertion site to prevent extensive bleeding.

Blood typing

All donated blood is typed, which means that it is analyzed to determine which of several major and minor blood types (also called blood groups) it belongs to. Blood types are genetically determined. The major types are classified by the ABO system. This system groups blood with reference to two substances in the red blood cells called antigen A and antigen B. The four ABO blood types are A, B, AB, and O. Type A blood has the A antigen, type B has the B antigen, type AB has both, and type O has neither. These four types of blood are further classified by the Rh factor. The Rh, or rhesus factor, is also an antigen in the red blood cells. A person who has the Rh factor is Rh positive; a person who does not have the factor is Rh negative. If a person has red blood cells with both the B and the Rh antigens, that person is said to have a B positive (B+) blood type. Blood types determine which kinds of donated blood a patient can receive. Generally, patients are limited to receiving only blood of the exact same ABO and Rh type as their own. For example, a person with B+ blood can receive blood or blood cells only from another person with B+ blood. An exception is blood type O. Individuals with type O blood are called universal donors, because people of all blood types can accept their blood.

Blood can also be typed with reference to several other minor antigens, such as Kell, Kidd, Duffy, and Lewis. These minor antigens can become important when a patient has received many transfusions. These patients tend to build up an immune response to the minor blood groups that do not match their own. They may have an adverse reaction upon receiving a transfusion with a mismatched minor blood group. A third group of antigens that may cause a reaction are residues from the donor's plasma attached to the RBCs. To eliminate this problem, the RBCs are rinsed to remove plasma residues. These rinsed cells are called washed RBCs.

Other transfusion procedures

Autologous transfusion is a procedure in which patients donate blood for their own use. Patients who are to undergo surgical procedures requiring a blood transfusion may choose to donate several units of blood ahead of time. The blood is stored at the hospital for the patient's exclusive use. Autologous donation assures that the blood type is an exact match. It also assures that no infection will be transmitted through the blood transfusion. Autologous donation accounts for 5% of blood use in the United States each year.

Directed donors are family or friends of the patient who needs a transfusion. Some people think that family and friends provide a safer source of blood than the general blood supply. Studies do not show that directed donor blood is any safer. Blood that is not used for the identified patient becomes part of the general blood supply.

Apheresis is a special procedure in which only certain specific components of a donor's blood are collected. The remaining blood fractions are returned to the

donor. A special blood-processing instrument is used in apheresis. It fractionates the blood, saves the desired component, and pumps all the other components back into the donor. Because donors give only part of their blood, they can donate more frequently. For example, people can give almost ten times as many platelets by apheresis as they could give by donating whole blood. The donation process takes about one to two hours.

Preparation

The first step in blood donation is the taking of the donor's medical history. Blood donors are questioned about their general health, their lifestyle, and any medical conditions that might disqualify them. These conditions include hepatitis, AIDS, cancer, heart disease, asthma, malaria, bleeding disorders, and high blood pressure. Screening prevents people from donating who might transmit diseases or whose medical condition would place them at risk if they donated blood. Some geographical areas or communities have a high rate of hepatitis or AIDS. Blood collection in most of these areas has been discontinued indefinitely.

The blood pressure, temperature, and pulse of donors are taken to ensure that they are physically able to donate blood. One pint (450 mL) of blood is usually withdrawn, although it is possible to donate smaller amounts. The average adult male has 10–12 pints of blood in his body; the average adult female has 8–9 pints in hers. Within hours after donating, most people's bodies have replaced the fluid lost with the donated blood, which brings their blood volume back to normal. Replacement of the blood cells and platelets, however, can take several weeks. Pregnant women and people with low blood pressure or anemia should not donate blood or should limit the amount of blood they give. Generally,

QUESTIONS
TO ASK THE DOCTOR

- Why is a transfusion recommended for my condition?
- Do I have the option of donating my own blood for future use?
- Will I need a transfusion of whole blood or blood components?
- What alternatives to blood transfusion are available to me?

people are allowed to donate blood only once every two months. This restriction ensures the health of the donor and discourages people from selling their blood. The former practice of paying donors for blood has essentially stopped. Donors who sell blood tend to be at high risk for the transmission of bloodborne diseases.

Aftercare

Recipients of blood transfusion are monitored during and after the transfusion for signs of an adverse reaction. Blood donors are generally given fluids and light refreshments to prevent such possible side effects as dizziness and nausea. They are also asked to remain in the donation area for 15–20 minutes after giving blood to make sure that they are not likely to faint when they leave.

Risks

Risks for donors

For donors, the process of giving blood is very safe. Only sterile equipment is used and there is no chance of catching an infection from the equipment. There is a slight chance of infection at the puncture site if the skin is not properly washed before the collection needle is inserted. Some donors feel lightheaded when they sit up or stand for the first time after donating. Occasionally, a donor will faint. Donors are encouraged to drink plenty of liquids to replace the fluid lost with the donated blood. It is important to maintain the fluid volume of the blood so that the blood pressure will remain stable. Strenuous **exercise** should be avoided for the rest of the day. It is normal to feel some soreness or to find a small bluish bruise at the site of the needle insertion. Most donors have very slight symptoms or no symptoms at all after giving blood.

Risks for recipients

A number of precautions must be taken for transfusion recipients. Donated blood must be matched with the recipient's blood type, as incompatible blood types can cause a serious adverse reaction (transfusion reaction). Blood is introduced slowly by gravity flow directly into the veins (intravenous infusion) so that medical personnel can observe the patient for signs of adverse reactions. People who have received many transfusions may develop an immune response to some factors in foreign blood cells (see below). This immune reaction must be evaluated before the patient is given new blood.

Adverse reactions to mismatched blood (transfusion reaction) is a major risk of blood transfusion. Transfusion reaction occurs when antibodies in the recipient's blood react to foreign blood cells introduced by the transfusion. The antibodies bind to the foreign cells and destroy them. This destruction is called a hemolytic reaction. In addition, a transfusion reaction may also cause a hypersensitivity of the immune system that may in turn result in tissue damage within the patient's body. The patient may also have an allergic reaction to mismatched blood.

The first symptoms of transfusion reaction are a feeling of general discomfort and anxiety. Breathing difficulties, flushing, and a sense of pressure in the chest or back pain may also be present. Evidence of a hemolytic reaction can be seen in the urine, which will be colored from the hemoglobin leaking from the destroyed red blood cells. Severe hemolytic reactions are occasionally fatal. Reactions to mismatches of minor factors are milder. These symptoms include itchiness, dizziness, fever, headache, rash, and swelling. Sometimes the patient will experience breathing difficulties and muscle spasms. Most adverse reactions from mismatched blood are not life-threatening.

Infectious diseases can also be transmitted through donated blood and constitute another major risk of blood transfusion. The infectious diseases most often acquired from blood transfusion in the United States are hepatitis and HIV.

Patients who are given too much blood can develop high blood pressure, a concern for people who have heart disease. Very rarely, an air embolism is created when air is introduced into a patient's veins through the tubing used for intravenous infusion. The danger of embolism is greatest when infusion is begun or ended. Care must be taken to ensure that all air is bled out of the tubing before infusion begins, and that the infusion is stopped before air can enter the patient's blood system.

Normal results

Most individuals will feel only a slight sting from the needle used during the blood donation process, and will not experience any side effects after the procedure is over. Plasma is regenerated by the body within 24 hours,

KEY TERMS

ABO blood groups—A system in which human blood is classified according to the A and B antigens found in red blood cells. Type A blood has the A antigen; type B has the B antigen, AB has both, and O has neither.

Antibody—A simple protein produced by the body to destroy bacteria, viruses, or other foreign bodies. The production of each antibody is triggered by a specific antigen.

Antigen—A substance that stimulates the immune system to manufacture antibodies (immunoglobulins). The function of antibodies is to fight off such intruder cells as bacteria or viruses. Antigens stimulate the blood to fight other blood cells that have the wrong antigens. If a person with blood type A is given a transfusion with blood type B, the A antigens will fight the foreign blood cells as though they were an infectious agent.

Apheresis—A procedure in which whole blood is withdrawn from a donor, a specific blood component is separated and collected, and the remainder is reinfused into the patient.

Autologous blood—The patient's own blood, drawn and set aside before surgery for use during surgery in case a transfusion is needed.

Fractionation—The process of separating the various components of whole blood.

Hemoglobin—The red pigment in red blood cells that transports oxygen.

Hemolysis—The destruction of red blood cells through disruption of the cell membrane, resulting in the release of hemoglobin. A hemolytic transfusion reaction is one that results in the destruction of red blood cells.

Immunoglobulin—An antibody.

Infusion—Introduction of a substance directly into a vein or tissue by gravity flow.

Injection—Forcing a fluid into the body by means of a needle and syringe.

Plasma—The liquid portion of blood, as distinguished from blood cells. Plasma constitutes about 55% of blood volume.

Platelets—Disk-shaped structures found in blood that play an active role in blood clotting. Platelets are also known as thrombocytes.

Rh (rhesus) factor—An antigen present in the red blood cells of 85% of humans. A person with Rh factor is Rh positive (Rh+); a person without it is Rh negative (Rh-). The Rh factor was first identified in the blood of a rhesus monkey.

Serum (plural, sera)—The clear fluid that separates from blood when the blood is allowed to clot completely. Blood serum can also be defined as blood plasma from which fibrinogen has been removed.

and red blood cells within a few weeks. Patients who receive a blood transfusion will usually experience mild or no side effects.

Morbidity and mortality rates

The risk of acquiring an infectious disease from a blood transfusion is very low. The risk of HIV transmission is one in 450,000 to 660,000 units of blood; hepatitis B virus (HBV), one in 137,000 units; and hepatitis C virus (HCV), one in 1,000,000 units. Bacterial contamination (a cause of infection) is identified in one in 4,200 transfusions. Approximately one in 25,000 individuals who receive a blood transfusion will develop a hemolytic reaction; the risk of a fatal hemolytic reaction is one in 160,000.

Alternatives

There are several alternatives to blood transfusion as of 2003. These include:

• Volume expanders. Certain fluids (saline, Ringer's lactate solution, dextran, etc.) may be used to increase the patient's blood volume without adding additional blood cells.

• Blood substitutes. Much research is currently being done into compounds that can replace some or all of the functions of blood components. One such compound, called HBOC-201 or Hemopure, is hemoglobin derived from bovine (cow) blood. Hemopure shows promise as a substitute for red blood cell transfusion.

• Bloodless surgery. It may be possible to avoid excessive blood loss through careful planning prior to surgery. Specialized instruments can minimize the amount of blood lost during a procedure. It is also possible to collect some of the blood lost during surgery and reinfuse it into the patient at the end of the operation.

See also Blood donation and registry; Bloodless surgery.

Resources

BOOKS

Berkow, Robert, ed. *Merck Manual of Medical Information.* Whitehouse Station, NJ: Merck Research Laboratories, 1997.

Lefevre, Patrice, and Pascale Poullin. "Current Information on Risks of Allogenic Blood Transfusion." In *Transfusion Medicine and Alternatives to Blood Transfusion.* Chatillon, France: Network for Advancement of Transfusion Alternatives, 2000.

ORGANIZATIONS

American Association of Blood Banks (AABB). 8101 Glenbrook Road, Bethesda, MD 20814-2749. (301) 907-6977. <www.aabb.org>.

American Red Cross (ARC) National Headquarters. 431 18th Street, NW. Washington, DC 20006. (202) 303-4498. <www.redcross.org>.

America's Blood Centers. 725 15th St., NW, Suite 700, Washington, DC 20005. (202) 393-5725. <www.americasblood.org>.

National Blood Data Resource Center (NBDRC). 8101 Glenbrook Road, Bethesda, MD 20814-2749. (301) 215-6506. <www.nbdrc.org>.

OTHER

American Association of Blood Banks. *Facts about Blood and Blood Banking.* Bethesda, MD: American Association of Blood Banks, June 2002 [cited February 27, 2003]. <www.aabb.org/All_About_Blood/FAQs/aabb_faqs.htm>.

"Hemopure (HBOC-201) Shows Promise as Alternative to Red Blood Cell Transfusion in Elective Orthopedic Surgery." *Doctor's Guide,* January 28, 2002 [cited February 27, 2003]. <www.pslgroup.com/dg/21371a.htm>.

National Blood Data Resource Center. *National Blood Data Resource Center: FAQs.* Bethesda, MD: National Blood Data Resource Center, 2002 [cited February 27, 2003]. <www.nbdrc.org/faqs.htm>.

John T. Lohr, PhD
Stephanie Dionne Sherk

Transplant surgery

Definition

Transplant surgery is the surgical removal of an organ(s), tissue, or blood products from a donor and surgically placing or infusing them into a recipient.

Purpose

Transplant surgery is a treatment option for diseases or conditions that have not improved with other medical treatments and have led to organ failure or injury. Transplant surgery is generally reserved for people with end-stage disease who have no other options.

The decision to perform transplant surgery is based on the patient's age, general physical condition, diagnosis and stage of the disease. Transplant surgery is not recommended for patients who have liver, lung, or kidney problems; poor leg circulation; cancer; or chronic infections.

Demographics

The typical cut-off age for a transplant recipient ranges from 40–55 years; however, a person's general health is usually a more important factor. In addition, the percentage of transplant recipients over age 50 has increased since 1996.

On average, 66 people receive transplants every day from either a living or deceased donor. In 2002, about 24,500 transplants were performed in the United States:

- 14,400 kidney transplants
- 5300 liver transplants
- 2200 heart transplants
- 1000 lung transplants
- 900 kidney/pancreas transplants
- 550 pancreas transplants
- 104 intestine transplants
- 31 heart/lung transplants

The national waiting list for most transplanted organs continues to grow every year, even though the number of recipients waiting for a heart transplant has leveled off in recent years, and the waiting list for heart-lung transplants has decreased over the past few years. As of April 2003, there were about 81,000 eligible recipients waiting for an organ transplant in the United States.

Description

Organ donors

Organ donors are classified as living donors or cadaveric (non-living) donors. All donors are carefully screened to make sure there is a suitable blood type match and to prevent any transmissible diseases or other complications.

LIVING DONORS. Living donors may be family members or biologically unrelated to the recipient. From 1992 to 2001, the number of biologically unrelated living donors increased tenfold. Living donors must be physically fit, in good general health, and have no existing disorders such as diabetes, high blood pressure, cancer, kidney disease, or heart disease. About 25% of all the organs transplanted in 2002 came from living donors. Organs that can be donated from living donors include:

• Single kidneys. In 2002, 52% of all kidney transplants came from living donors. There is little risk in living with one kidney because the remaining kidney compensates for and performs the work of both.

• Liver. Living donors can donate segments of the liver because the organ can regenerate and regain full function. The number of living donor liver transplants has doubled since 1999.

• Lung. Living donors can donate lobes of the lung although lung tissue does not regenerate.

• Pancreas. Living donors can donate a portion of the pancreas even though the gland does not regenerate.

Organs donated from living donors eliminate the need to place the recipient on the national waiting list. Transplant surgery can be scheduled at a mutually acceptable time rather than performed under emergency conditions. In addition, the recipient can begin taking immunosuppressant medications two days before the transplant surgery to prevent the risk of rejection. Living donor transplants are often more successful than cadaveric donor transplants because there is a better tissue match between the donor and recipient. The living donor's medical expenses are usually covered by the organ recipient's insurance company, but the amount of coverage may vary.

CADAVERIC OR DECEASED DONORS. Organs from cadaveric donors come from people who have recently died and have willed their organs before death by signing an organ donor card, or are brain-dead. The donor's family must give permission for organ donation at the time of death or diagnosis of brain death. Cadaveric donors may be young adults with traumatic head injuries, or older adults suffering from a stroke. The majority of deceased donors are older than the general population.

Transplant procedures

ORGAN HARVESTING. Harvesting refers to the process of removing cells or tissues from the donor and preserving them until they are transplanted. If the donor is deceased, the organ or tissues are harvested in a sterile **operating room**. They are packed carefully for transportation and delivered to the recipient via ambulance, helicopter or airplane. Organs from deceased donors should be transplanted within a few hours of harvesting. After the recipient is notified that an organ has become available, he or she should not eat or drink anything.

When the organ is harvested from a living donor, the recipient's transplant surgery follows immediately after the donor's surgery. The recipient and the donor should not eat or drink anything after midnight the evening before the scheduled operation.

PREOPERATIVE PROCEDURES. After arriving at the hospital, the recipient will have a complete physical and such other tests as a **chest x ray**, blood tests, and an electrocardiogram (EKG) to evaluate his or her fitness for surgery. If the recipient has an infection or major medical problem, or if the donor organ is found to be unacceptable, the operation will be canceled.

The recipient will be prepared for surgery by having the incision site shaved and cleansed. An intravenous tube (IV) will be placed in the arm to deliver medications and fluids, and a sedative will be given to help the patient relax.

TRANSPLANT SURGERY. After the patient has been brought to the operating room, the anesthesiologist will administer a general anesthetic. A central venous catheter may be placed in a vein in the patient's arm or groin. A breathing tube will be placed in the patient's throat. The breathing tube is attached to a mechanical ventilator that expands the lungs during surgery.

The patient will then be connected to a heart-lung bypass machine, also called a cardiopulmonary bypass pump, which takes over for the heart and lungs during the surgery. The heart-lung machine removes carbon dioxide from the blood and replaces it with oxygen. A tube is inserted into the patient's aorta to carry the oxygenated blood from the bypass machine back to the heart for circulation to the body. A nasogastric tube is placed to drain stomach secretions, and a urinary catheter is inserted to drain urine during the surgery.

The surgeon carefully removes the diseased organ and replaces it with the donor organ. The blood vessels of the donated organ are connected to the patient's blood vessels, allowing blood to flow through the new organ.

Diagnosis/Preparation

Pre-transplant evaluation

Several tests are performed before the transplant surgery to make sure that the patient is eligible to receive the organ and to identify and treat any problems ahead of time. The more common pre-transplant tests include:

• tissue typing

• blood tests

• chest x ray

• pulmonary function tests

• computed tomography (CT) scan

• heart function tests (electrocardiogram, echocardiogram, and cardiac catheterization)

WHO PERFORMS THE PROCEDURE AND WHERE IS IT PERFORMED?

A transplant surgeon, along with a multidisciplinary team of transplant specialists, should perform the transplant surgery. Transplant surgeons are usually board-certified by the American Board of Surgery, as well as certified by the medical specialty board or boards related to the type of organ transplant performed. Members of transplant teams include infectious disease specialists, pharmacologists, psychiatrists, advanced care registered nurses and transplant coordinators in addition to the surgeons and anesthesiologists.

Organ transplants are performed in special transplant centers, which should be members of the United Network for Organ Sharing (UNOS) as well as state-level accreditation organizations.

• sigmoidoscopy

• bone densitometry test

The pre-transplant evaluation usually includes a dietary and social work assessment. In addition, the patient must undergo a complete dental examination to reduce the risk of infection from bacteria in the mouth.

Insurance considerations

Organ transplantation is an expensive procedure. Insurance companies and health maintenance organizations (HMOs) may not cover all costs. Many insurance companies require precertification letters of medical necessity. As soon as transplantation is discussed as a treatment option, the patient should contact his or her insurance provider as soon as possible to determine what costs will be covered.

Patient education and lifestyle changes

Before undergoing transplant surgery, the transplant team will ensure that the patient understands the potential benefits and risks of the procedure. In addition, a team of health care providers will review the patient's social history and psychological test results to ensure that he or she is able to comply with the regimen that is needed after transplant surgery. An organ transplant requires major lifestyle changes, including dietary adjustments, complex drug treatments and frequent examinations. The patient must be committed to making these changes in order to become a candidate for transplant. Most transplant centers have extensive patient education programs.

Smoking cessation is an important consideration for patients who use tobacco. Many transplant programs require the patient to be a nonsmoker for a certain amount of time (usually six months) before he or she is eligible to participate in the pre-transplant screening evaluation. The patient must also be committed to avoid tobacco products after the transplant.

Informed consent

Patients are legally required to sign an **informed consent** form prior to transplant surgery. Informed consent signifies that the patient is a knowledgeable participant in making healthcare decisions. The doctor will discuss all of the following with the patient before he or she signs the form: the nature of the surgery; reasonable alternatives to the surgery; and the risks, benefits, and uncertainties of each option. Informed consent also requires the doctor to make sure that the patient understands the information that has been given.

Finding a donor

After the patient has completed the pre-transplant evaluation and has been approved for transplant surgery, the next step is locating a donor. Organs from cadaveric donors are located through a computerized national waiting list maintained by the United Network for Organ Sharing (UNOS) to assure equal access to and fair distribution of organs. When a deceased organ donor is identified, a transplant coordinator from an organ procurement organization enters the donor's data in the UNOS computer. The computer then generates a list of potential recipients. This list is called a match run. Factors affecting a potential organ recipient's ranking on the match run list include: tissue match, blood type, size of the organ, length of time on the waiting list, immune status, and the geographical distance between the recipient and donor. For some transplants, such as heart, liver, and intestinal segments, the degree of medical urgency is also taken into consideration.

The organ is offered to the transplant team of the first person on the ranked waiting list. The recipient must be healthy enough to undergo surgery, available, and willing to receive the organ transplant immediately. The matching process involves cross matching, performing an antibody screen and a host of other tests.

Donor searching can be a long and stressful process. A supportive network of friends and family is important to help the patient cope during this time. The health care provider or social worker can also put the patient in touch with support groups for transplant patients.

Contact and travel arrangements

The patient must be ready to go to the hospital as soon as possible after being notified that an organ is available. A suitcase should be kept packed at all times. Transportation arrangements should be made ahead of time. If the recipient lives more than a 90-minute drive from the transplant center, the transplant coordinator will help make transportation arrangements for the recipient and one friend or family member.

Because harvested organs cannot be preserved for more than a few hours, the transplant team must be able to contact the patient at all times. Some transplant programs offer a pager rental service, to be used only for receiving "the call" from the transplant center. The patient should clear travel plans with the transplant coordinator before taking any trips.

Blood donation and conservation

Some transplant centers allow patients to donate their own blood before surgery, which is known as autologous donation. Autologous blood is the safest blood for **transfusion**, since there is no risk of disease transmission. Preoperative donation is an option for patients receiving an organ from a living donor, since the surgery can be scheduled in advance. In autologous donation, the patient donates blood once a week for one to three weeks before surgery. The blood is separated and the blood components needed are reinfused during the operation.

In addition to preoperative donation, there are several techniques for minimizing the patient's blood loss during surgery:

- Intraoperative blood collection: the blood lost during surgery is processed, and the red blood cells are reinfused during or immediately after surgery.

- Immediate preoperative hemodilution: the patient donates blood immediately before surgery to decrease the loss of red blood cells during the operation. The patient is then given fluids to restore the volume of the blood.

- Postoperative blood collection: blood lost from the incision following surgery is collected and reinfused after the surgical site has been closed.

Aftercare

Inpatient recovery

A transplant recipient can expect to spend three to four weeks in the hospital after surgery. Immediately following the operation, the patient is transferred to an **intensive care unit** (ICU) for close monitoring of his or her **vital signs**. When the patient's condition is stable, he or she is transferred to a hospital room, usually in a specialized transplant

unit. The IV in the patient's arm, the urinary catheter, and a dressing over the incision remain in place for several days. A chest tube may be placed to drain excess fluids. Special stockings may be placed on the patient's legs to prevent blood clots in the deep veins of the legs. A breathing aid called an incentive spirometer is used to help keep the patient's lungs clear and active after surgery.

Medications to relieve pain will be given every three to four hours, or through a device known as a PCA (patient-controlled anesthesia). The PCA is a small pump that delivers a dose of medication into the IV when the patient pushes a button. The transplant recipient will also be given immunosuppressive medications to prevent the risk of organ rejection. These medications are typically taken by the recipient for the rest of his or her life.

A two to four-week waiting period is necessary before the transplant team can evaluate the success of the procedure. Visitors are limited during this time to minimize the risk of infection. The patient will be given intravenous antibiotic, antiviral and antifungal medications, as well as blood and platelet transfusions to help fight off infection and prevent excessive bleeding. Blood tests are performed daily to monitor the patient's kidney and liver function as well as his or her nutritional status. Other tests are performed as needed.

Outpatient recovery

After leaving the hospital, the transplant recipient will be monitored through home or outpatient visits for as long as a year. Medication adjustments are often necessary, but barring complications, the recipient can return to normal activities about 6–8 months after the transplant.

Proper outpatient care includes:

- taking medications exactly as prescribed
- attending all scheduled follow-up visits
- contacting the transplant team at the first signs of infection or organ rejection
- having blood drawn regularly
- following dietary and **exercise** recommendations
- avoiding rough contact sports and heavy lifting
- taking precautions against infection
- avoiding pregnancy for at least a year

Risks

Short-term risks following an organ transplant include pneumonia and other infectious diseases; excessive bleeding; and liver disorders caused by blocked blood vessels. In addition, the new organ may be rejected, which means that the patient's immune system is attacking the new organ. Characteristic signs of rejection include fever, rash, diarrhea, liver problems, and a compromised immune system. Transplant recipients are given immunosuppressive medications to minimize the risk of rejection. In most cases, the patient will take these medications for the rest of his or her life.

Long-term risks include an elevated risk of cancer, particularly skin cancer. An estimated 6–8% of transplant patients develop cancer over their lifetime as compared to less than 1% in the general population.

Normal results

In a successful organ transplant, the patient returns to a more nearly normal lifestyle with increased strength and stamina.

Morbidity and mortality rates

Mortality figures for transplant surgery include recipients who die before a match with a suitable donor can be found. About 17 patients die every day in the United States waiting for a transplant. In 2001, over 6000 patients died because the organ they needed was not donated in time.

The Scientific Registry of Transplant Recipients gives the first-year survival rates for transplant surgery as follows:

- 97% of pancreas transplant recipients
- 95% of kidney transplant and kidney/pancreas recipients
- 90% of autologous bone marrow transplant patients
- 86% of liver transplant patients
- 85% of heart transplant patients
- 77% of lung transplant patients
- 70% of allogeneic bone marrow transplant patients

Three-year survival rates are as follows:

- about 91% for kidney transplant patients
- about 87% for pancreas and kidney/pancreas transplant patients
- about 80% for liver transplant patients
- about 79% for heart transplant patients
- about 59% for lung transplant patients

Alternatives

Clinical trials

Available alternatives to transplant surgery depend upon the individual patient's diagnosis and severity of illness. Some patients may be eligible to participate in clinical trials, which are research programs that evaluate a new medical treatment, drug or device. Information on current clinical trials is available from the National Institutes of Health (NIH) clinical trials web site: lt;www.clinicaltrials.gov> or by calling the NIH at (888) FIND-NLM [(888) 346-3656] or (301) 594-5983.

Complementary and alternative (CAM) therapies

Complementary therapies can be used along with standard treatments to help alleviate the patient's pain; strengthen muscles; and decrease depression, anxiety and stress. Before trying a complementary treatment, however, patients should check with their doctors to make sure that it will not interfere with standard therapy or cause harm. Alternative approaches that have helped transplant recipients maintain a positive mental attitude both before and after surgery include meditation, biofeedback, and various relaxation techniques. Massage therapy, music therapy, aromatherapy, and hydrotherapy are other types of treatment that can offer patients some pleasant sensory experiences as well as relieve pain. Acupuncture has been shown in a number of NIH-sponsored studies to be effective in relieving nausea and headache as well as chronic muscle and joint pain. Some insurance carriers cover the cost of acupuncture treatments.

Resources

BOOKS

"Transplantation." Section 12, Chapter 149 in *The Merck Manual of Diagnosis and Therapy*, edited by Mark H. Beers,

Antibody—A substance produced by the immune system in response to specific antigens, thereby helping the body fight infection and foreign substances. An antibody screen involves mixing the white blood cells of the donor with the serum of the recipient to determine if antibodies in the recipient react with the antigens of the donor.

Autologous blood—The patient's own blood, drawn and set aside before surgery for use during surgery in case a transfusion is needed.

Bone densitometry test—A test that quickly and accurately measures the density of bone.

Brain death—Irreversible cessation of brain function. Patients with brain death have no potential capacity for survival or for recovery of any brain function.

Cadaveric donor—An organ donor who has recently died of causes not affecting the organ intended for transplant.

Compatible donor—A person whose tissue and blood type are the same as the recipient's.

Confirmatory typing—Repeat tissue typing to confirm the compatibility of the donor and patient before transplant

Donor—A person who supplies organ(s), tissue or blood to another person for transplantation.

Harvesting—The process of removing tissues or organs from a donor and preserving them for transplantation.

Hemodilution—A technique in which the fluid content of the blood is increased without increasing the number of red blood cells.

HLA (human leuckocyte antigen)—A group of protein molecules located on bone marrow cells that can provoke an immune response. A donor's and a recipient's HLA types should match as closely as possible to prevent the recipient's immune system from attacking the donor's marrow as a foreign material that does not belong in the body.

Immunosuppression—The use of medications to suppress the immune system to prevent organ rejection.

Organ procurement—The process of donor screening, and the evaluation, removal, preservation and distribution of organs for transplantation.

Pulmonary function test—A test that measures the capacity and function of the lungs as well as the blood's ability to carry oxygen. During the test, the patient breathes into a device called a spirometer.

Rejection—An immune response that occurs when a transplanted organ is viewed as a foreign substance by the body. If left untreated, rejection can lead to organ failure and even death.

MD, and Robert Berkow, MD. Whitehouse Station, NJ: Merck Research Laboratories, 1999.

ORGANIZATIONS

American Council on Transplantation. P.O. Box 1709, Alexandria, VA 22313. (800) ACT-GIVE (800-228-4483).

Children's Organ Transplant Association, Inc. 2501 COTA Drive, Bloomington, IN 47403. (800) 366-2682. <www.cota.org>.

Coalition on Donation. 700 North 4th Street, Richmond, VA 23219. (804)782-4920. E-mail: coalition@shareyourlife.org. <www.shareyourlife.org>.

Division of Organ Transplantation, Health Resources and Services Administration (HRSA). 5600 Fishers Lane, Rm. 14-45, Rockville, MD 20857. 301-443-3376. comments @hrsa.gov. <www.hrsa.gov>.

National Foundation for Transplants. 1102 Brookfield, Suite 200, Memphis, TN 38110. (800) 489-3863 or (901) 684-1697. <www.transplants.org>

National Heart, Lung and Blood Institute (NHLBI) Information Center. P. O. Box 30105, Bethesda, MD 20824-0105. (301) 251-2222. <www.nhlbi.nih.gov>.

National Organ and Tissue Donation Initiative. <www.organ donor.gov/>. Provides information and resources on organ donation and transplantation issues.

National Transplant Assistance Fund 3475 West Chester Pike, Suite 230, Newtown Square, PA 19073. (800) 642-8399 or (610) 353-1616. <www.transplantfund.org/>

Partnership for Organ Donation. Two Oliver Street, Boston, MA 02109. (617) 482-5746. E-Mail: info@organdona tion.org. <www.organdonation.org/>

Transplant Foundation. 8002 Discovery Drive, Suite 310 Richmond, VA 23229. (804) 285-5115. E-Mail: otfnatl@aol .com.

Transplant Recipients International Organization. International Headquarters: 2117 L Street NW, Suite 353, Washington, DC 20037. (800) TRIO-386. E-Mail: triointl@aol.com. <www.trioweb.org>.

United Network for Organ Sharing (UNOS). 700 North 4th Street, Richmond, VA 23219. (800) 24-DONOR (800-243-6667). <www.unos.org>. Provides general information on transplants, current statistics and listings of transplant centers.

OTHER

CenterSpan. <www.centerspan.org>. Features Transplant News Network, an on-line broadcasting service that publishes monthly news reports on recent developments in transplant medicine.

Scientific Registry of Transplant Recipients. <www.ustransplant.org>.

TransWeb. <www.transweb.org>.

Angela M. Costello

Transposition of the great arteries *see* **Heart surgery for congenital defects**

Transurethral bladder resection

Definition

Transurethral bladder resection is a surgical procedure used to view the inside of the bladder, remove tissue samples, and/or remove tumors. Instruments are passed through a cystoscope (a slender tube with a lens and a light) that has been inserted through the urethra into the bladder.

Purpose

Transurethral resection is the initial form of treatment for bladder cancers. The procedure is performed to remove and examine bladder tissue and/or a tumor. It may also serve to remove lesions, and it may be the only treatment necessary for noninvasive tumors. This procedure plays both a diagnostic and therapeutic role in the treatment of bladder cancers.

Demographics

Bladder cancer is the sixth most commonly diagnosed malignancy in the United States. According to the American Cancer Society, about 57,400 new cases of bladder cancer will be diagnosed in the United States in 2003.

Industrialized countries such as the United States, Canada, France, Denmark, Italy, and Spain have the highest incidence rates for bladder cancer. Rates are lower in England, Scotland, and Eastern Europe. The lowest rates occur in Asia and South America.

Smoking is a major risk factor for bladder cancer; it increases one's risk by two to five times and accounts for

WHO PERFORMS THE PROCEDURE AND WHERE IS IT PERFORMED?

Transurethral bladder resections are usually performed in a hospital by a urologist, a medical doctor who specializes in the diagnosis and treatment of diseases of the urinary systems in men and women, and treats structural problems and tumors or stones in the urinary system. Urologists can prescribe medications and perform surgery. If a transurethral bladder resection is required by a female patient, and there are complicating factors, a urogynecologist may perform the surgery. Urogynecologists treat urinary problems involving the female reproductive system.

approximately 50% of bladder cancers found in men and 30% found in women. If cigarette smokers quit, their risk declines in two to four years. Exposure to a variety of industrial chemicals also increases the risk of developing this disease. Occupational exposures may account for approximately 25% of all urinary bladder cancers.

The incidence of bladder cancer in the white population is almost twice that of the black population, and is more than 2.5 times more likely to be diagnosed in men than women. For other ethnic and racial groups in the United States, the incidence of bladder cancer falls between that of whites and blacks.

There is a greater incidence of bladder cancer with advancing age. Of newly diagnosed cases in both men and women, approximately 80% occur in people aged 60 years and older.

Description

Cancer begins in the lining layer of the bladder and grows into the bladder wall. Transitional cells line the inside of the bladder. Cancer can begin in these lining cells.

During transurethral bladder resection, a cystoscope is inserted through the urethra into the bladder. A clear solution is infused to maintain visibility, and the tumor or tissue to be examined is cut away using an electric current. A biopsy is taken of the tumor and muscle fibers in order to evaluate the depth of tissue involvement, while avoiding perforation of the bladder wall. Every attempt is made to remove all visible tumor tissue, along with a small border of healthy tissue. The resected tissue is examined under the microscope for diagnostic purposes. An indwelling catheter may be inserted to ensure adequate drainage of the bladder postoperatively. At this time, interstitial radiation therapy may be initiated if necessary.

Diagnosis/Preparation

If there is reason to suspect a patient may have bladder cancer, the physician will use one or more methods to determine if the disease is actually present. The doctor first takes a complete medical history to check for risk factors and symptoms, and does a **physical examination**. An examination of the rectum and vagina (in women) may also be performed to determine the size of a bladder tumor and to see if, and how far, it has spread. If bladder cancer is suspected, the following tests may be performed:

• biopsy

• **cystoscopy**

• urine cytology

• bladder washings

• urine culture

• intravenous pyelogram

• retrograde pyelography

• bladder tumor marker studies

Most of the time, the cancer begins as a superficial tumor in the bladder. Blood in the urine is the usual warning sign. Based on how they look under the microscope, bladder cancers are graded using Roman numerals 0 through IV. In general, the lower the number, the less the cancer has spread. A higher number indicates greater severity of cancer.

Because it is not unusual for people with one bladder tumor to develop additional cancers in other areas of the bladder or elsewhere in the urinary system, the doctor may biopsy several different areas of the bladder lining. If the cancer is suspected to have spread to other organs in the body, further tests will be performed.

Because different types of bladder cancer respond differently to treatment, the treatment for one patient could be different from that of another person with bladder cancer. Doctors determine how deeply the cancer has spread into the layers of the bladder in order to decide on the best treatment.

Standard with any surgical procedure, the patient is asked to sign a consent form after a thorough explanation of the planned procedure.

Aftercare

As with any surgical procedure, blood pressure and pulse will be monitored. Urine is expected to be blood-tinged in the early postoperative period. Continuous

QUESTIONS TO ASK THE DOCTOR

• What benefits can I expect from this operation?

• What are the risks of this operation?

• What are the normal results of this operation?

• What happens if this operation does not go as planned?

• Are there any alternatives to this surgery?

• What is the expected recovery time?

bladder irrigation (rinsing) may be used for approximately 24 hours after surgery. Most operative sites should be completely healed in three months. The patient is followed closely for possible recurrence with visual examination, using a special viewing device (cystoscope) at regular intervals. Because bladder cancer has a high rate of recurrence, frequent screenings are recommended. Normally, screenings would be needed every three to six months for the first three years, and every year after that, or as the physician considers necessary. Cystoscopy can catch a recurrence before it progresses to invasive cancer, which is difficult to treat.

Risks

All surgery carries some risk due to heart and lung problems or the anesthesia itself, but these risks are generally extremely small. The risk of death from general anesthesia for all types of surgery, for example, is only about one in 1,600. Bleeding and infection are other risks of any surgical procedure. If bleeding becomes a complication, bladder irrigation may be required postoperatively, during which time the patient's activity is limited to bed rest. Perforation of the bladder is another risk, in which case the urinary catheter is left in place for four to five days postoperatively. The patient is started on antibiotic therapy preventively. If the bladder is lacerated accompanied by spillage of urine into the abdomen, an abdominal incision may be required.

Normal results

The results of transurethral bladder resection will depend on many factors, including the type of treatment used, the stage of the patient's cancer before surgery, complications during and after surgery, the age and overall health of the patient, as well as the recurrence of the disease at a later date. The chances for survival are improved if the cancer is found and treated early.

KEY TERMS

Biopsy—The removal and microscopic examination of a small sample of body tissue to see whether cancer cells are present.

Bladder irrigation—To flush or rinse the bladder with a stream of liquid (as in removing a foreign body or medicating).

Bladder washings—A procedure in which bladder washing samples are taken by placing a salt solution into the bladder through a catheter (tube) and then removing the solution for microscopic testing.

Bladder tumor marker studies—A test to detect specific substances released by bladder cancer cells into the urine using chemical or immunologic (using antibodies).

Chemotherapy—The treatment of cancer with anti-cancer drugs.

Cystoscopy—A procedure in which a slender tube with a lens and a light is placed into the bladder to view the inside of the bladder and remove tissue samples.

Immunotherapy—A method of treating allergies in which small doses of substances that a person is allergic to are injected under the skin.

Interstitial radiation therapy—The process of placing radioactive sources directly into the tumor. These radioactive sources can be temporary (removed after the proper dose is reached) or permanent.

Intravenous pyelogram—An x ray of the urinary system after injecting a contrast solution that enables the doctor to see images of the kidneys, ureters, and bladder.

Metastatic—A change of position, state, or form; as a transfer of a disease-producing agency from the site of disease to another part of the body; a secondary growth of a cancerous tumor.

Noninvasive tumors—Tumors that have not penetrated the muscle wall and/or spread to other parts of the body.

Radiation therapy—The use of high-dose x rays to destroy cancer cells.

Retrograde pyelography—A test in which dye is injected through a catheter placed with a cystoscope into the ureter to make the lining of the bladder, ureters, and kidneys easier to see on x rays.

Urine culture—A test which tests urine samples in the lab to see if bacteria are present.

Ureters—Two thin tubes that carry urine downward from the kidneys to the bladder.

Urethra—The small tube-like structure that allows urine to empty from the bladder.

Urine cytology—The examination of the urine under a microscope to look for cancerous or precancerous cells.

Morbidity and mortality rates

After a diagnosis of bladder cancer, up to 80% of patients with superficial tumors survive for at least five years. The five-year survival rate may be as high as 75% for patients whose tumors have invaded the bladder muscle. The five-year survival rates are 40% or less for patients with more-invasive tumors or metastatic tumors. The five-year survival rate refers to the percentage of patients who live at least five years after their cancer is found, although many people live much longer. Five-year relative survival rates do not take into account patients who die of other diseases. Every person's situation is unique and the statistics cannot predict exactly what will happen in every case; these numbers provide an overall picture.

Mortality rates are two to three times higher for men than women. Although the incidence of bladder cancer in the white population exceeds those of the black population, black women die from the disease at a greater rate. This is due to a larger proportion of these cancers being diagnosed and treated at an earlier stage in the white population. The mortality rates for Hispanic and Asian men and women are only about one-half those for whites and blacks. Over the past 30 years, the age-adjusted mortality rate has decreased in both races and genders. This may be due to earlier diagnosis, better therapy, or both.

Of the 57,400 cases of bladder cancer diagnosed each year in the United States, approximately 12,500 will die.

Alternatives

Surgery, radiation therapy, immunotherapy, and chemotherapy are the main types of treatment for cancer of the bladder. One type of treatment or a combination of these treatments may be recommended, based on the stage of the cancer.

After the cancer is found and staged, the cancer care team discusses the treatment options with the patient. In choosing a treatment plan, the most significant factors to consider are the type and stage of the cancer. Other factors to consider include the patient's overall physical health, age, likely side effects of the treatment, and the personal preferences of the patient.

In considering treatment options, a **second opinion** may provide more information and help the patient feel more confident about the treatment plan chosen.

Alternative methods are defined as unproved or disproved methods, rather than evidence-based or proven methods to prevent, diagnose, and treat cancer. For some cancer patients, conventional treatment is difficult to tolerate and they may decide to seek a less unpleasant alternative. Others are seeking ways to alleviate the side effects of conventional treatment without having to take more drugs. Some do not trust traditional medicine, and feel that with alternative medicine approaches, they are more in control of making decisions about what is happening to their bodies.

A cancer patient should talk to the doctor or nurse before changing the treatment or adding any alternative methods. Some methods can be safely used along with standard medical treatment. Others may interfere with standard treatment or cause serious side effects.

The American Cancer Society (ACS) encourages people with cancer to consider using methods that have been proven effective or those that are currently under study. They encourage people to discuss all treatments they may be considering with their physician and other health care providers. The ACS acknowledges that more research is needed regarding the safety and effectiveness of many alternative methods. Unnecessary delays and interruptions in standard therapies could be detrimental to the success of cancer treatment.

At the same time, the ACS acknowledges that certain complementary methods such as aromatherapy, biofeedback, massage therapy, meditation, tai chi, or yoga may be very helpful when used in conjunction with conventional treatment.

Resources

BOOKS

Hanno, Philip M., S. Bruce Malkowicz, and Alan J. Wein, (editors). *Clinical Manual of Urology,* 3rd ed. Philadelphia: McGraw-Hill, Inc., 2001.

Hicks, M. *Bladder Cancer.* Cambridge, UK: Cambridge University Press, 2004.

Schoenberg, Mark P. *The Guide to Living with Bladder Cancer.* Baltimore, MA: Johns Hopkins University Press, 2001.

PERIODICALS

Bach, Peter B., Deborah Schrag, Otis W. Brawley, Aaron Galaznik, Sofia Yakren, and Colin B. Begg. "Survival of Blacks and Whites after a Cancer Diagnosis." *Journal of American Medical Association* 285 (2001): 324–328.

Smith, Shannon D., Marcia A. Wheeler, Janet Plescia, John W. Colberg, Robert M. Weiss, and Dario C. Altieri. "Urine Detection of Surviving and Diagnosis of Bladder Cancer." *Journal of American Medical Association* 285 (2001): 324–328.

ORGANIZATIONS

American Cancer Society. 1599 Clifton Road, N.E., Atlanta, GA 30329-4251. (800) 227-2345. <http://www.cancer.org>.

American Foundation for Urologic Disease. 1128 North Charles St., Baltimore, MD 21201. (410) 468-1800. (800) 242-2383. Fax: (410) 468-1808. E-Mail: <admin@afud.org>. <http://www.afud.org/>.

National Cancer Institute Public Inquiries Office. Suite 3036A. 6116 Executive Boulevard, MSC8322. Bethesda, MD 20892-8322. (800) 422-6237. <http://www.nci.nih.gov>.

National Comprehensive Cancer Network. 50 Huntingdon Pike, Suite 200, Rockledge PA 19046. (215) 728-4788. Fax: (215) 728-3877. Email: <information@nccn.org>. <http://www.nccn.org/>.

National Institutes of Health (NIH), Department of Health and Human Services. 9000 Rockville Pike. Bethesda, MD 20892.

OTHER

Aetna InteliHealth Inc. *Bladder Cancer,* 2003 [cited April 24, 2003] <http://www.intelihealth.com/>.

American Cancer Society, Inc. (ACS) *Cancer Refererence Information,* 2003 [cited April 24, 2003] <http://www3.cancer.org/cancerinfo>.

Kathleen D. Wright, RN
Crystal H. Kaczkowski, MSc

Transurethral resection of the prostate

Definition

Transurethral resection of the prostate (TURP) is a surgical procedure by which portions of the prostate gland are removed through the urethra.

Purpose

The prostate is a gland that is part of the male reproductive system. It consists of three lobes, and surrounds the neck of the bladder and urethra (tube that channels urine from the bladder to the outside through the tip of

WHO PERFORMS
THE PROCEDURE AND
WHERE IS IT PERFORMED?

Transurethral resection of the prostate is performed in hospitals by experienced urologic surgeons who are specialized in prostate disorders and in performing the TURP procedure.

the penis). The prostate weighs approximately one ounce (28 g), and is walnut-shaped. It is partly muscular and partly glandular, with ducts opening into the urethra. It secretes an antigen called prostate-specific antigen (PSA), and a slightly alkaline fluid that forms part of the seminal fluid (semen) that carries sperm.

A common prostate disorder is called benign prostatic hyperplasia (BPH) or benign prostatic enlargement (BPE). BPH is due to hormonal changes in the prostate, and is characterized by the enlargement or overgrowth of the gland as a result of an increase in the number of its constituent cells. BPH can raise PSA levels two to three times higher than normal. Men with increased PSA levels have a higher chance of developing prostate cancer. BPH usually affects the innermost part of the prostate first, and enlargement frequently results in a gradual squeezing of the urethra at the point where it runs through the prostate. The squeezing sometimes causes urinary problems, such as difficulty urinating. BPH may progress to the point of generating a dense capsule that blocks the flow of urine from the bladder, resulting in the inability to completely empty the bladder. Eventually, this could lead to bladder and kidney malfunction.

Transurethral resection of the prostate (TURP) is the treatment of choice for BPH, and the most common surgery performed for the condition. "Transurethral" refers to the procedure being performed through the urethra. "Resection " refers to surgical removal.

Demographics

Prostate disease usually occurs in men over age 40. BPH eventually develops in approximately 80% of all men. Prostate cancer occurs in one out of 10 men. In the United States, more than 30,000 men die of prostate cancer each year.

Description

TURP is a type of transurethral surgery that does not involve an external incision. The surgeon reaches the prostate by inserting an instrument through the urethra.

In addition to TURP, two other types of transurethral surgery are commonly performed, transurethral incision of the prostate (TUIP), and transurethral laser incision of the prostate (TULIP). The TUIP procedure widens the urethra by making small cuts in the bladder neck (where the urethra and bladder meet), and in the prostate gland itself. In TULIP, a laser beam directed through the urethra melts the tissue.

The actual TURP procedure is simple. It is performed under general or local anesthesia. After an IV is inserted, the surgeon first examines the patient with a cystoscope, an instrument that allows him or her to see inside the bladder. The surgeon then inserts a device up the urethra via the penis opening, and removes the excess capsule material that has been restricting the flow of urine. The density of the normal prostate differs from that of the restricting capsule, making it relatively easy for the surgeon to tell exactly how much to remove. After excising the capsule material, the surgeon inserts a catheter into the bladder through the urethra for the subsequent withdrawal of urine.

Diagnosis/Preparation

BPH symptoms include:

• increase in urination frequency, and the need to urinate during the night

• difficulty starting urine flow

• a slow, interrupted flow and dribbling after urinating

• sudden, strong urges to pass urine

• a sensation that the bladder is not completely empty

• pain or burning during urination

In evaluating the prostate gland for BPH, the physician usually performs a complete **physical examination** as well as the following procedures:

• Digital rectal examination (DRE). Recommended annually for men over the age of 50, the DRE is an examination performed by a physician who feels the prostate through the wall of the rectum. Hard or lumpy areas may indicate the presence of cancer.

• Prostate-specific antigen (PSA) test. Also recommended annually for men over the age of 50, the PSA test measures the levels of prostate-specific antigen secreted by the prostate. It is normal to observe small quantities of PSA in the blood. PSA levels vary with age, and tend to increase gradually in men over age 60. They also tend to rise as a result of infection (prostatitis), BPH, or cancer.

If the results of the DRE and PSA tests are indicative of a significant prostate disorder, the examining

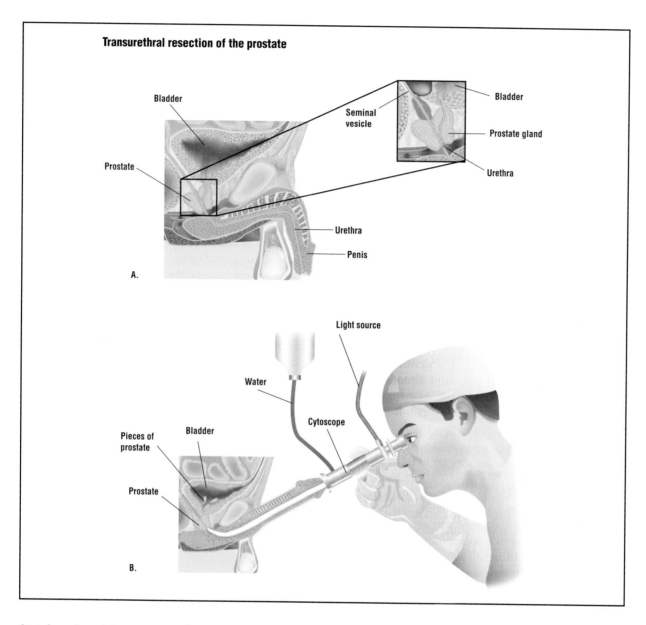

Transurethral resection of the prostate

A.
Bladder
Seminal vesicle
Prostate
Bladder
Prostate gland
Urethra
Urethra
Penis

B.
Light source
Water
Cytoscope
Pieces of prostate
Bladder
Prostate

An enlarged prostate can cause urinary problems due to its location around the male urethra (A). In TURP, the physician uses a cystoscope to gain access to the prostate through the urethra (B). The prostate material that has been restricting urine flow is cut off in pieces, which are washed into the bladder with water from the scope (B). *(Illustration by GGS Inc.)*

physician usually refers the patient to a urologist, a physician who specializes in diseases of the urinary tract and male reproductive system. The urologist performs additional tests, including blood and urine studies, to establish a diagnosis.

To prepare for TURP, patients should:

• Select an experienced TURP surgeon to perform the procedure.

• Purchase a mild natural bulk-forming laxative.

• Wear loose clothing on the morning of surgery.

• Ask friends or family to be available for assistance after surgery.

• Schedule a week off from work.

• Get sufficient sleep on the night before surgery.

Aftercare

When the patient awakens in the **recovery room** after the procedure, he already has a catheter in his penis, and is receiving pain medication via the IV line inserted prior to surgery.

The initial recovery period lasts approximately one week, and includes some pain and discomfort from the urinary catheter. Spastic convulsions of the bladder and prostate are expected as they respond to the surgical changes. The following medications are commonly prescribed after TURP:

• B&O suppository (Belladonna and Opium). This medication has the dual purpose of providing pain relief and reducing the ureteral and bladder spasms that follow TURP surgery. It is a strong medication that must be used only as prescribed.

• Bulk-forming laxative. Because of the surgical trauma and large quantities of liquids that patients are required to drink, they may need some form of laxative to promote normal bowel movements.

• Detrol. This pain reliever is not as strong as B&O. There may be wide variations in its effectiveness and the patient's response. It also controls involuntary bladder contractions.

• Macrobid. This antibiotic helps prevent urinary tract infections.

• Pyridium. This medication offers symptomatic relief from pain, burning, urgency, frequency, and other urinary tract discomfort.

When discharged from the hospital, patients are advised to:

• Refrain from alcoholic beverages.

• Avoid sexual activities for a few weeks.

• Avoid driving a car for a week or more.

• Keep domestic activities to a minimum.

• Avoid weight lifting or strenuous exercise.

• Check their temperature and report any fever to the physician.

• Practice good hygiene, especially of the hands and penis.

• Drink plenty of liquids.

Risks

Serious complications are less common for prostate surgery patients because of advances in operative methods. Nerve-sparing surgical procedures help prevent permanent injury to the nerves that control erection, as well as injury to the opening of the bladder. However, there are risks associated with prostate surgery. The first is the possible development of incontinence, the inability to control urination, which may result in urine leakage or dribbling, especially just after surgery. Normal control usually returns within several weeks or months after surgery, but some patients have become permanently in-

continent. There is also a risk of impotence, the inability to achieve penile erection. For a month or so after surgery, most men are not able to become erect. Eventually, approximately 40–60% of men will be able to have an erection sufficient for sexual intercourse. They no longer ejaculate semen because removal of the prostate gland prevents that process. This effect is related to many factors, such as overall health and age. Other risks associated with TURP include:

• blood loss requiring transfusion

• postoperative urinary tract infection

• unsatisfactory long-term outcome

TURP syndrome effects 2–6% of TURP patients. Symptoms may include temporary blindness due to irrigation fluid entering the bloodstream. On very rare occasions, this can lead to seizures, coma, and even death. The syndrome may also include toxic shock due to bacteria entering the bloodstream, as well as internal hemorrhage.

Normal results

TURP patients usually notice urine flow improvement as soon as the catheter is removed. Other improvements depend on the condition of the patient's prostate before TURP, his age, and overall health status. Patients are told to expect the persistance of some pre-surgery symptoms. In fact, some new symptoms may appear following TURP, such as occasional blood and tissue in the urine, bladder spasms, pain when urinating, and difficulty judging when to urinate. TURP represents a major adaptation for the body, and healing requires some time. Full recovery may take up to one year. Patients are almost always satisfied with their TURP outcome, and the adaptation to new symptoms is offset by the disappearance of previous problems. For example, most patients no longer have to take daily prostate medication, and quickly learn to gradually increase the time between urinating while enjoying uninterrupted and more restful sleep at night.

Normal post-operative symptoms include:

• urination at night and reduced flow

• mild burning and stinging sensation while urinating

• reduced semen at ejaculation

• bladder control problems

• mild bladder spams

• fatigue

• urination linked to bowel movements

To eliminate these symptoms, patients are advised to:

• Exercise.

- Retrain their bladder

- Take all medications that were prescribed after TURP

- Inform themselves via support groups or pertinent reading

- Get plenty of rest to facilitate the post-surgery healing process

Morbidity and mortality rates

TURP reduces symptoms in 88% of BPH patients. TURP mortality rates are 0.2%, but they can be as high as 10% in patients over 80 years of age. Following surgery, inadequate relief of BPH symptoms occurs in 20–25% of patients, and 15–20% require another operation within 10 years. Urinary incontinence affects 2–4%, and 5–10% of TURP patients become impotent.

Alternatives

Conventional surgical alternatives for BPH patients include:

- Interstitial laser coagulation. In this procedure, a laser beam inserted in the urethra via a catheter heats and destroys the extra prostate capsule tissue.

- Transurethral needle ablation (TUNA). This technique was approved by the FDA in 1996. It uses radio waves to heat and destroy the enlarged prostate through needles positioned in the gland. It is generally less effective than TURP for reducing symptoms and increasing urine flow.

- Transurethral electrovaporization. This procedure is a modified version of TURP, and uses a device that produces electronic waves to vaporize the enlarged prostate.

- Photoselective vaporization of the prostate (PVP). This procedure uses a strong laser beam to vaporize the tissue in a 20–50 minute outpatient operation.

- Transurethral incision of the prostate (TUIP). In this procedure, a small incision is made in the bladder, followed by a few cuts into the sphincter muscle to release some of the tension.

- Transurethral microwave thermotherapy (TUMT). TUMT uses microwave heat energy to shrink the enlarged prostate through a probe inserted into the penis to the level of the prostate. This outpatient procedure takes about one hour. The patient can go home the same day, and is able to resume normal activities within a day or two. TUMT does not lead to immediate improvement, and it usually takes up to four weeks for urinary problems to completely resolve.

QUESTIONS TO ASK THE DOCTOR

- What are the alternative treatments for benign prostatic hyperplasia?
- What are the risks involved with TURP?
- How long will it take to recover from the surgery?
- How painful is the TURP surgery?
- When and how often will the catheter require flushing?
- How long will it take to feel improvement?
- What are the post-operative problems?
- How will the surgery affect the ability to achieve erection?
- How many TURP procedures does the surgeon perform in a year?
- Will the surgery have to be repeated?

- Water-induced thermotherapy (WIT). WIT is administered via a closed-loop catheter system, through which heated water is maintained at a constant temperature. WIT is usually performed using only a local anesthetic gel to anesthetize the penis, and is very well tolerated. The procedure is FDA approved.

- Balloon dilation. In this procedure, a balloon is inserted in the urethra up to where the restriction occurs. At that point, the balloon expands to push out the prostate tissue and widen the urinary path. Improvements with this technique may only last a few years.

BPH patients have experienced improved prostate health from the following:

- Zinc supplements. This mineral plays an important role in prostate health because it decreases prolactin secretion and protects against heavy metals such as cadmium. Both prolactin and cadmium have been associated with BPH.

- Saw palmetto. Saw palmetto has long been used by Native Americans to treat urinary tract disturbances without causing impotence. It shows no significant side effects. A number of recent European clinical studies have also shown that fat soluble extracts of the berry help increase urinary flow and relieve other urinary problems resulting from BPH.

- Garlic. Garlic is believed to contribute to overall body and prostate health.

Tubal ligation

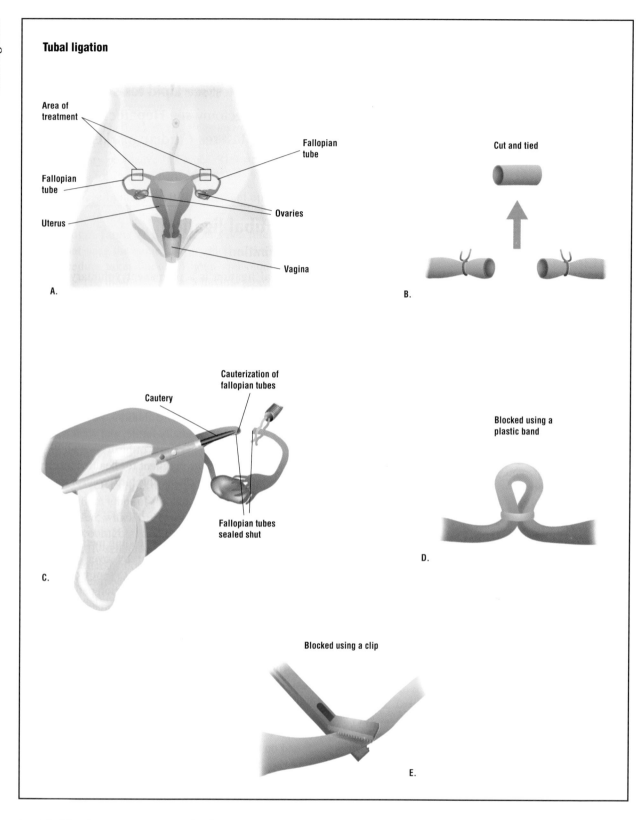

A.

Area of treatment

Fallopian tube

Fallopian tube

Ovaries

Uterus

Vagina

Cut and tied

B.

Cauterization of fallopian tubes

Cautery

Fallopian tubes sealed shut

C.

Blocked using a plastic band

D.

Blocked using a clip

E.

In a tubal ligation, a woman's reproductive organs are accessed by abdominal incision or laparoscopy (A). The fallopian tubes are cut and tied (B), cauterized (C), blocked with a silicone band (D), or clipped (E) to ensure sperm is not able to fertilize an egg. *(Illustration by GGS Inc.)*

thesia, or local anesthesia with sedation. The surgery can be performed on either hospitalized patients within 24 hours after childbirth or on outpatients. The woman can usually leave the hospital the same day.

Tubal ligation should be postponed if the woman is unsure about her decision. While the procedure is sometimes reversible, it should be considered permanent and irreversible. As many as 10% of sterilized women regret having had the surgery, and about 1% seek treatment to restore their fertility.

The most common surgical approaches to tubal ligation include **laparoscopy** and mini-laparotomy. In a laparoscopic tubal ligation, a long, thin telescope-like surgical instrument called a laparoscope is inserted into the pelvis through a small cut about 0.5 inches (1 cm) long near the navel. Carbon dioxide gas is pumped in to help move the abdominal wall to give the surgeon easier access to the tubes. Often the **surgical instruments** are inserted through a second incision near the pubic hair line. An instrument may be placed through the vagina to hold the uterus in place.

In a mini-laparotomy, a 1.2–1.6 in (3–4 cm) incision is made just above the pubic bone or under the navel. A larger incision, or laparotomy, is rarely used today. Tubal ligation can also be performed at the time of a **cesarean section**.

The tubal ligation itself is performed in several ways:

• Electrocoagulation. A heated needle connected to an electrical device is used to cauterize or burn the tubes. Electrocoagulation is the most common method of tubal ligation.

• Falope ring. In this technique, an applicator is inserted through an incision above the bladder and a plastic ring is placed around a loop of the tube.

• Hulka clip. The surgeon places a plastic clip across a tube held in place by a steel spring.

• Silicone rubber bands. A band placed over a tube forms a mechanical block to sperm.

Tubal ligation costs about $2,000 when performed by a private physician, but is less expensive when performed at a family planning clinic. Most insurance plans cover treatment costs.

Diagnosis/Preparation

Preparation for tubal ligation includes patient education and counseling. Before surgery, it is important that the woman understand the permanent nature of tubal ligation as well as the risks of anesthesia and surgery. Her medical history is reviewed, and a **physical examination** and laboratory testing are performed.

The patient is not allowed to eat or drink for several hours before surgery.

Aftercare

After surgery, the patient is monitored for several hours before she is allowed to go home. She is instructed on care of the surgical wound, and what signs to watch for, such as fever, nausea, vomiting, faintness, or pain. These signs could indicate that complications have occurred.

Risks

While major complications are uncommon after tubal ligation, there are risks with any surgical procedure. Possible side effects include infection and bleeding. After laparoscopy, the patient may experience pain in the shoulder area from the carbon dioxide used during surgery, but the technique is associated with less pain than mini-laparotomy, as well as a faster recovery period. Mini-laparotomy results in a higher incidence of pain, bleeding, bladder injury, and infection compared with laparoscopy. Patients normally feel better after three to four days of rest, and are able to resume sexual activity at that time.

The possibility for treatment failure is very low—fewer than one in 200 women (0.4%) will become pregnant during the first year after sterilization. Failure can happen if the cut ends of the tubes grow back together; if the tube was not completely cut or blocked off; if a plastic clip or rubber band has loosened or come off; or if the woman was already pregnant at the time of surgery.

Normal results

After having her tubes tied, a woman does not need to use any form of birth control to avoid pregnancy. Tubal ligation is almost 100% effective for the prevention of conception.

KEY TERMS

Contraception—The prevention of the union of the male's sperm with the female's egg.

Ectopic pregnancy—The implantation of a fertilized egg in a Fallopian tube instead of the uterus.

Electrocoagulation—The coagulation or destruction of tissue through the application of a high-frequency electrical current.

Female sterilization—The process of permanently ending a woman's ability to conceive by tying off or cutting apart the Fallopian tubes.

Laparoscopy—Abdominal surgery performed through a laparoscope, which is a thin telescopic instrument inserted through an incision near the navel.

Laparotomy—A procedure in which the surgeon opens the abdominal cavity to inspect the patient's internal organs.

Vasectomy—Surgical sterilization of the male, done by removing a portion of the tube that carries sperm to the urethra.

Morbidity and mortality rates

About 1–4% of patients experience complications following tubal ligation. There is a low risk (less than 1%, or seven per 1,000 procedures) of a later ectopic pregnancy. Ectopic pregnancy is a condition in which the fertilized egg implants in a place other than the uterus, usually in one of the fallopian tubes. Ectopic pregnancies are more likely to happen in younger women, and in women whose tubes were closed off by electrocoagulation.

Rarely, death may occur as a complication of general anesthesia if a major blood vessel is cut. The mortality rate of tubal ligation is about four in 100,000 sterilizations.

Alternatives

There are numerous options available to women who wish to prevent pregnancy. Oral contraceptives are the second most common form of contraception—the first being female sterilization—and have a success rate of 95–99.5%. Other methods of preventing pregnancy include **vasectomy** (99.9% effective) for the male partner; the male condom (86–97% effective); the diaphragm or cervical cap (80–94% effective); the female condom (80–95% effective); and abstinence.

See also Vasectomy.

Resources

BOOKS

"Family Planning: Sterilization." Section 18, Chapter 246 in *The Merck Manual of Diagnosis and Therapy*, edited by Mark H. Beers, MD, and Robert Berkow, MD. Whitehouse Station, NJ: Merck Research Laboratories, 1999.

PERIODICALS

Baill, I. C., V. E. Cullins, and S. Pati. "Counseling Issues in Tubal Sterilization." *American Family Physician* 67 (March 15, 2003): 1287-1294.

Kariminia, A., D. M. Saunders, and M. Chamberlain. "Risk Factors for Strong Regret and Subsequent IVF Request After Having Tubal Ligation." *Australian and New Zealand Journal of Obstetrics and Gynaecology* 42 (November 2002): 526-529.

ORGANIZATIONS

American College of Obstetricians and Gynecologists. 409 12th St., SW, P. O. Box 96920, Washington, DC 20090-6920. <www.acog.org>.

Planned Parenthood Federation of America, Inc. 810 Seventh Ave., New York, NY, 10019. (800) 669-0156. <www.plannedparenthood.org>

OTHER

Centers for Disease Control and Prevention. *Fact Sheet: Risk of Ectopic Pregnancy after Tubal Sterilization*, August 6, 2002 [cited March 1, 2003]. <www.cdc.gov/nccdphp/drh/mh_ectopic.htm>.

Planned Parenthood Federation of America. *All About Tubal Sterilization*. [cited March 1, 2003]. <www.plannedparenthood.org/bc/allabouttubal.htm>.

Planned Parenthood Federation of America. *Facts About Birth Control*, January 2001 [cited March 1, 2003]. <www.plannedparenthood.org/bc/bcfacts1.html>.

Mercedes McLaughlin
Stephanie Dionne Sherk

Tube-shunt surgery

Definition

Tube-shunt surgery, or Seton tube shunt glaucoma surgery, is a surgical method to treat glaucoma. Glaucoma is a potentially blinding disease affecting 2–3% of the United States population. The major known cause of glaucoma is a relative increase in intraocular pressure, or IOP. The purpose of glaucoma treatment, whether medical or surgical, is to lower the IOP.

Aqueous fluid is made continuously, and circulates throughout the eye before draining though channels in the eye's anterior chamber. When too much fluid is made, or it is not drained sufficiently, the IOP rises. This fluid build-up can lead to glaucoma. Normal intraocular pressure is under 21 mm/Hg. Glaucoma develops at IOPs higher than 21mm/Hg. However, approximately 20% of glaucoma patients never have pressures higher than 21 mm/Hg.

Seton tube implants are also called glaucoma drainage tubes or implants. The Seton implant is comprised of two parts:

• Tubing, a portion of which is implanted along the inside of the front of the eye. The distal (furthest from the center) end of the tubing protrudes through the anterior (front) or less commonly, the posterior (rear), chamber of the eye.

• An attached reservoir, called a plate, is placed under the conjunctiva of the eye at its equator, or midpoint.

Purpose

The function of the implant is to lower the intraocular pressure by filtering excess aqueous fluid out of the eye. During the first few weeks after surgery, a bleb of fibrous tissue and collagen forms around the plate of the implant. The formation of a filtration bleb is essential for filtering the excessive aqueous fluid. The thickness of the bleb, as well as the size or number of plates, determines the rate at which aqueous flows out of the anterior chamber of the eye. The excess aqueous fluid is shunted through the tubing of the implant, and passes through the space that develops between the bleb and the plate. By diffusion, the fluid flows into the capillaries where it exits the eye and enters general circulation. The IOP is lowered as a result of this decrease in fluid.

There are various types of implants used in glaucoma surgery. They fall into two categories: the non-valved (free flow implants) and valved (resisted-flow implants). One of the first free-flow implants was the Molteno implant, which consists of one or two polypropylene reser-

voirs connected to a silicone tube. The non-valved Baerveldt implant is larger than the Molteno, and is available in three sizes.

The restrictive implants, which include the Krupin and Ahmed implant, have valves that automatically close if the intraocular pressure is too low. This is important because in the first few weeks after surgery (before the bleb forms), the aqueous fluid can flow unimpeded through the implant. As a result, hypotony (low level of fluid in the eye) can develop.

Newer implants such as the Express shunt and the Gore-Tex tube shunt are in early stages of use.

Demographics

Seton tube implants are employed to treat all forms of glaucoma, but are primarily used in patients with elevated IOP despite aggressive medical treatment. They are also used when other types of surgery, such as conventional filtration, or **trabeculectomy**, have not been successful, or would not be recommended. A trabeculectomy should not be performed on patients with neovascular glaucoma, as well as those who have ocular complications caused by previous glaucoma surgeries.

Implants are often placed in the eyes of patients with uveitic glaucoma (fluctuating IOP). The surgeon implants a tube with a ligature, and manipulates the ligature to control pressure. Seton tubes are also used in young patients with aniridia, who often develop glaucoma. These tubes should not be used for patients who have silicon oil implants for the treatment of retinal detachment.

Description

A Seton implant is usually inserted under local anesthesia, but may be done under general anesthesia for an anxious patient or child. Since implantation may be

QUESTIONS TO ASK THE DOCTOR

- Which implant will be used?
- Is a tube implant the best surgical approach for this case?
- How many of these procedures has the surgeon performed?
- When will it be determined if the surgery has been successful?
- What are the risks for this surgery?
- Will glaucoma eye drops still be required after surgery?

painful for some children, drugs may be given intravenously during surgery.

After anesthesia is administered, the eye is draped and retractors are placed on the eye to hold it in place. An incision is made on the conjunctiva, a thin membrane layer that lies above the sclera (white of the eye). The implant plate is placed under the conjunctiva and sutured to the sclera, carefully avoiding damage to the recti muscles in the area. Incisions may be made in two quadrants of the eye if a double plate implant is inserted.

If the tubing is implanted into the anterior chamber, that portion of the eye is drained of excess fluid. If the tube is placed in the posterior chamber of the eye, all or part of the vitreous is removed. A needle puncture is made at the limbus where the cornea and the sclera meet, and the tubing is passed through this hole into one of the chambers of the eye. This opening is sealed with a donor scleral patch, which may be autologous (from the patient's own tissue). If a free-flow implant is used, the tubing is ligated with either a disposable suture, or the ligature is positioned such that it can be removed with a minor incision after a few weeks. As an alternative, the non-valved implant may be inserted in two stages. The plate is first implanted, and the tube is attached during a second surgery after the bleb has formed.

Diagnosis/Preparation

Prior to surgery, the patient's eye is examined with a slit-lamp biomicroscope. It is important that the conjunctiva in which the plate is placed is not scarred; that the cornea is clear; and that there are no attachments of the iris to the lens behind it or to the cornea in front of it. An ultrasound of pediatric patients is done to assess the size of the eye because not all implants are small enough to fit into a child's eye.

Antibiotic drops may be given for up to three days prior to surgery. The patient will continue most glaucoma medication until the day of surgery.

Informed consent must be given for the procedure. This includes consent for surgery and a list of risks for the Seton tube implant. It is important for the patient to understand that any vision loss acquired prior to surgery cannot be corrected.

Aftercare

For several weeks postoperatively, the patient is given topical **antibiotics** and steroids. In addition, oral steroids may be given to patients who had ocular inflammation prior to surgery. Some surgeons use atropine to maintain the eye in a temporary dilated state. Glaucoma medication may be continued for a few months due to possible IOP fluctuation during the early post-operative period. Follow-up visits are scheduled for one day after the surgery, weekly during the first month, twice a month during the second month, and again at three months. Patients can resume normal daily activities within a few days. The sutures may cause a foreign body sensation, which decreases as the stitches dissolve. This does not usually require treatment.

Aftercare in the surgeon's office involves monitoring for the signs of hypotony and lowered IOP. The treatment for post-operative hypotony is to tighten the tube of a non-valved implant. As the bleb forms, adjustments are made in the tubing ligature to increase flow through the ligature. If the pressure continues to rise, the tube may be blocked, and excess fluid may have to be tapped. Tube blockage may occasionally occur. Hypotony may also be caused by leakage from the conjunctival wound site.

Risks

This surgery has intraoperative and postoperative risks. During the procedure, an extraocular muscle can be severed. This is particularly true if the implant is placed in the inferior nasal section of the eye. Strabismus and double vision may follow. Also, the cornea may become scarred, hemorrhaging can occur within the eye, and the iris and lens can be damaged by the protruding tube.

Early post-operative complications include hyphema (blood clots in the anterior chamber of the eye), hypotony, tube obstruction, suture rupture with wound leakage, movement of the implanted plate, corneal edema, and detachment of the retina. Because of the position of the implant plate, retinal detachments are difficult to treat successfully if a Seton implant is present. Double vision during the early post-operative period

KEY TERMS

Anterior chamber—The front chamber of the eye bound by the cornea in front and the iris in the back. The anterior chamber is filled with aqueous humor. The drainage site for the aqueous fluid is in the anterior chamber.

Choroid—The middle, highly vascular layer of the eye that lies between the sclera and the retina.

Conjunctiva—A thin membrane covering the sclera (white of the eye).

Cornea—The clear part of the eye, surrounded by the sclera, through which light passes into the eye.

Glaucoma—A group of eye diseases, of which the primary feature is a relative elevation in the intraocular pressure, or IOP. The damage caused by pressure changes in the eye are potentially blinding.

IOP—A measure of the pressure in the eye. The gold standard for measurement of IOP is Goldmann tonometry.

Ophthalmologist—A physician with either an M.D. or D.O. degree, who has had residency training in the diagnosis and treatment of eye diseases.

Posterior chamber—The posterior part of the eye bound by the lens in front and the retina in back. The posterior chamber is filled with a jellylike substance called the vitreous.

Rectus muscles—The muscles responsible for movement of the eye.

Retina—The innermost layer in which the receptors for vision are located.

Sclera—The outer layer of the eye covering all of the front part of the eye, except for the cornea.

Seton tube—An implant placed in the eye that provides an alternative route for aqueous fluid drainage.

Strabismus—A condition in which the muscles of the eye do not work together, often causing double vision.

Vitrectomy—Removal of the vitreous jelly located in the posterior chamber.

---

may be due to swelling in the area, and often will resolve as the orbital edema decreases.

In the late post-surgical period, strabismus as well as orbital cellulitis, a condition that can spread to the central nervous system, can develop. Other long-term risks of glaucoma implant surgery include cataract formation, proptosis (bulging of the eye), and phthisis bulbi (a dangerous situation in which the eye is devoid of all fluid).

Surgical intervention is required for choroidal detachments, strabismus, and if tubing blocks or comes in contact with other structures of the eye, particularly the cornea. If the tube is blocked by blood clots, tissue plasminogen activator may dissolve them. A laser can cut strands of vitreous or iris that may clog the tubing. If bleb enlargement impinges on a muscle, causing strabismus, the implant may be removed and replaced with a smaller type. If the tubing continually rubs on the back or endothelium of the cornea, decomposition of the cornea is possible and a corneal transplant may be required if vision is comprised. In this case, the tubing will have to be relocated to the posterior chamber, and a vitrectomy performed.

Loss of vision is possible with this and all glaucoma surgery. For Seton tube implants, hypotony is the primary cause of vision loss. Other causes include retinal detachment, vitreous bleeding, and macular edema.

Normal results

Usually the IOP is lower within two weeks of Seton tube placement. At two months, the pressure is stabilized at 16–18 mm/Hg. Glaucoma medication must still be taken. The IOP in 85% of patients with a non-valved implant is lower than 21 mm/Hg without additional medication intervention. Only 50% of patients with a Krupin valve implant have an IOP lower than 21 mm/ Hg without added medical treatment.

Morbidity and mortality rates

For 70–90% of patients, the implant is functional one year after surgery. After three years, 60% remain functional. The failure rate for Seton implants is 4–8% per year, and differ for valved and non-valved implants. For the non-valved implants, the success rate is 90% at one year, but drops to 60% at two years. At least 66% of valved Seton tube implants are effective at one year, but this drops to 34% at six years. Choroidal detachment is a complication in one-third of these patients.

Strabismus is more common with the Krupin valve as opposed to the Ahmed valve, possibly because it is larger.

For high-risk glaucoma patients, the success rate for Seton tube surgery is approximately 50%. The rate of failure increases 10% with each year. High-risk patients include those who are aphakic (have no intraocular lens), have neovascular glaucoma (which develops from uncontrolled diabetes and hypertension), have congenital glaucoma, and who have had other unsuccessful glaucoma surgeries. Although the success rate for neovascular glaucoma is 56% at 18 months, eventually 31% of neovascular glaucoma patients will lose all vision except for light perception.

Alternatives

Trabeculectomy is another surgical filtration technique used to treat glaucoma. Trabeculectomy surgery is performed by making a flap in the sclera of the eye, which serves as an alternative drainage site for aqueous fluid. Patients who receive this treatment are not as high risk as those undergoing an implant procedure. Overall, they have a lower IOP, but may have more advanced glaucoma. If vascularization of the iris is present, as in neovascular glaucoma, a trabeculectomy is not performed. For patients who do not have neovascular glaucoma, the failure rate for trabeculotomy is similar to that of drainage tube implants.

Cyclodestruction is another alternative to Seton tube implants. Freezing temperatures or lasers are used to destroy the ciliary body, the part of the eye where the aqueous fluid is produced. When compared to the YAG laser cyclophotocoagulation, tube shunts are twice as successful.

Resources

BOOKS

Albert, Daniel M., M.D., M.S., et.al. *Ophthalmic Surgery Principles and Techniques* Malden, MA: Blackwell Science, 1999.

Albert, Daniel M., M.D., M.S., et.al. *Principles and Practice of Ophthalmology,* 2nd ed. Philadelphia, PA: W.B. Saunders Company, 2000.

Azuara-Blanco, M.D., Ph.D., Augusto, et.al. *Handbook of Glaucoma.* London, UK: Martin Dunitz Ltd., 2002.

Ritch, M.D., Robert, et.al. *The Glaucomas.* St Louis, MO: Mosby, 1996.

Shields, M.D. & M. Bruce. *Textbook of Glaucoma.* Baltimore, MD: Williams and Wilkins, 1998.

Weinreb, Robert, et.al. *Glaucoma in the 21st Century.* London, UK: Mosby International, 2000.

PERIODICALS

Arroyave, M.D., Claudia P., et.al. "Use of Glaucoma Drainage Devices in the Management of Glaucoma Associated with Aniridia." *American Journal of Ophthalmology* 135 (February 2003): 155-9.

Benz, M.D., Matthew S., et.al. "Retinal Detachment in Patients with a Preexisting Glaucoma Drainage Device." *Retina* 22 (June 2002): 283-7.

Garcia-Feijoo, M.D., Ph.D., J., et.al., "Peritubular Filtration as Cause of Severe Hypotony after Ahmed Valve Implantation for Glaucoma." *American Journal of Ophthalmology* 132 (October 2001): 571-2.

Nazemi, Paul P., et.al. "Migration of Intraocular Silicone Oil Into the Subconjunctival Space and Orbit Through an Ahmed Glaucoma Valve." *American Journal of Ophthalmology* 132 (December 2001): 929-31.

Netland, M.D. Peter A. and Lee, David A., M.D. "What's New in Glaucoma Research." *Review of Ophthalmology* (May 1999): 102-10.

OTHER

Glaucoma Associates of Texas, Drainage Implants. <http://www.glaucomaassociates.com/drainage-implants. html>.

Glaucoma Drainage Devices. <http://www.eyelink. com/Eye-Procedure.asp?EyeProcedureID=45>.

Martha Reilly, O.D.

Tube enterostomy

Definition

Tube enterostomy, or tube feeding, is a form of enteral or intestinal site feeding that employs a stoma or semi-permanent surgically placed tube to the small intestines.

Purpose

Many patients are unable to take in food by mouth, esophagus, or stomach. A number of conditions can render a person unable to take in nutrition through the normal pathways. Neurological conditions or injuries, injuries to the mouth or throat, obstructions of the stomach, cancer or ulcerative conditions of the gastrointestinal tract, and certain surgical procedures can make it impossible for a person to receive oral nutrition. Tube feeding is indicated for patients unable to ingest adequate nutrition by mouth, but who may have a cleared passage in the esophagus and stomach, and even partial functioning of gastrointestinal tract. Enteral nutrition procedures that utilize the gastrointestinal tract are preferred over intravenous feeding or parenteral nutrition because they maintain the function of the intestines, provide for immunity to infection, and avoid complications related to intravenous feeding.

Tube enterostomy, a feeding tube placed directly into the intestines or jejunum, is one such enteral procedure. It is used if the need for enteral feeding lasts longer than six weeks, or if it improves the outcomes of drastic surgeries such as removal or resection of the intestines.

Recently, it has become an important technique for use in surgery in which a gastroectomy—resection of the intestinal link to the esophagus—occurs. The procedure makes healing easier, and seeks to retain the patient's nutritional status and quality of life after reconstructive surgery. Some individuals have a tube enterostomy surgically constructed, and successfully utilize it for a long period of time.

There are a variety of enteral nutritional products, liquid feedings with the nutritional quality of solid food. Patients with normal gastrointestinal function can benefit from these products. Other patients must have nutritional counseling, monitoring, and precise nutritional diets developed by a health care professional.

Demographics

Tube enterostomy provides temporary enteral nutrition to patients with injuries as well as inflammatory, obstructive, and other intestinal, esophageal, and abdominal conditions. Other uses include patients with pediatric abnormalities, and those who have had surgery for cancerous tumors of the gastroesophageal junction (many of these cases are associated with Barrett's epithelium). Intestinal cancers in the United States have declined since the 1950s. However, this endemic form of gastric cancer is one of the most common causes of death from malignant disease, with an estimated 798,000 annual cases worldwide; 21,900 in the United States. As gastric cancer has declined, esophageal cancers have increased, requiring surgeries that resect and reconstruct the passage between the esophagus and intestine.

Description

Tube enterostomy refers to placement via a number of surgical approaches:

- laparoscopy
- esophagostomy (open surgery via the esophagus)
- stomach (**gastrostomy** or PEG)
- upper intestines or jejunum (jejunostomy)

The appropriate method depends on the clinical prognosis, anticipated duration of feeding, risk of aspirating or inhaling gastric contents, and patient preference. Whether through a standard operation or with laparoscopic surgical techniques, the surgeon fashions a stoma or opening into the esophagus, stomach or intestines, and inserts a tube from the outside through which nutrition will be introduced. These tubes are made of silicone or polyurethane, and contain weighted tips and insertion features that facilitate placement. The surgery is fairly simple to perform, and most patients have good outcomes with stoma placement.

WHO PERFORMS THE PROCEDURE AND WHERE IS IT PERFORMED?

Gastrointestinal surgeons and surgical oncologists perform this surgery in general hospital settings.

Diagnosis/Preparation

A number of conditions necessitate tube enterostomy for nutritional support. Many are chronic and require a complete medical evaluation including history, **physical examination**, and extensive imaging tests. Some conditions are critical or acute, and may emerge from injuries or serious inflammatory conditions in which the patient is not systematically prepared for the surgery. In many cases, the patient undergoing this type of surgery has been ill for a period of time. Sometimes the patient is a small child or adult who accidentally swallowed a caustic substance. Some are elderly patients who have obstructive carcinoma of the esophagus or stomach.

Optimal preparation includes an evaluation of the patient's nutritional status, and his or her potential requirement for blood transfusions and **antibiotics**. Patients who do not have gastrointestinal inflammatory or obstructive conditions are usually required to undergo bowel preparation that flushes the intestines of all material. The bowel preparation reduces the chances of infection.

The patient's acceptance of tube feeding as a substitute for eating is of paramount importance. Health care providers must be sensitive to these problems, and offer early assistance and feedback in the self-care that the tube enterostomy requires.

In preparation for surgery, patients learn that the tube enterostomy will be an artificial orifice placed outside the abdomen through which they will deliver their nutritional support. Patients are taught how to care for the stoma, cleaning and making sure it functions optimally. In addition, patients are prepared for the loss of the function of eating and its place in their lives. They must be made aware that their physical body will be altered, and that this may have social implications and affect their intimate activities.

Aftercare

Tube enterostomy requires monitoring the patient for infection or bleeding, and educating him or her on the proper use of the enterostomy. According to the type

QUESTIONS TO ASK THE DOCTOR

- How long will the tube enterostomy remain in place?
- How much assistance will be given in adjusting to the stoma and the special diet?
- If the condition does not improve, what other surgical alternatives are available?
- How long can a person live safely and comfortably with a tube enterostomy?

KEY TERMS

Enteral nutritional support—Nutrition utilizing an intact gastrointestinal tract, but bypassing another organ such as the stomach or esophagus.

Parenteral nutritional support—Intravenous nutrition that bypasses the intestines and its contribution to digestion.

Stoma—A portal fashioned from the side of the abdomen that allows for ingestion into or drainage out of the intestines or urinary tract.

Tube feeding—Feeding or nutrition through a tube placed into the body through the esophagus, nose, stomach, intestines, or via a surgically constructed artificial orifice called a stoma.

of surgery—minimally invasive or open surgery—it may take several days for the patient to resume normal functioning. Fluid intake and urinary output must be monitored to prevent dehydration.

Risks

Tube enterostomies are not considered high risk surgeries. Insertions have been completed in over 90% of attempts. Possible complications include diarrhea, skin irritation due to leakage around the stoma, and difficulties with tube placement.

Tube enterostomy is becoming more frequent due to great advances in minimally invasive techniques and new materials used for stoma construction. However, one recent radiograph study of 289 patients who had jejunostomy found that 14% of patients suffered one or more complications, 19% had problems related to the location or function of the tube, and 9% developed thickened small-bowel folds.

Normal results

Recovery without complications is the norm for this surgery. The greatest challenge is educating the patient on proper stoma usage and types of nutritional support that must be used.

Morbidity and mortality rates

Some feeding or tube stomas have the likelihood of complications. A review of 1,000 patients indicated that PEG tube placement has mortality in 0.5%, with major complications (stomal leakage, peritonitis [infection in the abdomen], traumatized tissue of the abdominal wall, and gastric [stomach] hemorrhage) in 1% of cases. Wound infection, leaks, tube movement or migration, and fever occurred in 8% of patients. In a review of seven published studies, re-

searchers found that a single intravenous dose of a broad-spectrum antibiotic was very effective in reducing infections with the stoma. Open surgery always carries with it a small percentage of cardiac complications, blood clots, and infections. Many gastric stoma patients have complicated diseases that increase the likelihood of surgical complications.

Alternatives

Oral routes are always the preferred method of providing nutritional intake. Intravenous fluid intake can be used as an eating substitute, but only for a short period of time. It is the preferred alternative when adequate protein and calories cannot be provided by oral or other enteral routes, or when the gastrointestinal system is not functioning.

Resources

BOOKS

Feldman, M.D., Mark. *Sleisenger & Fordtran's Gastrointestinal and Liver Disease,* 7th ed. Elsevier, 2002.

Townsend, Courtney M. *Sabiston Textbook of Surgery,* 16th ed. W. B. Saunders Company, 2001.

PERIODICALS

ASPEN Board of Directors and the Clinical Guidelines Task Force. "Guidelines for the Use of Parenteral and Enteral Nutrition in Adult and Pediatric Patients." *Journal of Parenteral Enteral Nutrition* 26, no.1 (Suppl) (January/February 2002).

Chin, A. and N.J. Espat. "Total Gastrectomy: Options for the Restoration of Gastrointestinal Continuity." *The Lancet Oncology* 4, no.5 (May 2003).

Marik, P.E. and G.P. Zaloga. "Early Enteral Nutrition in Acutely Ill Patients: A Systematic Review." *Critical Care Medicine* 29, no.12 (December 2001).

Mentec, H., et.al. "Upper Digestive Intolerance During Enteral Nutrition in Critically Ill Patients: Frequency, Risk Factors, and Complications." *Critical Care Medicine* 29, no.10 (October 2001).

ORGANIZATIONS

American Society Parenteral and Enteral Nutrition. 8630 Fenton St., Suite 412, Silver Springs, Maryland 20910. (301) 587-6315. Fax: (301) 587-2365. <www.clinnutr.org>.

United Ostomy Association, Inc. 19772 MacArthur Blvd., Suite 200, Irvine, CA 92612-2405. (800) 826-0826. <www.uoa.org>.

OTHER

Tube Feeding. Patient Handout, MDConsult,<www.MD Consult.com>.

Nancy McKenzie, Ph.D.

Tube feeding *see* **Tube enterostomy**

Tummy tuck *see* **Abdominoplasty**

Tumor marker tests

Definition

Tumor markers are a group of proteins, hormones, enzymes, receptors, and other cellular products that are overexpressed (produced in higher than normal amounts) by malignant cells. Tumor markers are usually normal cellular constituents that are present at normal or very low levels in the blood of healthy persons. If the substance in question is produced by the tumor, its levels will be increased either in the blood or in the tissue of origin.

Purpose

The majority of tumor markers are used to monitor patients for recurrence of tumors following treatment. In addition, some markers are associated with a more aggressive course and higher relapse rate and have value in staging and prognosis of the cancer. Most tumor markers are not useful for screening because levels found in early malignancy overlap the range of levels found in healthy persons. The levels of most tumor markers are elevated in conditions other than malignancy, and are therefore not useful in establishing a diagnosis.

Precautions

Tumor markers are sometimes elevated in nonmalignant conditions. Not every tumor will cause a rise in the level of its associated marker, especially in the early stages of some cancers. When a marker is used for cancer screening or diagnosis, the physician must confirm a positive test result by using imaging studies, tissue biopsies, and other procedures. False positive results may occur in laboratory tests when the patient has cross-reacting antibodies that interfere with the test.

Description

Physicians use changes in tumor marker levels to follow the course of a patient's disease, to measure the effect of treatment, and to check for recurrence of certain cancers. Tumor markers have been identified in several types of cancer, including malignant melanoma; multiple myeloma; and bone, breast, colon, gastric, liver, lung, ovarian, pancreatic, prostate, renal, and uterine cancers. Serial measurements of a tumor marker are often an effective means to monitor the course of therapy. Some tumor markers can provide physicians with information used in staging cancers, and some help predict the response to treatment. A decrease in the levels of the tumor marker during treatment indicates that the therapy is having a positive effect on the cancer, while an increase indicates that the cancer is growing and not responding to the therapy.

Types of tumor markers

There are five basic types of tumor markers.

ENZYMES. Many enzymes that occur in certain tissues are found in blood plasma at higher levels when the cancer involves that tissue. Enzymes are usually measured by determining the rate at which they convert a substrate to an end product, while most tumor markers of other types are measured by a test called an immunoassay. Some examples of enzymes whose levels rise in cases of malignant diseases are acid phosphatase, alkaline phosphatase, amylase, creatine kinase, gamma glutamyl transferase, lactate dehydrogenase, and terminal deoxynucleotidyl transferase.

TISSUE RECEPTORS. Tissue receptors, which are proteins associated with the cell membrane, are another type of tumor marker. These substances bind to hormones and growth factors, and therefore affect the rate of tumor growth. Some tissue receptors must be measured in tissue samples removed for a biopsy, while others are secreted into the extracellular fluid (fluid outside the cells) and may be measured in the blood. Some important receptor tumor markers are estrogen receptor, progesterone receptor, interleukin-2 receptor, and epidermal growth factor receptor.

ANTIGENS. Oncofetal antigens are proteins made by genes that are very active during fetal development but function at a very low level after birth. The genes become activated when a malignant tumor arises and produce large amounts of protein. Antigens comprise the largest class of tumor marker and include the tumor-associated glycoprotein antigens. Important tumor markers in this class are alpha-fetoprotein (AFP), carcinoembryonic antigen (CEA), prostate specific antigen (PSA), cathespin-D, HER-2/neu, CA-125, CA-19-9, CA-15-3, nuclear matrix protein, and bladder tumor-associated antigen.

ONCOGENES. Some tumor markers are the product of oncogenes, which are genes that are active in fetal development and trigger the growth of tumors when they are activated in mature cells. Some important oncogenes are BRAC-1, myc, p53, RB (retinoblastoma) gene (RB), and Ph[1] (Philadelphia chromosome).

HORMONES. The fifth type of tumor marker consists of hormones. This group includes hormones that are normally secreted by the tissue in which the malignancy arises as well as those produced by tissues that do not normally make the hormone (ectopic production). Some hormones associated with malignancy are adrenal corticotropic hormone (ACTH), calcitonin, catecholamines, gastrin, human chorionic gonadogropin (hCG), and prolactin.

Tumor markers in clinical use

Currently, there are over 60 analytes that are used as tumor markers. All of the enzymes and hormones mentioned above have been approved as tumor markers by the Food and Drug Administration (FDA), but most of the others are not; they have been designated for investigation purposes only. The following list describes the most commonly used tumor markers approved by the FDA for screening, diagnosis, or monitoring of cancer.

• Alpha-fetoprotein (AFP): AFP is a glycoprotein produced by the developing fetus, but its blood levels decline after birth. Healthy adults who are not pregnant rarely have detectable levels of AFP in their blood. The AFP test is primarily used for prenatal diagnoses of spina bifida and other abnormalities associated with cerebrospinal fluid leakage during embryonic development. In adult males and nonpregnant females, an AFP above 300 ng/L is often associated with cancer, although levels in this range may be seen in nonmalignant liver diseases. Levels above 1000 ng/L are almost always associated with cancer. AFP has been approved by the FDA for the diagnosis and monitoring of patients with non-seminoma testicular cancer. It is elevated in almost all yolk sac tumors and 80% of malignant liver tumors.

• CA-125: Measurement of this tumor marker is FDA-approved for the diagnosis and monitoring of women with ovarian cancer. Approximately 75% of persons with ovarian cancer shed CA-125 into the blood and

have elevated serum levels. This figure includes approximately 50% of persons with Stage I disease and 90% with Stage II or higher. Elevated levels of CA-125 are also found in approximately 20% of persons with pancreatic cancer. Other cancers detected by this marker include malignancies of the liver, colon, breast, lung, and digestive tract. Test results, however, are affected by pregnancy and menstruation. Benign diseases detected by the test include endometriosis, ovarian cysts, fibroids, inflammatory bowel disease, cirrhosis, peritonitis, and pancreatitis. CA-125 levels correlate with tumor mass; consequently, this test is used to determine whether recurrence of the cancer has occurred following chemotherapy. Some patients, however, have a recurrence of their cancer without a corresponding increase in the level of CA-125.

• Carcinoembryonic antigen (CEA): CEA is a glycoprotein that is part of the normal cell membrane. It is shed into blood serum and reaches very high levels in colorectal cancer. Over 50% of persons with breast, colon, lung, gastric, ovarian, pancreatic, and uterine cancer have elevated levels of CEA. CEA levels in plasma are monitored in patients with tumors that secrete this antigen to determine if **second-look surgery** should be performed. CEA levels may also be elevated in inflammatory bowel disease (IBD), pancreatitis, and liver disease. Heavy smokers and about 5% of healthy persons have elevated plasma levels of CEA.

• Prostate specific antigen (PSA): PSA is a small glycoprotein with protease activity that is specific for prostate tissue. The antigen is present in low levels in all adult males, which means that an elevated level may require additional testing to confirm that cancer is the cause. High levels are seen in prostate cancer, benign prostatic hypertrophy, and inflammation of the prostate. PSA is approved as a screening test for prostatic carcinoma. PSA has been found to be elevated in more than 60% of persons with Stage A and more than 70% with Stage B cancer of the prostate. It has replaced the use of prostatic acid phosphatase for prostate cancer screening because it is far more sensitive. Most PSA is bound to antitrypsins in plasma but some PSA circulates unbound to protein (free PSA). Persons with a borderline total PSA (between 4–10 ng/L), but who have a low free PSA are more likely to have malignant prostate disease.

• Estrogen receptor (ER): ER is a protein found in the nucleus of breast and uterine tissues. The level of ER in the tissue is used to determine whether a person with breast cancer is likely to respond to estrogen therapy with tamoxifen, which binds to the receptors blocking the action of estrogen. Women who are ER-negative have a greater risk of recurrence than women who are

ER-positive. Tissue levels are measured using one of two methods. The tissue can be homogenized into a cytosol, and an immunoassay used to measure the concentration of ER receptor protein. Alternatively, the tissue is frozen and thin-sectioned. An immunoperoxidase stain is used to detect and measure the estrogen receptors in the tissue.

• Progesterone receptor (PR): PR consists of two proteins, like the estrogen receptor, which are located in the nuclei of both breast and uterine tissues. PR has the same prognostic value as ER, and is measured by similar methods. Tissue that does not express the PR receptors is less likely to bind estrogen analogs used to treat the tumor. Persons who test negative for both ER and PR have less than a 5% chance of responding to endocrine therapy. Those who test positive for both markers have greater than a 60% chance of tumor shrinkage when treated with hormone therapy.

• Human chorionic gonadotropin (hCG): hCG is a glycoprotein produced by cells of the trophoblast and developing placenta. Very high levels are produced by trophoblastic tumors and choriocarcinoma. About 60% of testicular cancers secrete hCG. hCG is also produced less frequently by a number of other tumors. Some malignancies cause an increase in alpha and/or beta hCG subunits in the absence of significant increases in intact hCG. For this reason, separate tests have been developed for alpha and beta hCG, and most laboratories use these assays as tumor marker tests. Most EIA tests for pregnancy are specific for hCG, but detect the whole molecule and are called intact hCG assays.

• Nuclear matrix protein (NMP22) and bladder tumor-associated analytes (BTA): NMP22 is a structural nuclear protein that is released into the urine when bladder carcinoma cells die. Approximately 70% of bladder carcinomas are positive for NMP22. BTA is comprised of type IV collagen, fibronectin, laminin, and proteoglycan, which are components of the basement membrane that are released into the urine when bladder tumor cells attach to the basement membrane of the bladder wall. These products can be detected in urine using a mixture of antibodies to the four components. BTA is elevated in about 30% of persons with low-grade bladder tumors and over 60% of persons with high-grade tumors.

Preparation

Determination of the circulating level of tumor markers requires a blood test performed by a laboratory scientist. A nurse or phlebotomist usually draws the patient's blood; he or she ties a tourniquet above the patient's elbow, locates a vein near the inner elbow, cleanses the skin overlying the vein with an antiseptic solution, and in-

serts a sterile needle into that vein. The blood is drawn through the needle into an attached vacuum tube. Collection of a blood sample takes only a few minutes.

Tissue samples are collected by a physician at the time of surgical or needle biopsy. A urine sample is collected by the patient, using the midstream void technique.

Aftercare

Aftercare following a blood test consists of routine care of the area around the puncture site. Pressure is applied for a few seconds and the wound is covered with a bandage. If a bruise or swelling develops around the puncture site, the area is treated with a moist warm compress.

Risks

The risks associated with drawing blood include dizziness, bruising, swelling, or excessive bleeding from the puncture site. As previously mentioned, the results of blood tests should be interpreted with caution. A single test result may not yield clinically useful information. Several laboratory reports over a period of months may be needed to evaluate treatment and identify recurrence. Positive results must be interpreted cautiously because some tumor markers are increased in nonmalignant diseases and in a small number of apparently healthy persons. In addition false negative results may occur because the tumor does not produce the marker, and because levels seen in healthy persons may overlap those seen in the early stages of cancer. A false positive result occurs when the value is elevated even though cancer is not present. A false negative result occurs when the value is normal but cancer is present.

Normal results

Reference ranges for tumor markers will vary from one laboratory to another because different antibodies and calibrators are used by various test systems. The values below are representative of normal values or cutoffs for commonly measured tumor markers.

• Alpha-fetoprotein (AFP): Less than 15 ng/L in men and nonpregnant women. Levels greater than 1,000 ng/L indicate malignant disease (except in pregnancy).

• CA125: Less than 35 U/mL.

• Carcinoembryonic antigen (CEA): Less than 3 μg/L for nonsmokers and less than 5 μg/L for smokers.

• Estrogen receptor: Less than 6 fmol/mg protein is negative; greater than 10 fmol/mg protein is positive.

• Human chorionic gonadotropin (HCG): Less than 20 IU/L for males and non-pregnant females. Greater than 100,00 IU/L indicates trophoblastic tumor.

KEY TERMS

Analyte—A material or chemical substance subjected to analysis.

Antitrypsin—A substance that inhibits the action of trypsin.

Biopsy—The removal of living tissue from the body, done in order to establish a diagnosis.

Glycoprotein—Any of a group of complex proteins that consist of a carbohydrate combined with a simple protein. Some tumor markers are glycoproteins.

Immunoassay—A laboratory method for detecting the presence of a substance by using an antibody that reacts with it.

Multiple myeloma—An uncommon disease that occurs more often in men than in women and is associated with anemia, hemorrhage, recurrent infections and weakness. Ordinarily it is regarded as a malignant neoplasm that originates in bone marrow and involves mainly the skeleton.

Oncogene—A gene that is capable under certain conditions of triggering the conversion of normal cells into cancer cells.

Oncologist—A physician who specializes in the diagnosis and treatment of tumors.

Overexpression—Production in abnormally high amounts.

Serum (plural, sera)—The clear, pale yellow liquid part of blood that separates from a clot when the blood coagulates.

Staging—The classification of cancerous tumors according to the extent of the tumor.

Substrate—A substance acted upon by an enzyme.

• Progesterone receptor: Less than 6 fmol/mg protein is negative. Greater than 10 fmol/mg protein is positive.

• Prostate specific antigen (PSA): Less than 4 ng/L.

Resources

BOOKS

Burtis, C.A., and E.R. Ashwood, eds. *Tietz Fundamentals of Clinical Chemistry*, 5th ed. Philadelphia, PA: Saunders, 2001.

Henry, J.B., ed. *Clinical Diagnosis and Management by Laboratory Methods*, 20th ed. Philadelphia, PA: Saunders, 2001.

"Tumor Immunology." Section 11, Chapter 143 in *The Merck Manual of Diagnosis and Therapy*, edited by Mark H. Beers, MD, and Robert Berkow, MD. Whitehouse Station, NJ: Merck Research Laboratories, 1999.

Wallach, Jacques. *Interpretation of Diagnostic Tests*, 7th ed. Philadelphia, PA: Lippincott Williams & Wilkens, 2000.

ORGANIZATIONS

American Cancer Society. 1599 Clifton Rd. NE, Atlanta, GA 30329-4251. (800) 227-2345. <www.cancer.org>.

American Society of Clinical Oncology (ASCO). 1900 Duke Street, Suite 200, Alexandria, VA 22314. (703) 299-0150. <www.asco.org>.

National Cancer Institute (NCI). NCI Public Inquiries Office, Suite 3036A, 6116 Executive Boulevard, MSC8332, Bethesda, MD 20892-8322. (800) 4-CANCER or (800) 332-8615 (TTY). <www.nci.nih.gov>.

United States Food and Drug Administration (FDA). 5600 Fishers Lane, Rockville, MD 20857-0001. (888) INFO-FDA. <www.fda.gov>.

OTHER

Abbott Laboratories. <www.abbottdiagnostics.com/medical_conditions/cancer/index.htm/>.

National Institutes of Health. <www.nlm.nih.gov/medlineplus/encyclopedia.html> [cited April 5, 2003].

Tumor Marker Tests. <www.secundus.vh.org/adult/patient/cancercenter/tumormarker/index.html> July, 2002 [cited April 4, 2003].

Victoria E. DeMoranville
Mark A. Best

Tumor removal

Definition

A tumor is an abnormal growth caused by the uncontrolled division of cells. Benign tumors do not have the potential to spread to other parts of the body (a process called metastasis) and are curable by surgical removal. Malignant or cancerous tumors, however, may metastasize to other parts of the body and will ultimately result in death if not successfully treated by surgery and/or other methods.

Purpose

Surgical removal is one of four main ways that tumors are treated. Chemotherapy, radiation therapy, and biological therapy are other treatment options. There are a number of factors used to determine which methods will best treat a tumor. Because benign tumors do not have the potential to metastasize, they are often treated successfully with surgical removal alone. Malignant tumors, however, are most often treated with a combination of surgery and chemotherapy and/or radiation therapy (in about 55% of cases). In some instances, non-curative surgery may make other treatments more effective. Debulking a cancer—making it smaller by surgical removal of a large part of it—is thought to make radiation and chemotherapy more effective.

Surgery is often used to accurately assess the nature and extent of a cancer. Most cancers cannot be adequately identified without examining a sample of the abnormal tissue under a microscope. Such tissue samples are procured during a surgical procedure. Surgery may also be used to determine exactly how far a tumor has spread.

There are a few standard methods of comparing one cancer to another for the purposes of determining appropriate treatments and estimating outcomes. These methods are referred to as staging. The most commonly used method is the TNM system.

- "T" stands for *tumor* and reflects the size of the tumor.

- "N" represents the spread of the cancer to lymph *nodes*, largely determined by those nodes removed at surgery that contain cancer cells. Since cancers spread mostly through the lymphatic system, this is a useful measure of a cancerís ability to disperse.

- "M" refers to *metastasis* and indicates if metastases are present and how far they are from the original cancer.

Staging is particularly important with such lymphomas as Hodgkin's disease, which may appear in many places in the lymphatic system. Surgery is a useful tool for staging such cancers and can increase the chance of a successful cure, since radiation treatment is often curative if all the cancerous sites are located and irradiated.

Demographics

The American Cancer Society estimates that approximately one million cases of cancer are diagnosed in the United States each year. Seventy-seven percent of cancers are diagnosed in men and women over the age of 55, although cancer may affect individuals of any age. Men develop cancer more often than women; one in two men will be diagnosed with cancer during his lifetime, compared to one in three women. Cancer affects individuals of all races and ethnicities, al-

though incidence may differ among these groups by cancer type.

WHO PERFORMS THE PROCEDURE AND WHERE IS IT PERFORMED?

Tumors are usually removed by a general surgeon or surgical oncologist. The procedure is frequently done in a hospital setting, but specialized outpatient facilities may sometimes be used.

Description

Surgery may be used to remove tumors for diagnostic or therapeutic purposes.

Diagnostic tumor removal

A biopsy is a medical procedure that obtains a small piece of tissue for diagnostic testing. The sample is examined under a microscope by a doctor who specializes in the effects of disease on body tissues (a pathologist) to detect any abnormalities. A definitive diagnosis of cancer cannot be made unless a sample of the abnormal tissue is examined histologically (under a microscope).

There are four main biopsy techniques used to diagnose cancer. These include:

- Aspiration biopsy. A needle is inserted into the tumor and a sample is withdrawn. This procedure may be performed under local anesthesia or with no anesthesia at all.

- Needle biopsy. A special cutting needle is inserted into the core of the tumor and a core sample is cut out. Local anesthesia is most often administered.

- Incisional biopsy. A portion of a large tumor is removed, usually under local anesthesia in an outpatient setting.

- Excisional biopsy. An entire cancerous lesion is removed along with surrounding normal tissue (called a clear margin). Local or general anesthesia may be used.

Therapeutic tumor removal

Once surgical removal has been decided, a surgical oncologist will remove the entire tumor, taking with it a large section of the surrounding normal tissue. The healthy tissue is removed to minimize the risk that abnormal tissue is left behind.

When surgical removal of a tumor is unacceptable as a sole treatment, a portion of the tumor is removed to debulk the mass; this is called cytoreduction. Cytoreductive surgery aids radiation and chemotherapy treatments by increasing the sensitivity of the tumor and decreasing the number of necessary treatment cycles.

In some instances the purpose of tumor removal is not to cure the cancer, but to relieve the symptoms of a patient who cannot be cured. This approach is called palliative surgery. For example, a patient with advanced cancer may have a tumor causing significant pain or bleeding; in such a case, the tumor may be removed to ease the patient's pain or other symptoms even though a cure is not possible.

Seeding

The surgical removal of malignant tumors demands special considerations. There is a danger of spreading cancerous cells during the process of removing abnormal tissue (called seeding). Presuming that cancer cells can implant elsewhere in the body, the surgeon must minimize the dissemination of cells throughout the operating field or into the blood stream.

Special techniques called block resection and no-touch are used. Block resection involves taking the entire specimen out as a single piece. The no-touch technique involves removing a specimen by handling only the normal tissue surrounding it; the cancer itself is never touched. These approaches prevent the spread of cancer cells into the general circulation. Pains are taken to clamp off the blood supply first, preventing cells from leaving by that route later in the surgery.

Diagnosis/Preparation

A tumor may first be palpated (felt) by the patient or by a health care professional during a **physical exami-** **nation**. A tumor may be visible on the skin or protrude outward from the body. Still other tumors are not evident until their presence begins to cause such symptoms as weight loss, fatigue, or pain. In some instances, tumors are located during routine tests (e.g. a yearly mammogram or Pap test).

Aftercare

Retesting and periodical examinations are necessary to ensure that a tumor has not returned or metastasized after total removal.

Risks

Each tumor removal surgery carries certain risks that are inherent to the procedure. There is always a risk of misdiagnosing a cancer if an inadequate sample was procured during biopsy, or if the tumor was not properly located. There is a chance of infection of the surgical site, excessive bleeding, or injury to adjacent tissues. The possibility of metastasis and seeding are risks that have to be considered in consultation with an oncologist.

Normal results

The results of a tumor removal procedure depend on the type of tumor and the purpose of the treatment. Most benign tumors can be removed successfully with no risk of the abnormal cells spreading to other parts of the body and little risk of the tumor returning. Malignant tumors are considered successfully removed if the entire tumor can be removed, if a clear margin of healthy tissue is removed with the tumor, and if there is no evidence of metastasis. The normal results of palliative tumor removal are a reduction in the patient's symptoms with no impact on survival.

Morbidity and mortality rates

The recurrence rates of benign and malignant tumors after removal depend on the type of tumor and its location. The rate of complications associated with tumor removal surgery differs by procedure, but is generally very low.

Alternatives

If a benign tumor shows no indication of harming nearby tissues and is not causing the patient any symptoms, surgery may not be required to remove it. Chemotherapy, radiation therapy, and biological therapy are treatments that may be used alone or in conjunction with surgery.

Resources

BOOKS

Abeloff, Martin D., James O. Armitage, Allen S. Lichter, and John E. Niederhuber. "Cancer Management." *Clinical On-*

cology, 2nd ed. Philadelphia, PA: Churchill Livingstone, Inc., 2000.

"Principles of Cancer Therapy: Surgery." Section 11, Chapter 144 in *The Merck Manual of Diagnosis and Therapy*, edited by Mark H. Beers, MD, and Robert Berkow, MD. Whitehouse Station, NJ: Merck Research Laboratories, 1999.

ORGANIZATIONS

American Cancer Society. 1599 Clifton Rd. NE, Atlanta, GA 30329-4251. (800) 227-2345. <www.cancer.org>.

National Cancer Institute (NCI). NCI Public Inquiries Office, Suite 3036A, 6116 Executive Boulevard, MSC8332, Bethesda, MD 20892-8322. (800) 4-CANCER or (800) 332-8615 (TTY). <www.nci.nih.gov>.

Society of Surgical Oncologists. 85 West Algonquin Rd., Suite 550, Arlington Heights, IL 60005. (847) 427-1400. <www.surgonc.org>.

OTHER

American Cancer Society. *All About Cancer: Detailed Guide*, 2003 [cited April 9, 2003]. <www.cancer.org/docroot/CRI/CRI_2_3.asp>.

J. Ricker Polsdorfer, MD
Stephanie Dionne Sherk

TURP *see* **Transurethral resection of the prostate**

Tylenol *see* **Acetaminophen**

Tympanoplasty

Definition

Tympanoplasty, also called eardrum repair, refers to surgery performed to reconstruct a perforated tympanic membrane (eardrum) or the small bones of the middle ear. Eardrum perforation may result from chronic infection or, less commonly, from trauma to the eardrum.

Purpose

The tympanic membrane of the ear is a three-layer structure. The outer and inner layers consist of epithelium cells. Perforations occur as a result of defects in the middle layer, which contains elastic collagen fibers. Small perforations usually heal spontaneously. However, if the defect is relatively large, or if there is a poor blood supply or an infection during the healing process, spontaneous repair may be hindered. Eardrums may also be perforated as a result of trauma, such as an object in the ear, a slap on the ear, or an explosion.

The purpose of tympanoplasty is to repair the perforated eardrum, and sometimes the middle ear bones (ossicles) that consist of the incus, malleus, and stapes. Tympanic membrane grafting may be required. If needed, grafts are usually taken from a vein or fascia (muscle sheath) tissue on the lobe of the ear. Synthetic materials may be used if patients have had previous surgeries and have limited graft availability.

Demographics

In the United States, ear disorders leading to hearing loss affect all ages. Over 60% of the population with hearing loss is under the age of 65, although nearly 25% of those above age 65 have a hearing loss that is considered significant. Causes include: birth defect (4.4%), ear infection (12.2%), ear injury (4.9%), damage due to excessive noise levels (33.7%), advanced age (28%), and other problems (16.8%).

Description

There are five basic types of tympanoplasty procedures:

- Type I tympanoplasty is called myringoplasty, and only involves the restoration of the perforated eardrum by grafting.

- Type II tympanoplasty is used for tympanic membrane perforations with erosion of the malleus. It involves grafting onto the incus or the remains of the malleus.

- Type III tympanoplasty is indicated for destruction of two ossicles, with the stapes still intact and mobile. It involves placing a graft onto the stapes, and providing protection for the assembly.

- Type IV tympanoplasty is used for ossicular destruction, which includes all or part of the stapes arch. It involves placing a graft onto or around a mobile stapes footplate.

- Type V tympanoplasty is used when the footplate of the stapes is fixed.

Depending on its type, tympanoplasty can be performed under local or general anesthesia. In small perforations of the eardrum, Type I tympanoplasty can be easily performed under local anesthesia with intravenous sedation. An incision is made into the ear canal and the remaining eardrum is elevated away from the bony ear canal, and lifted forward. The surgeon uses an operating microscope to enlarge the view of the ear structures. If the perforation is very large or the hole is far forward and away from the view of the surgeon, it may be necessary to perform an incision behind the ear. This elevates the entire outer ear forward, providing access to the perforation. Once the hole is fully exposed, the perforated remnant is rotated forward, and the bones of hearing are inspected. If scar tissue is present, it is removed either with micro hooks or laser.

Tissue is then taken either from the back of the ear, the tragus (small cartilaginous lobe of skin in front the ear), or from a vein. The tissues are thinned and dried. An absorbable gelatin sponge is placed under the eardrum to support the graft. The graft is then inserted underneath the remaining eardrum remnant, which is folded back onto the perforation to provide closure. Very thin sheeting is usually placed against the top of the graft to prevent it from sliding out of the ear when the patient sneezes.

If it was opened from behind, the ear is then stitched together. Usually, the stitches are buried in the skin and do not have to be removed later. A sterile patch is placed on the outside of the ear canal and the patient returns to the **recovery room**.

Diagnosis/Preparation

The examining physician performs a complete physical with diagnostic testing of the ear, which includes an audiogram and history of the hearing loss, as well as any vertigo or facial weakness. A microscopic exam is also performed. Otoscopy is used to assess the mobility of the tympanic membrane and the malleus. A fistula test can be performed if there is a history of dizziness or a marginal perforation of the eardrum.

Preparation for surgery depends upon the type of tympanoplasty. For all procedures, however; blood and urine studies, and hearing tests are conducted prior to surgery.

Aftercare

Generally, the patient can return home within two to three hours. **Antibiotics** are given, along with a mild pain reliever. After 10 days, the packing is removed and the ear is evaluated to see if the graft was successful. Water is kept away from the ear, and nose blowing is discouraged. If there are allegies or a cold, antibiotics and a decongestant are usually prescribed. Most patients can return to work after five or six days, or two to three weeks if they perform heavy physical labor. After three weeks, all packing is completely removed under the operating microscope. It is then determined whether or not the graft has fully taken.

Post-operative care is also designed to keep the patient comfortable. Infection is generally prevented by soaking the ear canal with antibiotics. To heal, the graft must be kept free from infection, and must not experience shearing forces or excessive tension. Activities that change the tympanic pressure are forbidden, such as sneezing with the mouth shut, using a straw to drink, or heavy nose blowing. A complete hearing test is performed four to six weeks after the operation.

Tympanoplasty

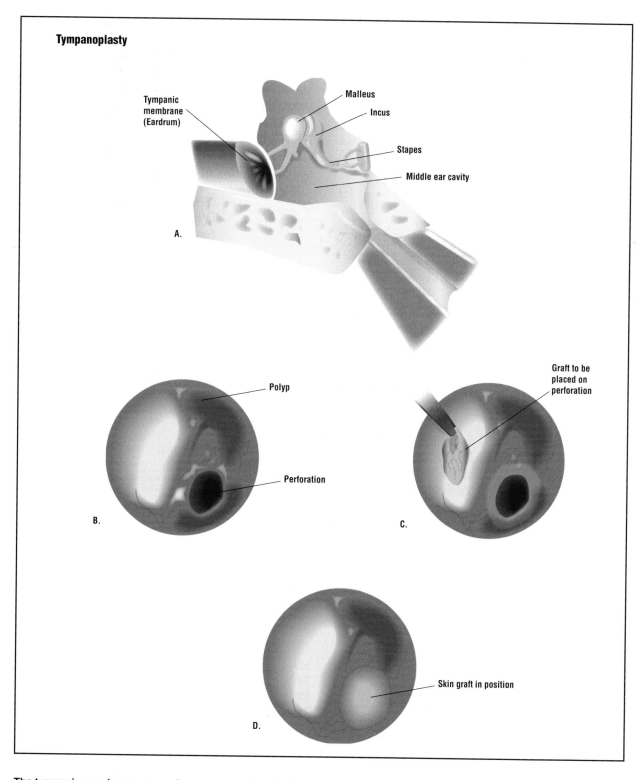

The tympanic membrane, or ear drum, may need surgical repair when punctured (A). During a type I tympanoplasty, a perforation in the ear drum is visualized (B). A tissue graft is placed over the perforation (C) and held in place by the existing ear drum (D). *(Illustration by GGS Inc.)*

QUESTIONS TO ASK THE DOCTOR

- Are there any other options aside from tympanoplasty?
- How will the surgery impact hearing?
- How long will it take to recover from the surgery?
- What are the possible complications?
- How many tympanoplasty surgeries does the surgeon perform each year?
- How successful is tympanoplasty in restoring normal hearing?

Risks

Possible complications include failure of the graft to heal, causing recurrent eardrum perforation; narrowing (stenosis) of the ear canal; scarring or adhesions in the middle ear; perilymph fistula and hearing loss; erosion or extrusion of the prosthesis; dislocation of the prosthesis; and facial nerve injury. Other problems such as recurrence of cholesteatoma, may or may not result from the surgery.

Tinnitus (noises in the ear), particularly echo-type noises, may be present as a result of the perforation itself. Usually, with improvement in hearing and closure of the eardrum, the tinnitus resolves. In some cases, however, it may worsen after the operation. It is rare for the tinnitus to be permanent after surgery.

Normal results

Tympanoplasty is successful in over 90% of cases. In most cases, the operation relieves pain and infection symptoms completely. Hearing loss is minor.

Morbidity and mortality rates

There can be imbalance and dizziness immediately after this procedure. Dizziness, however, is uncommon in tympanoplasties that only involve the eardrum. Besides failure of the graft, there may be further hearing loss due to unexplained factors during the healing process. This occurs in less than 5% of patients. A total hearing loss from tympanoplasty surgery is rare, occurring in less than 1% of operations. Mild postoperative dizziness and imbalance can persist for about a week after surgery. If the ear becomes infected after surgery, the risk of dizziness increases. Generally, imbalance and dizziness completely disappears after a week or two.

Alternatives

Myringoplasty is another operative procedure used in the reconstruction of a perforation of the tympanic membrane. It is performed when the middle ear space, its mucosa, and the ossicular chain are free of active infection. Unlike tympanoplasty, there is no direct inspection of the middle ear during this procedure.

See also Mastoidectomy.

Resources

BOOKS

Fisch, H. and J. May. *Tympanoplasty, Mastoidectomy, and Stapes Surgery.* New York: Thieme Medical Pub., 1994.

Roland, P. S. *Tympanoplasty: Repair of the Tympanic Membrane.* Continuing Education Program (American Academy of Otolaryngology-Head and Neck Surgery Foundation). Alexandria, VA: American Academy of Otolaryngology, 1994.

Tos, M. *Manual of Middle Ear Surgery: Approaches, Myringoplasty, Ossiculoplasty and Tympanoplasty.* New York: Thieme Medical Pub., 1993.

PERIODICALS

Downey, T. J., A. L. Champeaux, and A. B. Silva. "AlloDerm Tympanoplasty of Tympanic Membrane Perforations." *American Journal of Otolaryngology* 24 (January/February 2003): 6-13.

Duckert, L. G., K. H. Makielski, and J. Helms. "Prolonged Middle Ear Ventilation with the Cartilage Shield T-tube Tympanoplasty." *Otology & Neurotology* 24 (March 2003): 153-7.

Oshima, T., Y. Kasuya, Y. Okumura, E. Terazawa, and S. Dohi. "Prevention of Nausea and Vomiting with Tandospirone in Adults after Tympanoplasty." *Anesthesia & Analgesia* 95 (November 2002): 350-1.

Sheahan, P., T. O'Dwyer, and A. Blayney. "Results of Type 1 Tympanoplasty in Children and Parental Perceptions of Outcome of Surgery." *Journal of Laryngology & Otology* 116 (June 2002): 430-4.

Uzun, C., M. Velepic, D. Manestar, D. Bonifacic, and T. Braut. "Cartilage Palisade Tympanoplasty, Diving and Eustachian Tube Function." *Otology & Neurotology* 24 (March 2003): 350-1.

ORGANIZATIONS

American Academy of Otolaryngology - Head and Neck Surgery. One Prince Street, Alexandria, VA 22314. (703) 806-4444. <www.entnet.org>.

American Hearing Research Foundation. 55 E. Washington St., Suite 2022, Chicago, IL 60602. (312) 726-9670. <http://www.american-hearing.org/>

OTHER

"Perforated Ear Drums." *Audiology Net.* <www.voice-center.com/tmperf.html>.

Tympanoplasty animation. *Otolaryngology Houston:* <www.ghorayeb.com/TympanoplastyPictures.html>.

KEY TERMS

Audiogram—A test of hearing at a range of sound frequencies.

Epithelium—The covering of internal and external surfaces of the body, including the lining of vessels and other small cavities. It consists of cells joined by small amounts of cementing substances.

Fistula test—Compression or rarefaction of the air in the external auditory canal.

Mastoid process—The nipple-like projection of part of the temporal bone (the large irregular bone situated in the base and side of the skull).

Mastoidectomy—Hollowing out the mastoid process by curretting, gouging, drilling, or otherwise removing the bony partitions forming the mastoid cells.

Myringoplasty—Surgical restoration of a perforated tympanic membrane by grafting.

Ossicles—Small bones of the middle ear, called stapes, malleus, and incus.

Ossiculoplasty—Surgical insertion of an implant to replace one or more of the ear ossicles. Also called ossicular replacement.

Otoscopy—Examination of the ear with an otoscope, an instrument designed to evaluate the condition of the ear.

Tinnitus—Noises or ringing in the ear.

"What is Tympanolasty?" *PennHealth.* <www.pennhealth.com/health/hi_files/balance/hi13.html>.

Monique Laberge, Ph.D.

Type and screen

Definition

Blood typing is a laboratory test that identifies blood group antigens (substances that stimulate an immune response) belonging to the ABO blood group system. The test classifies blood into four groups designated A, B, AB, and O. Antibody screening is a test to detect atypical antibodies in the serum that may have been formed as a result of **transfusion** or pregnancy. An antibody is a protein produced by lymphocytes (nongranular white blood cells) that binds to an antigen, facilitating its removal by phagocytosis (or engulfing by macrophages) or lysis (cell rupture or decomposition). The type and screen (T&S) is performed on persons who may need a transfusion of blood products. These tests are followed by the compatibility test (cross-match). This test insures that no antibodies are detected in the recipient's serum that will react with the donor's red blood cells.

Purpose

Blood typing and screening are most commonly performed to ensure that a person who needs a transfusion will receive blood that matches (is compatible with) his or her own; and that clinically significant antibodies are identified if present. People must receive blood of the same blood type; otherwise, a severe transfusion reaction may result.

Prenatal care

Parents who are expecting a baby have their blood typed to diagnose and prevent hemolytic disease of the newborn (HDN), a type of anemia also known as erythroblastosis fetalis. Babies who have a blood type different from their mother's are at risk for developing this disease.

Determination of paternity

A child inherits factors or genes from each parent that determine his or her blood type. This fact makes blood typing useful in paternity testing. The blood types of the child, mother, and alleged father are compared to determine paternity.

Forensic investigations

Legal investigations may require typing of blood or such other body fluids as semen or saliva to identify criminal suspects. In some cases typing is used to identify the victims of crime or major disasters.

Description

Blood typing and screening tests are performed in a blood bank laboratory by technologists trained in blood bank and transfusion services. The tests are performed on blood after it has been separated into cells and serum (the yellow liquid left after the blood cells are removed). Costs for both tests are covered by insurance when the tests are determined to be medically necessary.

Blood bank laboratories are usually located in blood center facilities, such as those operated by the American Red Cross, that collect, process, and supply blood that is donated. Blood bank laboratories are also found in most hospitals and other facilities that prepare blood for transfusion. These laboratories are regulated by the United States Food and Drug Administration (FDA) and are inspected and accredited by a professional association such as the American Association of Blood Banks (AABB).

Blood typing and screening tests are based on the reaction between antigens and antibodies. An antigen can be anything that triggers the body's immune response. The body produces a special protein called an antibody that has a uniquely shaped site that combines with the antigen to neutralize it. A person's body normally does not produce antibodies against its own antigens.

The antigens found on the surface of red blood cells are important because they determine a person's blood type. When red blood cells having a certain blood type antigen are mixed with serum containing antibodies against that antigen, the antibodies combine with and stick to the antigen. In a test tube, this reaction is visible as clumping or aggregating.

Although there are over 600 known red blood cell antigens organized into 22 blood group systems, routine blood typing is usually concerned with only two systems: the ABO and Rh blood group systems. Antibody screening helps to identify antibodies against several other groups of red blood cell antigens.

Blood typing

THE ABO BLOOD GROUP SYSTEM. In 1901, Karl Landsteiner, an Austrian pathologist, randomly combined the serum and red blood cells of his colleagues. From the reactions he observed in test tubes, he developed the ABO blood group system. This discovery earned him the 1930 Nobel Prize in Medicine. A person's ABO blood type—A, B, AB, or O—is based on the presence or absence of the A and B antigens on his red blood cells. The A blood type has only the A antigen and the B blood type has only the B antigen. The AB blood type has both A and B antigens, and the O blood type has neither the A nor the B antigen.

By the time a person is six months old, he or she will have developed antibodies against the antigens that his or her red blood cells lack. That is, a person with A blood type will have anti-B antibodies, and a person with B blood type will have anti-A antibodies. A person with AB blood type will have neither antibody, but a person with O blood type will have both anti-A and anti-B antibodies. Although the distribution of each of the four ABO blood types varies among racial groups, O is the most common and AB is the least common in all groups.

FORWARD AND REVERSE TYPING. ABO typing is the first test done on blood when it is tested for transfusion. A person must receive ABO-matched blood because

ABO incompatibilities are the major cause of fatal transfusion reactions. To guard against these incompatibilities, typing is done in two steps. In the first step, called forward typing, the patient's blood is mixed with serum that contains antibodies against type A blood, then with serum that contains antibodies against type B blood. A determination of the blood type is based on whether or not the blood clots in the presence of these sera.

In reverse typing, the patient's blood serum is mixed with blood that is known to be type A and type B. Again, the presence of clotting is used to determine the type.

An ABO incompatibility between a pregnant woman and her baby is a common cause of HDN but seldom requires treatment. This is because the majority of ABO antibodies are IgM, which are too large to cross the placenta. It is the IgG component that may cause HDN, and this is most often present in the plasma of group O mothers.

Paternity testing compares the ABO blood types of the child, mother, and alleged father. The alleged father cannot be the biological father if the child's blood type requires a gene that neither he nor the mother have. For example, a child with blood type B whose mother has blood type O requires a father with either AB or B blood type; a man with blood type O cannot be the biological father.

In some people, ABO antigens can be detected in body fluids other than blood, such as saliva, sweat, or semen. People whose body fluids contain detectable amounts of antigens are known as secretors. ABO typing of these fluids provides clues in legal investigations.

THE RH BLOOD GROUP SYSTEM. The Rh, or Rhesus, system was first detected in 1940 by Landsteiner and Wiener when they injected blood from rhesus monkeys into guinea pigs and rabbits. More than 50 antigens have since been discovered that belong to this system, making it the most complex red blood cell antigen system.

In routine blood typing and cross-matching tests, only one of these 50 antigens, the D antigen, also known as the Rh factor or $Rh_o[D]$, is tested for. If the D antigen is present, that person is Rh-positive; if the D antigen is absent, that person is Rh-negative.

Other important antigens in the Rh system are C, c, E, and e. These antigens are not usually tested for in routine blood typing tests. Testing for the presence of these antigens, however, is useful in paternity testing, and in cases in which a technologist screens blood to identify unexpected Rh antibodies or find matching blood for a person with antibodies to one or more of these antigens.

Unlike the ABO system, antibodies to Rh antigens don't develop naturally. They develop only as an immune response after a transfusion or during pregnancy. The incidence of the Rh blood types varies between

Recipient's blood			Reactions with donor's red blood cells			
ABO antigens	ABO antibodies	ABO blood type	Donor type O cells	Donor type A cells	Donor type B cells	Donor type AB cells
None	Anti-A Anti-B	O				
A	Anti-B	A				
B	Anti-A	B				
A & B	None	AB				

Compatible   Not compatible

Blood typing is a laboratory test done to discover a person's blood type. If the person needs a blood transfusion, cross-matching is done following blood typing to locate donor blood that the person's body will accept. *(Illustration by Electronic Il-lustrators Group.)*

racial groups, but not as widely as the ABO blood types: 85% of whites and 90% of blacks are Rh-positive; 15% of whites and 10% of blacks are Rh-negative.

The distribution of ABO and Rh blood groups in the overall United States population is as follows:

• O Rh-positive, 38%

• O Rh-negative, 7%

• A Rh-positive, 34%

• A Rh-negative, 6%

• B Rh-positive, 9%

• B Rh-negative, 2%

• AB Rh-positive, 3%

• AB Rh-negative, 1%

In transfusions, the Rh system is next in importance after the ABO system. Most Rh-negative people who receive Rh-positive blood will develop anti-D antibodies. A later transfusion of Rh-positive blood may result in a severe or fatal transfusion reaction.

Rh incompatibility is the most common and severe cause of HDN. This incompatibility may occur when an Rh-negative mother and an Rh-positive father have an Rh-positive baby. Cells from the baby can cross the placenta and enter the mother's bloodstream, causing the mother to make anti-D antibodies. Unlike ABO antibodies, the structure of anti-D antibodies makes it likely that they will cross the placenta and enter the baby's bloodstream. There, they can destroy the baby's red blood cells, causing a severe or fatal anemia.

The first step in preventing HDN is to find out the Rh types of the expectant parents. If the mother is Rh-negative and the father is Rh-positive, the baby is at risk for developing HDN. The next step is performing an antibody screen of the mother's serum to make sure she doesn't already have anti-D antibodies from a previous pregnancy or transfusion. Finally, the Rh-negative mother is given an injection of Rh immunoglobulin (RhIg) at 28 weeks of gestation and again after delivery, if the baby is Rh positive. The RhIg attaches to any Rh-positive cells from the baby in the mother's bloodstream, preventing them from triggering anti-D antibody production in the mother. An Rh-negative woman

FREQUENCY (%) OF ABO AND Rh BLOOD TYPES IN U.S. POPULATION						
Racial Group	**ABO Blood Type**				**Rh Blood Type**	
	O	*A*	*B*	*AB*	*Positive*	*Negative*
Whites	45%	40%	11%	4%	85%	15%
Blacks	49%	27%	20%	4%	90%	10%

(Illustration by Standley Publishing. Courtesy of Gale Group.)

should also receive RhIg following a miscarriage, abortion, or ectopic pregnancy.

OTHER BLOOD GROUP SYSTEMS. Several other blood group systems may be involved in HDN and transfusion reactions, although they are much less common than ABO and Rh incompatibilities. Some of the other groups are the Duffy, Kell, Kidd, MNS, and P systems. Tests for antigens from these systems are not included in routine blood typing, but they are commonly used in paternity testing.

Like Rh antibodies, antibodies in these systems do not develop naturally, but as an immune response after transfusion or during pregnancy. An antibody screening test is done before a cross-match to check for unexpected antibodies to antigens in these systems. A person's serum is mixed in a test tube with commercially prepared cells containing antigens from these systems. If hemagglutination, or clumping, occurs, the antibody is identified.

Antibody screening

Antibody screening is done to look for unexpected antibodies to other blood groups, such as certain Rh (e.g. E, e, C, c), Duffy, MNS, Kell, Kidd, and P system antigens. The recipient's serum is mixed with screening reagent red blood cells. The screening reagent red blood cells are cells with known antigens. This test is sometimes called an indirect antiglobulin or Coombs test. If an antibody to an antigen is present, the mixture will cause agglutination (clumping) of the red blood cells or cause hemolysis (breaking of the red cell membrane). If an antibody to one of these antigens is found, only blood without that antigen will be compatible in a cross-match. This sequence must be repeated before each transfusion a person receives.

Testing for infectious disease markers

As of 2003, pretransfusion testing includes analyzing blood for the following infectious disease markers:

• Hepatitis B surface antigen (HBsAg). This test detects the outer envelope of the heptatitis B virus.

• Antibodies to the core of the hepatitis B virus (Anti-HBc). This test detects an antibody to the hepatitis B virus that is produced during and after an infection.

• Antibodies to the hepatitis C virus (Anti-HCV).

• Antibodies to human immunodeficiency virus, types 1 and 2 (Anti-HIV-1, -2).

• HIV-1 p24 antigen. This test screens for antigens of HIV-1. The advantage of this test is that it can detect HIV-1 infection a week earlier than the antibody test.

• Antibodies to human T-lymphotropic virus, types I and II (Anti-HTLV-I, -II). In the United States, HTLV infection is most common among intravenous drug users.

• Syphilis. This test is performed to detect evidence of infection with the spirochete *Treponema pallidum*.

• Nucleic acid amplification testing (NAT). NAT uses a new form of blood testing technology that directly detects the genetic material of the HCV and HIV viruses.

• Confirmatory tests. These are done to screen out false positives.

Cross-matching

Cross-matching is the final step in pretransfusion testing. It is commonly referred to as compatibility testing, or "type and cross." Before blood from a donor and the recipient are cross-matched, both are ABO and Rh typed. To begin the cross-match, a unit of blood from a donor with the same ABO and Rh type as the recipient is selected. Serum from the patient is mixed with red blood cells from the donor. The cross-match can be performed either as a short (5–10 min) incubation intended only to verify ABO compatibility or as a long (45 min) incubation with an antihuman globulin test intended to verify compatibility for all other red cell antigens. If clumping occurs, the blood is not compatible; if clumping does not occur, the blood is compatible. If an unexpected antibody is found in either the patient or the donor, the blood bank does further testing to ensure that the blood is compatible.

In an emergency, when there is not enough time for blood typing and cross-matching, O red blood cells may be given, preferably Rh-negative. O-type blood is called the universal donor because it has no ABO antigens for a patient's antibodies to combine with. In contrast, AB blood type is called the universal recipient because it has no ABO antibodies to combine with the antigens on transfused red blood cells. If there is time for blood typing, red blood cells of the recipient type (type-specific cells) are given. In either case, the cross-match is continued even though the transfusion has begun.

Autologous donation

The practice of collecting a patient's own blood prior to **elective surgery** for later transfusion is called autologous donation. Since the safest blood for transfusion is the patient's own, autologous donation is particularly useful for patients with rare blood types. Two to four units of blood are collected several weeks before surgery, and the patient is given iron supplements to build up his or her hemoglobin levels.

Preparation

To collect the 10 mL of blood needed for these tests, a healthcare worker ties a tourniquet above the patient's elbow, locates a vein near the inner elbow, cleans the skin overlying the vein, and inserts a needle into that vein. The blood is drawn through the needle into an attached vacuum tube. Collection of the sample takes only a few minutes.

Blood typing and screening must be done three days or less before a transfusion. A person does not need to change diet, medications, or activities before these tests. Patients should tell their health care provider if they have received a blood transfusion or a plasma substitute during the last three months, or have had a radiology procedure using intravenous contrast media. These can give false clumping reactions in both typing and cross-matching tests.

Aftercare

The possible side effects of any blood collection are discomfort, bruising, or excessive bleeding at the site where the needle punctured the skin, as well as dizziness or fainting. Bruising and bleeding is reduced if pressure is applied with a finger to the puncture site until the bleeding stops. Discomfort can be treated with warm packs to the puncture site.

Risks

Aside from the rare event of infection or bleeding, there are no risks from blood collection. Blood transfu-

sions, however, always have the risk of an unexpected transfusion reaction. These complications may include an acute hemolytic transfusion reaction (AHTR), which is most commonly caused by ABO incompatibility. The patient may complain of pain, difficult breathing, fever and chills, facial flushing, and nausea. Signs of shock may appear, including a drop in blood pressure and a rapid but weak pulse. If AHTR is suspected, the transfusion should be stopped at once.

Other milder transfusion reactions include a delayed hemolytic transfusion reaction, which may occur one to two weeks after the transfusion. It consists of a slight fever and a falling **hematocrit**, and is usually self-limited. Patients may also have allergic reactions to unknown components in donor blood.

Normal results

The blood type is labeled as A+, A-, B+, B-, O+, O-, AB+, or AB-, based on both the ABO and Rh systems. If antibody screening is negative, only a cross-match is necessary. If the antibody screen is positive, then blood that is negative for those antigens must be identified. The desired result of a cross-match is that compatible donor blood is found. Compatibility testing procedures are designed to provide the safest blood product possible for the recipient, but a compatible cross-match is no guarantee that an unexpected adverse reaction will not appear during the transfusion.

Except in an emergency, a person cannot receive a transfusion without a compatible cross-match result. In rare cases, the least incompatible blood has to be given.

See also Blood donation and registry; Transfusion.

Resources

BOOKS

Beadling, Wendy V., Laura Cooling, and John B. Henry. "Immunohematology." In *Clinical Diagnosis and Management by Laboratory Methods*, 20th ed., edited by John B. Henry. Philadelphia: W. B. Saunders Company, 2001.

Boral, Leonard I., Edward D. Weiss, and John B. Henry. "Transfusion Medicine." In *Clinical Diagnosis and Management by Laboratory Methods*, 20th ed. Edited by John B. Henry. Philadelphia: W. B. Saunders Company, 2001.

Daniels, Geoff. *Human Blood Groups.* Oxford, UK: Blackwell, 1995.

Issitt, Peter D. and David J. Anstee *Applied Blood Group Serology*, 4th ed. Durham, NC: Montgomery Scientific Publications, 1998.

Triulzi, Darrell J., ed. *Blood Transfusion Therapy: A Physician's Handbook*, 7th ed. Bethesda: American Association of Blood Banks, 2002.

KEY TERMS

ABO blood type—Blood type based on the presence or absence of the A and B antigens on the red blood cells. There are four types: A, B, AB, and O.

Acute hemolytic transfusion reaction (AHTR)—A severe transfusion reaction with abrupt onset, most often caused by ABO incompatibility. Symptoms include difficulty breathing, fever and chills, pain, and sometimes shock.

Antibody—A protein produced by B-lymphocytes that binds to an antigen facilitating its removal by phagocytosis or lysis.

Antigen—Any substance that stimulates the production of antibodies and combines specifically with them.

Autologous donation—Donation of the patient's own blood, made several weeks before elective surgery.

Blood bank—A laboratory that specializes in blood typing, antibody identification, and transfusion services.

Blood type—Any of various classes into which human blood can be divided according to immunological compatibility based on the presence or absence of certain antigens on the red blood cells. Blood types are sometimes called blood groups.

Cross-match—A laboratory test done to confirm that blood from a donor and blood from the recipient are compatible. Serum from each is mixed with red blood cells from the other and observed for hemagglutination.

Ectopic pregnancy—The implantation of a fertilized egg in a woman's fallopian tube instead of the uterus.

Gene—A piece of DNA, located on a chromosome, that determines how such traits as blood type are inherited and expressed.

Hemagglutination—The clumping of red blood cells due to blood type incompatibility.

Hematocrit—The proportion of the volume of a blood sample that consists of red blood cells. It is expressed as a percentage.

Indirect Coombs' test—A test used to screen for unexpected antibodies against red blood cells. The patient's serum is mixed with reagent red blood cells, incubated, washed, tested with antihuman globulin, and observed for clumping.

Lysis—Destruction or decomposition.

Pathologist—A doctor who specializes in the study of diseases. The ABO blood groups were discovered by an Austrian pathologist.

Rh blood type—In general, refers to the blood type based on the presence or absence of the D antigen on the red blood cells. There are, however, other antigens in the Rh system.

Serum (plural, sera)—The clear, pale yellow liquid that separates from a clot when blood coagulates.

Tourniquet—A thin piece of tubing or other device used to stop bleeding or control circulation by compressing the blood vessels in an arm or leg. Health care professionals apply a tourniquet before drawing blood.

Transfusion—The therapeutic introduction of blood or a blood component into a patient's bloodstream.

ORGANIZATIONS

American Association of Blood Banks (AABB). 8101 Glenbrook Road, Bethesda, MD 20814. (301) 907-6977. <www.aabb.org> [cited March 15, 2003].

American College of Obstetricians and Gynecologists. 409 12th Street SW, Washington, DC 20024-2188. (202) 638-5577. <www.acog.org> [cited April 4, 2003].

American Red Cross Blood Services. 430 17th Street NW, Washington, DC 20006. (202) 737-8300. <www.redcross.org>[cited March 15, 2003].

OTHER

American Association of Blood Banks. *All About Blood.* Bethesda, MD: American Association of Blood Banks, <www.aabb.org/All_About_Blood/FAQs/aabb_faqs.htm> June 2002. [cited April 7, 2003].

Mark A. Best

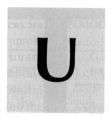

UGI *see* **Upper GI exam**

Ulcer surgery *see* **Vagotomy**

Ultrasonic lithotripsy *see* **Lithotripsy**

Umbilical hernia repair

Definition

An umbilical hernia repair is a surgical procedure performed to fix a weakness in the abdominal wall or to close an opening near the umbilicus (navel) that has allowed abdominal contents to protrude. The abdominal contents may or may not be contained within a membrane or sac. The medical name for a hernia repair is herniorraphy.

Purpose

Umbilical hernias are usually repaired either to relieve discomfort or to prevent complications. It is not always necessary to fix an umbilical hernia. If the person is not in pain, the hernia is often not repaired. Complications may develop if pressure inside the abdomen resulting from daily activity pushes the abdominal contents further through the opening. They may then become twisted or strangulated. Strangulation is a condition in which the circulation to a section of the intestine (or other part of the body) is cut off by compression or constriction; it can cause extreme pain. If the strangulation persists, the tissue can die from lack of blood supply and lead to an infection.

Demographics

An umbilical hernia can occur in both men and women, and can occur at any age, although it is often present at birth. Umbilical hernias are found in about 20% of

newborns, especially in premature infants. Umbilical hernias are more common in male than in female infants; with regard to race, they are eight times more common in African Americans than in Caucasians or Hispanics. While umbilical hernia is not a genetically determined condition, it tends to run in families. In the adult population, umbilical hernias are more common in overweight persons with weak abdominal muscles, and in women who are either pregnant or have borne many children. People with liver disease or fluid in the abdominal cavity are also at higher risk of developing an umbilical hernia.

Description

Repair of an abdominal hernia involves a cut, or incision, in the umbilical area. Most herniorraphies take about two hours to complete. After the patient has been given a sedative, the anesthesiologist will administer a local, spinal, or general anesthetic. The type of anesthesia used depends on the patient's age, general health, and complexity of the procedure. The incision is usually made underneath the belly button. The herniated tissues are isolated and pushed back inside the abdominal cavity. A hernia repair may be done using traditional open surgery or with a laparoscope. A laparoscopic procedure is performed through a few very small incisions. The hole in the abdominal wall may be closed with sutures, or by the use of a fine sterile surgical mesh. The mesh provides additional strength. Some surgeons may choose to use the mesh when repairing a larger hernia. A hernia repair done with a mesh insert is called a tension-free procedure because the surgeon does not have to put tension on the layer of muscle tissue in order to bring the edges of the hole together.

Diagnosis/Preparation

Diagnosis

In children, umbilical hernias are often diagnosed at birth, usually when the doctor feels a lump in the area around the belly button. The hernia may also be diag-

Umbilical hernia repair

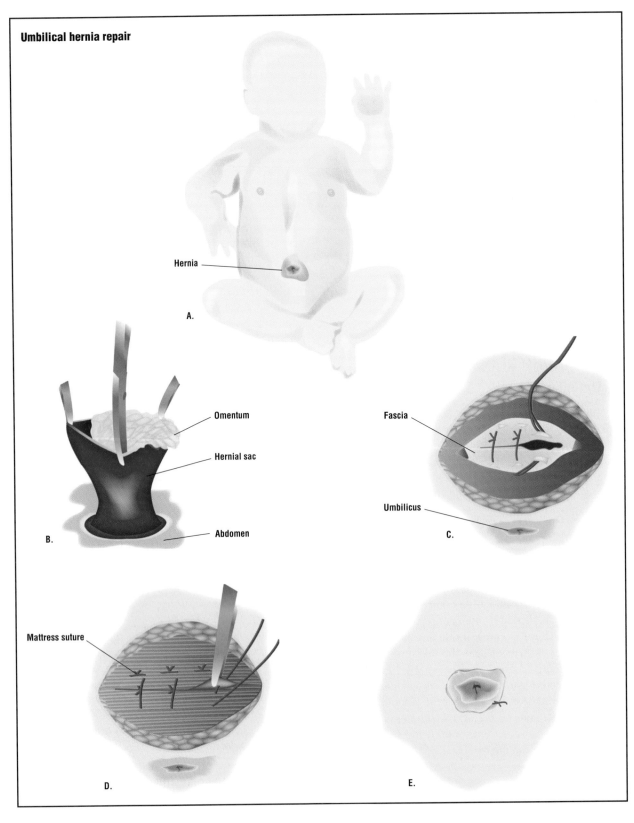

A.

Hernia

B.

Omentum

Hernial sac

Abdomen

C.

Fascia

Umbilicus

D.

Mattress suture

E.

Baby with an umbilical hernia (A). To repair, the hernia is cut open (B), and the contents replaced in the abdomen. Connecting tissues, or fascia, are sutured closed (D), and the skin is repaired (D). *(Illustration by GGS Inc.)*

nosed if the child is crying from pain, because the crying will increase the pressure inside the abdomen and make the hernia more noticeable.

Umbilical hernias in adults occur more often in pregnant women and obese persons with weak stomach muscles. They may develop gradually without producing any discomfort, but the patient may see a bulge in the abdomen while bathing or getting dressed. Other patients consult their doctor because they have felt the tissues in the abdomen suddenly give way when they are having a bowel movement. In an office examination, the patient may be asked to lie down, lift the head, and cough. This action increases pressure inside the abdomen and causes the hernia to bulge outward.

A hernia that has become incarcerated or strangulated is a medical emergency. Its symptoms include:

- nausea
- vomiting
- abdominal swelling or distension
- pale complexion
- weakness or dizziness
- extreme pain

When a hernia is present at birth, some surgeons may opt for a "wait and see" approach, as umbilical hernias in children often close by themselves with time. If the hernia has not closed by the time the child is three or four years old, then surgery is usually considered. If the hernia is very large, surgery may be recommended.

Repair of an umbilical hernia in an adult is usually considered **elective surgery**. The patient's surgeon may recommend the procedure, however, on the grounds that hernias in adults do not close by themselves and tend to grow larger over time.

Preparation

Adults scheduled for a herniorraphy are given standard blood tests and a **urinalysis**. They should not eat breakfast on the morning of the procedure, and they should wear loose-fitting, comfortable clothing that they can easily pull on after the surgery without straining their abdomen.

Aftercare

Aftercare will depend in part on the invasiveness of the surgery, whether laparoscopic or open; the type of anesthesia; the patient's age; and his or her general medical condition. Immediately after the procedure, the person will be taken to the recovery area of the surgical center, where nurses will monitor the patient for signs of ex-

cessive bleeding, infection, uncontrolled pain, or shock. Hernia repairs are usually performed on an outpatient basis, which means that the patient can expect to go home within a few hours of the surgery. Adult patients, however, should arrange to have a friend or relative drive them home. If possible, someone should stay with them for the first night.

The nurses will provide the patient with instructions on **incision care**. The specific instructions will depend on the type of surgery and the way in which the incision was closed. Sometimes a see-through dressing is placed on the wound that the patient can remove about three days after the procedure. It may be necessary to keep the dressing dry until some healing has taken place. Very small incisions may be closed with Steri-strips rather than sutures.

Risks

There are surgical and anesthesia-related risks with all surgical procedures. The primary surgical risks include bleeding and infection. Anesthesia-related risks include reactions to the specific anesthetic agents that are used; interactions with over-the-counter and herbal preparations; and respiratory problems. The greatest risk associated with umbilical hernia is missing the diagnosis. Additional risks include the formation of scar tissue and recurrence of the hernia.

Normal results

Umbilical hernia repair is usually considered an uncomplicated procedure with a relatively short recovery period. A study reported in the December 2002 issue of the American Journal of Surgery found that patients who had laparoscopic surgery with the use of a surgical mesh had fewer complications and reoccurrences of a hernia than those with the traditional open surgery. However, laparoscopic surgery took somewhat longer to perform, possibly because the laparoscopic approach is often used for larger repairs.

Morbidity and mortality rates

In general, there are few complications with hernia repair in children. The most serious complication is surgical injury to the bladder or intestine; fortunately, this complication is very rare—about one in 1000 patients. The recurrence rate is between 1% and 5%; recurrence is more likely in patients with very large hernias. The rate of infection is less than 1%. In the adult population, a November 2001 study reported in the *American Journal of Surgery* found a 5% mortality in elderly patients undergoing emergency hernia repairs.

Alternatives

There are no medical or surgical alternatives to an umbilical hernia repair other than watchful waiting. Since umbilical hernias present at birth often close on their own, intervention can often be delayed until the child is several years old. There is some risk that the hernia will enlarge, however, which increases the risk of incarceration or strangulation.

Resources

BOOKS

"Congenital Anomalies: Gastrointestinal Defects." Section 19, Chapter 261 in *The Merck Manual of Diagnosis and Therapy*, edited by Mark H. Beers, MD, and Robert Berkow, MD. Whitehouse Station, NJ: Merck Research Laboratories, 1999.

Delvin, David. *Coping with a Hernia*. London, UK: Sheldon Press, 1998.

PERIODICALS

Manthey, David, MD. "Hernias." *eMedicine*, June 22, 2001 [June 6, 2003]. <www.emedicine.com/EMERG/topic251.htm>.

Wright, B.E., et al. "Is Laparoscopic Umbilical Hernia Repair with Mesh a Reasonable Alternative to Conventional Repair?" *American Journal of Surgery* 184 (December 2002): 505-508.

ORGANIZATIONS

American Academy of Family Physicians. 11400 Tomahawk Creek Parkway, Leawood, KS 66211-2672. (913) 906-6000. <www.aafp.org>. E-mail: fp@aafp.org

American Academy of Pediatrics. 141 Northwest Point Boulevard, Elk Grove Village, IL 60007-1098. (847) 434-4000; FAX: (847) 434-8000. <www.aap.org>. E-mail: kidsdoc@aap.org

American College of Surgeons. 633 North St. Clair Street, Chicago, IL 60611-3231. (312) 202-5000; FAX: (312) 202-5001. <www.facs.org>.

OTHER

American College of Surgeons. *About Hernia Repair*. <www.facs.org/public_info/operation/hernrep.pdf>.

Esther Csapo Rastegari, R.N., B.S.N., Ed.M.

Undescended testicle repair *see* **Orchiopexy**

Upper GI exam

Definition

An upper GI examination is a fluoroscopic examination (a type of x ray imaging) of the upper gastrointestinal tract, including the esophagus, stomach, and upper small intestine (duodenum).

Purpose

An upper GI series is frequently requested when a patient experiences unexplained symptoms of abdominal pain, difficulty in swallowing (dysphagia), regurgitation, diarrhea, or unexplained weight loss. It is used to help diagnose disorders and diseases of, or related to, the upper gastrointestinal tract. Some of these conditions are: hiatal hernia, diverticula, tumors, obstruction, gastroesophageal reflux disease, pulmonary aspiration, and inflammation (e.g., ulcers, enteritis, and Crohn's disease).

Glucagon, a medication sometimes given prior to an upper GI procedure, may cause nausea and dizziness. It is used to relax the natural movements of the stomach, which will enhance the overall study.

Description

An upper GI series takes place in a hospital or clinic setting, and is performed by an x ray technologist and a radiologist. Before the test begins, the patient is sometimes given a glucagon injection, a medication that slows stomach and bowel activity, to provide the radiologist with a clear picture of the gastrointestinal tract. In order to further improve the upper GI picture clarity, the patient may be given a cup of fizzing crystals to swallow, which distends the esophagus and stomach by producing gas.

Once these preparatory steps are complete, the patient stands against an upright x ray table, and a fluoroscopic screen is placed in front of him or her. The patient will be asked to drink from a cup of flavored barium sulfate, a thick and chalky-tasting liquid, while the radiologist views the esophagus, stomach, and duodenum on the fluoroscopic screen. The patient will be asked to change positions frequently to coat the entire surface of the gastrointestinal tract with barium, move overlapping loops of bowel to isolate each segment, and provide multiple views of each segment. The technician or radiologist may press on the patient's abdomen to spread the barium throughout the folds within the lining of the stomach. The x ray table will also be moved several times throughout the procedure. The radiologist will ask the patient to hold his or her breath periodically while exposures are taken. After the radiologist completes his or her

portion of the exam, the technologist takes three to six additional films of the GI tract. The entire procedure takes approximately 15–30 minutes.

In addition to the standard upper GI series, a physician may request a detailed small bowel follow-through (SBFT), which is a timed series of films. After the preliminary upper GI series is complete, the patient will drink additional barium sulfate, and will be escorted to a waiting area while the barium moves through the small intestines. X rays are initially taken at 15-minute intervals until the barium reaches the colon (the only way to be sure the terminal ileum is fully seen is to see the colon or ileocecal valve). The interval may be increased to 30 minutes, or even one hour if the barium passes slowly. Then the radiologist will obtain additional views of the terminal ileum (the most distal segment of the small bowel, just before the colon). This procedure can take from one to four hours.

Esophageal radiography, also called a barium esophagram or a barium swallow, is a study of the esophagus only, and is usually performed as part of the upper GI series (sometimes only a barium swallow is done). It is commonly used to diagnose the cause of difficulty in swallowing (dysphagia), and to detect a hiatal hernia. The patient drinks a barium sulfate liquid, and sometimes eats barium-coated food while the radiologist examines the swallowing mechanism on a fluoroscopic screen. The test takes approximately 30 minutes.

Preparation

Patients must not eat, drink, or smoke for eight hours prior to undergoing an upper GI examination. Longer dietary restrictions may be required, depending on the type and diagnostic purpose of the test. Patients undergoing a small bowel follow-through exam may be asked to take **laxatives** the day before to the test. Patients are required to wear a hospital gown, or similar attire, and to remove all jewelry, to provide the camera with an unobstructed view of the abdomen.

Aftercare

No special aftercare treatment or regimen is required for an upper GI series. The patient may eat and drink as soon as the test is completed. The barium sulfate may make the patient's stool white for several days, and can cause constipation; therefore patients are encouraged to drink plenty of water to eliminate it from their system.

Risks

Because the upper GI series is an x ray procedure, it does involve minor exposure to ionizing radiation. Un-

KEY TERMS

Crohn's disease—A chronic, inflammatory bowel disease usually affecting the ileum, colon, or both.

Diverticula—Pouch-like herniations through the muscular wall of an organ such as the stomach, small intestine, or colon.

Enteritis—Inflammation of the mucosal lining of the small intestine.

Gastroesophageal reflux disease—A painful, chronic condition in which stomach acid flows back into the esophagus causing heartburn and, in time, erosion of the esophageal lining.

Hiatal hernia—Protrusion of the stomach up through the diaphragm.

less the patient is pregnant, or multiple radiological or fluoroscopic studies are required, the small dose of radiation incurred during a single procedure poses little risk. However, multiple studies requiring fluoroscopic exposure that are conducted in a short time period have been known, on very rare occasions, to cause skin death (necrosis) in some individuals. This risk can be minimized by careful monitoring and documentation of cumulative radiation doses.

Normal results

A normal upper GI series shows a healthy, normally functioning, and unobstructed digestive tract. Hiatal hernia, obstructions, inflammation (including ulcers or polyps of the esophagus, stomach, or small intestine), or irregularities in the swallowing mechanism are just a few of the possible abnormalities that may appear on an upper GI series. Additionally, abnormal peristalsis, or digestive movements of the esophagus, stomach, and small intestine can often be visualized on the fluoroscopic part of the exam, and in the interpretation of the SBFT.

Resources

BOOKS

Ross, Linda, ed. *Gastrointestinal Diseases and Disorders Sourcebook,* Vol. 16. Detroit: Omnigraphics, 1996.

PERIODICALS

Newman, J. "Radiographic and Endoscopic Evaluation of the Upper GI Tract." *Radiology Technology* 69 (January/February 1998): 213-26.

Debra Novograd, B.S., R.T.(R)(M)
Lee A. Shratter, M.D.

Ureteral stenting

Definition

A ureteral stent is a thin, flexible tube threaded into the ureter to help urine drain from the kidney to the bladder or to an external collection system.

Purpose

Urine is normally carried from the kidneys to the bladder via a pair of long, narrow tubes called ureters (each kidney is connected to one ureter). A ureter may become obstructed as a result of a number of conditions including kidney stones, tumors, blood clots, postsurgical swelling, or infection. A ureteral stent is placed in the ureter to restore the flow of urine to the bladder. Ureteral stents may be used in patients with active kidney infection or with diseased bladders (e.g., as a result of cancer or radiation therapy). Alternatively, ureteral stents may be used during or after urinary tract surgical procedures to provide a mold around which healing can occur, to divert the urinary flow away from areas of leakage, to manipulate kidney stones or prevent stone migration prior to treatment, or to make the ureters more easily identifiable during difficult surgical procedures. The stent may remain in place on a short-term (days to weeks) or long-term (weeks to months) basis.

Demographics

Chronic blockage of a ureter affects approximately five individuals out of every 1,000; acute blockage affects one out of every 1,000. Bilateral obstruction (blockage to both ureters) is more rare; chronic blockage affects one individual per 1,000 people, and acute blockage affects five per 10,000.

Description

The size, shape, and material of the ureteral stent to be used depends on the patient's anatomy and the reason why the stent is required. Most stents are 5–12 inches (12–30 cm) in length, and have a diameter of 0.06–0.2 inches (1.5–6 mm). One or both ends of the stent may be coiled (called a pigtail stent) to prevent it from moving out of place; an open-ended stent is better suited for patients who require temporary drainage. In some instances, one end of the stent has a thread attached to it that extends through the bladder and urethra to the outside of the body; this aids in stent removal. The stent material must be flexible, durable, non-reactive, and radiopaque (visible on an x ray).

The patient is usually placed under general anesthesia for stent insertion; this ensures the physician that the patient will remain relaxed and will not move during the procedure. A cystoscope (a thin, telescope-like instrument) is inserted into the urethra to the bladder, and the opening to the ureter to be stented is identified. In some instances, a guide wire is inserted into the ureter under the aid of a fluoroscope (an imaging device that uses x rays to visualize structures on a fluorescent screen). The guide wire provides a path for the placement of the stent, which is advanced over the wire. Once the stent is in place, the guide wire and cystoscope are removed. Patients who fail this method of ureteral stenting may have the stent placed percutaneously (through the skin), into the kidney, and subsequently into the ureter.

A stent that has an attached thread may be pulled out by a physician in an office setting. **Cystoscopy** may also be used to remove a stent.

Diagnosis/Preparation

A number of different technologies aid in the diagnosis of ureteral obstruction. These include:

- cystoscopy (a procedure in which a thin, tubular instrument is used to visualize the interior of the bladder)

- ultrasonography (an imaging technique that uses high-frequency sounds waves to visualize structures inside the body)

- computed tomography (an imaging technique that uses x rays to produce two-dimensional cross-sections on a viewing screen)

- pyelography (x rays taken of the urinary tract after a contrast dye has been injected into a vein or into the kidney, ureter, or bladder)

Prior to ureteral stenting, the procedure should be thoroughly explained by a medical professional. No food or drink is permitted after midnight the night before surgery. The patient wears a hospital gown during the procedure. If the stent insertion is performed with the aid of a cystoscope, the patient will assume a position that is typically used in a gynecological exam (lying on the back, with the legs flexed and supported by stirrups).

Aftercare

Stents must be periodically replaced to prevent fractures within the catheter wall or build-up of encrustation. Stent replacement is recommended approximately every six months; more often in patients who form stones.

Risks

Complications associated with ureteral stenting include:

- bleeding (usually minor and easily treated, but occasionally requiring transfusion)

- catheter migration or dislodgement (may require readjustment)

- coiling of the stent within the ureter (may cause lower abdominal pain or flank pain on urination, urinary frequency, or blood in the urine)

- introduction or worsening of infection

- penetration of adjacent organs (e.g., bowel, gallbladder, or lungs)

Normal results

Normally, a ureteral stent re-establishes the flow of urine from the kidney to the bladder. Postoperative urine flow will be monitored to ensure the stent has not been dislodged or obstructed.

Morbidity and mortality rates

Serious complications occur in approximately 4% of patients undergoing ureteral stenting, with minor complications in another 10%.

KEY TERMS

Acute—A condition that has a short but severe course.

Chronic—A condition that is persistent or recurs frequently.

Cystoscopy—Examination or treatment of the interior of the urinary bladder by looking through a special instrument with reflected light.

Kidney stones—Small, solid masses that form in the kidney.

Urethra—The tube through which urine travels from the bladder to the outside of the body.

Alternatives

If a ureter is obstructed and ureteral stenting is not possible, a **nephrostomy** may be performed. During this procedure, a tube is placed through the skin on the patient's back, into the area of the kidney that collects urine. The tube may be connected to an external drainage bag. In other cases, the tube is connected directly from the kidney to the bladder.

Resources

BOOKS

Su, Li-Ming & R. Ernest Sosa. "Ureteroscopy and Retrograde Ureteral Access." (Chapter 97) In *Campbell's Urology,* 8th ed., edited by Patrick C. Walsh. Philadelphia: Elsevier Science, 2002.

ORGANIZATIONS

American Urological Association. 1120 North Charles Street, Baltimore, MD 21201. (410) 727-1100. <http://www.auanet.org>.

OTHER

"Extrinsic Obstruction of the Ureter." *UrologyHealth.org.* [cited May 19, 2003] <http://www.urologyhealth.org/adult/index.cfm?cat=01&topic=93>.

Sutherland, Suzette E. and Martin I. Resnick. "Urinary Tract Obstruction." *eMedicine.* May 6, 2002 [cited May 19, 2003] <http://www.emedicine.com/med/topic2782.htm>.

Kathleen D. Wright, R.N.
Stephanie Dionne Sherk

Ureterosigmoidoscopy

Definition

Ureterosigmoidoscopy is a surgical procedure that treats urinary incontinence by joining the ureters to the lower colon, thereby allowing urine to evacuate through the rectum.

Purpose

The surgery is indicated when there is resection (surgical cutting and/or removal), malformation, or injury to the bladder. The bladder disposes of wastes passed to it from the kidneys, which is the organ that does most of the blood filtering and retaining of needed glucose, salts, and minerals.

Wastes from the kidneys drip through the ureters to the bladder, and on to the urethra where they are expelled via urination. Waste from the kidneys is slowed or impaired when the bladder is diseased because of ulcerative, inflammatory, or malignant conditions; is malformed; or if it has been removed. In these cases, the kidney is unable to outflow the wastes, resulting in hydronephrosis, (distention of the kidneys). Over time, this leads to kidney deterioration. Saving the kidneys by bladder diversion is as important as restoring urinary continence.

The surgical techniques for urinary and fecal diversion fall into two categories: continent diversion and conduit diversion. In continent diversion, an internal reservoir for urine or feces is created, allowing natural evacuation from the body. In urinary and fecal conduit diversion, a section of existing tissue is altered to serve as a passageway to an external reservoir or ostomy. Both continent and conduit diversions reproduce bladder or colon function that was impaired due to surgery, obstruction, or a neurogenically created condition. Both the continent and conduit diversion methods have been used for years, with advancements in minimally invasive surgical techniques and biochemical improvements in conduit materials and ostomy appliances.

Catherization was the original solution for urinary incontinence, especially when major organ failure or removal was involved. But catherization was found to have major residual back flow of urine into the kidneys over the long term. With the advent of surgical anatomosis—the grafting of vascularizing tissue for the repair and expansion of organ function—and with the ability to include flap-type valves to prevent back-up into the kidneys, major continent restoring procedures have become routine in **urologic surgery**. Catherization has been replaced as a permanent remedy for persistent incontinence. Continent surgical procedures developed since the 1980s offer the possibility of safely retaining natural evacuation functions in both colonic (intestinal) and urinary systems.

Quality of life issues associated with urinary diversion are increasingly important to patients and, along with medical requirements, put an optimal threshold on the requirements for the surgical procedure. The bladder substitute or created reservoir must offer the following advantages:

- maintain continence
- maintain sterile urine
- empty completely
- protect the kidneys
- prevent absorption of waste products
- maintain quality of life

Ureterosigmoidoscopy is one of the earliest continent diversions for a resected bladder, bladder abnormalities, and dysfunction. It is one of the more difficult surgeries, and has significant complications. Ureterosigmoidoscopy does have a major benefit; it allows the natural expelling of wastes without the construction of a stoma—an artificial conduit—by using the rectum as a urinary reservoir. When evacuation occurs, the urine is passed along with the fecal matter.

Ureterosigmoidoscopy is a single procedure, but there are additional refinements that allow rectal voiding of urine. A procedure known as the Mainz II pouch has undergone many refinements in attempts to lessen the complications that have traditionally accompanied uretersigmoidoscopy. This surgery is indicated for significant and serious conditions of the urinary tract including:

- Cancer or ulceration of the bladder that necessitates a radical **cystectomy** or removal of the bladder, primarily occurring in adults, particularly those of advanced age.
- Various congenital abnormalities of the bladder in infants, especially eversion of part or all of the bladder. Eversion (or exotrophy) is a malformation of the bladder in which the wall adjacent to the abdomen fails to close. In some children, the bladder plate may be too small to fashion a closure.

Demographics

Bladder cancer affects over 50,000 people annually in the United States. The average age at diagnosis is 68 years. It accounts for approximately 10,000 deaths per year. Bladder cancer is the fifth leading cause of cancer deaths among men older than 75 years. Male bladder cancer is three times more prevalent than female bladder cancer.

In the United States, radical cystectomy (total removal of the bladder) is the standard treatment for muscle-invading bladder cancer. The operation usually involves removal of the bladder (with oncology staging) and pelvic lymph node, and prostate and seminal conduits with a form of urinary diversion. Uretersigmoscopy is one option that restores continence.

Pediatric ureterosigmoidoscopy is performed primarily for bladder abnormalities occuring at birth. Classic bladder exstrophy occurs in 3.3 per 100,000 births, with a male to female ratio of 3:1 (6:1 in some studies).

Description

The most basic ureterosigmoidoscopy modification is the Mainz II pouch. There is a 6 cm cut along antimesenteric border of the colon, both on the proximal and distal sides of the rectum/sigmoid colon junction. The ureters are drawn down into the colon. A special flap technique is applied by folding the colon to stop urine from refluxing back to the kidneys. After the colon is closed, the result is a small rectosigmoid reservoir that holds urine without refluxing it back to the upper urinary tract. Some variations of the Mainz II pouch include the construction of a valve, as in the Kock pouch, that confines urine to the distal segment of the colon.

Ureterosigmoidoscopy is typically performed in patients with complex medical problems, often those who have had numerous surgeries. Ureterosigmoidoscopy as a continent diversion technique relies heavily upon an intact and functional rectal sphincter. The treatment of pediatric urinary incontinence due to bladder eversion or other anatomical anomalies is a technical challenge, and is not always the first choice of surgeons. In Europe, early urinary diversion with ureterosigmoidoscopy is used widely for most exstrophy patients. Its main advantage is the possibility for spontaneous emptying by evacuation of urine and stool.

Diagnosis/Preparation

A number of tests are performed as part of the pre-surgery diagnostic workup for bladder conditions such as cancer, ulcerative or inflammatory disease, or pediatric abnormalities. Tests may include:

- cystoscopy (bladder inspection with a laparoscope)
- CT scan
- liver function
- renal function
- rectal sphincter function evaluation (The rectal sphincter will be a critical ingredient in urination after the

KEY TERMS

Bladder exstrophy—One of many bladder and urinary congenital abnormalities. Occurs when the wall of the bladder fails to close in embryonic development and remains exposed to the abdominal wall.

Conduit diversion—A surgical procedure that restores urinary and fecal continence by diverting these functions through a constructed conduit leading to an external waste reservoir (ostomy).

Cystectomy—The surgical resection of part or all of the bladder.

Urinary continent diversion—A surgical procedure that restores urinary continence by diverting urinary function around the bladder and into the intestines, thereby allowing for natural evacuation through the rectum or an implanted artificial sphincter.

surgery, and it is important to determine its ability to function. Adult patients are often asked to have an oatmeal enema and sit upright for a period of time to test sphincter function.)

In adult patients, a discussion of continent diversion is conducted early in the diagnostic process. Patients are asked to consider the possibility of a conduit urinary diversion if the ureterosigmoidoscopy proves impossible to complete. Educational sessions on specific conduit alternatives take place prior to surgery. Topics include options for placement of a stoma, and appliances that may be a part of the daily voiding routine after surgery. Many doctors provide a stomal therapist to consult with the patient.

Aftercare

After surgery, patients may remain in the hospital for a few days to undergo blood, renal, and liver tests, and monitoring for fever or other surgical complications. In pediatric patients, a cast keeps the legs abducted (apart) and slightly elevated for three weeks. Bladder and kidneys are fully drained via multiple catheters during the first few weeks after surgery. **Antibiotics** are continued after surgery. Permanent follow-up with the urologist is essential for proper monitoring of kidney function.

Normal results

Good results have been reported, especially in children; however, ureterosigmoidoscopy offers some severe morbid complications. Post-surgical bladder function and continence rates are very high. However, many newly created reservoirs do not function normally; some deteriorate over time, creating a need for more than one diversion surgery. Many patients have difficulty voiding after surgery. Five-year survival rates for bladder surgery patients are 50–80%, depending on the grade, depth of bladder penetration, and nodal status.

Morbidity and mortality rates

The continence success rate with ureterosigmoidoscopy and its variants is higher than 95% for exstrophy; however, long-term malignancy rates are quite high. Adenocarcinoma is the most common of these malignancies, and may be caused by chronic irritation and inflammation of exposed mucosa of the exostrophic bladder. In one series of studies, adenocarcinoma was reported in more than 10% of patients. However, the malignancy is actually higher in untreated patients whose bladders are left exposed for years before surgery.

Upper urinary tract deterioration is a potential complication, caused by reflux of urine back to the kidneys, resulting in febrile infections.

Alternatives

Other options include construction of a full neo-bladder in certain carefully defined circumstances, and bladder enhancement for congenitally shortened or abnormal bladders. Surgical bladder resection is often followed by continent operations using other parts of the colon, and by various conduit surgeries that utilize an external ostomy appliance.

See also Ureterostomy, cutaneous.

Resources

BOOKS

"Continent Urinary Diversion." In Walsh, P. *Campbell's Urology* 8th ed. Elsevier, 2002.

"Pediatric Urology: Continent Urinary Diversion." In Walsh, P. *Campbell's Urology,* 8th ed. Elsevier, 2002.

PERIODICALS

Stehr, M. "Selected Secondary Reconstructive Procedures for Improvement of Urinary Incontinence in Bladder Exstrophy and Neurogenic Bladder Dysfunction in Childhood." *Wiener Medizinische Wochenschr* 150, no.11 (January 1, 2000): 245-8.

Yerkes, B. and H.M. Snyder, H.M. "Exstrophy and Epispadias." *Pediatrics/Urology* 3, no.5 (May 6, 2002). Available at: <www.author.eMedicine.com>.

ORGANIZATIONS

American Academy of Pediatrics. 141 Northwest Point Boulevard; Elk Grove Village, IL 60007-1098. (847) 434-4000. Fax: (847) 434-8000. <www.aap.org>.

National Institutes of Diabetes & Digestive & Kidney Disease. <www.niddk.nih.gov/tools/mail.htm>.

OTHER

Girgin, C., et.al. "Comparison of Three Types of Continent Urinary Diversions in a Single Center." *Digital Urology Journal* <www.duj.com>.

Nancy McKenzie, Ph.D.

Ureterostomy, cutaneous

Definition

A cutaneous ureterostomy, also called ureterocutaneostomy, is a surgical procedure that detaches one or both ureters from the bladder, and brings them to the surface of the abdomen with the formation of an opening (stoma) to allow passage of urine.

Purpose

The bladder is the membranous pouch that serves as a reservoir for urine. Contraction of the bladder results in urination. A ureterostomy is performed to divert the flow of urine away from the bladder when the bladder is not functioning or has been removed. The following conditions may result in a need for ureterostomy.

- bladder cancer
- spinal cord injury
- malfunction of the bladder
- birth defects, such as spina bifida

Demographics

Bladder disorders afflict millions of people in the United States. According to the American Cancer Society (ACS), there were 54,200 new cases of bladder cancer in

WHO PERFORMS THE PROCEDURE AND WHERE IS IT PERFORMED?

Ureterostomy is performed in a hospital setting by experienced surgeons trained in urology, the branch of medicine concerned with the diagnosis and treatment of diseases of the urinary tract and urogenital system. Specially trained nurses called wound ostomy continence nurses (WOCN) are commonly available for consultation in most major medical centers.

1999, with approximately 12,100 deaths from the disease. Bladder cancer incidence is steadily rising, and by 2010 it is projected to increase by 28% for both men and women.

Description

Urostomy is the generic name for any surgical procedure that diverts the passage of urine by re-directing the ureters (fibromuscular tubes that carry the urine from the kidney to the bladder). There are two basic types of urostomies. The first features the creation of a passage called an "ileal conduit." In this procedure, the ureters are detached from the bladder and joined to a short length of the small intestine (ileum). The other type of urostomy is cutaneous ureterostomy. With this technique, the surgeon detaches the ureters from the bladder and brings one or both to the surface of the abdomen. The hole created in the abdomen is called a stoma, a reddish, moist abdominal protrusion. The stoma is not painful; it has no sensation. Since it has no muscles to regulate urination, urine collects in a bag.

There are four common types of ureterostomies:

- Single ureterostomy. This procedure brings only one ureter to the surface of the abdomen.

- Bilateral ureterostomy. This procedure brings the two ureters to the surface of the abdomen, one on each side.

- Double-barrel ureterostomy. In this approach, both ureters are brought to the same side of the abdominal surface.

- Transuretero ureterostomy (TUU). This procedure brings both ureters to the same side of the abdomen, through the same stoma.

Diagnosis/Preparation

Ureterostomy patients may have the following tests and procedures as part of their diagnostic work-up:

QUESTIONS
TO ASK THE DOCTOR

- Why is ureterostomy required?
- What type will be performed?
- How long will it take to recover from the surgery?
- When can normal activities be resumed?
- How many ureterostomies does the surgeon perform each year?
- What are the possible complications?

- Renal function tests; blood, urea, nitrogen (BUN); and creatinine.

- Blood tests, **complete blood count** (CBC) and electrolytes.

- Imaging studies of the ureters and renal pelvis. These studies characterize the ureters, and define the surgery required to obtain adequate ureteral length.

The quality, character, and usable length of the ureters is usually assessed using any of the following tests:

- Intravenous pyelogram (IVP). A special diagnostic test that follows the time course of excretion of a contrast dye through the kidneys, ureters, and bladder after it is injected into a vein.

- Retrograde pyelogram (RPG). x ray study of the kidney, focusing on the urine-collecting region of the kidney and ureters.

- Antegrade nephrostogram.

- CT scan. A special imaging technique that uses a computer to collect multiple x ray images into a two-dimentional cross-sectional image.

- MRI with intravenous gadolinium. A special technique used to image internal stuctures of the body, particularly the soft tissues. An MRI image is often superior to a routine x ray image.

The pre-surgery evaluation also includes an assessment of overall patient stability. The surgery may take from two to six hours, depending on the health of the ureters, and the experience of the surgeon.

Aftercare

After surgery, the condition of the ureters is monitored by IVP testing, repeated postoperatively at six months, one year, and then yearly.

Following ureterostomy, urine needs to be collected in bags. Several designs are available. One popular type features an open bag fitted with an anti-reflux valve, which prevents the urine from flowing back toward the stoma. A urostomy bag connects to a night bag that may be attached to the bed at night. Urostomy bags are available as one- and two-piece bags:

- One-piece bags: The adhesive and the bag are welded together. The advantage of using a one-piece appliance is that it is easy to apply, and the bag is flexible and soft.

- Two-piece bags: The bag and the adhesive are two separate components. The adhesive does not need to be removed frequently from the skin, and can remain in place for several days while the bag is changed as required.

Risks

The complication rate associated with ureterostomy procedures is less than 5–10%. Risks during surgery include heart problems, pulmonary (lung) complications, development of blood clots (thrombosis), blocking of arteries (embolism), and injury to adjacent structures, such as bowel or vascular entities. Inadequate ureteral length may also be encountered, leading to ureteral kinking and subsequent obstruction. If plastic tubes need inserting, their malposition can lead to obstruction and eventual breakdown of the opening (anastomosis). Anastomotic leak is the most frequently encountered complication.

Normal results

Normal results for a ureterostomy include the successful diversion of the urine pathway away from the bladder, and a tension-free, watertight opening to the abdomen that prevents urinary leakage.

Morbidity and mortality rates

The outcome and prognosis for ureterostomy patients depends on a number of factors. The highest rates of complications exist for those who have pelvic cancer or a history of radiation therapy.

In one study, a French medical team followed 69 patients for a minimum of one year (an average of six years) after TUU was performed. They reported one complication per four patients (6.3%), including a case requiring open drainage, prolonged urinary leakage, and common ureteral death (necrosis). Two complications occurred three and four years after surgery. The National Cancer Institute performed TUU for pelvic malignancy in 10 patients. Mean follow-up was 6.5 years. Complications include common ureteral narrowing (one patient); subsequent kidney removal, or **nephrectomy** (one pa-

KEY TERMS

Anastomosis—An opening created by surgical, traumatic, or pathological means between two separate spaces or organs.

Cecum—The pouch-like start of the large intestine (colon) at the end of the small intestine.

Gastrointestinal (GI) tract—The entire length of the digestive tract, from the stomach to the rectum.

Ileum—The last portion of the small intestine that communicates with the large intestine.

Large intestine—Also called the colon, this structure has six major divisions: cecum, ascending colon, transverse colon, descending colon, sigmoid colon, and rectum.

Ostomy—General term meaning a surgical procedure in which an artificial opening is formed to either allow waste (stool or urine) to pass from the body, or to allow food into the GI tract. An ostomy can be permanent or temporary, as well as single-barreled, double-barreled, or a loop.

Small intestine—The small intestine consists of three sections: duodenum, jejunum, and ileum.

Spina bifida—A congenital defect in the spinal column, characterized by the absence of the vertebral arches through which the spinal membranes and spinal cord may protrude.

Stent—A tube made of metal or plastic that is inserted into a vessel or passage to keep it open and prevent closure.

Stoma—A surgically created opening in the abdominal wall.

Ureter—The fibromuscular tube that transports the urine from the kidney to the bladder.

---

tient); recurrence of disease with ureteral obstruction (one patient); and disease progression in a case of inflammation of blood vessels, or vasulitis (one patient). One patient died of sepsis (infection in the bloodstream) due to urine leakage at the anastomosis, one died after a heart attack, and three died from metastasis of their primary cancer.

Alternatives

There are several alternative surgical procedures available:

- Ileal conduit urostomy, also known as "Bricker's loop." The two ureters that transport urine from the kidneys are detached from the bladder, and then attached so that they will empty through a piece of the ileum. One end of the ileum piece is sealed off and the other end is brought to the surface of the abdomen to form the stoma. It is the most common technique used for urinary diversion.

- Cystostomy. The flow of urine is diverted from the bladder to the abdominal wall. It features placement of a tube through the abdominal wall into the bladder, and is indicated in cases of blockage or stricture of the ureters. It can be temporary or permanent.

- Indiana pouch. A pouch is constructed using the end part of the ileum and the first part of the large intestine (cecum). The remaining ileum is first attached to the large intestine to maintain normal digestive flow. A pouch is then created from the removed cecum, and the attached ileum is brought to the surface of the abdominal wall to create a stoma.

- Percutaneous **nephrostomy**. A nephrostomy is created when the flow of urine is diverted directly from the kidneys to the abdominal wall. Tubes are placed within the kidney to collect the urine as it is generated, and transport it to the abdominal wall. This procedure is usually temporary; however, it may be permanent for cancer patients.

See also Nephrostomy; Open prostatectomy; Transurethral resection of the prostate.

Resources

BOOKS

Door Mullen, B. & K. A. McGinn. *The Ostomy Book: Living Comfortably With Colostomies, Ileostomies, and Urostomies.* Boulder, CO: Bull Publishing Co., 1992.

Jeter, K. F. *Urostomy Guide.* Irvine, CA: American Urological Association, code 05-006.

PERIODICALS

Cedillo, U., C. Gracida, R. Espinoza, and J. Cancino. "Vesical Augmentation and Continent Ureterostomy in Kidney Transplant Patients." *Transplant Proceedings* 34 (November 2002): 2541-2.

Hiratsuka, Y., T. Ishii, H. Taira, and A. Okadome. "Simple Correction of Ureteral Stomal Stenosis for Cutaneous Ureterostomy." *International Journal of Urology* 10 (March 2003): 180-1.

Purohit, R. S., and P. N. Bretan, Jr. "Successful Long-term Outcome Using Existing Native Cutaneous Ureterostomy for Renal Transplant Drainage." *Journal of Urology* 163 (February 2000): 446-9.

Yoshimura, K., S. Maekawa, K. Ichioka, N. Terada, Y. Matsuta, K. Okubo, and Y. Arai. "Tubeless Cutaneous Ureterostomy: The Toyoda Method Revisited." *Journal of Urology* 165 (March 2001): 785-8.

ORGANIZATIONS

American Urological Association (AUA). 1120 North Charles Street, Baltimore, MD 21201. (410) 727-1100. <www.auanet.org>.

United Ostomy Association (UOA). 19772 MacArthur Blvd., #200, Irvine, CA 92612-2405. (800) 826-0826. <www.uoa.org>.

Monique Laberge, Ph.D.

Uric acid tests *see* **Kidney function tests**

Urinalysis

Definition

A urinalysis is a group of manual and/or automated qualitative and semi-quantitative tests performed on a urine sample. A routine urinalysis usually includes the following tests: color, transparency, specific gravity, pH, protein, glucose, ketones, blood, bilirubin, nitrite, urobilinogen, and leukocyte esterase. Some laboratories include a microscopic examination of urinary sediment with all routine urinalysis tests. If not, it is customary to perform the microscopic exam, if transparency, glucose, protein, blood, nitrite, or leukocyte esterase is abnormal.

Purpose

Routine urinalyses are performed for several reasons:

• general health screening to detect renal and metabolic diseases

• diagnosis of diseases or disorders of the kidneys or urinary tract

• monitoring of patients with diabetes

In addition, quantitative urinalysis tests may be performed to help diagnose many specific disorders, such as endocrine diseases, bladder cancer, osteoporosis, and porphyrias (a group of disorders caused by chemical imbalance). Quantitative analysis often requires the use of a timed urine sample. The urinary microalbumin test measures the rate of albumin excretion in the urine using laboratory tests. This test is used to monitor the kidney function of persons with diabetes mellitus. In diabetics, the excretion of greater than 200 µg/mL albumin is predictive of impending kidney disease.

Precautions

Voided specimens

All patients should avoid intense athletic training or heavy physical work before the test, as these activities may cause small amounts of blood to appear in the urine. Many urinary constituents are labile, and samples should be tested within one hour of collection or refrigerated. Samples may be stored at 36–46°F (2–8°C) for up to 24 hours for chemical urinalysis tests; however, the microscopic examination should be performed within four hours of collection, if possible. To minimize sample contamination, women who require a urinalysis during menstruation should insert a fresh tampon before providing a urine sample.

Over two dozen drugs are known to interfere with various chemical urinalysis tests. These include:

• ascorbic acid

• chlorpromazine

• L-dopa

• nitrofurantoin (Macrodantin, Furadantin)

• penicillin

• phenazopyridine (Pyridium)

• rifampin (Rifadin)

• tolbutamide

The preservatives that are used to prevent loss of glucose and cells may affect biochemical test results. The use of preservatives should be avoided whenever possible in urine tests.

Description

Routine urinalysis consists of three testing groups: physical characteristics, biochemical tests, and microscopic evaluation.

Physical tests

The physical tests measure the color, transparency (clarity), and specific gravity of a urine sample. In some cases, the volume (daily output) may be measured. Color and transparency are determined from visual observation of the sample.

COLOR. Normal urine is straw yellow to amber in color. Abnormal colors include bright yellow, brown, black (gray), red, and green. These pigments may result from medications, dietary sources, or diseases. For example, red urine may be caused by blood or hemoglobin, beets, medications, and some porphyrias. Black-gray urine may result from melanin (melanoma) or homogentisic acid (alkaptonuria, a result of a metabolic disorder).

Bright yellow urine may be caused by bilirubin (a bile pigment). Green urine may be caused by biliverdin or certain medications. Orange urine may be caused by some medications or excessive urobilinogen (chemical relatives of urobilinogen). Brown urine may be caused by excessive amounts of prophobilin or urobilin (a chemical produced in the intestines).

TRANSPARENCY. Normal urine is transparent. Turbid (cloudy) urine may be caused by either normal or abnormal processes. Normal conditions giving rise to turbid urine include precipitation of crystals, mucus, or vaginal discharge. Abnormal causes of turbidity include the presence of blood cells, yeast, and bacteria.

SPECIFIC GRAVITY. The specific gravity of urine is a measure of the concentration of dissolved solutes (substances in a solution), and it reflects the ability of the kidneys to concentrate the urine (conserve water). Specific gravity is usually measured by determining the refractive index of a urine sample (refractometry) or by chemical analysis. Specific gravity varies with fluid and solute intake. It will be increased (above 1.035) in persons with diabetes mellitus and persons taking large amounts of medication. It will also be increased after radiologic studies of the kidney owing to the excretion of x ray contrast dye. Consistently low specific gravity (1.003 or less) is seen in persons with diabetes insipidus. In renal (kidney) failure, the specific gravity remains equal to that of blood plasma (1.008–1.010) regardless of changes in the patient's salt and water intake. Urine volume below 400 mL per day is considered oliguria (low urine production), and may occur in persons who are dehydrated and those with some kidney diseases. A volume in excess of 2 liters (slightly more than 2 quarts) per day is considered polyuria (excessive urine production); it is common in persons with diabetes mellitus and diabetes insipidus.

Biochemical tests

Biochemical testing of urine is performed using dry reagent strips, often called dipsticks. A urine dipstick consists of a white plastic strip with absorbent microfiber cellulose pads attached to it. Each pad contains the dried reagents needed for a specific test. The person performing the test dips the strip into the urine, lets it sit for a specified amount of time, and compares the color change to a standard chart.

Additional tests are available for measuring the levels of bilirubin, protein, glucose, ketones, and urobilinogen in urine. In general, these individual tests provide greater sensitivity; they therefore permit detection of a lower concentration of the respective substance. A brief description of the most commonly used dry reagent strip tests follows.

pH: A combination of pH indicators (methyl red and bromthymol blue) react with hydrogen ions (H^+) to produce a color change over a pH range of 5.0 to 8.5. pH measurements are useful in determining metabolic or respiratory disturbances in acid-base balance. For example, kidney disease often results in retention of H^+ (reduced acid excretion). pH varies with a person's diet, tending to be acidic in people who eat meat but more alkaline in vegetarians. pH testing is also useful for the classification of urine crystals.

Protein: Based upon a phenomenon called the "protein error of indicators," this test uses a pH indicator, such as tetrabromphenol blue, that changes color (at constant pH) when albumin is present in the urine. Albumin is important in determining the presence of glomerular damage. The glomerulus is the network of capillaries in the kidneys that filters low molecular weight solutes such as urea, glucose, and salts, but normally prevents passage of protein or cells from blood into filtrate. Albuminuria occurs when the glomerular membrane is damaged, a condition called glomerulonephritis.

Glucose (sugar): The glucose test is used to monitor persons with diabetes. When blood glucose levels rise above 160 mg/dL, the glucose will be detected in urine. Consequently, glycosuria (glucose in the urine) may be the first indicator that diabetes or another hyperglycemic condition is present. The glucose test may be used to screen newborns for galactosuria and other disorders of carbohydrate metabolism that cause urinary excretion of a sugar other than glucose.

Ketones: Ketones are compounds resulting from the breakdown of fatty acids in the body. These ketones are produced in excess in disorders of carbohydrate metabolism, especially Type 1 diabetes mellitus. In diabetes, excess ketoacids in the blood may cause life-threatening acidosis and coma. These ketoacids and their salts spill into the urine, causing ketonuria. Ketones are also found in the urine in several other conditions, including fever; pregnancy; glycogen storage diseases; and weight loss produced by a carbohydrate-restricted diet.

Blood: Red cells and hemoglobin may enter the urine from the kidney or lower urinary tract. Testing for blood in the urine detects abnormal levels of either red cells or hemoglobin, which may be caused by excessive red cell destruction, glomerular disease, kidney or urinary tract infection, malignancy, or urinary tract injury.

Bilirubin: Bilirubin is a breakdown product of hemoglobin. Most of the bilirubin produced in humans is conjugated by the liver and excreted into the bile, but a very small amount of conjugated bilirubin is reabsorbed and reaches the general circulation to be excreted in the urine. The normal level of urinary bilirubin is below the detection limit of the test. Bilirubin in the urine is derived from the liver, and a positive test indicates hepatic disease or hepatobiliary obstruction.

Specific gravity: Specific gravity is a measure of the ability of the kidneys to concentrate urine by conserving water.

Nitrite: Some disease bacteria, including the lactose-positive *Enterobactericeae, Staphylococcus, Proteus, Salmonella,* and *Pseudomonas* are able to reduce nitrate in urine to nitrite. A positive test for nitrite indicates bacteruria, or the presence of bacteria in the urine.

Urobilinogen: Urobilinogen is a substance formed in the gastrointestinal tract by the bacterial reduction of conjugated bilirubin. Increased urinary urobilinogen occurs in prehepatic jaundice (hemolytic anemia), hepatitis, and other forms of hepatic necrosis that impair the circulation of blood in the liver and surrounding organs. The urobilinogen test is helpful in differentiating these conditions from obstructive jaundice, which results in decreased production of urobilinogen.

Leukocytes: The presence of white blood cells in the urine usually signifies a urinary tract infection, such as cystitis, or renal disease, such as pyelonephritis or glomerulonephritis.

Microscopic examination

A urine sample may contain cells that originated in the blood, the kidney, or the lower urinary tract. Microscopic examination of urinary sediment can provide valuable clues regarding many diseases and disorders involving these systems.

The presence of bacteria or yeast and white blood cells helps to distinguish between a urinary tract infection and a contaminated urine sample. White blood cells are not seen if the sample has been contaminated. The presence of cellular casts (casts containing RBCs, WBCs, or epithelial cells) identifies the kidneys, rather than the lower urinary tract, as the source of such cells. Cellular casts and renal epithelial (kidney lining) cells are signs of kidney disease.

The microscopic examination also identifies both normal and abnormal crystals in the sediment. Abnormal crystals are those formed as a result of an abnormal metabolic process and are always clinically significant. Normal crystals are formed from normal metabolic processes; however, they may lead to the formation of renal calculi, or kidney stones.

Preparation

A urine sample is collected in an unused disposable plastic cup with a tight-fitting lid. A randomly voided

sample is suitable for routine urinalysis, although the urine that is first voided in the morning is preferable because it is the most concentrated. The best sample for analysis is collected in a sterile container after the external genitalia have been cleansed using the midstream void (clean-catch) method. This sample may be cultured if the laboratory findings indicate bacteruria.

To collect a sample using the clean-catch method:

• Females should use a clean cotton ball moistened with lukewarm water (or antiseptic wipes provided with collection kits) to cleanse the external genital area before collecting a urine sample. To prevent contamination with menstrual blood, vaginal discharge, or germs from the external genitalia, they should release some urine before beginning to collect the sample.

• Males should use a piece of clean cotton moistened with lukewarm water or antiseptic wipes to cleanse the head of the penis and the urethral meatus (opening). Uncircumcised males should draw back the foreskin. After the area has been thoroughly cleansed, they should use the midstream void method to collect the sample.

• For infants, a parent or health care worker should cleanse the baby's outer genitalia and surrounding skin. A sterile collection bag should be attached to the child's genital area and left in place until he or she has urinated. It is important to not touch the inside of the bag, and to remove it as soon as a specimen has been obtained.

Urine samples can also be obtained via bladder catheterization, a procedure used to collect uncontaminated urine when the patient cannot void. A catheter is a thin flexible tube that a health care professional inserts through the urethra into the bladder to allow urine to flow out. To minimize the risk of infecting the patient's bladder with bacteria, many clinicians use a Robinson catheter, which is a plain rubber or latex tube that is removed as soon as the specimen is collected. If urine for culture is to be collected from an indwelling catheter, it should be aspirated (removed by suction) from the line using a syringe and not removed from the bag in order to avoid contamination.

Suprapubic bladder aspiration is a collection technique sometimes used to obtain urine from infants younger than six months or urine directly from the bladder for culture. The doctor withdraws urine from the bladder into a syringe through a needle inserted through the skin.

Aftercare

The patient may return to normal activities after collecting the sample and may start taking any medications that were discontinued before the test.

Acidosis—A condition of the blood in which bicarbonate levels are below normal.

Alkalosis—A condition of the blood and other body fluids in which bicarbonate levels are higher than normal.

Bilirubin—A yellow bile pigment found as sodium (soluble) bilirubinate, or as an insoluble calcium salt found in gallstones.

Biliverdin—A green bile pigment formed from the oxidation of heme, which is a bilin with a structure almost identical to that of bilirubin.

Cast—An insoluble gelled protein matrix that takes the form of the renal tubule in which it was deposited. Casts are washed out by normal urine flow.

Catheter—A thin flexible tube inserted through the urethra into the bladder to allow urine to flow out.

Clean-catch specimen—A urine specimen that is collected from the middle of the urine stream after the first part of the flow has been discarded.

Cystine—An amino acid normally reabsorbed by the kidney tubules. Cystinuria is an inherited disease in which cystine and some other amino acids are not reabsorbed by the body in normal amounts. Cystine crystals then form in the kidney, which leads to obstructive renal failure.

Epithelium—A general term for the layer of cells that lines blood vessels or small body cavities.

Ketones—Substances produced during the breakdown of fatty acids. They are produced in excessive amounts in diabetes and certain other abnormal conditions.

pH—A chemical symbol that denotes the acidity or alkalinity of a fluid, ranging from 1 (more acid) to 14 (more alkaline).

Meatus—A general term for an opening or passageway in the body. The urethral meatus should be cleansed before a urine sample is collected.

Porphyrias—A group of disorders involving heme biosynthesis, characterized by excessive excretion of polyphrins. The porphyrias may be either inherited or acquired (usually from the effects of certain chemical agents).

Trichomonads—Parasitic protozoa commonly found in the digestive and genital tracts of humans and other animals. Some species cause vaginal infections in women characterized by itching and a frothy discharge.

Turbidity—The degree of cloudiness of a urine sample (or other solution).

Urethra—The tube that carries urine from the bladder to the outside of the body.

Urinalysis (plural, urinalyses)—The diagnostic testing of a urine sample.

Voiding—The medical term for emptying the bladder or urinating.

Risks

There are no risks associated with voided specimens. The risk of bladder infection from catheterization with a Robinson catheter is about 3%.

Normal results

Normal urine is a clear straw-colored liquid, but may also be slightly hazy. It has a slight odor, and some laboratories will note strong or atypical odors on the urinalysis report. A normal urine specimen may contain some normal crystals as well as squamous or transitional epithelial cells from the bladder, lower urinary tract, or vagina. Urine may contain transparent (hyaline) casts, especially if it was collected after vigorous **exercise**. The presence of hyaline casts may be a sign of kidney disease, however, when the cause cannot be attributed to exercise, running, or medications. Normal urine contains a small amount of urobilinogen, and may contain a few RBCs and WBCs. Normal urine does *not* contain detectable amounts of glucose or other sugars, protein, ketones, bilirubin, bacteria, yeast cells, or trichomonads. Normal values used in many laboratories are given below:

• Glucose: negative (quantitative less than 130 mg/day or 30 mg/dL).

• Bilirubin: negative (quantitative less than 0.02 mg/dL).

• Ketones: negative (quantitative 0.5–3.0 mg/dL).

• pH: 5.0–8.0.

• Protein: negative (quantitative 15–150 mg/day, less than 10 mg/dL).

• Blood: negative.

• Nitrite: negative.

• Specific gravity: 1.015–1.025.

- Urobilinogen: 0–2 Ehrlich units (quantitative 0.3–1.0 Ehrlich units).

- Leukocyte esterase: negative.

- Red blood cells: 0–2 per high power field.

- White blood cells: 0–5 per high power field (0–10 per high power field for some standardized systems).

Resources

BOOKS

Chernecky, Cynthia C, and Barbara J. Berger. *Laboratory Tests and Diagnostic Procedures*, 3rd ed. Philadelphia, PA: W. B. Saunders Company, 2001.

Henry, J.B. *Clinical Diagnosis and Management by Laboratory Methods*, 20th ed. Philadelphia, PA: W.B. Saunders Company, 2001.

Kee, Joyce LeFever. *Handbook of Laboratory and Diagnostic Tests*, 4th ed. Upper Saddle River, NJ: Prentice Hall, 2001.

Wallach, Jacques. *Interpretation of Diagnostic Tests*, 7th ed. Philadelphia, PA: Lippincott Williams & Wilkens, 2000.

ORGANIZATIONS

American Association of Kidney Patients. 100 S. Ashley Drive, Suite 280, Tampa, FL 33260. (800) 749-2257. <www.aakp.org>.

American Kidney Fund. 6110 Executive Blvd., Suite 1010, Rockville, MD 20852. (301) 881-3052. <www.akfinc.org>.

American Medical Technologists. 710 Higgins Road, Park Ridge, IL 60068-5765. (847) 823-5169. <www.amt1.com>.

American Society for Clinical Pathology (ASCP). 2100 West Harrison Street, Chicago, Il 60612-3798. (312) 738-1336. <www.ascp.org>.

National Kidney and Urologic Diseases Information Clearinghouse. 3 Information Way, Bethesda, MD 20892-3580.

OTHER

National Institutes of Health. <www.nlm.nih.gov/medline plus/encyclopedia.html> [cited April 4, 2003].

Victoria E. DeMoranville
Mark A. Best

Urinary anti-infectives

Definition

Urinary anti-infectives are medicines used to treat or prevent infections of the urinary tract, which is the passage through which urine flows from the kidneys out of the body.

Purpose

Normally, no bacteria or other disease-causing organisms live in the bladder. Likewise, the urethra—the tube-like structure that carries urine from the bladder to the outside of the body—usually contains either no bacteria or not enough to cause problems. But the bladder, urethra, and other parts of the urinary tract may become infected when disease-causing organisms enter it from other body regions or from outside the body. Urinary anti-infectives are used to treat such infections.

Although many **antibiotics** and some **sulfonamides** are equally effective in treating urinary tract infections, urinary anti-infectives have the advantage of being active only in the urinary tract. This means they are less likely to cause development of resistant microorganisms, or cause diarrhea by destroying the bacteria in the large intestine.

Some urinary anti-infectives have been used to prevent urinary tract infections, but the evidence that they are effective for this purpose is limited.

Description

Commonly used urinary anti-infectives include methenamine (Urex, Hiprex, Mandelamine); nalidixic acid (NegGram); and nitrofurantoin (Macrobid, Furatoin, and other brands). Nalidixic acid belongs to a group of synthetic antibacterial drugs known as quinolones. The first quinolone to be approved for clinical use, nalidixic acid has been used to treat urinary tract infections since 1967. Nitrofurantoin is also a synthetic antibacterial medication.

Urinary anti-infectives are available only with a physician's prescription. They come in capsule, tablet, granular, and liquid forms.

Recommended dosage

Methenamine

For adults and children 12 years and over, the usual dosage is 1 gram, taken either twice a day or four times a day, depending on the form of the medication that the doctor prescribes. For children aged six to 12 years, the dosage ranges from 500 mg taken two to four times a day to 1 gram taken twice a day, again depending on the form of the drug. A physician must determine the dose for children under six years.

Urinary anti-infectives will not work properly unless the urine is acidic, with a pH reading of 5.5 or lower. The physician who prescribes the medicine will explain how to test the urine's acidity. He or she may suggest dietary changes that will make the urine more acidic, such as eating more protein; drinking cranberry juice; eating plums and prunes while avoiding most other fruits; and cutting down on milk and other dairy products. The patient should also avoid taking antacids.

Nalidixic acid

The recommended dosage of this drug for adults and children 12 years and older is 1 gram every six hours. If the medicine is taken for more than one or two weeks, the dosage may be decreased to 500 mg every six hours. A physician must determine the correct dosage for children three months to 12 years old. Children under three months should not take nalidixic acid because it causes bone problems in young animals and could have the same effect in young children.

Nitrofurantoin

CAPSULES, TABLETS, OR LIQUID. The usual dose for adults and adolescents is 50–100 mg every six hours.

EXTENDED-RELEASE CAPSULES. For adults and children 12 years and older, the usual dosage is 100 mg every 12 hours for seven days.

A physician must determine the correct dose of all forms of nitrofurantoin for children one month and older according to the child's body weight. Children under one month should not be given this medicine.

Precautions

Methenamine

Methenamine may produce adverse effects in some patients with systemic disorders. For example, it may worsen the symptoms of people with severe liver disease. People who are dehydrated or who have severe kidney disease may be more likely to have side effects that affect the kidneys.

Nalidixic acid

Some people feel drowsy, dizzy, or less alert than usual when using this drug. Nalidixic acid may also cause blurred vision or other visual problems. Because of these possible side effects, anyone who takes nalidixic acid should not drive, operate machinery, or do anything else that might be dangerous until they have found out how the drugs affect them.

Nalidixic acid may increase sensitivity to sunlight. Even brief exposure to sunlight may cause a severe sunburn or a rash. Patients treated with this medication should avoid sun exposure, especially during high sun (between 10 A.M. and 3 P.M.). They should wear a hat or scarf and tightly woven clothing that covers the arms and legs; use a sunscreen with a sun protection factor (SPF) of at least 15; protect the lips with a lip balm containing sun block; and avoid the use of tanning beds, tanning booths, and sunlamps.

Diabetic patients should be aware that nalidixic acid may cause false results on some urine sugar tests. They should check with a physician before making any changes in their diet or diabetes medicine based on the results of a urine test.

In laboratory studies, nalidixic acid has been found to interfere with bone development in young animals. The drug's effects have not been studied in pregnant women, but because of its effects in animals, it is not recommended for use during pregnancy.

This medicine does not cause problems in most nursing babies whose mothers are taking it during lactation. However, nursing babies with glucose-6-phosphate dehydrogenase (G6PD) deficiency (an inherited disorder that affects mainly black males) may have blood problems if their mothers take nalidixic acid.

People with certain medical conditions may be more likely to have particular side effects if they take this medicine. For example, people with a history of seizures or severe hardening of the arteries in the brain may be more likely to have side effects that affect the nervous system. People with glucose-6-phosphate dehydrogenase (G6PD) deficiency are more likely to have side effects that affect the blood. In addition, people with liver disease or severe kidney disease are at increased risk of having any of the drug's possible side effects.

Nitrofurantoin

Pregnant women should not take this medicine within two weeks of their delivery date. They should not use it during labor and delivery, as this could cause problems in the baby.

Women who are breastfeeding should check with their physicians before using this medicine. It passes into breast milk and could cause problems in nursing babies whose mothers take it. This is especially true of babies with glucose-6-phosphate dehydrogenase (G6PD) deficiency. The medicine also should not be given directly to babies up to one month of age, as they are particularly sensitive to its effects.

Older people may be more likely to have side effects when taking nitrofurantoin, because they are more sensitive to the drug's effects.

Taking nitrofurantoin may cause problems for people with certain medical conditions. Side effects may be greater, for example, in people with lung disease or nerve damage. In people with kidney disease, the medicine may not work as well as it should, but may cause more side effects. Those with glucose-6-phosphate dehydrogenase (G6PD) deficiency who take nitrofurantoin may develop anemia.

Diabetic patients should be aware that this medicine may cause false results on some urine sugar tests. They should check with a physician before making any changes in diet or diabetes medicine based on the results of a urine test.

General precautions for all urinary anti-infectives

The symptoms of a urinary tract infection should improve within a few days of starting to take a urinary anti-infective. If they do not, or if they become worse, the patient should consult a physician right away. Patients who need to take this medicine for long periods should see their doctors regularly, so that the their improvement and any side effects can be monitored.

Anyone who has had unusual reactions to urinary anti-infectives in the past should let his or her physician know before taking the drugs again. The physician should also be told about any allergies to foods, dyes, preservatives, or other substances. Patients taking nalidixic acid should tell their physicians if they have ever had reactions to such other quinolones as cinoxacin (Cinobac), ciprofloxacin (Cipro), enoxacin (Penetrex), norfloxacin (Noroxin), or ofloxacin (Floxin), all of which are also used to treat or prevent infections. Anyone taking nitrofurantoin should let the physician know if he or she has had an unusual reaction to such drugs as furazolidone (Furoxone) or nitrofurazone (Furacin).

Side effects

Methenamine

Nausea and vomiting are not common but may occur. These side effects do not need medical attention unless they are severe. One side effect that should be brought to a physician's attention immediately is a skin rash.

Nalidixic acid

Some side effects are fairly minor and are likely to go away as the body adjusts to the drug. These include dizziness, drowsiness, headache, nausea or vomiting, stomach pain and diarrhea. Unless these problems continue or are bothersome, they do not need medical attention.

Other side effects, however, should have prompt medical attention. Anyone who has such visual symptoms as blurred vision, double vision, decreased vision, changes in color vision, seeing halos around lights, or increased glare from lights should consult a physician immediately.

Nitrofurantoin

This medicine may discolor the urine, causing it to turn reddish-yellow or brown. Patients should not be concerned about this change in color. Other possible side effects that do not need medical attention unless they are severe include pain in the stomach or abdomen; stomach upset; diarrhea; loss of appetite; and nausea or vomiting.

Anyone who has chest pain, breathing problems, fever, chills, or a cough while taking nitrofurantoin should consult their physician immediately.

General advice on side effects for all urinary anti-infectives

Other side effects are possible when taking any urinary anti-infective. Anyone who has unusual symptoms while taking this type of medication should get in touch with his or her physician.

Interactions

Methenamine

Certain medicines may make methenamine less effective. These include thiazide **diuretics** (water pills) and medicines that make the urine less acid, such as antacids; bicarbonate of soda (baking soda); and the drugs acetazolamide (Diamox), dichlorphenamide (Daranide), and methazolamide (Neptazane), which are used to treat glaucoma, epilepsy, altitude sickness, and other conditions.

Nalidixic acid

People who are taking blood thinners (anticoagulants) may be more likely to have bleeding problems if they take this medicine.

Nitrofurantoin

Nitrofurantoin may interact with many other medicines. For example, taking nitrofurantoin with certain drugs that include methyldopa (Aldomet), sulfonamides (sulfa drugs), vitamin K, and diabetes medicines taken by mouth may increase the chance of side effects that affect the blood. General side effects are more likely in people who take nitrofurantoin with the gout drugs probenecid (Benemid) or sulfinpyrazone (Anturane). The risk of side effects that involve the nervous system is higher in people who take nitrofurantoin with such drugs as lithium (Lithane); disulfiram (Antabuse); other anti-infectives; and the cancer drugs cisplatin (Platinol) and vincristine (Oncovin). Patients who have been vaccinated with DPT (diphtheria, tetanus, and pertussis) within the last 30 days or are vaccinated after taking nitrofurantoin are also more likely to have side effects that affect the nervous system. Because of the many possible interactions, anyone taking nitrofurantoin should be sure to consult a physician before combining it with any other medicine.

Laxatives containing psyllium and other bulk-forming substances may interfere with the body's absorption

KEY TERMS

Altitude sickness—A set of symptoms that people who normally live at low altitudes may have when they climb mountains or travel to high altitudes. The symptoms include nosebleed, nausea, and shortness of breath.

Anemia—A low level of hemoglobin in the blood.

Anticoagulant—A type of medication given to prevent the formation of blood clots. Anticoagulants are sometimes called blood thinners.

Bacteria—Microscopically small one-celled forms of life that cause many diseases and infections.

Glaucoma—A condition in which fluid pressure in the eye is abnormally high. If not treated, glaucoma may lead to blindness.

Glucose-6-phosphate dehydrogenase (G6PD) deficiency—An inherited disorder in which the body lacks an enzyme that normally protects red blood cells from toxic chemicals. When people with this condition take certain drugs, their red blood cells break down, causing anemia. This may also happen when they have a fever or an infection. The condition usually occurs in males. About 10% of

black males have it, as do a small percentage of people from the Mediterranean region.

Granule—A small grain or pellet. Medicines that come in granule form are usually mixed with liquids or sprinkled on food before they are taken.

Hemoglobin—The reddish-colored compound in blood that carries oxygen from the lungs throughout the body and brings waste carbon dioxide from the cells to the lungs, where it is released

pH—A measure of the acidity or alkalinity of a substance or compound. The pH scale ranges from 0 to 14. Values below 7 are acidic; values above 7 are alkaline.

Psyllium—A herb whose seeds contain a water-soluble fiber that adds bulk to the contents of the digestive tract. The bulk helps to prevent constipation. Laxatives containing psyllium may interfere with the body's absorption of urinary anti-infectives.

Quinolones—A group of synthetic antibacterial drugs originally derived from quinine. Nalidixic acid is the first quinolone that was approved for clinical use.

Seizure—A sudden attack, spasm, or convulsion.

---

of nitrofurantoin. Patients with constipation who are taking nitrofurantoin should consult their doctor before taking an over-the-counter laxative.

General advice about drug interactions

Not every drug that may interact with a urinary anti-infective is listed here. Patients should check with a physician or pharmacist before combining a urinary anti-infective with any other prescription or nonprescription (over-the-counter) medicine.

Patients who are taking any kind of herbal preparation or other alternative medicine should give their doctor and pharmacist a list of all the compounds that they use on a regular basis. Most of these preparations are unlikely to interact with urinary anti-infectives, but there is much that is still unknown about possible interactions between standard prescription medications and alternative medicines.

Resources

BOOKS

"Antibacterial Drugs: Miscellaneous Antibiotics." Section 13, Chapter 153 in *The Merck Manual of Diagnosis and Therapy*, edited by Mark H. Beers, MD, and Robert Berkow,

MD. Whitehouse Station, NJ: Merck Research Laboratories, 1999.

"Antibacterial Drugs: Quinolones." Section 13, Chapter 153 in *The Merck Manual of Diagnosis and Therapy*, edited by Mark H. Beers, MD, and Robert Berkow, MD. Whitehouse Station, NJ: Merck Research Laboratories, 1999.

Wilson, Billie Ann, RN, PhD, Carolyn L. Stang, PharmD, and Margaret T. Shannon, RN, PhD. *Nurses Drug Guide 2000*. Stamford, CT: Appleton and Lange, 1999.

PERIODICALS

Cunha, B. A. "Antibiotic side effects." *Medical Clinics of North America* 85 (January 2001): 149-185.

Emmerson, A. M., and A. M. Jones. "The Quinolones: Decades of Development and Use." *Journal of Antimicrobial Chemotherapy* 51 (May 2003): Supplement 1, 13-20.

ORGANIZATIONS

American Society of Health-System Pharmacists (ASHP). 7272 Wisconsin Avenue, Bethesda, MD 20814. (301) 657-3000. <www.ashp.org>.

United States Food and Drug Administration (FDA). 5600 Fishers Lane, Rockville, MD 20857-0001. (888) INFO-FDA. <www.fda.gov>.

Nancy Ross-Flanigan
Sam Uretsky, PharmD

Urinary artificial sphincter see **Artificial sphincter insertion**

Urinary catheterization, female see **Catheterization, female**

Urinary catheterization, male see **Catheterization, male**

Urinary diversion see **Ureterostomy, cutaneous**

Urinary diversion surgery see **Ileal conduit surgery**

Urobilinogen test see **Urinalysis**

Urologic surgery

Definition

Urologic surgery is the integration of surgical activities for the pelvis—the colon, urogenital, and gynecological organs—primarily for the treatment of obstructions, dysfunction, malignancies, and inflammatory diseases. Common urologic operations include:

- renal (kidney) surgery
- kidney removal (**nephrectomy**)
- surgery of the ureters, including ureterolithotomy or removal of calculus (stones) in the ureters
- bladder surgery
- pelvic lymph node dissection
- prostatic surgery, removal of the prostate
- testicular (scrotal) surgery
- urethra surgery
- surgery to the penis

Purpose

Conditions that commonly dictate a need for urologic surgery include neurogenic sources like spinal cord injury; injuries to the pelvic organs; chronic digestive and urinary diseases; as well as prostate infections and inflammations. There are many other common chronic and malignant diseases that can benefit from resection, surgical augmentation, or surgery to clear obstructions. These conditions impact the digestive, renal, and reproductive systems.

Most organs are susceptible to cancer in the form of tumors and invasion of the surrounding tissue. Urologic malignancies are on the rise. Other conditions that are seen more frequently include kidney stones, diseases and infections; pancreatic diseases; ulcerative colitis; penile dysfunction; and infections of the genitourinary tract.

Urologic surgery has been revolutionized by striking advances in urodynamic diagnostic systems. Changes in these areas have been particularly beneficial for urologic surgery: laparascopy, endoscopic examination for colon cancer, implantation procedures, and imaging techniques. These procedural and imaging advances have brought the field of urology to a highly active and innovative stage, with new surgical options created each year.

Demographics

According to the National Kidney Foundation, kidney and urologic diseases affect at least 5% of the American population, and cause over 260,000 deaths. As the population ages, these conditions are expected to increase, especially among ethnic minorities who have a disproportionate share of urologic diseases. Major urologic surgery includes radical and partial resections for malignant and benign conditions; and implantation and diversion surgeries.

Cancer

Prostate cancer is the most common cancer affecting males in the United States. One in 10 men will have the disease at some time in his life. It is, however, treated successfully with surgery.

According to the Urological Foundation, more than 50,000 new cases of bladder cancer are detected each year. In the United States, bladder cancer is the fourth most common cancer in men and the ninth most common for women.

Kidney cancer occurs in 30,000 patients per year, with about 11,000 deaths. It is the eighth most common cancer in men and the tenth most common cancer in women. Renal cell carcinoma makes up 85% of all kidney tumors. In adults ages 50–70 years, kidney cancer occurs twice as often in men as women. At the time of diagnosis, metastasis is present in 25–30% of patients with renal cell carcinoma.

Other conditions

Enlarged prostate (benign prostate hyperplasia, or BPH) is very common, and often treated with surgery. Interstitial cystitis (bladder infection of unknown origin) often affects women with severe pain and incontinence. The condition, like other forms of severe incontinence, requires surgery.

Incontinence is an increasingly diagnosed problem among the aging population in the United States, and is gaining recognition for its highly debilitating effects both in its fecal and urinary forms. According to the National Institute of Diabetes & Digestive & Kidney Diseases (NIDDK), more than 6.5 million Americans have fecal incontinence. Fecal incontinence affects people of all ages; many cases are never reported. Women are five times more likely than men to have fecal incontinence. This is primarily due to obstetric injury, especially with forceps delivery and anal sphincter laceration.

More than 13 million people in the United States experience urinary incontinence. Community based studies reveal that 30% of patients are over the age of 65, and 63% are female. According to one study published in the *American Journal of Gastroenterology,* only 34% of incontinent patients have ever mentioned their problem to a physician, even though 23% wear absorbent pads, 12% take medications, and 11% lead lives restricted by their incontinence.

Many surgical procedures are now available to correct both fecal and urinary incontinence. They include retropubic slings for urinary incontinence, artificial sphincter implants for urinary and fecal incontinence, and bladder and colon diversion surgeries for restoration of voiding and waste function with an outside appliance called an ostomy. Kidney surgery and transplantation account for a large segment of urologic surgery. Benign conditions include sexual dysfunction, kidney stones, and fertility issues.

Description

Until the late twentieth century, urological operations usually involved open abdominal surgery with full incision, lengthy hospital stays, and long recovery periods. Today, surgery is less traumatic, with shortened hospitalizations. Minimally invasive surgeries are the norm in many cases, with new laparascopic procedures developed each year. Laparoscopic surgery is effective for many kidney tumors and kidney removal (nephrectomy), lymph node excision, prostate and ureteral cancers, as well as incontinence, urological reconstruction, kidney stones, and some cases of bladder dysfunction.

Diagnosis/Preparation

Testing is often required to determine if a patient is better suited for open or laparscopic surgery. Blood tests for some cancers, as well as function tests for the affected organs, will be required. Radiographic or ultrasound techniques are helpful in providing images of abnormalities.

Cystoscopy is often used with bladder and urethra surgery. In this procedure, a thin telescope-like instrument is inserted directly into the bladder. Disorders of

the colon may be studied with endoscopes, imaging instruments inserted directly into the colon. Urodynamic studies of the bladder and sphincter determine how the bladder fills and empties. Digital rectal exams diagnose prostatic disorders. In this procedure, the physician feels the prostate with a gloved, lubricated finger inserted into the rectum.

Aftercare

Hospital stays range from one day to one week, depending upon the level of organ involvement and type of urologic surgery (open versus laparoscopic). Major urologic surgeries may require stents (temporary diversion of urine or feces) and catheters that are removed after surgery. Some surgeries are staged in two parts to accommodate the removal of diseased tissue, and the augmentation or reconstruction to replace function. Laparoscopic surgery patients benefit from shorter hospital stays, more rapid recovery, and possibly lower morbidity rates than open surgery procedures. This is increasingly true for prostate cancer surgeries.

Risks

The risks of urologic surgery vary with the type of surgical procedure (open or laparacopic), and the extent of organ involvement. According to one study of 2,407 urologic surgeries in four centers, the overall complication rate was 4.4%, with a mortality rate of 0.08%.

Open surgery poses the standard surgery and anesthetic risks associated with strain on the heart and lungs. Risks of infection at the wound site accompany all surgeries, open and laparoscopic. The risk of injury to adjacent organs is higher in laparoscopic surgery. Kidney removal and transplantation have many risks because of the extent of the surgery, as do surgeries of the colon, bladder, and prostate.

Significant gains have been made in prostate surgery. Urinary control issues following prostate

KEY TERMS

Genitourinary reconstruction—Surgery that corrects birth defects or the results of disease that involve the genitals and urinary tract, including the kidneys, ureters, bladder, urethra, and the male and female genitals.

Nephrectomy—Surgical removal of a kidney.

Neurogenic bladder—Bladder dysfunction caused by neurological diseases that alter the brain's messages to the bladder.

Prostatectomy—Prostate cancer surgery that includes partial or complete removal of the prostate.

surgery, especially radical prostatectomy, have improved. However, postoperative urinary incontinence remains a significant risk, with 27% of patients in one study reporting the need for some kind of leakage protection. In the same study, only 14.2% of previously potent men reported the ability to achieve and maintain a postoperative erection that is sufficient for sexual intercourse. Urologic surgeons are well versed in the risks and benefits of the surgeries they perform, and they expect to be asked questions related to these issues.

Normal results

The expected surgery result is a topic that the urologic surgeon and patient should address prior to surgery. It is important that the patient understands the issues of recovery, rehabilitation, training or retraining, and the limitations surgery may offer for basic daily functions and enjoyment. Results of urologic surgery are individual, and depend upon the health of the patient and his or her motivation to deal with postoperative recovery issues and changes to organ function brought about by the surgery.

Alternatives

Many urological diseases can be dealt with through diet, weight loss, and lifestyle changes. These modifications are especially significant in preventing and treating conditions of the urinary tract. Obesity and nutrition play a significant role in urologic diseases, and impact many urologic cancers, inflammatory and ulcerative conditions, incontinence, and sexual dysfunction.

Medical interventions are another form of treatment, particularly for infectious and inflammatory urologic conditions. They are particularly useful along with special adjunctive surgical procedures for the treatment of incontinence and painful bladder and kidney conditions. While many cancers must be treated surgically, prostate cancer is often treated with a "wait and see" approach due to its slow rate of growth. There is an increasing trend for men with slow-growing prostate cancers to have regular check-ups instead of immediate treatment.

See also Open prostatectomy; Transurethral resection of the prostate; Ureterostomy.

Resources

BOOKS

Walsh, P. *Campbell's Urology.* 8th ed. Elsevier Science, 2002.

PERIODICALS

Hedican, S.P. "Laparoscopy in Urology." *Surgical Clinics of North America* 80, no.5 (October 1, 2000): 1465-85.

Leng, W. and E.J. McGuire. "Reconstructive Urology Surgical Craft: Laparoscopic Live Donor Nephrectomy." *Urologic Clinics of North America* 26, no.1 (February 1999).

Leung, A.K.H., et.al. "Critical Care and the Urologic Patient." *Critical Care Clinics* 19, no.1 (January 2003).

ORGANIZATIONS

American Society of Nephrology. 1725 Eye Street, NW Suite 510,Washington, DC 20006. (202) 659-0599. Fax: (202) 659-0709.

American Society of Transplantation. 236 Route 38 West, Suite 100, Moorestown, NJ 08057. (856) 608-1104. Fax: (856) 608-1103. <www.a-s-t.org>.

National Institute of Diabetes and Digestive and Kidney Diseases. National Institutes of Health, Information Office. 31 Center Drive, MSC 2560, Building 31, Room 9A-04,Bethesda, MD 20892-2560. (800) 860-8747, (800) 891-5389, (800) 891-5390, (301) 496-3583. Fax: (301) 496-7422. <www.niddk.nih.gov/>.

National Kidney Foundation. Director of Communications, 30 East 33rd Street, New York, NY 10016. (800) 622-9010, (212) 889-2210. Fax: (212) 689-9261. <www.kidney.org>.

OTHER

"Resource Guide: Prostate Cancer." American Foundation for Urologic Diseases.

Nancy McKenzie, Ph.D.

Uterine fibroid removal *see* Myomectomy

Uterine stimulants

Definition

Uterine stimulants (uterotonics) are medications given to cause a woman's uterus to contract, or to increase the frequency and intensity of the contractions. These drugs are used to induce (start) or augment (speed) labor; facilitate uterine contractions following a miscarriage; induce abortion; or reduce hemorrhage following childbirth or abortion. The three uterotonics used most frequently are the oxytocins, prostaglandins, and ergot alkaloids. Uterotonics may be given intravenously (IV), intramuscularly (IM), as a vaginal gel or suppository, or by mouth.

Purpose

Uterine stimulants are used to induce, or begin, labor in certain circumstances when the mother's labor has not started naturally. These circumstances may include the mother's being past her due date; that is, the pregnancy has lasted longer than 40 weeks. Labor is especially likely to be induced if tests indicate a decrease in the volume of amniotic fluid. Uterotonics may also be used in cases of premature rupture of the membranes; preeclampsia (elevated blood pressure in the later stages of pregnancy); diabetes; and intrauterine growth retardation (IUGR), if these conditions require delivery before labor has begun. These medications may be recommended if the expectant mother lives a great distance from the healthcare facility and there is concern for either her or her baby's safety if she were unable to reach the facility once labor begins.

Uterine stimulants are also used in the augmentation of existing contractions, to increase their strength and frequency when labor is not progressing well.

According to the American College of Obstetrics and Gynecology (ACOG), the 1990s saw an increase in the rate of induced labor—from 9% of deliveries to 18%. The ACOG reported in May 2001 that the increase in the rate of Caesarian sections seen over the same period of time was not due to the induction process but to such other factors as the condition of the mother's cervix at the time of induction and whether the pregnancy was the woman's first.

Precautions

It is important to establish a clear baseline of **vital signs** before a woman is given any uterine stimulant. Consistent reevaluation and documentation of vital signs permit faster recognition of an abnormal change in a woman's condition. Documentation includes the time and dosage of any medications given, as well as a record of any side effects. A faster pulse and a drop in blood pressure signal a potential hemorrhage. When oxytocin is given intravenously, it must be diluted in IV fluid and never given as a straight IV. PGs should not be administered if there is any question about the condition of the fetus—for example, an abnormal fetal heart rate tracing. Methergine should never be given intravenously, and never to a woman with hypertension (high blood pressure).

Description

Oxytocin

Oxytocin is a naturally occurring hormone used to induce labor. The production and secretion of natural oxytocin is stimulated by the pituitary gland. It is also available in synthetic form under the trade names of Pitocin and Syntocinon.

Oxytocin is used in a contraction **stress test** (CST). A CST is done prior to the onset of labor to evaluate the fetus's ability to withstand the contractions of the uterus. To avoid the possibility of exogenous (introduced) oxytocin putting the woman into labor, she may instead be asked to stimulate her nipples to release her natural oxytocin. A negative, or normal, CST result is three contractions within a 10-minute period with no abnormal slowing of the fetal heart rate (FHR). The CST occasionally produces false positives, however.

Oxytocin may be used in the treatment of a miscarriage to assure that all the products of conception (POC) are expelled from the uterus. If the fetus died but was not expelled, a prostaglandin (PGE_2) may be given to ripen the cervix to facilitate a dilatation and evacuation, or to encourage uterine contractions. The prostaglandin may be administered either in gel form or as a vaginal suppository.

In a routine delivery, oxytocin may be given to the mother after the placenta has been delivered in order to help the uterus contract and minimize bleeding. It is also used to treat uterine hemorrhage. While hemorrhage occurs in about 4% of vaginal deliveries and 6% of Caesarian deliveries, it accounts for about 35% of maternal deaths due to bleeding during pregnancy. If the bleeding started at the placental detachment site, contractions of the uterus help to close off the blood vessels and thereby stop excessive bleeding. Additional medications may be used, including PGF2$_{alpha}$ (Hemabate), misoprostol (Cytotec), or the ergot alkaloid methylergonovine (Methergine).

Prostaglandins

Prostaglandins (PGs) play a major role in stimulating the uterine contractions at the beginning of labor. Research indicates that PGs are also involved in the transition from the early phase of labor to the later stages. In addition, PGs may be used to ripen the cervix prior to induction. Administration of prostaglandins is sometimes sufficient to stimulate labor, and the woman needs no further medication for labor to progress. There are many PGs used in medicine, but the most significant are PGE$_1$, PGE$_2$, and PGF2$_{alpha}$. Researchers are investigating which prostaglandins are the most effective for specific purposes. For example, PGE$_2$ in the form of dinoprostone (Cervidil and Prepidil) has proved to be superior to the PGF series for cervical ripening. Misoprostol (Cytotec), a synthetic form of PGE$_1$, is also effective in cervical ripening and labor induction, while the PGF2$_{alpha}$ analogue, carboprost (Prostin 15-M, or Hemabate), is the preferred prostaglandin for stimulating the uterus.

Ergot alkaloids

Ergot alkaloids are derived from a fungus, *Claviceps purpurea*, which grows primarily on rye grain. The fungus forms a hard blackish body known as a sclerotium, which contains alkaloid compounds that can be used to treat migraine headache. Ergot by itself, however, is toxic to the central nervous system of humans and animals, producing irritability, spasms, cramps, and convulsions. Because of its potentially harmful side effects, one ergot-based drug (Ergonovine or Ergotrate) was taken off the American market in 1993. Methylergonovine maleate (Methergine) is now the only ergot derivative in use in the United States. It is given only as a uterine stimulant to control PPH. Because of the risk of complications, and because the use of Methergine is contraindicated in many women, it has largely been replaced by the PGs as a second-line uterotonic.

Preparation

A health care professional should review information about a medication or procedure with the pregnant woman before administering it to make sure that she understands what will happen during the procedure or the potential side effects of the medication. The patient should inform the doctor or nurse about any allergies to medications, as well as any side effects she may have experienced previously.

If the patient is anxious about induction of labor or augmentation of contractions, the nurse or doctor should discuss these concerns and relieve the patient's anxiety.

Aftercare

The expectant mother should be monitored closely during induction of labor or cervical ripening. The FHR and uterine contractions are usually monitored for an hour after induction. Frequent checks of the patient's vital signs alert the nurse to any potential complications.

Risks

Oxytocin

Oxytocin takes effect rapidly when it is given intravenously. Individual responses to oxytocin vary considerably; for this reason, the drug dosage is usually increased slowly and incrementally. Oxytocin can cause hyperstimulation of the uterus, which in turn can place the fetus at risk for asphyxia. Hyperstimulation is defined as more than five contractions in 10 minutes; contractions lasting longer than 60 seconds, and increased uterine tonus either with or without significant decrease in FHR. Uterine rupture has also been linked to oxytocin administration, particularly when the drug is given for four hours or longer.

Oxytocin has a mild antidiuretic effect that is usually dose-related; it can lead to water intoxication (hyponatremia). Onset occurs gradually and may go unnoticed. Signs of water intoxication may include reduced urine output, confusion, nausea, convulsions, and coma. Expectant mothers receiving oxytocin should have their blood pressure monitored closely, as both hypotension and hypertension can occur.

Although the subject remains controversial, some evidence suggests oxytocin increases the incidence of neonatal jaundice. Although oxytocin may increase the risk of uterine rupture in women who were delivered by Caesarian section in a previous pregnancy, contraindications to the use of the drug are virtually the same as contraindications for labor. Other side effects of oxytocin include nausea, vomiting, cardiac arrhythmias, and fetal bradycardia (slowing of the heartbeat). When used judiciously, oxytocin is a very effective medication for the progression of labor.

Prostaglandins

PGs have significant systemic side effects. These include headache, nausea, diarrhea, tachycardia (rapid heartbeat), vomiting, chills, fever, sweating, hypertension, and hypotension (low blood pressure). There is also an in-

KEY TERMS

Alkaloid—Any of a group of bitter-tasting alkaline compounds that contain nitrogen and are commonly found in plants. Alkaloids derived from ergot can be used as uterine stimulants.

Antidiuretic—A medication or other compound that suppresses the production of urine.

Cesarian section—An incision made through the wall of a pregnant woman's abdomen and uterus in order to deliver the fetus. The origin of the name is unclear, but it has been associated with the tradition that Julius Caesar was delivered by this method. It is commonly abbreviated as "C-section."

Cyanosis—A bluish discoloration of the skin and mucous membranes caused by low levels of oxygen in the blood.

Ergot alkaloids—Compounds derived from a fungus, *Claviceps purpurea*, which grows on rye plants and forms a hard blackish body. Ergot itself is toxic.

Hemorrhage—The loss of an excessive amount of blood in a short period of time. After childbirth, a loss of more than 500 mL over a 24-hour period is considered a postpartum hemorrhage.

Induce—To begin or start.

Miscarriage—The loss of a fetus before it is viable, usually between the third and seventh months of pregnancy. A miscarriage is sometimes called a spontaneous abortion.

Postpartum—After childbirth or after delivery.

Prostaglandins—A group of unsaturated fatty acids involved in the contraction of smooth muscle, control of body temperature, and other body functions.

Vital signs—Measurements of a patient's essential body functions, usually defined as pulse rate, breathing rate, and body temperature.

creased risk of uterine hyperstimulation and uterine rupture. $PGF2_{alpha}$ (carboprost—Prostin 15-M or Hemabate) can cause hypotension, pulmonary edema, and intense bronchospasms in women with asthma. Because carboprost stimulates the production of steroids, it may be contraindicated in women with disorders of the adrenal gland. When used for abortion, it may result in sufficient blood loss to cause anemia, which may make a **transfusion** necessary. Medical problems (or a history) of diabetes, epilepsy, heart or blood vessel disease, jaundice, kidney disease, or liver disease should be brought to the attention of the health care practitioner before the patient is given carboprost. The use of this PG has been reported to increase the fluid pressure in the eyes in women with glaucoma; however, this side effect is fortunately rare.

Ergot alkaloids

Ergot alkaloids have an alpha-adrenergic action with a vasoconstrictive effect, which means that they cause the blood vessels to become narrower. These drugs can cause hypertension, cardiovascular changes, cyanosis, muscle pain, tingling, other symptoms associated with decreased blood circulation, and severe uterine cramping. The health care professional should be informed of other medications taken by the patient. The presence or history of such medical problems as angina, hypertension, stroke, infection, kidney and liver disease, and Raynaud's phenomenon may be contraindications to the use of ergot alkaloids.

Normal results

The normal results of uterine stimulants, when administered in appropriate circumstances and correct dosages, are preparation of the cervix for childbirth; induction or stimulation of uterine contractions to produce a safe delivery of a newborn; encouragement of a complete spontaneous or induced abortion; elimination of blood clots or other tissue debris from the uterus; and the slowing or cessation of hemorrhage following childbirth or abortion.

Normal results would include the achievement of these outcomes without significant side effects for the mother or fetus.

Resources

BOOKS

Creasy, Robert K., and Robert Resnik. *Maternal-Fetal Medicine*, 4th ed. Philadelphia, PA: W. B. Saunders Company, 1999.

Rakel, Robert A., MD, ed. *Conn's Current Therapy 2000*. Philadelphia, PA: W. B. Saunders Company, 2000.

Scott, James. *Danforth's Obstetrics and Gynecology*, 8th ed. Philadelphia, PA: Lippincott Williams & Wilkins, 1999.

Wilson, Billie Ann, RN, PhD, Carolyn L. Stang, PharmD, and Margaret T. Shannon, RN, PhD. *Nurses Drug Guide 2000*. Stamford, CT: Appleton and Lange, 1999.

ORGANIZATIONS

American College of Obstetricians and Gynecologists (ACOG). 409 12th St. SW, PO Box 96920, Washington, DC 20090-6920. <www.acog.com>.

United States Food and Drug Administration (FDA). 5600 Fishers Lane, Rockville, MD 20857-0001. (888) INFO-FDA. <www.fda.gov>.

Esther Csapo Rastegari, R.N., B.S.N., Ed.M.
Sam Uretsky, PharmD

Uterus removal *see* **Hysterectomy**

Uvulopalatoplasty *see* Snoring surgery

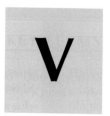

Vagal nerve stimulation

Definition

Vagal nerve stimulation is a treatment for epilepsy in which an electrode is implanted in the neck to deliver electrical impulses to the vagus nerve.

Purpose

Vagal nerve stimulation is an alternative to medication or surgical removal of brain tissue in controlling epileptic seizures. The seizures of epilepsy are caused by uncontrolled electrical discharges spreading through the brain. Anti-seizure drugs interrupt this process by reducing the sensitivity of individual brain cells to stimulation. Brain surgery for epilepsy either removes the portion of the brain where seizures originate, or cuts nerve fibers to prevent the nerve impulses that occur during a seizure from spreading to other parts of the brain. Vagal nerve stimulation uses a different approach; it provides intermittent electrical stimulation to a nerve outside the brain—the vagus, or tenth cranial nerve, which influences certain patterns of brain activity.

The vagus nerve is a major connection between the brain and the rest of the body. It carries sensory information from the body to the brain, and motor commands from the brain to the body. The vagus is involved in complex control loops between these destinations; its precise pathways and mechanisms are still not fully understood. It is also not known how stimulation of the vagus nerve works to reduce seizure activity—it may stimulate inhibitory pathways that prevent the brain's electrical activity from getting out of control, interrupt some feedback loops that worsen seizures, or act in some other fashion.

Vagal nerve stimulation has been effective in reducing seizure frequency in patients whose seizures are not controlled by drugs, and who are either not candidates for other types of brain surgery or who have chosen not to undergo these procedures.

Demographics

Epilepsy affects about 1% of people in the general worldwide population. Approximately 40% of patients do not respond well to medications, however, and so may be candidates for surgical treatment. Vagus nerve stimulation was first performed in the United States in 1988 and received final approval by the United States Food and Drug Administration (FDA) in July 1997. Approximately 10,000 people worldwide have had stimulators implanted as of 2003; about a fifth of these patients are children 12 years old and younger.

Description

The vagal nerve stimulator has two parts: an electrode that wraps around the left vagus nerve in the neck; and a pulse generator, which is implanted under the skin below the collarbone. The two parts are connected by a wire. Stimulation is performed only on the left vagal nerve, as the right vagal nerve helps control the heartbeat.

Surgery to implant a VNS device takes about two hours. A neurosurgeon implants the electrode and generator while the patient is under general anesthesia. A vertical incision is made in the left side of the neck, and the helical electrode is attached to the nerve itself. A second incision is made on the left side of the chest below the collarbone, and the pulse generator (a disc about 2 in [5 cm] in diameter) is implanted under the skin. The connecting wire is threaded around the muscles and bones to join the elec-

QUESTIONS TO ASK THE DOCTOR

- What will the procedure cost? Will my insurance cover the cost?
- How often will I need to return to have the stimulator adjusted?
- Will my medication dosages be reduced after this procedure?
- How long will the procedure take?
- How many VNS devices have you implanted? What is your success rate?

trode and generator. The generator makes a small bulge under the skin but is hidden by clothing after the operation.

Before the neurosurgeon closes the incisions, he or she tests the VNS device to make sure it is working, and programs it to deliver the lowest amount of stimulation. The device is usually timed to stimulate the vagus nerve for 30 seconds every five minutes.

Diagnosis/Preparation

A candidate for vagal nerve stimulation will have had many tests already to determine the focal point of seizure activity. Preoperative tests include neuroimaging as well as psychological tests to determine the patient's cognitive (thinking) strengths and weaknesses.

The patient must be fully informed about VNS—how it works, its advantages and disadvantages, what will happen during surgery—before the operation is scheduled. A video as well as written material about VNS is available to view and discuss with the doctor.

Aftercare

Implantation of the stimulator in an adult may be performed as either an outpatient or inpatient procedure. In the latter case, the patient will remain in the hospital overnight for monitoring of heart function and other **vital signs**. Children who are receiving a VNS are usually scheduled for an overnight stay. Pain medication is given as needed.

The stimulation parameters are adjustable, and the neurologist may require several visits to find the right settings. Settings are adjusted with a magnetic wand that delivers commands to the stimulator's computer chip. The patient may be taught how to use a magnet to temporarily increase stimulation, to prevent a seizure, or to abort it once it begins.

The VNS generator is powered by a battery that lasts several years. It is replaced during an outpatient procedure under local anesthesia.

Risks

The most common adverse effects from vagal nerve stimulation are a hoarse voice, cough, headache, and ear pain. These side effects can be reduced by adjusting the stimulation settings, and may subside on their own over time. Infection and device malfunction are possible though rare.

Patients who have had a VNS implanted must avoid strong magnets, which may affect the stimulator settings. Areas with warning signs posted regarding **pacemakers** should be avoided. The patient should consult with the neurologist and the neurosurgeon about other hazards.

Normal results

Approximately half of all patients who have received vagal nerve stimulation experience about a 50% reduction in seizures. Another 9% of patients obtain complete relief from seizures. Most patients who continue to take antiseizure medications can reduce their dosage, however, which offers some relief from the side effects of these drugs.

Morbidity and mortality rates

Vagal nerve stimulation is a relatively safe procedure, with no deaths attributed to the stimulation as of 2003. Pilot studies of 300 patients that were done prior to FDA approval of VNS reported the following complication rates: hoarseness, 37% of patients; coughing, 14%; voice alteration, 13%; chest pain, 12%; and nausea, 2%.

Alternatives

Some candidates for vagal nerve stimulation are also likely to be candidates for a **corpus callosotomy**, temporal lobectomy, or other surgical procedures.

See also Hemispherectomy.

Resources

BOOKS

Devinsky, O. *A Guide to Understanding and Living with Epilepsy.* Philadelphia: E. A. Davis, 1994.

"Seizure Disorders." Section 14, Chapter 172 in *The Merck Manual of Diagnosis and Therapy*, edited by Mark H. Beers, MD, and Robert Berkow, MD. Whitehouse Station, NJ: Merck Research Laboratories, 1999.

PERIODICALS

Rielo, Diego, MD, and Selim R. Benbadis, MD. "Vagus Nerve Stimulation." *eMedicine*, April 12, 2002 [June 10, 2003]. <www.emedicine.com/neuro/topic559.htm>.

KEY TERMS

Epilepsy—The name for a group of syndromes characterized by periodic temporary disturbances of brain function. The symptoms of an epileptic seizure may include loss of consciousness, abnormal movements, falling, emotional reactions, and disturbances of sight or hearing.

Helical—Having a spiral shape.

Neurologist—A physician who specializes in diagnosing and treating disorders of the nervous system.

Seizure—A single episode of epilepsy. Seizures are also called convulsions or fits.

Vagus nerve—The tenth cranial nerve, running from the head through the neck and chest into the abdomen. Intermittent electrical stimulation of the vagus nerve can help to control epileptic seizures.

ORGANIZATIONS

American Association of Neurological Surgeons (AANS). 5550 Meadowbrook Drive, Rolling Meadows, IL 60008. (847) 378-0500. <www.neurosurgery.org>.

Epilepsy Foundation. 4351 Garden City Drive, Landover, MD 20785-7223. (800) 332-1000. <www.epilepsyfoundation.org>.

Richard Robinson

Vaginal wall repair *see* **Colporrhaphy**

Vaginotomy *see* **Colpotomy**

Vagotomy

Definition

Vagotomy is the surgical cutting of the vagus nerve to reduce acid secretion in the stomach.

Purpose

The vagus nerve trunk splits into branches that go to different parts of the stomach. Stimulation from these branches causes the stomach to produce acid. Too much stomach acid leads to ulcers that may eventually bleed and create an emergency situation.

A vagotomy is performed when acid production in the stomach can not be reduced by other means. The purpose of the procedure is to disable the acid-producing capacity of the stomach. It is used when ulcers in the stomach and duodenum do not respond to medication and changes in diet. It is an appropriate surgery when there are ulcer complications, such as obstruction of digestive flow, bleeding, or perforation. The frequency with which elective vagotomy is performed has decreased in the past 20 years as it has become clear that the primary cause of ulcers is an infection by a bacterium called *Helicobacter pylori*. Drugs have become increasingly effective in treating ulcers. However, the number of vagotomies performed in emergency situations has remained about the same.

A vagotomy procedure is often performed in conjunction with another gastrointestinal surgery, such as partial removal of the stomach (**antrectomy** or subtotal **gastrectomy**).

Demographics

Gastric (peptic) ulcers are included under the general heading of gastrointestinal (GI) diseases. GI disorders affect an estimated 25–30% of the world's population. In the United States, 60 million adults experience gastrointestinal reflux at least once a month, and 25 million adults suffer daily from heartburn. Left untreated, these conditions often evolve into ulcers. Four million people have active peptic ulcers; about 350,000 new cases are diagnosed each year. Four times as many duodenal ulcers as gastric ulcers are diagnosed. The first-degree relatives of patients with duodenal ulcer have a two to three times greater risk of developing duodenal ulcer. Relatives of gastric ulcer patients have a similarly increased risk of developing a gastric ulcer.

Description

A vagotomy can be performed using closed (laparoscopic) or open surgical technique. The indications for a laparoscopic vagotomy are the same as open vagotomy.

There are four basic types of vagotomy procedures:

- Truncal or total abdominal vagotomy. The main vagal trunks are divided, and surgery is accompanied by a drainage procedure, such as **pyloroplasty**.

- Selective (total gastric) vagotomy. The main vagal trunks are dissected to the point where the branch leading to the biliary tree divides, and there is a cut at the section of vagus close to the hepatic branch. This procedure is rarely indicated or performed.

- Highly selective vagotomy (HSV). HSV selectively deprives the parietal cells of vagal nerves, and reduces

Vagotomy

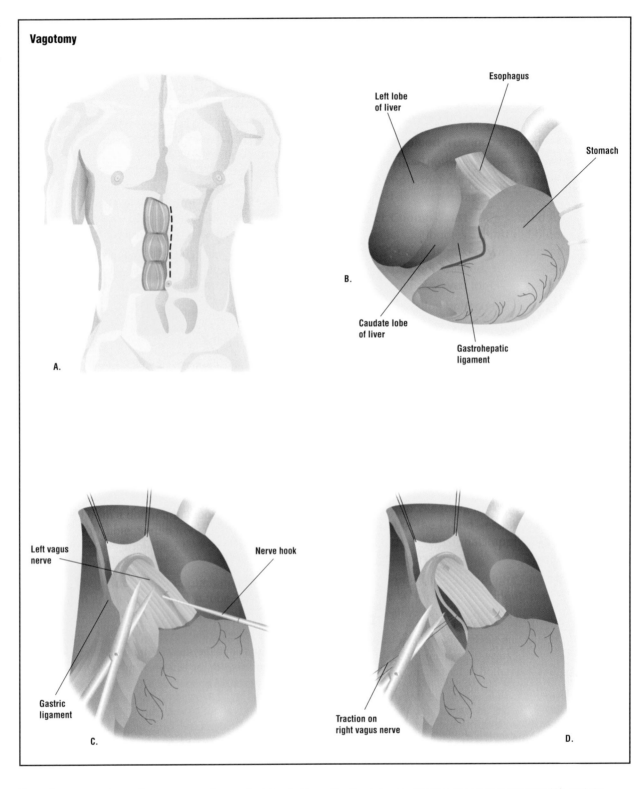

To perform a vagotomy, the surgeon makes an incision in the patient's abdomen (A). The stomach is located (B), and the vagus nerves are cut in turn (C and D). *(Illustration by GGS Inc.)*

their sensitivity to stimulation and the release of acid. It does not require a drainage procedure. The branches of Latarjet's nerve are divided from the esophagogastric junction to the crow's foot along the lesser curvature of the stomach.

• Thoracoscopic vagotomy. Performed through the third, sixth, and seventh left intercostal spaces, the posterior vagus trunk is isolated, clipped, and a segment excised.

A vagotomy is performed under general anesthesia. The surgeon makes an incision in the abdomen and locates the vagus nerve. Either the trunk or the branches leading to the stomach are cut. The abdominal muscles are sewn back together, and the skin is closed with sutures.

Often, other gastrointestinal surgery is performed (e.g., part of the stomach may be removed) at the same time. Vagotomy causes a decrease in peristalsis, and a change in the emptying patterns of the stomach. To ease this, a pyloroplasty is often performed to widen the outlet from the stomach to the small intestine.

Diagnosis/Preparation

A gastroscopy and x rays of the gastrointestinal system determine the position and condition of the ulcer. Standard preoperative blood and urine tests are done. The patient discusses with the anesthesiologist any medications or conditions that might affect the administration of anesthesia.

Aftercare

Patients who have had a vagotomy stay in the hospital for about seven days. Nasogastric suctioning is required for the first three or four days. A tube is inserted through the nose and into the stomach. The stomach contents are then suctioned out. Patients eat a clear liquid diet until the gastrointestinal tract regains function. When patients return to a regular diet, spicy and acidic foods should be avoided.

It takes about six weeks to fully recover from the surgery. The sutures that close the skin can be removed in seven to 10 days. Patients are encouraged to move around soon after the operation to prevent the formation of deep vein blood clots. Pain medication, stool softeners, and **antibiotics** may be prescribed following the operation.

Risks

Standard surgical risks, such as excessive bleeding and infection, are potential complications. In addition, the emptying patterns of the stomach are changed. This can lead to dumping syndrome and diarrhea. Dumping syndrome is a condition in which the patient experiences

palpitations, sweating, nausea, cramps, vomiting, and diarrhea shortly after eating.

The following complications are also associated with vagotomy surgery:

• Gastric or esophageal perforation. May occur from an electrocautery injury or by clipping the branch of the nerve of Latarjet.

• Delayed gastric emptying. Most common after truncal and selective vagotomy, particularly if a drainage procedure is not performed.

People who use alcohol excessively, smoke, are obese, and are very young or very old are at higher risk for complications.

Normal results

Normal recovery is expected for most patients. Ulcers recur in about 10% of those who have vagotomy without stomach removal. Recurrent ulcers are also found in 2–3% of patients who have some portion of their stomach removed.

Morbidity and mortality rates

In the United States, approximately 3,000 deaths per year are due to duodenal ulcer and 3,000 to gastric ulcer. There has been a marked decrease in reported hospitalization and mortality rates for gastric ulcer.

Alternatives

The preferred short-term treatment for gastric ulcers is drug therapy. A recent review surveying medical articles published from 1977 to 1994 concluded that drugs such as cimetidine, ranitidine, famotidine, H2 blockers, and sucralfate were efficient, with omeprazole considered the "gold standard" for active gastric ulcer treatment. Surgical intervention, however, is recommended for people who do not respond to medical therapy.

Resources

BOOKS

Ansolon, K. B. *Developmental Technology of Gastrectomy & Vagotomy.* Rockville, MD: Kabel Publishers, 1995.

Kral, J. *Vagal Nerve Function.* New York: Elsevier Science Ltd., 1984.

"Stomach and Duodenum." In *Current Surgical Diagnosis and Treatment,* 10th ed. Edited by Lawrence W. Day. Stamford: Appleton & Lange, 1994.

PERIODICALS

Chang, T. M., D.C. Chan, Y.C. Liu, S.S. Tsou, and T. H. Chen. "Long-term Results of Duodenectomy with Highly Selective Vagotomy in the Treatment of Complicated Duodenal Ulcers." *American Journal of Surgery* 181 (April 2001): 372-6.

Gilliam, A. D., W.J. Speake, and D. N. Lobo. "Current Practice of Emergency Vagotomy and Helicobacter Pylori Eradication for Complicated Peptic Ulcer in the United Kingdom." *British Journal of Surgery* 90 (January 2003): 88-90.

Saindon, C. S., F. Blecha, T.I. Musch, D.A. Morgan, R.J. Fels, and M. J. Kenney. "Effect of Cervical Vagotomy on Sympathetic Nerve Responses to Peripheral Interleukin-1beta." *Autonomic Neuroscience* 87 (March 2001): 243-8.

ORGANIZATIONS

American College of Surgeons. 633 N. Saint Clair St., Chicago, IL 60611. (312) 202-5000. <www.faacs.org>.

Society of American Gastrointestinal Endoscopic Surgeons. 2716 Ocean Park Boulevard, Suite 3000, Santa Monica, CA 90405. (310) 314-2404. <www.sages.org>.

OTHER

"Laparoscopic Vagotomy." *SAGES web center.* <www.sages.org/primarycare/chapter19.html>.

Tish Davidson, A.M.
Monique Laberge, Ph.D.

Valvuloplasty, balloon *see* **Balloon valvuloplasty**

Varicose vein sclerotherapy *see* **Sclerotherapy for varicose veins**

Vascular study *see* **Angiography**

Vascular surgery

Definition

Vascular surgery is the treatment of surgery on diagnosed patients with diseases of the arterial, venous, and lymphatic systems (excluding the intracranial and coronary arteries).

Purpose

Vascular surgery is indicated when a patient has vascular disease that cannot be treated by less invasive, nonsurgical treatments. The purpose of vascular surgery is to treat vascular diseases, which are diseases of the arteries and veins. Arterial disease is a condition in which blood clots, arteriosclerosis, and other vascular conditions occur in the arteries. Venous disease involves problems that occur in the veins. Some vascular conditions occur only in arteries, others occur only in the veins, and some affect both veins and arteries.

Demographics

As people age, vascular diseases are very common. Since they rarely cause symptoms in the early stages, many people do not realize that they suffer from these diseases. Of the eight million people in the United States who may have peripheral vascular disease (PVD), a large percentage are males. In the majority of cases, the blockage is caused by one or more blood clots that travel to the lungs from another part of the body. Factors that increase the chances of vascular disease include:

• increasing age (which results in a loss of elasticity in the veins and their valves)

• a family history of heart or vascular disease

• illness or injury

• pregnancy

• prolonged periods of inactivity sitting, standing, or bed rest

• smoking

• obesity

• hypertension, diabetes, high cholesterol, or other conditions that affect the health of the cardiovascular system

• lack of **exercise**

Description

Vascular surgery involves techniques relating to endovascular surgeries including: balloon **angioplasty** and/or stenting, aortic and peripheral vascular endovascular stent/graft placement, thrombolysis, and other adjuncts for vascular reconstruction.

The vascular system is the network of blood vessels that circulate blood to and from the heart and lungs. The circulatory system (made up of the heart, arteries, veins, capillaries, and the circulating blood) provides nourishment to the body's cells and removes their waste. The arteries carry oxygenated blood from the heart to the cells. The veins return the blood from the cells back to the lungs for reoxygenation and recirculation by the heart. The aorta is the largest artery leaving the heart; it then subdivides into smaller arteries going to every part of the body. The arteries, as they narrow, are connected to smaller vessels called capillaries. In these capillaries, oxygen and nutrients are released from the blood into the cells, and cellular wastes are collected for the return trip. The capillaries then connect to veins, which return the blood back to the heart.

The aorta stems from the heart, arches upward, and then continues down through the chest (thorax) and the abdomen. The iliac arteries, which branch out from the aorta, provide blood to the pelvis and legs. The thoracic

section of the aorta supplies blood to the upper body, as it continues through the chest. The abdominal section of the aorta, which supplies blood to the lower body, continues through the abdomen.

Vascular diseases are usually caused by conditions that clog or weaken blood vessels, or damage valves that control the flow of blood in and out of the veins, thus robbing them of vital blood nutrients and oxygen. A few common diseases affecting the arteries are peripheral vascular disease (PVD), carotid artery disease, and aortic aneurysms (AAA).

Surgery is used to treat specific diseased arteries, such as atherosclerosis, to help prevent strokes or heart attacks, improve or relieve angina or hypertension, remove aneurysms, improve claudication, and save legs that would otherwise have to be amputated. The choices involve repairing the artery, bypassing it, or replacing it.

As people age, atherosclerosis, commonly called hardening of the arteries, occurs with the constant passage of blood through the arteries. It can take on a number of forms, of which atherosclerosis (hardening of the innermost portion) is the most common. This occurs when fatty material containing cholesterol or calcium (plaque) is deposited on the innermost layer of the artery. This causes a narrowing of the inside diameter of the blood vessel. Eventually, the artery becomes so narrow that a blood clot (thrombus) forms, and blocks blood flow to an entire portion of the body. This condition is called PVD or peripheral arterial disease. In another form of atherosclerosis, a rough area or ulcer forms in the diseased interior of the artery. Blood clots then tend to develop on this ulcer, break off, and travel further along, forming a blockage where the arteries get narrower. A blockage resulting from a clot formed elsewhere in the body is called an embolism.

People who have few areas affected by PVD may be treated with angioplasty by opening up the blood vessel with a balloon placed on the end of a catheter. A stent is often used with angioplasty to help keep the artery open. The type of surgery used to treat PVD is based upon the size and location of the damaged artery. The following are surgery techniques used for severe PVD:

- Bypass surgery is preferred for people who have many areas of blockage or a long, continuous blockage.

- Aortobifemoral bypass is used for PVD affecting the major abdominal artery (aorta) and the large arteries that branch off of it.

- In a technique called thromboendarterectomy, the inner diseased layers of the artery are removed, leaving the relatively normal outer coats of the artery.

- Resection involves a technique to remove a diseased artery following an aneurysm; a bypass is created with a synthetic graft.

- In a bypass graft, a vein graft from another part of the body or a graft made from artificial material is used to create a detour around a blocked artery.

- Tibioperoneal bypass is used for PVD affecting the arteries in the lower leg or foot.

- Femoropopliteal (fem-pop) bypass surgery is used for PVD affecting the arteries above and below the knee.

- Embolectomy is a technique in which an embolic clot on the wall of the artery is removed, using an inflatable balloon catheter.

- Thrombectomy is a technique in which a balloon catheter is inserted into the affected artery beyond a blood clot. The balloon is then inflated and pulled back, bringing the clot with it.

An aneurysm occurs when weakened blood vessels bulge like balloons as blood flows through them. Once they have grown to a certain size, there is a risk of rupture and life-threatening bleeding. There are two types of aortic aneurysms: abdominal aortic aneurysm (AAA) and thoracic aortic aneurysm. This classification is based on where the aneurysm occurs along the aorta. Aneurysms are more common in the abdominal section of the aorta than the thoracic section.

Most blood clots originate in the legs, but they can also form in the veins of arms, the right side of the heart, or even at the tip of a catheter placed in a vein. The following venous disease conditions usually occur in the veins of the legs:

- varicose veins
- phlebitis
- venous stasis disease
- deep vein thrombosis (DVT)
- claudication
- blood clots

Carotid artery disease is a condition in which the arteries in the neck that supply blood to the brain become clogged; this condition can cause a stroke.

Lymphatic obstruction involves blockage of the lymph vessels, which drain fluid from tissues throughout the body and allow immune cells to travel where they are needed. Some of the causes of lymphatic obstruction (also known as swelling of the lymph passages), include infections such as chronic cellulitis, or parasitic infections such as filariasis, trauma, tumors, certain surgeries including mastectomy, and radiation therapy. There are rare forms of congenital lymphedema that probably result from abnormalities in the development of the lymphatic vessels. Most patients with lymphedema will not need surgery, as the symptoms are usually managed by other techniques. Surgical therapy for lymphedema includes removal of tissue containing abnormal lymphatics, and less commonly, transplant of tissue from areas with normal lymphatic tissues to areas with abnormal lymphatic drainage. In rare cases, bypass of abnormal lymphatic tissue is attempted, sometimes using vein grafts.

Other examples of vascular surgery include:

- cerebral aneurysm
- acute arterial and graft occlusion
- carotid endarterectomy
- endovascular grafting
- vasculogenic erectile dysfunction
- renal artery aneurysm
- surgery on varicose veins
- lower extremity amputation

Diagnosis/Preparation

In order for a patient to be diagnosed with a vascular disease, they must be clinically evaluated by a vascular surgeon, which includes a history and **physical examination**. A vascular surgeon also treats vascular disorders by non-operative means, including drug therapy and risk factor management.

The symptoms produced by atherosclerosis, thrombosis, embolisms, or aneurysms depend on the particular artery affected. These conditions can sometimes cause pain, but often there are no symptoms at all.

A physician has many ways of feeling, hearing, measuring, and even seeing arterial blockages. Many arteries in the body can be felt or palpated. A doctor can feel for a pulse in an area he or she believes afflicted. Usually the more advanced the arteriosclerosis, the less pulse in a given area.

As the artery becomes blocked, it can cause a noise very much like water roaring over rocky rapids. Your physician can listen to this noise (bruit) directly, or can use special amplification systems to hear the noise.

There are other tests that can be done to determine if arterial blood flow is normal:

- ankle-brachial index (ABI) test
- arteriogram
- segmental pressure test
- ultrasound scan
- magnetic resonance imaging
- computed tomography scan
- angiography
- lymphangiography
- lymphoscintigraphy
- plethysmography
- duplex ultrasound scanning

There may be no symptoms of vascular disease caused by blood clots until the clot grows large enough to block the flow of blood through the vein. The following symptoms may then come on suddenly:

- pain
- sudden swelling in the affected limb
- reddish blue discoloration
- enlargement of the superficial veins
- skin that is warm to the touch

The physician will probably do an evaluation of all organ systems including the heart, lungs, circulatory system, kidneys, and the gastrointestinal system. The decision whether to have surgery or not is based on the outcome of these evaluations.

For high-risk patients undergoing vascular surgery, research has shown that taking oral beta-blockers one to two weeks before surgery and continuing for at least two weeks after the operation can significantly reduce the chance of dying or having a heart attack. Scientists suspect that the drug improves oxygen balance in the wall of the heart and stabilizes plaques in the arteries.

Aftercare

The length of time in intensive care and hospitalization will vary with each surgery, as will the recovery

QUESTIONS TO ASK THE DOCTOR

- Can my vascular disease be controlled with lifestyle changes?
- If a procedure is required, am I a candidate for a less invasive, interventional radiology treatment?
- What are the risks and benefits of this operation?
- What are the normal results of this operation?
- What happens if this operation does not go as planned?
- What is the expected recovery time?

time, depending on numerous factors. Because surgery for an AAA is more serious, the patient can expect to be in intensive care for 24 hours, and in the hospital for five to 10 days, providing the patient was healthy and had a smooth operative and postoperative course. If there are complications, the hospital stay will likely increase. It may take as long as six months to fully recover from surgery for an AAA.

Living a "heart-healthy lifestyle" is the best way of preventing and controlling vascular disease: do not smoke; eat nutritious foods low in fat; exercise; maintain a healthy weight; and control risk factors such as high blood pressure, high cholesterol, diabetes, hypertension, and other factors that contribute to vascular disease.

Medications that may be used to treat PVD include:

- aspirin and other antiplatelet medications to treat leg pain
- statins to lower cholesterol levels
- medications to control high blood pressure
- medications to control diabetes
- anticoagulants are rarely, but not generally, used to treat PVD unless the person is at an increased risk for forming blood clots

Risks

All surgeries carry some risks. There is a risk of infection whenever incisions are required. Operations in the chest or those that involve major blood vessels carry a higher risk of complications. Patients who smoke, have high blood pressure, chronic lung or kidney disease, or other illnesses are at greater risk of complications during and after surgery. Other risks of vascular surgery include:

- bleeding

Ankle-brachial index (ABI) test—A means of checking the blood pressure in the arms and ankles using a regular blood pressure cuff and a special ultrasound stethoscope (Doppler). The pressure in the ankle is compared to the pressure in the arm.

Aorta—A large, elastic artery beginning at the upper part of the left ventricle of the heart that becomes the main trunk of the arterial system.

Aortic aneurysms—Occurs when an area in the aorta (the main artery of the heart) is weakened and bulges like a balloon.

Arteriogram—A test to check the blood pressure at several points in the leg by using a blood pressure cuff and a Doppler. The patient is then asked to walk on a treadmill, after which the ankle pressure is taken again to determine if the pressure decreased after walking.

Abdominal aortic aneurysm—Occurs when an area in the aorta (the main artery of the heart) is weakened and bulges like a balloon. The abdominal section of the aorta supplies blood to the lower body.

Aneurysm—A weakening of the artery wall, due to atherosclerosis, causing a bulge which can rupture, and lead to thrombosis or embolism.

Angiography or angiogram—An x ray exam of the arteries and veins (blood vessels) to diagnose blockages and other blood vessel problems.

Atherosclerosis—A form of arteriosclerosis affecting the innermost area of the artery; a series of calcified deposits that can close down the vessel.

Arteriogram—An x ray picture of an artery achieved by injecting an opaque dye with a needle or tube into the affected artery.

Artery—A blood vessel conveying blood in a direction away from the heart.

Bruit—A roaring sound created by a partially blocked artery.

Capillary—Smallest extremity of the arterial vessel, where oxygen and nutrients are released from the blood into the cells, and cellular waste is collected.

Carotid artery—Major artery leading to the brain, blockages of which can cause temporary or permanent strokes.

Carotid artery disease—A condition in which the arteries in the neck that supply blood to the brain become clogged, causing the danger of a stroke.

Carotid endarterectomy—A surgical technique for removing intra-arterial obstructions of the internal carotid artery.

Cerebral aneurysm—The dilation, bulging, or ballooning out of part of the wall of a vein or artery in the brain.

Cholesterol—An abundant fatty substance in animal tissues. High levels in the diet are a factor in the cause of atherosclerosis.

Claudication—Attacks of lameness of pain chiefly in the calf muscles, brought on by walking because of a lack of oxygen reaching the muscle.

Computed tomography scan—A special type of x ray that can produce detailed pictures of structures inside the body.

Collaterals—Alternate pathways for arterial blood.

Claudication—Blockage in the arteries supplying the legs with blood can cause muscle discomfort after walking.

- failed or blocked grafts

- heart attack or stroke

- leg swelling if a leg vein is used

- people over 65 years are at greater risk for brain impairment after major surgery

- the more damaged the circulatory system is before surgery, the higher susceptibility to mental decline after vascular surgery

- impotence

The patient should discuss risks with their surgeon after careful review of the patient's medical history and a physical examination.

Normal results

The success rate for vascular surgery varies depending on a number of factors which may influence the decision on whether to have surgery or not, as well as the results.

The chance that an aneurysm will rupture generally increases with the size of the aneurysm; AAAs smaller than 1.6 in (4 cm) in diameter have up to a 2% risk of rupture while ones larger than 2 in (5 cm) in diameter have a 22% risk of rupture within two years.

Arterial bypass surgery and peripheral bypass surgery have very good success rates. Most of those who undergo AAA surgery recover well, except in the

KEY TERMS (contd.)

Coronary—Of or relating to the heart.

Embolism—Obstruction or closure of a vessel by a transported clot of foreign matter.

Endovascular grafting—A procedure which involves the insertion of a delivery catheter through a groin artery into the abdominal aorta under fluoroscopic guidance.

Intracranial—Existing or occurring within the cranium; or affecting or involving intracranial structures.

Lower extremity amputation—To cut a limb from the body.

Lymphangiography—Injection of dye into lymphatic vessels followed by x rays of the area. It is a difficult procedure, as it requires surgical isolation of the lymph vessels to be injected.

Lymphoscintigraphy—A technique in which a radioactive substance that concentrates in the lymphatic vessels is injected into the affected tissue and mapped using a gamma camera, which images the location of the radioactive tracer.

Magnetic resonance imaging—A noninvasive diagnostic technique that produces computerized images of internal body tissues and is based on nuclear magnetic resonance of atoms within the body induced by the application of radio waves.

Plethysmography—A test in which a patient sits inside a booth called a plethysmograph and breathes through a mouthpiece, while pressure and air flow measurements are collected to measure the total lung volume.

Pulmonary embolism—A blocked artery in the lung.

Renal artery aneurysm—An aneurysm relating to, involving, or located in the region of the kidneys.

Thoracic aortic aneurysm—Occurs when an area in the thoracic section of the aorta (the chest) is weakened and bulges like a balloon. The thoracic section supplies blood to the upper body.

Thrombus—A blood clot that may form in a blood vessel or in one of the cavities of the heart.

Thrombosis—The formation or presence of a blood clot within a blood vessel.

Thrombolysis—A treatment that opens up blood flow and may prevent permanent damage to the blood vessels.

Ulcer—A lesion or rough spot formed on the surface of an artery.

Vascular—Relating to the blood vessels.

Ultrasound scan—The scan produces images of arteries on a screen and is used to evaluate the blood flow, locate blockages, and measure the size of the artery.

Vasculogenic erectile dysfunction—The inability to attain or sustain an erection satisfactory for coitus, due to atherosclerotic disease of penile arteries, inadequate impedance of venous outflow (venous leaks), or a combination of both.

Venous stasis disease—A condition in which there is pooling of blood in the lower leg veins that may cause swelling and tissue damage, and lead to painful sores or ulcers.

Varicose veins—Twisted, enlarged veins near the surface of the skin, which develop most commonly in the legs and ankles.

---

case of a rupture. Most patients who have a ruptured aortic aneurysm die. Surgery for an already ruptured aneurysm is not usually successful, due to excessive, rapid blood loss.

Surgical therapy for lymphedema has met with limited success, and requires significant experience and technical expertise.

Morbidity and mortality rates

Peripheral vascular disease affects 10 million people in the United States, including 5% of those over 50. Only a quarter of PVD sufferers are receiving treatment. More than five million people in the United States develop DVT each year. More than 600,000 Americans experience a pulmonary embolism every year. Of those, approximately 200,000 people die from the condition.

Alternatives

There a few alternatives to treating vascular disease, although extensive research has not been done. Acupuncture is used to aid in hypertension and chelation therapy is thought to stabilize the effects of vascular disease. The focus should be on maintaining a proper diet and being aware of a family history of vascular disease so as to catch it as early as possible.

Resources

BOOKS

Cameron, John L. *Current Surgical Therapy.* 7th ed. Philadelphia: Mosby, 2002.

Hoballah, Jamal J. *Vascular Reconstructions: Anatomy, Exposures, and Techniques.* Berlin: Springer Verlag, 2000.

PERIODICALS

Abir, Farshad, Iannis Kakisis, and Bauer Sumpio. "Do Vascular Surgery Patients need a Cardiology Work-up? A Review of Pre-operative Cardiac Clearance Guidelines in Vascular Surgery." *European Journal of Vascular and Endovascular Surgery* 25, no. 2 (2003): 110–117.

Moore, Wesley S., M.D., G. Patrick Clagett, M.D., Frank J. Veith, M.D., Gregory L. Moneta, M.D., Marshall W. Webster, M.D. et al. "Guidelines for Hospital Privileges in Vascular Surgery: An Update by an Ad Hoc Committee of the American Association for Vascular Surgery and the Society for Vascular Surgery." *Journal of Vascular Surgery* 36, no. 6 (2002): 1276–1282.

ORGANIZATIONS

American Board of Vascular Surgery (ABVS). 900 Cummings Center. #221-U Beverly, MA 01915. <http://aavs.vascularweb.org>.

The National Heart, Lung and Blood Institute. 6701 Rockledge Drive, P.O. Box 30105, Bethesda, MD 20824-0105. (301) 592-8573. E-mail: <nhlbiinfo@rover.nhlbi.nih.gov>, <http://www.nhlhi.nih.gov>.

National Institutes of Health (NIH), Department of Health and Human Services. 9000 Rockville Pike. Bethesda, MD 20892.

The Society for Vascular Surgery. 900 Cummings Center, #221-U Beverly, MA 01915. <http://svs.vascularweb.org>.

Society of Interventional Radiology. 10201 Lee Highway, Suite 500. Fairfax, VA. 22030. (800) 488-7284. E-mail: <info@sirweb.org>,<http://www.sirweb.org/index.shtml>.

The U.S. Department of Health and Human Services. 200 Independence Avenue, S.W., Washington, D.C. 20201. (877) 696-6775.

Valley Baptist Heart and Vascular Institute. 2101 Pease Street, P.O. Drawer 2588. Harlingen, TX 78550. (956) 389-4848.

OTHER

Society of Interventional Radiology. *Vascular Diseases.* 2003 [cited May 29, 2003]. <http://www.sirweb.org/patPub/vascularTreatments.shtml>.

Crystal H. Kaczkowski, MSc

Vasectomy

Definition

A vasectomy is a surgical procedure performed on adult males in which the vasa deferentia (tubes that carry sperm from the testicles to the seminal vesicles) are cut,

---

WHO PERFORMS THE PROCEDURE AND WHERE IS IT PERFORMED?

Vasectomy is a minor procedure that can be performed in a clinic or doctor's office on an outpatient basis. The procedure is generally performed by a urologist, who is a medical doctor who has completed specialized training in the diagnosis and treatment of diseases of the urinary tract and genital organs.

---

tied, cauterized (burned or seared), or otherwise interrupted. The semen no longer contains sperm after the tubes are cut, so conception cannot occur. The testicles continue to produce sperm, but they die and are absorbed by the body.

Purpose

The purpose of the vasectomy is to provide reliable contraception. Research indicates that the level of effectiveness is 99.6%. Vasectomy is the most reliable method of contraception and has fewer complications and a faster recovery time than female sterilization methods.

The cost of a vasectomy ranges between $400 and $550 in most parts of the United States. Some insurance plans will cover the cost of the procedure.

Demographics

Approximately 500,000 vasectomies are performed annually in the United States. About one out of every six men over the age of 35 has had a vasectomy. Higher vasectomy rates are associated with higher levels of education and income.

Description

Vasectomies are often performed in the doctor's office or an outpatient clinic using local anesthesia. The area around the patient's scrotum (the sac containing the testicles that produce sperm) will be shaved and cleaned with an antiseptic solution to reduce the chance of infection. A small incision is made into the scrotum. Each of the vasa deferentia (one from each testicle) is tied in two places with nonabsorbable (permanent) sutures and the tube is severed between the ties. The ends may be cauterized (burned or seared) to decrease the chance that they will leak or grow back together.

"No scalpel" vasectomies are gaining in popularity. Instead of an incision, a small puncture is made into the

Vasectomy

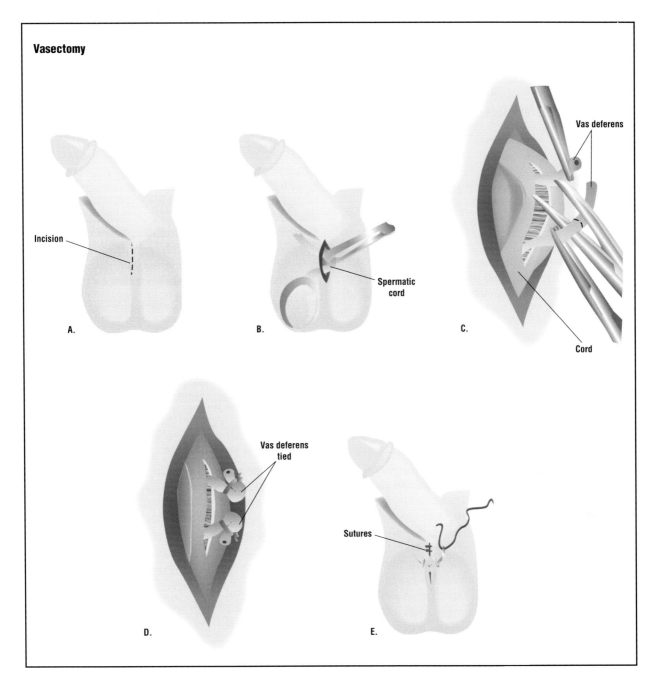

In a vasectomy, an incision is made in the man's scrotum. The spermatic cord is pulled out (B) and incised to expose the vas deferens, which is then severed (C). The ends may be cauterized or tied off (D). After the procedure is repeated on the opposite cord, the scrotal incision is closed (E). *(Illustration by GGS Inc.)*

scrotum. The vasa deferentia are cut and sealed in a manner similar to that described above. No stitches are necessary and the patient has less pain. Other advantages include less damage to the tissues, less bleeding, less risk of infection, and less discomfort after the procedure. The no-scalpel method has been used in the United States since 1990; as of 2003, about 30% of vasectomies are performed with this technique.

The patient is not sterile immediately after the procedure is finished. Men must use other methods of contraception until two consecutive semen analyses confirm that there are no sperm present in the ejaculate. It takes about four to six weeks or 15–20 ejaculations to clear all of the sperm from the tubes.

In some cases vasectomies may be reversed by a procedure known as a **vasovasostomy**. In this procedure,

QUESTIONS TO ASK THE DOCTOR

- How often do you perform vasectomies?
- What is your rate of complications?
- How long will the procedure take?
- What will the procedure cost? Will my insurance cover the cost?
- Do you perform vasectomy reversal? What is your success rate?

the surgeon reconnects the ends of the severed vasa deferentia. A vasectomy should be considered permanent, however, as there is no guarantee of successful reversal. Vasovasostomies are successful in approximately 40–50% of men.

Diagnosis/Preparation

No special physical preparation is required for a vasectomy. The physician will first assess the patient's general health in order to identify any potential problems that could occur. The doctor will then explain the possible risks and side effects of the procedure. The patient is asked to sign a consent form which indicates that he understands the information he has received, and gives the doctor permission to perform the operation.

Aftercare

Following the surgery, ice packs are often applied to scrotum to decrease pain and swelling. A dressing (or athletic supporter) which supports the scrotum can also reduce pain. Mild over-the-counter pain medication such as **aspirin** or **acetaminophen** (Tylenol) should be able to control any discomfort. Activities may be restricted for one to two days, and sexual intercourse for three to four days.

Risks

There are very few risks associated with vasectomy other than infection, bruising, epididymitis (inflammation of the tube that carries the sperm from the testicle to the penis), and sperm granulomas (collections of fluid that leaks from a poorly sealed or tied vas deferens). These complications are easily treated if they do occur. Patients do not experience difficulty achieving an erection, maintaining an erection, or ejaculating. There is no decrease in the production of the male hormone (testosterone), and the patient's sex drive and ability are not al-

tered. Vasectomy is safer and less expensive than **tubal ligation** (sterilization of a female by cutting the Fallopian tubes to prevent conception).

According to both the World Health Organization (WHO) and the National Institutes of Health (NIH), there is no evidence that a vasectomy will increase a man's long-term risk of testicular cancer, prostate cancer, or heart disease.

Normal results

Vasectomies are 99% successful in preventing conception. As such, male sterilization is one of the most effective methods of contraception available to consumers.

Morbidity and mortality rates

Complications occur in approximately 5% of vasectomies. The rates of incidence of some of the more common complications are:

- mild bleeding into the scrotum: one in 400
- major bleeding into the scrotum: one in 1000
- infection: one in 100
- epididymitis: one in 100
- sperm granuloma: one in 500
- persistent pain: one in 1,000

Fournier gangrene is a very rare but possible complication of vasectomy in which the lining of tissue underneath the skin of the scrotum becomes infected (a condition called fasciitis). Fournier gangrene progresses very rapidly and is treated with aggressive antibiotic therapy and surgery to remove necrotic (dead) tissue. Despite treatment, a mortality rate of 45% has been reported for this condition.

Alternatives

There are numerous options available to couples who are interested in preventing pregnancy. The most common methods are female sterilization, oral contraceptives, and the male condom. Female sterilization has a success rate of 99.5%; oral contraceptives, 95–99.5%; and the male condom, 86–97%.

Resources

BOOKS

"Family Planning: Sterilization." Section 18, Chapter 246 in *The Merck Manual of Diagnosis and Therapy*, edited by Mark H. Beers, MD, and Robert Berkow, MD. Whitehouse Station, NJ: Merck Research Laboratories, 1999.

KEY TERMS

Ejaculation—The act of expelling the sperm through the penis during orgasm. The fluid that is released is called the ejaculate.

Epididymitis—Inflammation of the small tube that rests on top of the testicle and is part of the system that carries sperm from the testicle to the penis. The condition can be successfully treated with antibiotics if necessary.

Scrotum—The sac that contains the testicles.

Sperm granuloma—A collection of fluid that leaks from an improperly sealed or tied vas deferens. They usually disappear on their own, but can be drained if necessary.

Testicles—The two egg-shaped organs found in the scrotum that produce sperm.

Tubal ligation—A surgical procedure in which the fallopian tubes are tied in two places and cut between. This prevents eggs from moving from the ovary to the uterus.

Vas deferens (plural, vasa deferentia)—The Latin name for the duct that carries sperm from the testicle to the epididymis. In a vasectomy, a portion of each vas deferens is removed to prevent the sperm from entering the seminal fluid.

Vasovasostomy—A surgical procedure that is done to reverse a vasectomy by reconnecting the ends of the severed vasa deferentia.

PERIODICALS

Hartanto, Victor, Eric Chenven, David DiPiazza, et al. "Fournier Gangrene Following Vasectomy." *Infections in Urology* 14, no.3 (2001): 80-82.

ORGANIZATIONS

Alan Guttmacher Institute. 1120 Connecticut Ave., NW, Suite 460, Washington, DC 20036. (202) 296-4012. <www.agi-usa.org>.

Planned Parenthood Federation of America. 810 Seventh Ave., New York, NY 10019. (212) 541-7800. <www.planned-parenthood.org>.

OTHER

The Alan Guttmacher Institute. "Contraceptive Use." 1999 [cited February 28, 2003]. <http://www.agi-usa.org/pubs/fb_contr_use.html>.

"Facts About Birth Control." *Planned Parenthood Federation of America.* January 2001 [cited February 28, 2003]. <http:// www.plannedparenthood.org/bc/bcfacts1.html>.

"Facts About Vasectomy Safety." *National Institute of Child Health and Human Development.* September 3, 2002 [cited February 28, 2003]. <www.nichd.nih.gov/publications/ pubs/vasect.htm>.

"Vasectomy: Questions and Answers." *EngenderHealth.* 2000 [cited February 28, 2003]. <www.engenderhealth.org/wh/fp/cvas2.html>.

VasectomyMedical.com. February 4, 2003 [cited February 28, 2003]. <http://www.vasectomymedical.com>.

Donald G. Barstow, RN
Stephanie Dionne Sherk

Vasectomy reversal *see* **Vasovasostomy**

Vasovasostomy

Definition

A vasovasostomy is a surgical procedure in which the effects of a **vasectomy** (male sterilization) are reversed. During a vasectomy, the vasa deferentia, which are ducts that carry sperm from the testicles to the seminal vesicles, are cut, tied, cauterized (burned or seared), or otherwise interrupted. A vasovasostomy creates an opening between the separated ends of each vas deferens so that the sperm may enter the semen before ejaculation.

Purpose

The purpose of a vasovasostomy is to restore a man's fertility, whereas a vasectomy, or male sterilization, is performed to provide reliable contraception (birth control). Research indicates that the level of effectiveness in preventing pregnancy is 99.6%. Vasectomy is the most reliable method of contraception and has less risk of complications and a faster recovery time than female sterilization methods.

In many cases, a vasectomy can be reversed. Vasectomy reversal does not, however, guarantee a successful pregnancy. The longer the time elapsed since a man has had a vasectomy, the more difficult the reversal and the lower the success rate. The rate of sperm return if a vasovasostomy is performed within three years of a vasectomy is 97%; this number decreases to 88% three to eight years after vasectomy, 79% by nine to 14 years, and 71% after 15 years. In addition, other factors affect the success rate of vasectomy reversal, including the age of the female partner, her fertility potential, the method of reversal used, and the experience of the surgeon performing the procedure.

Vasovasostomies are also performed in men who are sterile because of genital tract obstructions rather than

Vasovasostomy

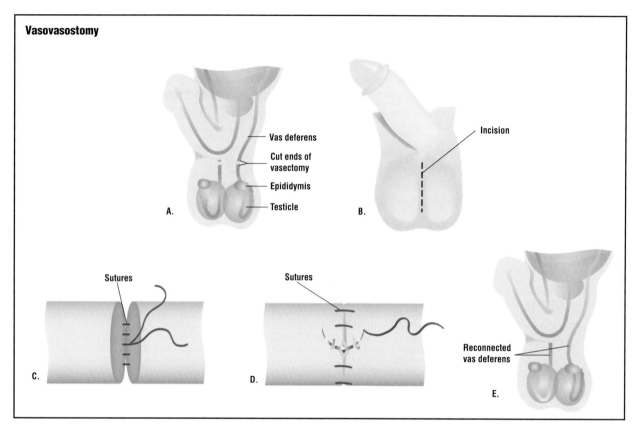

In a vasovasostomy, the surgeon makes an incision in scrotum at the site of the vasectomy scar (B). The spermatic cords are located, and the two vas deferens are reconnected with two layers of suture (C and D). *(Illustration by GGS Inc.)*

prior vasectomies. A vasovasostomy may also be performed on occasion to relieve pain associated with post-vasectomy pain syndrome.

Demographics

An estimated 5% of men who have had a vasectomy later decide that they would like to have children. Some reasons for wanting a vasectomy reversal include death of a child, death of a spouse, divorce, or experiencing a change in circumstances so that having more children is possible. One study found that divorce was the most commonly reported reason for a vasovasostomy and that the average age of men requesting a vasovasostomy is approximately 40 years.

About 7.4% of infertile men have primary genital tract obstructions caused by trauma, gonorrhea or other venereal infections, or congenital malformations of the vasa deferentia. Many of these men are good candidates for surgical treatment of their infertility.

Description

Most surgeons prefer to have the patient given either a continuous anesthetic block or general anesthesia because of the length of time required for the operation. A vasovasostomy generally takes two to three hours to perform, depending on the complexity of the surgery and the experience of the operating physician. More complex surgeries may take as long as five hours. The advantage of general anesthesia is that the patient remains unconscious for the duration of the surgery, which ensures that he remains comfortable. Regional anesthesia, such as a spinal block, allows the patient to remain awake during the procedure while blocking pain in the area of the surgery.

After an adequate level of anesthesia has been reached, the surgeon will make an incision from the top of one side of the scrotum, sometimes moving upward as far as several inches (centimeters) into the abdominal area. A similar incision will then be made on the other side of the scrotum. The vasa deferentia will be identified and isolated from surrounding tissue. Fluid will be removed from the testicular end of each vas deferens and analyzed for presence of sperm. If sperm are found, then a simpler procedure to connect the cut ends of the vasa deferentia will be performed. If no sperm are found, a more complex procedure called a vasoepididymostomy or epididymovasostomy (in which the vas deferens is attached to the epididymis, a structure in which the sperm mature and are stored) may be more successful in restoring sperm flow.

There are two techniques that may be used to reconnect the cut ends of the vasa deferentia. A single-layer closure involves stitching the outer layer of each cut end of the tube together with a very fine suture thread. This procedure takes less time but is often less successful in restoring sperm flow. A double-layer closure, however, involves stitching the inner layer of each cut end of the tube first, and then stitching the outer layer. After reconnection is established, the vasa deferentia are returned to their anatomical place and the scrotal incisions closed.

Diagnosis/Preparation

Before a vasovasostomy is performed, the patient will undergo a preoperative assessment, including a **physical examination** of the scrotum. This evaluation will allow the surgeon to determine what sort of vasectomy reversal should be performed and how extensive the surgery might be. A medical history will be taken. The physician will review the patient's medical records in order to determine how the patient's vasectomy was performed; if large portions of the vasa deferentia were removed during surgery, the vasectomy reversal will be more complicated and may have a lower chance of success. The patient's partner should also undergo a fertility assessment, including a gynecologic exam, to assess her reproductive health.

Some surgeons prefer to give the patient a broad-spectrum antibiotic about half an hour before surgery as well as a mild sedative.

Aftercare

After the procedure the patient will be transferred to a **recovery room** where he will remain for approximately three hours. The patient will be asked to void urine before discharge. Pain medication is prescribed and usually required for one to three days after the procedure. **Antibiotics** may be given after the procedure as well as beforehand to prevent infection. Ice packs applied to the scrotum will help to decrease swelling and discomfort. Heavy lifting, **exercise**, and sexual activity should be avoided for up to four weeks while the vasovasostomy heals.

Patients are usually allowed to return to work within three days. They may shower within two days after surgery, but should avoid soaking the incision (by taking a tub bath or going swimming) for about two weeks. The surgeon will schedule the patient for an incision check about a week after surgery and a semen analysis three months later.

Risks

The complications that most commonly occur after vasovasostomy include swelling, bruising, and symptoms associated with anesthesia (nausea, headache, etc.). There is a risk of low sperm count if the operation is done inadequately or if scarring partially blocks the channel inside the vasa deferentia. Less common complications are infection or severe hematoma (collection of blood under the skin). The most serious potential complication of a vasovasostomy is testicular atrophy (wasting away), which may result from damage to the spermatic artery during the procedure.

Normal results

If a successful vasectomy reversal has been performed, the average time to achieving pregnancy after the procedure is one year, with most pregnancies occurring within the first two years. A good sperm count usually returns within three to six months.

Morbidity and mortality rates

The chance that the vasa deferentia will become obstructed after a successful reversal is approximately 10%. Some doctors recommend that patients bank their sperm as a precautionary measure. Scrotal hematoma occurs in 1–2% of patients after vasovasostomy, and infection in less than 1%.

Alternatives

A vasoepididymostomy may be performed if the physician determines that a vasovasostomy will be insufficient in restoring sperm flow. The determining factor is usually the absence of sperm or fluid in the testicular end of the cut vas deferens (which is found during surgery), although a swollen or blocked epididymis found during a preoperative scrotal examination may also indicate a vasoepididymostomy will be necessary.

There are some options available to men and their partners who are seeking to conceive after a vasectomy but wish to avoid vasectomy reversal. As sperm are no longer present in the man's ejaculate, they may be retrieved from the testicle or epididymis by extraction (removal of tissue) or aspiration (removed by a needle). The sperm may then be incubated with a female egg under carefully controlled conditions, then transferred to the female uterus once fertilization has occurred; this process is called **in vitro fertilization** (IVF). A process called intracytoplasmic sperm injection (ICSI) may be used to improve the success rate of IVF; in this procedure, a single sperm is injected into the female egg.

Resources

BOOKS

"Family Planning: Sterilization." Section 18, Chapter 246 in *The Merck Manual of Diagnosis and Therapy*, edited by Mark H. Beers, MD, and Robert Berkow, MD. Whitehouse Station, NJ: Merck Research Laboratories, 1999.

PERIODICALS

Sabanegh, Edmund, MD. "Vasovasostomy and Vasoepididymostomy." *eMedicine*, February 13, 2002 [June 5, 2003]. <www.emedicine.com/med/topic3090.htm>.

Schroeder-Printzen, I., T. Diemer, and W. Weidner. "Vasovasostomy." *Urologia Internationalis* 70, no. 2 (2003): 101-107.

ORGANIZATIONS

American Board of Urology (ABU). 2216 Ivy Road, Suite 210, Charlottesville, VA 22903. (434) 979-0059. <www.abu.org>.

Center for Male Reproductive Medicine. 2080 Century Park East, Suite 907, Los Angeles, CA 90067. (310) 277-2873. <www.malereproduction.com>.

OTHER

"Alternatives to Vasectomy Reversal." *VasectomyMedical.com*. December 3, 2002 [cited March 22, 2003]. <www.vasectomy medical.com/vasectomy-reversal-alternatives.html>.

Fisch, Harry. *The Patient's Guide to Vasectomy Reversal*. [cited March 22, 2003]. <www.cpmcnet.columbia.edu/dept/urology/infertility.html>.

Silber, Sherman J. *Microscopic Vasectomy Reversal*. 2002 [cited March 22, 2003]. <www.infertile.com/treatmnt/treats/mvr/mvr.htm>.

"Vasectomy Reversal." *Center for Male Reproductive Medicine*. [cited March 22, 2003]. <www.malereproduction.com/08_vasectomyrev.html>.

Stephanie Dionne Sherk

Vein ligation and stripping

Definition

Vein ligation and stripping is a surgical approach to the treatment of varicose veins. It is also sometimes called phlebectomy. Ligation refers to the surgical tying off of a large vein in the leg called the greater saphenous

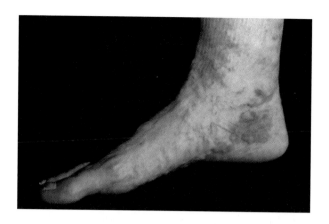

vein, while stripping refers to the removal of this vein through incisions in the groin area or behind the knee. If some of the valves in the saphenous vein are healthy, the weak portion of the vein can be closed off by ligation. If the entire vein is weak, it is closed off and pulled downward and out through an incision made below it. Tying and removal of the greater saphenous vein is done to reduce the pressure of blood flowing backward through this large vein into the smaller veins that feed into it.

Phlebectomy is one of the oldest forms of treatment for varicose veins; the earliest description of it was written by Aulus Cornelius Celsus, a Roman historian of medicine, in A.D. 45. The first description of a phlebectomy hook comes from a textbook on surgery published in 1545. The modern technique of ambulatory (outpatient) phlebectomy was developed around 1956 by a Swiss dermatologist named Robert Muller. As of 2003, surgical ligation and stripping of the saphenous vein is performed less frequently because of the introduction of less invasive forms of treatment.

Purpose

The purpose of vein ligation and stripping is to reduce the number and size of varicose veins that cannot be treated or closed by other measures. The reasons for **vascular surgery** in general include:

- Improvement of the appearance of the legs. Large varicose veins are considered disfiguring by many people.

- Relief from pain, leg cramps, and fatigue that may be associated with varicose veins.

- Treatment of skin problems that may develop as complications of varicose veins. These include chronic eczema, skin ulceration, external bleeding, and abnormal pigmentation of the skin.

- Prevention of such disorders as thrombophlebitis and pulmonary blood clots.

Demographics

The World Health Organization (WHO) estimates that about 25% of adults around the world have some type of venous disorder in the legs. The proportion of the general population with varicose veins is higher, however, in the developed countries. The American College of Phlebology (ACP), which is a group of dermatologists, plastic surgeons, gynecologists, and general surgeons with special training in the treatment of venous disorders, states that more than 80 million people in the United States suffer from varicose veins. In the past, the female to male ratio has been close to four to one, but this figure is changing due to the rapid rise in obesity among adult males in the past two decades.

Varicose veins on a man's leg. *(Photograph by Keith, Custom Medical Stock Photo. Reproduced by permission.)*

Varicose veins are more common in middle-aged and elderly adults than in children or young adults. Although varicose veins tend to run in families, they do not appear to be associated with specific racial or ethnic groups.

Description

Causes of varicose veins

To understand why surgical treatment of varicose veins is sometimes necessary, it is helpful to start with a brief description of the venous system in the human body. The venous part of the circulatory system returns blood to the heart to be pumped to the lungs for oxygenation, in contrast to the arterial system, which carries oxygenated blood away from the heart to be distributed throughout the body. Veins are more likely than arteries to expand or dilate if blood volume or pressure increases, because they consist of only one layer of tissue; this is in contrast to arteries, in which there are three layers.

There are three major categories of veins: superficial veins, deep veins, and perforating veins. All varicose veins are superficial veins; they lie between the skin and a layer of fibrous connective tissue called fascia, which cover and support the muscles and the internal organs. The deep veins of the body lie within the muscle fascia. This distinction helps to explain why a superficial vein can be removed or closed without damage to the deep circulation in the legs. Perforating veins are veins that connect the superficial and deep veins.

Veins contain one-way valves that push blood inward and upward toward the heart against the force of gravity when they are functioning normally. The blood pressure in the superficial veins is usually low, but if it rises and remains at a higher level over a period of time, the valves in the veins begin to fail. The blood flows backward and collects in the lower veins, and the veins dilate, or expand. Veins that are not functioning properly are said to be incompetent. As the veins expand, they become more noticeable under the surface of the skin. Small veins, or capillaries, often appear as spider-shaped or tree-like networks of reddish or purplish lines under the skin. The medical term for these is telangiectasias, but they are commonly known as spider veins or thread veins. Larger veins that form flat, blue-green networks often found behind the knee are called reticular varicosities. True varicose veins are formed when the largest superficial veins become distorted and twisted by a long-term rise in blood pressure in the legs.

The most important veins in the lower leg are the two saphenous veins—the greater saphenous vein, which runs from the foot to the groin area, and the short saphenous vein, which runs from the ankle to the knee. It is thought that varicose veins develop when the valves at the top of the greater saphenous vein fail, allowing more blood to flow backward down the leg and increase the pressure on the valves in the smaller veins in turn. The practice of ligation and stripping of the greater saphenous vein is based on this hypothesis.

Some people are at increased risk for developing varicose veins. These risk factors include:

• Sex. Females in any age group are more likely than males to develop varicose veins. It is thought that female sex hormones contribute to the development of varicose veins by making the veins dilate more easily. Many women experience increased discomfort from varicose veins during their menstrual periods.

• Genetic factors. Some people have veins with abnormally weak walls or valves. They may develop varicose veins even without a rise in blood pressure in the superficial veins. This characteristic tends to run in families.

• Pregnancy. A woman's total blood volume increases during pregnancy, which increases the blood pressure in the venous system. In addition, the hormonal changes of pregnancy cause the walls and valves in the veins to soften.

• Using birth control pills.

• Obesity. Excess body weight increases the pressure on the veins.

• Occupational factors. People who have jobs that require standing or sitting for long periods of time—without the opportunity to walk or move around—are more likely to develop varicose veins.

Ambulatory phlebectomy

Ambulatory phlebectomy is the most common surgical procedure for treating medium-sized varicose veins, as of early 2003. It is also known as stab avulsion or micro-extraction phlebectomy. An ambulatory phlebectomy is performed under local anesthesia. After the patient's leg has been anesthetized, the surgeon makes a series of very small vertical incisions 1–3 mm in length along the length of the affected vein. These incisions do not require stitches or tape closure afterward. Beginning with the more heavily involved areas of the leg, the surgeon inserts a phlebectomy hook through each micro-incision. The vein segment is drawn through the incision, held with a mosquito clamp, and pulled out through the incision. This technique requires the surgeon to be especially careful when removing varicose veins in the ankle, foot, or back of the knee.

After all the vein segments have been removed, the surgeon washes the patient's leg with hydrogen peroxide and covers the area with a foam wrap, several layers of cotton wrap, and an adhesive bandage. A compression stocking is then drawn up over the wrapping. The bandages are removed three to seven days after surgery, but the compression stocking must be worn for another two to four weeks to minimize bruising and swelling. The patient is encouraged to walk around for 10–15 minutes before leaving the office; this mild activity helps to minimize the risk of a blood clot forming in the deep veins of the leg.

Transilluminated powered phlebectomy

Transilluminated powered phlebectomy (TIPP) is a newer technique that avoids the drawbacks of stab avulsion phlebectomy, which include long operating times, the risk of scar formation, and a relatively high risk of infection developing in the micro-incisions. Transilluminated powered phlebectomy performed with an illuminator and a motorized resector. After the patient has been anesthetized with light general anesthesia, the surgeon makes only two small incisions: one for the illuminating device and the other for the resector. After making the first incision and introducing the illuminator, the surgeon uses a technique called tumescent anesthesia to plump up the tissues around the veins and make the veins easier to remove. Tumescent anesthesia was originally developed for **liposuction**. It involves the injection of large quantities of a dilute anesthetic into the tissues surrounding the veins until they become firm and swollen.

After the tumescent anesthesia has been completed, the surgeon makes a second incision to insert the resector, which draws the vein by suction toward an inner blade. The suction then removes the tiny pieces of venous tissue left by the blade. After all the clusters of varicose veins have been treated, the surgeon closes the two small incisions with a single stitch or Steri-Strips. The incisions are covered with a gauze dressing and the leg is wrapped in a sterile compression dressing.

Vein ligation and stripping

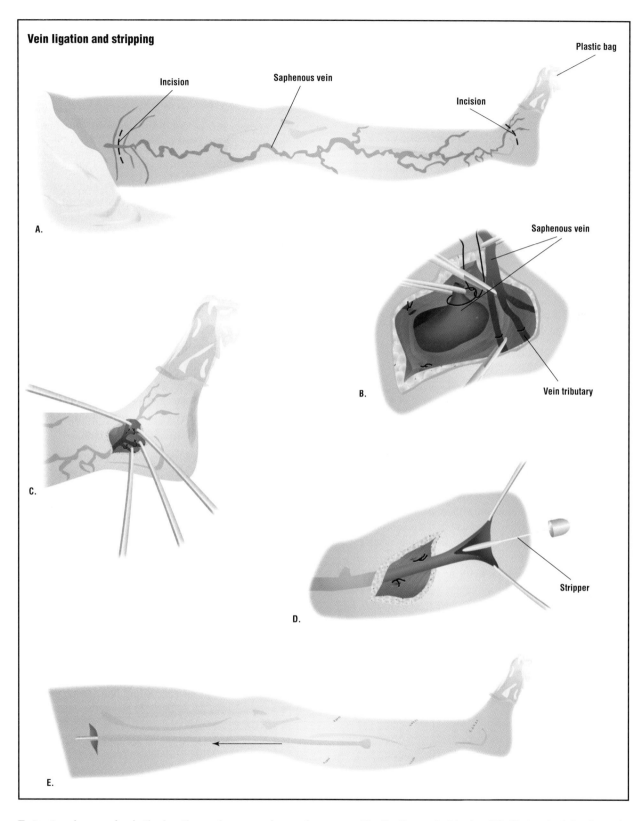

A.

B.

C.

D.

E.

To treat varicose veins in the leg, the saphenous vein may be removed by ligation and stripping (A). First an incision is made in the upper thigh, and the saphenous vein is separated from its tributaries (B). Another incision is made above the foot (C). The lower portion of the vein is cut, and a stripper is inserted into the vein (D). The stripper is pulled through the vein and out the incision in the upper thigh (E). *(Illustration by GGS Inc.)*

Diagnosis/Preparation

Diagnosis

Vein ligation and stripping and ambulatory phlebectomies are considered elective procedures; they are not performed on an emergency basis. The process of diagnosis may begin with the patient's complaints about the appearance of the legs or of pain and cramps, as well as with the physician's observations. It is important to note that there is no correlation between the size or number of a patient's varicose veins and the amount of pain that is experienced. Some people have experience considerable discomfort from fairly small varices, while others may have no symptoms from clusters of extremely swollen varicose veins. If the patient mentions pain, burning sensations, or other physical symptoms, the doctor will need to rule out other possible causes, such as nerve root irritation, osteoarthritis, diabetic neuropathy, or problems in the arterial circulation. Relief of pain when the leg is elevated is the most significant diagnostic sign of varicose veins.

After taking the patient's medical history and a family history of venous disorders, the doctor examines the patient from the waist down to note the location of varicose veins and to palpate (touch with gentle pressure) for signs of other venous disorders. Palpation helps the doctor locate both normal and abnormal veins; further, some varicose veins can be detected by touch even though they cannot be seen through the skin. Ideally, the examiner will have a small raised platform for the patient to stand on during the **physical examination**. The doctor will ask the patient to turn slowly while standing, and will be looking for scars or other signs of trauma, bulges and areas of discoloration in the skin, or other indications of chronic venous insufficiency. While palpating the legs, the doctor will note areas of unusual warmth or soreness, cysts, and edema (swelling of the soft tissues due to fluid retention). Next, the doctor will percuss certain parts of the legs where the larger veins lie closer to the surface. By gently tapping or thumping on the skin over these areas, the doctor can feel if there are any fluid waves in the veins and determine whether further testing for venous insufficiency is required.

The next stage of the diagnostic examination is an evaluation of the valves in the patient's greater saphenous vein. The doctor places a tourniquet around the patient's upper thigh while the patient is lying on the examination table with the leg raised. The patient is then asked to stand on the floor. If the valves in this vein are working properly, the lower superficial veins should not fill up rapidly as long as the tourniquet remains tied. This test is known as Trendelenburg's test. It has, however, been largely replaced by the use of duplex Doppler ultrasound—which maps the location of the varicose veins in the patient's leg and provides information about the condition of the valves in the veins. Most insurance companies now also require a Doppler test before authorizing surgical treatment. The doctor's findings will determine whether the greater saphenous vein will require ligation and stripping or endovenous ablation before smaller varicose veins can be treated.

Some disorders or conditions are contraindications for vascular surgery. They include:

- Cellulitis and other infectious diseases of the skin.
- Severe edema associated with heart or kidney disease. These disorders should be brought under control before a phlebectomy is performed.
- Uncontrolled diabetes.
- Disorders that affect the immune system, including HIV infection.
- Severe heart or lung disorders.

Preparation

Patients preparing for vascular surgery are asked to discontinue **aspirin** or aspirin-related products for a week before the procedure. They should not eat or drink after midnight on the day of surgery. They should not apply any moisturizers, creams, tanning lotions, or sunblock to the legs on the day of the procedure.

A patient scheduled for an ambulatory phlebectomy should arrive at the surgical center about an hour and a half before the procedure. All clothing must be removed before changing into a hospital gown. The patient is asked to walk up and down in the room or hallway for about 20 minutes to make the veins stand out. The surgeon marks the outlines of the veins with an indelible ink marker on the patient's legs while he or she is standing up. An ultrasound may be done at this point to verify the location and condition of the veins. The patient is then taken into the **operating room** for surgery.

Although patients are encouraged to walk around for a few minutes after an ambulatory phlebectomy, they should make arrangements for a friend or relative to drive them home from the surgical facility.

Aftercare

Surgical ligation and stripping of the greater saphenous vein usually requires an overnight stay in the hospital and two to eight weeks of **recovery at home** afterward.

Aftercare following surgical treatment of varicose veins includes wearing medical compression stockings that apply either 20–30 mmHg or 30–40 mmHg of pressure for two to six weeks after the procedure. Wearing compression stockings minimizes the risk of edema, discoloration, and pain. Fashion support stockings are a less acceptable alternative because they do not apply enough pressure to the legs.

The elastic surgical dressing applied at the end of an ambulatory phlebectomy should be left in place after returning home. Mild pain-killing medications may be taken for discomfort.

The patient is advised to watch for redness, swelling, pus, fever, and other signs of infection.

Patients are encouraged to walk, ride a bicycle, or participate in other low-impact forms of **exercise** (such as yoga, and tai chi) to prevent the formation of blood clots in the deep veins of the legs. They should lie down with the legs elevated above heart level for 15 minutes at least twice a day, and use a foot stool when sitting to keep the legs raised.

Risks

Vein ligation and stripping carries the same risks as other surgical procedures under general anesthesia, such as bleeding, infection of the incision, and an adverse reaction to the anesthetic. Patients with leg ulcers or fungal infections of the foot are at increased risk of developing infections in the incisions following surgical treatment of varicose veins.

Specific risks associated with vascular surgery include:

• Deep venous thrombosis.

• Bruising. Bruising is the most common complication of phlebectomies, but heals itself in a few days or weeks.

• Scar formation. Phlebectomy has been found to produce permanent leg scars more frequently than sclerotherapy.

• Injury to the saphenous nerve. This complication results in numbness, tingling, or burning sensations in the area around the ankle. It usually goes away without further treatment within six to 12 months.

• Seromas. A seroma is a collection of uninfected blood serum or lymphatic fluid in the tissues. Seromas usually resolve without further treatment, but can be drained by the surgeon, if necessary.

• Injury to the arteries in the thigh and groin area. This complication is extremely rare, but it can have serious consequences. One example is **amputation** of the leg.

• Leg swelling. This complication is caused by disruption of the lymphatic system during surgery. This lasts about two to three weeks and can be managed by wearing compression stockings.

• Recurrence of smaller varicose veins.

WHO PERFORMS THE PROCEDURE AND WHERE IS IT PERFORMED?

Surgical treatment of varicose veins is usually performed by general surgeons or by vascular surgeons, who are trained in the diagnosis and medical management of venous disorders as well as surgical treatment of them. Most vascular surgeons have completed five years of residency training in surgery after medical school, followed by one to two years of specialized fellowship training.

Phlebectomies and endovenous ablation treatments are performed in **ambulatory surgery centers** as outpatient procedures. Ligation and stripping of the greater saphenous vein, however, is more commonly performed in a hospital as an inpatient operation.

Normal results

Normal results of vein ligation and stripping, or ambulatory phlebectomy, include reduction in the size and number of varicose veins in the leg. About 95% of patients also experience significant relief of pain.

Morbidity and mortality rates

The mortality rate following vein ligation and stripping has been reported to be one in 30,000. The incidence of deep venous thrombosis (DVT) following vascular surgery is estimated to be 0.6%

Alternatives

Conservative treatments

Patients who are experiencing discomfort from varicose veins may be helped by any or several of the following approaches:

• Exercise. Walking or other forms of exercise that activate the muscles in the lower legs can relieve aching and cramping because these muscles keep the blood moving through the leg veins. One specific exercise that is often recommended is repeated flexing of the ankle joint. Flexing the ankles five to 10 times every few minutes and walking around for one to two minutes every half hour throughout the day helps to prevent the venous congestion that results from sitting or standing in one position for hours at a time.

QUESTIONS TO ASK THE DOCTOR

- Can my varicose veins be treated without ligation and stripping?
- Am I a candidate for treatment with EVLT or radiofrequency ablation?
- What specific technique(s) do you perform most frequently?
- Which treatment technique(s) do you recommend and why?

- Avoiding high-heeled shoes. Shoes with high heels do not allow the ankle to flex fully when the patient is walking. This limitation of the range of motion of the ankle joint makes it more difficult for the leg muscles to contract and force venous blood upwards toward the heart.

- Elevating the legs for 15–30 minutes once or twice a day. This change of position is frequently recommended for reducing edema of the feet and ankles.

- Wearing compression hosiery. Compression benefits the leg veins by reducing inflammation as well as improving venous outflow. Most manufacturers of medical compression stockings now sell some relatively sheer hosiery that looks attractive in addition to providing support.

- Medications. Drugs that have been used to treat the discomfort associated with varicose veins include **nonsteroidal anti-inflammatory drugs** (NSAIDs) and preparations of vitamins C and E. One prescription medication that is sometimes given to treat circulatory problems in the legs and feet is pentoxifylline, which improves blood flow in the smaller capillaries. Pentoxifylline is sold under the brand name Trendar®.

If appearance is the patient's primary concern, varicose veins can be partially covered with specially formulated cosmetics that come in a wide variety of skin tones. Some of these preparations are available in waterproof formulations for use during swimming and other athletic activities.

Endovenous ablation

Endovenous ablation refers to two newer and less invasive methods for treating incompetent saphenous veins. In the Closure(R) method, which was approved by the Food and Drug Administration (FDA) in 1999, the surgeon passes a catheter into the lumen of the saphenous vein. The catheter is connected to a radiofrequency gener-

ator and delivers heat energy to the vein through an electrode in its tip. As the tissues in the wall of the vein are heated, they shrink and coagulate, closing and sealing the vein. Radiofrequency ablation of the saphenous vein has been demonstrated to be safe and at least as effective as surgical stripping of the vein; in addition, patients can return to work the next day. Its chief risk is loss of feeling in a patch of skin about the size of a quarter above the knee. This numbness usually resolves in about six months.

Endovenous laser treatment, or EVLT, uses a laser instead of a catheter with an electrode to heat the tissues in the wall of an incompetent vein in order to close the vein. Although EVLT appears to be as safe and effective as radiofrequency ablation, patients experience more discomfort and bruising afterward; most require two to three days of recovery at home after laser treatment.

Sclerotherapy

Sclerotherapy is a treatment method in which irritating chemicals in liquid or foam form are injected into spider veins or smaller reticular varicosities to close them off. The chemicals cause the vein to become inflamed, and leads to the formation of fibrous tissue and closing of the lumen, or central channel of the vein. Sclerotherapy is sometimes used in combination with other techniques to treat larger varicose veins.

Complementary and alternative (CAM) treatments

According to Dr. Kenneth Pelletier, former director of the program in complementary and alternative treatments at Stanford University School of Medicine, horse chestnut extract works as well as compression stockings when used as a conservative treatment for varicose veins. Horse chestnut (*Aesculus hippocastanum*) preparations have been used in Europe for some years to treat circulatory problems in the legs; most recent research has been carried out in Great Britain and Germany. The usual dosage is 75 mg twice a day, at meals. The most common side effect of oral preparations of horse chestnut is occasional indigestion in some patients.

See also Sclerotherapy for varicose veins.

Resources

BOOKS

Pelletier, Kenneth R., M.D. *The Best Alternative Medicine*, Part II, "CAM Therapies for Specific Conditions: Varicose Veins." New York: Simon & Schuster, 2002.

"Varicose Veins." Section 16, Chapter 212 in *The Merck Manual of Diagnosis and Therapy*, edited by Mark H. Beers, M.D., and Robert Berkow, M.D. Whitehouse Station, NJ: Merck Research Laboratories, 1999.

KEY TERMS

Ablation—The destruction or removal of a body part. Saphenous ablation refers to several techniques for closing and destroying the greater saphenous vein without cutting or stripping.

Edema—The presence of abnormally large amounts of fluid in the soft tissues of the body.

Endovascular—Inside a blood vessel. Endovascular treatments of varicose veins are those that are performed inside the veins.

Incompetent—In a medical context, insufficient. An incompetent vein is one that is not performing its function of carrying blood back to the heart.

Ligation—The act of tying off a blood vessel.

Lumen—The channel or cavity inside a tube or hollow organ of the body.

Palpation—Examining by touch as part of the process of physical diagnosis.

Percussion—Thumping or tapping a part of the body with the fingers for diagnostic purposes.

Phlebectomy—Surgical removal of a vein or part of a vein.

Phlebology—The study of veins, their disorders, and their treatments. A phlebologist is a doctor who specializes in treating spider veins, varicose veins, and associated disorders.

Saphenous veins—Two large superficial veins in the leg that may be treated by ligation and stripping as therapy for varicose veins. The greater saphenous vein runs from the foot to the groin area, while the short saphenous vein runs from the ankle to the knee.

Sclerose—To harden or undergo hardening. Sclerosing agents are chemicals that are used in sclerotherapy to cause swollen veins to fill with fibrous tissue and close down.

Seroma—A collection of blood serum or lymphatic fluid in body tissues. It is an occasional complication of vascular surgery.

Telangiectasia—The medical term for the visible discolorations produced by permanently swollen capillaries and smaller veins.

Thrombophlebitis—The inflammation of a vein associated with the formation of blood clots.

Trendelenburg's test—A test that measures the speed at which the lower leg fills with blood after the leg has first been raised above the level of the heart. It is named for Friedrich Trendelenburg (1844–1924), a German surgeon.

Tumescent anesthesia—A type of local anesthesia originally developed for liposuction in which a large volume of diluted anesthetic is injected into the tissues around the vein until they become tumescent (firm and swollen).

Varicose—Abnormally enlarged and distended.

Varix (plural, varices)—The medical term for an enlarged blood vessel.

Vein ligation and stripping

PERIODICALS

Bergan, J. J., N. H. Kumins, E. L. Owens, and S. R. Sparks. "Surgical and Endovascular Treatment of Lower Extremity Venous Insufficiency." *Journal of Vascular and Interventional Radiology* 13 (June 2002): 563-568.

Brethauer, S. A., J. D. Murray, D. G. Hatter, et al. "Treatment of Varicose Veins: Proximal Saphenofemoral Ligation Comparing Adjunctive Varicose Phlebectomy with Sclerotherapy at a Military Medical Center." *Vascular Surgery* 35 (January-February 2001): 51-58.

de Roos, K. P., F. H. Nieman, and H. A. Neumann. "Ambulatory Phlebectomy Versus Compression Sclerotherapy: Results of a Randomized Controlled Trial." *Dermatologic Surgery* 29 (March 2003): 221-226.

Feied, Craig, M.D., Robert Weiss, M.D., and Robert B. Hashemiyoon, M.D. "Varicose Veins and Spider Veins." *eMedicine*, November 20, 2001 [cited April 10, 2003]. <www.emedicine.com/derm/topic475.htm>.

MacKay, D. "Hemorrhoids and Varicose Veins: A Review of Treatment Options." *Alternative Medicine Review* 6 (April 2001): 126-140.

Min, R. J., S. E. Zimmet, M. N. Isaacs, and M. D. Forrestal. "Endovenous Laser Treatment of the Incompetent Greater Saphenous Vein." *Journal of Vascular and Interventional Radiology* 12 (October 2001): 1167-1171.

Pittler, M. H., and E. Ernst. "Horse-Chestnut Seed Extract for Chronic Venous Insufficiency. A Criteria-Based Systematic Review." *Archives of Dermatology* 134 (November 1998): 1356-1360.

Proebstle, T. M., D. Gul, A. Kargl, and J. Knop. "Endovenous Laser Treatment of the Lesser Saphenous Vein with a 940-nm Diode Laser: Early Results." *Dermatologic Surgery* 29 (April 2003): 357-361.

Ramelet, A. A. "Phlebectomy. Technique, Indications and Complications." *International Angiology* 21 (June 2002): 46-51.

GALE ENCYCLOPEDIA OF SURGERY

1537

Weiss, Robert, and Albert-Adrien Ramelet. "Varicose Veins Treated with Ambulatory Phlebectomy." *eMedicine*, May 29, 2002 [cited April 13, 2003]. <www.emedicine.com/derm/ topic748.htm>.

Zotto, Lisa M., RN. "Treating Varicose Veins with Transilluminated Powered Phlebectomy." *AORN Journal* 76 (December 2002): 981-990.

ORGANIZATIONS

American Academy of Dermatology. 930 East Woodfield Rd., PO Box 4014, Schaumburg, IL 60168. (847) 330-0230. <www.aad.org>.

American Association for Vascular Surgery (AAVS). 900 Cummings Center, #221-U, Beverly, MA 01915. <www.aavs.vascularweb.org>.

American College of Phlebology. 100 Webster Street, Suite 101, Oakland, CA 94607-3724. (510) 834-6500. <www.phlebology.org>.

Peripheral Vascular Surgery Society (PVSS). 824 Munras Avenue, Suite C, Monterey, CA 93940. (831) 373-0508. <www.pvss.org>.

OTHER

Bergan, John J., M.D. *Surgery of Varicose Veins*. [cited April 13, 2003] <www.phlebology.org/surgery.html>.

Feied, Craig, M.D. *Venous Anatomy and Physiology*. [cited April 10, 2003] <www.phlebology.org/syllabus1.htm>.

Fronek, Helane S., M.D. *Conservative Therapy for Venous Disease*. [cited April 10, 2003] <www.phlebology.org/syllabus4.htm>.

Fronek, Helane S., M.D. *Functional Testing for Venous Disease*. [cited April 10, 2003] <www.phlebology.org/syllabus3.htm>.

Marley, Wayne, M.D. *Physical Examination of the Phlebology Patient*. [cited April 10, 2003] <www.phlebology.org/syllabus2.htm>.

Olivencia, José A., M.D. *Ambulatory Phlebectomy*. [cited April 13, 2003] <www.phlebology.org/amphlebec.html>.

Weiss, Robert, M.D. *Radiofrequency Endovenous Occlusion (Closure(R) Technique)*. [cited April 13, 2003] <www.phlebology.org/closure.htm>.

Rebecca Frey, Ph.D.

Venography *see* **Phlebography**

Venous thrombosis prevention

Definition

Venous thrombosis prevention is a means to prevent blood clots from forming in veins within the body.

Purpose

Different preventative methods can also maintain normal blood flow and therefore enable oxygen and nutrients to reach the cells of the body. Blood clots can be painful and can cause serious damage to tissues and organs. Sometimes, they can cause rapid death. Blood clot prevention can enhance blood flow and can save lives.

Description

Blood clots can form in any vein within the body. Deep vein thrombosis (DVT) can be quite serious. DVT occurs when a blood clot forms in the legs or pelvis. If it is large enough, it can block the blood flow within the vein, cutting off oxygen to the tissues. An embolus or a clot that breaks away from the wall of the blood vessel can travel into the lung, the heart, or the brain where it can disrupt the normal functioning of these organs and become life-threatening. Some blood clots distend the walls of the blood vessel, creating a sac called an aneurysm. Sometimes the aneurysm bursts, causing blood to leak out. If this occurs within the brain, the heart, or the lungs, it can be fatal.

Venous thrombosis can occur for several reasons. The patient may have disease within the blood vessels such as an inflammation of the walls of the vein (phlebitis) or hereditary blood clotting disorders. The patient may also develop blood clots because of other medical conditions such as heart disease, heart failure, stroke, or cancer. They can also occur after surgery or prolonged bed rest or inactivity. People who smoke and take oral contraceptives may be more susceptible to blood clots.

Pulmonary embolism is one of the most common, but highly fatal, blood clots that patients experience. The American Heart Association estimates 600,000 people in the United States develop pulmonary embolisms each year, with 10% of those ending in death. Sometimes there is little or no warning, causing sudden death. About 90% of these embolisms are the result of DVT that forms in the legs or the pelvis and moves into the lung and blocks the pulmonary artery. Most often the DVT occurs in the recovery period after surgery, though there is an alarming trend of DVT events that are the result of airline travel. In 1999, nearly 2,000 Americans, many of them young and fit, died from travel-related DVT strokes. In 2003, NBC reporter David Bloom, who was embedded with the United States Army as he covered the war in Iraq, died of a pulmonary embolism due to his riding in a cramped position for long hours over several days.

Prevention methods

There are several methods physicians use to prevent blood clots. Some use medications, others use mechanical means, and still others require behavioral changes, or a combination of all of these.

Heparin and other blood thinners

Anticoagulants (blood thinners) such as heparin are often prescribed as prophylactics for venous thrombosis. These drugs decrease the clotting ability of the blood. There has been very good success combining heparin and pneumatic compressions stockings, especially for colorectal and cardiac surgery patients.

There are some precautions, however, for using this drug. People who have had an unusual reaction to the drug should not take it, as well as those with allergies to beef and pork. Women who are pregnant and nursing should only use with caution. In addition, certain medications should not be used with heparin. They include **aspirin**, hyperthyroid medication, and drugs for pain or inflammation.

Mechanical leg pumps (pneumatic compression stockings)

Mechanical stimulation of the calf muscles of the leg can help stimulate blood flow. Many hospitals require all surgery patients, especially those who have abdominal or cardiac surgery, to wear pneumatic compression stockings. These devices wrap around the lower leg from ankle to the knee, some reach as high as the thigh. When plugged in and turned on, a pneumatic device pumps air into chambers within the stocking, which gently tighten around the legs for a few seconds and then are released. This pulsing massage keeps the blood flowing and discourages venous thrombosis.

Compression stockings

Often physicians recommend compression stockings for patients to prevent DVT and edema, and to treat varicose veins and phlebitis. Graduated compression stockings apply more pressure at the ankle and less up the leg and closer to the knee. This pressure prevents backflow of blood and clot formation.

Exercise

Sitting for long periods or being confined to bed after surgery or during a long illness can slow blood flow, allowing clots to form. As soon as possible after surgery, the patient should move the legs, stand, and begin taking short walks. Travelers or people who work sitting at a desk or computer for several hours at a time should take breaks every hour to get up and move around. While sitting in the confines of an airplane or lying in bed, specific exercises, such as ankle circles or leg lifts, can be done also.

KEY TERMS

Aneurysm—A sac created by the distention of the walls of a blood vessel.

Embolus—A clot that breaks away from the wall of the blood vessel and travels throughout the body.

Phlebitis—An inflammation of the walls of a vein.

Venous thrombosis—A blood clot in the vein.

Fluids

It is important not to restrict fluids when recovering from surgery, traveling, or working for long periods in a seated position. Not only will the body be kept hydrated but drinking fluids will help prevent venous thrombosis. Drinking fluids keeps the blood liquid and moving, discouraging clot formation. Travelers should drink something every hour. This may be difficult since some air carriers may not have frequent beverage service.

Preparation

The most important preparation that the patient can do is discuss his or her own personal risk of developing blood clots with a physician. If medication is given, the patient should be instructed how to take it and what side effects to look for. Special exercises should be explained to the patient, and a daily walk should be encouraged.

Normal results

Any of these prevention methods can help a patient avoid having a blood clot after surgery or during long periods of inactivity, such as bed rest or while traveling. Travelers and sedentary workers may find moving around and drinking fluids are the best methods for them to prevent blood clots. For patients recovering from surgery, however, a combination of methods is usually necessary. Pneumatic compression pumps with or without a round of heparin may be the best option for surgery patients.

Resources

PERIODICALS

Ball, Kay. "Deep Vein Thrombosis and Airline Travel—The Deadly Duo." *AORN Journal* 77 (February 2003): 346–354.

Dalen, James E. "Pulmonary Embolism: What Have We Learned Since Virchow? Treatment and Prevention." *Chest* 122 (November 2002): 1801–1818.

Henderson, C. W. "Blood Thinner Helps Treat Clots in Legs and Lungs." *Drug Week* (February 23, 2001): 8.

Monari, Gina-Louise. "Thrombosis Education." *Med Ad News* 21 (October 2002): 74–75.

Ramos, Roque, Bakr I. Salem, Maria P. De Pawlikowski, Cordie Coordes, Stephen Eisenberg, and Ronald Leidenfrost. "The Efficacy of Pneumatic Compression Stockings in the Prevention of Pulmonary Embolism after Cardiac Surgery." *Chest* 109 (January 1996): 82–86.

ORGANIZATIONS

American Heart Association. 7272 Greenville Avenue, Dallas, TX 75231. (800) 242-8721. <http://www.americanheart.org>.

OTHER

Wille-Jørgensen, P, M. S. Rasmussen, B. R. Andersen, and L. Borly. "Heparins and Mechanical Methods for Thromboprophylaxis in Colorectal Surgery." *The Cochrane Library.* Update Software, 2003.

Janie Franz

Ventilation *see* **Mechanical ventilation**

Ventricular assist device

Definition

A ventricular assist device (VAD) is a battery-operated mechanical system consisting of a blood pump and a control unit used for temporary support of blood circulation. The VAD decreases the workload of the heart while maintaining adequate blood flow and blood pressure.

Purpose

A VAD is a temporary life-sustaining device. VADs can replace the left ventricle (LVAD), the right ventricle (RVAD), or both ventricles (BIVAD). They are used when the heart muscle is damaged and needs to rest in order to heal, or when blood flow from the heart is inadequate. In November 2002, the Food and Drug Administration (FDA) approved the use of one type of LVAD as a form of permanent treatment for patients who are ineligible for a heart transplant. VADs can also be used as a bridge in patients awaiting **heart transplantation** or in patients whose bodies have rejected a transplanted heart.

Examples of patients who might be candidates for a VAD are those who:

• have suffered a massive heart attack

• cannot be weaned from heart-lung bypass after treatment with intravenous fluids, medications, and insertion of a balloon pump in the aorta

WHO PERFORMS THE PROCEDURE AND WHERE IS IT PERFORMED?

A VAD is implanted by a cardiothoracic surgeon. A cardiothoracic surgeon is a physician who has completed medical school followed by an internship and residency program for specialized training in cardiac and **thoracic surgery**.

VADs are implanted in hospitals that are equipped to handle cardiopulmonary bypass procedures, with surgeons that have been trained in the specific techniques required by a given type of VAD. The cost of supplies and the special training required limit the type and number of devices that can be implanted in a specific hospital. Patients are transported to specialized transplant centers for continued support and treatment if their heart function is not expected to return to normal.

• have an infection in the heart wall that does not respond to conventional treatment

• are awaiting a heart transplant and are unresponsive to drug therapy and intravenous fluids

• are undergoing high-risk procedures to clear blockages in a coronary artery

Although one in five people suffer left-side ventricular failure, only a minority are candidates for VADs. To be considered for a VAD, patients must meet specific criteria with regard to blood flow, blood pressure, and general health.

Demographics

About 40,000 people in the United States need a heart from a compatible donor, but only 2,200 donor hearts become available each year; hence there is a great need for mechanical devices that can keep patients alive during the wait for transplantation.

VADs are available to all patients in cardiovascular crisis, but their use is contraindicated in patients with:

• irreversible renal failure

• severe peripheral vascular disease

• irreversible brain damage

• cancer that has spread (metastasized)

• severe liver disease

• blood clotting disorders

- severe lung disease
- infections that do not respond to **antibiotics**
- advanced age

Description

A VAD is selected based on specific patient criteria, including the patient's size; the length of time that support will be needed; the amount of support (total or partial) required; and the type of flow desired (pulsatile or continuous). Different heart problems require different types of flow.

A VAD is implanted under general anesthesia in a hospital **operating room**. After the patient has been anesthetized, the surgeon makes an incision in the chest. He or she then inserts a catheter into the jugular vein in the neck. The catheter is threaded through the pulmonary artery, which carries blood from the right ventricle of the heart to the lungs. The catheter is used to measure the oxygen levels in the blood and to administer medications. A urinary catheter is also inserted and used to measure the output of urine. The surgeon sutures the catheters in place, then attaches tubing to connect the catheters to the VAD's pump. Once the pump is turned on, blood flows out of the diseased ventricle and into the pump. The blood is then returned to the proper artery; an LVAD is connected to the aorta, which leaves the heart from the left ventricle, whereas an RVAD is connected to the pulmonary artery. After the VAD has been implanted, the surgeon closes the incisions in the heart and the chest wall. The complete operation may take several hours.

Preparation

VADs are used in patients who have not benefited from other forms of treatment for heart disease. In order to evaluate a patient's eligibility for a VAD, the doctor will use **cardiac catheterization** to demonstrate poor cardiac function and make pressure measurements of the chambers in the patient's heart. Blood samples are drawn in order to measure the levels of blood cells and electrolytes in the patient's circulation. Monitoring of the heart includes an electrocardiogram (EKG) as well as measurements of arterial and venous blood pressures.

Aftercare

After a VAD implant, the patient is monitored in an **intensive care unit** (ICU) with follow-up laboratory studies. He or she will remain in the hospital for at least five to seven days. A breathing tube may be left in place until the patient is awake and able to breathe comfortably. Anticoagulant (blood thinning) medications are given to prevent the formation of blood clots, and antibiotics are given to prevent infections.

QUESTIONS TO ASK THE DOCTOR

- What types of VAD are available for implant at your institution?
- Which of these devices have you been trained to implant?
- What is the success rate for VAD patients at your hospital?
- What institutions are available for transport for patients waiting for a heart transplant?

Patients are slowly and gradually weaned from the VAD, except for those patients awaiting a heart transplant or approved for long-term use of the VAD. As the patient improves, he or she will begin a regular **exercise** program. Some VADs require drive lines connected to the control console that penetrate the chest or abdominal cavity. These connections must be cleansed and bandaged to prevent infection of the device. With appropriate training, the patient can continue treatment at home, returning to the hospital only when necessary.

Fully implanted VADs do not require the patient to remain connected to a bedside control console and power unit. He or she will need to carry battery packs in a waistband or shoulder harness, however. In addition, some fully implanted VADs require the patient to plug a cord attached to their body into an electrical outlet at night.

Risks

VAD insertion carries risks of severe complications. Bleeding from the surgery is common; it occurs in as many as 30–50% of patients. Other complications include the development of blood clots; partial paralysis of the diaphragm; respiratory failure; kidney failure; failure of the VAD; damage to the coronary blood vessels; stroke; and infection.

An additional risk is physical dependency on the device. If VADs are inserted in both ventricles, the heart may become so dependent that the patient cannot be weaned from ventricular support.

In addition to physical complications, many patients find that their emotions and cognitive functions are affected by the implantation procedure. Depression, mood swings, and memory loss are not unusual in patients with VADs.

KEY TERMS

Anticoagulant—A type of medication given to prevent the formation of blood clots in the circulatory system.

Aorta—The main artery in humans and other mammals, arising from the left ventricle of the heart.

Artery—A blood vessel that carries blood from the heart to other parts of the body.

Coronary blood vessels—The arteries and veins that supply blood to the heart muscle.

Pulmonary artery—The major artery that carries blood from the right ventricle of the heart to the lungs.

Ventricles—The two thickly walled lower chambers of the heart that receive blood from the upper chambers and send it into the major arteries.

Normal results

Because VADs are used in the treatment of critically ill patients, outcomes vary widely according to the state of the patient's health before treatment. The signs of a successful implant include normal cardiac output with normal blood pressure and systemic and pulmonary vascular resistance.

If the patient is a candidate for a heart transplant, a successful VAD transplant may allow him or her to continue treatment at home. The goal of this extended support is to survive the wait for a donor organ. As many as 5% of patients with implanted VADs may recover an adequate level of heart muscle function, however, and avoid the need for a heart transplant.

Resources

BOOKS

Hensley, Frederick A., et al., eds. *A Practical Approach to Cardiac Anesthesia*, 3rd ed. Philadelphia, PA: Lippincott Williams & Wilkins, 2003.

"Ventricular Assist Device." In *The Patient's Guide to Medical Tests*, ed. Barry L. Zaret et al. Boston, MA: Houghton Mifflin, 1997.

PERIODICALS

Rose, Eric A., Annetine C. Gelijns, Alan J. Moskowitz, et al. "Long-Term Use of a Left-Ventricular Assist Device for End-Stage Heart Failure." *New England Journal of Medicine* 345 (November 15, 2001): 1435-1443.

ORGANIZATIONS

American Association for Thoracic Surgery (AATS). 900 Cummings Center, Suite 221-U, Beverly, MA 01915. (978) 927-8330. <www.aats.org>.

American Heart Association (AHA), National Center. 7272 Greenville Avenue, Dallas, TX 75231. (800) 242-8721. <www.americanheart.org>.

United States Food and Drug Administration (FDA). 5600 Fishers Lane, Rockville, MD 20857-0001. (888) INFO-FDA. <www.fda.gov>.

OTHER

Department of Biological and Agricultural Engineering, New York State University. *Ventricular Assist Devices*. <www.bae.ncsu.edu>

Tish Davidson, A.M.
Allison J Spiwak, MSBME

Ventricular shunt

Definition

A ventricular shunt is a tube that is surgically placed in one of the fluid-filled chambers inside the brain (ventricles). The fluid around the brain and the spinal column is called cerebrospinal fluid (CSF). When infection or disease causes an excess of CSF in the ventricles, the shunt is placed to drain it and thereby relieve excess pressure.

Purpose

A ventricular shunt relieves hydrocephalus, a condition in which there is an increased volume of CSF within the ventricles. In hydrocephalus, pressure from the CSF usually increases. It may be caused by a tumor of the brain or of the membranes covering the brain (meninges), infection of or bleeding into the CSF, or inborn malformations of the brain. Symptoms of hydrocephalus may include headache, personality disturbances and loss of intellectual abilities (dementia), problems in walking, irritability, vomiting, abnormal eye movements, or a low level of consciousness.

Normal pressure hydrocephalus (a condition in which the volume of CSF increases without an increase in pressure) is associated with progressive dementia, problems walking, and loss of bladder control (urinary incontinence). Even though CSF is not thought to be under increased pressure in this condition, it may also be treated by ventricular shunting.

Demographics

The congenital form of hydrocephalus is believed to occur at an incidence of approximately one to four out of every 1,000 births. The incidence of acquired hydrocephalus is not exactly known. The peak ages for the development of hydrocephalus are in infancy, between four and eight years, and in early adulthood. Normal pressure hydrocephalus generally occurs in patients over the age of 60.

Description

The ventricular shunt tube is placed to drain fluid from the ventricular system in the brain to the cavity of the abdomen or to the large vein in the neck (jugular vein). Therefore, surgical procedures must be done both in the brain and at the drainage site. The tubing contains valves to ensure that fluid can only flow out of the brain and not back into it. The valve can be set at a desired pressure to allow CSF to escape whenever the pressure level is exceeded.

A small reservoir may be attached to the tubing and placed under the scalp. This reservoir allows samples of CSF to be removed with a syringe to check the pressure. Fluid from the reservoir can also be examined for bacteria, cancer cells, blood, or protein, depending on the cause of hydrocephalus. The reservoir may also be used to inject **antibiotics** for CSF infection or chemotherapy medication for meningeal tumors.

Diagnosis/Preparation

The diagnosis of hydrocephalus should be confirmed by diagnostic imaging techniques, such as computed tomography scan (CT scan) or **magnetic resonance imaging** (MRI), before the shunting procedure is performed. These techniques will also show any associated brain abnormalities. CSF should be examined if infection or tumor of the meninges is suspected. Patients with dementia or mental retardation should undergo neuropsychological testing to establish a baseline psychological profile before the shunting procedure.

As with any surgical procedure, the surgeon must know about any medications or health problems that may increase the patient's risk. Because infections are both common and serious, antibiotics are often given before and after surgery.

Aftercare

To avoid infections at the shunt site, the area should be kept clean. CSF should be checked periodically by the doctor to be sure there is no infection or bleeding into the shunt. CSF pressure should be checked to be sure the shunt is operating properly. The eyes should be examined regularly because shunt failure may damage the nerve to the eyes (optic nerve). If not treated promptly, damage to the optic nerve causes irreversible loss of vision.

Risks

Serious and long-term complications of ventricular shunting are bleeding under the outermost covering of the brain (subdural hematoma), infection, stroke, and shunt failure. When a shunt drains to the abdomen (ventriculoperitoneal shunt), fluid may accumulate in the abdomen or abdominal organs may be injured. If CSF pressure is lowered too much, patients may have severe headaches, often with nausea and vomiting, whenever they sit up or stand.

Normal results

After shunting, the ventricles get smaller within three or four days. This shrinkage occurs even when hydrocephalus has been present for a year or more. Clinically detectable signs of improvement occur within a few weeks. The cause of hydrocephalus, duration of hydrocephalus before shunting, and associated brain abnormalities affect the outcome.

Of patients with normal pressure hydrocephalus who are treated with shunting, 25–80% experience long-term improvement. Normal pressure hydrocephalus is more likely to improve when it is caused by infection of or bleeding into the CSF than when it occurs without an underlying cause.

KEY TERMS

Cerebrospinal fluid—Fluid bathing the brain and spinal cord.

Computed tomography (CT) scan—An imaging technique in which cross-sectional x rays of the body are compiled to create a three-dimensional image of the body's internal structures.

Dementia—Progressive loss of mental abilities.

Magnetic resonance imaging (MRI)—An imaging technique that uses a large circular magnet and radio waves to generate signals from atoms in the body. These signals are used to construct images of internal structures.

Morbidity and mortality rates

Complications of shunting occur in 30% of cases, but only 5% are serious. Infections occur in 5–10% of patients, and as many as 80% of shunts develop a mechanical problem at some point and need to be replaced.

Alternatives

In some cases of hydrocephalus, certain drugs may be administered to temporarily decrease the amount of CSF until surgery can be performed. In patients with hydrocephalus caused by a tumor, removal of the tumor often cures the buildup of CSF. Approximately 25% of patients respond to therapies other than shunt placement.

Patients with normal pressure hydrocephalus may experience a temporary improvement in walking and mental abilities upon the temporary drainage of a moderate amount of CSF. This improvement may be an indication that shunting will improve their condition.

Resources

BOOKS

Aldrich, E. Francois, Lawrence S. Chin, Arthur J. DiPatri, and Howard M. Eisenberg. "Hydrocephalus." In *Sabiston Textbook of Surgery,* edited by Courtney M. Townsend Jr. 16th ed. Philadelphia: W. B. Saunders Company, 2001.

Golden, Jeffery A., and Carsten G. Bonnemann. "Hydrocephalus." In *Textbook of Clinical Neurology,* edited by Christopher G. Goetz and Eric J. Pappert. Philadelphia: W. B. Saunders Company, 1999.

PERIODICALS

Hamid, Rukaiya K. A., and Philippa Newfield. "Pediatric Neuroanesthesia: Hydrocephalus." *Anesthesiology Clinics of North America* 19, no. 2 (June 1, 2001): 207–18.

ORGANIZATIONS

American Academy of Neurology. 1080 Montreal Ave., St. Paul, MN 55116. (800) 879-1960. <http://www.aan.com>.

OTHER

Dalvi, Arif. "Normal Pressure Hydrocephalus." *eMedicine,* January 14, 2002 [cited May 21, 2003]. <http://www.emedicine.com/neuro/topic277.htm>.

Hord, Eugenia-Daniela. "Hydrocephalus." *eMedicine,* January 14, 2002 [cited May 21, 2003]. <http://www.emedicine.com/neuro/topic161.htm>.

Sgouros, Spyros. "Management of Spina Bifida, Hydrocephalus, and Shunts." *eMedicine,* May 14, 2003. [cited May 21, 2003]. <http://www.emedicine.com/ped/topic2976.htm>.

Laurie Barclay, MD
Stephanie Dionne Sherk

Vertical banded gastroplasty

Definition

Vertical banded gastroplasty, or VBG, is an elective surgical procedure in which the stomach is partitioned with staples and fitted with a plastic band to limit the amount of food that the stomach can hold at one time. Gastroplasty is a term that comes from two Greek words, *gaster* or "stomach," and *plassein*, "to form or shape." "Stomach stapling," also known as VBG, is part of a relatively new surgical subspecialty called bariatric surgery. The word "bariatric" is also derived from two Greek words, *barys*, which means "heavy," and *iatros*, which means "healer." A restrictive bariatric procedure, VBG controls the amount of food that the stomach can hold—in contrast to malabsorptive surgeries, in which the food is rerouted within the digestive tract to prevent complete absorption of the nutrients in the food.

Purpose

The purpose of VBG is the treatment of morbid (unhealthy) obesity. It is one of the first successful procedures in bariatric surgery. VBG was developed in its present form in 1982 by Dr. Edward E. Mason, a professor of surgery at the University of Iowa.

Bariatric surgery in general is important in the management of severe obesity because it is the only one as of 2003 that has demonstrated long-term success in the majority of patients. Weight reduction diets, **exercise** programs, and appetite suppressant medications have had a very low long-term success rate in managing morbid obesity. Most people who try to lose weight on reduced-calorie diets regain two-thirds of the weight lost within one year; within five years, they have gained more weight in addition to all the weight they had lost previously. Appetite suppressants often have undesirable or harmful side effects as well as having a low rate of long-term effectiveness; in 1997 the Food and Drug Administration (FDA) banned the sale of fenfluramine and phentermine ("fen-phen") when they were discovered to cause damage to heart valves.

Obesity is a major health problem not only because it is widespread in the American population—as of 2003, 33% of adults in the United States meet the National Institutes of Health (NIH) criteria for obesity—but because it greatly increases a person's risk of developing potentially life-threatening disorders. Obesity is associated with type 2 (non-insulin-dependent) diabetes, hypertension, abnormal blood cholesterol levels, liver disease, coronary artery disease, sleep apnea syndrome, and certain types of cancer. In addition to these disorders, obesity is a factor in what have been called lifestyle-limiting conditions. These conditions are not life-threatening, but they can have a great impact on a people's day-to-day lives, particularly in their relationships and in the working world. Lifestyle-limiting conditions related to obesity include osteoarthritis and gout; urinary stress incontinence; heartburn; skin disorders caused by heavy perspiration accumulating in folds of skin; leg swelling and varicose veins; gallstones; and abdominal hernias. Obese women frequently suffer from irregular menstrual periods and infertility. Finally, societal prejudice against obese people is widespread and frequently mentioned as a source of acute psychological distress. Surgical treatment of obesity has been demonstrated to relieve emotional pain as well as to reduce risks to the patient's physical health.

Demographics

Like other procedures in bariatric surgery, VBG is performed only on patients who are severely or morbidly obese by NIH standards. Severe obesity is presently defined as a body mass index (BMI) of 35 or higher. Nonetheless, it is the epidemic with the greatest prevalence in the United States as of 2003. One out of every 20 adults, or 15 million people, have a BMI greater than 35.

At present, few figures are available regarding the number of VBGs performed in the United States each year compared with other types of obesity surgery. The International Bariatric Surgery Registry (IBSR) at the University of Iowa is presently compiling a database to monitor the outcomes of different procedures and to analyze statistical data about patients undergoing obesity surgery. In 2000, the IBSR analyzed data on a group of

14,641 people who had had obesity surgery as of 1998. The patients weighed an average of 280 lb (127 kg) at the time of surgery and had an average BMI of 46. Slightly less than 20% of the patients had BMIs between 35 and 39.9; 76.1% had BMIs of 40 or higher.

Description

There are two major types of VBG—open, which is the older of the two procedures; and the laparoscopic VBG, which is performed through very small incisions, with the help of special instruments.

Open vertical banded gastroplasty

The open VBG is done under general anesthesia. In most cases, it takes one to two hours to perform. The surgeon makes an incision several inches long in the patient's upper abdomen. After cutting through the layers of tissue over the stomach, the surgeon cuts a hole or "window" into the upper part of the stomach a few inches below the esophagus. The second step involves placing a line of surgical staples from the window in the direction of the esophagus, which creates a small pouch at the upper end of the stomach. The surgeon must measure the size of this pouch very carefully; when completed, it is about 10% of the size of a normal stomach and will hold about a tablespoon of solid food.

After forming the pouch and checking its size, the surgeon takes a band made out of polypropylene plastic and fits it through the window around the outlet of the stomach pouch. The vertical band is then stitched into place. Because the polypropylene does not stretch, it holds food in the stomach longer, which allows the patient to feel full on only a small amount of food.

Following the placement of the band, the surgeon will check to make sure that there is no leakage around the window and the line of surgical staples. The area of surgery will then be washed out with a sterile saline solution and the incision closed.

Laparoscopic vertical banded gastroplasty

A laparoscopic vertical banded gastroplasty, or LVBG, is performed with the help of a bariatric laparoscope. A laparoscope is a small (10 mm in diameter) tube that holds a fiberoptic cable that allows the surgeon to view the inside of the abdominal cavity on a high-resolution video screen and record the operation on a video recorder. In a laparoscopic VBG, the surgeon makes three small incisions on the left side of the abdomen for inserting the laparoscope, and a fourth incision about 2.5 in (14 cm) long on the right side. The formation of the stomach pouch and insertion of the plastic band are done through these small incisions. Because it is more difficult for the surgeon to maneuver the instruments through the small openings, an LVBG takes longer than an open VBG, about two to four hours.

A laparoscopic VBG requires that the surgeon spend more training and practice than with an open VBG. As of 2003, about 90% of VBGs performed in the United States are done as open procedures. In the event of complications developing during a laparoscopic VBG, the surgeon usually completes the operation using the open procedure.

Diagnosis/Preparation

Diagnosis

DETERMINATION OF OBESITY. The diagnosis of a patient for bariatric surgery begins with measuring the degree of the patient's obesity. This measurement is crucial because the NIH and almost all health insurers have established specific limits for approval of bariatric procedures.

The obesity guidelines that are cited most often were drawn up by Milliman and Robertson, a nationally recognized company that establishes medical need for a wide variety of procedures for health insurers. The Milliman and Robertson criteria for a patient to qualify for weight loss surgery are as follows:

- be least 100 lb (45 kg) over ideal weight, as defined by life insurance tables; have a BMI of 40 or higher; or have a BMI over 35 with a coexisting serious medical condition (for example: severe diabetes or coronary artery disease)

- demonstrate failure to lose or regain of weight despite having tried a multidisciplinary weight control program

- have another cause of obesity, such as an endocrine disorder

- have attained full adult growth

The patient must be treated not only by a doctor with special training in obesity surgery, but in a comprehensive program that includes preoperative psychological screening and medical examination; nutritional counseling; exercise counseling; and participation in support groups

There are several ways to measure obesity. Some are based on the relationship between a person's height and weight. The older measurements of this correlation are the so-called "height-weight" tables that listed desirable weights for a given height. The limitation of height-weight tables is that they do not distinguish between weight of human fatty tissue and weight of lean muscle tissue—many professional athletes and body builders are overweight by the standards of these tables. A more ac-

curate measurement of obesity is body mass index, or BMI. The BMI is an indirect measurement of the amount of body fat. The BMI is calculated in English measurements by multiplying a person's weight in pounds by 703.1, then dividing that number by the person's height in inches squared. A BMI between 19 and 24 is considered normal; 25–29 is overweight; 30–34 is moderately obese; 35–39 is severely obese; and 40 or higher is defined as morbidly obese.

More direct methods of measuring body fat include measuring the thickness of the skinfold at the back of the upper arm, and bioelectrical impedance analysis (BIA). Bioelectrical impedance measures the total amount of water in the body, using a special instrument that calculates the different degrees of resistance to a mild electrical current in different types of body tissue. Fatty tissue has a higher resistance to the current than body tissues containing larger amounts of water. A higher percentage of body water indicates a greater amount of lean tissue.

PSYCHOLOGICAL EVALUATION. Psychiatric and psychological screening before a VBG is done to evaluate the patient's emotional stability and to ensure the expectations of the results of weight loss are not unrealistic. Because of social prejudice against obesity, some obese people who have felt isolated from others or suffered job discrimination come to think of weight loss surgery as a magical or quick solution to all the problems in their lives. In addition, the surgeon will want to make sure that the patient understands the long-term lifestyle adjustments that are necessary after surgery, and that the patient is committed to making those changes. A third reason for a psychological assessment before a VBG is to determine whether the patient's eating habits are compulsive; these would be characterized by the persistent and irresistible impulse to eat with unknown or unconscious purpose. Compulsive eating is not a reason for not having weight loss surgery, but it does mean that the psychological factors contributing to the patient's obesity will also require treatment.

OTHER TESTS AND EXAMINATIONS. Patients must have a complete **physical examination** and blood tests before being considered for a VBG. Some bariatric surgeons will not accept patients with histories of major psychiatric illness; alcohol or drug abuse; previous abdominal surgery; or collagen vascular diseases, which include systemic lupus erythematosus (SLE) and rheumatoid arthritis. Many will not accept patients younger than 16 or older than 55, although some surgeons report successful VBGs in patients over 70. In any event, the patient will need to provide documentation of physical condition, particularly comorbid diseases or disorders, to their insurance company.

Preparation

Preparation for bariatric surgery requires more attention to certain matters than most other forms of surgery requiring hospitalization.

HEALTH INSURANCE ISSUES. Both bariatric surgeons and people who have had weight loss surgery report that obtaining preauthorization for a VBG from insurance companies is a lengthy, complicated, and frequently frustrating process. Insurance companies tend to reflect the prejudices against obese people that exist in the wider society. Although this situation is slowly changing because of increasingly widespread recognition of the high costs of obesity-related diseases, people considering a VBG should start early to secure approval for their operation. The American Obesity Association (AOA) has a pamphlet entitled, *Weight Management and Health Insurance*, a useful guide to the process of getting coverage for weight loss surgery. The pamphlet is available for free download from the AOA Web site.

LIFESTYLE CHANGES. A VBG requires a period of **recovery at home** after **discharge from the hospital**. Since the patient's physical mobility will be limited, the following should be done before the operation:

• Arrange for leave from work, assistance at home, help with driving, and similar tasks and commitments.

• Obtain a handicapped parking permit.

• Check the house or apartment thoroughly for needed adjustments to furniture, appliances, lighting, and personal conveniences; specific recommendations include the purchase of a shower chair and toilet seat lift. People recovering from bariatric surgery must minimize bending, stooping, and any risk of falling. There are good guides available written by people who have had weight loss surgery that describe household safety and comfort considerations in further detail.

• Stock up on prescription medications, nonperishable groceries, cleaning supplies, and similar items to minimize shopping. Food items should include plenty of clear liquids (juices, broth, soups) and soft foods (oatmeal and other cooked cereals, gelatin dessert mixes).

• Have a supply of easy-care clothing with elastic waistbands and simple fasteners. Shoes should be slip-ons or fastened with Velcro.

• Take "before" photographs prior to the operation, and make a written record of body measurements. These should include measurements of the neck, waist, wrist, widest part of hips, bust or chest, knees, and ankles, as well as shoe size. The preoperation photographs and measurements help to document the rate and amount of weight lost. Patients who have had weight loss surgery also point out that these records serve to boost morale

WHO PERFORMS THE PROCEDURE AND WHERE IS IT PERFORMED?

A VBG is performed in a hospital whether the operation is an open or a laparoscopic gastroplasty. It is done by a bariatric surgeon, who is a medical doctor (MD) or doctor of osteopathy (DO) who has completed at least three years' training in **general surgery** after medical school and internship. Most bariatric surgeons have had additional training in gastrointestinal or biliary surgery before completing a fellowship in bariatric surgery with an experienced practitioner in this subspecialty. Because laparoscopic VBGs require more experience on the surgeon's part and take longer to perform, there are fewer surgeons who perform laparoscopic procedures. A survey done in 2000 by the American Society for Bariatric Surgery (ASBS) found that about 90% of bariatric surgeons perform open VBGs; only about 10% use the laparoscopic technique.

In addition to demonstrating the technical skills necessary to perform a VBG, bariatric surgeons seeking hospital privileges must show that they are competent to provide the psychological and nutritional assessments and counseling included in weight loss surgery programs.

by allowing the patient to measure progress in losing weight after the surgery.

PRE-OPERATION CLASSES AND SUPPORT GROUPS. In line with the Milliman and Robertson guidelines, most bariatric surgeons now have "preop" classes and ongoing support groups for patients scheduled for VBG and other types of bariatric surgery. Facilitators of these classes can answer questions regarding preparation for the operation and what to expect during recovery, particularly about changes in eating patterns. In addition, they provide opportunities for patients to share concerns and experiences. Patients who have attended group meetings for weight loss surgery often report that simply sharing accounts of the effects of severe obesity on their lives strengthened their resolve to have the operation. In addition, clinical studies indicate that patients who have attended preop classes are less anxious before surgery and generally recover more rapidly.

MEDICAL PREPARATION. Patients scheduled for a gastroplasty are advised to eat lightly the day before surgery. The surgeon will provide specific instructions about taking medications prescribed for other health conditions. The patient will be given preoperation medications that usually include a laxative to clear the lower digestive tract, an anti-nausea drug, and an antibiotic to lower the risk of infection. Some surgeons ask patients to shower on the morning of their surgery with a special antiseptic skin cleanser.

Aftercare

Aftercare following a gastroplasty has long-term as well as short-term aspects.

Short-term aftercare

Patients who have had an open VBG usually remain in the hospital for four to five days after surgery; those who have had a laparoscopic VBG may return home after two to three days. Aftercare in the hospital typically includes:

- Pain medication. After returning from surgery, patients are given a patient-controlled anesthesia, or PCA device. The PCA is a small pump that delivers a dose of medication into the IV when the patient pushes a button.

- Clear fluids. Inpatient food is limited to a liquid diet following a VBG.

- Oxygen treatment and breathing exercises to get the patient's lungs back into shape. Patients are encouraged to get out of bed and walk around as soon as possible to prevent pneumonia.

- Regular change of surgical dressings. Patients may be given additional dressings for use at home, if needed.

Long-term aftercare

Long-term aftercare includes several adjustments to the patient's lifestyle:

- Slow progression from consuming foods and liquids to eating a normal diet. For the first two weeks after surgery, the patient is limited to liquids and foods that have been pureed in a blender. The reintroduction of solid foods takes place gradually over several months. In addition, patients sometimes have unpredictable reactions to specific foods; most of these resolve over time.

- Lifelong changes in eating habits. Patients who have had a VBG must learn to chew food thoroughly and to eat slowly to reduce the risk of nausea and vomiting. They must also be careful to avoid eating too many soft foods or sweets, to reduce the risk of regaining weight.

- A minimum of five years of follow-up visits to the surgeon to monitor weight maintenance and other health concerns. Patients considering bariatric surgery should choose a surgeon with whom they feel comfortable, as

they are making a long-term commitment to aftercare with this professional.

- Ongoing support group meetings to deal with the physical and psychological aftereffects of surgery and weight loss.

- Beginning and maintaining an appropriate exercise program.

Risks

Patients who undergo a VBG are at risk for some of the same complications that may follow any major operation, including death, pulmonary embolism, the formation of blood clots in the deep veins of the leg, and infection of the surgical incision. These risks are increased for severely obese patients; for example, the risk of infection is about 10% for obese patients compared to 2% for patients of normal weight. With specific regard to VBGs, recent studies indicate that the risks of complications after surgery are about the same for open and laparoscopic VBGs.

Specific risks of VBGs

Specific risks associated with vertical banded gastroplasty include:

- Incisional hernia. An incisional hernia is the protrusion of a loop or piece of tissue through a reopened incision. It results from the stress placed on the stitches holding the incision closed in extremely obese patients. Most can be repaired by resuturing the incision. Incisional hernias are more likely to occur with open VBGs than with laparoscopic procedures.

- Dehiscence. Dehiscence is the medical term for splitting open; it can occur in a VBG if the staples forming the pouch at the upper end of the stomach come loose.

- Nausea and vomiting. Nausea and vomiting usually result from eating more food than the stomach pouch can hold, or eating the food too quickly. In most cases, the vomiting disappears as the patient learns different eating habits.

- Formation of a stricture at the site of the plastic band. A stricture is an abnormal narrowing of a body canal or opening. It is also called a stenosis.

- Damage to the spleen. The spleen lies very close to the stomach and can be injured in the process of bariatric surgery. In most cases it can be repaired during the operation.

Long-term risks

The long-term risks of vertical banded gastroplasty include:

- Regaining weight. Patients who have had a VBG are more likely to regain lost weight than those who have had **gastric bypass** surgery. This is partly because the patient's digestive tract continues to absorb nutrients in food in normal fashion. Because the stomach pouch in a VBG is small, many patients are tempted to eat ice cream and high-calorie liquids that pass quickly through the pouch. A 10-year follow-up study of 70 patients who had had a VBG found that only 20% (14) of the patients had lost and kept off the loss of 50% of their excess body weight.

- Ongoing vomiting and heartburn. About 20% of patients with VBGs report long-term digestive difficulties.

- Psychological problems. Some people have difficulty adjusting to the changes in their outward appearance and to others' changed reactions to them. Others experience feelings of depression, which are thought to be related to biochemical changes resulting from the weight loss.

Normal results

The most rapid weight loss following a VBG takes place in the first six months. It usually takes between 18 and 24 months after the operation for patients to lose 50% of their excess body weight, which is the measurement used to define success in bariatric surgery. At this point, most patients feel much better physically and psychologically; diabetes, high blood pressure, urinary stress incontinence, and other complications associated with severe obesity have either improved or completely resolved.

The primary drawback of VBG is its relatively high rate of failure in maintaining the patient's weight loss over a five-year period. For this reason, some bariatric surgeons recommend VBGs for patients at the lower end of the severe obesity spectrum—those with BMIs between 35 and 40. The chief advantage of VBGs over malabsorptive types of weight loss surgery is that there is little risk of malnutrition or vitamin deficiencies.

Although bariatric surgeons advise patients to wait for two years after a VBG to have plastic surgery procedures, it is not unusual for patients to require operations to remove excess skin from the upper arms, abdomen, and other parts of the body that had large accumulations of fatty tissue.

Morbidity and mortality rates

According to the American Society of Bariatric Surgery, mortality following a VBG is about 5%. The rates of postsurgical complications are about 6% for leaks leading to infection and a need to reoperate; 4% for dehiscence; 1% for injury to the spleen; and 1% for pulmonary embolisms.

QUESTIONS TO ASK THE DOCTOR

- Do I meet the eligibility criteria for bariatric surgery?
- Would you recommend a vertical banded gastroplasty (VBG) for me, or a gastric bypass operation?
- Am I a candidate for a laparoscopic VBG?
- How long have you been practicing bariatric surgery?
- How many VBGs do you perform each year?

Alternatives

Established surgical alternatives

The primary restrictive alternative to a VBG is implanting a Lap-Band, which is an adjustable band that the surgeon positions around the upper end of the stomach to form the small pouch instead of using staples. The Lap-Band was approved by the Food and Drug Administration (FDA) for use in the United States in 2001. It can be implanted with the laparoscopic technique. When the band is in place, it is inflated with saline solution. It can be tightened or loosened after the operation through a portal under the skin. Although the Lap-Band eliminates the risk of dehiscence, it produces such side effects as vomiting, heartburn, abdominal cramps, or enlargement of the stomach pouch due to the band's slipping out of place. In one American study, 25% of patients eventually had the band removed.

The other major type of obesity surgery combines restriction of the size of the stomach with a malabsorptive approach. The combination surgery that is considered the safest and performed most frequently in the United States is the Roux-en-Y gastric bypass. In this procedure, the surgeon forms a stomach pouch and then divides the small intestine, connecting one part of it to the new pouch and reconnecting the other portion to the intestines at some distance from the stomach. The food bypasses the section of the stomach and the small intestine, where most nutrients are absorbed. The procedure takes its name from Cesar Roux, a Swiss surgeon who first performed it, and the "Y" shape formed by the reconnected intestines.

Experimental procedures

A newer technique in obesity surgery is known as gastric pacing. In gastric pacing, the surgeon implants

KEY TERMS

Appetite suppressant—A medication given to reduce the desire to eat.

Bariatrics—The branch of medicine that deals with the prevention and treatment of obesity and related disorders.

Body mass index (BMI)—A measurement that has replaced weight as the preferred determinant of obesity. The BMI can be calculated (in English units) as 703.1 times a person's weight in pounds divided by the square of the person's height in inches.

Comorbid—A term applied to a disease or disorder that occurs at the same time as another disease condition. There are a number of health problems that are comorbid with obesity.

Dehiscence—A separation or splitting apart. In a vertical banded gastroplasty, dehiscence refers to the coming apart of the line of staples used to form the stomach pouch.

Gastric pacing—An experimental form of obesity surgery in which electrodes are implanted in the muscle of the stomach wall. Electrical stimulation paces the timing of stomach contractions so that the patient feels full on less food.

Hernia—The protrusion of a loop or piece of tissue through an incision or abnormal opening in other tissues. Incisional hernias sometimes occur after open VBGs.

Laparoscope—An instrument that allows a doctor to look inside the abdominal cavity. A less invasive form of VBG can be performed with the help of a laparoscope.

Malabsorptive—A type of bariatric surgery in which a part of the stomach is partitioned off and connected to a lower portion of the small intestine in order to reduce the amount of nutrients that the body absorbs from the food.

Morbid—Unwholesome or bad for health. Morbid obesity is a condition in which the patient's weight is a very high risk to his or her health. The NIH (National Institutes of Health) prefers the term "severely obese" to "morbidly obese."

Obesity—Excessive weight gain due to accumulation of fat in the body, sometimes defined as a BMI (body mass index) of 30 or higher, or body weight greater than 30% above one's desirable weight on standard height-weight tables.

Prevalence—The number of cases of a disease or disorder that are present in a given population at a specific time.

Restrictive—A type of bariatric surgery that works by limiting the amount of food that the stomach can hold. Vertical banded gastroplasty is a restrictive procedure.

Sleep apnea syndrome—A disorder in which the patient's breathing temporarily stops at intervals during the night due to obstruction of the upper airway. People with sleep apnea syndrome do not get enough oxygen in their blood and often develop heart problems.

Stricture—An abnormal narrowing of a body canal or opening. Sometimes strictures form near the plastic band in a VBG. A stricture may also be called a stenosis.

---

electrodes in the muscle of the stomach wall that deliver a mild electrical current. These electrical impulses regulate the pace of stomach contractions so that the patient feels full on smaller amounts of food. Preliminary results from a team of Italian researchers on patients followed since 1995 indicate that gastric pacing is both safe and effective.

Resources

BOOKS

Boasten, Michelle. *Weight Loss Surgery: Understanding and Overcoming Morbid Obesity.* Akron, OH: FBE Service Network & Network Publishing, 2002.

Flancbaum, Louis, MD, with Erica Manfred and Deborah Biskin. *The Doctor's Guide to Weight Loss Surgery.* West Hurley, NY: Fredonia Communications, 2001.

"Nutritional Disorders: Obesity." Section 1, Chapter 5 in *The Merck Manual of Diagnosis and Therapy*, edited by Mark H. Beers, MD, and Robert Berkow, MD. Whitehouse Station, NJ: Merck Research Laboratories, 1999.

PERIODICALS

Balsiger, B. M., J. L. Poggio, J. Mai, et al. "Ten and More Years After Vertical Banded Gastroplasty as Primary Operation for Morbid Obesity." *Journal of Gastrointestinal Surgery* 4 (November-December 2000): 598-605.

Buchwald, H. "A Bariatric Surgery Algorithm." *Obesity Surgery* 12 (December 2002): 733-746.

Buchwald, H., and J. N. Buchwald. "Evolution of Operative Procedures for the Management of Morbid Obesity 1950–2000." *Obesity Surgery* 12 (October 2002): 705-717.

Cigaina, V. "Gastric Pacing as Therapy for Morbid Obesity:

Preliminary Results." *Obesity Surgery* 12 (April 2002), Supplement 1: 12S-16S.

Cummings, S., E. S. Parham, and G. W. Strain. "Position of the American Dietetic Association: Weight Management." *Journal of the American Dietetic Association* 102 (August 2002): 1145-1155.

Davila-Cervantes, A., D. Borunda, G. Dominguez-Cherit, et al. "Open Versus Laparoscopic Vertical Banded Gastroplasty: A Randomized Controlled Double-Blind Trial." *Obesity Surgery* 12 (December 2002): 812-818.

Fisher, B. L., and P. Schauer. "Medical and Surgical Options in the Treatment of Severe Obesity." *American Journal of Surgery* 184 (December 2002): 9S-16S.

Guisado, J. A., F. J. Vaz, J. Alarcon, et al. "Psychopathological Status and Interpersonal Functioning Following Weight Loss in Morbidly Obese Patients Undergoing Bariatric Surgery." *Obesity Surgery* 12 (December 2002): 835-840.

Magnusson, M., J. Freedman, E. Jonas, et al. "Five-Year Results of Laparoscopic Vertical Banded Gastroplasty in the Treatment of Massive Obesity." *Obesity Surgery* 12 (December 2002): 826-830.

Schauer, P. R., and S. Ikramuddin. "Laparoscopic Surgery for Morbid Obesity." *Surgical Clinics of North America* 81 (October 2001): 1145-1179.

Shai, I., Y. Henkin, S. Weitzman, and I. Levi. "Long-Term Dietary Changes After Vertical Banded Gastroplasty: Is the Trade-Off Favorable?" *Obesity Surgery* 12 (December 2002): 805-811.

Sugerman, H. J., E. L. Sugerman, E. J. DeMaria, et al. "Bariatric Surgery for Severely Obese Adolescents." *Journal of Gastrointestinal Surgery* 7 (January 2003): 102-108.

ORGANIZATIONS

American Obesity Association (AOA). 1250 24th Street NW, Suite 300, Washington, DC 20037. (202) 776-7711 or (800) 98-OBESE. <www.obesity.org>.

American Society of Bariatric Physicians. 5453 East Evans Place, Denver, CO 80222-5234. (303) 770-2526. <www.asbp.org>.

American Society for Bariatric Surgery. 7328 West University Avenue, Suite F, Gainesville, FL 32607. (352) 331-4900. <www.asbs.org>.

International Bariatric Surgery Registry (IBSR). University of Iowa Hospitals and Clinics, 200 Hawkins Drive, Iowa City, IA 52242. (800) 777-8442. <www.uihealthcare.com>.

Weight-control Information Network (WIN). 1 WIN Way, Bethesda, MD 20892-3665. (202) 828-1025 or (877) 946-4627.

OTHER

FDA Talk Paper. *FDA Approves Implanted Stomach Band to Treat Severe Obesity.* T01-26, June 5, 2001 [cited March 18, 2003]. <www.fda.gov/bbs/topics/ANSWERS/2001/ANS0 1087.html>.

MacGregor, Alex, MD. *The Story of Surgery for Obesity.* <www.asbs.org/html/story>.

NIH Consensus Statement Online. *Gastrointestinal Surgery for Severe Obesity*, March 25–27, 1991 [cited March 16, 2003]; 9 (1): 1-20.

Rebecca Frey, Ph.D.

Vital signs

Definition

Vital signs, or signs of life, include the following objective measures for a person: temperature, respiratory rate, heart beat (pulse), and blood pressure. When these values are not zero, they indicate that a person is alive. All of these vital signs can be observed, measured, and monitored. This will enable the assessment of the level at which an individual is functioning. Normal ranges of measurements of vital signs change with age and medical condition.

Purpose

The purpose of recording vital signs is to establish a baseline on admission to a hospital, clinic, professional office, or other encounter with a health care provider. Vital signs may be recorded by a nurse, physician, physician's assistant, or other health care professional. The health care professional has the responsibility of interpreting data and identifying any abnormalities from a person's normal state, and of establishing if current treatment or medications are having the desired effect.

Abnormalities of the heart are diagnosed by analyzing the heartbeat (or pulse) and blood pressure. The rate, rhythm and regularity of the beat are assessed, as well as the strength and tension of the beat, against the arterial wall.

Vital signs are usually recorded from once hourly to four times hourly, as required by a person's condition.

The vital signs are recorded and compared with normal ranges for a person's age and medical condition. Based on these results, a decision is made regarding further actions to be taken.

All persons should be made comfortable and reassured that recording vital signs is normal part of health checks, and that it is necessary to ensure that the state of their health is being monitored correctly. Any abnormalities in vital signs should be reported to the health care professional in charge of care.

Description

Temperature

Temperature is recorded to check for fever (pyrexia or a febrile condition), or to monitor the degree of hypothermia.

Manufacturer guidelines should be followed when recording a temperature with an electronic **thermometer**. The result displayed on the liquid crystal display (LCD) screen should be read, then recorded in a person's medical record. Electronic temperature monitors do not have to be cleaned after use. They have protective guards that are discarded after each use. This practice ensures that infections are not spread.

An alcohol or mercury thermometer can be used to monitor a temperature by three methods:

• Axillary, under the armpit. This method provides the least accurate results.

• Orally, under the tongue. This method is never used with infants or very young children because they may accidentally bite or break the thermometer. They also have difficulty holding oral thermometers under their tongues long enough for their temperatures to be accurately measured.

• Rectally, inserted into the rectum. This method provides the most accurate recording of recording the temperature. It is most often used for infants. A recent study reported that rectal thermometers were more accurate than ear thermometers in detecting high fevers. With the ability to detect low-grade fevers, rectal thermometers can be useful in discovering serious illnesses, such as meningitis or pneumonia. The tip of a rectal thermometer is usually blue, which distinguishes it from the silver tip of an oral, or axillary thermometer.

To record the temperature using an alcohol or mercury thermometer, one should shake down the thermometer by holding it firmly at the clear end and flicking it quickly a few times, with the silver end pointing downward. The health care provider who is taking the temperature should confirm that the alcohol or mercury is below a normal body temperature.

To record an axillary temperature, the silver tip of the thermometer should be placed under the right armpit. The arm clamps the thermometer into place, against the chest. The thermometer should stay in place for three to four minutes. After the appropriate time has elapsed, the thermometer should be removed and held at eye level. During this waiting period, the body temperature will be measured The alcohol or mercury will have risen to a mark that indicates the temperature of a person.

To record an oral temperature, the axillary procedure should be followed, except that the silver tip of the thermometer should be placed beneath the tongue for three to four minutes, then read as described previously.

In both cases, the thermometer should be wiped clean with an antiseptic and stored in an appropriate container to prevent breakage.

To record a rectal temperature, a rectal thermometer should be shaken down, as described previously. A small amount of water-based lubricant should be placed on the colored tip of the thermometer. Infants must be placed on their stomachs and held securely in place. The tip of

the thermometer is inserted into the rectum no more than 0.5 in (1.3 cm) and held there for two to three minutes. The thermometer is removed, read as before, and wiped with an antibacterial wipe. It is then stored in an appropriate container to prevent breakage, because ingestion of mercury can be fatal.

Respiratory rate

An examiner's fingers should be placed on the person's wrist, while the number of breaths or respirations in one minute is recorded. Every effort should be made to prevent people from becoming aware that their breathing is being checked. Respiration results should be noted in the medical chart.

Heart beat (pulse)

The pulse can be recorded anywhere that a surface artery runs over a bone. The radial artery in the wrist is the point most commonly used to measure a pulse. To measure a pulse, one should place the index, middle, and ring fingers over the radial artery. It is located above the wrist, on the anterior or front surface of the thumb side of the arm. Gentle pressure should be applied, taking care to avoid obstructing blood flow. The rate, rhythm, strength, and tension of the pulse should be noted. If there are no abnormalities detected, the pulsations can be counted for half a minute, and the result doubled. However, any irregularities discerned indicate that the pulse should be recorded for one minute. This will eliminate the possibility of error. Pulse results should be noted in the health chart.

Blood pressure

To record blood pressure, a person should be seated with one arm bent slightly, and the arm bare or with the sleeve loosely rolled up. With an aneroid or automatic unit, the cuff is placed level with the heart and wrapped around the upper arm, one inch above the elbow. Following the manufacturer's guidelines, the cuff is inflated and then deflated while an attendant records the reading.

If the blood pressure is monitored manually, a cuff is placed level with the heart and wrapped firmly but not tightly around the arm one inch above the elbow over the brachial artery. Wrinkles in the cuff should be smoothed out. Positioning a **stethoscope** over the brachial artery in front of the elbow with one hand and listening through the earpieces, the cuff is inflated well above normal levels (to about 200 mmHg), or until no sound is heard. Alternatively, the cuff should be inflated 10 mm Hg above the last sound heard. The valve in the pump is slowly opened. Air is allowed to escape no faster than 5 mmHg per second to deflate the pressure in the cuff to the point where a clicking sound is heard over the brachial artery. The reading of the gauge at this point is recorded as the systolic pressure.

The sounds continue as the pressure in the cuff is released and the flow of blood through the artery is no longer blocked. At this point, the noises are no longer heard. The reading of the gauge at this point is noted as the diastolic pressure. "Lub-dub" is the sound produced by the normal heart as it beats. Every time this sound is detected, it means that the heart is contracting once. The noises are created when the heart valves click to close. When one hears "lub," the atrioventricular valves are closing. The "dub" sound is produced by the pulmonic and aortic valves.

With children, the clicking noise does not disappear but changes to a soft muffled sound. Because sounds continue to be heard as the cuff deflates to zero, the reading of the gauge at the point where the sounds change is recorded as the diastolic pressure.

Blood pressure readings are recorded with the systolic pressure first, then the diastolic pressure (e.g., 120/70).

Blood pressure should be measured using a cuff that is correctly sized for the person being evaluated. Cuffs that are too small are likely to yield readings that can be 10 to 50 millimeters (mm) Hg too high. Hypertension (high blood pressure) may be incorrectly diagnosed.

Preparation

As there may be no recorded knowledge of a person's previous vital signs for comparison, it is important that a health care professional be aware that there is a wide range of normal values that can apply to persons of different ages. The health care professional should obtain as detailed a medical history from the person as soon as possible. Any known medical or surgical history, prior measurements of vital signs, and details of current medications should be recorded, as well. Physical exertion prior to measurement of vital signs, such as climbing stairs, may affect the measurements. This should be avoided immediately before the measurement of one's blood pressure. Tobacco, caffeinated drinks, and alcohol should be avoided for 30 minutes prior to recording.

A person should be sitting down or lying comfortably to ensure that the readings are taken in a similar position each time. There should be little excitement, which can affect the results. The equipment required include a watch with a second hand, an electronic or other form of thermometer, an electronic or manual **sphygmomanometer** with an appropriate sized cuff, and a stethoscope.

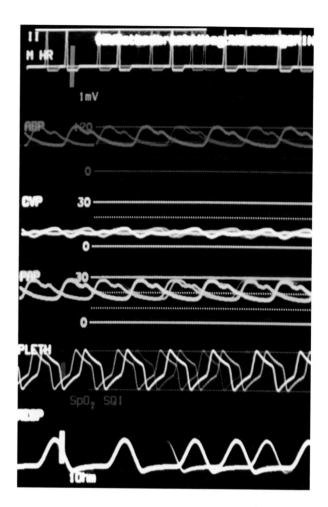

Normal vital signs, from the top: heart rate, arterial blood pressure (ABP), central venous pressure (CVP), pulmonary artery pressure (PAP), blood oxygen (PLETH), and respiration rate. *(Photograph by James King-Holmes. Science Source/Photo Researchers. Reproduced by permission.)*

Normal results

A normal body temperature taken orally is 98.6°F (37°C), with a range of 97.8–99.1°F (36.5–37.2°C). A fever is a temperature of 101°F (38.3°C) or higher in an infant younger than three months or above 102°F (38.9°C) for older children and adults. Hypothermia is recognized as a temperature below 96°F (35.5°C).

Respirations are quiet, slow, and shallow when the adult is asleep, and rapid, deeper, and noisier during and after activity.

Average respiration rates at rest are:

• infants, 34–40 per minute

• children five years of age, 25 per minute

• older children and adults, 16–20 per minute

Tachypnea is rapid respiration above 20 per minute.

The strength of a heart beat is raised during conditions such as fever and lowered by conditions such as shock or elevated intracranial pressure. The average heart rate for older children (aged 12 and older) and adults is approximately 72 beats per minute (bpm). Tachycardia is a pulse rate over 100 bpm, while bradycardia is a pulse rate of under 60 bpm.

Blood pressure is recorded for older children and adults. A normal adult blood pressure reading is 120/80.

See also Physical examination.

Resources

BOOKS

Bickley, L. S., P. G., Szilagyi. J. G. Stackhouse. *Bates' Guide to Physical Examination & History Taking, 8th edition.* Philadelphia: Lippincott Williams & Wilkins, 2002.

Chan, P. D., and P. J. Winkle. *History and Physical Examination in Medicine, 10th ed.* New York: Current Clinical Strategies, 2002.

Seidel, Henry M. *Mosby's Physical Examination Handbook, 4th ed.* St. Louis: Mosby-Year Book, 2003.

Swartz, Mark A., and William Schmitt. *Textbook of Physical Diagnosis: History and Examination, 4th edition.* Philadelphia: Saunders, 2001.

PERIODICALS

Ahmed A. M. "Deficiences of Physical Examination Among Medical Students." *Saudi Medical Journal* 24, no. 1 (2003): 108-111.

ORGANIZATIONS

American Academy of Family Physicians, 11400 Tomahawk Creek Parkway, Leawood, KS 66211-2672. (913) 906-6000. E-mail: <fp@aafp.org>. <http://www.aafp.org>.

American Academy of Pediatrics, 141 Northwest Point Boulevard, Elk Grove Village, IL 60007-1098. 847) 434-4000. Fax: (847) 434-8000. E-mail: <kidsdoc@aap.org>. <http://www.aap.org/default.htm>.

American College of Physicians. 190 N. Independence Mall West, Philadelphia, PA 19106-1572. (800) 523-1546, x2600 or (215) 351-2600. <http://www.acponline.org>.

OTHER

Karolinska Institute. [cited March 1, 2003] <http://isp.his.ki.se/text/physical.htm>.

Loyola University Chicago Stritch School of Medicine. [cited March 1, 2003] <http://www.meddean.luc.edu/lumen/MedEd/MEDICINE/PULMONAR/PD/Pdmenu.htm>.

National Library of Medicine. [cited March 1, 2003] <http://www.nlm.nih.gov/medlineplus/ency/article/002274.htm>.

Review of Systems School of Medical Transcription. [cited March 1, 2003] <http://www.mtmonthly.com/studentcorner/cpe.htm>.

L. Fleming Fallon, Jr., M.D., DrPH

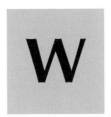

W

Water pills *see* Diuretics

Webbed finger or toe repair

Definition

Webbed finger or toe repair refers to corrective or reconstructive surgery performed to repair webbed fingers or toes, also called syndactyly. The long and ring fingers or the second and third toes are most often affected. Generally, syndactyly repairs are done between the ages of six months and two years.

Purpose

Webbing, or syndactyly, is a condition characterized by the incomplete separation or union of two or more fingers or toes, and usually only involves a skin connection between the two (simple syndactyly), but may—rarely—also include fusion of bones, nerves, blood vessels, and tendons in the affected digits (complex syndactyly). Webbing may extend partially up between the digits, frequently just to the first joint, or may extend the entire length of the digits. Polysyndactyly describes both webbing and the presence of an extra number of fingers or toes. The condition usually develops within six weeks after birth. Syndactyly can also occur in victims of fires, as the intense heat can melt the skin and fuse the epidermis and dermis of the phalanges, fingers, or toes. Burn victim syndactyly is always less invasive because bone fusion is not present in these cases. The purpose of repair surgery is to improve the appearance of the hand or foot and to prevent progressive deformity from developing as the child grows.

Demographics

In the United States, approximately one infant in every 2,000 births is born with webbed fingers or toes.

Both hands are involved in 50% of cases; the middle finger and ring finger in 41%; the ring finger and little finger in 27%; the index finger and middle finger in 23%; and the thumb and index finger in 9%.

Description

Polydactyly can be corrected by surgical removal of the extra digit or partial digit. Syndactyly can also be corrected surgically. This is usually accomplished with the addition of a skin graft from the groin.

There are several ways to perform this type of surgery; the design of the operation depends both on the features of the hand or foot and the surgeon's experience. The surgery is usually performed with zigzag cuts that cross back and forth across the fingers or toes so that the scars do not interfere with growth of the digits.

The procedure is performed under general anesthesia. The skin areas to be repaired are marked and the surgeon then proceeds to incise the skin, lifting small flaps at the sides of the fingers or toes and in the web. These flaps are sutured into position, leaving absent areas of skin. These areas may be filled in with full thickness skin grafts, usually taken from the skin in the groin area.

Webbed finger repair

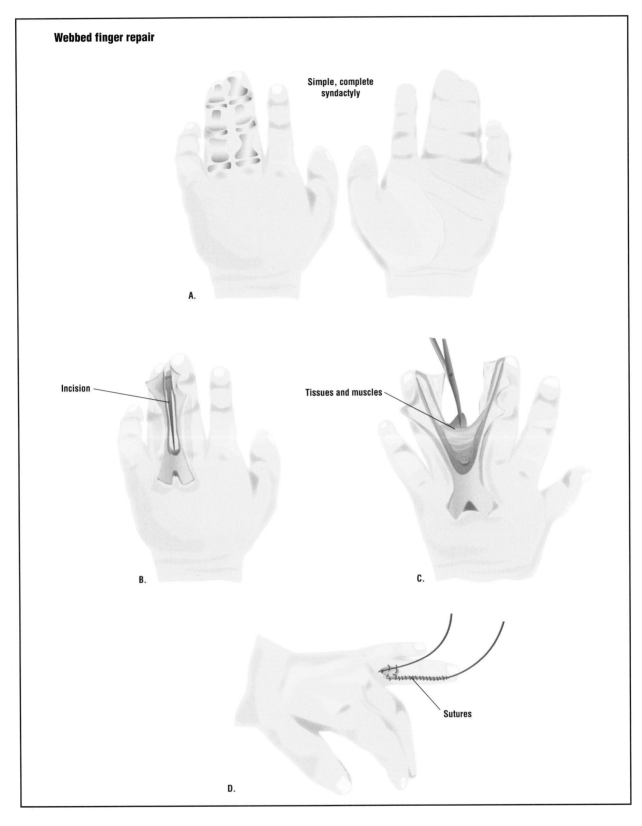

Simple, complete
syndactyly

A.

Incision

B.

Tissues and muscles

C.

Sutures

D.

This webbed finger shows a simple, complete syndactyly, meaning the bones for two fingers are complete, and only the soft tissues form the webbed section (A). To repair this, an incision is made in the skin of the webbing (B). Tissues and muscles are severed (C), and the two separated fingers are stitched (D). *(Illustration by GGS Inc.)*

The hand or foot is then immobilized with bulky dressings, or a cast. Webbed or toe repair surgery usually takes two to four hours.

Diagnosis/Preparation

Syndactyly may be diagnosed during an examination of an infant or child, with the aid of x rays. In its most common form, it is seen as webbing between the second and third toes. This form is often inherited. Syndactyly can also occur as part of a pattern of other congenital defects involving the skull, face, and bones.

An infant with webbed fingers or toes may have other symptoms that, when observed together, define a specific syndrome or medical condition. For example, syndactyly is a characteristic of Apert syndrome, Poland syndrome, Jarcho-Levin syndrome, oral-facial-digital syndrome, Pfeiffer syndrome, and Edwards syndrome. Diagnosis of a syndrome is made on family history, medical history, and thorough physical evaluation. The medical history questions documenting the condition in detail usually include:

• Which fingers (toes) are involved?

• Are any other family members affected by the same condition?

• What other symptoms or abnormalities are also present?

To prepare for surgery, seven to 10 days before surgery, the child visits the family physician or pediatrician for a general **physical examination** and blood tests. The child cannot have solid food after midnight before surgery. Breast milk, formula, or milk (no pablum or other cereal may be added) up to six hours before the scheduled start of surgery is allowed, and then only clear fluids up to three hours before surgery. Thereafter, the child may not have anything else to eat or drink.

Aftercare

Hospital stays of one or two days are common for webbed finger or toe repair surgery. There is usually some swelling and bruising. Pain medications are given to alleviate any discomfort. The bandages must be kept clean and dry and must remain for two to three weeks for proper healing and protection. Skin grafts and the hand or foot may become very dry, so it is encouraged to dampen them with a good moisturizer such as Lubriderm or Nivea. Small children with hand syndactylies may have a cast put on that extends above the flexed elbow. Sometimes, the cast extends beyond the fingers or toes. This protects the repaired areas from trauma.

The treating physician should be informed of any post-operative swelling, severe pain, fever, or fingers that tingle, are numb, or have a bluish discoloration.

> ## QUESTIONS TO ASK THE DOCTOR
>
> • What will happen during the surgery?
> • Does my baby have any other birth defect?
> • How long will it take to recover from surgery?
> • Will my baby have normal fingers/toes?
> • How many webbed finger/toe repair surgeries do you perform each year?
> • Will the syndactyly return?

Risks

Webbed finger or toe repair surgery carries the risks associated with any anesthesia, such as adverse reactions to medications, breathing problems, and sore throat from intubation. Risks associated with any surgery are excessive bleeding and infection.

Specific risks associated with the repair surgery include possible loss of skin graft and circulation damage from the cast or bandages.

Normal results

The results of webbed finger or toe repair depend on the degree of fusion of the digits and the repair is usually successful. When joined fingers share a single fingernail, the creation of two normal-looking nails is rarely possible. One nail will look more normal than the other. Some children may require a second surgery, depending on the type of syndactyly. If polydactyly or syndactyly are just cosmetic and not symptomatic of a condition or disorder, the outcome of surgery is usually very good. If it is symptomatic, the outcome will rely heavily on the management of the disorder.

Alternatives

Syndactyly does not generally pose any health risk, so that it is not mandatory that the repair be performed. However, if the thumb is joined, or if the fingers are joined out toward their tips, they will grow in a progressively worsening bend over time.

See also Cleft lip repair; Club foot repair.

Resources

BOOKS

Jones, Kenneth Lyons. *Smith's Recognizable Patterns of Human Malformation*. 5th ed. Philadelphia: W.B. Saunders, 1997.

to an electrical current in different types of body tissue. Fatty tissue has a higher resistance to the current than body tissues containing larger amounts of water. A higher percentage of body water indicates a greater amount of lean tissue.

Eating disorders

Eating disorders are a group of psychiatric disturbances defined by unhealthy eating or weight management practices. Anorexia nervosa is an eating disorder in which persons restrict their food intake severely, refuse to maintain a normal body weight, and express intense fear of becoming obese. Bulimia nervosa is a disorder marked by episodes of binge eating followed by attempts to avoid weight gain from the food by abusing **laxatives**, forcing vomiting, or overexercising. A third type, binge eating disorder, is found in some obese people, as well as in people of normal weight. In binge eating disorder, the person has an eating binge but does not try to get rid of the food after eating it. Although most patients diagnosed with anorexia or bulimia are women, 40% of patients with binge eating disorder are men.

Purpose

The purpose of weight management is to help each patient achieve and stay at the best weight possible the context of overall health, occupation, and living situation. A second purpose is the prevention and treatment of diseases and disorders associated with obesity or with eating disorders. These disorders include depression and other psychiatric disturbances, in addition to the physical problems associated with nutritional disorders.

Demographics and statistics

Obesity has become a major public health concern in the United States in the last decade. As of 2003, obesity ranks second only to smoking as a major cause of preventable deaths. It is estimated that 300,000 people die in the United States each year from weight-related causes. The proportion of overweight adults in the general population has continued to rise since the 1960s. About 34% of American adults, or 58 million people, are overweight, compared with 25% in 1980. In addition, there has been a 42% increase in the rate of childhood obesity since 1980.

The prevalence of obesity in the United States varies somewhat according to sex, age, race, and socioeconomic status. Among adults, 35% of women are considered obese, compared to 31% of men. The rate of obesity increases as people get older; those aged 55 or older are more than twice as likely to be obese as those in their twenties. African American men have the same rate of obesity as Caucasian men; however, African American women are almost twice as likely as Caucasian women to be obese by the time they reach middle age. The same ratio holds true for socioeconomic status; people in the lowest third of the income and educational level distribution are twice as likely to be obese as those with more education and higher income.

From the economic standpoint, obesity costs the United States over $100 billion each year. This amount includes the direct costs of hospital care and medical services, which come to $45.8 billion annually, or 6.8% of all health care costs. Another $18.9 billion represents the indirect costs of obesity, such as disabilities related to overweight or work days lost to obesity-related illnesses.

Obesity is considered responsible for:

- 88–97% of cases of type 2 diabetes
- 57–70% of cases of coronary heart disease
- 70% of gallstone attacks
- 35% of cases of hypertension
- 11% of breast cancers
- 10% of colon cancers

In addition, obesity intensifies the pain of osteoarthritis and gout; increases the risk of complications in pregnancy and childbirth; contributes to depression and other mental disorders; and makes a person a poor candidate for surgery. Many surgeons refuse to operate on patients who weigh more than 300 lb (136 kg).

Although fewer people suffer from eating disorders than from obesity, the National Institutes of Mental Health (NIMH) reports that 10 million adults in the United States meet the diagnostic criteria for anorexia or bulimia. Although eating disorders are stereotyped as affecting only adolescent or college-aged women, as of 2003 at least 10% of people with eating disorders are males—and the proportion of males to females is rising. Moreover, the number of women over 45 years of age who are diagnosed with eating disorders is also rising; many doctors attribute this startling new trend to fear of aging, as well as fear of obesity.

The long-term health consequences of eating disorders include gum disease and loss of teeth, irregular heart rhythm, disturbances in the chemical balance of the blood, and damage to the digestive tract. At least 50,000 people die each year in the United States as the direct result of an eating disorder; anorexia is the leading cause of death in women between the ages of 17 and 25.

Description

To understand the goals and structure of nutritionally sound weight management programs, it is helpful to look first as the causes of being overweight, obesity, and eating disorders.

Causes of nutrition-related disorders

GENETIC/BIOLOGIC. Studies of twins separated at birth and research with genetically altered mice have shown that there is a genetic component to obesity. Some researchers think that there are also genetic factors involved in eating disorders.

LIFESTYLE-RELATED. The ready availability of relatively inexpensive, but high-caloric snacks and "junk food" is considered to contribute to the high rates of obesity in developed countries. In addition, the fast pace of modern life encourages people to select quick-cooking processed foods that are high in calories, rather than making meals that are more healthful but take longer to prepare. Lastly, changes in technology and transportation patterns mean that people today do not do as much walking or hard physical labor as earlier generations did. This sedentary, or inactive lifestyle makes it easier for people to gain weight.

SOCIOCULTURAL. In recent years, many researchers have examined the role of advertising and the mass media in encouraging unhealthy eating patterns. On the one hand, advertisements for such items as fast food, soft drinks, and ice cream, often convey the message that food can be used to relieve stress, reward, or comfort oneself, or substitute for a fulfilling human relationship. On the other hand, the media also portray unrealistic images of human physical perfection. Their emphasis on slenderness as essential to beauty, particularly in women, is often cited as a major factor in the increase of eating disorders over the past three decades.

Another sociocultural factor that contributes to obesity among some Hispanic and Asian groups is the belief that children are not healthy unless they look plump. Overfeeding in infancy and early childhood, unfortunately, makes weight management in adolescence and adult life much more difficult.

MEDICATIONS. Recent research has found that a number of prescription medications can contribute to weight gain. These drugs include steroid hormones, antidepressants, benzodiazepine tranquilizers, lithium, and antipsychotic medications.

Aspects of weight management

Since the late 1980s, nutritionists and health care professionals had come to recognize that successful weight management programs have three characteristics, as follows:

- They present weight management as a lifetime commitment to healthful patterns of eating and **exercise**, rather than emphasize strict dieting alternating with carelessness about eating habits.

- They are tailored to each person's age, general health, living situation, and other individual characteristics.

- They recognize that the emotional, psychological, and spiritual facet of human life are as important to maintaining a healthy lifestyle as the medical and nutritional facets.

Nutrition

The nutritional aspect of weight management programs includes education about healthful eating, as well as modifying the person's food intake.

DIETARY REGULATION. Most weight-management programs are based on a diet that supplies enough vitamins and minerals; 50–63 grams of protein each day; an adequate intake of carbohydrates (100 g) and dietary fiber (20–30 g); and no more than 30% of each day's calories from fat. Good weight-management diets are intended to teach people how to make wise food choices and to encourage gradual weight loss. Some diets are based on fixed menus, while others are based on food exchanges. In a food-exchange diet, a person can choose among several items within a particular food group when following a menu plan. For example, if a person's menu plan allows for two items from the vegetable group at lunch, they can have one raw and one cooked vegetable, or one serving of vegetable juice along with another vegetable. More detailed information about these and other weight-management diets is available in a booklet from the Weight Information Network of the National Institutes of Health, called *Weight Loss for Life*, listed under "Resources" below.

NUTRITIONAL EDUCATION. Nutritional counseling is important to successful weight management because many people, particularly those with eating disorders, do not understand how the body uses food. They may also be trying to manage their weight in unhealthy ways. One recent study of adolescents found that 32% of the females and 17% of the males were using such potentially dangerous methods of weight control as smoking, fasting, over-the-counter diet pills, or laxatives.

Exercise

Regular physical exercise is a major part of weight management because it increases the number of calories used by the body and because it helps the body to replace fat with lean muscle tissue. Exercise also serves to lower emotional stress levels and to promote a general sense of well-being. People should consult a doctor before beginning an exercise program, however, to make sure that the activity that interests them is safe relative to any other health problems they may have. For example, people with osteoarthritis should avoid high-impact sports that are hard on the knee and ankle joints. Good choices for most people include swimming, walking, cycling, and stretching exercises.

Psychological/psychiatric

Both obesity and eating disorders are associated with a variety of psychiatric disorders, most commonly major depression and substance abuse. Almost all obese people feel harshly judged and criticized by others, and fear of obesity is a major factor in the development of both anorexia and bulimia. Many people find medications and/or psychotherapy to be a helpful part of a weight management program.

MEDICATIONS. In recent years, doctors have been cautious about prescribing appetite suppressants, which are drugs given to reduce the desire for food. In 1997, the Food and Drug Administration (FDA) banned the sale of two drugs: fenfluramine (known as "fen-phen") and phentermine when they were discovered to cause damage to heart valves. A newer appetite suppressant, known as sibutramine, has been approved as safe. Another new drug that is sometimes prescribed for weight management is called orlistat. It works by lowering the amount of dietary fat that is absorbed by the body. However, it can cause significant diarrhea.

People with eating disorders are sometimes given antidepressant medications, most often fluoxetine (Prozac) or venlafaxine, to relieve the symptoms of depression or anxiety that often accompany eating disorders.

COGNITIVE-BEHAVIORAL THERAPY. Cognitive-behavioral therapy (CBT) is a form of psychotherapy that has been shown to be effective in reinforcing the changes in food selection and eating patterns that are necessary to successful weight management. In this form of therapy, patients learn to modify their eating habits by keeping diaries and records of what they eat, what events or feelings trigger overeating, and any other patterns that they notice about their choice of foods or eating habits. They also examine their attitudes toward food and weight management, and work to change any attitudes that are self-defeating or interfere with a healthy lifestyle. Most CBT programs also include nutritional education and counseling.

WEIGHT-MANAGEMENT GROUPS. Many doctors and nutritional counselors suggest that patients attend a weight-management group for social support. Social support is essential in weight management, because many who suffer from obesity or an eating disorder struggle with intense feelings of shame. Many isolate themselves from others because they are afraid of being teased or criticized for their appearance. Such groups as Overeaters Anonymous (OA) or Take Off Pounds Sensibly (TOPS) help members in several ways: They help to reduce the levels of shame and anxiety that most members feel; they teach strategies for coping with setbacks in weight management; they provide settings for making new friends; and they help people learn to handle problems in their workplace or in relationships with family members.

Surgical

As of 2003, bariatric surgery is the most successful approach to weight management for people who are morbidly obese (BMI of 40 or greater), or severely obese with additional health complications. Surgical treatment of obesity usually results in a large weight loss that is successfully maintained for longer than five years. The most common surgical procedures for weight management are **vertical banded gastroplasty** (VBG), sometimes referred to as "stomach stapling," and **gastric bypass**. Vertical banded gastroplasty works by limiting the amount of food the stomach can hold, while gastric bypass works by preventing normal absorption of the nutrients in the food.

Complementary and alternative medicine (CAM) approaches

Some forms of complementary and alternative medicine are beneficial additions to weight management programs.

MOVEMENT THERAPIES. Movement therapies include a number of forms of exercise, such as tai chi, yoga, dance therapy, Trager work, and the Feldenkrais method. Many of these approaches help people improve their posture and move their bodies more easily as well as keeping active. Tai chi and yoga, for example, are good for people who must avoid high-impact physical workouts. Yoga can also be adapted to a person's individual needs or limitations with the help of a qualified teacher following a doctor's recommendations. Books and videos on yoga and weight management are available through most bookstores or the American Yoga Association.

SPIRITUAL AND RELIGIOUS PRACTICE. Prayer, meditation, and regular religious worship have been linked to reduced emotional stress in people struggling with weight issues. In addition, many people find that spiritual practice helps them to keep a healthy perspective on weight management, so that it does not crowd out other important interests and concerns in their lives.

HERBAL PREPARATIONS. The one type of alternative treatment that people should be extremely cautious about

KEY TERMS

Anorexia nervosa—An eating disorder marked by refusal to eat, intense fear of obesity, and distortions of body image.

Appetite suppressant—A medication given to reduce the desire to eat.

Bariatrics—The branch of medicine that deals with the prevention and treatment of obesity and related disorders.

Binge—A time-limited bout of excessive indulgence in eating; consuming a larger amount of food within a limited period of time than most people would eat in similar circumstances.

Binge eating disorder—An eating disorder in which the person binges but does not try to get rid of the food afterward by vomiting, using laxatives, or exercising.

Body mass index (BMI)—A measurement that has replaced weight as the preferred determinant of obesity. The BMI can be calculated (in English units) as 703.1 times a person's weight in pounds divided

by the square of the person's height in inches.

Bulimia nervosa—An eating disorder marked by episodes of binge eating followed by purging, overexercising, or other behaviors intended to prevent weight gain.

Ephedra—A herb used in traditional Chinese medicine to treat asthma and hay fever. It should never be used for weight management.

Obesity—Excessive weight gain due to accumulation of fat in the body, sometimes defined as a BMI of 30 or higher, or body weight greater than 30% above one's desirable weight on standard height-weight tables.

Prevalence—The number of cases of a disease or disorder that are present in a given population at a specific time.

Sedentary—Characterized by inactivity and lack of exercise. A sedentary lifestyle is a major risk factor for becoming overweight or obese.

making part of a weight management program is over-the-counter herbal preparations advertised as "fat burners," muscle builders, or appetite suppressants. Within a two-week period in early 2003, the national media carried accounts of death or serious illness from taking these substances. One is ephedra, a herb used in traditional Chinese medicine that can cause strokes, heart attacks, seizures, and psychotic episodes. The other is usnic acid, a compound derived from lichens that can cause liver damage.

Normal results

As of 2003, much more research needs to be done to improve the success of weight management programs. A position paper published by the American Dietetic Association in the summer of 2002 summarizes the present situation: "Although our knowledge base has greatly expanded regarding the complex causation of increased body fat, little progress has been made in long-term maintenance interventions, with the exception of surgery." Most adults in weight maintenance programs find it difficult to change eating patterns learned over a lifetime. Furthermore, their efforts are all too often undermined by friends or relatives, as well as by media messages that encourage overeating or the use of food as a mood-enhancing drug. More effective weight mainte-

nance programs may well depend on broad-based changes in society.

Resources

BOOKS

American Psychiatric Association. "Eating Disorders." In *Diagnostic and Statistical Manual of Mental Disorders*, 4th edition, text revision. Washington, DC: American Psychiatric Association, 2000.

Brownell, Kelly, Ph.D., and Judith Rodin, Ph.D. *The Weight Maintenance Survival Guide*. Dallas, TX: Brownell & Hager Publishing Co., 1990.

Flancbaum, Louis, M.D., with Erica Manfred and Deborah Biskin. *The Doctor's Guide to Weight Loss Surgery*. West Hurley, NY: Fredonia Communications, 2001.

Hornbacher, Marya. *Wasted: A Memoir of Anorexia and Bulimia*. New York: Harper Perennial Editions, 1999.

" Nutritional Disorders: Obesity." Section 1, Chapter 5 in *The Merck Manual of Diagnosis and Therapy*, edited by Mark H. Beers, M.D., and Robert Berkow, M.D. Whitehouse Station, NJ: Merck Research Laboratories, 1999.

Pelletier, Kenneth R., M.D. "CAM Therapies for Specific Conditions: Obesity." In *The Best Alternative Medicine*, Part II. New York: Simon & Schuster, 2002.

PERIODICALS

Bellafante, Ginia. " When Midlife Seems Just An Empty Plate." *New York Times*, March 9, 2003 [cited March 12, 2003]. <www.nytimes.com/2003/03/09/health.html>.

Chass, Murray. "Pitcher's Autopsy Points to Ephedra As One Factor." *New York Times*, March 14, 2003 [cited March 14, 2003]. <www.nytimes.com/2003/03/14/sports/baseball/14BASE.html>.

Cummings, S., E. S. Parham, and G. W. Strain. "Position of the American Dietetic Association: Weight Management." *Journal of the American Dietetic Association* 102 (August 2002): 1145-1155.

Davis, R. B., and L. W. Turner. "A Review of Current Weight Management: Research and Recommendations." *Journal of the American Academy of Nurse Practitioners* 13 (January 2001): 15-19.

Drohan, S. H. "Managing Early Childhood Obesity in the Primary Care Setting: A Behavior Modification Approach." *Pediatric Nursing* 28 (November-December 2002): 599-610.

Grady, Denise. "Seeking to Shed Fat, She Lost Her Liver." *New York Times*, March 4, 2003 [cited March 4, 2003]. <www.nytimes.com/2003/03/04/health.html>.

Hanif, M. W., and S. Kumar. "Pharmacological Management of Obesity." *Expert Opinion on Pharmacotherapy* 3 (December 2002): 1711-1718.

Lowry, R., D. A. Galuska, J. E. Fulton, et al. "Weight Management Goals and Practices Among U. S. High School Students: Associations with Physical Activity, Diet, and Smoking." *Journal of Adolescent Health* 31 (August 2002): 133-144.

Malhotra, S., K. H. King, J. A. Welge, et al. "Venlafaxine Treatment of Binge-Eating Disorder Associated with Obesity: A Series of 35 Patients." *Journal of Clinical Psychiatry* 63 (September 2002): 802-806.

Riebe, D., G. W. Greene, L. Ruggiero, et al. "Evaluation of a Healthy-Lifestyle Approach to Weight Management." *Preventive Medicine* 36 (January 2003): 45-54.

ORGANIZATIONS

American Dietetic Association. (800) 877-1600. <www.eatright.org>.

American Obesity Association (AOA). 1250 24th Street NW, Suite 300, Washington, DC 20037. (202) 776-7711 or (800) 98-OBESE. <www.obesity.org>.

American Society for Bariatric Surgery. 7328 West University Avenue, Suite F, Gainesville, FL 32607. (352) 331-4900. <www.asbs.org>.

American Yoga Association. <www.americanyogaassociation.org>.

Overeaters Anonymous (OA). World Service Office, P. O. Box 44020, Rio Rancho, NM 87174-4020. (505) 891-2664. <www.oa.org>.

Shape Up America! c/o WebFront Solutions Corporation, 15757 Crabbs Branch Way, Rockville, M. D. 20855. (301) 258-0540. <www.shapeup.org>.

Weight-control Information Network (WIN). 1 WIN Way, Bethesda, MD 20892-3665. (202) 828-1025 or (877) 946-4627.

OTHER

National Institutes of Health, National Institute of Diabetes & Digestive & Kidney Diseases (NIDDK). *Choosing a Safe and Successful Weight-Loss Program.* Bethesda, MD: NIDDK, 1998. NIH Publication No. 94-3700.

National Institutes of Health, National Institute of Diabetes & Digestive & Kidney Diseases (NIDDK). *Do You Know the Health Risks of Being Overweight?* Bethesda, MD: NIDDK, 2001. NIH Publication No. 98-4098.

National Institutes of Health, National Institute of Diabetes & Digestive & Kidney Diseases (NIDDK). *Weight Loss for Life.* Bethesda, MD: NIDDK, 2002. NIH Publication No. 98-3700.

Rebecca Frey, Ph.D.

White blood cell count and differential

Definition

A white blood cell (WBC) count determines the concentration of white blood cells in the patient's blood. A differential determines the percentage of each of the five types of mature white blood cells.

Purpose

This test is included in general health examinations and to help investigate a variety of illnesses. An elevated WBC count occurs in infection, allergy, systemic illness, inflammation, tissue injury, and leukemia. A low WBC count may occur in some viral infections, immunodeficiency states, and bone marrow failure. The WBC count provides clues about certain illnesses, and helps physicians monitor a patient's recovery from others. Abnormal counts which return to normal indicate that the condition is improving, while counts that become more abnormal indicate that the condition is worsening. The differential will reveal which WBC types are affected most. For example, an elevated WBC count with an absolute increase in lymphocytes having an atypical appearance is most often caused by infectious mononucleosis. The differential will also identify early WBCs which may be reactive (e.g., a response to acute infection) or the result of a leukemia.

Precautions

Many medications affect the WBC count. Both prescription and non-prescription drugs including herbal supplements should be noted. Normal values for both the WBC count and differential are age-related.

Sources of error in manual WBC counting are due largely to variance in the dilution of the sample and the distribution of cells in the chamber, as well as the small

KEY TERMS

Band cell—An immature neutrophil at the stage just preceding a mature cell. The nucleus of a band cell is unsegmented.

Basophil—Segmented white blood cell with large dark blue-black granules that releases histamine in allergic reactions.

Cytoplasm—The part of a cell outside of the nucleus, like the egg white.

Differential—Blood test that determines the percentage of each type of white blood cell in a person's blood.

Eosinophil—Segmented white blood cell with large orange-red granules that increases in response to parasitic infections and allergic reactions.

Lymphocyte—Mononuclear white blood cell that is responsible for humoral (antibody mediated) and cell mediated immunity.

Monocyte—Mononuclear phagocytic white blood cell that removes debris and microorganisms by phagocytosis and processes antigens for recognition by immune lymphocytes.

Nucleus—The part of a cell that contains the DNA, such as an egg yolk.

Neutrophil—Segmented white blood cell normally comprising 50–70% of the total. The cytoplasm contains both primary and secondary granules that take up both acidic and basic dyes of the Wright stain. Neutrophils remove and kill bacteria by phagocytosis.

Phagocytosis—A process by which a white blood cell envelopes and digests debris and microorganisms to remove them from the blood.

number of WBCs that are counted. For electronic WBC counts and differentials, interference may be caused by small fibrin clots, nucleated red blood cells (RBCs), platelet clumping, and unlysed RBCs. Immature WBCs and nucleated RBCs may cause interference with the automated differential count. Automated cell counters may not be acceptable for counting WBCs in other body fluids, especially when the number of WBCs is less than 1000/μL or when other nucleated cell types are present.

Description

White cell counts are usually performed using an automated instrument, but may be done manually using a microscope and a counting chamber, especially when counts are very low, or if the patient has a condition known to interfere with an automated WBC count.

An automated differential may be performed by an electronic cell counter or by an image analysis instrument. When the electronic WBC count is abnormal or a cell population is flagged, meaning that one or more of the results is atypical, a manual differential is performed. The WBC differential is performed manually by microscopic examination of a blood sample that is spread in a thin film on a glass slide. White blood cells are identified by their size, shape, and texture.

The manual WBC differential involves a thorough evaluation of a stained blood film. In addition to determining the percentage of each mature white blood cell, the following tests are preformed as part of the differential:

- Evaluation of RBC morphology is performed. This includes grading of the variation in RBC size (anisocytosis) and shape (poikilocytosis); reporting the type and number of any abnormal or immature RBCs; and counting the number of nucleated RBCs per 100 WBCs.

- An estimate of the WBC count is made and compared with the automated or chamber WBC count. An estimate of the platelet count is made and compared with the automated or chamber platelet count. Abnormal platelets, such as clumped platelets or excessively large platelets, are noted on the report.

- Any immature WBCs are included in the differential count of 100 cells, and any inclusions or abnormalities of the WBCs are reported.

Preparation

This test requires a 3.5 mL sample of blood. Vein puncture with a needle is usually performed by a nurse or phlebotomist, a person trained to draw blood. There is no restriction on diet or physical activity.

Aftercare

Discomfort or bruising may occur at the puncture site. Pressure to the puncture site until the bleeding stops reduces bruising; warm packs relieve discomfort. Some people feel dizzy or faint after blood has been drawn and should be allowed to lie down and relax until they are stable.

Risks

Other than potential bruising at the puncture site, and/or dizziness, there are no complications associated with this test.

Normal results

Normal values vary with age. White blood cell counts are highest in children under one year of age and then decrease somewhat until adulthood. The increase is largely in the lymphocyte population. Adult normal values are shown below.

- WBC count: 4,500–11,000/μL

- polymorphonuclear neutrophils: 1800–7800/μL; (50–70%)

- band neutrophils: 0–700/μL; (0–10%)

- lymphocytes: 1000–4800/μL; (15–45%)

- monocytes: 0–800/μL; (0–10%)

- eosinophils: 0–450/μL; (0–6%)

- basophils: 0–200/μL; (0–2%)

Resources

BOOKS

Chernecky, Cynthia C., and Barbara J. Berger. *Laboratory Tests and Diagnostic Procedures,* 3rd ed. Philadelphia, PA: W. B. Saunders Company, 2001.

Henry, J. B. *Clinical Diagnosis and Management by Laboratory Methods,* 20th ed. Philadelphia, PA: W.B. Saunders Company, 2001.

Kee, Joyce LeFever. *Handbook of Laboratory and Diagnostic Tests,* 4th ed. Upper Saddle River, NJ: Prentice Hall, 2001.

Wallach, Jacques. *Interpretation of Diagnostic Tests,* 7th ed. Philadelphia, PA: Lippincott Williams & Wilkens, 2000.

OTHER

National Institutes of Health. [cited April 5, 2003] <http://www.nlm.nih.gov/medlineplus/encyclopedia.html>.

Victoria E. DeMoranville
Mark A. Best

Wound care

Definition

A wound is a disruption in the continuity of cells—anything that causes cells that would normally be connected to become separated. Wound healing is the restoration of that continuity. Several effects may result with the occurrence of a wound: immediate loss of all or part of organ functioning, sympathetic stress response, hemorrhage and blood clotting, bacterial contamination, and death of cells. The most important factor in minimizing these effects and promoting successful care is careful asepsis, which can be accomplished using aseptic techniques when treating a wound.

Description

Wound healing is a biological process that begins with trauma and ends with scar formation. There are two types of tissue injury: full and partial thickness. Partial thickness injury is limited to the epidermis and superficial dermis, with no damage to the dermal blood vessels. Healing occurs by regeneration of other tissues. Full thickness injury involves loss of the dermis extends to deeper tissue layers, and disrupts dermal blood vessels. Wound healing involves the synthesis of several types of tissue and scar formation.

The three phases of repair are lag, proliferative, and remodeling. Directly after injury, hemostasis is achieved with clot formation. The fibrin clot acts like a highway for the migration of cells into the wound site. Within the first four hours of injury, neutrophils begin to appear. These inflammatory cells kill microbes, and prevent the colonization of the wound. Next the monocyte, or macrophage, appears. Functions of these cells include the killing of microbes, the breakdown of wound debris, and the secretion of cytokines that initiate the proliferative phase of repair. Synthetic cells, or fibroblasts, proliferate and synthesize new connective tissue, replacing the transitional fibrin matrix. At this time, an efficient nutrient supply develops through the arborization (terminal branching) of adjacent blood vessels. This ingrowth of new blood vessels is called angiogenesis. This new and very vascular connective tissue is referred to as granulation tissue.

The first phase of repair is called the lag or inflammatory phase. The inflammatory response is dependent on the depth and volume of tissue loss from the injury. Characteristics of the lag phase include acute inflammation and the initial appearance and infiltration of neutrophils. Neutrophils protect the host from microorganisms and infection. If inflammation is delayed or stopped, the wound becomes susceptible to infection and closure is delayed.

The proliferative phase is the second phase of repair and is anabolic in nature. The lag and remodeling phase are both catabolic processes. The proliferative phase generates granulation tissue. In this process, acute inflammation releases cytokines, promoting fibroblast infiltration of the wound site, then creating a high density of cells. Collagen is the major connective tissue protein produced and released by fibroblasts. The connective tissue physically supports the new blood vessels that form and endothelial cells promote ingrowth of new vessels. These new blood vessels are necessary to meet the nutritional needs of the wound healing process. The mark of wound closure is when a new epidermal cover seals the defect. The process of wound healing continues beneath the new surface. This is the remodeling or maturation phase and is the third phase in healing.

The first principle of wound care is the removal of nonviable tissue, including necrotic (dead) tissue, slough, foreign debris, and residual material from dressings. Removal of nonviable tissue is referred to as **debridement**; removal of foreign matter is referred to as cleansing. Chronic wounds are colonized with bacteria, but not necessarily infected. A wound is colonized when a limited number of bacteria are present in the wound and are of no consequence in the healing process. A wound is infected when the bacterial burden overwhelms the immune response of the host and bacteria grow unchecked. Clinical signs of infection are redness of the skin around the wound, purulent (pus-containing) drainage, foul odor, and edema.

The second principle of wound care is to provide a moist environment. This has been shown to promote re-epithelialization and healing. Exposing wounds to air dries the surface and may impede the healing process. Gauze dressings provide a moist environment provided they are kept moist in the wound. These are referred to as wet-to-dry dressings. Generally, a saline-soaked gauze dressing is loosely placed into the wound and covered with a dry gauze dressing to prevent drying and contamination. It also supports autolytic debridement (the body's own capacity to lyse and dissolve necrotic tissue), absorbs exudate, and traps bacteria in the gauze, which are removed when the dressing is changed.

Preventing further injury is the third principle of wound care. This involves elimination or reduction of the condition that allowed the wound to develop. Factors that contribute to the development of chronic wounds include losses in mobility, mental status changes, deficits of sensation, and circulatory deficits. Patients must be properly positioned to eliminate continued pressure to the chronic wound. Pressure reducing devices, such as mattresses, cushions, supportive boots, foam wedges, and fitted shoes can be used to keep pressure off wounds.

Providing nutrition, specifically protein for healing, is the fourth principle of healing. Protein is essential for wound repair and regeneration. Without essential amino acids, angiogenesis, fibroblast proliferation, collagen synthesis, and scar remodeling will not occur. Amino acids also support the immune response. Adequate amounts of carbohydrates and fats are needed to prevent the amino acids from being oxidized for caloric needs. Glucose is also needed to meet the energy requirements of the cells involved in wound repair. Albumin is the most important indicator of malnutrition because it is sacrificed to provide essential amino acids if there is inadequate protein intake.

Diagnosis/Preparation

Effective wound care begins with an assessment of the entire patient. This includes obtaining a complete **health history** and a physical assessment. Assessing the patient assists in identifying causes and contributing factors of the wound. When examining the wound, it is important to document its size, location, appearance, and the surrounding skin. The health care professional also examines the wound for exudate, necrotic tissue, signs of infection, and drainage, and documents how long the patient has had the wound. It is also important to know what treatment, if any, the patient has previously received for the wound.

Actual components of wound care include cleaning, dressing, determining frequency of dressing changes, and reevaluation. Dead tissue and debris can impede healing: the goal of cleaning the wound is its removal. When cleaning the wound, protective goggles should be worn and sterile saline solution should be used. Providone iodine, sodium hypochlorite, and hydrogen peroxide should never be used, as they are toxic to cells.

Gentle pressure should be used to clean the wound if there is no necrotic tissue. This can be accomplished by utilizing a 60 cc catheter tip syringe to apply the cleaning solution. If the wound has necrotic tissue, more pressure may be needed. Whirlpools can also be used for wounds having a thick layer of exudate. At times, chemical or surgical debridement may be needed to remove debris.

Dressings are applied to wounds for the following reasons: to provide the proper environment for healing, to absorb drainage, to immobilize the wound, to protect the wound and new tissue growth from mechanical injury and bacterial contamination, to promote hemostasis, and to provide mental and physical patient comfort. There are several types of dressings and most are designed to maintain a moist wound bed:

• Alginate: Made of non-woven fibers derived from seaweed, alginate forms a gel as it absorbs exudate. It is used for wounds with moderate-to-heavy exudate or drainage, and is changed every 12 hours to three days, depending on when the exudate penetrates the secondary dressing.

• Composite dressings: Combining physically distinct components into a single dressing, composite dressings provide bacterial protection, absorption, and adhesion. The frequency of dressing changes vary.

• Foam: Made from polyurethane, foam comes in various thicknesses having different absorption rates. It is used for wounds with moderate-to-heavy exudate or drainage. Dressing change is every three to seven days.

• Gauze: Available in a number of forms including sponges, pads, ropes, strips, and rolls, gauze can be impregnated with petroleum, antimicrobials, and saline. Frequent changes are needed because gauze has limited moisture retention and properties, and there is little protection from contamination. With removal of a dried dressing, there is a risk of wound damage to the healing skin surrounding the wound. Gauze dressings are changed two to three times a day.

• Hydrocolloid: Made of gelatin or pectin, hydrocolloid is available as a wafer, paste, or powder. While absorbing exudate, the dressing forms a gel. Hydrocolloid dressings are used for light-to-moderate exudate or drainage. This type of dressing is not used for wounds with exposed tendon or bone, third-degree burns, or in the presence of bacterial, fungal, or viral infection or active cellulitis or vasculitis because it is almost totally occlusive. Dressings are changed every three to seven days.

• Hydrogel: Composed primarily of water, hydrogel dressings are used for wounds with minimal exudate. Some are impregnated in gauze or non-woven sponge. Dressings are changed one or two times a day.

• Transparent film: An adhesive, waterproof membrane that keeps contaminants out while allowing oxygen and water vapor to cross through, it is used primarily for wounds with minimal exudate. It is also used as a secondary material to secure non-adhesive gauzes. Dressings are changed every three to five days if the film is used as a primary dressing.

In cases where a wound is particularly severe, large, or if it is a third degree burn, cellular wound healing products may be used to close the wound and speed recovery. In some cases (i.e., a third-degree burn), a skin graft will often be used. Although most surgeons prefer to use skin donated from another person (known as cadaver skin, or human allograft), skin donations are not always available. They must rely on more recent products available, such as cellular wound dressings, for the treatment of burns. For **skin grafting** of full-thickness burn wounds, surgeons use healthy skin from another part of the person's own body (autografting) as a permanent treatment. Surgeons may use cellular wound dressings as a temporary covering when the skin damage is so extensive that there is not enough healthy skin available

to graft initially. This helps prevent infection and fluid loss until autografting can be performed.

The survival rate for burn patients has increased considerably through the process of quickly removing dead tissue and immediately covering the wound. Burns covering half the body were routinely fatal 20 years ago but today, even people with extensive and severe burns have a good chance of survival, according to the American Burn Association.

Cellular wound dressings

In recent years, the technology of burn and wound care using cellular wound dressings and grafts are helping to transform the treatment of burns and chronic wounds by decreasing the risk of infection, protecting against fluid loss, requiring fewer skin grafts, and promoting and speeding the healing process. These dressings provide a cover that keeps fluids from evaporating and prevents blood from oozing out once the dead skin has been removed. Some of these products grow in place and expand natural skin when it heals.

Cellular wound dressings may look and feel like skin, but they do not function totally like skin because they are missing hair follicles, sweat glands, melanocytes, and Langerhans' cells. Some cellular wound dressings have a synthetic top layer structured like an epidermis. It peels away over time, or is replaced with healthy skin through skin grafting. How these products are involved in wound repair is a subject of great scientific interest; it is known that they promote a higher rate of healing than does standard wound care.

People with severe wounds, chronic wounds, burns, and ulcers can benefit from cellular wound dressings. Several artificial skin products are available for non-healing wounds or burns such as: Apligraft® (Norvartis), Demagraft®, Biobrane®, Transcyte® (Advance Tissue Science), Integra® Dermal Regeneration Template® (from Integra Life Sciences Technology), and OrCel®.

• Apligraf is a two-layer wound dressing that contains live human skin cells combined with cow collagen. It delivers live cells from a different donor (circumcised infant foreskin). Thousands of pieces of Apligraf are produced in the laboratory from one small patch of cells from a single donor.

• Dermagraft is made from human cells placed on a dissolvable mesh material. The mesh material is gradually absorbed and the human cells grow and replace the damaged skin after being placed on the wound or ulcer.

• Biobrane is used as a temporary dressing for a variety of wounds, including ulcers, lacerations, and full-thickness burns. It may also be used on wounds that develop on

KEY TERMS

Allograft—Skin donated from another person to treat burns.

Asepsis—Freedom from infection or infectious material; also, the absence of viable pathogenic organisms. Asepsis can be accomplished using aseptic techniques, which are the use of surgical practices that restrict microorganisms in the environment and prevent contamination of the surgical wound; they include sterilization of instruments and the wearing of sterile caps, gloves, and masks.

Anabolic—Metabolic processes characterized by the conversion of simple substances into more complex compounds.

Cadaver skin—Skin donated from another person to treat burns.

Catabolic—Metabolic processes characterized by the release of energy through the conversion of complex compounds into simple substances.

Cytokine—A protein that regulates the duration and intensity of the body's immune response.

Dermis—The thick layer of skin below the epidermis.

Epidermis—The outermost layer of the skin.

Exudate—Fluid, cells, or other substances that are slowly discharged by tissue, especially due to injury or inflammation.

Fibrin—The fibrous protein of blood clots.

Fibroblast—An undifferentiated connective tissue cell that is capable of forming collagen fibers.

Hemostasis—Slowing down or stopping bleeding.

Langerhans' cells—Cells in the epidermis that help protect the body against infection.

Melanocytes—Cells within the epidermis that give skin its color

Neutrophil—A type of white blood cell.

Scar—Scar tissue is the fibrous tissue that replaces normal tissue destroyed by injury or disease.

areas from which healthy skin is transplanted to cover damaged skin. It consists of an ultrathin silicone film and nylon fabric. As the wound heals, or until autografting becomes possible, the Biobrane is trimmed away.

• TransCyte is used as a temporary covering over full thickness and some partial thickness burns until autografting is possible, as well as a temporary covering for some burn wounds that heal without autografting. It consists of human cells from circumcised infant foreskin, and grown on nylon mesh, combined with a synthetic epidermal layer. TransCyte starts with living cells, but these cells die when it is shipped in a frozen state to burn treatment facilities. The product is then thawed and stretched over a burn site. In one to two weeks, the TransCyte starts peeling off, and the surgeon trims it away as it peels.

• Integra Dermal Regeneration Template is used to treat full thickness and some partial thickness burns. Integra consists of two layers; the bottom layer, made of shark cartilage and collagen from cow tendons, acts as a matrix onto which a person's own cells migrate over two to three weeks. A new dermis is created as the cells gradually absorb the cartilage and collagen. The top layer is a protective silicone sheet that is peeled off after several weeks, while the bottom layer is a permanent cover. A very thin layer of the person's own skin is then grafted onto the neo-dermis.

• OrCel is also made from circumcised infant foreskin, grown on a cow collagen matrix, and used to treat donor sites in burn patients. It is also used to help treat epidermolysis bullosa, a rare skin condition in children.

To ensure the safety and quality of products such as cellular wound dressings, the Food and Drug Administration (FDA) has initiated a new regulatory system.

Risks

• Hematoma: dressings should be inspected for hemorrhage at intervals during the first 24 hours after surgery. A large amount of bleeding is to be reported to a health care professional immediately. Concealed bleeding sometimes occurs in the wound, beneath the skin. If the clot formed is small, it will be absorbed by the body, but if large, the wound bulges and the clot must be removed for healing to continue.

• Infection: The second most frequent nosocomial (hospital-acquired) infection in hospitals is surgical wound infections with *Staphylococcus aureus*, *Escherichia coli*, and *Pseudomonas aeruginosa*. Prevention is accomplished with meticulous wound management. Cellulitis is a bacterial infection that spreads into tissue planes; systemic **antibiotics** are usually prescribed to treat it. If the infection is in an arm or leg, elevation of

GALE ENCYCLOPEDIA OF SURGERY **1569**

the limb reduces dependent edema and heat application promotes blood circulation. Abscess is a bacterial infection that is localized and characterized by pus. Treatment consists of surgical drainage or excision with the concurrent administration of antibiotics.

• Dehiscence (disruption of the surgical wound) and evisceration (protrusion of wound contents): This condition results from sutures giving way, infection, distention, or cough. Dehiscence results in pain; the surgeon is called immediately. Prophylactically, an abdominal binder may be utilized.

• Keloid: refers to excessive growth of scar tissue. Careful wound closure, hemostasis, and pressure support are used to ward off this complication.

Normal results

The goals of wound care include reducing risks that inhibit wound healing, enhancing the healing process, and lowering the incidence of wound infections.

Resources

BOOKS

Dipietro, Luisa A. and Aime L. Burns, eds. *Wound Healing: Methods and Protocols (Methods in Molecular Medicine Ser).* Totowa, NJ: Humana Press, 2003.

Herndon, David, ed. *Total Burn Care,* 2nd ed. London: W. B. Saunders Co., 2001.

Hess, Cathy Thomas. *Clinical Guide to Wound Care,* 4th ed. Philadelphia, PA: Lippincott Williams & Wilkins, 2002.

Hess, Cathy Thomas and Richard Salcido. *Wound Care,* 3rd ed. Springhouse, PA: Springhouse Pub Co., 2000.

PERIODICALS

Collins, Nancy. "Obesity and Wound Healing." *Advances in Wound Care* 16, no 1. (January/February 2003): 45.

Collins, Nancy. "Vegetarian Diets and Wound Healing." *Advances in Wound Care* 16, no. 2 (March/April 2003): 65.

McGuckin, Maryanne, Robert Goldman, Laura Bolton, and Richard Salcido. "The Clinical Relevance of Microbiology in Acute and Chronic Wounds." *Advances in Wound Care* 16, no 1. (January/February 2003): 12.

Trent, Jennifer T., and Robert S. Kirsner. "Wounds and Malignancy." *Advances in Wound Care* 16, no 1. (January/February 2003): 31.

ORGANIZATIONS

American Burn Association. 625 N. Michigan Ave., Suite 1530, Chicago, IL 60611. (800) 548-2876. Fax: (312) 642.9130. E-mail: info@ameriburn.org. <http://www.ameriburn.org>.

American Diabetes Association. 1701 North Beauregard Street, Alexandria, VA 22311. (800) 342-2383. E-Mail: AskADA @diabetes.org. <http://www.diabetes.org>.

American Professional Wound Care Association (APWCA). Suite #A1-853 Second Street Pike, Richboro, PA 18954.

(215) 364-4100. Fax: (215) 364-1146. E-mail: wounds @erols.com. < http://www.apwca.org>.

National Institutes of Health. 9000 Rockville Pike, Bethesda, MD 20892. (301) 496-4000. Email: NIHInfo@OD.NIH .GOV. <http://www.nih.gov>.

OTHER

Lippincott Williams & Wilkins. *Advances in Skin & Wound Care* 2003. [cited April 9, 2003]. <http://www.aswcjournal. com/>.

René A. Jackson, RN
Crystal H. Kaczkowski, M. Sc.

Wound culture

Definition

A wound culture is a diagnostic laboratory test in which microorganisms—such as bacteria or fungi from an infected wound, are grown in the laboratory on nutrient-enriched substance called media—then identified. Wound cultures always include aerobic (with oxygen) culture, but direct smear evaluation by Gram stain and anaerobic (without oxygen) culture are not performed on every wound. These tests are performed when indicated or requested by the physician.

Purpose

The purpose of a wound culture is to isolate and identify bacteria or fungi causing an infection of the wound. Only then can **antibiotics** that will be effective in destroying the organism can be identified.

Preparation

A biopsy sample is usually preferred by clinicians, but this is a moderately invasive procedure and may not always be feasible. The health-care professional prepares the patient by cleansing the affected area with a sterile solution, such as saline. **Antiseptics** such as ethyl alcohol are not recommended, because they kill bacteria and cause the culture results to be negative. The patient is given a local anesthetic and the tissue is removed by the practitioner, who uses a cutting sheath. Afterwards, pressure is applied to the wound to control bleeding.

Needle aspiration is less invasive and is a good technique to use in wounds where there is little loss of skin, such as in the case of puncture wounds. The skin around the wound is cleaned with an antiseptic to kill bacteria on the skin's surface, and a small needle is inserted. To obtain a sample of the fluid to be biopsied, the clinician pulls back on the plunger, then changes the angle of the needle two or three times to remove fluid from different areas of the wound. This procedure may be painful for the patient, so many initial cultures are done with the swab technique. After completion of any of the three procedures, the wound should be cleaned thoroughly and bandaged.

Description

Wounds are injuries to body tissues caused by physical trauma or disease processes that may include surgery, diabetes, burns, punctures, gunshots, lacerations, bites, bed sores, and broken bones. Types of wounds may include:

• Abraded or abrasion: Caused by scraping, such as falling on concrete.

• Contused or contusion: A bruise or bleeding into the tissue.

• Incised or incision: A wound formed by a clean cut, as by a sharp instrument like a knife.

• Lacerated or laceration: A wound caused by heavy pressure, causing tearing of the skin or other tissues.

• Nonpenetrating: An injury caused without disruption of the surface of the body. These wounds are usually in the thorax or abdomen and can also be termed blunt trauma wounds.

• Open: A wound in which tissues are exposed to the air.

• Penetrating: Disruption of the body surface and extension into the underlying tissue.

• Perforating: A wound with an exit and an entry, such as a gunshot wound.

• Puncture: A wound formed when something goes through the skin and into the body tissues. This wound has a very small opening, but can be very deep.

The chance of a wound becoming infected depends on the nature, size, and depth of the wound; its proximity to and involvement of nonsterile areas, such as the skin and gastrointestinal (GI) tract; the opportunity for organisms from the environment to enter the wound; and the immunologic, nutritional, and general health status of the person. In general, acute (sudden onset) wounds are more prone to infection than chronic (long-lasting) wounds. Wounds with a large loss of body surface, such as abrasions, are also easily infected. Puncture wounds can permit the growth of microorganisms because there is a break in the skin with minimal bleeding; they are also difficult to clean. Deep wounds, closed off from oxygen, are an ideal breeding environment for anaerobic infections. Foul-smelling odors, gas, or dead tissue at the infection site are signs of an infection caused by anaerobic bacte-

ria. Surgical wounds can also cause infection by introducing bacteria from one body compartment into another.

Diagnosing infection in a wound may be difficult. One of the chief signs the clinician looks for is slow healing. Within hours of injury, most wounds display a release of fluid, called exudate. This fluid contains compounds that aid in healing, and is normal. It should not be present 48–72 hours after injury. Exudate indicative of infection may be thicker than the initial exudate and may also be purulent (containing pus) and foul smelling. Clinicians will look at color, consistency, and the amount of exudate to monitor early infection. In addition, infected wounds may display skin discoloration, swelling, warmth to touch and an increase in pain.

Wound infection prevents healing, and the bacteria or yeast can spread from wounds to other body parts, including the blood. Infection in the blood is termed septicemia and can be fatal. Symptoms of a systemic infection include a fever and rise in white blood cells (WBCs), along with confusion and mental status changes in the elderly. It is important to treat the infected wound early with a regimen of antibiotics to prevent further complications.

Wound infections often contain multiple organisms, including both aerobic and anaerobic gram-positive cocci and gram-negative bacilli and yeast. The most common pathogens isolated from wounds are *Streptococcus* group A, *Staphylococcus aureus*, *Escherichia coli*, *Proteus*, *Klebsiella*, *Pseudomonas*, *Enterobacter*, Enterococci, *Bacteroides*, *Clostridium*, *Candida*, *Peptostreptococcus*, *Fusobacterium*, and *Aeromonas*.

The tissue used for the tests is obtained by three different methods: tissue biopsy, needle aspiration, or the swab technique. The biopsy method involves the removal of tissue from the wound using a cutting sheath. The swab technique is most commonly used, but contains the least amount of specimen.

Wound specimens are cultured on both nonselective enriched and selective media. Cultures are examined each day for growth and any colonies are Gram stained and subcultured (i.e., transferred) to appropriate media. The subcultured isolates are tested via appropriate biochemical identification panels to identify the species present. Organisms are also tested for antibiotic susceptibility. The selection of antibiotics for testing depends on the organism isolated.

Normal results

The initial Gram-stain result is available the same day, or in less than an hour, if requested by the doctor. An early report, known as a preliminary report, is usually available after one day. After that, preliminary reports

KEY TERMS

Aerobe—Bacteria that require oxygen to live.

Agar—A gelatinous material extracted from red algae that is not digested by bacteria. It is used as a support for growth in plates.

Anaerobe—Bacteria that live only where there is no oxygen.

Antibiotic—A medicine that can be used topically or taken orally, intramuscularly, or intravenously to limit the growth of bacteria.

Antimicrobial—A compound that prevents the growth of microbes which may include bacteria, fungi, and viruses.

Antimycotic—A medicine that can be used to kill yeast and fungus.

Antiseptic—A compound that kills all bacteria, also known as a bactericide.

Broth—A growth mixture for bacteria. Different compounds, such as sugars or amino acids, may be added to increase the growth of certain organisms. Also known as media.

Exudate—Any fluid that has been released by tissue or its capillaries due to injury or inflammation.

Normal flora—The mixture of bacteria normally found at specific body sites.

Purulent—Containing, consisting of or forming pus.

Pus—A fluid that is the product of inflammation and infection containing white blood cells and debris of dead cells and tissue.

will be posted whenever an organism is identified. Cultures showing no growth are signed out after two to three days unless a slow-growing mycobacterium or fungus is found. These organisms take several weeks to grow and are held for four to six weeks. The final report includes complete identification, an estimate of the quantity of the microorganisms, and a list of the antibiotics to which each organism is sensitive and resistant.

Risks

The physician may choose to start the person on an antibiotic before the specimen is collected for culture. This may alter results, since antibiotics in the person's system may prevent microorganisms present in the wound from growing in culture. In some cases, the patient may begin antibiotic treatment after the specimen is collected. The antibiotic chosen may or may not be appropriate for one or more organisms recovered by culture.

Clinicians must be very careful when finishing a wound culture collection to make ensure that the wound has been cleaned thoroughly and is bandaged properly. It is important to watch for bleeding and further infection from the procedure. In addition, patients may be in pain from the manipulation, so giving pain-killing drugs, such as **acetaminophen**, may be advised.

Resources

BOOKS

Henry, John B. *Clinical Diagnosis and Management by Laboratory Methods*, 20th ed. Philadelphia: W. B. Saunders Company, 2001

ORGANIZATIONS

The Wound Healing Society. 13355 Tenth Ave., Suite 108, Minneapolis, MN 55441-5554. [cited April 4, 2003] <http://www.woundheal.org/>.

OTHER

National Institutes of Health. [cited April 5, 2003] <http://www.nlm.nih.gov/medlineplus/encyclopedia.html>.

Jane E. Phillips, Ph.D.
Mark A. Best, M.D.

Wrist replacement

Definition

Wrist replacement surgery is performed to replace a wrist injured or damaged beyond repair. An artificial wrist joint replacement is implanted.

Purpose

Traumatic injuries or severe degenerative diseases affecting the wrist (such as osteoarthritis and rheumatoid arthritis with bony destruction) may require replacement of the painful wrist joint with an artificial wrist joint. The purpose of wrist replacement surgery is to restore wrist motion for activities of daily living and non-contact sports. A wrist replacement recovers lost strength by restoring length to the muscles and tendons of the fingers and wrist, maintains a useful arc of motion and provides the stability required for an active life.

Description

Surgery to replace a wrist starts with an incision through the skin on the back of the wrist. The surgeon then moves the tendons extending over the back of the wrist out of the way to access the joint capsule on the back of the wrist joint, which is then opened to expose the wrist joint area. A portion of the carpal bones and the end of the radius and ulna are then removed from the wrist to allow room for the new artificial wrist joint. The bones of the hand and the radius bone of the forearm are prepared with the use of special instruments to form holes in the bones; the stems of the artificial joint components can then fit in. Next, the components are inserted into the holes. After obtaining a proper fit, the surgeon verifies the range of motion of the joint to ensure that it moves correctly. Finally, the surgeon cements the two sides of the joint and replaces the tendons back into their proper position before closing the wound.

A total wrist replacement implant consists of the following components:

- An ellipsoid head that simulates the curvature of the natural wrist joint and allows for a functional range of motion. This ensures that the patient may flex and extend the wrist and move it side-to-side.

- An offset radial stem that anchors the implant in the forearm. The special shape of this component is designed to assist the function of the tendons used to extend the wrist and to ensure the stability of the implant.

- An elongated radial tray surface with a molded bearing usually made of polyethylene. This component is required to distribute forces over the entire surface of the artificial joint.

- A fixation stem that is secured to the patient's bone to add stability and eliminate rotation of the artificial joint within the bone.

- A curved metacarpal stem that secures the artificial wrist within the hand.

Diagnosis/Preparation

The orthopedic surgeon who will perform the surgery will usually require a complete **physical examination** of the patient by the primary care physician to ensure that the patient will be in the best possible condition to undergo the surgery. The patient may also need to see the physical therapist responsible for managing rehabilitation after wrist replacement. The therapist prepares the patient before surgery to ensure readiness for rehabilitation post-surgery. The purpose of the preoperative examination is also for the physician to pre-record a baseline of information that will include measurements of the patient's current pain levels, functional wrist capacity, and the range of motion and strength of each hand.

Before surgery, patients are advised to take all of their normal medications, with the exception of blood thinners such as **aspirin**, ibuprofen, and other anti-inflammatory drugs that may cause greater blood loss during surgery. Patients may eat as they please the night before surgery, including solid food, until midnight. After midnight, patients should not eat or drink anything unless told otherwise by their doctor.

Aftercare

Following surgery, the patient's wrist, hand, and lower arm are placed into a bulky bandage and a splint. A small plastic tube may be inserted to drain any blood that gathers under the incision to prevent excessive swelling (hematoma). The tube is usually removed within 24 hours. Sutures may be removed 10–14 days after surgery.

Risks

Some of the most common risks associated with wrist replacement surgery are:

• Infection. Infection can be a very serious complication following wrist replacement surgery. Infection following wrist replacement occurs in approximately 1–2% of cases. Some infections may appear before the patient leaves the hospital, while others may not become apparent for months, or even years, after surgery.

• Loosening. There is also a risk that the artificial joints may eventually fail, due to a loosening process where the metal or cement meets the bone. There have been great advances in extending how long an artificial joint will last, but most will eventually loosen and require revision surgery. The risk of loosening is much greater in younger, more active people. A loose artificial wrist is a problem because of the resulting pain. Once the pain becomes unbearable, another operation is usually required to either revise the wrist replacement or perform a wrist fusion.

• Nerve injury. All of the nerves and blood vessels that go to the hand travel across the wrist joint. Wrist replacement surgery is performed very close to these structures, introducing a risk of injury either to the nerves or the blood vessels.

Normal results

Wrist replacement surgery often succeeds at restoring wrist function. On average, a wrist replacement is expected to last for 10–15 years.

Alternatives

An alternative to wrist replacement is wrist fusion (arthrodesis). Wrist fusion surgery eliminates pain by allowing the bones that make up the joint to grow together, or fuse, into one solid bone. The surgery reduces pain, but also reduces the patient's ability to move the wrist. Wrist fusions were very common before the invention of artificial joints, and they are still performed often.

See also Arthroplasty.

Resources

BOOKS

Ferlic, D. C. *A Colour Atlas of Joint Replacement of the Wrist and Hand (Single Surgical Procedures, 41).* St. Louis: Year Book Medical Pub, 1986.

Gilula, L. A. *Imaging of the Wrist and Hand.* Philadelphia: W B Saunders, 1996.

Weinzweig, J., ed. *Hand & Wrist Surgery Secrets.* New York: Hanley & Belfus, 2000.

PERIODICALS

Courtman, N. H., D. H., Sochart. I. A., Trail. and J. K. Stanley. "Biaxial Wrist Replacement. Initial Results in the Rheumatoid Patient." *The Journal of Hand Surgery: Jour-*

KEY TERMS

Arthritis—An inflammatory condition that affects joints

Carpal bones—Eight wrist bones arranged in two rows that articulate proximally with the radius and indirectly with the ulna, and distally with the five metacarpal bones.

Metacarpal bones—Five cylindrical bones extending from the wrist to the fingers.

Osteoarthritis—Non-inflammatory degenerative joint disease occurring mostly in older persons accompanied by pain and stiffness, especially after prolonged activity.

Radius—One of the two forearm bones. The largest portion of the radius is at the wrist joint where it articulates with the carpal bones of the hand. Above, the radius articulates with the humerus at the elbow joint.

Rheumatoid arthritis—Chronic inflammatory disease in which there is destruction of joints.

Tendon—A fibrous, strong, connective tissue that connects muscle to bone.

Ulna—One of the two bones of the forearm. The largest section articulates with the humerus at the elbow joint and the smallest portion of the ulna articulates with the carpal bones in the wrist.

---

nal of the British Society for Surgery of the Hand 24 (February 1999): 32-34.

Cuenod, P., E. Charriere, and M. Y. Papaloizos. "A mechanical comparison of bone-ligament-bone autografts from the wrist for replacement of the scapholunate ligament." *Journal of Hand Surgery (American)* 27 (November 2002): 985-990.

Takwale, V. J., D., Nuttall. I. A., Trail. and J. K. Stanley. "Biaxial total wrist replacement in patients with rheumatoid arthritis. Clinical review, survivorship and radiological analysis." *Journal of Bone and Joint Surgery (British)* 84 (July 2002): 692-699.

Meuli, H. C. "Recent literature on total wrist replacement not carefully reviewed." *The Journal of Hand Surgery: Journal of the British Society for Surgery of the Hand* 24 (October 1999): 635.

ORGANIZATIONS

The American Academy of Orthopaedic Surgeons (AAOS). 6300 North River Road, Rosemont, Illinois 60018-4262. (847) 823-7186; (800) 346-AAOS. <www.aaos.org>.

OTHER

"Wrist Replacement." *University of Maryland Information Page.* <www.wristreplacement.com/>.

"Wrist Joint Replacement (Arthroplasty)." *AAOS.* <orthoinfo. aaos.org/fact/thr_report.cfm?Thread_ID=347&topcategory =Hand>.

Monique Laberge, Ph.D.

GLOSSARY

A

ABDOMEN The portion of the body that lies between the thorax and the pelvis. It contains a cavity with many organs.

ABDOMINAL AORTIC ANEURYSM Aneurysm that involves the descending aorta from the diaphragm to the split at the iliac arteries.

ABDOMINAL DISTENSION Swelling of the abdominal cavity that creates painful pressure on the internal organs.

ABDOMINAL HERNIA A defect in the abdominal wall through which the abdominal organs protrude.

ABLATION To remove or destroy tissue or a body part, such as by burning or cutting.

ABLATION THERAPY A procedure used to treat arrhythmias, especially atrial fibrillation. During the procedure, a catheter (small, flexible tube) is inserted in a vein and threaded to the heart. High-frequency electrical energy is delivered through the catheter to disconnect the pathway causing the abnormal heart rhythm in the heart.

ABO ANTIGEN Protein molecules located on the surfaces of red blood cells that determine a person's blood type: A, B, or O.

ABO BLOOD GROUPS A system in which human blood is classified by whether the red blood cells contain A or B antigens. Type A blood has the A antigen; type B has the B antigen, AB has both, and O has neither.

ABO BLOOD TYPE Blood type based on the presence or absence of the A and B antigens on the red blood cells.

ABSCESS A localized collection of pus in the skin or other body tissue caused by infection.

ACCESS SITE The vein tapped for vascular access in hemodialysis treatments. For patients with temporary treatment needs, access to the bloodstream is gained by inserting a catheter into the subclavian vein near the patient's collarbone. Patients in long-term dialysis require stronger, more durable access sites, called fistulas or grafts, that are surgically created.

ACCESSORY ORGAN A lump of tissue adjacent to an organ that is similar to it, but which serves no important purpose, if it is functional at all. While not necessarily harmful, such organs can cause problems if they grow too large or become cancerous. In any case, their presence points to an underlying abnormality in the parent organ.

ACETABULAR DYSPLASIA A type of arthritis resulting in a shallow hip socket.

ACETABULUM The large cup-shaped cavity at the junction of pelvis and femur (thigh bone).

ACETAMINOPHEN A drug used for pain relief as well as to decrease fever. A common trade name for the drug is Tylenol.

ACETIC ACID A colorless liquid present in vinegar that is used as an astringent in medicine.

ACHALASIA An esophageal disease of unknown cause, in which the lower sphincter or muscle is unable to relax normally, resulting in obstruction, either partial or complete.

ACIDOSIS A disturbance of the balance of acid to base in the body causing an accumulation of acid or loss of alkali (base). Blood plasma normally has a pH of 7.35-7.45. Alkaline blood has a pH value greater than pH 7.45. When the blood pH value is less than 7.35, the patient is in acidosis. There are two types of acidosis: metabolic and respiratory.

ACQUIRED IMMUNODEFICIENCY SYNDROME (AIDS) An infectious disease caused by the human immunodeficiency virus (HIV). A person infected with HIV gradually loses immune function, becoming less able to resist other infections and certain cancers.

ACROMIOCLAVICULAR DISLOCATION Disruption of the normal articulation between the acromion and the collarbone. The acromioclavicular joint (AC joint) is normally stabilized by several ligaments that can be torn in the process of dislocating the AC joint.

ACROMIOCLAVICULAR (AC) JOINT The shoulder joint. Articulation and ligaments between the collarbone and the acromion of the shoulder blade.

ACROMION The triangular projection of the spine of the shoulder blade that forms the point of the shoulder and articulates with the collarbone.

ACTINIC KERATOSIS A crusty, scaly pre-cancerous skin lesion caused by damage from the sun.

ACTIVATED PARTIAL THROMBOPLASTIN TIME Partial thromboplastin time test that uses activators to shorten the clotting time, making it more useful for heparin monitoring.

ACTIVITIES OF DAILY LIVING (ADLS) The activities performed during the course of a normal day such as eating, bathing, dressing, toileting, etc.

ACUPUNCTURE Based on the same traditional Chinese medical foundation as acupressure, acupuncture uses sterile needles inserted at specific points to treat certain conditions or relieve pain.

ACUTE Refers to a disease or symptom that has a sudden onset and lasts a relatively short period of time.

ACUTE HEMOLYTIC TRANSFUSION REACTION (AHTR) A severe transfusion reaction with abrupt onset, most often caused by ABO incompatibility. Symptoms include difficulty breathing, fever and chills, pain, and sometimes shock.

ACUTE OTITIS MEDIA Inflammation of the middle ear with signs of infection lasting less than three months.

ACUTE PAIN Pain in response to injury or another stimulus that resolves when the injury heals or the stimulus is removed.

ADDICTION The state of being both physically and psychologically dependent on a substance.

ADENOCARCINOMA A malignant tumor that arises within the tissues of a gland and retains its glandular structure.

ADENOIDS Common name for the pharyngeal tonsils, which are lymph masses in the wall of the air passageway (pharynx) just behind the nose.

ADENOMA A type of noncancerous (benign) tumor that often involves the overgrowth of certain cells found in glands. These tumors can secrete hormones or cause changes in hormone production in nearby glands.

ADHESION An abnormal union or attachment of two areas of tissue.

ADHESIONS Web-like scar tissue that may develop as a result of endometriosis and bind organs to one another.

ADJUVANT THERAPY A treatment that is intended to aid primary treatment.

ADRENAL GLANDS A pair of endocrine glands (glands that secrete hormones directly into the bloodstream) that are located on top of the kidneys. The outer tissue of the glands (cortex) produces several steroid hormones, while the inner tissue (medulla) produces the hormones epinephrine (adrenaline) and norepinephrine.

ADRENERGIC Refers to neurons (nerve cells) that use catecholamines as neurotransmitters at a synapse.

ADSORPTION The binding of a chemical (e.g., drug or poison) to a solid material such as activated charcoal or clay.

ADVANCE DIRECTIVE A general term for two types of documents, living wills and medical powers of attorney, that allow people to give instructions about health care in the event that they cannot speak for themselves.

AEROBIC BACTERIA Bacteria that require oxygen to live and grow.

AEROBIC EXERCISE Exercise training that is geared to provide a sufficient cardiovascular overload to stimulate increases in cardiac output.

AFFERENT Refers to peripheral nerves that transmit signals to the spinal cord and the brain. These nerves carry out sensory function.

AGAR A gel made from red algae that is used to culture certain disease agents in the laboratory.

AIRWAY The passageway through the mouth, nose, and throat that allows air to enter and leave the lungs; the term can also refer to a tube or other artificial device used to create an air passageway into and out of the lungs when the patient is under general anesthesia or unable to breathe properly.

ALGORITHM A procedure or formula for solving a problem. It is often used to refer to a sequence of steps used to program a computer to solve a specific problem.

ALKALOID A type of chemical commonly found in plants and often having medicinal properties.

ALKALOSIS A condition of the blood and other body fluids in which bicarbonate levels are higher than normal.

ALLELE Types of genes that occupy the same site on a chromosome.

ALLOGENEIC Refers to bone marrow transplants between two different, genetically dissimilar people.

ALLOGRAFT Tissue that is taken from one person's body for transplantation to another person.

ALLOPLAST An implant made of an inert foreign material such as silicone or hydroxyapatite.

ALOPECIA The loss of hair, or baldness.

ALPHA FETOPROTEIN (AFP) A substance produced by a fetus' liver that can be found in the amniotic fluid and in the mother's blood. Abnormally high levels of this substance suggests there may be defects in the fetal neural tube, a structure that will include the brain and spinal cord when completely developed. AFP may also be found at elevated levels in the blood of adults with liver, testicular, and ovarian cancer.

ALTITUDE SICKNESS A set of symptoms that people who normally live at low altitudes may have when they travel to high altitudes. The symptoms include nosebleed, nausea, and shortness of breath.

ALZHEIMER'S DISEASE A progressive, neurodegenerative disease characterized by loss of function and death of nerve cells in several areas of the brain, leading to loss of mental functions such as memory and learning.

AMBULATE To move from place to place.

AMBULATORY CARE An outpatient facility; designed for patients who don't require inpatient hospital treatment or care.

AMBULATORY MONITORING Electrocardiogram (ECG) recording over a prolonged period during which the patient can move around.

AMBULATORY SURGERY Surgery done on an outpatient basis; the patient goes home the same day.

AMBULATORY SURGERY CENTER An outpatient facility with at least two operating rooms, either connected or not connected to a hospital.

AMINE A chemical compound that contains NH_3 as part of its structure.

AMNIOCENTESIS A procedure performed at 16-18 weeks of pregnancy in which a needle is inserted through a woman's abdomen into her uterus to draw out a small sample of the amniotic fluid from around the baby for analysis. Either the fluid itself or cells from the fluid can be used for a variety of tests to obtain information about genetic disorders and other medical conditions in the fetus.

AMNIOTIC MEMBRANE The thin tissue that creates the walls of the amniotic sac.

ANAEROBIC An organism that grows and thrives in an oxygen-free environment.

ANALGESICS A class of pain-relieving medicines, including aspirin and Tylenol.

ANALYTE A material or chemical substance subjected to analysis.

ANAPHYLACTIC SHOCK A potentially fatal allergic reaction to a substance that causes a severe drop in blood pressure, swelling of the respiratory tract with associated breathing problems, rash, and possible convulsions.

ANASTOMOSIS The surgical union of parts and especially hollow tubular parts.

ANDROGENS Hormones (specifically testosterone) responsible for male sex characteristics.

ANEMIA A condition in which there is an abnormally low number of red blood cells in the bloodstream. It may be due to loss of blood, an increase in red blood cell destruction, or a decrease in red blood cell production. Major symptoms are paleness, shortness of breath, unusually fast or strong heart beats, and tiredness.

ANENCEPHALY A genetic defect resulting in the partial to complete absence of the brain and malformation of the brainstem.

ANESTHESIA Treatment with medicine that causes a loss of feeling, especially pain. Local anesthesia numbs only part of the body; general anesthesia causes loss of consciousness.

ANESTHESIOLOGIST A medical specialist who has special training and expertise in the delivery of anesthetics.

ANESTHESIOLOGY The branch of medicine that specializes in the study of anesthetic agents, their effects on patients, and their proper use and administration.

ANESTHESIST A nurse trained in anesthesiology who, working as an assistant to a anesthesiologist, administers the anesthesia in surgery and monitors the patient after surgery.

ANESTHETIC A drug that causes a loss of feeling, especially of pain. Some anesthetics also cause a loss of consciousness.

ANEURYSM A weakened area in the wall of a blood vessel which causes an outpouching or bulge. Aneurysms may be fatal if these weak areas burst, resulting in uncontrollable bleeding.

ANGINA Angina pectoris, or chest pain, caused by an insufficient supply of oxygen and decreased blood flow to the heart muscle. Angina is frequently the first sign of coronary artery disease.

ANGIOEDEMA Patches of circumscribed swelling involving the skin and its subcutaneous layers, the mucous membranes, and sometimes the organs frequently caused by an allergic reaction to drugs or food. Also called angioneurotic edema, giant urticaria, Quincke's disease, or Quincke's edema.

ANGIOGRAM An x ray of a blood vessel after a special radiopaque dye has been injected into it.

ANGIOGRAPHY Radiographic examination of blood vessels after injection with a radiopaque contrast substance or dye.

ANGIOMATOUS MALFORMATIONS Tumors in blood vessels.

ANGIOPLASTY A medical procedure in which a catheter, or thin tube, is threaded through blood vessels. The catheter is used to place a balloon or stent (a small metal rod) at a narrowed or blocked area and expand it mechanically.

ANGIOTENSIN-CONVERTING ENZYME (ACE) IN-HIBITOR A drug that relaxes blood vessel walls and lowers blood pressure.

ANGLE (EYE) The open point in the anterior chamber of the eye at which the iris meets the cornea.

ANGLE CLOSURE A blockage of the angle of the eye, causing an increase in pressure in the eye and possible glaucoma.

ANION An ion with a negative charge.

ANKLE-BRACHIAL INDEX (ABI) TEST A means of checking the blood pressure in the arms and ankles using a regular blood pressure cuff and a special ultrasound stethoscope (Doppler). The pressure in the ankle is compared to the pressure in the arm.

ANKYLOSING SPONDYLITIS A type of arthritis that causes gradual loss of flexibility in the spinal column. It occurs most commonly in males between 16 and 35.

ANNULUS A ring-shaped structure.

ANOMALY A marked deviation from normal structure or function, particularly as the result of congenital defects.

ANOREXIA NERVOSA An eating disorder marked by an unrealistic fear of weight gain, self-starvation, and distortion of body image. It most commonly occurs in adolescent females.

ANTIARRHYTHMIC Medication used to treat abnormal heart rhythms.

ANTIBIOTICS Drugs that are designed to kill or inhibit the growth of the bacteria that cause infections.

ANTIBODY A special protein made by the body's immune system as a defense against foreign material (bacteria, viruses, etc.) that enters the body. It is uniquely designed to attack and neutralize the specific antigen that triggered the immune response.

ANTICHOLINERGIC DRUGS Drugs that block the action of the neurotransmitter acetylcholine. They are used to lessen muscle spasms in the intestines, lungs, bladder, and eye muscles.

ANTICOAGULANT DRUGS Drug used to prevent clot formation or to prevent a clot that has formed from enlarging. Anticoagulant drugs inhibit clot formation by blocking the action of clotting factors or platelets. They fall into three groups: inhibitors of clotting factor synthesis, inhibitors of thrombin, and antiplatelet drugs.

ANTIDIURETIC DRUGS Medications that suppress the production of urine.

ANTIEMETIC DRUGS Medications that help control nausea; also called an antinausea drug.

ANTIGEN A substance (usually a protein) identified as foreign by the body's immune system, triggering the release of antibodies as part of the body's immune response.

ANTIHISTAMINE DRUGS A drug used to treat allergic conditions that blocks the effects of histamine, a substance in the body that causes itching, vascular changes, and mucus secretion when released by cells.

ANTIMICROBIAL A substance that acts to inhibit the growth of harmful microorganisms, or acts to destroy them.

ANTIMYCOTIC DRUGS Medication that can be used to kill yeast and fungus.

ANTIPLATELET DRUGS Drugs that inhibit platelets from aggregating to form a plug. They are used to prevent clotting and alter the natural course of atherosclerosis.

ANTISEPTIC A substance that inhibits the growth and reproduction of microorganisms.

ANTITHROMBIN Any substance that counters the effect of thrombin, an enzyme that converts fibrinogen into fibrin, leading to blood coagulation.

ANTRECTOMY A surgical procedure for ulcer disease in which the antrum, a portion of the stomach, is removed.

ANTROSTOMY The drainage of a sinus cavity.

ANTRUM The cavity of a sinus.

ANUS The opening at the end of the intestine through which solid waste (stool) passes as it leaves the body.

ANXIETY Worry or tension in response to real or imagined stress, danger, or dreaded situations. Physical reactions, such as fast pulse, sweating, trembling, fatigue, and weakness, may accompany anxiety.

ANXIOLYTICS A medication that helps to relieve anxiety.

AORTA The main artery located above the heart that pumps oxygenated blood out into the body. The aorta is the largest artery in the body.

AORTIC VALVE The valve between the heart's left ventricle and ascending aorta that prevents regurgitation of blood back into the left ventricle.

APHAKIC Having no lens in the eye.

APHERESIS Extraction of a specific component from donated blood, with the remainder returned to the donor.

APICOECTOMY Also called root canal. In this dental procedure, the root tip of a tooth is accessed in the bone and a small amount is shaved away. The diseased tissue is removed and a filling is placed to reseal the canal.

APLASTIC ANEMIA A disorder in which the bone marrow greatly decreases or stops production of blood cells.

APNEA The temporary absence of breathing. Sleep apnea consists of repeated episodes of temporary suspension of breathing during sleep.

APPENDECTOMY Surgical removal of the appendix.

APPENDIX The worm-shaped pouch attached to the cecum, the beginning of the large intestine.

APPETITE SUPPRESSANT Drugs that decrease feelings of hunger. Most work by increasing levels of serotonin or catecholamine, chemicals in the brain that control appetite.

AQUEOUS HUMOR A transparent liquid, contained within the eye, that is composed of water, sugars, vitamins, proteins, and other nutrients.

AREFLEXIA A condition in which the body's normal reflexes are absent. It is one of the objectives of general anesthesia.

ARGON A colorless, odorless gas.

ARRHYTHMIA Any deviation from a normal heart beat.

ARTERIAL BLOOD GAS TEST A blood test that measures oxygen and carbon dioxide in the blood.

ARTERIAL EMBOLISM A blood clot arising from another location that blocks an artery.

ARTERIAL LINE A catheter inserted into an artery and connected to a physiologic monitoring system to allow direct measurement of oxygen, carbon dioxide, and invasive blood pressure.

ARTERIOGRAM A diagnostic test that involves viewing the arteries and/or attached organs by injecting a contrast medium, or dye, into the artery and taking an x ray.

ARTERIOLE The smallest type of artery.

ARTERIOSCLEROSIS A chronic condition characterized by thickening, loss of elasticity, and hardening of the arteries and the build-up of plaque on the arterial walls. Arteriosclerosis can slow or impair blood circulation. It includes atherosclerosis, but the two terms are often used synonymously.

ARTERIOVENOUS MALFORMATION An abnormal tangle of arteries and veins in which the arteries feed directly into the veins without a normal intervening capillary bed.

ARTERY A blood vessel that carries blood away from the heart to the cells, tissues, and organs of the body.

ARTHRITIS A painful condition that involves inflammation of one or more joints.

ARTHRODESIS A procedure that is sometimes used as an alternative to knee revision surgery, in which the joint is first fixed in place with a surgical nail and then fused as new bone tissue grows in.

ARTHROGRAPHY An imaging technique that entails injecting contrast dye into a joint and then taking an x ray.

ARTHROPLASTY The surgical reconstruction or replacement of a joint.

ARTHROSCOPE An instrument for the visual examination of the interior of a joint.

ARTHROSCOPY Examination of a joint with an arthroscope or joint surgery using an arthroscope.

ARTHROSIS A disease of a joint.

ARTIFICIAL SPHINCTER An implanted device that functions to control the opening and closing of the urethral or anal canal for the expelling of urine or feces, respectively.

ASCITES An abnormal accumulation of fluid within the abdominal cavity.

ASEPTIC Sterile; containing no microorganisms, especially no bacteria.

ASPIRATE To remove a fluid or air from a body cavity by suction often using a needle.

ASPIRATION The process of removing fluids or gases from the body by suction. Also refers to the inhalation of food or liquids into the lungs.

ASTIGMATISM An eye condition in which the cornea doesn't focus light properly on the retina, resulting in a blurred image.

ATELECTASIS Partial or complete collapse of the lung, usually due to a blockage of the air passages with fluid, mucus or infection.

ATHERECTOMY A non-surgical technique for treating diseased arteries with a rotating device that cuts or shaves away obstructing material inside the artery.

ATHEROMA A collection of plaque (lesion) blocking a portion of an artery.

ATHEROSCLEROSIS A disease process whereby plaques of fatty substances are deposited inside arteries, reducing the inside diameter of the vessels and eventually causing damage to the tissues located beyond the site of the blockage.

ATRESIA The congenital absence of a normal body opening or duct.

ATRIA The right and left upper chambers of the heart.

ATRIAL FIBRILLATION A type of heart arrhythmia in which the upper chamber of the heart quivers instead of pumping in an organized way. In this condition, the upper chambers (atria) of the heart do not completely empty when the heart beats, which can allow blood clots to form.

ATRIAL FLUTTER A type of abnormal heart rhythm characterized by rapid pulsation of the upper chamber of the heart that interferes with normal function. In atrial flutter, the heart beats regularly, but much more rapidly than normal.

ATRIOVENTRICULAR NODE (AV NODE) A highly specialized area of the heart muscle which transmits electrical impulses.

ATROPHY The progressive wasting and loss of function of any part of the body.

AUDIOGRAM A chart or graph of the results of a hearing test conducted with audiographic equipment. The chart reflects the softest (lowest volume) sounds that can be heard at various frequencies or pitches.

AUDIOLOGIST A person with a degree and/or certification in the areas of identification and measurement of hearing impairments and rehabilitation of those with hearing problems.

AURICLE The external structure of the ear.

AUSCULTATION The process of listening to sounds that are produced in the body. Direct auscultation uses the ear alone, such as when listening to the grating of a moving joint. Indirect auscultation involves the use of a stethoscope to amplify the sounds from within the body, like a heartbeat.

AUTOGRAFT Tissue that is taken from one part of a person's body and transplanted to a different part of the same person.

AUTOIMMUNE DISORDER One of a group of disorders, like rheumatoid arthritis and systemic lupus erythematosus, in which the immune system is overactive and has lost the ability to distinguish between self and non-self. The body's immune cells turn on the body, attacking various tissues and organs.

AUTOLOGOUS Refers to blood or tissue from the same person. An autologous breast reconstruction uses the woman's own tissues. An autologous blood transfusion is blood removed from a person and then transfused back to the same person at a later time.

AUTOLOGOUS BLOOD The patient's own blood, drawn and set aside before surgery for use during surgery in case a transfusion is needed.

AUTONOMIC NERVOUS SYSTEM The part of the nervous system that controls so-called involuntary functions, such as heart rate, salivary gland secretion, respiratory function, and pupil dilation.

AUTOTRANSFUSION A technique for recovering blood during surgery, separating and concentrating the red blood cells, and reinfusing them in the patient. Autotransfusion is also known as blood salvage.

AUXILIARY HOSPITAL SERVICES A term used broadly to designate such nonmedical services as financial services, birthing classes, support groups, etc. that are instituted in response to consumer demand.

AVASCULAR NECROSIS A disorder in which bone tissue dies and collapses following the temporary or permanent loss of its blood supply. It is also known as osteonecrosis.

AVULSION The forcible separation of a piece from the entire structure.

AXILLARY Located in or near the armpit.

AXILLARY VEIN A blood vessel that takes blood from tissues back to the heart to receive oxygenated blood.

B

B CELL A type of white blood cell derived from bone marrow. B cells are sometimes called B lymphocytes. They secrete antibodies and have a number of other complex functions within the human immune system.

BACTERIA Singular, bacterium; tiny, one-celled forms of life that cause many diseases and infections.

BALANCED ANESTHESIA The use of a combination of inhaled and intravenous drugs in anesthetizing patients.

BALLOON ANGIOPLASTY A surgical procedure in which a balloon catheter is used to flatten plaque against an artery wall.

BAND An immature neutrophil.

BARIATRIC SURGERY Weight loss surgery, such as gastric bypass.

BARIATRICS The branch of medicine that deals with the prevention and treatment of obesity and related disorders.

BARIUM ENEMA X RAY An x-ray procedure that involves the administration of barium into the intestines by a tube inserted into the rectum. Barium is a chalky substance that enhances the visualization of the gastrointestinal tract on x-ray.

BARIUM SULFATE A chemical compound used in certain radiological studies to enhance visualization of anatomical structures.

BARIUM SWALLOW Barium is used to coat the throat in order to take x-ray pictures of the tissues lining the throat.

BAROTRAUMA Ear pain caused by unequal air pressure on the inside and outside of the ear drum. Barotrauma, which is also called pressure-related ear pain or barotitis media, is the most common reason for myringotomies in adults.

BARRETT'S SYNDROME Also called Barrett's esophagus or Barrett's epithelia, this is a condition where the squamous epithelial cells that normally line the esophagus are replaced by thicker columnar epithelial cells.

BASAL CELL CANCER The most common form of skin cancer; it usually appears as one or several nodules having a central depression. It rarely spreads (metastasizes), but is locally invasive.

BASOPHIL White blood cell that increases in response to parasitic infections and allergic reactions.

BENIGN In medical usage, benign is the opposite of malignant. It describes an abnormal growth that is stable, treatable, and generally not life-threatening.

BENIGN PROSTATIC HYPERTROPHY (BPH) An enlargement of the prostate, most commonly seen in men over 50, that is not cancerous. However, it may cause problems with urinating or other symptoms. It is also known as benign prostatic hyperplasia.

BETA BLOCKERS The popular name for a group of drugs that are usually prescribed to treat heart conditions, but that also are used to reduce the physical symptoms of anxiety and phobias, such as sweating and palpitations.

BEVEL The slanted opening on one side of the tip of a needle.

BEZOAR A collection of foreign material, usually hair or vegetable fibers or a mixture of both, that may occasionally occur in the stomach or intestines and block the passage of food.

BILATERAL Occurring on two sides. For example, a patient with bilateral retinoblastoma has this retinal tumor in both eyes.

BILATERAL CLEFT LIP Cleft that occurs on both sides of the lip.

BILE A bitter yellow-green substance produced by the liver. Bile breaks down fats in the small intestine so that they can be used by the body. It is stored in the gallbladder and passes from the gallbladder through the common bile duct to the top of the small intestine (duodenum) as needed to digest fat.

BILE DUCTS Tubes that carry bile, a thick yellow-green fluid that is made by the liver, stored in the gallbladder, and helps the body digest fats.

BILIARY Of bile or of the gallbladder and bile ducts that transport bile and make up the biliary system or tract.

BILIRUBIN A reddish yellow pigment formed from the breakdown of red blood cells, and metabolized by the liver. When levels are abnormally high, it causes the yellowish tint to eyes and skin known as jaundice. Levels of bilirubin in the blood increase in patients with liver disease, blockage of the bile ducts, and other conditions.

BINGE A pattern of eating marked by episodes of rapid consumption of large amounts of food; usually food that is high in calories.

BINGE EATING DISORDER An eating disorder in which the person binges but does not try to get rid of the food afterward by vomiting, using laxatives, or exercising.

BIOLOGICAL TISSUE VALVE An autograft is a valve that comes from the patient, usually the pulmonary valve. An autologous pericardial valve is constructed from the patient's pericardium at the time of surgery. Homograft (or allograft) valve that is harvested from a human cadaver. Porcine heterograft is a pig tissue valve that is sterilized.

BIOMECHANICS The application of mechanical laws to the structures in the human body, such as measuring the force and direction of stresses on a joint.

BIOPSY The surgical removal and microscopic examination of living tissue for diagnostic purposes or to follow the course of a disease. Most commonly the term refers to the collection and analysis of tissue from a suspected tumor to establish malignancy.

BLADDER The muscular sac which receives urine from the kidneys, stores it, and ultimately works to remove it from the body during urination.

BLADDER EXSTROPHY One of many bladder and urinary congenital abnormalities. Occurs when the wall of the bladder fails to close in embryonic development and remains exposed to the abdominal wall.

BLADDER IRRIGATION To flush or rinse the bladder with a stream of liquid (as in removing a foreign body or medicating).

BLADDER TUMOR MARKER STUDIES A test to detect specific substances released by bladder cancer cells into the urine using chemical or immunologic (using antibodies).

BLADDER WASHINGS A procedure in which bladder washing samples are taken by placing a salt solution into the bladder through a catheter (tube) and then removing the solution for microscopic testing.

BLANK If an individual has inherited the same HLA antigen from both parents, the HLA typing is designated by the shared HLA antigen followed by a "blank"(−).

BLAST CELLS Blood cells in the early stage of cellular development.

BLAST CRISIS Stage of chronic myelogenous leukemia where large quantities of immature cells are produced by the bone marrow and is not responsive to treatment.

BLEB A thin-walled auxiliary drain created on the outside of the eyeball during filtering surgery for glaucoma. It is sometimes called a filtering bleb.

BLEEDING DISORDER Any disorder related to problems in the clotting mechanism of the blood.

BLEPHAROPLASTY Surgical reshaping of the eyelid.

BLOOD BANK A laboratory that specializes in blood typing, antibody identification, and transfusion services.

BLOOD PRESSURE The pressure of the blood in the cardiovascular system measured in millimeters of mercury.

BLOOD TYPE Blood categories based on the presence or absence of certain antigens on the red blood cells.

BLOOD UREA NITROGEN (BUN) A test used to measure the blood level of urea nitrogen, an end product of protein metabolism formed in the liver. This waste product is normally filtered by the kidneys and patients with kidney normally have high BUN levels.

BODY DYSMORPHIC DISORDER A psychiatric disorder marked by preoccupation with an imagined physical defect.

BODY MASS INDEX (BMI) A measurement that has replaced weight as the preferred determinant of obesity. The BMI can be calculated (in English units) as 703.1 times a person's weight in pounds divided by the square of the person's height in inches.

BOLUS A mass of food ready to be swallowed, or a preparation of medicine to be given by mouth or IV all at once rather than gradually.

BONE DENSITOMETRY TEST A test that quickly and accurately measures the density of bone.

BONE MARROW The spongy tissue inside the large bones in the body that is responsible for making the red blood cells, most white blood cells, and platelets.

BONE MARROW BIOPSY A procedure in which a needle is inserted into the large bones of the hip or breastbone and a small piece of marrow is removed for microscopic examination.

BONE MARROW TRANSPLANTATION A medical procedure in which a quantity of bone marrow is extracted through a needle from a donor, and then passed into a patient to replace the patient's diseased or absent bone marrow.

BONE MORPHOGENETIC PROTEINS A family of substances in human bones and blood that encourage the process of bone formation.

BONE SPUR Also called an osteophyte, it is an outgrowth or ridge that forms on a bone.

BONY LABYRINTH A series of cavities contained in a capsule inside the temporal bone of the skull. The endolymph-filled membranous labyrinth is suspended in a fluid inside the bony labyrinth.

BORBORYGMI Sounds created by the passage of food, gas, or fecal material in the stomach or intestines.

BOTULINUM TOXIN A potent bacterial toxin or poison made by *Clostridium botulinum*; causes paralysis in high doses, but is used medically in small, localized doses to treat disorders associated with involuntary muscle contraction and spasms, in addition to strabismus.

BOUGIE A mercury-filled dilator in the shape of a cylinder or tapered cylinder. Bougies come in a range of different sizes.

BOWEL LUMEN The space within the intestine.

BRACHYTHERAPY A method of treating cancers, such as prostate cancer, involving the implantation near the tumor of radioactive seeds.

BRADYCARDIA A slow heart rate, usually under 60 beats per minute.

BRAIN DEATH Irreversible cessation of brain function. Patients with brain death have no potential capacity for survival or for recovery of any brain function.

BRCA1 OR BRCA2 GENETIC MUTATION A genetic mutation that predisposes otherwise healthy women to breast cancer.

BREAST AUGMENTATION To increase the size of breasts.

BREAST BIOPSY A procedure in which suspicious breast tissue is removed and examined by a pathologist for cancer or other disease. The breast tissue may be obtained by open surgery or through a needle.

BREATHING RATE The number of breaths per minute.

BREECH PRESENTATION The condition in which the baby enters the birth canal with its buttocks or feet first.

BRONCHI Singular, bronchus; the large tubular passages that carry air to the lung and allow air to be expelled from the lungs.

BRONCHIECTASIS A disorder of the bronchial tubes marked by abnormal stretching, enlargement, or destruction of the walls. Bronchiectasis is usually caused by recurrent inflammation of the airway.

BRONCHIOLES Small airways extending from the bronchi into the lobes of the lungs.

BRONCHITIS Inflammation of the air passages of the lungs.

BRONCHOALVEOLAR LAVAGE A procedure for obtaining a sample of cells from the airways by introducing and then removing a fluid through a flexible tube into a section of the lung, while the rest of the lung is isolated by an inflated balloon. It is used to diagnose lung diseases.

BRONCHODILATORS Drugs that help open the bronchial tubes (airways) of the lungs, allowing more air to flow through them.

BRONCHOPLEURAL FISTULA An abnormal connection between an air passage and the membrane that covers the lungs.

BRONCHOSCOPY A procedure in which a hollow tube (bronchoscope) is inserted into the airway to allow visual examination of the larynx, trachea, bronchi, and bronchioles. It is also used to collect specimens for biopsy or culturing, and to remove airway obstructions.

BRONCHOSPASM A spasmodic contraction of the muscles that line the two branches of the trachea that lead into the lungs, causing difficulty in breathing. Bronchospasm is a common complication in heavy smokers under anesthesia.

BROTH A growth mixture for bacteria. Different compounds, such as sugars or amino acids, may be added to increase the growth of certain organisms. Also known as media.

BRUIT A roaring sound created by a partially blocked artery.

BRUNESCENT Developing a brownish or amber color over time. Nuclear cataracts are sometimes called brunescent.

BUCCAL SULCUS Groove in the upper part of the upper jaw (where there are teeth).

BUERGER'S DISEASE An episodic disease that causes inflammation and blockage of the veins and arteries of the limbs. It tends to be present almost exclusively on men under age 40 who smoke, and may require amputation of the hand or foot.

BULIMIA NERVOSA An eating disorder characterized by binge eating and inappropriate compensatory behavior, such as vomiting, misusing laxatives, or excessive exercise.

BUNION A swelling or deformity of the big toe, characterized by the formation of a bursa and a sideways displacement of the toe.

BURCH PROCEDURE A surgical procedure, also called retropubic colposuspension, in which the neck of the bladder is suspended from nearby ligaments with sutures. It is performed to treat urinary incontinence.

BURSA A closed sac lined with a synovial membrane and filled with fluid, usually found in areas subject to friction, such as where a tendon passes over a bone.

BURSITIS Inflammation of a bursa, a fluid-filled cavity or sac. In the body, bursae are located at places where friction might otherwise develop.

C

CADAVER The human body after death.

CADAVER ORGAN An organ from a brain-dead organ donor used for purposes of transplantation.

CALCIUM-CHANNEL BLOCKERS Drugs that block the entry of calcium into the muscle cells of small blood vessels (arterioles) and keep them from narrowing. They are used to treat high blood pressure.

CALCULUS Any type of hard concretion (stone) in the body, but usually found in the gallbladder, pancreas, and kidneys. They are formed by the accumulation of excess mineral salts and other organic material such as blood or mucous. Calculi (pl.) can cause problems by lodging in and obstructing the proper flow of fluids, such as bile to the intestines or urine to the bladder. In dentistry, calculus refers to a hardened yellow or brown mineral deposit from unremoved plaque, also called tartar.

CALDWELL-LUC PROCEDURE A surgical procedure where the maxillary sinus is entered by making an opening under the upper lip above the teeth.

CALLUS Thickened skin due to chronic rubbing or irritation.

CANCER A disease caused by uncontrolled growth of the body's cells.

CANCER STAGING A surgical procedure to remove a lymph node and examine the cells for cancer. It determines the extent of the cancer and how far it has spread.

CANINES The two sharp teeth located next to the front incisor teeth in mammals that are used to grip and tear.

CANKER SORE A blister-like sore on the inside of the mouth that can be painful but is not serious.

CANNULA A tube inserted into a cavity to serve as a channel for the transport of fluid.

CAPILLARIES The tiniest blood vessels with the smallest diameter. These vessels receive blood from the arterioles and deliver blood to the venules. In the lungs, capillaries are located next to the alveoli so that they can pick up oxygen from inhaled air.

CAPSULAR CONTRACTURE Thick scar tissue around a breast implant, which may tighten and cause discomfort and/or firmness.

CAPSULORRHEXIS The creation of a continuous circular tear in the front portion of the lens capsule during cataract surgery to allow for removal of the lens nucleus.

CAPSULOTOMY A procedure that is sometimes needed after ECCE to open a lens capsule that has become cloudy.

CARBOHYDRATES Compounds, such as cellulose, sugar, and starch, that contain only carbon, hydrogen, and oxygen, and are a major part of the diets of people and other animals.

CARBON DIOXIDE A heavy, colorless gas that dissolves in water.

CARCINOMA The common medical term for cancer.

CARCINOMA IN SITU Cancer that is confined to the cells in which it originated and has not spread to other tissues.

CARDIAC ANGIOGRAPHY A procedure used to visualize blood vessels of the heart. A catheter is used to inject a dye into the vessels, so that the vessels can imaged by x ray.

CARDIAC ARREST Temporary or permanent cessation of the heartbeat.

CARDIAC ARRHYTHMIA An irregular heart rate (frequency of heartbeats) or rhythm (the pattern of heartbeats).

CARDIAC CATHETER Long, thin, flexible tube that is threaded into the heart through a blood vessel.

CARDIAC CATHETERIZATION A procedure to passes a catheter through a large vein into the heart and its vessels for the purpose of diagnosing coronary artery disease, assessing injury or disease of the aorta, or evaluating cardiac function.

CARDIAC MARKER A substance in the blood whose level rises following a myocardial infarction (heart attack).

CARDIAC TAMPONADE Compression and restriction of the heart that occurs when the pericardium fills with blood or fluid. This increase in pressure outside the heart interferes with heart function and can result in shock and/or death.

CARDIOLOGIST A physician who specializes in diagnosing and treating heart diseases.

CARDIOMYOPATHY A disease of the heart muscle.

CARDIOPULMONARY Relating to the heart and lungs.

CARDIOPULMONARY BYPASS Mechanically circulating the blood with a heart-lung machine that bypasses the heart and lungs.

CARDIOPULMONARY RESUSCITATION (CPR) An emergency procedure designed to stimulate breathing and blood flow through a combination of chest compressions and rescue breathing. It is used to restore circulation and prevent brain death to a person who has collapsed, is unconscious, is not breathing, and has no pulse.

CARDIOVASCULAR Relating to the heart and blood vessels.

CARDIOVERSION An electrical shock delivered to the heart to restore a normal rhythm.

CARDIOVERTER A device to apply electric shock to the chest to convert an abnormal heartbeat into a normal heartbeat.

CAROTID ARTERY One of the major arteries supplying blood to the head and neck.

CARPAL BONES Eight wrist bones arranged in two rows that articulate proximally with the radius and indirectly with the ulna, and distally with the five metacarpal bones.

CARTILAGE A tough, elastic connective tissue found in the joints, outer ear, nose, larynx, and other parts of the body.

CASE MANAGER A health-care professional who can provide assistance with a patient's needs beyond the hospital.

CAST An insoluble gelled protein matrix that takes the form of the renal tubule in which it was deposited. Casts are washed out by normal urine flow.

CATABOLISM A process of metabolism that breaks down complex substances into simple ones.

CATARACT A condition in which the lens of the eye turns cloudy and interferes with vision.

CATEGORICALLY NEEDY A term that describes certain groups of Medicaid recipients who qualify for the basic mandatory package of Medicaid benefits. There are categorically needy groups that states participating in Medicaid are required to cover, and other groups that the states have the option to cover.

CATGUT The oldest type of absorbable suture. In spite of its name, catgut is made from collagen derived from sheep or cattle intestines. Synthetic absorbable sutures have been available since the 1980s.

CATHARSIS Therapeutic discharge of emotional tension by recalling past events.

CATHARTIC COLON A poorly functioning colon, resulting from the chronic abuse of stimulant cathartics.

CATHERIZATION The process of inserting a hollow tube into a body cavity or blood vessel.

CATHETER A thin, hollow tube inserted into the body at specific points in order to inject or withdraw fluids from the body.

CATHETERIZATION The process of inserting a hollow tube into a body cavity or blood vessel.

CATION An ion with a positive charge.

CAUDA EQUINA The roots of the spinal nerves controlling movement and sensation in the legs. These nerve roots are located in the lower spine and resemble a horse's tail (*cauda equina* in Latin).

CAUSALGIA A severe burning sensation sometimes accompanied by redness and inflammation of the skin. Causalgia is caused by injury to a nerve outside the spinal cord.

CAUTERIZE To damage with heat or cold so that tissues shrink. It is an effective way to stop bleeding or destroy tissue.

CECUM The beginning of the large intestine and the place where the appendix attaches to the intestinal tract.

CELLULITE Dimpled skin that is caused by uneven fat deposits beneath the surface.

CENTRAL NERVOUS SYSTEM Part of the nervous system consisting of the brain, cranial nerves, and spinal cord. The brain is the center of higher processes, such as thought and emotion and is responsible for the coordination and control of bodily activities and the interpretation of information from the senses. The cranial nerves and spinal cord link the brain to the peripheral nervous system, that is the nerves present in the rest of body.

CENTRAL VENOUS LINE A catheter inserted into a vein and connected to a physiologic monitoring system to directly measure venous blood pressure.

CEPHALOPELVIC DISPROPORTION The condition in which the baby's head is too large to fit through the mother's pelvis.

CEREBRAL ANEURYSM An abnormal, localized bulge in a blood vessel that is usually caused by a congenital weakness in the wall of the vessel.

CEREBRAL CORTEX The thin, convoluted surface of the brain consisting mainly of nerve cell bodies. This brain region is responsible for reasoning, mood, and perception.

CEREBRAL PALSY A nonprogressive movement disability caused by abnormal development of or damage to motor control centers of the brain.

CEREBROSPINAL FLUID The clear, normally colorless fluid that fills the brain cavities (ventricles), the subarachnoid space around the brain, and the spinal cord and acts as a shock absorber.

CEREBROVASCULAR ACCIDENT Brain hemorrhage, also known as a stroke.

CERVICAL CRYOTHERAPY Surgery performed after a biopsy has confirmed abnormal cervical cells (dysplasia).

CERVIX A small, cylindrical structure about an inch or so long and less than an inch around that makes up the lower part and neck of the uterus. The cervix separates the body and cavity of the uterus from the vagina.

CESAREAN SECTION Delivery of a baby through an incision in the mother's abdomen instead of through the vagina; also called a C-section.

CHARCOT ARTHROPATHY Also called neuropathic arthropathy, a condition in which the shoulder joint is destroyed following loss of its nerve supply.

CHEMICAL PEEL A skin treatment that uses the application of chemicals, such as phenol or trichloractic acid (TCA), to remove the uppermost layer of skin.

CHEMOPREVENTION The use of drugs, vitamins, or other substances to reduce the risk of developing cancer or of the cancer returning.

CHEMOTHERAPY Any treatment of an illness with chemical agents. The term is usually used to describe the treatment of cancer with drugs that inhibit cancer growth or destroy cancer cells.

CHEST TUBE A tube inserted into the chest to drain fluid and air from around the lungs.

CHEST X RAY A diagnostic procedure in which a very small amount of radiation is used to produce an image of the structures of the chest (heart, lungs, and bones) on film.

CHILD LIFE SPECIALIST A person who has had specific training in the care of children, including understanding growth and development specific to each age range and how to talk to children of different ages.

CHIROPRACTIC A method of treatment based on the interactions of the spine and the nervous system. Chiropractors adjust or manipulate segments of the patient's spinal column in order to relieve pain.

CHOLECYSTECTOMY Surgical removal of the gallbladder.

CHOLECYSTITIS Inflammation of the gallbladder, usually due to infection

CHOLELITHIASIS Also known as gallstones, these hard masses are formed in the gallbladder or passages, and can cause severe upper right abdominal pain radiating to the right shoulder, as a result of blocked bile flow.

CHOLELITHOTOMY A surgical procedure to remove gallstones through an incision in the gallbladder.

CHOLESTASIS A blockage in the flow of bile.

CHOLESTEROL A steroid fat found in animal foods that is also produced in the human body from saturated fat. Cholesterol is used to form cell membranes and process hormones and vitamin D. High cholesterol levels contribute to the development of atherosclerosis.

CHORDAE TENDINEAE The strands of connective tissue that connect the mitral valve to the papillary muscle of the heart's left ventricle.

CHORDEE A condition associated with hypospadias in which the penis bends downward during erections.

CHORIOAMNIONITIS Infection of the amniotic sac.

CHORIONIC VILLUS SAMPLING (CVS) A procedure used for prenatal diagnosis at 10-12 weeks gestation. Under ultrasound guidance a needle is inserted either through the mother's vagina or abdominal wall and a sample of the chorionic membrane. These cells are then tested for chromosome abnormalities or other genetic diseases.

CHOROID In the human eye, the thin layer of tissue that lies between the sclera and the retina. The choroid is rich in blood vessels that nourish the retina and the dark pigments of the choroid absorb light rays so that they are not reflected back out of the eye.

CHROMOSOME A microscopic thread-like structure found within each cell of the human body and consisting of a complex of proteins and DNA. Humans have 46 chromosomes arranged into 23 pairs. Chromosomes contain the genetic information necessary to direct the development and functioning of all cells and systems in the body.

CHRONIC Refers to a disease or condition that progresses slowly but persists or recurs over time.

CHRONIC KIDNEY FAILURE End-stage renal disease (ESRD); chronic kidney failure is diagnosed as ESRD when kidney function falls to 5-10% of capacity.

CHRONIC MYELOGENOUS LEUKEMIA Chronic leukemia is a cancer in which too many white blood cells are made in the bone marrow. Chronic myelogenous leukemia, also called chronic myelocytic leukemia, involve the overproduction and accumulation of granulocytes.

CHRONIC OTITIS MEDIA Inflammation of the middle ear with signs of infection lasting three months or longer.

CHRONIC PAIN Pain that lasts over a prolonged period and threatens to disrupt daily life.

CILIA Tiny hairlike projections on certain cells within the body. Cilia produce lashing or whipping movements to direct or cause motion of substances or fluids within the body. Within the respiratory tract, the cilia act to move mucus along, in an effort to continually flush out and clean the respiratory tract.

CILIARY BODY A structure in the eye that joins the iris with the choroid and containing muscles that permit the focusing of the lens.

CIRCUMCISION A surgical procedure, usually with religious or cultural significance, where the prepuce or skin covering the tip of the penis on a boy, or the clitoris on a girl, is cut away.

CIRRHOSIS A chronic degenerative disease of the liver, in which normal cells are replaced by fibrous tissue and normal liver function is disrupted. The most common symptoms are mild jaundice, fluid collection in the tissues, mental confusion, and vomiting of blood.

CLASSIC INCISION In a cesarean section, an incision made vertically along the uterus; this kind of incision makes a larger opening but also creates more bleeding, a greater chance of infection, and a weaker scar.

CLAUDICATION Cramping or pain in a leg caused by poor blood circulation. This condition is frequently caused by hardening of the arteries (atherosclerosis). Intermittent claudication occurs only at certain times, usually after exercise, and is relieved by rest.

CLEAN CATCH SPECIMEN A urine specimen that is collected from the middle of the urine stream after the first part of the flow has been voided.

CLEFT PALATE A congenital malformation in which there is an abnormal opening in the roof of the mouth that allows the nasal passages and the mouth to be improperly connected.

CLINICAL BREAST EXAM An examination of the breast and surrounding tissue by a physician, who is feeling for lumps and looking for other signs of abnormality.

CLINICAL NURSE SPECIALISTS Nurses with advanced training as well as a master's degree.

CLOT A soft, semi-solid mass that forms when blood coagulates.

COAGULATION CASCADE The sequence of biochemical activities, involving clotting factors, that stops bleeding by forming a clot.

COAGULOPATHY A disorder in which blood is either too slow or too quick to coagulate (clot).

COARCTATION OF THE AORTA A congenital defect in which severe narrowing or constriction of the aorta obstructs the flow of blood.

COATS' DISEASE A chronic and progressive disorder of the retina marked by exudative RD. It is named for George Coats (1876-1915), a British ophthalmologist. It occurs most frequently in preadolescent boys and young adults.

COCHLEA The hearing part of the inner ear. This snail-shaped structure contains fluid and thousands of microscopic hair cells tuned to various frequencies, in addition to the organ of Corti (the receptor for hearing).

CO-INSURANCE The percentage of health care charges that an insurance company pays after the beneficiary pays the deductible. Most co-insurance percentages are 70–90%.

COLD SORE A small blister on the lips or face caused by a virus. Also called a fever blister.

COLECTOMY The surgical removal of the colon or part of the colon.

COLITIS Inflammation of the colon (large intestine).

COLLAGEN The main supportive protein of cartilage, connective tissue, tendon, skin, and bone.

COLON The part of the large intestine that extends from the cecum to the rectum. The sigmoid colon is the area of the intestine just above the rectum; linking the descending colon with the rectum. It is shaped like the letter S.

COLONOSCOPE A thin, flexible, hollow, lighted tube that in inserted through the rectum into the colon to enable the doctor to view the entire lining of the colon.

COLONOSCOPY An examination of the lining of the colon performed with a colonoscope.

COLORECTAL CANCER Cancer of the large intestine, or colon, including the rectum (the last 16 in of the large intestine before the anus).

COLOSTOMY A surgical procedure in which an opening is made in the wall of the abdomen to allow a part of the large intestine (the colon) to empty outside the body. Colostomies are usually required because portions of the intestine have been removed or an intestinal obstruction exists.

COLPORRHAPHY A surgical procedure in which the vagina is sutured.

COLPOSCOPY A diagnostic procedure using a hollow, lighted tube (colposcope) to examine the vagina and cervix.

COLUMELLA The strip of skin running from the tip of the nose to the upper lip, which separates the nostrils.

COMA A condition of deep unconsciousness from which the person cannot be aroused

COMMISSURES The normal separations between the valve leaflets.

COMMON BILE DUCT The branching passage through which bile, a necessary digestive enzyme, travels from the liver and gallbladder into the small intestine. Digestive enzymes from the pancreas also enter the intestines through the common bile duct.

COMORBID A term applied to a disease or disorder that occurs at the same time as another disease condition. There are a number of health problems that are comorbid with obesity.

COMPATIBLE DONOR A person whose tissue and blood type are the same as the recipient's.

COMPLETE BLOOD COUNT (CBC) A routine analysis performed on a sample of blood taken from the patient's vein with a needle and vacuum tube. The measurements taken in a CBC include a white blood cell count, a red blood cell count, the red cell distribution width, the hematocrit (ratio of the volume of the red blood cells to the blood volume), and the amount of hemoglobin (the blood protein that carries oxygen).

COMPOUND FRACTURE A fracture in which the broken end or ends of the bone have torn through the skin. Compound fractures are also known as open fractures.

COMPUTED TOMOGRAPHY (CT) An imaging technique in which cross-sectional x rays of the body are compiled to create a three-dimensional image of the body's internal structures; also called computed axial tomography.

CONCEPTION The union of egg and sperm to form a fetus.

CONCHA The hollow shell-shaped portion of the external ear.

CONDITIONING Process of preparing a patient to receive bone marrow donation, often through the use of chemotherapy and radiation therapy.

CONDUCTIVE HEARING LOSS A type of medically treatable hearing loss in which the inner ear is usually normal, but there are specific problems in the middle or outer ears that prevent sound from getting to the inner ear in a normal way.

CONDUIT DIVERSION A surgical procedure that restores urinary and fecal continence by diverting these functions through a constructed conduit leading to an external waste reservoir (ostomy).

CONFIRMATORY TYPING Repeat tissue typing to confirm the compatibility of the donor and patient before transplant.

CONGENITAL Present at birth.

CONGENITAL HEART DEFECTS Abnormal formation of structures of the heart or of its major blood vessels that is present at birth.

CONJUNCTIVA The mucous membrane that covers the white part of the eyes (sclera) and lines the eyelids.

CONJUNCTIVITIS Inflammation of the conjunctiva, the mucous membrane covering the white part of the eye (sclera) and lining the inside of the eyelids also called pinkeye.

CONNECTIVE TISSUE A group of tissues responsible for support throughout the body; includes cartilage, bone, fat, tissue underlying skin, and tissues that support organs, blood vessels, and nerves throughout the body.

CONSERVATION SURGERY Surgery that preserves the aesthetics of the area undergoing an operation.

CONSTRICT To squeeze tightly, compress, draw together.

CONSULTATION Evaluation by an outside expert or specialist, someone other than the primary care provider.

CONTAMINATION Passage of an infectious organism, such as a virus, from an infected person to an object or into the food or water supply, so that the infection may be passed on to another person.

CONTINUITY Uninterrupted and successive.

CONTINUOUS POSITIVE AIRWAY PRESSURE (CPAP) A ventilation system that blows a gentle stream of air into the nose to keep the airway open.

CONTRACEPTION The prevention of the union of the male's sperm with the female's egg.

CONTRACTURE A tightening or shortening of muscles that prevents normal movement of the associated limb or other body part.

CONTRAST AGENT Also called a contrast medium, this is usually a barium or iodine dye that is injected into the area under investigation. The dye makes the interior body parts more visible on an x-ray film.

COR PULMONALE Enlargement of the right ventricle of the heart caused by pulmonary hypertension that may result from emphysema or bronchiectasis; eventually, the condition leads to congestive heart failure.

CORACOID PROCESS A long curved projection from the scapula overhanging the glenoid cavity; it provides attachment to muscles and ligaments of the shoulder and back region.

CORN A horny thickening of the skin on a toe, caused by friction and pressure from poorly fitted shoes or stockings.

CORNEA The clear, dome-shaped outer covering of the eye that lies in front of the iris and pupil. The cornea lets light into the eye.

CORNEAL TOPOGRAPHY Mapping the cornea's surface with a specialized computer that illustrates corneal elevations.

CORONARY ARTERY DISEASE A narrowing or blockage, due to atherosclerosis, of the arteries that provide oxygen and nutrients to the heart. When blood flow is cut off, a heart attack results. Also called coronary occlusive artery disease.

CORONARY BLOOD VESSELS The arteries and veins involved in the coronary circulation. The coronary arteries supply blood to the heart muscle and the coronary veins drain blood from the heart muscle.

CORONARY BYPASS SURGERY Surgery in which a section of blood vessel is used to bypass a blocked coronary artery and restore an adequate blood supply to the heart muscle.

CORTICOSTEROIDS A group of hormones produced naturally by the adrenal gland or manufactured synthetically. They are often used to treat inflammation. Examples include cortisone and prednisone.

CORTISONE Glucocorticoid produced by the adrenal cortex in response to stress. Cortisone is a steroid with anti-inflammatory and immunosuppressive properties.

COSMETIC SURGERY Surgery that is intended to improve a patient's appearance or correct disfigurement. It is also called aesthetic surgery.

COUCHING The oldest form of cataract surgery, in which the lens is dislocated and pushed backward into the vitreous body with a lance.

C-PAP MACHINE A continuous positive airway pressure machine used at night to alleviate sleep apnea. A mask is placed over the nose and room air is blown into the patient's airway, keeping the airway from collapsing, and alleviating snoring and periods of stopping breathing during the night.

CRANIOSYNOSTOSIS A premature closure of one or more of the joints (fissures) between the bones of the skull, which causes an abnormally shaped skull.

CRANIOTOMY A surgical incision into the skull.

CRANIUM Skull; the bony framework that holds the brain.

CREATININE The metabolized by-product of creatine, an organic acid that assists the body in producing muscle contractions. Creatinine is found in the bloodstream and in muscle tissue. It is removed from the blood by the kidneys and excreted in the urine. Higher than normal levels of this substance may indicate kidney disease.

CREATININE CLEARANCE RATE The clearance of creatinine from the plasma compared to its appearance in the urine. Since there is no reabsorption of creatinine, this measurement can estimate kidney filtration rate.

CREMASTERIC REFLEX A reflex in which the cremaster muscle, which covers the testes and the spermatic cord, pulls the testicles back into the scrotum. It is important for a doctor to distinguish between an undescended testicle and a hyperactive cremasteric reflex in small children.

CRICOID CARTILAGE A ring-shaped piece of cartilage that forms the lower and rear parts of the voice box or larynx; it is sometimes called the annular cartilage because of its shape.

CRICOTHYROID MEMBRANE The piece of connective tissue that lies between the thyroid and cricoid cartilages.

CRICOTHYROIDOTOMY An emergency tracheotomy that consists of a cut through the cricothyroid membrane to open the patient's airway as fast as possible. Also called cricothyrotomy.

CRITICAL CARE The multidisciplinary health care specialty that provides care to patients with acute, life-threatening illness or injury.

CROHN'S DISEASE A chronic, inflammatory disease, primarily involving the small and large intestine, but which can affect other parts of the digestive system as well.

CROSSMATCH A laboratory test to determine if patient and donor blood or tissues are compatible.

CROWN The natural part of the tooth covered by enamel. A restorative crown is a protective shell that fits over a tooth.

CRYOANESTHESIA The use of the numbing effects of cold as a surgical anesthetic. For dermabrasion, this involves the spraying of a cold-inducing chemical on the area being treated.

CRYOGEN A substance, such as liquid nitrogen, that induces freezing and is used in cryotherapy treatment to destroy diseased tissue.

CRYOPEXY Reattachment of a detached retina by freezing the tissue behind the tear with nitrous oxide.

CRYOPROSTATECTOMY Freezing of the prostate through the use of liquid nitrogen probes guided by transrectal ultrasound of the prostate.

CRYOTHERAPY The use of a very low-temperature probe to freeze and thereby destroy tissue. Cryotherapy is used in the treatment skin lesions, Parkinson's disease, some cancers, retinal detachment, and cataracts. Also called cryosurgery.

CRYPTORCHIDISM Undescended testes, a condition in which a boy is born with one or both testicles in the lower abdomen rather than the scrotum.

CUL-DE-SAC The closed end of a pouch.

CULDOCENTESIS Removal of material from the pouch of Douglas, a deep peritoneal recess between the uterus and the upper vaginal wall, by means of puncture of the vaginal wall.

CULTURE A test in which a sample of body fluid is placed on materials specially formulated to grow microorganisms. A culture is used to learn what type of bacterium is causing infection.

CUPID'S BOW Double curve of the upper lip.

CURETTE Also spelled curet; a small loop or scoop-shaped surgical instrument with sharpened edges that can be used to remove tissue, growths, or debris.

CUSHING'S DISEASE A hormonal disorder caused by an abnormally high level of cortisol, a corticosteroid hormone that is produced by the adrenal glands. It is most commonly caused by taking medications containing the hormone over a long period of time or more rarely by a pituitary or adrenal gland tumor that stimulates the body to produce excessive amounts of cortisol.

CUTANEOUS SQUAMOUS CELL CARCINOMA Malignant skin tumor of the epidermis or its appendages.

CYANOSIS A bluish tinge to the skin that can occur when the blood oxygen level drops too low.

CYANOTIC Marked by a bluish tinge to the skin that occurs when the blood oxygen level drops too low. It is one of the types of congenital heart disease.

CYST An abnormal sac or enclosed cavity in the body filled with liquid or partially solid material. Also refers to a protective, walled-off capsule in which an organism lies dormant.

CYSTIC FIBROSIS A hereditary genetic disorder that occurs most often in Caucasians. It affects the body's ability to move salt and water in and out of cells. This defect causes the lungs and pancreas to secrete thick mucus, blocking passageways and preventing their proper function.

CYSTOSCOPE A pencil-thin instrument that allows viewing and treatments inside the urinary system.

CYSTOSCOPY A diagnostic procedure in which a hollow lighted tube (cystoscope) is used to look inside the bladder and the urethra.

CYTOKINES Chemicals made by the cells that act on other cells to stimulate or inhibit their function. They are important controllers of immune functions.

CYTOMEGALOVIRUS (CMV) A common human virus causing mild or no symptoms in healthy people, but permanent damage or death to an infected fetus, a transplant patient, or a person with HIV.

CYTOPLASM The part of a cell that is outside the nucleus, like the white of an egg.

D

DACRON A synthetic polyester fiber used to surgically repair damaged sections of heart muscle and blood vessel walls.

DEBRIDEMENT The surgical removal of dead tissue and/or foreign bodies from a wound or cut.

DECOMPRESSION A decrease in pressure from the surrounding water that occurs with decreasing diving depth.

DEEP VEIN THROMBOSIS The development or presence of a blood clot in a vein deep within the leg. Deep vein thrombosis can lead to pulmonary embolism if untreated.

DEFECATION The act of having a bowel movement or the passage of feces through the anus.

DEFIBRILLATION A procedure to stop the type of irregular heart beat called ventricular fibrillation, usually by using electric shock.

DEFIBRILLATOR A device that delivers a controlled electric shock to the heart muscle through the chest wall in order to restore a normal heart rate.

DEHISCENCE Separation of a surgical incision or rupture of a wound closure.

DEHYDRATION An excessive loss of water from the body. It may follow vomiting, prolonged diarrhea, or excessive sweating.

DELTOID MUSCLE Muscle that covers the prominence of the shoulder.

DEMENTIA Loss of memory and other higher functions, such as thinking or speech, lasting six months or more.

DEMYELINATION Disruption or destruction of the myelin sheath, leaving a bare nerve. It results in a slowing or stopping of the impulses that travel along that nerve.

DERMABRASION A technique for removing the upper layers of skin with planing wheels powered by compressed air.

DERMIS The basal layer of skin; it contains blood and lymphatic vessels, nerves, glands, and hair follicles.

DETOXIFICATION The process of physically eliminating drugs and/or alcohol from the system of a substance-dependent individual.

DETRUSOR MUSCLE Muscle of the bladder wall.

DEVIATED SEPTUM A shift in the position of the nasal septum, the partition that divides the two nasal cavities.

DIABETES MELLITUS The clinical name for common diabetes. It is a chronic disease characterized by the inability of the body to produce or respond properly to insulin, a hormone required by the body to convert glucose to energy.

DIABETIC RETINOPATHY A condition seen most frequently in individuals with poorly controlled diabetes mellitus where the tiny blood vessels to the retina, the tissues that sense light at the back of the eye, are damaged. This damage causes blurred vision, sudden blindness, or black spots, lines, or flashing light in the field of vision.

DIAGNOSTIC WINDOW A cardiac marker's timeline for rising, peaking, and returning to normal after a heart attack.

DIALYSATE A chemical bath used in dialysis to draw fluids and toxins out of the bloodstream and supply electrolytes and other chemicals to the bloodstream.

DIALYSIS A process of filtering and removing waste products from the bloodstream, it is used as a treatment for patients whose kidneys do not function properly. Two main types are hemodialysis and peritoneal dialysis.

DIALYSIS PRESCRIPTION The general parameters of dialysis treatment that vary according to each patient's individual needs. Treatment length, type of dialyzer and dialysate used, and rate of ultrafiltration are all part of the dialysis prescription.

DIALYZER An artificial kidney usually composed of hollow fiber which is used in hemodialysis to eliminate waste products from the blood and remove excess fluids from the bloodstream.

DIAPHRAGM The thin layer of muscle that separates the chest cavity containing the lungs and heart from the abdominal cavity containing the intestines and digestive organs. This term is also used for a dome-shaped device used to cover the back of a woman's vagina during intercourse in order to prevent pregnancy.

DIASTOLIC The phase of blood circulation in which the heart's pumping chambers (ventricles) are being filled with blood. During this phase, the ventricles are at their most relaxed, and the pressure against the walls of the arteries is at its lowest.

DIATHERMY Also called electrocautery, this is a procedure uses heat generated by electric current to destroy abnormal cells. It is gradually being replaced by cryosurgery, lasers, or loop electrosurgical excision (LEEP).

DIETHYLSTILBESTROL (DES) A synthetic estrogen drug that is used to treat a number of hormonal conditions. It was linked to several serious birth defects and disorders of the reproductive system in daughters of women who took DES. In 1971, the FDA suggested it not be used during pregnancy and banned its use in 1979 as a growth promoter in livestock.

DIFFERENTIAL A blood test that determines the percentage of each type of white blood cell in a person's blood.

DIGESTIVE TRACT The stomach, intestines, and other parts of the body through which food passes. Also called the gastrointestinal tract or the alimentary canal.

DIGIT A finger or a toe.

DIGITAL RECTAL EXAMINATION A type of phyical examination in which the physician inserts a gloved, lubricated index finger into the rectum to check for any abnormalities.

DILATION AND CURETTAGE (D & C) A procedure performed under anesthesia during which the cervix is opened more (or dilated) and tissue lining the uterus is scraped out with a metal, spoon-shaped instrument (curette) or a suction tube. The procedure can be used to diagnose a problem, to remove growths (polyps), or to terminate a pregnancy.

DIMINISHED CHEST EXPANSION A decease in the chest expansion due to an inability of the lungs to fully inspire and expire air.

DIRECTED DONATION Blood donated by a patient's family member or friend, to be used by the patient.

DISCHARGE PLANNER A health care professional who helps patients arrange for health and home care needs after they go home from the hospital.

DIURETIC DRUGS A group of medications that increase the amount of urine produced and relieve excess fluid buildup in body tissues. Diuretics may be used in treating high blood pressure, lung disease, premenstrual syndrome, and other conditions.

DIVERTICULITIS Inflammation of the diverticula (small outpouchings) along the wall of the colon, the large intestine.

DIVERTICULOSIS A condition in which the colon (large intestine) develops a number of outpouchings or sacs.

DIVERTICULUM Plural, diverticula; an outpouching in a tubular organ caused when the inner, lining layer bulges out (herniates) through the outer, muscular layer. Diverticula are present most often in the colon (large intestine), but are also found in the stomach and the small intestine.

DOMINANT HAND The hand that the individual prefers to use for most activities, especially writing.

DONOR A person who donates an organ or tissue for transplantation.

DOPPLER ECHOCARDIOGRAPHY A testing technique that uses Doppler ultrasound technology to evaluate the pattern and direction of blood flow in the heart.

DOWN SYNDROME A chromosomal disorder caused by an extra copy or a rearrangement of chromosome 21. Children with Down syndrome have varying degrees of mental retardation and may have heart defects.

DRESSING A bandage, gauze pad, or other material placed over a wound or incision to cover and protect it.

DRY EYE Corneal dryness due to insufficient tear production.

DRY SOCKET A painful condition following tooth extraction in which a blood clot does not properly fill the empty socket, leaving the bone underneath exposed to air and food.

DUANE SYNDROME A hereditary congenital syndrome in which the affected eye shows a limited capacity to move and deficient convergence with the other eye.

DUCTOGRAM A test used for imaging the breast ducts and diagnosing the cause of abnormal nipple discharges.

DUMPING SYNDROME A complex physical reaction to food passing too quickly from the stomach into the small intestine, characterized by sweating, nausea, abdominal cramps, dizziness, and other symptoms.

DUODENECTOMY Excision of the duodenum.

DUODENUM The first of the three segments of the small intestine. The duodenum is about 10 in (25 cm) long and connects the stomach and the jejunum.

DURA MATER The strongest and outermost of three membranes that protect the brain, spinal cord, and nerves of the cauda equina.

DURABLE MEDICAL POWER OF ATTORNEY A legal document that empowers a person to make medical decisions for the patient should the patient be unable to make the decisions.

DYSMENORRHEA Painful menstruation.

DYSMOTILITY A lack of normal muscle movement (motility), especially in the esophagus, stomach, or intestines.

DYSPHAGIA Difficulty in swallowing.

DYSPLASIA Abnormal changes in cells.

DYSPNEA Difficulty in breathing, usually associated with heart or lung diseases.

DYSTOCIA Failure to progress in labor, either because the cervix will not dilate (expand) further or because the head does not descend through the mother's pelvis after full dilation of the cervix.

E

EALES DISEASE A disorder marked by recurrent hemorrhages into the retina and vitreous body. It occurs most often in males between the ages of 10 and 25.

EAR MOLDING A non-surgical method for treating ear deformities shortly after birth with the application of a mold held in place by tape and surgical glue.

ECHOCARDIOGRAM A record of the internal structures of the heart obtained from beams of ultrasonic waves directed through the wall of the chest.

ECHOCARDIOGRAPHY A non-invasive technique, using ultrasound waves, used to look at the various structures and functions of the heart.

ECTOPIC Out of place or located away from the normal position.

ECTOPIC BEAT Abnormal heart beat arising elsewhere than from the sinoatrial node.

ECTOPIC PARATHYROID TISSUE Parathyroid tissue located in an abnormal place.

ECTOPIC PREGNANCY A pregnancy that develops outside of the mother's uterus, such as in the fallopian tube. Ectopic pregnancies often cause severe pain in the lower abdomen and are potentially life-threatening because of the massive blood loss that may occur as the developing embryo/fetus ruptures and damages the tissues in which it has implanted.

ECTROPION A complication of blepharoplasty, in which the lower eyelid is pulled downward, exposing the conjunctival tissue below.

EDEMA The presence of abnormally large amounts of fluid in the intercellular tissue spaces of the body.

EDTA A colorless compound used to keep blood samples from clotting before tests are run.

EFFUSION The escape of fluid from blood vessels or the lymphatic system and its collection in a cavity.

EJACULATION The process by which semen (made up in part of prostatic fluid) is ejected by the erect penis.

EJECTION FRACTION The fraction of all blood in the ventricle that is ejected at each heartbeat. It is one of the most important measures of the heart's performance.

ELECTIVE Referring to a surgical procedure that is a matter of choice; an elective operation may be beneficial to the patient but is not urgently needed.

ELECTROCARDIOGRAM (ECG, EKG) A record of the electrical activity of the heart, with each wave being labeled as P, Q, R, S, and T waves. It is often used in the diagnosis of cases of abnormal cardiac rhythm and myocardial damage.

ELECTROCARDIOGRAPHY A test that uses electrodes attached to the chest with an adhesive gel to transmit the electrical impulses of the heart muscle to a recording device.

ELECTROCAUTERY The cauterization of tissue using electric current to generate heat.

ELECTROCOAGULATION The coagulation or destruction of tissue through the application of a high-frequency electrical current.

ELECTRODE A medium for conducting an electrical current.

ELECTRODESSICATION To make dry, dull, or lifeless with the use of electrical current.

ELECTROENCEPHALOGRAM (EEG) A record of the tiny electrical impulses produced by the brain's activity picked up by electrodes placed on the scalp. By measuring characteristic wave patterns, the EEG can help diagnose certain conditions of the brain.

ELECTROMYOGRAPHY (EMG) A diagnostic test that records the electrical activity of muscles. In the test, small electrodes are placed on or in the skin; the patterns of electrical activity are projected on a screen or over a loudspeaker. This procedure is used to test for muscle disorders, including muscular dystrophy.

ELECTRON One of the small particles that make up an atom. An electron has the same mass and amount of charge as a positron, but the electron has a negative charge.

ELECTRONYSTAGMOGRAPHY A method for measuring the electricity generated by eye movements. Electrodes are placed on the skin around the eye and the individual is subjected to a variety of stimuli so that the quality of eye movements can be assessed.

ELECTROPHYSIOLOGY STUDY A test that monitors the electrical activity of the heart in order to diagnose arrhythmia. An electrophysiology study measures electrical signals through a cardiac catheter that is inserted into an artery in the leg and guided up into the atrium and ventricle of the heart.

ELECTROSURGICAL DEVICE A medical device that uses electrical current to cauterize or coagulate tissue during surgical procedures; often used in conjunction with laparoscopy.

EMASCULATION Another term for castration of a male.

EMBOLISM A blood clot, air bubble, or mass of foreign material that travels and blocks the flow of blood in an artery. When blood supply to a tissue or organ is blocked by an embolism, infarction, or death of the tissue the artery feeds, occurs. Without immediate and appropriate treatment, an embolism can be fatal.

EMBOLIZATION A technique to stop or prevent hemorrhage by introducing a foreign mass, such as an air-filled membrane (balloon), into a blood vessel to block the flow of blood. This term also refers to an alternative to splenectomy that involves injecting silicone or a similar substances into the splenic artery to shrink the size of the spleen.

EMBOLUS Plural, emboli. An embolus is something that blocks the blood flow in a blood vessel. It may be a gas bubble, a blood clot, a fat globule, a mass of bacteria, or other foreign body that forms somewhere else and travels through the circulatory system until it gets stuck.

EMESIS BASIN A basin used to collect a patient's sputum or vomit.

EMPHYSEMA A chronic respiratory disease that involves the destruction of air sac walls to form abnormally large air sacs that have reduced gas exchange ability and that tend to retain air within the lungs. Symptoms include labored breathing, the inability to forcefully blow air out of the lungs, and an increased susceptibility to respiratory tract infections. Emphysema is usually caused by smoking.

EMPYEMA The collection of pus in a body cavity, particularly the lung or pleural cavity.

ENCEPHALITIS Inflammation of the brain, usually caused by a virus. The inflammation may interfere with normal brain function and may cause seizures, sleepiness, confusion, personality changes, weakness in one or more parts of the body, and even coma.

ENDEMIC Natural to or characteristic of a particular place, population, or climate.

ENDOCARDITIS Inflammation of the inner membrane lining heart and/or of the heart valves caused by infection.

ENDOCRINE Refers to glands that secrete hormones circulated in the bloodstream or lymphatic system.

ENDOCRINE SYSTEM A group of ductless glands and parts of glands that secrete hormones directly into the bloodstream or lymphatic system to control metabolic activity. Pituitary, thyroid, adrenals, ovaries, and testes are all part of the endocrine system.

ENDOCRINOLOGIST A physician who specializes in treating patients who have diseases of the thyroid, parathyroid, adrenal glands, and/or the pancreas.

ENDODONTIC Pertaining to the inside structures of the tooth, including the dental pulp and tooth root, and the periapical tissue surrounding the root.

ENDODONTIST A dentist who specializes in diagnosing and treating diseases of the pulp and other inner structures of the tooth.

ENDOLYMPH The watery fluid contained in the membranous labyrinth of the inner ear.

ENDOMETRIAL POLYP A growth in the lining of the uterus (endometrium) that may cause bleeding and can develop into cancer.

ENDOMETRIOSIS A condition in which the tissue that normally lines the uterus (endometrium) grows in other areas of the body, causing pain, irregular bleeding, and frequently, infertility.

ENDOMYOCARDIAL BIOPSY Removal of a small sample of heart tissue to check it for signs of damage caused by organ rejection.

ENDOPHTHALMITIS Inflammation of the eyeball.

ENDORPHINS A group of chemicals resembling opiates that are released in the body in response to trauma or stress. Endorphins react with opiate receptors in the brain to reduce pain sensations.

ENDOSCOPE A medical instrument that can be passed into an area of the body (the bladder or intestine, for example) to allow visual examination of that area. The endoscope usually has a fiber-optic camera that allows a greatly magnified image to be shown on a television screen viewed by the operator. Many endoscopes also allow the operator to retrieve a small sample (biopsy) of the area being examined, to more closely view the tissue under a microscope.

ENDOSCOPIC RETROGRADE CHOLANGIOPANCRE-ATOGRAPHY A diagnostic procedure in which a flexible tube with a light transmitter (endoscope) is inserted down the throat and into the pancreatic and bile ducts. A contrast dye is instilled directly into the ducts and a series of x-ray images are taken. This procedure is used to diagnose and treat blockages of the bile and pancreatic ducts.

ENDOSCOPIC ULTRASOUND A medical procedure in which sound waves are sent to an organ or other body structure by an ultrasound probe attached to the end of an endoscope. The pattern of echoes generated by the reflected sound waves are translated into an image of the organ by a computer.

ENDOSCOPY Visual examination of an organ or body cavity using an endoscope, a thin, tubular instrument containing a camera and light source. Many endoscopes also allow the retrieval of a small sample (biopsy) of the area being examined, in order to more closely view the tissue under a microscope.

ENDOTRACHEAL Placed within the trachea, also known as the windpipe.

ENDOTRACHEAL TUBE A hollow tube that is inserted into the trachea (windpipe) through the nose or mouth. It is used to administer anesthesia, to deliver oxygen under pressure, or to deliver medications (e.g. surfactants).

END-STAGE HEART FAILURE Severe heart disease that does not respond adequately to medical or surgical treatment.

ENEMA The introduction of water or another liquid into the bowels through a tube inserted into the anus. Enemas are used to treat constipation and for other purposes.

ENOPHTHALMOS A condition in which the eye falls back into the socket and inhibits proper eyelid function.

ENTERAL NUTRITION Liquid nutrition provided through tubes that enter the gastrointestinal tract, usually through the mouth or nose.

ENTEROSTOMAL THERAPIST A specialized counselor, usually a registered nurse, who provides ostomy patients with education and counseling before surgery. After surgery, the therapist helps the patient learn to take care of the stoma and appliance, and offers long-term emotional support.

ENTITLEMENT A program that creates a legal obligation by the federal government to any person, business, or government entity that meets the legally defined criteria. Medicare is an entitlement for eligible individuals.

ENUCLEATION Surgical removal of the eyeball.

ENZYME A protein that catalyzes a biochemical reaction without changing its own structure or function.

EOSINOPHIL A type of white blood cell containing granules that can be stained by eosin (a chemical that produces a red stain). Eosinophils increase in response to parasitic infections and allergic reactions.

EPHEDRA A herb used in traditional Chinese medicine to treat asthma and hay fever. It should never be used for weight management.

EPIDERMIS The outermost layer of the human skin.

EPIDIDYMIS A small, coiled tube connected to each testis where sperm mature and are stored. The epididymis empties into the vase deferens or sperm duct.

EPIDIDYMITIS Inflammation of the epididymis, a small, coiled tube that is part of the system that carries sperm from the testes to the penis. The condition can be successfully treated with antibiotics if necessary.

EPIDURAL ANESTHESIA A type of anesthesia in which a local anesthetic is injected into the epidural space of the spinal cord to numb the nerves leading to the lower half of the body.

EPIDURAL SPACE The space immediately surrounding the outermost membrane (dura mater) of the spinal cord.

EPIGLOTTIS A leaf-like piece of cartilage extending upwards from the larynx, which can close like a lid over the trachea to prevent the airway from receiving any food or liquid being swallowed.

EPIKERATOPHAKIA A procedure in which the donor cornea is attached directly onto the host cornea.

EPILEPSY A neurological disorder characterized by recurrent seizures with or without a loss of consciousness.

EPINEPHRINE A hormone produced by the adrenal medulla. It is important in the response to stress and partially regulates heart rate and metabolism. It is also called adrenaline.

EPITHELIAL CELLS Cells that cover body surfaces, line body cavities, and form glands.

EPITHELIUM The layer of cells that covers body surfaces, lines body cavities, and forms glands.

ERBIUM:YAG A crystal made of erbium, yttrium, aluminum, and garnet that produces light that is well absorbed by the skin, so it is used for laser skin resurfacing treatments.

ERUPTION The process of a tooth breaking through the gum tissue to grow into place in the mouth.

ERYTHEMA A diffuse red and inflamed area of the skin.

ERYTHROPOIETIN A hormone produced by the kidneys that stimulates the production of red blood cells by bone marrow.

ESCHAR A hardened, black crust or scab that may form over a wound. For example, in scrub typhus, an eschar forms over the initial sore from the chigger bite.

ESOPHAGEAL VARIX Plural: esophageal varices; an enlarged vein of the esophagus.

ESOPHAGECTOMY Surgical removal of the esophagus.

ESOPHAGITIS Inflammation of the esophagus.

ESOPHAGUS The muscular tube that leads from the back of the throat to the entrance of the stomach. It is coated with mucus and surrounded by muscles, and pushes food to the stomach by sequential waves of contraction.

ESTATE PLANNING Preparation of a plan of administration and disposition of one's property before or after death, including will, trusts, gifts, and power of attorney.

ESTROGEN Female hormone produced mainly by the ovaries and released by the follicles as they mature. Responsible for female sexual characteristics, estrogen stimulates and triggers a response from at least 300 tissues. After menopause, the production of the hormone gradually stops.

ETHMOID SINUSES Paired labyrinth of air cells between nose and eyes.

EUSTACHIAN TUBE A thin tube between the middle ear and the pharnyx. Its purpose is to equalize pressure on either side of the ear drum.

EUTHANASIA To bring about the death of another person who is suffering from an incurable disease or condition.

EVENT RECORDER A small machine, worn by a patient usually for several days or weeks, that is activated by the patient to record his or her EKG when a symptom is detected.

EXCIMER LASER An instrument that is used to vaporize tissue with a cold, coherent beam of light with a single wavelength in the ultraviolet range.

EXCISION The process of excising, removing completely, or amputating.

EXOPHTHALMOS A condition in which the eyes stick out of their sockets and inhibit proper eyelid function.

EXTRACORPOREAL Outside of, or unrelated to, the body.

EXTRACORPOREAL CIRCUIT The path the hemodialysis patient's blood takes outside of the body. It typically consists of plastic tubing, a hemodialysis machine, and a dialyzer.

EXTRACORPOREAL SHOCK WAVE LITHOTRIPSY (ESWL) This is a technique that uses high-pressure waves similar to sound waves that can be "focused" on a very small area, thereby fracturing small solid objects such as gallstones, kidney stones, etc. The small fragments can pass more easily and harmlessly into the intestine or can be dissolved with medications.

EXTRACTION The removal of a tooth from its socket in the bone.

EXTRACTION SITE The empty tooth socket following removal of the tooth.

EXTRAOCULAR MUSCLES The muscles (lateral rectus, medial rectus, inferior rectus, superior rectus, superior oblique, and inferior oblique) that move the eyeball.

EXUDATE Cells, protein, fluid, or other materials that pass through cell or blood vessel walls. Exudates may accumulate in the surrounding tissue or may be discharged outside the body.

F

FACE LIFT Plastic surgery performed to remove sagging skin and wrinkles from the patient's face.

FALLOPIAN TUBES The pair of narrow tubes leading from a woman's ovaries to the uterus. After an egg is released from the ovary during ovulation, fertilization (the union of sperm and egg) normally occurs in the fallopian tubes.

FALSE NEGATIVE A test result that falsely shows the absence of a disease or condition when the disease or condition actually is present.

FALSE POSITIVE A test result that falsely shows the presence of a disease or condition when the disease or conditon is not present.

FASCIA The sheet of connective tissue that covers the body under the skin and envelops every muscle, bone, nerve, gland, organ, and blood vessel. Fascia helps the body to retain its basic shape.

FATIGUE Loss of energy, tiredness.

FECAL INCONTINENCE Inability to control bowel movements.

FECAL OCCULT BLOOD TEST A blood test that chemically checks the stool for hidden (occult) blood.

FEDERAL POVERTY LEVEL (FPL) The definition of poverty provided by the federal government, used as the reference point to determine Medicaid eligibility for certain groups of beneficiaries. The FPL is adjusted every year to allow for inflation.

FEMALE STERILIZATION The process of permanently ending a woman's ability to conceive by tying off or severing the fallopian tubes.

FEMORAL ARTERY An artery located in the groin area that is the most frequently accessed site for arterial puncture in angiography.

FEMUR The thigh bone.

FIBER Carbohydrate material in food that cannot be digested.

FIBEROPTICS In medicine, fiberoptics uses glass or plastic fibers to transmit light through a specially designed tube. The tube is inserted into organs or body cavities where it transmits a magnified image of the internal body structures.

FIBRILLATION Rapid, uncoordinated contractions of the upper or the lower chambers of the heart.

FIBRIN The last step in the blood coagulation process. Fibrin forms strands that add bulk to a forming blood clot to hold it in place and help "plug" an injured blood vessel wall.

FIBRINOGEN A type of blood protein called a globulin that interacts with thrombin to form fibrin.

FIBROBLASTS A type of undifferentiated cell found in connective tissue.

FIBROID TUMOR A non-cancerous (benign) growth in the uterus. Fibroids occur in 30-40% of women over age 40, and do not need to be removed unless they are causing symptoms that interfere with a woman's normal activities. Also called a uterine fibroid.

FIBROSIS The formation of fibrous, or scar, tissue which may follow inflammation and destruction of normal tissue.

FIBROUS CONNECTIVE TISSUE Dense tissue found in various parts of the body containing very few living cells.

FINE NEEDLE ASPIRATION BIOPSY A procedure using a thin needle to remove fluid and cells from a lump in the breast.

FINGER STICK A technique for collecting a very small amount of blood from the fingertip area.

FISTULA An abnormal channel that connects two organs or connects an organ to the skin.

FLAP A section of tissue moved from one area of the body to another.

FLOATERS Translucent specks that float across the visual field, due to small objects floating in the vitreous humor.

FLOW METER Device for measuring the rate of a gas (especially oxygen) or liquid.

FLUORESCEIN DYE A fluorescent yellow-orange chemical used to aid in examinations of various structures of the eye.

FLUOROSCOPE A device used in some radiology procedures that provides immediate images and motion on a screen much like those seen at airport baggage security stations. It is often used to visualize the placement of a catheter in a the patient's artery during cardiac catheterization.

FLUOROSCOPY An x-ray procedure that produces immediate images and motion on a screen. The images look like those seen at airport baggage security stations.

FOLEY CATHETER A two-channel catheter with a balloon on the bladder end of one channel. Once inflated, the balloon keeps the catheter securely in the bladder. The other channel of the catheter facilitates the flow of urine out of the bladder.

FORAMEN A small opening or passage.

FORCED EXPIRATORY VOLUME The maximum amount of air expired in one second.

FORESKIN A covering fold of skin over the tip of the penis.

FRACTIONATION A procedure for dividing a dose of radiation into smaller treatment doses. Also, a laboratory test or process in which blood or another fluid is broken down into its components.

FREE FLAP A section of tissue detached from its blood supply, moved to another part of the body, and reattached by microsurgery to a new blood supply.

FREQUENCY Sound, whether traveling through air or the human body, produces vibrations—molecules bouncing into each other—as the sound wave travels along. The frequency of a sound is the number of vibrations per second. Within the audible range, frequency means pitch—the higher the frequency, the higher a sound's pitch.

FUCHS' DYSTROPHY A hereditary disease of the inner layer of the cornea. Treatment requires penetrating keratoplasty. The lens of the eye may also be affected and require surgical replacement at the same time as the cornea.

FUNGAL Caused by a fungus.

FUNGUS A member of a group of simple organisms that are related to yeast and molds.

G

GADOLINIUM A very rare metallic element useful for its sensitivity to electromagnetic resonance, among other things. Traces of it can be injected into the body to enhance the pictures produced by magnetic resonance imaging.

GAIT Walking motions.

GALLBLADDER A small, pear-shaped organ located on the under surface of the right lobe of the liver. It is connected by a series of ducts (tube-like channels) to the liver, pancreas, and duodenum (first part of the small intestine). The gallbladder receives bile from the liver, and concentrates and stores it. After a meal, bile is squeezed out of the gallbladder into the intestine, where it aids in digestion of food.

GAMETE INTRAFALLOPIAN TRANSFER (GIFT) An assisted reproductive technique where eggs are taken from a woman's ovaries, mixed with sperm, and then deposited into the woman's fallopian tube in the hope that fertilization will occur.

GAMMA RAY Short wavelength, high energy electromagnetic radiation emitted by radioactive substances.

GANGRENE Decay or death of body tissue because the blood supply is cut off. Tissues that have died in this way must be surgically removed.

GANTRY A name for the couch or table used in a computed tomography scan. The patient lies on the gantry while it slides into the x-ray scanner.

GASTRIC ULCER An ulcer (sore) of the stomach, duodenum, or other part of the gastrointestinal system. Though the causes are not fully understood, they include excessive secretion of gastric acid, stress, heredity, the use of certain drugs (especially acetylsalicylic acid and nonsteroidal anti-inflammatory drugs), and the presence of the bacterium *Helicobacter pylori* in the gastrointestinal tract. Also called a peptic ulcer.

GASTRIN A hormone secreted in the stomach that is involved in the production of gastric acid. Overproduction of gastric acid contributes to gastric (peptic) ulcer formation.

GASTROENTEROLOGIST A physician who specializes in diseases of the digestive system.

GASTROENTEROLOGY The branch of medicine that specializes in the diagnosis and treatment of disorders affecting the stomach and intestines.

GASTROESOPHAGEAL REFLUX DISEASE (GERD) A disorder of the lower end of the esophagus in which the lower esophageal sphincter does not open and close normally. As a result the acidic contents of the stomach can flow backward into the esophagus and irritate the tissues.

GASTROINTESTINAL The digestive organs and structures, including the stomach and intestines.

GASTROINTESTINAL TUBE A tube surgically inserted into the stomach for feeding a patient who is unable to eat by mouth.

GASTROJEJUNOSTOMY A surgical procedure where the stomach is surgically connected to the jejunum (small intestine).

GENDER IDENTITY DISORDER (GID) A strong and lasting cross-gender identification and persistent discomfort with one's biological gender (sex) role. This discomfort must cause a significant amount of distress or impairment in the functioning of the individual.

GENDER REASSIGNMENT SURGERY The surgical alteration and reconstruction of a person's sex organs to resemble those of the other sex as closely as possible; it is sometimes called sex reassignment surgery.

GENE A building block of inheritance, which contains the instructions for the production of a particular protein, and is made up of a molecular sequence found on a section of DNA. Each gene is found on a precise location on a chromosome.

GENERAL ANESTHESIA Deep sleep induced by a combination of medicines that allows surgery to be performed.

GENERAL SURGEON A physician who has special training and expertise in performing a variety of surgical operations.

GENERALIZED INFECTION An infection that has entered the bloodstream and has general systemic symptoms such as fever, chills, and low blood pressure.

GENETIC Refers to genes, the basic units of biological heredity, which are contained on the chromosomes.

GENITAL Refers to the sexual or reproductive organs that are visible outside the body.

GESTATIONAL AGE The estimated age of a fetus expressed in weeks, calculated from the first day of the last normal menstrual period.

GIGANTISM Excessive growth, especially in height, resulting from overproduction of growth hormone during childhood or adolescence by a pituitary tumor. Untreated, the tumor eventually destroys the pituitary gland, resulting in death during early adulthood.

GINGIVITIS Inflammation of the gums in which the margins of the gums near the teeth are red, puffy, and bleeding. It is most often due to poor dental hygiene.

GLANS The cone-shaped tip of the penis.

GLAUCOMA A common eye disease characterized by increased fluid pressure in the eye that damages the optic nerve, which carries visual impulses to the brain. Glaucoma can be caused by another eye disorder, such as a tumor or congenital malformation, or can appear without obvious cause, but if untreated it generally leads to blindness.

GLENOID CAVITY The hollow cavity in the head of the shoulder blade that receives the head of the humerus to make the glenohumeral or shoulder joint.

GLOMERULONEPHRITIS An inflammation of the filtering units of the kidney (glomeruli). The condition hinders removal of waste products, salt, and water from the bloodstream, leading to serious complications. It is the most common cause of renal failure.

GLOTTIS The opening between the vocal cords at the upper part of the larynx.

GLUCOSE A simple sugar that serves as the body's main source of energy.

GLUCOSE-6-PHOSPHATE DEHYDROGENASE (G6PD) DEFICIENCY A sex-linked hereditary disorder in which the body lacks an enzyme that normally protects red blood cells from toxic chemicals. When people with this condition take certain drugs, their red blood cells break down, causing anemia.

GOITER Chronic enlargement of the thyroid gland.

GONADOTROPHIN Hormones that stimulate the ovary and testicles.

GONIOSCOPE An instrument used to examine the anterior chamber of the eye. It consists of a magnifier and a lens equipped with mirrors, which sits on the patient's cornea during the examination.

GONIOSCOPY A technique for examining the angle between the iris and the cornea with the use of a special mirrored lens applied to the cornea.

GONORRHEA A sexually transmitted disease that causes infection in the genital organs and may cause disease in other parts of the body.

GRAFT A transplanted organ or other tissue.

GRAFT-VERSUS-HOST DISEASE A life-threatening complication of certain grafts, especially bone marrow transplants, in which the donated tissue triggers an immune reaction against the recipient's body.

GRANULE A small grain or pellet. Medicines that come in granule form usually are mixed with liquids or sprinkled on food before they are taken.

GRANULOCYTE Any of several types of white blood cells that have granules in their cell substance. Neutrophils are the most common type of granulocyte.

GRAVEL The debris which is formed from a fragmented kidney stone.

GUIDE WIRE A wire that is inserted into an artery to guide a catheter to a certain location in the body.

GUIDED IMAGERY The use of relaxation and mental visualization to improve mood and/or physical well-being.

GUILLAIN-BARRÉ SYNDROME Progressive and usually reversible paralysis or weakness of multiple muscles usually starting in the lower extremities and often ascending to the muscles involved in respiration. The syndrome is due to inflammation and loss of the myelin covering of the nerve fibers, often associated with an acute infection. Also called acute idiopathic polyneuritis.

GUTTA PERCHA An inert latex-like substance used for filling root canals.

GYNECOMASTIA Overly developed or enlarged breasts in a male.

H

HAIR FOLLICLE The root of a hair (that portion of a hair below the skin surface) together with its epithelial and connective tissue coverings.

HALF-LIFE The time required for half of the atoms in a radioactive substance to decay.

HALLUCINATION A false or distorted perception of objects, sounds, or events that seems real. Hallucinations usually result from drugs or mental disorders.

HARMONIC SCALPEL A scalpel that uses ultrasound technology to seal tissues while it is cutting.

HEAD-UPRIGHT TILT TABLE TEST A test used to determine the cause of fainting spells. During the test, the patient is tilted at different angles on special table for a period time. During the test, the patient's heart rhythm, blood pressure, and other measurements are evaluated with changes in position.

HEART MONITOR LEADS Sticky pads placed on the chest to monitor the electrical activity of the heart. The pads are connected to an electrocardiogram machine.

HEARTBURN A burning sensation in the chest that can extend to the neck, throat, and face. It is the primary symptom of gastroesophageal reflux (the movement of stomach acid into the esophagus).

HELICOBACTER PYLORI A gram-negative rod-shaped bacterium that lives in the tissues of the stomach and causes inflammation of the stomach lining.

HEMAGGLUTINATION The clumping or clustering of red blood cells caused by certain viruses, antibodies, or other substances.

HEMATEMESIS Vomit that contains blood, usually seen as black specks in the vomitus.

HEMATOCRIT A measure of the percentage of red blood cells in the total volume of blood in the human body.

HEMATOLOGIST A medical specialist who specializes diseases and disorders of the blood and blood-forming organs.

HEMATOMA A localized collection of blood, often clotted, in body tissue or an organ, usually due to a break or tear in the wall of blood vessel.

HEMOCHROMATOSIS An inherited blood disorder that causes the body to retain excessive amounts of iron. This iron overload can lead to serious health consequences, including painful joints, diabetes, and liver damage, if the iron concentration is not lowered.

HEMODILUTION A technique in which the fluid content of the blood is increased without increasing the number of red blood cells.

HEMOGLOBIN An iron-containing pigment of red blood cells composed of four amino acid chains (alpha, beta, gamma, delta) that delivers oxygen from the lungs to the cells of the body and carries carbon dioxide from the cells to the lungs.

HEMOLYSIS The process of breaking down of red blood cells. As the cells are destroyed, hemoglobin, the component of red blood cells which carries the oxygen, is liberated.

HEMOPTYSIS Coughing up blood from the respiratory tract.

HEMORRHAGE Severe, massive bleeding that is difficult to control. The bleeding may be internal or external.

HEMORRHAGIC STROKE A disruption of the blood supply to the brain caused by bleeding into the brain.

HEMOSTASIS The stopping of bleeding..

HEMOTHORAX An accumulation of blood and fluid in the pleural cavity, usually as a result of trauma.

HEPARIN An organic acid that occurs naturally in the body and prevents blood clots. Heparin is also made synthetically and can be given as an anticoagulant treatment.

HEPATIC ARTERY The blood vessel supplying arterial blood to the liver.

HEPATITIS An inflammation of the liver, with accompanying liver cell damage or cell death, caused most frequently by viral infection, but also by certain drugs, chemicals, or poisons. May be either acute (of limited duration) or chronic (continuing). Symptoms include jaundice, nausea, vomiting, loss of appetite, tenderness in the right upper abdomen, aching muscles, and joint pain. In severe cases, liver failure may result.

HEPATOCELLULAR CARCINOMA A dangerous cancer of the liver that may develop in patients who have had hepatitis, sometimes as much as 20 or 30 years earlier. Also called hepatoma.

HEPATOCYTE A liver cell.

HEREDITARY Something which is inherited, that is passed down from parents to offspring. In biology and medicine, the word pertains to inherited genetic characteristics.

HEREDITARY SPHEROCYTOSIS An inherited blood disorder in which the red blood cells are relatively fragile and are damaged or destroyed when they pass through the spleen.

HERNIA A rupture in the wall of a body cavity, through which an organ may protrude.

HERNIATED DISK A blisterlike bulging or protrusion of the contents of the disk out through the fibers that normally hold them in place. It is also called a ruptured disk, slipped disk, or displaced disk.

HERNIORRHAPHY Surgical repair of a hernia.

HETEROTOPIC BONE Bone that develops as an excess growth around the hip joint following surgery.

HIATAL HERNIA A condition in which part of the stomach protrudes through the diaphragm into the chest cavity.

HIGH-DENSITY LIPOPROTEIN A cholesterol-poor protein-rich lipoprotein of blood plasma correlated with reduced risk of atherosclerosis.

HIRSUTISM An abnormal growth of hair on the face and other parts of the body caused by an excess of androgens.

HISTOCOMPATIBILITY A measure of the similarity of the antigens that characterizes how well the recipient and tissue donor are matched.

HISTOCOMPATIBILITY ANTIGENS Genetically determined antigens on the surface of body tissues. These antigens are particularly important in organ and tissue transplantation.

HLA TYPE Refers to the unique set of proteins called human leukocyte antigens. These proteins are present on each individual's cell and allow the immune system to recognize "self" from "foreign." HLA type is particularly important in organ and tissue transplantation.

HODGKIN'S DISEASE One of two general types of lymphoma (cancers that arise in the the lymphatic system and can invade other organs), Hodgkin's disease is characterized by lymph node enlargement and the presence of a large polyploid cells called Reed-Sternberg cells.

HOLISTIC A practice of medicine that focuses on the whole patient, and addresses the social, emotional, and spiritual needs of a patient as well as their physical treatment.

HOLTER MONITOR A small machine, worn by a patient usually for 24 hours, that continuously records the patient's electrocardiogram during usual daily activity.

HOMOCYSTEINE An sulfur-containing amino aid.

HORMONE A chemical messenger secreted by a gland or organ and released into the bloodstream. It travels via the bloodstream to distant cells where it exerts an effect.

HOSPICE A system of care for terminally ill persons. Hospice care is designed to keep the patient comfortable and to maintain an acceptable quality of life throughout the dying process.

HOST The organism in which a parasite lives, is nourished, grows, and reproduces.

HUMAN CHORIONIC GONADOTROPIN (HCG) A hormone produced by the placenta during pregnancy.

HUMAN LEUCKOCYTE ANTIGEN (HLA) A group of protein molecules located on bone marrow cells that can provoke an immune response. A donor's and a recipient's HLA types should match as closely as possible to prevent the recipient's immune system from attacking the donor's marrow as a foreign material that does not belong in the body.

HUMAN PAPILLOMA VIRUS (HPV) A virus that causes common warts of the hands and feet, as well as lesions in the genital and vaginal area. More than 50 types of HPV have been identified, some of which are linked to cancerous and precancerous conditions, including cancer of the cervix.

HUMERUS The bone of the upper arm.

HYDROCELE A collection of fluid between two layers of tissue surrounding the testicle; the most common cause of painless scrotal swelling.

HYDROCEPHALUS An abnormal accumulation of cerebrospinal fluid within the brain. This accumulation can be harmful by pressing on brain structures, and damaging them.

HYDROGEN The simplest, most common element known in the universe. It is composed of a single electron (negatively charged particle) circling a nucleus consisting of a single proton (positively charged particle). It is the nuclear proton of hydrogen that makes MRI possible by reacting resonantly to radio waves while aligned in a magnetic field.

HYDROXYAPATITE A calcium phosphate complex that is the primary mineral component of bone.

HYPERCHOLESTEROLEMIA A condition characterized by the presence of excessively high levels of cholesterol in the blood.

HYPERGLYCEMIA A condition characterized by excessively high levels of glucose in the blood. It occurs when the body does not have enough insulin or cannot use the insulin it does have to turn glucose into energy.

HYPERHIDROSIS Excessive sweating. Hyperhidrosis can be caused by heat, overactive thyroid glands, strong emotion, menopause, or infection.

HYPEROPIA The inability to see near objects as clearly as distant objects, and the need for accommodation to see objects clearly.

HYPEROSMOTIC DRUGS A class of glaucoma drugs that increase the osmotic pressure in the blood, which then pulls water from the eye into the blood.

HYPERPARATHYROIDISM An abnormal endocrine condition characterized by overactivity of the parathyroid glands. Symptoms include generalized aches and pains, depression, and abdominal pain.

HYPERTENSION Abnormally high arterial blood pressure, which if left untreated can lead to heart disease and stroke.

HYPERTHYROIDISM A condition characterized by abnormal over-functioning of the thyroid glands. Patients are hypermetabolic, lose weight, are nervous, have muscular weakness and fatigue, sweat more, and have increased urination and bowel movements. Also called thyrotoxicosis.

HYPERTROPHIC Refers to an increase in the size of a tissue or organ due to the enlargement of its cells rather than to cell multiplication.

HYPERTROPHY An increase in the size of a tissue or organ brought about by the enlargement of its cells rather than cell multiplication.

HYPHEMA Bleeding inside the anterior chamber of the eye.

HYPNOSIS The technique by which a trained professional induces a trance-like state of extreme relaxation and suggestibility in a patient. Hypnosis is used to treat amnesia and identity disturbances that occur in dissociative disorders.

HYPNOTICS A class of drugs that are used as a sedatives and sleep aids.

HYPOCHROMIC A descriptive term applied to a red blood cell with a decreased concentration of hemoglobin.

HYPOGLYCEMIA A condition characterized by abnormally low levels of glucose in the blood.

HYPOKALEMIA A condition characterized by a deficiency of potassium in the blood.

HYPOPARATHYROIDISM A condition caused by insufficient production of parathyroid hormone, which results in low levels of blood calcium.

HYPOPITUITARISM A condition characterized by underactivity of the pituitary gland.

HYPOSPADIAS A congenital abnormality of the penis in which the urethral opening is located on the underside of the penis rather than at its tip.

HYPOTENSION Low blood pressure.

HYPOTHERMIA A serious condition in which body temperature falls below 95°F (35°C). It is usually caused by prolonged exposure to the cold.

HYPOTHYROIDISM A disorder in which the thyroid gland produces too little thyroid hormone causing a de-

crease in the rate of metabolism with associated effects on the reproductive system. Symptoms include fatigue, difficulty swallowing, mood swings, hoarse voice, sensitivity to cold, forgetfulness, and dry/coarse skin and hair.

HYPOXEMIA A condition characterized by an abnormally low amount of oxygen in the arterial blood. It is the major consequence of respiratory failure, when the lungs no longer are able to perform their chief function of gas exchange.

HYPOXIA A condition characterized by insufficient oxygen in the cells of the body.

HYSTERECTOMY Surgical removal of the uterus.

I

IATROGENIC A condition that is caused by the diagnostic procedures or treatments administered by medical professionals. Iatrogenic conditions may be caused by any number of things including contaminated medical instruments or devices, contaminated blood or implants, or contaminated air within the medical facility.

IDIOPATHIC Refers to a disease or condition of unknown origin.

IDIOPATHIC THROMBOCYTOPENIA PURPURA A bleeding disorder caused by an abnormally low level of platelets in a patient's blood. Also called immune thrombocytopenic purpura.

ILEUM The third segment of the small intestine, connecting the jejunum and the large intestine.

ILEUS An obstruction of the intestines usually caused by the absence of peristalsis.

ILIAC ARTERY Large blood vessel in the pelvis that leads into the leg.

IMMUNE RESPONSE A physiological response of the body controlled by the immune system that involves the production of antibodies to fight off specific foreign substances or agents (antigens).

IMMUNE SYSTEM The system of specialized organs, lymph nodes, and blood cells throughout the body that work together to defend the body against foreign invaders (bacteria, viruses, fungi, etc.).

IMMUNOASSAY A laboratory method for detecting the presence of a substance by using an antibody that reacts with it.

IMMUNOCOMPROMISED A state in which the immune system is suppressed or not functioning properly.

IMMUNODEFICIENCY A condition in which the body's immune response is damaged, weakened, or is not functioning properly.

IMMUNOGLOBULIN (IG) An antibody formed by mature B cells in response to foreign proteins (antigens) in the body. There are five types of immunoglobulins, but the major one is gamma globulin or immunoglobulin G.

IMMUNOSUPPRESSANT Any chemical substance that suppresses the natural functioning of the immune system.

IMMUNOSUPPRESSION Techniques used to prevent transplant graft rejection by the recipient's immune system.

IMMUNOSUPPRESSIVE Any agent that suppresses the immune response of an individual.

IMMUNOSUPPRESSIVE DRUGS Medications given to transplant recipients to prevent their immune systems from attacking the transplanted organs.

IMMUNOTHERAPY A mode of cancer treatment in which the immune system is stimulated to fight the cancer.

IMPACTED TOOTH Any tooth that is prevented from reaching its normal position in the mouth by another tooth, bone, or soft tissue.

IMPACTION GRAFTING The use of crushed bone from a donor to fill in the central canal of the femur during hip revision surgery.

IMPLANTABLE CARDIOVERTER-DEFIBRILLATOR A device placed in the body to deliver an electrical shock to the heart in response to a serious abnormal rhythm.

INCARCERATED HERNIA A hernia of the bowel that can not return to its normal place without manipulation or surgery.

INCARCERATION The abnormal confinement of a section of the intestine or other body tissues. A femoral hernia may lead to incarceration of part of the intestine.

INCENTIVE SPIROMETER Device that is used postoperatively to prevent lung collapse and promote maximum inspiration. The patient inhales until a preset volume is reached, then sustains the volume by holding his or her breath for three to five seconds.

INCISION The medical term for a cut made by a surgeon into a tissue or organ.

INCISIONAL HERNIA Hernia occuring at the site of a prior surgery.

INCONTINENCE A condition characterized by the inability to control urination or bowel functions.

INCUS The middle of the three bones of the middle ear. It is also known as the anvil.

INDEMNITY Protection, as by insurance, against damage or loss.

INFARCTION Death of tissue due to inadequate blood supply.

INFECTIOUS DISEASE TEAM A team of physicians who help control the hospital environment to protect patients against harmful sources of infection.

INFERIOR VENA CAVA The large vein that returns blood to the heart from the lower half of the body.

INFERTILITY The inability of a man and woman to conceive a child after 12 months of unprotected sexual intercourse.

INFLAMMATION Pain, redness, swelling, and heat that develop in response to tissue irritation or injury. It usually is caused by the immune system's response to the the body's contact with a foreign substance, such as an allergen or pathogen.

INFLAMMATORY BOWEL DISEASE A chronic inflammatory disease that can affect any part of the gastrointestinal tract. Ulcerative colitis and Crohn's disease are both inflammatory bowel diseases.

INFORMED CONSENT An educational process between health care providers and patients intended to instruct the patient about the nature and purpose of the procedure or treatment, the risks and benefits of the procedure, and alternatives, including the option of not proceeding with the test or treatment.

INFUSION Introduction of a substance directly into a vein or tissue by gravity flow.

INGUINAL Referring to the groin area.

INGUINAL HERNIA An opening, weakness, or bulge in the lining tissue of the abdominal wall in the groin area, with protrusion of the large intestine.

INJECTION Forcing a fluid into the body by means of a needle and syringe.

INJECTION SNOREPLASTY A technique for reducing snoring by injecting a chemical that forms scar tissue near the base of the uvula, helping to anchor it and reduce its fluttering or vibrating during sleep.

INNER EAR The interior section of the ear, where sound vibrations and information about balance are translated into nerve impulses.

INOTROPIC DRUGS Medications used to stimulate the heart beat.

INPATIENT SURGERY Surgery that requires an overnight stay of one or more days in the hospital.

INSUFFLATION Inflation of the abdominal cavity using carbon dioxide; performed prior to laparoscopy to give the surgeon space to maneuver surgical equipment.

INTEGUMENT The skin.

INTERMITTENT CATHETERIZATION Periodic catheterization to facilitate urine flow.

INTERMITTENT CLAUDICATION Cramp-like leg pain and weakness caused by poor circulation of blood to leg muscles and brought on by walking.

INTERSTITIAL CYSTITIS A chronic inflammatory condition of the bladder involving symptoms of bladder pain, frequent urination, and burning during urination.

INTERSTITIAL LUNG DISEASE A group of more than 150 chronic lung diseases characterized by scarring or fibrosis of the lungs. The most common symptoms are a dry, non-productive cough and shortness of breath with exercise. The causes include exposure to a foreign substance (such as asbestos or silica), infection, circulatory impairment, or an inherited condition.

INTERSTITIAL RADIATION THERAPY The process of placing radioactive sources directly into the tumor. These radioactive sources can be temporary (removed after the proper dose is reached) or permanent.

INTESTINAL PERFORATION A hole in the intestinal wall.

INTESTINES Also called the bowels and divided into the large and small intestine, they extend from the stomach to the anus, where waste products exit the body. The small intestine is about 20 ft (6.1 m) long and the large intestine, about 5 ft (1.5 m) long.

INTRA-ABDOMINAL PRESSURE Pressure that occurs within the abdominal cavity. Pressure in this area builds up with coughing, crying, and the pressure exerted when bearing down with a bowel movement.

INTRACRANIAL Refers to the area within the skull or cranium.

INTRACYTOPLASMIC SPERM INJECTION A process used to inject a single sperm into each egg before the fertilized eggs are put back into the woman's body. It may be used if the male has a low sperm count.

INTRAOCULAR LENS (IOL) A small, plastic device that is usually implanted in the lens capsule of the eye to correct vision after the lens of the eye is removed. This is the implant is used in cataract surgery.

INTRAOCULAR PRESSURE (IOP) The pressure inside the eye as measured by tonometry.

INTRATHECAL Introduced into or occurring in the space under the arachnoid membrane that covers the brain and spinal cord.

INTRAVENOUS Into a vein; a needle is inserted into a vein in the back of the hand, inside the elbow, or some other location on the body. Fluids, nutrients, and drugs can be injected.

INTRAVENOUS PYELOGRAM (IVP) X rays of the kidneys, ureters, and bladder using a contrast agent that is excreted by the kidneys into the urine. IVPs are most often done to assess structural abnormalities or obstruction to urine flow.

INTRAVENOUS SEDATION A method of injecting a fluid sedative into the blood through the vein.

INTRAVENTRICULAR HEMORRHAGE A condition in which blood vessels within the brain burst and bleed into the hollow chambers (ventricles) normally reserved for cerebrospinal fluid and into the tissue surrounding them.

INTRINSIC SPHINCTER DEFICIENCY One of the major factors in stress incontinence. Loss of support of the urethra causes the internal sphincter muscles to be unable to keep the bladder neck closed due to lack of contractive ability.

INTUBATION A procedure in which a tube is inserted through the mouth and into the trachea to keep the airway open and to help a patient breathe.

INTUSSUSCEPTION The slipping or telescoping of one part of the intestine into the section next to it.

INVASIVE Characterized by a tendency to spread or intrude. An invasive diagnostic test cuts through healthy tissue. An invasive cancer is one that spreads into the tissue surrounding the original tumor.

INVASIVE SURGERY Surgery that involves making an incision in the patient's body and inserting instruments or other medical devices into it.

IONIZING RADIATION Radiation that can damage living tissue by disrupting and destroying individual cells at the molecular level. All types of nuclear radiation—x rays, gamma rays, and beta rays—are potentially ionizing. Sound waves physically vibrate the material through which they pass, but do not ionize it.

IRIDECTOMY Removal of a portion of the iris.

IRIDOPLASTY Surgery to alter the iris.

IRIDOTOMY A procedure in which a laser is used to make a small hole in the iris to relieve fluid pressure in the eye.

IRIS The circular membrane that forms the colored portion of the eye and expands or contracts around the pupil.

ISCHEMIA A decrease in the blood supply to an area of the body caused by obstruction or constriction of blood vessels.

ISCHEMIC Refers to ischemia, a decrease in the blood supply to an area of the body caused by obstruction or constriction of blood vessels.

ISLETS OF LANGERHANS Clusters of cells in the pancreas that produce the hormones insulin and glucagon.

ISOENZYME One of a group of enzymes that catalyze the same reaction but are differentiated by variations in their physical properties.

J

JAUNDICE A condition in which the skin and whites of the eyes take on a yellowish color due to an increase of bilirubin (a compound produced by the liver) in the blood. Also called icterus.

JEJUNOSTOMY A surgical procedure that creates an opening through the abdominal wall to the middle portion of the small intestine (jejunum).

JUGULAR VEIN Major vein of the neck that returns blood from the head to the heart.

K

KEGEL EXERCISES A series of contractions and relaxations of the muscles in the perineal area. These exercises are thought to strengthen the pelvic floor and may help prevent urinary incontinence in women. Also called pubococcygeal exercises or pelvic muscle exercises.

KELOID An unusual or abnormal growth of scar tissue.

KERATINOCYTE A cell found in the epidermis. The keratinocytes at the outer surface of the epidermis are dead and form a tough protective layer. The cells underneath divide to replenish the supply.

KERATOCONUS An eye condition in which the central part of the cornea bulges outward, interfering with normal vision. Usually both eyes are affected.

KERATOMETER A device that measures the curvature of the cornea. It is used to determine the correct power for an IOL prior to cataract surgery.

KETONES Poisonous acidic chemicals produced by the body when fat instead of glucose is burned for energy. Breakdown of fat occurs when not enough insulin is present to channel glucose into body cells.

KETOSIS An abnormal increase in ketones in the body, usually found in people with uncontrolled diabetes mellitus.

KIDNEY STONE A hard mass that occurs in the kidney, a kidney stone can cause pain, bleeding, obstruction, or infection. Stones are primarily made up of calcium. Also called a renal calculus.

KNEE SURGERY Refers primarily to knee repair, replacement or revision of parts of the knee, both tissue and bond, and includes both arthroscopic and open surgeries.

L

LABIAL Referring to the lips.

LACERATION A cut or separation of skin or other tissue by a tremendous force, producing irregular edges. Also called a tear.

LAMINAE The broad plates of bone on the upper surface of the vertebrae that fuse together at the midline to form a bony covering over the spinal canal.

LAMINECTOMY A surgical procedure in which the surgeon cuts through the covering of a vertebra to reach a herniated disk in order to remove it.

LAMINOTOMY A less invasive alternative to a laminectomy in which a hole is drilled through the lamina.

LAPAROSCOPE An optical or fiberoptic instrument that is inserted by incision in the abdominal wall and is used to view the interior of the peritoneal cavity.

LAPAROSCOPIC CHOLECYSTECTOMY Removal of the gallbladder using a laparoscope, a fiberoptical instrument inserted through the abdomen.

LAPAROSCOPY A surgical procedure in which a small incision is made, usually in the navel, through which a viewing tube (laparoscope) is inserted. This allows the doctor to examine abdominal and pelvic organs. Other small incisions can be made to insert instruments to perform procedures. Laparoscopy is done to diagnose conditions or to perform certain types of surgeries.

LARGE CORE NEEDLE BIOPSY A procedure using a thicker needle to remove a core of tissue, about the size of a grain of rice, from the breast.

LARYNGECTOMY Surgical removal of the larynx to treat cancer.

LARYNGOSCOPE An endoscope that is used to examine the interior of the larynx.

LARYNGOSCOPY A medical procedure that uses flexible, lighted, narrow tubes inserted through the mouth or nose to examine the larynx and other areas deep inside the neck.

LARYNGOSPASM Spasmodic closure of the larynx.

LARYNX Also known as the voice box, the larynx is the part of the airway that lies between the pharynx and the trachea. It is composed of cartilage that contains the apparatus for voice production—the vocal cords and the muscles and ligaments that move the cords.

LASER A device that concentrates electromagnetic radiation into a narrow beam and treats tissue quickly without heating surrounding areas.

LASER PERIPHERAL IRIDOTOMY A procedure that uses a laser to create a drainage hole in the iris to allow the fluid to drain from the eye.

LASER SKIN RESURFACING The use of laser light to remove the uppermost layer of skin. Two types of lasers commonly used in this manner are CO_2 and Erbium.

LASER THERAPY A cancer treatment that uses a laser beam (a narrow beam of intense light) to kill cancer cells.

LASER-ASSISTED IN-SITU KERATOMILEUSIS (LASIK) A procedure that uses a cutting tool and a laser to modify the cornea and correct moderate to high levels of myopia (nearsightedness).

LATERAL RELEASE SURGERY Release of tissues in the knee that keep the kneecap from tracking properly in its groove (sulcus) in the femur; by realigning or tightening tendons, the kneecap can be forced to track properly.

LE FORT FRACTURE A term that refers to a system for classifying fractures of the facial bones into three groups according to the region affected.

LEAD An electrode that is attached to the skin to record electrical activity.

LEGG-CALVE-PERTHES DISEASE (LCP) A disorder in which the femoral head deteriorates within the hip joint as a result of insufficient blood supply.

LEGIONNAIRES' DISEASE A type of pneumonia caused by *Legionella* bacteria.

LEIOMYOSARCOMA A malignant tumor of smooth muscle origin. Smooth muscle is the major structural component of most hollow internal organs and the walls of blood vessels. Can occur almost anywhere in the body, but is most frequent in the uterus and gastrointestinal tract.

LENS The transparent, elastic, curved structure behind the iris (colored part of the eye) that helps focus light on the retina. Also refers to any device that bends light waves.

LEUKEMIA A cancer of the blood-forming organs (bone marrow and lymph system) characterized by an abnormal increase in the number of white blood cells in the tissues. There are many types of leukemias and they are classified according to the type of white blood cell involved.

LICENSED PRACTICAL NURSE (LPN) A person who is licensed to provide basic nursing care under the supervision of a physician or a registered nurse.

LIFE SUPPORT Methods of replacing or supporting a failing bodily function, such as using mechanical ventilation to support breathing. In treatable or curable conditions, life support is used temporarily to aid healing, until the body can resume normal functioning.

LIGAMENT A type of tough, fibrous tissue that connects bones or cartilage and provides support and strength to joints.

LIGAMENTA FLAVA Singular, ligamentum flavum. A series of bands of tissue that are attached to the vertebrae in the spinal column. They help to hold the spine straight and to close the spaces between the laminar arches. The Latin name means "yellow band(s)."

LIGATION Tying off a blood vessel or other structure with cotton, silk, or some other material. Rubber band ligation is one approach to treating internal hemorrhoids.

LIPIDS Organic compounds not soluble in water, but soluble in fat solvents such as alcohol. Lipids are stored in the body as energy reserves and are also important components of cell membranes.

LIPOMA A usually benign tumor of fatty tissue.

LIPOPROTEIN A lipid and protein chemically bound together, which aids in tansfer of the lipid in and out of cells, across the wall of the intestine, and through the bloodstream. There are five major types of lipoproteins.

LIPOSHAVING Liposhaving involves removing fat that lies closer to the skins surface by using a needle-like instrument that contains a sharp-edged shaving device.

LIPOSUCTION A surgical technique for removing fat from under the skin by vacuum suctioning.

LITHOTRIPSY A nonsurgical technique for removing gallstones by breaking them apart with high-frequency sound waves.

LIVING WILL A legal document detailing a person's wishes during the end of life, to be carried out by designated decision makers.

LOBECTOMY A surgical procedure that removes one lobe of the thyroid.

LOCAL ANESTHETIC Medication applied topically to the skin or administered through an injection that deadens a specific part of the body and inhibits the sensation of pain without causing the patient to lose consciousness.

LOCALIZED INFECTION An infection that is limited to a specific part of the body and has local symptoms.

LONG-TERM CARE Residential care over a period of time. A nursing home is a type of long-term care facility that offers nursing care and assistance with daily living tasks.

LONG-TERM CARE (LTC) INSURANCE A type of private health insurance intended to cover the cost of long-term nursing home or home health care.

LOOP ELECTROCAUTERY EXCISION PROCEDURE (LEEP) A procedure for diagnosing and treating cervical abnormalities that uses a thin wire loop that emits a low-voltage high-frequency radio wave to excise tissue. It is considered better than either lasers or electrocautery because it can both diagnose and treat precancerous cells or early stage cancer at the same time.

LOUPE A convex lens used to magnify small objects at very close range. It may be held on the hand, mounted on eyeglasses, or attached to a headband.

LOW TRANSVERSE INCISION A type of incision made horizontally across the lower end of the uterus to perform a cesarean section. This kind of incision is preferred because it results in reduced blood loss and a decreased chance of rupture.

LOW-DENSITY LIPOPROTEIN (LDL) A type of lipoprotein that consists of about 50% cholesterol and is associated with an increased risk of CAD.

LUMBAR Referring to the part of the back between the chest and the pelvis.

LUMBAR VERTEBRAE The vertebrae of the lower back below the level of the ribs.

LUMEN The inner cavity or canal of a tube-shaped organ, such as the bowel.

LUMPECTOMY A surgical procedure in which the cancerous tumor in the breast is removed together with a small rim of normal tissue.

LUPUS ERYTHEMATOSUS A chronic inflammatory disease in which inappropriate immune system reactions cause abnormalities in the blood vessels and connective tissue.

LUXATE To loosen or dislocate the tooth from the socket.

LYMPH Clear, slightly yellow fluid carried by a network of thin tubes to every part of the body. Cells that fight infection are carried in the lymph.

LYMPH NODE DISSECTION The surgical removal of an anatomic group of lymph nodes.

LYMPH NODES Small, bean-shaped collections of tissue located throughout the lymphatic system. They produce cells and proteins that fight infection and filter lymph. Nodes are sometimes called lymph glands.

LYMPHATIC SYSTEM A network composed of vessels, lymph nodes, the tonsils, the thymus gland, and the spleen. It is responsible for transporting fluid and nutrients to the bloodstream and for maturing certain blood cells that are part of the body's immune system.

LYMPHEDEMA Swelling caused by an accumulation of fluid from faulty lymph drainage.

LYMPHOCYTE A type of white blood cell that participates in the immune response. The two main groups are the B cells that have antibody molecules on their surface and T cells that destroy antigens.

LYMPHOID TISSUE Any tissue relating to the lymphatic system.

LYMPHOMA A diverse group of cancers of the lymphatic system characterized by abnormal growth of lymphatic cells. Two general types are commonly recognized—Hodgkin's disease and non-Hodgkin's lymphoma.

LYMPHOPROLIFERATIVE An increase in the number of lymphocytes. Lymphocytes are a white blood cell (WBC) formed in lymphatic tissue throughout the body—in the lymph nodes, spleen, thymus, tonsils, Peyer patches, and sometimes in bone marrow. In normal adults, they comprise approximately 22%–28% of the total number of leukocytes in the circulating blood.

LYMPHOSCINTIGRAPHY A technique in which a radioactive substance that concentrates in the lymphatic vessels is injected into the affected tissue and mapped using a gamma camera, which images the location of the radioactive tracer.

M

MACROCYTIC A descriptive term applied to a larger than normal red blood cell.

MACROMASTIA Excessive size of the breasts.

MACROPHAGE A large white blood cell that engulfs and digests foreign invaders, such as bacteria and viruses, in an attempt to stop them from causing disease within the body.

MACULA The central part of the retina where the rods and cones are densest.

MACULAR DEGENERATION A condition usually associated with age in which the area of the retina called the macula is impaired due to hardening of the arteries (arteriosclerosis). This condition interferes with vision.

MAGNETIC FIELD The three-dimensional area surrounding a magnet, in which its force is active. During MRI, the patient's body is permeated by the force field of a superconducting magnet.

MAGNETIC RESONANCE IMAGING (MRI) An imaging technique that uses a large circular magnet and radio waves to generate signals from atoms in the body. These signals are used to construct detailed images of internal body structures and organs, including the brain.

MALABSORPTION Absorption of fewer calories.

MALABSORPTIVE A type of bariatric surgery in which a part of the stomach is partitioned off and connected to a lower portion of the small intestine in order to reduce the amount of nutrients that the body absorbs from the food.

MALIGNANCY A locally invasive and destructive growth.

MALIGNANT Cells that have been altered such that they have lost normal control mechanisms and are capable of local invasion and spread to other areas of the body. Often used to describe a cancer.

MALIGNANT HYPERTHERMIA A type of reaction (probably with a genetic origin) that can occur during general anesthesia and in which the patient experiences a high fever, muscle rigidity, and irregular heart rate and blood pressure.

MALLEUS One of the three bones of the middle ear. It is also known as the hammer.

MALOCCLUSION The misalignment of opposing teeth in the upper and lower jaws.

MALPRACTICE A doctor or lawyer's failure in his or her professional duties through ignorance, negligence, or criminal intent.

MAMMARY ARTERY A chest wall artery that descends from the aorta and is commonly used for bypass grafts.

MAMMARY HYPERPLASIA Increased size of the breast.

MAMMOGRAPHY X-ray imaging of the breast that can often detect lesions in the tissue too small or too deep to be felt.

MAMMOPLASTY A surgical procedure performed to change the size of the breasts.

MANDIBLE The lower jaw, a U-shaped bone attached to the skull at the temporomandibular joints.

MANNITOL A type of diuretic.

MARFAN SYNDROME An inherited disorder of the connective tissue that causes abnormalities of the patient's eyes, cardiovascular system, and musculoskeletal system. Major indicators are excessively long arms and legs, lax joints, and vascular defects.

MASTECTOMY, MODIFIED RADICAL A surgical procedure involving a total mastectomy with axillary lymph node dissection, but with preservation of the pectoral muscles.

MASTECTOMY, RADICAL A surgical procedure in which the breast, pectoral muscles, axillary lymph nodes, and associated skin and subcutaneous tissue are removed.

MASTECTOMY, SIMPLE A surgical procedure in which only the breast tissue, nipple, and a small portion of the overlying skin are removed.

MASTOID ANTRUM A cavity in the temporal bone of the skull, communicating with the mastoid cells and with the middle ear.

MASTOID BONE The prominent bone behind the ear that projects from the temporal bone of the skull.

MASTOID PROCESS The protrusions of bone behind the ears at the base of the skull.

MASTOIDITIS An inflammation of the bone behind the ear (the mastoid bone) caused by an infection spreading from the middle ear to the cavity in the mastoid bone.

MASTOPEXY Surgical procedure to lift a breast. It may be used on the opposite breast to achieve symmetrical appearance with a reconstructed breast.

MATCH How similar the HLA type (out of a possible six antigens) is between the donor and the recipient.

MATERNAL BLOOD SCREENING Screening that is normally done early in pregnancy to test for a variety of conditions. Abnormal amounts of certain proteins in a pregnant woman's blood raise the probability of fetal defects. Amniocentesis is recommended if such a probability occurs.

MAXILLA The bone of the upper jaw which serves as a foundation of the face and supports the orbits.

MAXILLARY SINUSES Sinuses located in the cheek under the eye next to the ethmoid sinus.

MEAN CORPUSCULAR HEMOGLOBIN (MCH) A measurement of the average weight of hemoglobin in a red blood cell.

MEAN CORPUSCULAR HEMOGLOBIN CONCENTRATION (MCHC) A measurement of the average concentration of hemoglobin in a red blood cell.

MEAN CORPUSCULAR VOLUME (MCV) A measurement of the average volume of a red blood cell.

MEAN PLATELET VOLUME (MPV) A measurement of the average volume of a platelet.

MECHANICAL VALVE There are three types of mechanical valves: ball valve, disk valve, and bileaflet valve.

MEDIASTINOSCOPY A medical procedure that allows the doctor to see the areas of the mediastinum, the cavity behind the breastbone the lies between the lungs, using a thin, lighted, hollow tube-shaped instrument (a mediastinoscope). The organs in the mediastinum include the heart and its vessels, the lymph nodes, trachea, esophagus, and thymus.

MEDIASTINUM The area between the lungs, bounded by the spine, breastbone, and diaphragm. The organs in the mediastinum include the heart and its vessels, the lymph nodes, trachea, esophagus, and thymus.

MEDICAID The federally funded program in the United States for state-operated programs that provide medical assistance to permanently disabled patients and to low-income people.

MEDICALLY NEEDY A term that describes a group whose coverage is optional with the states because of high medical expenses. These persons meet category requirements of Medicaid (they are children or parents or elderly or disabled) but their income is too high to qualify them for coverage as categorically needy.

MEDICARE The federally-funded national health insurance program in the United States for all people over the age of 65.

MEDICARE PART A Hospital insurance provided by Medicare, provided free to persons aged 65 and older.

MEDICARE PART B Medical insurance provided by Medicare that requires recipients to pay a monthly premium. Part B pays for some medical services Part A does not.

MEDIGAP A group of 10 standardized private health insurance policies intended to cover the coinsurance and deductible costs not covered by Medicare.

MEGACOLON Abnormal dilation of the colon.

MELANOCYTE The type of skin cell that creates melanin.

MELANOMA A malignant tumor arising from the melanocytic system of the skin and other organs.

MENGHINI NEEDLE A special needle used to obtain a sample of liver tissue.

MENIERE'S DISEASE A disease of the inner ear, marked by recurrent episodes of loss of balance (vertigo), hearing loss, and roaring in the ears (tinnitus) lasting several hours. Its cause is unknown.

MENINGES The three-layer membranous covering of the brain and spinal cord, composed of the dura mater, arachnoid, and pia mater. It provides protection for the brain and spinal cord, as well as housing many blood vessels and participating in the appropriate flow of cerebrospinal fluid.

MENINGITIS An infection or inflammation of the membranes that cover the brain and spinal cord. It is usually caused by bacteria or a virus.

MENISCUS One of two crescent-shaped pieces of cartilage attached to the upper surface of the tibia. The menisci act as shock absorbers within the knee joint.

METABOLISM The sum of all chemical reactions that occur in the body resulting in growth, transformation of foodstuffs into energy, waste elimination, and other bodily functions. These include processes that break down substances to yield energy and processes that build up other substances necessary for life.

METABOLITES Substances produced by metabolism or by a metabolic process.

METASTATIC The term used to describe a secondary cancer, or one that has spread from one area of the body to another.

METHOTREXATE A drug that interferes with cell growth and is used to treat rheumatoid arthritis as well as various types of cancer. Side-effects may include mouth sores, digestive upsets, skin rashes, and hair loss. Since this drug can supress an infant's immune system, it should not be taken by nursing mothers.

MICROCYTIC A descriptive term applied to a smaller than normal red blood cell.

MICRODERMABRASION A technique for skin resurfacing that uses abrasive crystals passed through a hand piece to even out skin irregularities.

MICROKERATOME A precision surgical instrument that can slice an extremely thin layer of tissue from the surface of the cornea.

MICROORGANISM An organism that is too small to be seen with the naked eye, such as a bacterium, virus, or fungus.

MICROSURGERY Surgery on small body structures or cells performed with the aid of a microscope and other specialized instruments.

MIDDLE EAR The cavity or space between the eardrum and the inner ear. It includes the eardrum, the three little bones (hammer, anvil, and stirrup) that transmit sound to the inner ear, and the eustachian tube, which connects the inner ear to the nasopharynx (the back of the nose).

MINIGRAFT/MICROGRAFT Transplantation of a small number of hair follicles, as few as one to three hairs, into a transplant site.

MINIMALLY INVASIVE SURGERY Surgical techniques, especially the use of small instruments and tiny video cameras, that allow surgery to take place without a full operative wound.

MIOTIC A drug that causes pupils to contract.

MISCARRIAGE Loss of the embryo or fetus and other products of pregnancy before the twentieth week. Often, early in a pregnancy, if the condition of the baby and/or the mother's uterus are not compatible with sustaining life, the pregnancy stops, and the contents of the uterus are expelled. For this reason, miscarriage is also referred to as spontaneous abortion.

MITRAL VALVE The heart valve that allows blood to flow from the left atrium to the left ventricle and prevents it from flowing backwards from the left ventricle into the left atrium. Also known as the bicuspid valve.

MIXED DENTITION A mix of both baby teeth and permanent teeth.

MIXED LYMPHOCYTE CULTURE A test that measures the level of reactivity between donor and recipient lymphocytes.

MOHS' MICROGRAPHIC SURGERY A surgical technique in which successive rings of skin tissue are removed and examined under a microscope to ensure that no cancer is left.

MONOCHORIONIC PREGNANCY A pregnancy in which twin fetuses share a placenta.

MONOCYTE A large white blood cell that is formed in the bone marrow and spleen. About 4% of the white blood cells in normal adults are monocytes. Monocytes increase in response to a variety of conditions including severe infections. They remove debris and microorganisms by phagocytosis.

MORBIDLY OBESE A term defining individuals who are more than 100 lb (45 kg) over their ideal body weight.

MORPHOLOGY Literally, the study of form. In medicine, morphology refers to size, shape, and structure rather than function.

MORTALITY The death rate, which reflects the number of deaths per unit of population in any specific region, age group, disease, or other classification, usually expressed as deaths per 1,000, 10,000, or 1,000,000.

MOTILITY The movement or capacity for movement of an organism or body organ. Indigestion is sometimes caused by abnormal patterns in the motility of the stomach.

MOUTHGUARD A plastic device that protects the upper teeth from injury during athletic events.

MUCOCILIARY Involving cilia of the mucous membranes of the respiratory system.

MUCOUS MEMBRANE The moist lining of a body cavity or structure, such as the nose or digestive tract.

MUCUS The thick fluid produced by the mucous membranes that line many body cavities and structures. It contains mucin, white blood cells, water, inorganic salts, and shed cells, and it serve to lubricate body parts and to trap particles of dirt or other contaminants.

MULTIPLE MYELOMA A cancer of a certain kind of white blood cell, called a plasma cell. It is the second most-common cancer of the blood.

MULTIPLE SCLEROSIS A progressive, autoimmune disease of the central nervous system characterized by damage to the myelin sheath that covers nerves. The disease, which causes progressive paralysis, is marked by periods of exacerbation and remission.

MURMUR An abnormal heart sound that can indicate a valve dysfunction.

MYCOBACTERIA A group of bacteria that includes *Mycobacterium tuberculosis*, the bacterium that causes tuberculosis, and other forms that cause related illnesses.

MYELOGRAM An x-ray image of the spinal cord, spinal canal, and nerve roots taken with the aid of a contrast dye.

MYELOMA Cancer that arises in the bone marrow and involves plasma cells, a type of white blood cell.

MYELOMENINGOCELES (MMC) A protrusion in the vertebral column containing spinal cord and meninges.

MYOCARDIAL INFARCTION The technical term for heart attack. Myocardial means heart muscle and infarction means death of tissue from lack of oxygen. It is characterized, in most cases, by severe, unremitting chest pain.

MYOGLOBIN A protein that holds oxygen in heart and skeletal muscle. Myoglobin levels rise after damage to either of these muscle types.

MYOMA A benign, fibroid tumor of the uterus.

MYOPIA Nearsightedness, a vision problem in which distant objects appear blurry. Myopia results when the cornea is too steep or the eye is too long and the light doesn't focus properly on the retina.

MYRINGOPLASTY Surgical restoration of a perforated tympanic membrane by grafting.

MYRINGOTOMY A surgical procedure in which an incision is made in the ear drum to allow fluid or pus to escape from the middle ear.

N

NARCOTIC A drug derived from opium or compounds similar to opium. Such drugs are potent pain relievers and can affect mood and behavior. Long-term use of narcotics can lead to dependence and tolerance.

NASAL CANNULA A piece of flexible plastic tubing with two small clamps that fit into the nostrils and provide supplemental oxygen flow.

NASOGASTRIC TUBE A long, flexible tube inserted through the nasal passages, down the throat, and into the stomach.

NEARSIGHTEDNESS A condition in which one or both eyes cannot focus normally, causing objects at a distance to appear blurred and indistinct. Also called myopia.

NECESSARY SURGERY Surgery that is required for the continuance of life and its quality.

NECROSIS Localized tissue death due to disease or injury, such as a lack of oxygen supply to the tissues.

NEEDLE BIOPSY The procedure of using a large hollow needle to obtain a sample of intact tissue.

NEONATAL JAUNDICE A disorder in newborns where the liver is too premature to conjugate bilirubin, which builds up in the blood.

NEONATE A newborn infant, from birth until 28 days of age.

NEOPLASM An abnormal formation of new tissue. A neoplasm may be malignant or benign.

NEOVASCULAR GLAUCOMA A form of glaucoma that results from uncontrolled diabetes or hypertension.

NEPHRECTOMY A surgical procedure in which the kidney is removed.

NEPHROLOGIST A doctor specializing in kidney disease.

NEPHROSCOPE An fiberoptic instrument that is inserted into the kidney through an incision in the back and used to locate kidney stones. The stones are broken up with high frequency sound waves and removed by suction through the scope.

NEPHROTOXIC Toxic, or damaging, to the kidney.

NEPHROTOXIN A substance that damages the kidneys.

NEUROBLASTOMA A type of cancer that originates in the adrenal glands or in nerve cells or tissue. Neuroblastomas occur most often in children.

NEUROFIBROMATOSIS A progressive genetic condition often including multiple café-au-lait spots, multiple raised nodules on the skin (neurofibromas), developmental delays, slightly larger head size, and freckles in the armpits, groin, and iris. Also known as von Recklinghausen's disease.

NEUROGENIC Caused by or originating in the nerves.

NEUROGENIC BLADDER A urinary problem of neurological origin in which there is abnormal emptying of the bladder with subsequent retention or incontinence of urine.

NEUROLOGIST A doctor who specializes in disorders of the nervous system, including the brain, spinal cord, and nerves.

NEUROMODULATION Electrical stimulation of a nerve for relief of pain.

NEUROPATHY A disease or abnormality of the peripheral nerves (the nerves outside the brain and spinal cord). Major symptoms include weakness, numbness, paralysis, or pain in the affected area.

NEUROSURGEON A surgeon who specializes in surgery of the nervous system, including the brain and nerves.

NEUROSURGERY Surgery performed on the brain.

NEUROTRANSMITTER A chemical messenger that transmits an impulse from one nerve cell to the next.

NEUTROPHIL The primary type of white blood cell involved in inflammation. Neutrophils are a type of granulocyte, also known as a polymorphonuclear leukocyte. They increase in response to bacterial infection and remove and kill bacteria by phagocytosis.

NICOTINE A colorless, oily chemical found in tobacco that makes people physically dependent on smoking. It is poisonous in large doses.

NITROUS OXIDE A colorless, sweet-smelling gas used by dentists for mild anesthesia. It is sometimes called laughing gas because it makes some patients feel giddy or silly.

NOCICEPTOR A nerve cell that is capable of sensing pain and transmitting a pain signal.

NONABLATIVE Not requiring removal or destruction of the epidermis. Some techniques for minimizing scars are nonablative.

NONINVASIVE Pertaining to a diagnostic procedure or treatment that does not require the skin to be broken or a body cavity to be entered.

NON-MYELOBLATIVE ALLOGENEIC BONE MARROW TRANSPLANT Also called "mini" bone marrow transplants. This type of bone marrow transplant involves receiving low-doses of chemotherapy and radiation therapy, followed by the infusion of a donor's bone marrow or peripheral stem cells. Mini transplants are still under investigation but are promising for the future.

NONPALPABLE Something that cannot be felt by hand. In cancer, growths that are nonpalpable are too small to be felt, but may be seen on ultrasound or mammogram.

NONPHARMACOLOGICAL Referring to therapy that does not involve drugs.

NONPROFIT HOSPITALS Hospitals that combine a teaching function with providing for uninsured within large, complex networks technically designated as nonprofit institutions. While the institution may be nonprofit, however, its services are allowed to make a profit.

NONSTEROIDAL ANTI-INFLAMMATORY DRUGS (NSAIDS) A group of drugs, including aspirin, ibuprofen, and naproxen, that are taken to reduce fever and inflammation and to relieve pain. They work primarily by interfering with the formation of prostaglandins, enzymes implicated in pain and inflammation.

NOREPINEPHRINE A hormone secreted by certain nerve endings of the sympathetic nervous system, and by the medulla (center) of the adrenal glands. Its primary function is to help maintain a constant blood pressure by stimulating certain blood vessels to constrict when the blood pressure falls below normal.

NORMAL FLORA The mixture of microorganisms normally found at specific body sites.

NORMOCHROMIC A descriptive term applied to a red blood cell with a normal concentration of hemoglobin.

NORMOCYTIC A descriptive term applied to a red blood cell of normal size.

NOSOCOMIAL INFECTION An infection acquired in a hospital setting.

NUCLEAR SCANNING A diagnostic technique that uses injected or ingested radioactive substances and a scanning device to gather information about various parts of the body.

NUCLEUS The central part of a cell that contains most of its genetic material, including chromosomes and DNA.

NURSE ANESTHETIST A registered nurse who has obtained advanced training in anesthesia delivery and patient care.

NYHA HEART FAILURE CLASSIFICATION A classification system for heart failure developed by the New York Heart Association. It includes the following four categories: I, symptoms with more than ordinary activity; II, symptoms with ordinary activity; III, symptoms with minimal activity; IV, symptoms at rest.

NYSTAGMUS An involuntary, rhythmic movement of the eyes.

O

OBESITY An abnormal accumulation of body fat, usually 20% or more over an individual's ideal body weight.

OBSTRUCTIVE SLEEP APNEA A potentially life-threatening condition characterized by episodes of breathing cessation during sleep alternating with snoring or disordered breathing. The low levels of oxygen in the blood of patients with OSA may eventually cause heart problems or stroke.

OCCLUSION The way upper and lower teeth fit together during biting and chewing. Also refers to the blockage of some area or channel of the body.

OCCULT Not visible or easily detected.

OCULAR HYPERTENSION A condition in which fluid pressure inside the eye is higher than normal but the optic nerve and visual fields are normal.

OCULAR MELANOMA A malignant tumor that arises within the structures of the eye. It is the most common eye tumor in adults.

OCULAR ORBIT The bony cavity containing the eyeball.

OINTMENT A thick, spreadable substance that contains medication and is meant to be used on the outside of the body.

OLIGOHYDRAMNIOS Low levels of amniotic fluid during pregnancy.

OMBUDSMAN A patient representative who investigates patient complaints and problems related to hospital service or treatment. He or she may act as a mediator between the patient, the family, and the hospital.

OMPHALOCELE A hernia that occurs at the navel.

ONCOGENE A gene that has to do with the regulation of cell growth. An alternation or abnormality of such a gene can produce cancer.

ONCOLOGIST A physician specializing in the diagnosis and treatment of cancer

ONCOLOGY The branch of medicine that deals with the diagnosis and treatment of cancer.

OOPHORECTOMY Surgical removal of the ovaries; often performed laparoscopically.

OPERATIVE NURSE A nurse specially trained to assist the surgeon and work in all areas of the surgical event to care for the patient.

OPHTHALMOLOGIST A physician who specializes in the anatomy and physiology of the eyes and in the diagnosis and treatment of eye diseases and disorders.

OPHTHALMOLOGY The medical specialty concerned with the anatomy and physiology of the eyes and the diagnosis and treatment of eye diseases and disorders.

OPHTHALMOSCOPE A medical instrument which shines a light through the pupil of the patient's eye and illuminates the retina (back) of the eye, allowing a visual examination of the interior of the eye.

OPIATE A drug that is derived from opium (i.e., morphine, hydromorphone, oxymorphone, heroin, codeine, hydrocodone, oxycodone) or that resembles these opium derivatives (e.g., meperidine). Commonly referred to as a narcotic.

OPIOID Any natural or synthetic substance that produces the same effects as an opiate, such as pain relief, sedation, constipation and respiratory depression. Some opioids are produced by the human body (e.g., endorphins), while others are produced in the laboratory (e.g., methadone).

OPTIC NERVE A bundle of nerve fibers that carries visual messages from the retina in the form of electrical signals to the brain.

OPTOMETRIST A health care professional who examines and tests the eyes for disease and treats visual disorders by prescribing corrective lenses and/or vision therapy. In many states, optometrists are licensed to use diagnostic and therapeutic drugs to treat certain ocular diseases.

ORAL AND MAXILLOFACIAL SURGEON A dentist who is trained to perform surgery to correct injuries, defects, or conditions of the mouth, teeth, jaws, and face.

ORBIT The eye socket which contains the eyeball, muscles, nerves, and blood vessels that serve the eye.

ORCHIECTOMY Surgical removal of one or both testes. Also called orchidectomy.

ORGANISM A single, independent unit of life, such as a bacterium, a plant, or an animal.

OROPHARYNX One of the three regions of the pharynx, the oropharynx is the region behind the mouth.

ORTHODONTIC TREATMENT The process of straightening teeth to correct their appearance and function.

ORTHOPEDIC SURGERY Surgical procedures performed on the supporting structures of the body—bones, joints, ligaments, and muscles.

ORTHOPEDICS A medical specialty concerned with treating diseases, injuries, and malformations of the bones and supporting structures, such as tendons, ligaments, and muscles.

ORTHOSIS An external device, such as a splint or a brace, that prevents or assists movement.

ORTHOTICS Mechanical devices or appliances that assist a motion or function or correct deformities of the musculoskeletal system.

OSMOLALITY A measure of the solute-to-solvent concentration of a solution. More specifically a measurement of urine concentration that depends on the number of particles dissolved in it.

OSSICLES The three small bones of the middle ear: the malleus (hammer), the incus (anvil) and the stapes (stirrup). These bones help carry sound from the eardrum to the inner ear.

OSTEOARTHRITIS A noninflammatory type of arthritis, usually occurring in older people, characterized by degeneration of cartilage, enlargement of the margins of the bones, and changes in the membranes in the joints. Also called degenerative arthritis.

OSTEOBLAST A bone-building cell.

OSTEOCLAST A large, multinuclear cell involved in the physiological destruction and absorption of bone.

OSTEOCONDUCTION Provision of a scaffold for the growth of new bone.

OSTEOCYTE A mature bone cell.

OSTEOGENESIS The growth of new bone.

OSTEOINDUCTION Acceleration of new bone formation by chemical means.

OSTEOLYSIS Dissolution and loss of bone resulting from inflammation caused by particles of polyethylene debris from a prosthesis.

OSTEOMALACIA A bone disease that occurs in adults due to a prolonged period of vitamin D deficiency. It is characterized by softening of the bone and is sometimes referred to as adult rickets.

OSTEOPATHY A system of medical practice that originally arose in the nineteenth century. Osteopathy now employs conventional methods of medical diagnosis and treatment while maintaining a particular emphasis on the interrelationship between the musculoskeletal system and the body's organs.

OSTEOPOROSIS Literally meaning "porous bones," this condition occurs when bones lose an excessive amount of their protein and mineral content, particularly calcium. Over time, bone mass and strength are reduced leading to increased risk of fractures.

OSTOMY A surgically-created opening in the abdomen for elimination of waste products (urine or stool).

OTITIS MEDIA Inflammation or infection of the middle ear space behind the eardrum. It commonly occurs in early childhood and is characterized by ear pain, fever, and hearing problems.

OTOLARYNGOLOGIST A doctor who is trained to treat injuries, defects, diseases, or conditions of the ear, nose, and throat. Also sometimes known as an otorhinolaryngologist.

OTOLOGIC Relating to the study, diagnosis, and treatment of diseases and disorders of the ear and related structures.

OTOSCLEROSIS A hereditary disorder characterized by an excessive growth in the bones of the middle ear, especially of the stapes, that interferes with the transmission of sound.

OTOSCOPE A hand-held instrument with a tiny light and a funnel-shaped attachment called an ear speculum, which is used to examine the ear canal and eardrum.

OUTPATIENT SURGERY Also called same-day or ambulatory surgery. The patient arrives for surgery and returns home on the same day.

OVARIAN CYST A sac containing fluid or semisolid material that develops in or on the surface of an ovary. Most are benign. An ovarian cyst can disappear without treatment or become painful and require surgical removal.

OVARY One of the two almond-shaped glands in the female reproductive system responsible for producing eggs and the sex hormones estrogen and progesterone.

OVULATION The monthly process by which an ovarian follicle ruptures releasing a mature egg cell.

OXIMETRY The measurement of the degree of oxygen saturation of circulating blood.

OXYGENATION Saturation with oxygen.

P

PACEMAKER A surgically implanted electronic device that regulates a slow or erratic heartbeat. The pacemaker sends electrical impulses via an insulated wire(s) to the chambers of the heart.

PAIN DISORDER A psychiatric disorder in which pain in one or more parts of the body is caused or made worse by psychological factors. The lower back is one of the most common sites for pain related to this disorder.

PALATE The roof of the mouth.

PALLIATIVE TREATMENT A type treatment that does not provide a cure, but eases the uncomfortable symptoms.

PALPATE To examine the body by touching or pressing with the fingers or the palm of the hand.

PALPEBRAL FISSURE The opening between the upper and lower eyelids.

PANCREAS A five-inch-long gland that lies behind the stomach and next to the duodenum. The pancreas releases glucagon, insulin, and some of the enzymes which aid digestion.

PANCREATICODUODENECTOMY Surgical removal of all or part of the pancreas along with the duodenum. Also known as "Whipple's procedure" or "Whipple's operation."

PANCREATITIS Inflammation of the pancreas, either acute (sudden and episodic) or chronic, usually caused by excessive alcohol intake or gallbladder disease.

PANIC DISORDER An anxiety disorder in which people have sudden and intense attacks of fear in certain situations. Symptoms such as shortness of breath, sweating, dizziness, chest pain, and extreme fear often accompany the attacks.

PAP TEST A screening test for precancerous and cancerous cells on the cervix. This simple test is done during a routine pelvic exam and involves scraping cells from the cervix. These cells are then stained and examined under a microscope. Also known as the Papanicolaou test.

PARACENTESIS A procedure in which fluid is drained from a body cavity by means of a catheter placed through an incision in the skin.

PARAQUAT A highly toxic restricted-use pesticide. Death following ingestion usually results from multiple organ failure.

PARASYMPATHETIC NERVOUS SYSTEM A part of the autonomic (involuntary) nervous system with nerves emerging from the brain or sacral region of the spinal cord. It slows heart rate, increases digestive and gland activity, and relaxes the sphincter muscles that close off body organs.

PARATHYROID GLANDS Two pairs of smaller glands that lie close to the lower surface of the thyroid gland. They secrete parathyroid hormone, which regulates the body's use of calcium and phosphorus.

PARAVAGINAL PROCEDURE A popular surgical procedure for stabilizing the urethra by a simple suturing of the urethra to supporting tissue.

PARENTERAL NUTRITIONAL SUPPORT Intravenous nutrition that bypasses the intestines and its contribution to digestion.

PARESTHESIA An abnormal sensation often described as burning, tickling, tingling, or "pins and needles."

PARIETAL CELLS Specific cells that line the inside of the stomach. These cells are responsible for secreting intrinsic factor and hydrochloric acid.

PARIETAL PERICARDIUM External or outer layer of the pericardial cavity.

PARONYCHIA Inflammation of the folds of skin that surround a nail.

PATELLA The kneecap.

PATELLECTOMY Surgical removal of the kneecap removal.

PATENT DUCTUS ARTERIOSUS A congenital defect in which the temporary blood vessel connecting the left pulmonary artery to the aorta in the fetus doesn't close after birth.

PATHOGEN Any disease-producing microorganism.

PATHOLOGIST A doctor who specializes in studying diseases. In particular, he/she examines the structural and functional changes in the tissues and organs of the body that are caused by disease or that cause disease themselves.

PATIENT SELF-DETERMINATION ACT (PSDA) Federal law that ensures that medical providers offer the option of medical directives to patients and include documents in their medical records.

PATIENT-CONTROLLED ANALGESIA An approach to pain management that allows the patient to control the timing of intravenous doses of analgesic drugs.

PECTUS CARINATUM An abnormality of the chest in which the sternum (breastbone) is pushed outward. It is sometimes called "pigeon breast."

PECTUS EXCAVATUM An abnormality of the chest in which the sternum (breastbone) sinks inward; sometimes called "funnel chest."

PEDIATRICS The medical specialty of caring for children.

PEDICLE FLAP Also called an attached flap. A section of tissue, with its blood supply intact, which is maneuvered to another part of the body.

PELVIC INFLAMMATORY DISEASE (PID) Any infection of the lower female reproductive tract (vagina and cervix) that spreads to the upper female reproductive tract (uterus, fallopian tubes, and ovaries). Symptoms include severe abdominal pain, high fever, and vaginal discharge. PID is the most common and most serious consequence of infection with sexually transmitted diseases in women and is a leading cause of female fertility problems.

PELVIC ORGANS The internal organs that are located within the confines of the pelvis. This includes the bladder and rectum in both sexes and the reproductive organs (uterus, ovaries, and fallopian tubes) in females.

PERCUSSION Thumping or tapping a part of the body with the fingers for diagnostic purposes.

PERCUTANEOUS Performed through the skin.

PERCUTANEOUS BIOPSY A biopsy in which a needle is inserted and a tissue sample removed through the skin.

PERCUTANEOUS TRANSLUMINAL CORONARY ANGIOPLASTY (PTCA) A cardiac intervention in which an artery blocked by plaque is dilated, using a balloon catheter to flatten the plaque and open the vessel; it is also called balloon angioplasty.

PERFORATION A hole.

PERFUSION LUNG SCAN A radiographic scan using a contrast dye to show the pattern of blood flow in the lungs.

PERINEAL AREA The genital area between the vulva and anus in a woman, and between the scrotum and anus in a man.

PERINEUM The area between the opening of the vagina and the anus in a woman, or the area between the scrotum and the anus in a man.

PERIODONTITIS Inflammation of the periodontium, the tissues that support and anchor the teeth. Without treatment it can destroy the structures supporting the teeth, including bone.

PERIPHERAL ARTERIAL DISEASE An occlusive disease of the arteries most often caused by progressive atherosclerosis.

PERIPHERAL BLOOD STEM CELL TRANSPLANT (PBSCT) A method for replacing blood-forming cells that are destroyed by cancer treatment. In PBSCT, peripheral blood stem cells obtained from ciculating blood are used for transplatation rather than bone marrow stem cells.

PERIPHERAL ENDARTERECTOMY The surgical removal of fatty deposits, called plaque, from the walls of arteries other than those of the heart and brain.

PERIPHERAL NERVES Nerves outside the brain and spinal cord that provide the link between the body and the central nervous system.

PERIPHERAL NERVOUS SYSTEM (PNS) The part of the nervous system that is outside the brain and spinal cord. Sensory, motor, and autonomic nerves are included. PNS nerves link the central nervous system with sensory organs, muscles, blood vessels, and glands.

PERIPHERAL VISION The ability to see objects that are not located directly in front of the eye. Peripheral vision allows people to see objects located on the side or edge of their field of vision.

PERISTALSIS Slow, rhythmic contractions of the muscles in a tubular organ, such as the intestines, that move the contents along.

PERITONEUM The transparent membrane lining the abdominal and pelvic cavities (parietal peritoneum) and the membrane forming the outer layer of the stomach and interstines (visceral peritoneum). Between the visceral and parietal peritoneums is a potential space called the peritoneal cavity.

PERITONITIS Inflammation of the peritoneum. It is most often due to bacterial infection, but can also be caused by a chemical irritant (such as spillage of acid from the stomach or bile from the gall bladder).

PERSONAL CARE ATTENDANT An employee hired either through a health-care facility, home care agency, or private agency to assist a patient in performing everyday activities.

PH A measurement of the acidity or alkalinity of a solution. Based on a scale of 14, a pH of 7.0 is neutral. A pH below 7.0 is an acid; the lower the number, the stronger the acid. A pH above 7.0 is a base; the higher the number, the stronger the base. Blood pH is slightly alkaline (basic) with a normal range of 7.36-7.44.

PHACOEMULSIFICATION A surgical procedure to remove a cataract using sound waves to disintegrate the lens which is then removed by suction.

PHAGOCYTOSIS A process by which certain cells envelope and digest debris and microorganisms to remove them from the blood.

PHARMACOLOGICAL Referring to therapy that relies on drugs.

PHARYNX The throat, a tubular structure that lies between the mouth and the esophagus.

PHENOTYPE The physical expression of an individual's genes.

PHENYLKETONURIA (PKU) A rare, inherited, metabolic disorder in which the enzyme necessary to break down and use phenylalanine, an amino acid necessary for normal growth and development, is lacking. As a result, phenylalanine builds up in the body causing mental retardation and other neurological problems.

PHEOCHROMOCYTOMA A tumor that originates from the adrenal gland's chromaffin cells, causing overproduction of catecholamines, powerful hormones that induce high blood pressure and other symptoms.

PHILTAL DIMPLE The skin or depression below the nose, extending to the upper lip in the midline.

PHIMOSIS A tightening of the foreskin that may close the opening of the penis.

PHLEBECTOMY Surgical removal of a vein or part of a vein.

PHLEBITIS Inflammation of a vein.

PHLEBOLOGY The study of veins, their disorders, and their treatments. A phlebologist is a doctor who specializes in treating spider veins, varicose veins, and associated disorders.

PHOBIA An intense and irrational fear of a specific object, activity, or situation that leads to avoidance.

PHOTOCOAGULATION A type of cancer treatment in which cancer cells are destroyed by an intense beam of laser light.

PHOTODYNAMIC THERAPY A novel mode of treatment in which a combination of special light rays and drugs are used to destroy the cancerous cells. First, the drugs, which make the cancerous cells more susceptible to the light rays, are administered. Then the light is shone on the target area to kill the cancer cells.

PHOTON A light particle.

PILES Another name for hemorrhoids.

PILOCARPINE Drug used to treat glaucoma.

PITUITARY GLAND The most important of the endocrine glands (glands that release hormones directly into the bloodstream), the pituitary is located at the base of the brain. Sometimes referred to as the "master gland," it regulates and controls the activities of other endocrine glands and many body processes including growth and reproductive function.

PLACENTA The organ that provides oxygen and nutrition from the mother to the unborn baby during pregnancy. The placenta is attached to the wall of the uterus and leads to the unborn baby via the umbilical cord.

PLACENTA PREVIA A condition in which the placenta totally or partially covers the cervix, preventing vaginal delivery.

PLACENTAL ABRUPTION An abnormal separation of the placenta from the uterus before the birth of the baby, with subsequent heavy uterine bleeding. Normally, the baby is born first and then the placenta is delivered within a half hour.

PLANTAR FASCIITIS An inflammation of the fascia on the bottom of the foot.

PLAQUE A deposit, usually of fatty material, on the inside wall of a blood vessel. Also refers to a small, round demyelinated area that develops in the brain and spinal cord of an individual with multiple sclerosis.

PLASMA A watery fluid containing proteins, salts, and other substances that carries red blood cells, white blood cells, and platelets throughout the body. Plasma makes up 50% of human blood.

PLASMA CELL A type of white blood cell that produces antibodies; derived from an antigen-specific B cell.

PLATELET A cell-like particle in the blood that plays an important role in blood clotting. Platelets are activated when an injury causes a blood vessel to break. They change shape from round to spiny, "sticking" to the broken vessel wall and to each other to begin the clotting process. In addition to physically plugging breaks in blood vessel walls, platelets also release chemicals that promote clotting.

PLEURAL CAVITY The area within the thorax that contains the lungs.

PLEURAL SPACE The potential area between the visceral and parietal layers of the pleurae.

PNEUMATIC RETINOPEXY Reattachment of a detached retina using an injected gas bubble to hold the retina against the back of the eye.

PNEUMOCYSTIS CARINII PNEUMONIA A severe lung infection caused by a fungus. The disease mainly affects people with weakened immune systems, such as people with AIDS.

PNEUMONIA An infection in which the lungs become inflamed. It can be caused by nearly any class of organism known to cause human infections, including bacteria, viruses, fungi, and parasites.

PNEUMOTHORAX A collection of air or gas in the chest or pleural cavity that causes part or all of a lung to collapse.

PODIATRIST A physician who specializes in the care and treatment of the foot.

PODIATRY A medical specialty concerned with treating diseases, injuries, and malformations of the feet.

POLAND SYNDROME A condition associated with chest wall deformities in which varying degrees of underdevelopment of one side of the chest and arm may occur.

POLIOMYELITIS A disorder caused by a viral infection (poliovirus) that can affect the whole body, including muscles and nerves.

POLYCYSTIC KIDNEY DISEASE A hereditary kidney disease that causes fluid- or blood-filled pouches of tissue called cysts to form on the tubules of the kidneys. These cysts impair normal kidney function.

POLYCYTHEMIA A condition characterized by an overabundance of red blood cells.

POLYCYTHEMIA VERA A chronic blood disorder marked by an abnormal increase in three types of blood cells produced by the bone marrow: red blood cells, white blood cells, and platelets. It is a myeloproliferative disorder, which means that the bone marrow produces too many cells too quickly.

POLYDACTYLY A developmental abnormality characterized by an extra digit on the hand or foot.

POLYP A growth that projects from the surface of any mucous membrane. Polyps are commonly found in the cervix, uterus, nose, bladder, intestines, and rectum.

POLYSOMNOGRAPHY An overnight series tests designed to evaluate a patient's basic physiological processes during sleep. Polysomnography generally includes monitoring of the patient's airflow through the nose and mouth, blood pressure, electrocardiographic activity, blood oxygen level, brain wave pattern, eye movement, and the movement of respiratory muscles and limbs

POLYSYNDACTYLY A condition involving both webbing and the presence of an extra number of fingers or toes.

PORPHYRIA Any of a group of inherited disorders of porphyrin metabolism characterized by excess pophyrins (various biologically active compounds with a distinct structure) in the urine and by extreme sensitivity to light.

PORPHYRIN An organic compound found in living things that founds the foundation structure for hemoglobin, chlorophyll, and other respiratory pigments. In humans, porphyrins combine with iron to form hemes.

PORTABLE CHEST X RAY An x ray procedure taken by equipment that can be brought to the patient. The resulting radiographs may not be as high in quality as stationary x ray radiographs, but allow a technologist to come to the bedridden patient.

PORTAL An entrance or a means of entrance.

PORTAL HYPERTENSION Increased pressure in the portal vein that forces the blood flow backward, causing the portal veins to enlarge and the emergence of bleeding varices across the esophagus and stomach from the pressure in the portal vein. Portal hypertension is most commonly caused by cirrhosis, but can also be seen in portal vein obstruction from unknown causes.

PORTAL VEIN The blood vessel carrying venous blood from the digestive organs to the liver.

PORTAL VEIN THROMBOSIS The development of a blood clot in the vein that brings blood into the liver. Untreated portal vein thrombosis causes portal hypertension.

POSITRON One of the small particles that make up an atom. A positron has the same mass and amount of charge as an electron, but the positron has a positive charge.

POSITRON EMISSION TOMOGRAPHY (PET) A computerized diagnostic technique that uses radioactive substances to examine structures of the body. When used to assess the brain, it produces a three-dimensional image that shows anatomy and function, including such information as blood flow, oxygen consumption, glucose metabolism, and concentrations of various molecules in brain tissue.

POSTERIOR CHAMBER The posterior part of the eye bound by the lens in front and the retina in back. The posterior chamber is filled with a jellylike substance called the vitreous.

POSTOPERATIVE CARE Medical care and support required after surgery to promote healing and recovery.

POSTPARTUM After childbirth.

POTASSIUM A mineral found in whole grains, meat, legumes, and some fruits and vegetables. Potassium is important for many body processes, including proper functioning of the nerves and muscles.

PREECLAMPSIA A condition that develops after the twentieth week of pregnancy and results in high blood pressure, fluid retention that doesn't go away, and large amounts of protein in the urine. Without treatment, it can progress to a dangerous condition called eclampsia, in which a woman goes into convulsions.

PREFERRED PROVIDER ORGANIZATION (PPO) Roster of professionals who have been approved to provide services to members of a particular managed care organization.

PREGNANCY CATEGORY A system of classifying drugs according to their established risks for use during pregnancy. Category A: Controlled human studies have demonstrated no fetal risk. Category B: Animal studies indicate no fetal risk, but no human studies, or adverse effects in animals, but not in well-controlled human studies. Category C: No adequate human or animal studies, or adverse fetal effects in animal studies, but no available human data. Category D: Evidence of fetal risk, but benefits outweigh risks. Category X: Evidence of fetal risk. Risks outweigh any benefits.

PREPUCE A fold of skin, such as the foreskin of the penis or the skin that surrounds the clitoris.

PRESBYOPIA A condition affecting people over the age of 40 where the system of accommodation that allows the eyes to focus on near objects fails to work because of age-related hardening of the lens of the eye.

PRESSURE ULCER Also known as a decubitus ulcer or bedsore, a pressure ulcer is an open wound that forms whenever prolonged pressure is applied to skin covering bony prominences of the body. Patients who are bedridden are at risk of developing pressure ulcers.

PREVALENCE The number of existing cases of a disease or event in a specific period of time.

PRIMARY CARE PHYSICIAN (PCP) A family practitioner, pediatrician, internist, or gynecologist who takes care of a patient's routine medical needs and refers him or her to a surgeon or other specialist when necessary.

PRIMARY SNORING Simple snoring; snoring that is not interrupted by episodes of breathing cessation.

PRIMARY TEETH A child's first set of teeth, sometimes called baby teeth.

PROCTOSIGMOIDOSCOPY A procedure in which a sigmoidoscope (an instrument consisting of a tube and a ligh) is used by a physician to visually examine the rectum and sigmoid colon.

PROGNOSIS The predicted outcome of a disease.

PROLAPSED CORD The umbilical cord is pushed into the vagina beside or ahead of the baby and becomes compressed, cutting off blood flow to the baby.

PROLAPSED UTERUS A uterus that has slipped out of place, sometimes protruding down through the vagina.

PRONATION The lowering of the inner edge of the foot by turning the entire foot outwards.

PROPHYLACTIC Preventing the spread or occurrence of disease or infection.

PROPHYLAXIS Protection against or prevention of a disease. Antibiotic prophylaxis is the use of antibiotics to prevent a possible infection.

PROSTAGLANDINS A group of hormonelike molecules that exert local effects on a variety of processes including fluid balance, blood flow, and gastrointestinal function. They may be responsible for the production of some types of pain and inflammation.

PROSTATE A donut-shaped gland in males below the bladder that contributes to the production of semen.

PROSTATECTOMY Prostate cancer surgery that includes partial or complete removal of the prostate.

PROSTHESIS An artificial replacement for a missing part of the body.

PROSTHETICS The branch of surgery concerned with the replacement of missing body parts with artificial substitutes.

PROTEIN An important building blocks of the body, a protein is a large, complex organic molecule composed of amino acids. It is involved in the formation of body structures and in controlling the basic functions of the human body.

PROTHROMBIN TIME A blood test that assesses the clotting ability of an individual's blood. It is used to monitor patients taking certain medications (warfarin) and to help diagnose clotting disorders.

PRUNE BELLY SYNDROME (PBS) A genetic disorder associated with abnormalities of human chromosomes 18 and 21. Male infants with PBS often have cryptorchidism along with other defects of the genitals and urinary tract. PBS is also known as triad syndrome and Eagle-Barrett syndrome.

PSEUDOPHAKIC BULLOUS KERATOPATHY Painful swelling of the cornea occasionally occurring after surgery to implant an artificial lens in place of a lens affected by cataract.

PSORIASIS A chronic, noncontagious skin disease that is marked by dry, scaly, and silvery patches of skin that appear in a variety of sizes and locations on the body.

PSYCHIATRIC NURSING The nursing specialty concerned with the prevention and treatment of mental disorders and their consequences.

PSYCHOACTIVE DRUG Any drug that affects the mind or behavior. There are five main classes of psychoactive drugs: opiates and opioids (e.g. heroin and methadone), stimulants (e.g. cocaine, nicotine), depressants (e.g. tranquilizers, antipsychotics, alcohol), hallucinogens (e.g. LSD), and marijuana and hashish.

PSYLLIUM The seeds of the fleawort plant, taken with water to produce a bland, jelly-like bulk which helps to move waste products through the digestive tract and prevent constipation.

PTOSIS The medical term for drooping of the upper eyelid.

PUBIS The anterior portion of the pelvis located in the anterior abdomen.

PULMONARY Referring to the lungs and respiratory system.

PULMONARY ARTERY An artery that carries blood from the heart to the lungs.

PULMONARY EMBOLISM Blockage of an artery in the lungs by foreign matter such as fat, tumor tissue, or a clot originating from a vein. A pulmonary embolism can be a very serious, and in some cases fatal, condition.

PULMONARY EMBOLUS Foreign matter such as fat, tumor tissue, or a clot originating from a vein that blocks an artery in the lungs.

PULMONARY FIBROSIS An end result of many forms of lung disease (especially chronic inflammatory conditions). Normal lung tissue is converted to scarred, "fibrotic" tissue that cannot carry out gas exchange.

PULMONARY FUNCTION TEST A group of procedures used to evaluate the function of the lungs and confirm the presence of certain lung disorders.

PULMONARY HYPERPLASIA Underdeveloped lungs.

PULMONARY HYPERTENSION A disorder in which the pressure in the blood vessels of the lungs is abnormally high.

PULMONARY REHABILITATION A program to treat chronic obstructive pulmonary disease (COPD), which generally includes education and counseling, exercise, nutritional guidance, techniques to improve breathing, and emotional support.

PULMONARY VALVE The valve located between the pulmonary artery and the right ventricle, which brings blood to the lungs.

PULMONARY VEIN ISOLATION A surgical procedure used to treat atrial fibrillation. During the procedure, a radio frequency probe, microwave probe, or cryoprobe is inserted and, under direct vision, used to create lesion lines in the heart to interrupt the conduction of abnormal impulses.

PULP The soft, innermost layer of a tooth that contains its blood vessels and nerves.

PULP CHAMBER The area within the natural crown of the tooth occupied by dental pulp.

PULPITIS Inflammation of the pulp of a tooth that involves the blood vessels and nerves.

PULSE OXIMETRY A non-invasive test in which a device that clips onto the finger measures the oxygen level in the blood.

PUPIL The black, circular opening in the center of the iris that allows light to pass through to the retina.

PURULENT Containing or producing pus.

PUS A thick, yellowish or greenish fluid composed of the remains of dead white blood cells, pathogens, and decomposed cellular debris. It is most often associated with bacterial infection.

PYLORUS The ring of muscle that controls the passage of material from the stomach into the small intestine.

PYREXIA A medical term meaning fever.

Q

QUADRICEPS, HIP FLEXORS, HAMSTRINGS Major muscles in the thigh area that affect knee mechanics.

R

RADIATION THERAPY A cancer treatment that uses high-energy rays or particles to kill or weaken cancer cells. Radiation may be delivered externally or internally via surgically implanted pellets. Also called radiotherapy.

RADIO WAVES Electromagnetic energy of the frequency range corresponding to that used in radio communications, usually 10,000 cycles per second to 300 billion cycles per second.

RADIOGRAPHICALLY DENSE Describes breast tissue whose details are difficult to see on an x ray.

RADIOGRAPHY Examination of any part of the body through the use of x rays. The process produces an image of shadows and contrasts on film.

RADIOLOGIST A medical doctor specially trained in radiology, the branch of medicine concerned with radioactive substances and their use for the diagnosis and treatment of disease.

RANGE OF MOTION (ROM) The range of motion of a joint from full extension to full flexion (bending) measured in degrees like a circle.

RAYNAUD'S DISEASE A vascular, or circulatory system, disorder which is characterized by abnormally cold hands and feet. This chilling effect is caused by constriction of the blood vessels in the extremities, and occurs when the hands and feet are exposed to cold weather. Emotional stress can also trigger the cold symptoms.

RECEPTOR A molecular structure in a cell or on the surface of a cell that allows binding of a specific substance that causes a specific physiologic response.

RECIPIENT A person who receives an organ or tissue transplant or a blood transfusion.

RECTUM The lower section of the large intestine in which feces collect for elimination through the anus.

RECURRENT LARYNGEAL NERVE One of two offshoots of the vagus nerve that connect to the larynx. It is located below the larynx.

RED BLOOD CELL Hemoglobin-containing blood cells that transport oxygen from the lungs to tissues. In the tissues, the red blood cells exchange their oxygen for carbon dioxide, which is brought back to the lungs to be exhaled. Also called an erythrocyte.

RED BLOOD CELL INDICES Measurements that describe the size and hemoglobin content of red blood cells. The indices are used to help in the differential diagnosis of anemia. Also called red cell absolute values or erythrocyte indices.

RED CELL DISTRIBUTION WIDTH (RDW) A measure of the variation in size of red blood cells.

REDUCTION The restoration of a body part to its original position after displacement, such as the reduction of a fractured bone by bringing ends or fragments back into original alignment. Also describes a chemical reaction in which one or more electrons are added to an atom or molecule.

REFLEX An involuntary response to a particular stimulus.

REFLUX The backward flow of a body fluid or secretion. Indigestion is sometimes caused by the reflux of stomach acid into the esophagus.

REGISTERED NURSE A graduate nurse who has passed a state nursing board examination and been registered and licensed to practice nursing.

REJECTION The process in which the immune system attacks tissue, such as a transplanted organ, it sees as foreign to the body.

REMISSION A disappearance of a disease and its symptoms. Complete remission means that all disease is gone. Partial remission means that the disease is significantly improved, but residual traces of the disease are still present. A remission may be due to treatment or may be spontaneous.

RENAL CELL CARCINOMA Cancer of the kidney.

RESECTION Surgically removing all or a significant part of an organ or other body structure.

RESISTANT ORGANISMS Organisms that are difficult to eradicate with antibiotics.

RESPIRATION The physical and chemical processes by which an organism acquires oxygen and releases carbon dioxide.

RESPIRATORY DISTRESS SYNDROME (RDS) Also known as hyaline membrane disease, this is a condition of premature infants in which the lungs are imperfectly expanded due to a lack of a substance (surfactant) on the lungs that reduces tension.

RESTENOSIS The narrowing of a blood vessel after it has been opened, usually by balloon angioplasty.

RESUSCITATION Bringing a person back to life or consciousness after he or she was apparently dead.

RETINA The inner, light-sensitive layer of the eye containing rods and cones. The retina transforms the image it receives into electrical signals that are sent to the brain via the optic nerve.

RETINAL DETACHMENT A serious vision disorder in which the light-detecting layer of cells inside the eye (retina) is separated from its normal support tissue and no longer functions properly.

RETINOBLASTOMA Malignant tumor of the retina.

RETINOPATHY OF PREMATURITY A condition in which the blood vessels in a premature infant's eyes do not develop normally. It can, in some cases, result in blindness.

RETROBULBAR HEMATOMA A rare complication of blepharoplasty, in which a pocket of blood forms behind the eyeball.

RETROGRADE PYELOGRAM An x-ray image of the kidneys produced by a technique in which radiopaque dye is injected into the kidneys from below, by way of the ureters. It is particularly useful in locating blockages and obstructions.

REVASCULARIZATION Restoring normal blood flow (circulation) in the body's vascular (veins and arteries) system.

REYE'S SYNDROME A serious, life-threatening illness in children, usually developing after a bout of flu or chickenpox, and often associated with the use of aspirin. Symptoms include uncontrollable vomiting, often with lethargy, memory loss, disorientation, or delirium. Swelling of the brain may cause seizures, coma, and in severe cases, death.

RH FACTOR An antigen present in the red blood cells of 85% of humans. A person with Rh factor is Rh positive (Rh+); a person without it is Rh negative (Rh-). The Rh factor was first identified in the blood of a rhesus monkey and is also known as the rhesus factor.

RH NEGATIVE Refers to blood lacking the Rh factor, genetically determined antigens in red blood cells that produce immune responses. If an Rh negative woman is pregnant with an Rh positive fetus, her body will produce antibodies against the fetus's blood, causing a disease known as Rh disease.

RHEUMATIC CARDITIS Inflammation of the heart muscle associated with acute rheumatic fever.

RHEUMATIC FEVER An illness that arises as a complication of an untreated or inadequately treated streptococcal infection of the throat. It ususally occurs among school-aged children and cause serious damage to the heart valves.

RHEUMATOID ARTHRITIS A chronic, autoimmune disease that causes inflammation and deformity of the joints. Other problems throughout the body may also develop including inflammation of the blood vessels, lung disease, blood disorders, and weakening of the bones.

RHINITIS Inflammation and swelling of the mucous membranes that line the nasal passages.

RHINOPLASTY Plastic surgery of the nose to repair it or change its shape.

RHYTIDECTOMY Literally meaning "wrinkle excision," this is another, misleading, term for face lift surgery.

ROCKY MOUNTAIN SPOTTED FEVER An infectious disease that is caused by *Rickettsia rickettsia* and spread by ticks. High fever, muscle pain, and spots on the skin are among the symptoms.

ROOT CANAL The space within a tooth that runs from the pulp chamber to the tip of the root.

ROOT CANAL TREATMENT The process of removing diseased or damaged pulp from a tooth, then filling and sealing the pulp chamber and root canals.

ROSACEA A chronic skin disease typically appearing in people aged 30-40. It is marked by redness of the face; flushing of the skin; and the presence of hard or pus-filled pimples and small, visible, spider-like veins called telangiectasias. In later stages, the face may swell and the nose may take on a bulb-like appearance called rhinophyma.

ROTOBLATION A non-surgical technique for treating diseased arteries in which a special catheter with a diamond-coated tip is guided to the point of narrowing in the artery, spins at high speeds, and grinds away the blockage or plaque on the artery walls.

RUPTURE A breaking apart of an organ or tissue.

S

SALICYLATES A group of drugs that includes aspirin and related compounds. Salicylates are used to relieve pain, reduce inflammation, and lower fever.

SALIVARY GLAND Three pairs of glands that secrete saliva into the mouth. Saliva is a fluid that contains the digestive enzyme salivary amylase, as well as mucus secretions that lubricate the mouth.

SALPINGECTOMY The surgical removal of a fallopian tube.

SANITATION The process of keeping drinking water, foods, or any anything else with which people come into contact free of microorganisms such as viruses.

SAPHENOUS VEINS Two large superficial veins in the leg that may be treated by ligation and stripping as therapy for varicose veins. The greater saphenous vein runs from the foot to the groin area, while the short saphenous vein runs from the ankle to the knee. They are also commonly used for bypass grafts.

SARCOIDOSIS A chronic disease that causes the formation of granulomas, masses resembling small tumors composed of clumps of immune cells, in any organ or tissue. Common sites include the lungs, spleen, liver, mucous membranes, skin, and lymph nodes.

SARCOMA A type of cancer that originates from connective tissue such as bone or muscle.

SCALING AND ROOT PLANING A dental procedure to treat gingivitis in which the teeth are scraped inside the gum area and the root of the tooth is planed to dislodge bacterial deposits.

SCHLEMM'S CANAL A reservoir deep in the front part of the eye where the fluid drained from the trabecular meshwork collects prior to being send out to systemic or general circulation.

SCIATICA Pain that radiates along the sciatic nerve, extending from the lower part of the spinal cord, down the back of the leg, to the foot.

SCLERA The tough, fibrous, white outer protective covering of the eyeball.

SCLEROSANT An irritating solution that stops bleeding by hardening the blood or vein it is injected into.

SCLEROSE To harden or undergo hardening. Sclerosing agents are chemicals that are used in sclerotherapy to cause swollen veins to fill with fibrous tissue and close down.

SCROTUM The external pouch containing the male reproductive glands (testes) and part of the spermatic cord.

SEDATIVE A medication that has a calming effect and may be used to treat nervousness or restlessness. Sometimes used as a synonym for hypnotic.

SEDENTARY Characterized by inactivity and lack of exercise. A sedentary lifestyle is a risk factor for high blood cholesterol levels.

SEIZURE A sudden attack, spasm, or convulsion.

SENTINEL LYMPH NODE The first lymph node to receive lymph fluid from a tumor. If the sentinel node is cancer-free, then it is likely that the cancerous cells have not metastasized.

SEPSIS A severe systemic infection in which bacteria have entered the bloodstream or body tissues.

SEPTAL DEFECT A hole in the septum, the muscle wall separating the right and left sides of the heart. Atrial septal defects are openings between the two upper heart chambers and ventricular septal defects are openings between the two lower heart chambers.

SEPTIC ARTHRITIS Another name for infectious arthritis, a serious infection of the joints characterized by pain, fever, occasional chills, inflammation and swelling in one or more joints, and a loss of function in the affected joints.

SEPTICEMIA A systemic infection due to the presence of bacteria and their toxins in the bloodstream. Septicemia is sometimes called blood poisoning.

SEPTUM A wall or partition. Often refers to the muscular wall dividing the left and right heart chambers or the partition in the nose that separates the two nostrils. Also refers to an abnormal fold of tissue down that center of the uterus that can cause infertility.

SEQUESTRATION AND MARGINATION The removal of neutrophils from circulating blood by cell changes that trap them in the lungs and spleen.

SERIAL X RAYS A number of x rays performed at set times in the disease progression or treatment intervals. The radiographs are compared to one another to track changes.

SERUM The fluid part of the blood that remains after blood cells, platelets, and fibrogen have been removed. Also called blood serum.

SEXUALLY TRANSMITTED DISEASE (STD) One of more than 20 diseases that is passed from one person to another through sexual intercourse or other intimate sexual contact. Also called a veneral disease.

SHINGLES An disease caused by an infection with the *Herpes zoster* virus, the same virus that causes chickenpox. Symptoms of shingles include pain and blisters along one nerve, usually on the face, chest, stomach, or back.

SHOCK A medical emergency in which the organs and tissues of the body are not receiving an adequate flow of blood. This deprives the organs and tissues of oxygen and allows the build-up of waste products. Shock can be caused by certain diseases, serious injury, or blood loss.

SHORT BOWEL SYNDROME A condition in which the bowel is not as long as normal, either because of surgery or because of a congenital defect. Because the bowel has less surface area to absorb nutrients, malabsorption syndrome can result from this condition.

SHUNT A passageway (or an artificially created passageway) that diverts blood flow from one main route to another. Also refers to a small tube placed in a ventricle of the brain to direct cerebrospinal fluid away from a blockage into another part of the body.

SICKLE CELL ANEMIA An inherited disorder in which red blood cells contain an abnormal form of hemoglobin, a protein that carries oxygen. The abnormal form of hemoglobin causes the red cells to become sickle-shaped. The misshapen cells may clog blood vessels, preventing

STROKE Interruption of blood flow to a part of the brain with consequent brain damage. A stroke may be caused by a blood clot or by hemorrhage due to a burst blood vessel. Also known as a cerebrovascular accident.

STROMA A term used to describe the supportive tissue surrounding a particular structure. An example is the tissue that surrounds and supports the actually functional lung tissue.

SUBARACHNOID Referring to the space underneath the arachnoid membrane, the middle of the three membranes that sheath the spinal cord and brain.

SUBARACHNOID HEMORRHAGE A collection of blood in the subarachnoid space, the space between the arachnoid and pia mater membranes that surround the brain. This space is normally filled with cerebrospinal fluid. A subarachnoid hemorrhage can lead to stroke, seizures, permanent brain damage, and other complications.

SUBCUTANEOUS Referring to the area beneath the skin.

SUBJECTIVE Influenced by personal opinion, bias, or experience; not reliably repeatable.

SUBSTRATE A substance acted upon by an enzyme.

SUPERIOR VENA CAVA The major vein that carries blood from the upper body to the heart.

SUPINE Lying on the back with the face upward.

SUPRAVENTRICULAR TACHYCARDIA A fast heart beat (exceeding 100 beats/minute) that originates in the area of the heart immediately above the ventricles.

SURFACTANT A protective film secreted by the alveoli in the lungs that reduces the surface tension of lung fluids, allowing gas exchange and helping maintain the elasticity of lung tissue. Premature infants may lack surfactant and are more susceptible to respiratory problems without it.

SURGICAL ALTERNATIVES Surgical options within a range of surgical procedures used to treat a specific condition.

SURGICENTER Another term for ambulatory surgical center.

SUTURES Materials used in closing a surgical or traumatic wound.

SWAN-GANZ CATHETER Also called a pulmonary artery catheter. This type of catheter is inserted into a large vessel in the neck or chest and is used to measure the amount of fluid in the heart and to determine how well the heart is functioning.

SYMPATHETIC NERVOUS SYSTEM The part of the autonomic nervous system whose neurons emerge through the ventral roots of the thoracic and two upper lumbar spinal nerves. It is concerned especially with preparing the body to react to situations of stress or emergency.

SYMPATHOMIMETIC Refers to a drug that mimics the effects of stimulation of organs and structures by the sympathetic nervous system.

SYNDACTYLY Fusion of two or more toes or fingers.

SYNDROME A group of signs and symptoms that collectively characterize a disease or disorder.

SYNERGISTIC Refers to a situation in which the combined action of two or more processes is greater than the sum of each acting separately.

SYNGENEIC Refers to a bone marrow transplant from one identical twin to the other.

SYNOVIAL FLUID A transparent fluid secreted by the membrane surrounding the joints that lubricates the joints and tendons.

SYNOVITIS Inflammation of the synovial membrane, the membrane that lines the inside of the articular capsule of a joint.

SYSTEMIC CIRCULATION Refers to the general blood circulation of the body, not including the lungs.

SYSTOLIC The phase of blood circulation in which the heart's pumping chambers (ventricles) are actively pumping blood. The ventricles are squeezing (contracting) forcefully, and the pressure against the walls of the arteries is at its highest.

T

T CELL A type of white blood cell that is produced in the bone marrow and matured in the thymus gland. It helps to regulate the immune system's response to infections or malignancy.

TACHYCARDIA A rapid heart beat, usually over 100 beats per minute.

TARDIVE DYSKINESIA Involuntary movements of the face and/or body which are a side effect of the long-term use of some older antipsychotic (neuroleptic) drugs. Tardive dyskinesia affects 15-20% of patients on long-term neuroleptic treatment.

TAY-SACHS DISEASE An inherited disease caused by a missing enzyme that is prevalent among the Ashkenazi

Jewish population of the United States. Infants with the disease are unable to process a certain type of fat which accumulates in nerve and brain cells, causing mental and physical retardation, and, finally, death.

TEACHING HOSPITALS Hospitals whose primary mission is training medical personnel in collaboration with (or ownership by) a medical school or research center.

TELANGIECTASIA Abnormal dilation of capillary blood vessels leading to the formation of skin lesions.

TEMPORAL LOBE EPILEPSY (TLE) The most common type of epilepsy, with elaborate and multiple sensory, motor, and psychic symptoms. A common feature is the loss of consciousness and amnesia during seizures. Other manifestations may include more complex behaviors like bursts of anger, emotional outbursts, fear, or automatisms.

TENDINITIS Inflammation of a tendon (a tough band of tissue that connects muscle to bone) that is often the result of overuse over a long period of time.

TENDON A tough cord of dense white fibrous connective tissue that connects a muscle with some other part, especially a bone, and transmits the force which the muscle exerts.

TESTES Singular, testis. The two egg-shaped male sex organs located in the scrotum that produce sperm and testosterone. Also called testicles.

TESTICULAR TORSION Twisting of the testicle around the spermatic cord, cutting off the blood supply to the testicle. It is considered a urologic emergency.

TESTOSTERONE Male hormone produced by the testes and (in small amounts) in the ovaries. Testosterone is responsible for some masculine secondary sex characteristics such as growth of body hair and deepening voice. It also is sometimes given as part of hormone replacement therapy to women whose ovaries have been removed.

TETANY A disorder of the nervous system characterized by muscle cramps, spasms of the arms and legs, and numbness of the extremities. It is a symptom of an abnormality in calcium metabolism.

TETRALOGY OF FALLOT A congenital heart defect in which the blood pumped through the body is not sufficiently oxygenated. It consists of four associated abnormalities (tetralogy): a large hole between the ventricles (ventricular septal defect), narrowing at or beneath the pulmonary valve (pulmonary stenosis), an overly muscular right ventricle, and a displacement of the aorta that allows oxygen-depleted blood to flow directly from the right ventricle to the aorta.

THALASSEMIA An inherited group of anemias occurring primarily among people of Mediterranean descent. They are caused by defective formation of part of the hemoglobin molecule.

THORACENTESIS A procedure in which fluid is withdrawn from the pleural cavity through a needle inserted between the ribs. The fluid may be withdrawn either for diagnostic testing or to drain the cavity. Also called a pleural fluid tap.

THORACIC Refers to the chest area. The thorax runs between the abdomen and neck and is encased in the ribs.

THORACIC VERTEBRAE The vertebrae in the chest region to which the ribs attach.

THORACOSCOPY Visual examination of the contents of the chest through a thin, lighted tube passed through a small incision.

THORACOTOMY A surgical opening in the chest.

THORAX The chest area, which runs between the abdomen and neck and is encased in the ribs.

THROMBIN An enzyme in blood plasma that helps to convert fibrinogen to fibrin during the last stage of the clotting process.

THROMBIN INHIBITOR A type of anticoagulant medication used to help prevent formation of harmful blood clots in the body by blocking the activity of thrombin.

THROMBOCYTE Another name for platelet.

THROMBOCYTOPENIA A persistent decrease in the number of blood platelets usually associated with hemorrhaging.

THROMBOCYTOSIS An abnormally high platelet count. It occurs in polycythemia vera and other disorders in which the bone marrow produces too many platelets.

THROMBOEMBOLISM A condition in which a blood vessel is blocked by a free-floating bood clot carried in the bloodstream. It can lead to infarction, or death of the surrounding tissue due to lack of blood supply.

THROMBOPHLEBITIS An inflammation of a vein, usually in the legs, accompanied by the formation of a blood clot.

THROMBOSIS The formation of a blood clot in a vein or artery that may obstruct local blood flow or may dislodge, travel downstream, and obstruct blood flow at a remote location. The clot or thrombus may lead to infarction, or death of tissue, due to a blocked blood supply.

THROMBUS A blood clot that forms within a blood vessel or the heart.

THYMUS GLAND An endocrine gland located in the upper chest just below the neck that functions as part of the lymphatic system. It coordinates the development of the immune system.

THYROID STORM An unusual complication of thyroid function that is sometimes triggered by the stress of thyroid surgery. It is a medical emergency.

TIBIA One of the two bones of the lower leg.

TINNITUS A noise, ranging from faint ringing or thumping to roaring, that originates in the ear, not in the environment.

TOCOLYTICS Drugs administered to stop or delay the onset of labor.

TOLERANCE A condition in which an addict needs higher doses of a substance to achieve the same effect previously achieved with a lower dose.

TONOMETRY The measurement of intraocular pressure.

TONSILLECTOMY A surgical procedure to remove the tonsils. A tonsillectomy is performed if the patient has recurrent sore throats or throat infections, or if the tonsils have become so swollen that the patient has trouble breathing or swallowing.

TONSILLITIS Inflammation of a tonsil, a small mass of tissue in the throat.

TONSILS Common name for the palatine tonsils, which are lymph masses in the back of the mouth, on either side of the tongue. Tonsils act like filters to trap bacteria and viruses.

TOPICAL Not ingested; applied to the outside of the body, for example to the skin, eye, or mouth.

TOTAL LUNG CAPACITY TEST A test that measures the amount of air in the lungs after a person has breathed in as much as possible.

TOURNIQUET Any device that is used to compress a blood vessel to stop bleeding or as part of collecting a blood sample. Phlebotomists usually use an elastic band as a tourniquet.

TRABECULAR MESHWORK A sponge-like tissue located near the cornea and iris that functions to drain the aqueous humor from the eye into the blood.

TRACHEA The windpipe. A tube composed of cartilage and membrane that extends from below the voice box into the chest where it splits into two branches, the bronchi, that lead to each lung.

TRACHEOSTOMY A procedure in which a small opening is made in the neck and into the trachea or windpipe. A breathing tube is then placed through this opening.

TRACHEOTOMY An surgical procedure in which the surgeon cuts directly through the patient's neck into the windpipe below a blockage in order to keep the airway open.

TRANQUILIZER A medication that has a calming effect and is used to treat anxiety and mental tension.

TRANSCONJUCTIVAL BLEPHAROPLASTY A type of blepharoplasty in which the surgeon makes no incision on the surface of the eyelid, but, instead, enters from behind to tease out the fat deposits.

TRANSDUCER A device that converts electrical signals into ultrasound waves and ultrasound waves back into electrical impulses.

TRANSESOPHAGEAL ECHOCARDIOGRAPHY A diagnostic test that uses an ultrasound device passed into the esophagus of the patient to create a clear image of the heart muscle.

TRANSFUSION The transfer of blood or blood components from one person to another. Transfusions can be direct, in which blood is transferred from the donor to the recipient; or indirect, in which the blood is taken from the donor, stored in a container, and then given to the recipient.

TRANSILLUMINATION A technique of checking for tooth decay by shining a light behind the patient's teeth. Decayed areas show up as spots or shadows.

TRANSPLANTATION The removal of tissue from one part of the body for implantation to another part of the body; or the removal of tissue or an organ from one individual and its surgical implantation in another individual.

TRANSPOSITION OF THE GREAT ARTERIES A reversal of the two great arteries of the heart, causing blood containing oxygen to be carried back to the lungs and blood that is lacking in oxygen to be transported throughout the body.

TRANSSEXUAL A person whose gender identity is opposite his or her anatomic sex.

TRANSURETHRAL RESECTION A surgical procedure to remove abnormal tissue from the bladder. The technique involves the insertion of an instrument called a cytoscope into the bladder through the urethra, and the removal of the tumor through it.

TRANSVERSE PRESENTATION An abnormal position of the fetus in which the baby is laying sideways across the cervix instead of head first.

TREACHER COLLINS SYNDROME A disorder that affects facial development and hearing, thought to be caused by a gene mutation on human chromosome 5. Treacher Collins syndrome is sometimes called mandibulofacial dysostosis.

TREMOR Involuntary shakiness or trembling.

TRENDELENBURG'S TEST A test that measures the speed at which the lower leg fills with blood after the leg has first been raised above the level of the heart. It is named for Friedrich Trendelenburg (1844-1924), a German surgeon.

TREPHINE A small surgical instrument that is rotated to cut a circular incision.

TRICUSPID VALVE The valve between the right atrium and the right ventricle of the heart.

TRIGLYCERIDE A substance formed in the body from fat in the diet. Triglycerides are the main fatty materials in the blood. Bound to protein, they make up high- and low-density lipoproteins (HDLs and LDLs). Triglyceride levels are important in the diagnosis and treatment of many diseases including high blood pressure, diabetes, and heart disease.

TROCAR A sharp pointed tube through which a needle can be inserted.

TUBAL LIGATION A surgical sterilization procedure in which the fallopian tubes are tied in two places and cut between. This prevents eggs from moving from the ovary to the uterus.

TUBERCULOSIS Tuberculosis (TB) is a potentially fatal contagious disease that can affect almost any part of the body, but is mainly an infection of the lungs. It is caused by a bacterial microorganism, the tubercle bacillus or *Mycobacterium tuberculosis*. Symptoms include fever, weight loss, and coughing up blood.

TUMESCENT TECHNIQUE The tumescent technique of liposuction involves swelling, or tumescing, the tissue with large volumes of dilute anesthetic.

TUMOR MARKERS Biochemicals produced by tumor cells or by the body in response to tumor cells. Their levels in the blood help evaluate people for certain kinds of cancer.

TUNICA The medical term for a membrane or piece of tissue that covers or lines a body part. The eyeball is surrounded by three tunicae.

TURBIDITY The cloudiness or lack of transparency of a solution, resulting from particles suspended in the fluid.

TURBINATE The ridge-shaped cartilage or soft bony tissue inside the nose.

TWILIGHT ANESTHESIA An intravenous mixture of sedatives and other medications that decreases patients' awareness of the procedure being performed.

TYMPANIC MEMBRANE The eardrum, a thin disc of tissue that separates the outer ear from the middle ear. It can rupture if pressure in the ear is not equalized during airplane ascents and descents.

TYMPANOSTOMY TUBE An ear tube. A tympanostomy tube is small tube made of metal or plastic that is inserted during myringotomy to ventilate the middle ear.

U

ULCER A site of damage to the skin or mucous membrane that is characterized by the formation of pus, death of tissue, and is frequently accompanied by an inflammatory reaction.

ULCERATION The formation of an ulcer, a site of damage to the skin or mucous membrane that is characterized by pus, death of tissue, and is frequently accompanied by an inflammatory reaction.

ULCERATIVE COLITIS A form of inflammatory bowel disease characterized by inflammation of the mucous lining of the colon, ulcerated areas of tissue, and bloody diarrhea.

ULTRASONOGRAM An image produced by ultrasonography, a procedure where high-frequency sound waves that cannot be heard by human ears are bounced off internal organs and tissues. These sound waves produce a pattern of echoes which are then used by the computer to create sonograms, or pictures of areas inside the body.

ULTRASONOGRAPHY A medical test in which sound waves are directed against internal structures in the body. As sound waves bounce off the internal structure, they create an image on a video screen. Ultrasonography is often used to diagnose fetal abnormalities, gallstones, heart defects, and tumors. Also called ultrasound imaging.

UMBILICAL CORD BLOOD TRANSPLANT A procedure in which the blood from a newborn's umbilical cord, which is rich in stem cells, is used as the donor source for bone marrow transplants. Currently, umbilical cord blood transplants are mainly used for sibling bone marrow transplants or to store blood for an anonymous donation.

UMBILICUS The navel or the point on the abdomen where the umbilical cord jointed the fetus.

UNILATERAL Refers to one side of the body or only one organ in a pair.

UREA A by-product of protein metabolism that is formed in the liver. Because urea contains ammonia, which is toxic to the body, it must be quickly filtered from the blood by the kidneys and excreted in the urine. Urea levels in the blood rise when kidney failure occurs.

URETER The tube that carries urine from the kidney to the bladder; each kidney has one ureter.

URETHRA A passageway from the bladder to the outside of the body for the discharge of urine. In the female this tube lies between the vagina and clitoris; in the male the urethra travels through the penis and opens at the tip. In males, seminal fluid and sperm also pass through the urethra.

URETHRITIS Inflammation of the urethra, the tube through which the urine moves from the bladder to the outside of the body.

URIC ACID A compound resulting from the body's breakdown of purine. It is normally present in human urine only in small amounts.

URINALYSIS A diagnostic physical, chemical, and microscopic examination of a urine sample (specimen). Specimens can be obtained by normal emptying of the bladder (voiding) or by a hospital procedure called catheterization.

URINARY INCONTINENCE Unintentional loss of urine that is sufficient enough in frequency and amount to cause physical and/or emotional distress in the person experiencing it. This situation becomes more common as people age, and is more common in women who have given birth to more than one child.

URINARY RETENTION The result of progressive obstruction of the urethra by an enlarging prostate, causing urine to remain in the bladder even after urination.

URINARY TRACT The system of organs that produces and expels urine from the body. This system begins at the kidneys, where the urine is formed; passes through the bladder; and ends at the urethra, where urine is expelled.

URINE The fluid excreted by the kidneys, stored in the bladder, then discharged from the body through the tube that carries urine from the bladder to the outside of the body (urethra).

UROLOGIST A physician who specializes in the anatomy, physiology, diseases, and care of the urinary tract (in men and women) and male rreproductive tract.

UROLOGY The branch of medicine that deals with disorders of the urinary tract in both males and females, and with the genital organs in males.

UTERINE PROLAPSE A condition characterized by bulging of the uterus into the vagina.

UTERUS The female reproductive organ that contains and nourishes a fetus from implantation until birth. Also called the womb.

UVEA The pigmented membrane that lines the back of the retina of the eye and extends forward to include the iris. The uvea is sometimes called the uveal tract and has three parts: the iris, the choroid, and the ciliary body.

UVEITIS Inflammation of all or part the uvea. The uvea is a continuous layer of tissue which consists of the iris, the ciliary body, and the choroid. The uvea lies between the retina and sclera.

UVULOPALATOPHARYNGOPLASTY (UPPP) A surgical procedure to remove excess tissue at the back of the throat to prevent it from closing off the airway during sleep.

V

VAGINA The tube-like passage from the vulva (a woman's external genital structures) to the cervix (the portion of the uterus that projects into the vagina). The vagina is also known as the birth canal, since it is the passage through which a baby passes at birth.

VAGOTOMY Cutting of the vagus nerve. If the vagus nerves are cut as they enter the stomach (truncal vagotomy), gastric secretions are decreased, as is intestinal motility (movement) and stomach emptying. In a selective vagotomy, only those branches of the vagus nerve are cut that stimulate the secretory cells.

VAGUS NERVE A cranial nerve, that is, a nerve connected to the brain. The vagus nerve has branches to most of the major organs in the body, including the larynx, throat, windpipe, lungs, heart, and most of the digestive system.

VALVE Tissue in the passageways between the heart's upper and lower chambers that controls the passage of blood and prevents regurgitation.

VAPORIZE To change a liquid or solid material or into a gaseous state.

VARICES Singular, varix. A type of varicose vein that develops in veins in the linings of the esophagus and upper stomach when these veins fill with blood and swell due to an increase in blood pressure in the portal veins.

VARICOSE VEINS The permanent enlargement and twisting of veins, usually in the legs. They are most often seen in people with occupations requiring long periods of standing, and in pregnant women.

VAS DEFERENS A tube that is a continuation of the epididymis. This tube transports sperm from the testis to the prostatic urethra.

VASCULAR Pertaining to blood vessels.

VASECTOMY Surgical sterilization of the male, done by removing a portion of the tube that carries sperm to the urethra.

VASOCONSTRICTION Constriction of a blood vessel.

VASOSPASM The constriction or narrowing of a blood vessel caused by a spasm of the smooth muscle of the vessel wall. In cases of hemorrhage, the constriction is prompted by chemical signals from the escaped blood as it breaks down.

VASOVAGAL REACTION A reaction due to the action of stimuli from the vagus nerve on blood vessels.

VBAC Vaginal birth after cesarean.

VEIN A blood vessel that returns oxygen-depleted blood from various parts of the body to the heart.

VENA CAVA The large vein that drains directly into the heart after gathering incoming blood from the entire body.

VENTILATOR A mechanical device that can take over the work of breathing for a patient whose lungs are injured or are starting to heal. Sometimes called a respirator.

VENTRICLE One of the two lower chambers of the heart that are involved in pumping blood. The right ventricle pumps blood into the lungs to receive oxygen. The left ventricle pumps blood into the circulation of the body to deliver oxygen to all of the body's organs and tissues.

VENTRICULAR FIBRILLATION An arrhythmia characterized by a very rapid, uncoordinated, ineffective series of contractions throughout the lower chambers of the heart. Unless stopped, these chaotic impulses are fatal.

VENTRICULAR TACHYCARDIA An arrhythmia characterized by a rapid heart beat that originates in one of the lower chambers (the ventricles) of the heart. To be classified as tachycardia, the heart rate is usually at least 100 beats per minute.

VERMILION BORDER The line between the lip and the skin.

VERTEBRAE Singular, vertebra. The individual bones of the spinal column that are stacked on top of each other. There is a hole in the center of each bone, through which the spinal cord passes.

VERTIGO A feeling of dizziness together with a sensation of movement and a feeling of rotating in space.

VIDEOSCOPE A surgical camera.

VITAL CAPACITY The largest amount of air expelled after a person's deepest inhalation.

VITAL SIGNS The basic indicators of a person's essential body functions, usually defined as the pulse, body temperature, and breathing rate. Also not strictly speaking a vital sign, blood pressure is usually included.

VITREOUS HUMOR The clear, gel-like substance that fills the eyeball behind the lens.

VOIDING Emptying the bladder or urinating.

VOLVULUS A twisting of the intestine that causes an obstruction.

VULVA The external genital organs of a woman, including the outer and inner lips, clitoris, and opening of the vagina.

W

WEGENER'S GRANULOMATOSIS A rare disease usually affecting males that causes the infiltration of inflammatory cells and tissue death in the lungs, kidneys, blood vessels, heart, and other tissues.

WITHDRAWAL SYMPTOMS A group of physical and/or mental symptoms that may occur when a person suddenly stops using a drug or other substance upon which he or she has become dependent.

WOLFF-PARKINSON-WHITE SYNDROME An abnormal, rapid heart rhythm, due to an extra pathway for the electrical impulses to travel from the atria to the ventricles.

X X Y

X RAY A form of electromagnetic radiation with shorter wavelengths than normal light. X rays can pene-

Glossary

trate most structures and are used in the diagnosis and treatment of diseases.

XENOGRAFT Tissue that is transplanted from one species to another (e.g., pigs to humans).

ZOLLINGER-ELLISON SYNDROME A rare condition characterized by severe and recurrent peptic ulcers in the stomach, duodenum, and upper small intestine, caused by a tumor, or tumors, usually found in the pancreas. The tumor secretes the hormone gastrin, which stimulates the stomach and duodenum to produce large quantities of acid, leading to ulceration.

ZYGOTE INTRAFALLOPIAN TUBE TRANSFER (ZIFT) An assisted reproductive technique in which the eggs are fertilized in a laboratory dish and then placed in the woman's fallopian tube in the hopes that pregnancy will result.

ORGANIZATIONS

The list of organizations is arranged in alphabetical order. Although the list is comprehensive, it is by no means exhaustive. It is a starting point for further information that can be used in conjunction with the Resources section of each main body entry, as well as other online and print sources. Email addresses and URLs listed were provided by the associations; Gale Group is not responsible for the accuracy of the addresses or the contents of the websites.

Academic Orthopaedic Society (AOS)
6300 N. River Rd., Suite 505
Rosemont, IL 60018
(847) 318-7330
<http://www.a-o-s.org>

Academy of General Dentistry
211 East Chicago Avenue
Chicago, IL 60611
(312) 440-4300
<http://www.agd.org>

Accreditation Association for Ambulatory Health Care (AAAHC)
3201 Old Glenview Road, Suite 300
Wilmette, IL 60091-2992
(847) 853-6060
<http://www.aahc.org>

Action on Smoking and Health
2013 H Street, NW
Washington, DC 20006
(202) 659-4310
<http://ash.org>

Adult Day Care Group
3 Ramsgate Ct.
Blue Bell, PA 19422
(610) 941-0340
Fax: (610) 834-0459
<http://www.libertynet.org/adcg>

Agency for Health Care Policy and Research (AHCPR), Publications Clearinghouse
P.O. Box 8547
Silver Spring, MD, 20907
(800) 358-9295
<http://www/ahcpr.gov>

Agency for Healthcare Research and Quality (AHRQ)
2101 East Jefferson St., Suite 501
Rockville, MD 20852
(301) 594-1364
<http://www.ahcpr.gov>

Alan Guttmacher Institute
1120 Connecticut Ave., NW, Suite 460
Washington, DC 20036
(202) 296-4012
<http://www.agi-usa.org>

Alexander Graham Bell Association for the Deaf
3417 Volta Place NW
Washington, DC 20007
(202) 337-5220
<http://www.agbell.org>

ALS Association
27001 Agoura Road, Suite 150
Calabasas Hills, CA 91301-5104
(800) 782-4747
<http://www.alsa.org>

Alzheimer's Association
919 North Michigan Avenue, Suite 100
Chicago, IL 60611-1676
(800) 272-3900
(312) 375-8700
Fax: (312) 335-1110
<http://www.alz.org>

America's Blood Centers
725 15th St., NW, Suite 700
Washington, DC 20005
(202) 393-5725
<http://www.americasblood.org>

American Academy of Allergy, Asthma and Immunology
611 East Wells Street
Milwaukee, WI 53202
(414) 272-6071
<http://www.aaaai.org>

American Academy of Anesthesiologist Assistants
P.O. Box 81362
Wellesley, MA 02481-0004
(800) 757-5858
<http://www.anesthetist.org>

American Academy of Audiology
11730 Plaza America Drive, Suite 300
Reston, VA 20190

(703) 790-8466
<http://www.audiology.org>

American Academy of Cosmetic Surgery
737 N. Michigan Ave., Suite 820
Chicago, IL 60611
(312) 981-6760
<http://www.cosmeticsurgery.org>

American Academy of Dermatology
930 N. Meacham Road, P.O. Box 4014
Schaumburg, IL 60168-4014
(847) 330-0230
Fax: (847) 330-0050
<http://www.aad.org/>

American Academy of Emergency Medicine (AAEM)
611 East Wells Street
Milwaukee, WI 53202
(800) 884-2236
<http://www.aaem.org>

American Academy of Facial Plastic and Reconstructive Surgery (AAFPRS)
310 South Henry Street
Alexandria, VA 22314
(703) 299-9291
Fax: (703) 299-8898
<http://www.facemd.org>

American Academy of Family Physicians
11400 Tomahawk Creek Parkway
Leawood, KS 66211-2672
(913) 906-6000
Email: fp@aafp.org
<http://www.aafp.org>

American Academy of Hospice and Palliative Medicine (AAHPM)
4700 West Lake Avenue
Glenview, IL 60025-1485
(847) 375-4712
<http://www.aahpm.org>

American Academy of Implant Dentistry
211 E. Chicago Avenue, Suite 750
Chicago, IL 60611
(312) 335-1550
Fax: (312) 335-9090
<http://www.aaid-implant.org>

American Academy of Medical Acupuncture (AAMA)
4929 Wilshire Boulevard, Suite 428
Los Angeles, CA 90010
(323) 937-5514
<http://www.medicalacupuncture.org>

American Academy of Neurological and Orthopaedic Surgeons (AANOS)
2300 South Rancho Drive, Suite 202
Las Vegas, NV 89102
(702) 388-7390
<http://www.aanos.org>

American Academy of Neurology
1080 Montreal Avenue
St. Paul, Minnesota 55116
(651) 695-1940
Fax: (651) 695-2791
Email: info@aan.org
<http://www.aan.com/>

American Academy of Ophthalmology
655 Beach Street, P.O. Box 7424
San Francisco, CA 94120-7424
(415) 561-8500
<http://www.aao.org>

American Academy of Orthopaedic Surgeons (AAOS)
6300 North River Rd. Suite 200
Rosemont, IL 60018
(847) 823-7186
(800) 346-2267
Fax: (847) 823-8125
<http://www.aaos.org>

American Academy of Otolaryngology—Head and Neck Surgery
One Prince St.
Alexandria, VA 22314-3357
(703) 836-4444
<http://www.entnet.org>

American Academy of Pediatric Dentistry
211 East Chicago Avenue, Ste. 700
Chicago, IL 60611-2616
(312) 337- 2169
Fax: 312-337-6329
<http://www.aapd.org>

American Academy of Pediatrics (AAP)
141 Northwest Point Boulevard

Elk Grove Village, IL 60007
(847) 434-4000
Fax: (847) 434-8000
Email: kidsdoc@aap.org.
<http://www.aap.org>

American Academy of Sleep Medicine (AASM)
One Westbrook Corporate Center, Suite 920
Westchester, IL 60154
(708) 492-0930
<http://www.aasmnet.org>

American Academy of Wound Management
1255 23rd St., NW
Washington, DC 20037
(202) 521-0368
<http://www.aawm.org>

American Association for Accreditation of Ambulatory Surgery Facilities (AAAASF)
1202 Allanson Road
Mundelein, IL 60060
(888) 545-5222

American Association for Cardiovascular and Pulmonary Rehabilitation (AACVPR)
7600 Terrace Avenue, Suite 203
Middleton, Wisconsin 53562
(608) 831-6989
Email: aacvpr@tmahq.com
<http://www.aacvpr.org>

American Association for Hand Surgery
20 North Michigan Avenue, Suite 700
Chicago, IL 60602
(321) 236-3307
Fax: (312) 782-0553
Email: contact@handssurgery.org
<http://www.handsurgery.org>

American Association for Respiratory Care
11030 Ables Lane
Dallas, TX 75229
(972) 243-2272
Email: info@aarc.org
<http://www.aarc.org>

American Association for Thoracic Surgery (AATS)
900 Cummings Center, Suite 221-U
Beverly, MA 01915
(978) 927-8330
<http://www.aats.org>

American Association for Vascular Surgery (AAVS)
900 Cummings Center, Suite 221-U
Beverly, MA 01915
<http://www.aavs.vascularweb.org>

American Association of Ambulatory Surgical Centers (AAASC)
P.O. Box 23220
San Diego, CA 92193
(800) 237-3768
<http://www.aaasc.org>

American Association of Blood Banks (AABB)
8101 Glenbrook Road
Bethesda, MD 20814-2749
(301) 907-6977
Fax: (301) 907-6895
<http://www.aabb.org>

American Association of Clinical Endocrinologists (AACE)
1000 Riverside Ave., Suite 205
Jacksonville, FL 32204
(904) 353-7878
<http://www.aace.com/>

American Association of Critical Care Nurses (ACCN)
101 Columbia
Aliso Viejo, CA 92656-4109
(800) 889-AACN [(800) 889-2226]
(949) 362-2000
<http://www.aacn.org>

American Association of Electrodiagnostic Medicine
421 First Avenue SW, Suite 300 East
Rochester, MN 55902
(507) 288-0100
Fax: (507) 288-1225
Email: aaem@aaem.net
<http://www.aaem.net/>

American Association of Endocrine Surgeons (AAES)
MetroHealth Medical Center, H920
2500 MetroHealth Drive
Cleveland, OH 44109-1908
(216) 778-4753
<http://www.endocrinesurgeons.org/gt;

American Association of Endodontists
211 E. Chicago Ave., Suite 1100
Chicago, IL 60611-2691
(800) 872-3636
(312) 266-7255
Fax: (866) 451-9020
(312) 266-9867
<http://www.aae.org>
Email: info@aae.org.

American Association of Gynecological Laparoscopists
13021 East Florence Avenue
Sante Fe Springs, CA 90670-4505
(800) 554-2245
<http://www.aagl.com/>

American Association of Immunologists (AAI)
9650 Rockville Pike
Bethesda, MD 20814
(301) 634-7178
<http://www.12.17.12.70/aai/default/asp>

American Association of Kidney Patients
3505 E. Frontage Rd., Suite 315
Tampa, FL 33607
(800) 749-2257
Email: <info@aakp.org>
<http://www.aakp.org>

American Association of Managed Care Nurses
P.O. Box 4975
Glen Allen, VA 23058-4975
(804) 747-9698
<http://www.aamcn.org/joinaamcn.htm>

American Association of Neurological Surgeons (AANS)
5550 Meadowbrook Drive, Rolling Meadows, IL 60008
(888) 566-AANS(2267)
Fax: (847) 378-0600
Email: info@aans.org
<http://www.neurosurgery.org/>

American Association of Nurse Anesthetists (AANA), Federal Government Affairs Office
412 1st Street, SE, Suite 12
Washington, DC 20003
(202) 484-8400
Fax: (202) 484-8408
Email: info@aanadc.com

American Association of Nurse Anesthetists (AANA)
222 South Prospect Avenue
Park Ridge, IL 60068-4001
(847) 692-7050
Fax: (847) 692-6968
Email: info@aana.com
<http://www.aana.com>

American Association of Oral and Maxillofacial Surgeons
9700 West Bryn Mawr Ave.
Rosemont, IL 60018-5701
(847) 678-6200
<http://www.aaoms.org>

American Association of Tissue Banks
1350 Beverly Road, Suite 220-A
McLean, VA 22101
(703) 827-9582
Fax: (703) 356-2198
Email: aatb@aatb.org
<http://www.aatb.org/menu.htm>

American Board of Anesthesiology
4101 Lake Boone Trail, Suite 510
Raleigh, North Carolina 27607-7506
(919) 881-2570
<http://www.abanes.org/>

American Board of Colorectal Surgeons (ABCRS)
20600 Eureka Rd., Ste. 600, Taylor, MI 48180
(734) 282-9400
<http://www.abcrs.org>

American Board of Medical Specialties (ABMS)
1007 Church Street, Suite 404, Evanston, IL 60201
(847) 491-9091
<http://www.abms.org/>

American Board of Obstetrics and Gynecology
2915 Vine Street, Suite 300, Dallas, TX 75204
(214) 871-1619
Fax: (214) 871-1943
Email: info@abog.org
<http://www.abog.org>

American Board of Oral and Maxillofacial Surgery
625 North Michigan Avenue, Suite 1820, Chicago, IL 60611
(312) 642-0070
Fax: (312) 642-8584
<http://www.aboms.org>

American Board of Plastic Surgery, Inc
Seven Penn Center, Suite 400, 1635 Market Street, Philadelphia, PA 19103-2204
(215) 587-9322
<http://www.abplsurg.org>

American Board of Registration of EEG and EP Technologists
PO Box 891663
Longwood, FL 32791
(407) 788-6308
<http://www.abret.org/index.htm>

American Board of Surgery (ABS)
1617 John F. Kennedy Boulevard, Suite 860
Philadelphia, PA 19103
(215) 568-4000
Fax: (215) 563-5718
<http://www.absurgery.org>

American Board of Urology (ABU)
2216 Ivy Road, Suite 210
Charlottesville, VA 22903
(434) 979-0059
<http://www.abu.org>

American Board of Vascular Surgery (ABVS)
900 Cummings Center, Suite 221-U
Beverly, MA 01915
<http://aavs.vascularweb.org>

American Burn Association
625 N. Michigan Ave., Suite 1530
Chicago, IL 60611
(800) 548-2876
Fax: (312) 642.9130
Email: info@ameriburn.org
<http://www.ameriburn.org>

American Cancer Society (ACS)
1599 Clifton Rd. NE
Atlanta, GA 30329-4251
(800) 227-2345
<http://www.cancer.org>

American Chiropractic Association
1701 Clarendon Blvd.
Arlington, VA 22209
(800) 986-4636
<http://www.amerchiro.org>

American Chronic Pain Association
P.O. Box 850
Rocklin, CA 95677-0850
(916) 632-0922
<http://members.tripod.com/~widdy/acpa.html>

American Cleft Palate-Craniofacial Association
104 South Estes Drive, Suite 204
Chapel Hill, NC 27514
(919) 933-9044
<http://www.cleftline.org>

American College of Cardiology
Heart House
9111 Old Georgetown Rd.
Bethesda, MD 20814-1699
(800) 253-4636, ext. 69
(301) 897-5400
<http://www.acc.org>

American College of Chest Physicians
3300 Dundee Road
Northbrook, Illinois 60062-2348
(847) 498-1400
<http://www.chestnet.org>

American College of Foot and Ankle Surgeons (ACFAS)
515 Busse Highway, Park Ridge, IL, 60068
(847) 292-2237
(800) 421-2237
<http://www.cmeonline.com/index.html>

American College of Gastroenterology (ACG)
4900-B South 31st Street
Arlington, VA 22206-1656
(703) 820-7400
Fax: (703) 931-4520
<http://www.acg.gi.org>

American College of Healthcare Executives
One North Franklin, Suite 1700
Chicago, IL 60606-4425
(312) 424-2800
Fax: 312-424-0023
<http://www.ache.org/>

American College of Nurse Practitioners
503 Capitol Ct. NE #300
Washington, DC 20002
(202) 546-4825
Email: acnp@nurse.org

American College of Nurse-Midwives
818 Connecticut Ave., NW, Suite 900
Washington, DC 20006
(202) 728-9860
<http://www.midwife.org>

American College of Obstetricians and Gynecologists (ACOG)
409 12th St. SW, PO Box 96920
Washington, DC 20090-6920
<http://www.acog.com>

American College of Phlebology
100 Webster Street, Suite 101
Oakland, CA 94607-3724
(510) 834-6500
<http://www.phlebology.org>

American College of Physicians
190 N. Independence Mall West
Philadelphia, PA 19106-1572
(800) 523-1546, ext. 2600
(215) 351-2600
<http://www.acponline.org>

American College of Radiology (ACR)
1891 Preston White Drive
Reston, VA 20191-4397
(800) 227-5463
<http://www.acr.org>

American College of Sports Medicine
401 West Michigan Street
Indianapolis, IN 46202-3233
(Mailing Address: P.O. Box 1440
Indianapolis, IN 46206-1440)
(317) 637-9200
Fax: (317) 634-7817
<http://www.acsm.org>

American College of Surgeons (ACS)
Office of Public Information

633 North Saint Clair Street
Chicago, IL 60611-3211
(312) 202-5000
<http://www.facs.org>

American Council on Transplantation
P.O. Box 1709
Alexandria, VA 22313
(800) ACT-GIVE (800-228-4483)

American Dental Association
211 E. Chicago Avenue
Chicago, IL 60611
(312) 440-2500
Fax: (312)440-7494
<http://www.ada.org>

American Diabetes Association
1701 North Beauregard Street
Alexandria, VA 22311
(800) 342-2383
Email: AskADA@diabetes.org
<http://www.diabetes.org>

American Foundation for Urologic Disease
1128 North Charles St.
Baltimore, MD 21201
(410) 468-1800
(800) 242-2383
Fax: (410) 468-1808
Email: admin@afud.org
<http://www.afud.org/>

American Gastroenterological Association (AGA)
4930 Del Ray Avenue
Bethesda, MD 20814
(301) 654-2055
<http://www.gastro.org>

American Health Lawyers Association
1025 Connecticut Avenue NW, Suite 600
Washington, DC 20036-5405
(202) 833-1100
<http://www.healthlawyers.org>

American Hearing Research Foundation
55 E. Washington St., Suite 2022
Chicago, IL 60602
(312) 726-9670
<http://www.american-hearing.org/>

American Heart Association
7272 Greenville Ave.
Dallas, TX 75231
(800) 242-8721
(214) 373-6300
<http://www.americanheart.org>

American Hospital Association, One North Franklin, Chicago, IL 60606-3421
(312) 422-3000
Fax: (312) 422-4796
<http://www.aha.org>

American Infertility Association
666 Fifth Avenue, Suite 278
New York, NY 10103
(718) 621-5083
Email: <info@americaninfertility.org>
<http://www.americaninfertility.org>

American Institute of Ultrasound in Medicine
14750 Sweiter Lane, Suite 100
Laurel, MD 20707-5906
(301) 498-4100
(800) 638-5352
<http://www.aium.org>

American Kidney Fund (AKF)
6110 Executive Boulevard, Suite 1010
Rockville, MD 20852
(800) 638-8299
Email: helpline@akfinc.org
<http://www.akfinc.org>

American Lithotripsy Society
305 Second Avenue, Suite 200,
Waltham, MA 02451

American Liver Foundation
75 Maiden Lane, Suite 603
New York, NY 10038
(800) 465-4837
(888) 443-7872
Fax: (212) 483-8179
Email: info@liverfoundation.org
<http://www.liverfoundation.org>

American Lung Association and American Thoracic Society
1740 Broadway
New York, NY 10019-4374
(800) 586-4872
(212) 315-8700
<http://www.lungusa.org> and
<http://www.thoracic.org>

American Medical Association
515 N. State Street
Chicago, IL 60610
(312) 464-5000
<http://www.ama-assn.org>

American Nurses Association
600 Maryland Avenue, SW, Suite 100 West
Washington, DC 20024
(800) 274-4262
<http://www.nursingworld.org>

American Obesity Association
1250 24th Street, NW, Suite 300

Washington, DC 20037
(202) 776-7711
<http://www.obesity.org>

American Optometric Association
243 North Lindbergh Blvd.
St. Louis, MO 63141
(314) 991-4100
<http://www.aoanet.org>

American Orthopaedic Foot and Ankle Society
2517 Eastlake Avenue E.
Seattle, WA 98102
(206) 223-1120
Fax: (206) 223-1178
Email: aofas@aofas.org
<http://www.aofas.org>

American Osteopathic Association (AOA)
142 East Ontario Street
Chicago, IL 60611
(800) 621-1773
(312) 202-8000
<http://www.aoa-net.org>

American Osteopathic College of Otolaryngology—Head and Neck Surgery
405 W. Grand Avenue
Dayton, OH 45405
(937) 222-8820
(800) 455-9404
Fax: (937) 222-8840
Email: info@aocoohns.org.

American Osteopathic College of Radiology
119 East Second St.
Milan, MO 63556
(660) 265-4011
<http://www.aocr.org>

American Pain Society
4700 West Lake Ave.
Glenview, IL 60025
(847) 375-4715
<http://www.ampainsoc.org>

American Pediatric Surgical Association (APSA)
60 Revere Drive, Suite 500
Northbrook, IL 60062
(847) 480-9576
<http://www.eapsa.org>

American Physical Therapy Association (APTA)
1111 North Fairfax Street
Alexandria, VA 22314
(703)684-APTA
(800) 999-2782
<http://www.apta.org>

American Podiatric Medical Association (APMA)
9312 Old Georgetown Road
Bethesda, MD 20814
(301) 571-9200
(800) 275-2762
Fax: (301) 530-2752
<http://www.apma.org>

American Professional Wound Care Association (APWCA)
Suite #A1-853 Second Street Pike
Richboro, PA 18954
(215) 364-4100
Fax: (215) 364-1146
Email: wounds@erols.com
<http://www.apwca.org>

American Prostate Society
P.O. Box 870
Hanover, MD 21076
(800) 308-1106
<http://www.ameripros.org>

American Psychiatric Association
1400 K Street NW
Washington, DC 20005
(888) 357-7924
Fax: (202) 682-6850
Email: apa@psych.org

American Psychological Association
750 First Street NW
Washington, DC 20002-4242
(800) 374-2721
(202) 336-5500
<http://www.apa.org/>

American Red Cross (ARC) National Headquarters
431 18th Street, NW
Washington, DC 20006
(202) 303-4498
<http://www.redcross.org>

American Registry of Diagnostic Medical Sonographers
600 Jefferson Plaza, Suite 360
Rockville, MD 20852-1150
(800) 541-9754
<http://www.ardms.org>

American Shoulder and Elbow Surgeons (ASES)
6300 North River Road, Suite 727
Rosemont, IL, 60018-4226
(847) 698-1629
<http://www.ases-assn.org>

American Sleep Apnea Association (ASAA)
1424 K Street NW, Suite 302
Washington, DC 20005
(202) 293-3650
<http://www.sleepapnea.org>

American Society for Aesthetic Plastic Surgery
11081 Winners Circle
Los Alamitos, CA 90720
(800) 364-2147
(562) 799-2356
<http://www.surgery.org>

American Society for Bariatric Surgery
7328 West University Avenue, Suite F
Gainesville, FL 32607
(352) 331-4900
<http://www.asbs.org>

American Society for Blood and Marrow Transplantation (ASBMT)
85 W. Algonquin Road, Suite 550
Arlington Heights, IL 60005
(847) 427-0224
Email: mail@asbmt.org.

American Society for Bone and Mineral Research
2025 M Street, NW, Suite 800
Washington, DC 20036-3309
(202) 367-1161
<http://www.asbmr.org/>

American Society for Clinical Pathology (ASCP)
2100 West Harrison Street
Chicago, Il 60612-3798
(312) 738-1336
<http://www.ascp.org>

American Society for Colposcopy and Cervical Pathology
20 West Washington St., Suite 1
Hagerstown, MD 21740
(301) 733-3640
<http://www.asccp.org/index.html>

American Society for Dermatologic Surgery (ASDS)
5550 Meadowbrook Dr., Suite 120
Rolling Meadows, IL 60008
(847) 956-0900
<http://www.asds-net.org>

American Society for Gastrointestinal Endoscopy
1520 Kensington Road, Suite 202
Oak Brook, IL 60523
(630) 573-0600
Fax: (630) 573-0691
Email: <info@asgeoffice.org>
<http://www.asge.org>

American Society for Laser Medicine and Surgery
2404 Stewart Square
Wausau, WI 54401
(715) 845-9283
<http://www.aslms.org>

American Society for Mohs Surgery
Private Mail Box 391
5901 Warner Avenue
Huntington Beach, CA 92649-4659
(714) 840-3065; (800) 616-ASMS
(2767)
<http://www.mohssurgery.org>

American Society for Reconstructive Microsurgery
20 North Michigan Ave., Suite 700
Chicago, IL 60602
(312) 456-9579
<http://www.microsurg.org>

American Society for Reproductive Medicine
1209 Montgomery Highway
Birmingham, AL 35216-2809
(205) 978-5000
<http://www.asrm.com>

American Society for Surgery of the Hand
6300 North River Road, Suite 600
Rosemont, IL 60018
(847) 384-1435
<http://www.assh.org>

American Society of Anesthesiologists/ASA
520 North Northwest Highway
Park Ridge, IL 60068-2573
(847) 825-5586
Fax: (847) 825-1692
Email: mail@asahq.org
<http://www.asahq.org>

American Society of Bariatric Physicians
5453 East Evans Place
Denver, CO 80222-5234
(303) 770-2526
<http://www.asbp.org>

American Society of Cataract and Refractive Surgery
4000 Legato Road, Suite 850
Fairfax, VA 22033-4055
(703) 591-2220
Email: ascrs@ascrs.org
<http://www.ascrs.org>

American Society of Clinical Oncology (ASCO)
1900 Duke Street, Suite 200
Alexandria, VA 22314
(703) 299-0150
<http://www.asco.org>

American Society of Colon and Rectal Surgeons
85 W. Algonquin Rd., Suite 550
Arlington Heights, IL 60005
(847) 290-9184
Fax: (847) 290-9203

Email: ascrs@fascrs.org
<http://www.fascrs.org>

American Society of Echocardiography
1500 Sunday Drive, Suite 102
Raleigh, NC 27607
(919) 787-5181
<http://asecho.org>

American Society of Electroneurodiagnostic Technologists Inc.
204 W. 7th
Carroll, IA 51401
(712) 792-2978
<http://www.aset.org/>

American Society of Extra-corporeal Technology
503 Carlisle Dr., Suite 125
Herndon, VA 20170
(703) 435-8556
<http://www.amsect.org>

American Society of Health-System Pharmacists (ASHP)
7272 Wisconsin Avenue
Bethesda, MD 20814
(301) 657-3000
<http://www.ashp.org>

American Society of Nephrology
1725 Eye Street, NW Suite 510
Washington, DC 20006
(202) 659-0599
Fax: (202) 659-0709.

American Society of PeriAnesthesia Nurses/ASPAN
10 Melrose Avenue, Suite 110
Cherry Hill, NJ 08003-3696
(877) 737-9696
Fax: (856) 616-9601
Email: aspan@aspan.org
<http://www.aspan.org>

American Society of Plastic Surgeons (ASPS)
444 East Algonquin Road
Arlington Heights, IL 60005
(847) 228-9900
<http://www.plasticsurgery.org>

American Society of Radiologic Technologists (ASRT)
15000 Central Avenue SE
Albuquerque, NM 87123-2778
(800) 444-2778
<http://www.asrt.org>

American Society of Transplantation
236 Route 38 West, Suite 100
Moorestown, NJ 08057
(856) 608-1104
Fax: (856) 608-1103
<http://www.a-s-t.org.>

American Society Parenteral and Enteral Nutrition
8630 Fenton St., Suite 412
Silver Springs, Maryland 20910
(301) 587-6315
Fax: (301) 587-2365
<http://www.clinnutr.org>

American Speech-Language-Hearing Association
10801 Rockville Pike
Rockville, MD 20852
(800) 638-8255
<http://www.asha.org>

American Urological Association (AUA)
1120 North Charles Street
Baltimore, MD 21201
(410) 727-1100
<http://www.auanet.org>

Anesthesia Patient Safety Foundation (APSF)
4246 Colonial Park Drive
Pittsburgh, PA 15227-2621
(412) 882-8040
<http://www.gasnet.org/societies/apsf>

Applied Biometrics
P.O. Box 3170
Burnsville, MN 55337
(952) 890-1123.

Arthritis Foundation
1300 W. Peachtree St.
Atlanta, GA 30309
(800) 283-7800
<http://www.arthritis.org>

Association of Perioperative Registered Nurses (AORN)
2170 South Parker Road, Suite 300
Denver, CO 80231-5711
(303) 755-6300
(800) 755-2676
<http://www.aorn.org>

Association of Surgical Technologists
7108-C South Alton Way, Suite 100
Englewood, CO 80112-2106
(800) 637-7433

Association of Thyroid Surgeons
717 Buena Vista St.
Ventura, CA 93001
Fax: (509) 479-8678
Email: info@thyroidsurgery.org

Association of Women's Health, Obstetric, and Neonatal Nurses
2000 L St., NW, Suite 740
Washington, DC 20036
(800) 673-8499
<http://www.awhonn.org>

Asthma and Allergy Foundation of America
1125 15th Street NW, Suite 502
Washington, DC 20005
(800) 727-8462
<http://www.aafa.org>

Better Hearing Institute
515 King Street, Suite 420
Alexandria, VA 22314
(703) 684-3391

BMT Infonet (Blood and Marrow Transplant Information Network)
2900 Skokie Valley Road, Suite B
Highland Park, IL 60035
(847) 433-3313, (888) 597-7674
Email: help@bmtinfonet.org
<http://www.bmtinfonet.org>

British Association of Oral and Maxillofacial Surgeons
Royal College of Surgeons
35-43 Lincoln's Inn Fields
London, UK WC2A 3PN
<http://www.baoms.org.uk>

Canadian Association of Gastroenterology (CAG)
2902 South Sheridan Way
Oakville, Ontario L6J 7L6
(888) 780-0007
(905) 829-2504
<http://www.cag-acg.org>

Canadian Institute for Health Information/Institut Canadien d'Information sur la Santé (CIHI)
377 Dalhousie Street, Suite 200
Ottawa, Ontario K1N 9N8
(613) 241-7860
<http://secure.cihi.ca/cihiweb>

Canadian Ophthalmological Society (COS)
610-1525 Carling Avenue, Ottawa ON K1Z 8R9 Canada
<http://www.eyesite.ca>

Canadian Prostate Cancer Network
P.O. Box 1253
Lakefield, Ontario K0L 2H0
(705) 652-9200
<http://www.cpcn.org>

Cancer Information Service, National Cancer Institute
Building 31, Room 10A19
9000 Rockville Pike
Bethesda, MD 20892
(800) 4-CANCER
<http://www.nci.nih.gov/cancerinfo/index.html>

Cancer support groups
<http://www.cancernews.com>

Cancercare
(800) 813-HOPE (4673)
<http://www.cancercare.org>

Cardiac Arrhythmia Research and Education Foundation (C.A.R.E.)
2082 Michelson Dr. #301
Irvine, CA 92612
(800) 404-9500
<http://www.longqt.com/>

Center for Biologics Evaluation and Research (CBER)
U.S. Food and Drug Administration (FDA)
1401 Rockville Pike
Rockville, MD 20852-1448
(800) 835-4709
(301) 827-1800
<http://www.fda.gov/cber>

Center for Devices and Radiological Health
United States Food and Drug Administration
1901 Chapman Ave.
Rockville, MD 20857
(301) 443-4109
<http://www.fda.gov/cdrh>

Center for Emergency Medicine
230 McKee Place, Suite 500
Pittsburgh, PA 15213
(412) 647-5300
<http://www.centerem.com>

Center for Fetal Diagnosis and Treatment
Children's Hospital of Philadelphia
34th Street and Civic Center Boulevard
Philadelphia, PA 19104-4399
(800) IN-UTERO
<http://fetalsurgery.chop.edu>

Center for Hip and Knee Replacement
Columbia University Department of Orthopaedic Surgery
Columbia Presbyterian Medical Center
622 West 168th Street, PH11-Center
New York, NY 10032
(212) 305-5974
<http://www.hipnknee.org>

Center for Male Reproductive Medicine
2080 Century Park East, Suite 907
Los Angeles, CA 90067
(310) 277-2873
<http://www.malereproduction.com>

Center for Medicare Advocacy
P.O. Box 350
Willimantic, CT 06226
(860) 456-7790
(202) 216-0028
<http://www.medicareadvocacy.org>

Center for Uterine Fibroids
Brigham and Women's Hospital
623 Thorn Building
20 Shattuck Street
Boston, MA 02115
(800) 722-5520
<http://www.fibroids.net>

Centers for Disease Control and Prevention (CDC)
1600 Clifton Road
Atlanta, GA 30333
(404) 639-3534
(800) 311-3435
<http://www.cdc.gov>

Centers for Disease Control and Prevention (CDC)
Cancer Prevention and Control Program
4770 Buford Highway, NE, MS K64
Atlanta, GA 30341
(888) 842-6355
<http://www.cdc.gov/cancer/comments.htm>

Centers for Disease Control and Prevention (CDC)
Division of Diabetes Translation
National Center for Chronic Disease Prevention and Health Promotion
4770 Buford Highway NE, TISB Mail Stop K-13
Atlanta, GA 30341-3724
(770) 488-5080
<http://www.cdc.gov/diabetes>

Centers for Disease Control and Prevention
Division of Reproductive Health
4770 Buford Highway, NE, Mail Stop K-20
Atlanta, GA 30341-3717
(770) 488-5200
<http://www.prochoice.org>

Centers for Medicare & Medicaid Services
7500 Security Boulevard
Baltimore, MD 21244-1850
(410) 786-3000
(877) 267-2323
<http://www.medicare.gov>

Children's Health Information Network
1561 Clark Drive
Yardley, PA 19067
(215) 493-3068
<http://www.tchin.org>

Children's Hospice International (CHI)
901 North Pitt Street, Suite 230
Alexandria, VA 22314
(703) 684-0330

(800) 2-4-CHILD
<http://www.chionline.org>

Children's Organ Transplant Association, Inc
2501 COTA Drive
Bloomington, IN 47403
(800) 366-2682
<http://www.cota.org>

Cleveland Clinic Heart Center
The Cleveland Clinic Foundation
9500 Euclid Avenue, F25
Cleveland, OH 44195
(800) 223-2273 ext. 46697
(216) 444-6697
<http://www.clevelandclinic.org/
heartcenter>

Coalition on Donation
700 North 4th Street
Richmond, VA 23219
(804)782-4920
Email: coalition@shareyourlife.org
<http://www.shareyourlife.org>

Cochlear Implant Club International
5335 Wisconsin Ave. NW, Suite 440
Washington, DC 20015-2052
(202) 895-2781
<http://www.cici.org>

Colorectal Cancer Network (CCNetwork)
P.O. Box 182
Kensington, MD 20895-0182
(301) 879-1500
Fax: (301) 879-1901
<http://www.colorectal-cancer.net>

Congenital Heart Anomalies Support, Education & Resources, Inc.
2112 North Wilkins Road
Swanton, OH 43558
(419) 825-5575
<http://www.csun.edu/~hfmth006/
chaser>

Council for Refractive Surgery Quality Assurance
8543 Everglade Drive
Sacramento, CA 95826-0769
(916) 381-0769
Email: info@usaeyes.org
<http://www.usaeyes.org>

Crohn's & Colitis Foundation of America Inc.
386 Park Avenue South, 17th floor
New York, NY 10016-8804
(800) 932-2423
(212) 685-3440
Fax: (212) 779-4098
Email: info@ccfa.org
<http://www.ccfa.org.>

DES Action USA
610 16th St., Ste. 301
Oakland, CA 94612
(510) 465-4011
<http://www.desaction.org>

Diabetic Retinopathy Foundation
350 North LaSalle, Suite 800
Chicago, IL 60610
<http://www.retinopathy.org>

e-Healthcare Solutions, Inc.
953 Route 202 North
Branchburg, NJ 08876
(908) 203-1350
Fax: (908) 203-1307
Email:info@e-healthcaresolutions.com
<http://www.digitalhealthcare.com/>

EA/TEF Child and Family Support Connection
111 West Jackson Blvd., Suite 1145
Chicago, IL 60604
(312) 987-9085
<http://www.eatef.org>

Endometriosis Association
8585 North 76th Place
Milwaukee, WI 53223
(414) 355-2200
<http://www.endometriosisassn.org>

Epilepsy Foundation
4351 Garden City Drive
Landover, MD 20785-7223
(800) 332-1000
<http://www.epilepsyfoundation.org/>

European Institute of Telesurgery
1, Place de l'Hôpital
F 67091 STRASBOURG Cedex
+33(0)388119000
<http://www.eits.org>

Extracorporeal Life Support Organization (ELSO)
1327 Jones Dr., Ste. 101
Ann Arbor, MI 48105
(734) 998-6600
<http://www.elso.med.umich.edu/>

Eye Bank Association of America
1015 Eighteenth Street NW, Suite 1010
Washington, DC 20036
(202) 775-4999
<http://www.restoresight.org>

FACES: The National Craniofacial Association
P.O. Box 11082
Chattanooga, TN 37401
(800) 332-2373
<http://www.faces-cranio.org>

Federal Drug Administration (FDA)
5600 Fishers Ln.

Rockville, MD 20857
(800) 532-4440
<http://www.fda.gov>

Federated Ambulatory Surgery Association (FASA)
700 North Fairfax Street, #306
Alexandria, VA 22314
(703) 836-8808
<http://www.fasa.org>

Federation of State Medical Boards of the United States, Inc.
P.O. Box 619850
Dallas, TX 75261-9850
(817) 868-4000
<http://www.fsmb.org>

Fetal Diagnosis & Therapy
Vanderbilt University Medical Center
B-1100 Medical Center North
Nashville, TN 37232
(615) 343-5227

Fetal Treatment Center
University of California San Francisco
513 Parnassus Ave., HSW 1601
San Francisco, CA 94143-0570
(800) RX-FETUS
<http://www.fetus.ucsf.edu>

Glaucoma Foundation
116 John Street, Suite 1605
New York, NY 10038
(212) 285-0080
(800) 452-8266
<http://www.glaucoma-foundation.org>

Glaucoma Research Foundation
490 Post Street, Suite 1427
San Francisco, CA 94102
(415) 986-3162
(800) 826-6693
<http://www.glaucoma.org>

Gynecologic Surgery Society
2440 M Street, NW, Suite 801
Washington, DC 20037
(202) 293-2046
<http://www.gynecologicsurgery
society.org>

Harry Benjamin International Gender Dysphoria Association, Inc. (HBIGDA)
1300 South Second Street, Suite 180
Minneapolis, MN 55454
(612) 625-1500
<http://www.hbigda.org>

Health Canada/Santé Canada
A.L. 0900C2
Ottawa, Ontario K1A 0K9
(613) 957-2991
<http://www.hc-sc.gc.ca>

**Health Care Financing
Administration**
United States Department of Health
and Human Services
200 Independence Avenue SW
Washington, DC 20201
<http://www.hcfa.gov>

**Health Insurance Association of
America**
1201 F Street, NW, Suite 500
Washington, DC 20004-1204
(202) 824-1600
Fax: (202) 824-1722
<http://www.hiaa.org/index_flash.cfm>

**Health Resources and Services
Administration (HRSA)**
5600 Fishers Lane, Rm. 14-45
Rockville, MD 20857
(301) 443-3376
Email:comments@hrsa.gov
<http://www.hrsa.gov>

Hearing Loss Link
2600 W. Peterson Ave., Ste. 202
Chicago, IL 60659
(312) 743-1032
(312) 743-1007 (TDD)

**Hepatitis Foundation International
(HFI)**
504 Blick Drive
Silver Spring, MD
20904-2901
(800) 891-0707
(301) 622-4200
Fax: (301) 622-4702
Email: hfi@comcast.net
<http://www.hepfi.org>

Hospice Foundation of America
2001 S. Street NW, Suite 300
Washington, DC 20009
(800) 854-3402
(202) 638-5419l
Fax: (202) 638-5312
Email: jon@hospicefoundation.org
<http://www.hospicefoundation.org>

**Illinois Nurses Association—
Advanced Practices Registered
Nurses (APRNs) Statistics**
105 W. Adams Suite 2101
Chicago, IL 60603
<http://www.illinoisnurses.org/aprn.
html>

Immune Tolerance Network (ITN)
5743 South Drexel Avenue, Suite 200
Chicago, IL 60637
(773) 834-5341
<http://www.immunetolerance.org>

**Institute for Bone and Joint
Disorders**
2222 East Highland Avenue
Phoenix, AZ 85016
(602) 553-3113
<http://www.ibjd.com>

Institute of Medicine (IOM)
The National Academies
500 Fifth Street, NW
Washington, DC 20001
<http://www.iom.edu>

**International Association of
Enterstomal Therapy**
27241 La Paz Road, Suite 121
Laguna Niguel, CA 92656
(714) 476-0268

**International Bariatric Surgery
Registry (IBSR)**
University of Iowa Hospitals and
Clinics
200 Hawkins Drive
Iowa City, IA 52242
(800) 777-8442
<http://www.uihealthcare.com>

**International Bone Marrow
Transplant Registry/Autologous
Blood and Marrow Transplant
Registry North America**
Health Policy Institute
Medical College of Wisconsin
8701 Watertown Plank Road
P.O. Box 26509
Milwaukee, WI 53226
(414) 456-8325
Email:ibmtr@mcw.edu

**International Cesarean Awareness
Network**
1304 Kingsdale Ave.
Redondo Beach, CA 90278
(310) 542-6400
<http://www.ican-online.org>

**International Council on Infertility
Information Dissemination, Inc.**
P.O. Box 6836
Arlington, VA 22206
(703) 379-9178
<http://www.inciid.org>

**International EECP Therapists
Association**
P.O. Box 650005
Vero Beach, FL 32965-0005
(800) 376-3321, ext. 140
<http://www.ietaonline.com>

**International Foundation for
Functional Gastrointestinal
Disorders (IFFGD)**
P.O. Box 170864
Milwaukee, WI 53217

(888) 964-2001
(414) 964-1799
Fax: (414) 964-7176
Email: iffgd@iffgd.org
<http://www.iffgd.org>

**International Radiosurgery Support
Association (IRSA)**
3005 Hoffman Street
Harrisburg, PA 17110
(717) 260-9808
<http://www.irsa.org>

Interstitial Cystitis Association
51 Monroe Street, Suite 1402
Rockville, MD 20850
(301) 610-5300
<http://www.ichelp.org>

Johns Hopkins Radiosurgery
Weinberg 1469, 600 North Wolfe Street
Baltimore, MD 21287
(410) 614-2886
<http://www.hopkinsmedicine.org/radi
osurgery/treatmentoptions/stereotact
icradiosurgery.cfm>

**Joint Commission on Accreditation
of Healthcare Organizations
(JCAHO)**
One Renaissance Boulevard
Oakbrook Terrace, IL 60181
(630) 792-5800
<http://www.jcaho.org>

Leukemia & Lymphoma Society, Inc.
1311 Mamaroneck Avenue
White Plains, NY 10605
(914) 949-5213
<http://www.leukemia-lymphoma.org>

Lipoplasty Society of North America
444 East Algonquin Road
Arlington Heights, IL 60005
(708) 228-9273
(800) 848-1991, ext. 1126
<http://www.lipoplasty.com/business/ls
na/index.htm>

**Lymphoma Research Foundation of
America**
8800 Venice Boulevard, Suite 207
Los Angeles, CA 90034
(800) 500-9976
(310) 204-7040
Email:helpline@lymphoma.org
<http://www.lymphoma.org>

**March of Dimes Birth Defects
Foundation**
1275 Mamaroneck Avenue
White Plains, NY
(914) 428-7100
<http://wwwmodimes.org>

Mayo Clinic
200 First St. SW
Rochester, MN 55905
(507) 284-2511
<http://www.mayoclinic.org>

Mayo Clinic
Division of Colon and Rectal Surgery
200 First St. SW
Rochester, MN 55905
(507) 284-2511
<http://www.mayoclinic.org/colo
   rectalsurgery-rst/laparoscopic
   surgery.html>

Midlife Women's Network
5129 Logan Ave. S.
Minneapolis, MN 55419
(800) 886-4354

Midwives Alliance of North America
4805 Lawrenceville Highway, Suite
   116-279
Lilburn, GA 30047
(888) 923-MANA
<http://www.mana.org>

Muscular Dystrophy Association
3300 E. Sunrise Drive
Tucson, AZ 85718
(800) 572-1717
<http://www.mdausa.org>

National Abortion Federation
1755 Massachusetts Ave., NW, Suite
   600
Washington, DC 20036
(202) 667-5881
<http://www.prochoice.org>

**National Adult Day Services
   Association**
8201 Greensboro Drive, Suite 300
McLean, VA 22102
(866) 890-7357
(703) 610-9035
Fax: (703) 610-9005
Email: info@nadsa.org

**National Alliance of Breast Cancer
   Organizations (NABCO)**
9 East 37th Street, 10th Floor
New York, NY 10016
(888) 80-NABCO
<http://www.nabco.org>

National Amputation Foundation
40 Church Street
Malverne, NY 11565
(516) 887-3600
<http://www.nationalamputation.org/>

**National Association for Continence
   (NAFC)**
P.O. Box 1019
Charleston, SC 29402-1019

(843) 377-0900
<http://www.nafc.org>

**National Association for Home Care
   and Hospice**
228 Seventh Street SE
Washington, DC 20003
(202) 547-7424
<http://www.nahc.org>

National Association for the Deaf
814 Thayer Ave.
Silver Spring, MD 20910
(301) 587-1788
(301) 587-1789 (TDD)
<http://www.nad.org>

**National Association for Women's
   Health**
300 W. Adams Street, Suite 328
Chicago, IL 60606-5101
(312) 786-1468
<http://www.nawh.org/>

**National Association of Emergency
   Medical Technicians (NAEMT)**
P.O. Box 1400
Clinton, MS 39060-1400
(800) 34-NAEMT
<http://www.naemt.org>

**National Association of Neonatal
   Nurses**
4700 West Lake Ave.
Glenview, IL 60025-1485
(847) 375-3660
(800) 451-3795
<http://www.nann.org>

**National Blood Data Resource
   Center (NBDRC)**
8101 Glenbrook Road
Bethesda, MD 20814-2749
(301) 215-6506
<http://www.nbdrc.org>

**National Blood Data Resource
   Center**
(301) 215-6506
<http://www.nbdrc.org>

**National Bone Marrow Transplant
   Link**
20411 W. 12 Mile Road, Suite 108
Southfield, MI 48076
(800) LINK-BMT (800-546-5268)
<http://comnet.org/nbmtlink/home2.
   html>

**National Cancer Institute (NCI) and
   Cancer Information Service (CIS)
   Office of Cancer Communications**
Bldg. 31, Room 10A16
Bethesda, MD 20892
(800) 4-CANCER
(800) 422-6237

Fax: (800) 624-2511
(301) 402-5874
Email:cancermail@cips.nci.nih.gov
<http://cancernet.nci.nih.gov>

**National Center for Complementary
   and Alternative Medicine
   (NCCAM) Clearinghouse**
P.O. Box 7923
Gaithersburg, MD 20898
(888) 644-6226
TTY: (866) 464-3615
Fax: (866) 464-3616
<http://www.nccam.nih.gov.>

**National Center on Sleep Disorders
   Research (NCSDR)**
Two Rockledge Centre, Suite 10038
6701 Rockledge Drive, MSC 7920
Bethesda, MD 20892-7920
(301) 435-0199
<http://www.nhlbi.nih.gov/about/ncsdr/
   index.htm>

**National Cholesterol Education
   Program**
National Heart, Lung, and Blood
   Institute (NHLBI)
National Institutes of Health
PO Box 30105
Bethesda, MD, 20824-0105
(301) 251-1222
<http://www.nhlbi.nih.gov/guidelines/
   cholesterol/atglance.pdf>

**National Chronic Pain Outreach
   Association, Inc.**
P.O. Box 274
Millboro, VA 24460-9606
(540) 597-5004

**National Committee for Quality
   Assurance**
2000 L St. NW
Washington, DC 20036
(202) 955-3500
<http://www.ncqa.org>

**National Comprehensive Cancer
   Network**
50 Huntingdon Pike, Suite 200
Rockledge PA 19046
(215) 728-4788
Fax: (215) 728-3877
Email: information@nccn.org
<http://www.nccn.org/>

**National Diabetes Information
   Clearinghouse (NDIC)**
1 Information Way
Bethesda, MD 20892-3560
(301) 907-8906
<http://www.niddk.nih.gov/health/
   diabetes/ndic.htm>

National Digestive Diseases Information Clearinghouse
2 Information Way
Bethesda, MD 20892-3570
Email:nddic@aerie.com
<http://www.niddk.nih.gov/Brochures/NDDIC.htm>

National Down Syndrome Society (NDSS)
666 Broadway
New York, NY 10012
(212) 460-9330
(800) 221-4602
<http://www.ndss.org>

National Eye Institute
2020 Vision Place
Bethesda, MD 20892-3655
(301) 496-5248
<http://www.nei.nih.gov>

National Foundation for Transplants
1102 Brookfield, Suite 200
Memphis, TN, 38110
(800) 489-3863
(901) 684-1697
<http://www.transplants.org>

National Head Injury Foundation, Inc.
(888) 222-5287
<http://www.nhif.org/home.html>

National Heart, Lung and Blood Institute (NHLBI)
6701 Rockledge Drive
P.O. Box 30105
Bethesda, MD 20824-0105
(301) 592-8573
<http://www.nhlhi.nih.gov/>

National Heart, Lung and Blood Institute (NHLBI)
Division of Blood Diseases and Resources
Two Rockledge Center, Suite 10138
6701 Rockledge Drive, MSC 7950
Bethesda, MD 20892-7950
<http://www.nhlbi.nih.gov/about/dbdr>

National Hospice and Palliative Care Organization (NHPCO)
1700 Diagonal Road, Suite 625
Alexandria, VA 22314
(703) 837-1500
(800) 658-8898 (Helpline)
<http://www.nhpco.org>

National Institute for Jewish Hospice (NIJH)
Cedars-Sinai Medical Center
444 South San Vincente Blvd., Suite 601
Los Angeles, CA 90048
(800) 446-4448
<http://www.jewishla.org>

National Institute of Arthritis and Musculoskeletal and Skin Diseases (NIAMS) Information Clearinghouse
National Institutes of Health
1 AMS Circle
Bethesda, MD 20892
(301) 495-4484
TTY: (301) 565-2966
<http://www.niams.nih.gov>

National Institute on Deafness and Other Communication Disorders (NIDCD)
National Institutes of Health
31 Center Drive, MSC 2320
Bethesda, MD 20892-2320
<http://www.nidcd.nih.gov>

National Institutes of Health
9000 Rockville Pike
Bethesda, MD 20892
(301) 496-4000
Email: NIHInfo@OD.NIH.GOV
<http://www.nih.gov/>

National Jewish Medical and Research Center
Lung-Line
14090 Jackson Street
Denver, Colorado 80206
<http://www.nationaljewish.org>

National Kidney and Urologic Diseases Information Clearinghouse
3 Information Way
Bethesda, MD 20892-3580
(800) 891-5390
(301) 654-4415
<http://www.niddk.nih.gov>

National Kidney Foundation
30 East 33rd Street, Suite 1100
New York, NY 10016
(800) 622-9010
(212) 889-2210
<http://www.kidney.org>

National Lung Health Education Program (NLHEP)
1850 High Street
Denver, CO 80218
<http://www.nlhep.org>

National Lymphedema Network
2211 Post St., Suite 404
San Francisco, CA 94115-3427
(800) 541-3259
(415) 921-1306
<http://www.wenet.net/~lymphnet>

National Marrow Donor Program
3001 Broadway Street NE, Suite 500
Minneapolis, MN 55413-1753
(800) 627-7692
<http://www.marrow.org>

National Organization for Rare Disorders (NORD)
55 Kenosia Avenue
P.O. Box 1968
Danbury, CT 06813-1968
(203) 744-0100
<http://www.rarediseases.org>

National Parkinson's Disease Foundation
Bob Hope Parkinson Research Center
1501 N.W. 9th Avenue, Bob Hope Road
Miami, FL 33136-1494
(305) 547-6666
(800) 327-4545
Fax: (305) 243-4403
<http://www.parkinson.org>

National Patient Advocate Foundation
753 Thimble Shoals Blvd, Suite A
Newport News, VA 23606
(800) 532-5274
Email: action@npaf.org
<http://www.npaf.org>

National Pressure Ulcer Advisory Panel
12100 Sunset Hills Road, Suite 130
Reston, VA 20190
(703) 464-4849
<http://www.npuap.org>

National Prison Hospice Association (NPHA)
P.O. Box 3769
Boulder, CO 80307-3769
(303) 544-5923
<http://www.npha.org>

National Scoliosis Foundation
5 Cabot Place
Stoughton, MA 020724
(800) 673-6922
<http://www.scoliosis.org>

National Stroke Association
9707 E. Easter Lane
Englewood, CO 80112
(800) Strokes
(303) 649-9299
<http://www.stroke.org>

National Transplant Assistance Fund
3475 West Chester Pike, Suite 230
Newtown Square, PA 19073
(800) 642-8399
(610) 353-1616
<http://www.transplantfund.org/>

New England Ophthalmological Society (NEOS)
P.O. Box 9165
Boston, MA 02114
(617) 227-6484
<http://www.neos-eyes.org/>

North American Society for Head and Neck Pathology
Department of Pathology
H179, P.O. Box 850
Milton S. Hershey Medical Center
Penn State University School of Medicine
Hershey, PA 17033
(717) 531-8246
<http://www.headandneckpathology.com/>

North American Society of Pacing and Electrophysiology
6 Strathmore Rd.
Natick, MA 01760-2499
(508) 647-0100
<http://www.naspe.org>

North American Spine Society
22 Calendar Court, 2nd Floor
LaGrange, IL 60525
(877) Spine-Dr
Email: info@spine.org
<http://www.spine.org>

Office of Rare Diseases (NIH)
6100 Executive Boulevard, Room 3A07, MSC 7518
Bethesda, Maryland 20892-7518
(301) 402-4336
<http://rarediseases.info.nih.gov/info-diseases.html>

Oral Cancer Foundation
3419 Via Lido, # 205
Newport Beach, CA 92663
(949) 646-8000
<http://www.oralcancer.org>

Orthopedic Trauma Association
6300 N. River Road, Suite 727
Rosemont, IL 60018-4226
(847) 698-1631
<http://www.ota.org/links.htm>

Overeaters Anonymous (OA)
World Service Office, P.O. Box 44020
Rio Rancho, NM 87174-4020
(505) 891-2664
<http://www.oa.org>

Partnership for Caring
1620 Eye St., NW, Suite 202
Washington, DC 20006
(202) 296-8071
(800) 989-9455
Fax: (202) 296-8352
<http://www.partnershipforcaring.org/>

Partnership for Organ Donation
Two Oliver Street
Boston, MA 02109
(617) 482-5746
E-Mail: info@organdonation.org
<http://www.organdonation.org/>

Periodontal (Gum) Diseases
National Institute of Dental and Craniofacial Research
National Institutes of Health
Bethesda, MD 20892-2190
(301) 496-4261
<http://www.nidcrinfo.nih.gov.>

Peripheral Vascular Surgery Society (PVSS)
824 Munras Avenue, Suite C
Monterey, CA 93940
(831) 373-0508
<http://www.pvss.org>

Physicians and Nurses for Blood Conservation (PNBC)
P.O. Box 217, 6-2400 Dundas Street West
Mississauga, Ontario L5K 2R8
(905) 608-1647
<http://www.pnbc.ca>

Planned Parenthood Federation of America, Inc.
810 Seventh Ave.
New York, NY 10019
(800) 669-0156
<http://www.plannedparenthood.org>

Prevent Blindness America
500 East Remington Road
Schaumburg, IL 60173
(800) 331-2020
<http://www.prevent-blindness.org>

Promoting Excellence in End of Life Care
RWJ Foundation National Program Office
c/o The Practical Ethics Center
The University of Montana
1000 East Beckwith Avenue
Missoula, Montana 59812
(406) 243-6601
Fax: (406) 243-6633
Email: excell@selway.umt.edu
<http://www.promotingexcellence.org/content/contactus.html>

Prune Belly Syndrome Network
P.O. Box 2125
Evansville, IN 47728-0125
<http://www.prunebelly.org>

Radiological Society of North America
820 Jorie Boulevard
Oak Brook, IL 60523-2251
(630) 571-2670
<http://www.rsna.org>

Rothman Institute of Orthopaedics
925 Chestnut Street
Philadelphia, PA 19107-4216
(215) 955-3458
<http://www.rothmaninstitute.com>

Rush Arthritis and Orthopedics Institute
1725 West Harrison Street, Suite 1055
Chicago, IL 60612
(312) 563-2420
<http://www.rush.edu>

Second Wind Lung Transplant Association, Inc
9030 West Lakeview Court
Crystal River, FL 34428
(888) 222-2690
<http://www.arthouse.com/secondwind>

Shape Up America!
c/o WebFront Solutions Corporation
15757 Crabbs Branch Way
Rockville, MD 20855
(301) 258-0540
<http://www.shapeup.org>

Shrine and Shriner's Hospitals
2900 Rocky Point Dr.
Tampa, FL 33607-1460
(813) 281-0300
<http://www.shrinershq.org/index.html>

Simon Foundation for Continence
P.O. Box 835
Wilmette, IL 60091
(800) 23-SIMON
(847) 864-3913
<http://www.simonfoundation.org>

Society for the Advancement of Blood Management (SABM)
350 Engle Street
Englewood, NJ 07631
(866) 894-3916
<http://www.sabm.org>

Society of American Gastrointestinal Endoscopic Surgeons
2716 Ocean Park Blvd., Suite 3000
Santa Monica, CA 90405
(310) 314-2404
Fax: (310) 314-2585
Email: sagesweb@sages.org
<http://www.sages.org>

Society of Critical Care Medicine (SCCM)
701 Lee Street, Suite 200
Des Plaines, IL 60016
(847) 827-6869
Fax: (847) 827-6869
<http://www.sccm.org>

Society of Diagnostic Medical Sonography
12770 Coit Road, Suite 708
Dallas, TX 75251-1319
(972) 239-7367
<http://www.sdms.org>

Society of Gastroenterology Nurses and Associates Inc.
401 North Michigan Avenue
Chicago, IL 60611-4267
(800) 245-7462
Fax: (312) 527-6658
<http://www.sgna.org>

Society of Gynecologic Oncologists
401 North Michigan Ave.
Chicago, IL 60611
(312) 644-6610
<http://www.sgo.org>

Society of Interventional Radiology
10201 Lee Highway, Suite 500
Fairfax, VA 22030
(800) 488-7284
Email: info@sirweb.org
<http://www.sirweb.org/index.shtml>

Society of Laparoendoscopic Surgeons
7330 SW 62nd Place, Suite 410
Miami, FL 33143-4825
(305) 665-9959
<http://www.sls.org>

Society of Nuclear Medicine (SNM)
1850 Samuel Morse Drive
Reston, VA 20190
(703) 708-9000
<http://www.snm.org>

Society for Pediatric Urology (SPU)
c/o HealthInfo
870 East Higgins Road, Suite 142
Schaumburg, IL 60173
<http://www.spuonline.org>

Society of Surgical Oncology
85 W. Algonquin Rd., Suite 550
Arlington Heights, IL 60005
(847) 427-1400
<http://www.surgonc.org>

Society for Technology in Anesthesia (STA)
PMB 300, 223 North Guadalupe
Santa Fe, NM 87501
(505) 983-4923
<http://www.anestech.org>

Society of Thoracic Surgeons
633 N. Saint Clair St., Suite 2320
Chicago, IL 60611-3658
(312) 202-5800
Fax: 312-202-5801
Email:sts@sts.org
<http://www.sts.org>

Society of Toxicology (SOT)
1767 Business Center Drive, Suite 302
Reston, VA 20190
(703) 438-3115
<http://www.toxicology.org>

Society of Urologic Nurses and Associates
East Holly Avenue, Box 56
Pitman, NJ 08071-0056
(609) 256-2335
<http://suna.inurse.com/>

Society for Vascular Surgery
900 Cummings Center
Beverly, MA 01915-1314
(978) 927-8330
<http://www.svs.vasculaweb.org>

Southern Thoracic Surgical Association
633 N. Saint Clair St., Suite 2320
Chicago, IL, 60611-3658
(800) 685-7872
<http://www.stsa.org/>

Spina Bifida Association of America
4590 MacArthur Boulevard, NW, Suite 250
Washington, DC 20007-4226
(800) 621-3141
(202)944-3285
Email:sbaa@sbaa.org
<http://www.sbaa.org>

Spine Center
1911 Arch St.
Philadelphia, PA 19103
(215) 665-8300
<http://www.thespinecenter.com>

Texas Heart Institute Heart Information Service
P.O. Box 20345
Houston, TX 77225-0345
(800) 292-2221
<http://www.tmc.edu/thi/his.html>

Tissue Adhesive Center
University of Virginia Health Sciences Center
MR4 Building, Room 3122
Charlottesville, VA 22908
(434) 243-0315
<http://www.hsc.virginia.edu/tac>

Transplant Foundation
8002 Discovery Drive, Suite 310
Richmond, VA 23229
(804) 285-5115
Email: otfnatl@aol.com

Transplant Recipients International Organization
2117 L Street NW, Suite 353
Washington, DC 20037
(800) TRIO-386
Email: triointl@aol.com
<http://www.trioweb.org/>

United Cerebral Palsy
1660 L Street, NW, Suite 700

Washington, DC 20036
(800) 872-5827
(202)776-0406
TTY: (202) 973-7197
Fax: (202) 776-0414
Email:webmaster@ucp.org
<http://www.UCP.org>

United Network for Organ Sharing (UNOS)
700 North 4th St.
Richmond, VA 23219
(888) 894-6361
<http://www.transplantliving.org>

United Ostomy Association (UOA)
19772 MacArthur Blvd., #200
Irvine, CA 92612-2405
(800) 826-0826
<http://www.uoa.org>

U.S. Administration on Aging (AOA)
United States Department of Health and Human Services
330 Independence Avenue, SW
Washington, DC 20201
(202) 619-0724
<http://www.aoa.gov>

U.S. Living Will Registry
523 Westfield Ave., P.O. Box 2789
Westfield, NJ 07091-2789
(800) LIV-WILL
(800) 548-9455
<http://www.uslivingwillregistry.com/>

United States Food and Drug Administration (FDA)
5600 Fishers Lane
Rockville, MD 20857-0001
(888) INFO-FDA
<http://www.fda.gov>

United States Renal Data System (USRDS)
Coordinating Center
The University of Minnesota
914 South 8th Street, Suite D-206
Minneapolis, MN 55404
(888) 99USRDS
<http://www.usrds.org>

University of Maryland Medical Center
R. Adams Cowley Shock Trauma Center
22 South Greene Street
Baltimore, MD 21201
(410) 328-2757
(800) 373-4111
<http://www.umm.edu/shocktrauma>

University of Michigan Kellogg Eye Center
Department of Ophthalmology and Visual Sciences

1000 Wall Street
Ann Arbor, MI 48105
(734) 763-1415
<http://www.kellogg.umich.edu>

Valley Baptist Heart and Vascular Institute
2101 Pease Street, P.O. Drawer 2588
Harlingen, TX 78550
(956) 389-4848

Vascular Birthmark Foundation
P.O. Box 106
Latham, NY 12110
(877) VBF-LOOK (daytime)
(877) VBF-4646 (evenings and
    weekends)
<http://www.birthmark.org>

Vascular Disease Foundation
3333 South Wadsworth Blvd. B104-37
Lakewood, CO 80227
(303) 949-8337
(866) PADINFO (723-4636)
<http://www.vdf.org>

Vestibular Disorders Association (VEDA)
PO Box 4467
Portland, OR 97208-4467
(800) 837-8428
<http://www.vestibular.org>

Visiting Nurse Associations of America
11 Beacon Street, Suite 910
Boston, MA 02108
(888) 866-8773
(617) 523-4042
Fax: (617) 227-4843
Email:vnaa@vnaa.org
<http://www.vnaa.org>

Washington Home Center for Palliative Care Studies(CPCS)
4200 Wisconsin Avenue, NW, 4th Floor
Washington, DC 20016
(202) 895-2625
Fax: (202) 966-5410
Email: info@medicaring.org
<http://www.medicaring.org>

WE MOVE, Worldwide Education and Awareness for Movement Disorders
204 West 84th Street
New York, NY 10024
(800) 437-MOV2
Fax: (212) 875-8389
<http://www.wemove.org>

Weight-Control Information Network (WIN)
1 WIN Way
Bethesda, MD 20892-3665
(202) 828-1025
(877) 946-4627

Wills Eye Hospital
840 Walnut Street
Philadelphia, PA 19107
(215) 928-3000
<http://www.willseye.org>

Wound Care Institute
1100 N.E. 163rd Street, Suite #101
North Miami Beach, FL 33162
(305) 919-9192
<http://woundcare.org>

Wound Healing Society
13355 Tenth Ave., Suite 108
Minneapolis, MN 55441-5554
<http://www.woundheal.org/>

Wound Ostomy and Continence Nurses Society
2755 Bristol Street, Suite 110
Costa Mesa, CA 92626
(714) 476-0268
<http://www.wocn.org>

Y-ME National Breast Cancer Organization
212 W. Van Buren St., Suite 500
Chicago, IL 60607-3908
(312) 986-8338
Fax: (312) 294-8597
(800) 221-2141 (English)
(800) 986-9505 (Español)
<http:// www.y-me.org>

Zen Hospice Project
273 Page Street
San Francisco, CA 94102
(415) 863-2910
<http://www.zenhospice.org>

INDEX

References to individual volumes are indicated by numbers (1, 2, or 3) followed by a colon. The numbers following the colon refer to page numbers. **Boldface** references indicate main topical essays. Illustrations are highlighted with an *italicized* page number; tables are also indicated with the page number followed by an *italicized* lowercase "t."

A

A-Line (R) monitor, 1:164
A-mode ultrasound, 1:3
A-scan measurement, 2:608, 3:1143
AAA. *See* Aortic aneurysm
AAAAPSF (American Association for Accreditation of Ambulatory Plastic Surgery Facilities), 1:38
AAAHC (Accreditation Association for Ambulatory Health Care), 1:540, 2:595
AABB (American Association of Blood Banks), 1:172, 175, 181, 196, 3:1439
AACS (American Academy of Cosmetic Surgery), 1:521, 549
AAFPRS (American Academy of Facial Plastic and Reconstructive Surgery), 3:1263
AAHPM (American Academy of Hospice and Palliative Medicine), 2:682–683
AARP (American Association of Retired Persons), 2:907
Aarskog syndrome, 1:301
Abbokinase. *See* Urokinase
ABC (Airway patency, Breathing and Circulation), 1:374
Abdominal aorta
    angiography of, 1:70
    peripheral endarterectomy of, 3:1129
    peripheral vascular bypass surgery of, 3:1132–1136
Abdominal aortic aneurysm
    emergency surgery for, 1:453
    endovascular stent surgery for, 1:466
    lithotripsy and, 2:884
    mortality from, 1:469
    repair of, 1:102, 103
    ultrasound for, 1:2, 3
Abdominal cerclage, 1:279
Abdominal hernia, 2:573
Abdominal hysterectomy, 1:332, 333, 2:708, 709, 3:1259
Abdominal injuries
    biliary stenting for, 1:160

exploratory laparotomy for, 2:838
ultrasound for, 1:1
Abdominal mass ultrasound, 1:1
Abdominal pain
    from lithotripsy, 2:884
    ultrasound for, 1:1, 3
Abdominal paravaginal repair, 1:397
Abdominal skin abdominoplasty, 1:7
Abdominal surgery
    incisional hernia repair for, 2:746–750
    myomectomy and, 2:999, 1000–1001
    oophorectomy and, 2:1039
    surgical oncology and, 3:1384
    See also Laparoscopy
Abdominal ultrasound, **1:1–5**, *2*
Abdominal wall defect repair, **1:5–7**
    See also Hernia repair
Abdominal wall defects, 1:5–7, 3:1116–1117
    See also Hernia
Abdominoplasty, **1:7–12**, *8, 11*
Aberrometer, 2:844
AbioCor artificial heart, 2:644
Ablating electrode catheters, 1:450
Ablation
    catheter, 1:449, 450, 451
    decentered, 2:846
    endometrial, 2:910
    LASIK and, 2:844
    for pain, 3:1085
    radiofrequency, 2:828, 937, 999, 3:1390
ABMS. *See* American Board of Medical Specialists
Abnormal heart rhythms. *See* Arrhythmia
ABO blood groups, 3:1440–1441
    blood donation, 1:174
    compatibility and, 3:1483
    defined, 3:1480, 1482
    for tissue compatibility testing, 2:691
    transfusion reaction and, 1:180
Abortion
    incomplete, 1:419, 421
    induced, **1:12–18**, *14*, 2:1034
    medical (drug-induced), 1:13–14

surgical, 1:15–16
    therapeutic, 1:13, 533
    See also Miscarriage
ABS. *See* American Board of Surgery
Abscess
    from anesthetics, 1:66
    brain, 1:369, 483, 2:1026
    debridement of, 1:406
    erythromycins for, 1:483
    incision and drainage, **1:18–21**, *19*
    lung, *1:19*, 2:904
    ovarian, 2:1038
    spinal epidural, 2:1026
    spleen, 3:1362
Absorbable sutures, 2:743, 972, 3:1374
Abuse
    child, 1:362
    elder, 2:1031–1032
Academy of Hospice Physicians, 2:682
Acardiac twins, 1:534
Accidents
    automobile, 1:363, 372
    children in, 3:1118–1119
Accreditation
    of ambulatory surgery centers, 1:38, 540, 2:579, 595, 1072, 3:1195
    of hospitals, 1:540, 3:1195
Accreditation Association for Ambulatory Health Care (AAAHC), 1:540, 2:595
Accupril. *See* Quinapril
Accutane. *See* Cis-retinoic acid
ACE II inhibitors, 1:89, 91
ACE inhibitors. *See* Angiotensin-converting enzyme inhibitors
Acebutolol, 1:89, 90*t*, 91
Acetabular dysplasia, 2:661, 662
Acetabulum, 2:661, 662, 664, 666
Acetaminophen, **1:21–23**
    for analgesia, 1:50, 51, 52, 3:1084, 1379
    with codeine, 1:359
    for colposcopy, 1:330
    for cryotherapy, 1:378
    for cyclocryotherapy, 1:389
    for cystoscopy, 1:400
    erythromycins and, 1:485
    eye muscle surgery and, 1:518
    for gingivectomy, 2:599

interferons and, 2:730
  for liver biopsy, 2:889
  in opioid analgesics, 1:53
  overdose, 1:22, 2:652, 886
  for tooth replantation, 3:1430
  after vasectomy, 3:1526
Acetazolamide, 2:608
  for closed-angle glaucoma, 2:773
  for glaucoma, 1:428
  for intraocular pressure, 2:851
Acetic acid, 2:859
Acetylsalicylic acid. *See* Aspirin
Achalasia, 1:492, 494, 2:583
Achilles tendon, 1:231, 3:1400, 1404
Acid-base balance tests, 1:446–449
Acid clearing test, 1:491
Acid perfusion test, 1:491
Acid reflux disease. *See* Gastroe-
  sophageal reflux disease
Acidosis, 1:447
AcipHex. *See* Rabeprazole
ACL. *See* Anterior cruciate ligament
  (ACL) injuries
Acne dermabrasion, 1:416–419
Acne scars, 3:1266
ACOG (American College of Obstetri-
  cians and Gynecologists), 1:287,
  3:1509
Acquired hernia, 2:753–755
Acquired immunodeficiency syndrome
  (AIDS), 3:1440, 1441
Acrocyanosis, 3:1128
Acromegaly, 3:1329
Acromioclavicular joint, 3:1308, 1312,
  1313, 1314
    See also Shoulder
Acrylic implants, 2:855, 856
Acrylic polymer cement, 2:666
ACTH (Adrenocorticotropic hormone),
  1:360
Acthar. *See* Adrenocorticotropic hor-
  mone
Actinic keratoses
    cryotherapy for, 1:377
    curettage and electrosurgery for,
    1:385–387
Actinomyces infections, 1:48
Activase. *See* Alteplase
Activated carbon, 2:652
Active immune therapy, 2:731
Activities of daily living, 2:678, 906,
  1030
Actrel. *See* Adrenocorticotropic hor-
  mone
Acupressure, 3:1084–1085
Acupuncture
    back pain, 2:826
    carpal tunnel syndrome, 1:261
    myringotomy, 2:1005, 1006
    pain, 3:1084–1085
    smoking cessation, 3:1339
    snoring, 3:1348
Acute care physiologic monitoring,
  2:760, 1046

Acute cholecystitis, 1:295, 296–297,
  2:558–559
Acute hemolytic transfusion reaction
  (AHTR), 3:1483
Acute normo-volemic hemodilution,
  1:135
Acute pain, 1:50, 67, 3:1083, 1086
Acute pancreatitis, 2:580
Acyclovir, 2:687
Adalat. *See* Nifedipine
Adam's apple, 1:374
Addiction
    analgesics and, 1:50, 51
    nicotine, 3:1241, 1338
    opioid analgesics and, 1:52, 3:1087,
    1185
    See also Alcoholism
Addisonian crisis, 1:360
Addison's disease, 1:359, 447, 2:647
Adenocarcinoma
    esophageal, 1:493, 494, 2:580, 3:1412
    of the lung, 3:1411–1412
    small intestine, 3:1333, 1335
    stomach, 2:566, 576
    urachus tube defects and, 3:1103
    ureterosigmoidoscopy and, 3:1494
Adenoidectomy, **1:23–26**, *24*, 1:433,
  434, 435, 2:1006
Adenoids
    chronic infection of, 1:24
    removal of, 1:23–26, *1:24*, 1:433,
    434, 435, 2:1006
    snoring and, 3:1345
Adenoma, pituitary, 2:697
Adenosine triphosphate (ATP), 1:240
Adhesions
    intestinal obstruction repair for,
    2:763
    lysis of, 2:764
    from myomectomy, 2:1001
    peritoneal dialysis and, 2:781
    second-look surgery for, 3:1288
Adhesive
    surgical, 2:703
    wound, 1:536–538
Administration on Aging, Ombudsmen
  Program, 2:908–909
Admission to the hospital, **1:26–28,**
  2:757, 956, 3:1169–1171
Adolescents
    bone marrow aspiration and biopsy
    for, 1:191
    fluoroquinolones for, 1:546
    liver transplantation for, 2:898, 899
    preparing for surgery, 3:1113
    rhinoplasty for, 3:1240
    spinal fusion for, 3:1353
Adoption, 1:18
Adoptive immunotherapy, 2:731–732
Adrenal crisis, 1:360
Adrenal gland hormones, 1:28, 30
Adrenal gland tumors, 1:28
Adrenalectomy, **1:28–32**, *29*
Adrenalin. *See* Epinephrine

Adrenergic drugs, **1:32–35**
Adrenergic nerve stimulation, 1:89
Adrenocorticoids, 1:153
Adrenocorticotropic hormone (ACTH),
  1:360
Adult day care, **1:35–37,** 2:908
Advance directives
    health care proxy and, 2:622–623
    hospital admissions and, 1:27,
    3:1170–1171
    power of attorney and, 3:1190
    preoperative, 3:1198, 1201
    purpose of, 1:404
    See also Do-not-resuscitate orders;
    Living wills
Adverse events, 2:959
Advertisements, 1:541, 3:1561
Advil. *See* Ibuprofen
AEDS (Automated external defibrilla-
  tors), 1:412
AER system, 1:228
Aerobic exercise, 1:508, 2:574
Aerophagia, 2:1075
Aesculus hippocastanum, 3:1284–1285
AESOP endoscopy, 3:1398
Aethoxysklerol, 3:1282
Afferent loop syndrome, 2:566
AFP. *See* Alpha-fetoprotein test
African Americans
    bladder cancer, 3:1452
    glaucoma, 3:1431
    umbilical hernia repair, 3:1485
Aganglionic megacolon, 3:1116
Age factors
    anesthesia, 1:57, 162
    bone marrow transplantation, 1:194
    carpal tunnel release, 1:257
    cartilage injuries, 2:801
    glaucoma, 3:1273
    hip revision surgery, 2:676
    hospital services and, 2:689
    knee arthroscopic surgery, 2:796
    knee injuries, 2:812
    lens opacification, 2:854–855
    low back pain, 2:820
    pain, 3:1082
    surgical risk, 1:403
Aged. *See* Elderly
Agency for Health Care Policy and Re-
  search
    on alternatives to surgery, 1:539
    on bedsores, 1:156
    HCUP Nationwide Inpatient Sam-
    ple, 2:1013–1014
    on medical errors, 2:962
    on urinary incontinence, 1:124–125,
    3:1330
Aggrastat. *See* Tirofiban
Aging
    cataracts and, 1:510, 511
    fractures and, 1:553, 555
    laser skin resurfacing for,
    2:857–859
    See also Age factors

AHF plasma, 1:173
AHTR (Acute hemolytic transfusion reaction), 3:1483
AIDS (Acquired immunodeficiency syndrome), 3:1440, 1441
Air pollution, 2:903, 3:1175
Airflow
    negative-pressure, 1:130
    positive-pressure, 1:129
Airway assessment
    for anesthesia, 1:57
    for snoring surgery, 3:1346
    spirometry tests for, 3:1358–1360
    stethoscope for, 3:1371, 1372
Airway management
    cricothyroidotomy for, 1:372–377
    laryngeal mask and, 1:62, 465
    lung biopsy for, 2:914
Airway obstruction, 3:1175
Airway puncture, emergency, **1:372–377**, *373*
AJWRB (Associated Jehovah's Witnesses for Reform on Blood), 1:180
Akinesis, 2:993
Alanine aminotransferase (ALT), 2:890–895
Alarms
    intensive care unit equipment, 2:762
    pulse oximeter, 3:1207–1208
Albumin
    fructosamine assay for, 2:605
    liver function tests for, 2:890–895
    surgical risk and, 1:403
Albuterol, 1:33, 3:1359
Alcohol antiseptics, 1:94
Alcohol injections, 1:391
Alcoholic beverages
    acetaminophen and, 1:22
    anticoagulants and, 1:87
    antinausea drugs and, 1:92
    arrhythmias and, 1:251, 2:940
    atherosclerosis prevention and, 1:469
    cephalosporins and, 1:269
    ophthalmologic surgery and, 2:1050
    opioid analgesics and, 1:53
    snoring and, 3:1343, 1345
    throat cancer and, 3:1147
    tongue cancer and, 2:601
Alcoholic liver disease, 2:892–894
Alcoholics Anonymous, 2:900
Alcoholism
    cataracts and, 1:511
    cirrhosis from, 3:1179
    confidentiality and, 3:1106–1107
    esophageal cancer and, 1:494
    fracture repair and, 1:555
    liver transplantation and, 2:895, 900
    magnesium and, 1:448
Aldactone. *See* Spironolactone
Aldatazide, 1:90*t*
Aldesleukin, 2:728, 729, 730–731
Aldomet. *See* Methyldopa
Aldrete scale, 3:1188

Aleve. *See* Naproxen
Alexander technique, 2:826
Alexandrite lasers, 3:1284
Alfa interferons, 2:729
Alfalfa, 1:34
Alferon, 2:729
Alginate dressings, 1:144, 145
Alimentary tract obstruction, 3:1116
Alka-Seltzer Original Effervescent Antacid Pain Reliever, 1:131
Alkaline phosphatase, 1:295, 2:892
Alkaline reflux gastritis, 2:577
Alkalosis, metabolic, 1:447
Alleles, 2:691, 692
Allergic rhinitis, 3:1305
Allergies
    adrenergic drugs for, 1:32, 33
    to anesthesia, 1:59
    to anticoagulants, 1:87
    to aspirin, 1:51, 132
    to azithromycin, 1:484
    to barbiturates, 1:152
    to cephalosporins, 1:269, 3:1206
    to clarithromycin, 1:484
    to contrast medium, 1:72, 237, 238, 3:1150
    cricothyroidotomy for, 1:374
    to diuretics, 1:429
    eosinophils and, 1:337
    to erythromycins, 1:484
    to fluoroquinolones, 1:547
    to immunosuppressant drugs, 2:734
    to iodine, 1:115, 237, 2:659
    to latex, 3:1192
    to NSAIDs, 2:1028
    to sclerosing agents, 3:1283
    to sulfonamides, 1:429, 3:1378
    to topical antibiotics, 1:85
Allogenic bone marrow transplantation, 1:194, 195, 197, 202
Allogenic transfusion, 1:134, 136
Allografts, 1:185, 187, 3:1325
Alloimmunization, 1:179
Alloplastic implants, 2:968
Allopurinol, 2:736, 1020
Alopecia, 2:613–615
Alozol. *See* Indapamide
Alpha-1 globulin, 2:893
Alpha-2 globulin, 2:893
Alpha/beta-adrenergic blockers, 1:89
Alpha coma, 1:445
Alpha-fetoprotein (AFP) test, 1:532
    amniocentesis and, 1:41
    for liver cancer, 2:892
    for spina bifida, 2:965
    tumor markers, 3:1470, 1471
Alpha-hydroxy acid, 3:1267
Alpha receptors, 1:33
Alpha waves, 1:444, 445
Alprazolam, 1:80, 93
ALS, mechanical ventilation for, 3:1436
ALT (Alanine aminotransferase), 2:890–895

Altace. *See* Ramipril
Altemeier procedure, 3:1223, 1224
Alteplase, 3:1417
Alternative medicine. *See* Complementary and alternative medicine
Alupent. *See* Albuterol
Alzheimer's disease, 1:444
AMA. *See* American Medical Association
Amalgams, 3:1245
Amantadine, 2:687, 3:1380
Ambiguous genitalia, 3:1305
Ambulatory esophageal pH monitoring, 1:490–493, 2:583, 584, 589
Ambulatory phlebectomy, 3:1532
Ambulatory surgery centers, **1:37–40,** 2:1071–1072
    accreditation of, 1:38, 540, 2:579, 595, 1072, 3:1195
    laser surgery in, 2:862
    operating rooms in, 2:1047–1048
    postoperative care in, 3:1187
    recovery rooms in, 3:1222
    selecting, 3:1195
    surgical teams in, 3:1386–1387
    See also Outpatient surgery
American Academy of Cosmetic Surgery (AACS), 1:521, 549
American Academy of Facial Plastic and Reconstructive Surgery (AAFPRS), 3:1263
American Academy of Family Physicians, 1:149, 461
American Academy of Hospice and Palliative Medicine (AAHPM), 2:682–683
American Academy of Ophthalmology, 2:842, 1048, 3:1158
American Academy of Orthopaedic Surgeons
    on arthroplasty, 1:116, 118
    on arthroscopic surgery, 1:121, 122
    on hip replacement, 2:665
    on knee injuries, 2:796, 812
    on knee replacement, 2:802
    on low back pain, 2:825
    on orthopedic surgeons, 2:1064
American Academy of Pediatrics
    on circumcision, 1:298
    on conscious sedation, 3:1293
    on subspecialists, 3:1115
American Academy of Sleep Medicine, 3:1346
American Association for Accreditation of Ambulatory Plastic Surgery Facilities (AAAAPSF), 1:38
American Association for the Study of Liver Diseases, 3:1138–1139
American Association of Blood Banks (AABB), 1:172, 175, 181, 196, 3:1439
American Association of Cancer Registries, 3:1382–1383

American Association of Endodontists, 3:1430

American Association of Retired Persons (AARP), 2:907

American Board of Eye Surgery, 1:474

American Board of Medical Specialists (ABMS)
  certification by, 1:540, 3:1165, 1195
  on general surgeons, 1:539
  on ophthalmology, 2:772
  on second opinions, 3:1291

American Board of Ophthalmology, 1:474

American Board of Plastic Surgeons, 1:9

American Board of Surgery (ABS), 1:206, 539, 3:1194, 1387

American Burn Association, 3:1326

American Burn Institute, 1:363

American Cancer Society
  on bladder cancer, 3:1450, 1453, 1495
  on breast cancer, 1:210, 2:912, 929
  on cancer demographics, 2:923
  on cervical cancer, 1:339–340
  demographics, 3:1473
  on laryngeal cancer, 2:839, 840
  on melanoma of the iris, 2:772
  on renal cell carcinoma, 2:1014

American Cleft Palate Association, 1:303

American College of Cardiology, 1:236
  on cardiac marker tests, 1:242
  on implantable cardioverter-defibrillator, 2:738
  on incisional hernia repair, 2:749–750

American College of Gastroenterology, 2:580

American College of Obstetricians and Gynecologists (ACOG), 1:287, 3:1509

American College of Phlebology, 3:1280, 1531

American College of Radiology, 2:931

American Council on Sports Medicine, 1:506

American Dental Association, 3:1429

American Diabetes Association, 2:603, 604, 605, 606

American Heart Association
  on angioplasties, 1:353
  on aortic aneurysm repair, 1:103
  on breast cancer, 3:1319
  on cardiac catheterization, 1:236
  on cardiac marker tests, 1:242
  on cardiopulmonary resuscitation, 1:246
  on cardiovascular disease, 1:442
  on coronary artery bypass graft surgery, 1:346
  on defibrillation, 1:412
  on endovascular stent surgery, 1:468
  on heart transplantation, 2:641
  on homocysteine, 1:241
  on lung cancer, 2:914

on pulmonary embolism, 3:1538
on renal cell carcinoma, 2:1015
on stroke, 1:256
on troponin levels, 1:241

American Hospital Association, 2:757, 3:1108–1109, 1167

American Journal of Gastroenterology, 3:1507

American Journal of Surgery, 3:1487

American Lung Association, 3:1175

American Medical Association (AMA)
  on advertisements, 1:541
  on certifying boards, 3:1165, 1195
  on managed care plans, 2:933

American Obesity Association (AOA), 2:572, 3:1547

American Orthopaedic Foot & Ankle Society, 1:231, 233

American Red Cross, 1:181, 3:1439, 1441, 1479

American Sleep Apnea Association, 3:1346

American Society for Aesthetic Plastic Surgery
  on cosmetic surgery, 1:521
  on dermabrasion, 1:416
  on laser skin resurfacing, 2:857–858

American Society for Bariatric Surgery (ASBS), 3:1547, 1549

American Society for Laser Medicine and Surgery, 2:862

American Society for Microbiology, 2:934–935

American Society of Anesthesiologists
  ambulatory surgery centers and, 1:39
  on anesthesiologists' role, 1:56, 67
  Committee on Transfusion Medicine, 1:180
  on general anesthesia, 1:59
  on safety, 1:403
  on transfusion safety, 1:180

American Society of Colon and Rectal Surgeons, 1:206

American Society of Plastic and Reconstructive Surgeons (ASPRS), 1:38
  on breast augmentation, 1:217
  on breast implants, 1:213
  on breast reconstruction, 1:217
  on breast reduction, 1:222–223
  on craniofacial reconstruction, 1:362
  on forehead lift, 1:549
  on hand surgery, 2:621
  on otoplasty, 2:1066–1067
  on spider veins, 3:1280

American Urological Association, 2:1012, 3:1254

Amgen, Inc., 3:1402

Amiloride, 1:428

Amino-Cerv cream, 1:282

Aminoglutethimide, 2:700

Aminoglycosides, 1:82, 83

Aminopenicillins, 1:81

Aminophylline, 1:547, 2:569

Aminotransferase, 1:295

Amitriptyline, 1:55, 3:1084

Ammonia tests, 2:891, 892–893

Amnesia, anesthesia and, 1:162

Amniocentesis, **1:40–43**
  for birth defects, 1:40–43, 532, 2:965
  for lipid tests, 2:875, 876
  ultrasound for, 2:876, 3:1120

Amniotic fluid, 1:488, 533

Amniotic fluid analysis. *See* Amniocentesis

Amniotic membranes, ruptured, 1:535

Amoxicillin, 1:81, 3:1206

Amphetamines, 1:63

Amphotericin B, 2:687

Ampicillin, 1:81, 3:1364

Ampulla of Vater, 2:557, 559

Amputation, **1:43–47**, *44*
  above the knee, *1:44*, 1:46
  for bedsores, 1:158
  demographics of, 1:545
  finger, 1:542–545, *1:543, 544,* 2:620, 621
  hand, 2:620, 621
  for limb length discrepancy, 2:867, 869
  vs. limb salvage, 2:872, 874
  penile, 1:300
  for peripheral artery disease, 3:1131, 1136
  replantation for, 2:973
  thumb, 1:542

Amyloidosis, 2:886

Anaerobic bacterial cultures, **1:47–50**

Anal cancer, 1:504

Anal electromyography, 1:126

Anal encirclement, 3:1223, 1224

Anal fissures, 1:318

Analgesics, **1:50–52**, 3:1185
  during anesthesia, 1:162
  for cholecystectomy, 1:296–297
  for endolymphatic shunt, 1:454
  for endometriosis, 2:835
  for hip pain, 2:671
  for knee pain, 2:807
  for lithotripsy, 2:884
  for low back pain, 2:824
  for mastoidectomy, 2:935
  for Maze procedure, 2:939
  multimodal, 3:1185–1186
  on-Q administration of, 3:1185
  preemptive, 3:1184
  for premedication, 1:61
  side effects of, 3:1186
  See also Opioid analgesics; Patient-controlled analgesia

Anaprox. *See* Naproxen

Anastomosis
  end-to-end, 2:764, 769, 972
  end-to-side, 2:972
  ileoanal, 1:318, **2:717–720**, *718,* 2:725, 726

orthoptic urethral, 2:713
pancreatic, 3:1093
rectal, 3:1225
Roux-en-Y, 2:571–572, 896
Anatomic hemispherectomy, 2:649
Ancef. *See* Cefazolin
Androgens
  cyclosporins and, 2:736
  erythromycins and, 1:485
  for gender reassignment, 3:1307
  lipid tests and, 2:876
  sulfonamides and, 3:1380
Anemia
  aplastic, 1:337
  bone marrow aspiration for, 1:192
  bone marrow biopsy for, 1:189
  causes of, 1:335, 336, 3:1228–1229
  complete blood count for, 1:334,
    335, 339
  from dialysis, 2:782
  hematocrit for, 2:647–648
  hemoglobin test for, 2:650–652
  hemolytic, 1:447, 2:604, 892
  hypochromic, 1:339, 3:1229
  iron-deficiency, 1:97, 336,
    3:1228–1229
  liver function tests for, 2:892, 894
  macrocytic, 1:336, 339,
    3:1228–1229
  megaloblastic, 2:892
  microcytic, 1:339
  normocytic, 1:339, 3:1228–1229
  postoperative, 1:182
  red blood cell indices for, 1:336,
    3:1228–1230
  sickle cell, 1:175, 339, 3:1362
Anesthesia
  age factors and, 1:57, 162
  allergies to, 1:59
  in ambulatory surgery centers, 1:38
  balanced, 1:162
  bispectral index for, 1:161–166
  complications from, 1:38, 67,
    403–404
  direct measurement of, 1:163
  EEG measurement of, 1:163–164
  evaluation for, **1:55–59**
  gender differences in, 1:162
  goals of, 1:162
  hemodynamic response to, 1:163
  indirect measurement of, 1:162–163
  mortality from, 1:38
  outpatient surgery and, 1:61, 2:690
  overdose, 1:60
  risks of, 1:403
  safety of, 3:1388
  spinal, 1:65, 66, 67, 279, 284, 286
  stages of, 1:60
  with tendon repairs, 3:1400
  twilight, 1:521, 2:858, **3:1292–1294**
  types of, 1:60–61, 3:1387
  See also General anesthesia; Local
    anesthesia; specific types of anes-
    thesia

Anesthesiologists, 1:56, **1:66–68,**
  2:961, 3:1387
Anesthetic depth, 1:161–162, 163
Anesthetics
  combinations of, 1:162
  dental, 1:61, 64, 65
  eye, 1:64, 65, 389, 2:1050, 3:1158
  gels, 1:266
  inhalation, 1:60, 162
  intravenous, 1:60–61, 162
  opioid analgesics and, 1:55
  street drugs and, 1:63
  topical, 1:64, 65, 2:656, 817
  toxicity from, 1:62
  types of, 1:60–61, 3:1387
Aneurysm
  angiography for, 1:69, *1:69,* 1:102
  berry, 1:271
  cerebral, *1:271,* 1:271–276, 369
  emergency surgery for, 1:452
  intracranial, 1:70, 2:1024–1025
  magnetic resonance angiography of,
    2:927
  obliteration, 1:271, 274
  re-bleeding, 1:273, 274
  ruptured, 1:271–272, 274
  thoracic, 1:101, 102, 103, 469
  unruptured, 1:273, 275
  See also Abdominal aortic
    aneurysm; Aortic aneurysm
Aneurysm repair, cerebral, **1:271–276,**
  272
Anexsia. *See* Hydrocodone-acetaminophen
Angel dust. *See* Phencyclidine
Angelica
  adrenergic drugs and, 1:34
  for atherosclerosis prevention,
    1:256, 469, 3:1132, 1136
Anger management, 1:540
Angina
  coronary artery bypass graft surgery
    for, 1:346, 351
  enhanced external counterpulsation
    for, 1:470–474
  heart transplantation and, 2:643
  non-surgical treatment of, 1:352
  from stress tests, 3:1376
Angiography, **1:68–72,** *69*
  for aortic aneurysm repair, 1:102
  cerebral, 1:69, *1:69,* 1:273
  computerized tomographic, 1:70
  coronary, 1:69–70, 235, 236, 348,
    2:976
  digital, 1:236, 255, 273
  fluorescein, 1:70, 71, 72, 2:774, 855
  fluoroscopic, 1:69, 273, 275
  hemangioma excision and, 2:645
  magnetic resonance, 2:925, 927,
    3:1130, 1135
  MUGA scan for, 2:992
  myocardial resection for, 2:997
  for peripheral artery disease, 3:1130

for peripheral vascular disease,
    3:1135
Angioma
  liver biopsy for, 2:888
  spider, 3:1282
Angioplasty, **1:72–75,** *73*
  for cerebral aneurysm repair, 1:274
  coronary stenting and, 1:353–357,
    1:354
  endovascular stent surgery and,
    1:467, 468
  indications for, 1:238
  vs. minimally invasive heart surgery,
    2:977–978
  percutaneous transluminal coronary,
    1:72, 74, 353, 2:628, 977–978
  for peripheral vascular disease,
    3:1520, 1521, 1523
  for TURP syndrome, 3:1457
  valvular, 1:141
  for vascular diseases, 3:1519
AngioSeal, 1:236
Angiotensin-converting enzyme (ACE)
  inhibitors
  for angina, 1:352
  aspirin and, 1:133
  for coronary artery disease, 1:472
  diuretics and, 1:429
  for hypertension, 1:89, 91
  laparoscopy and, 2:829
Angle closure glaucoma
  iridectomy for, 2:770–776
  laser iridotomy for, 2:848–854
  from scopolamine patches, 3:1287
Animal bites. *See* Bite injuries
Anions, 1:447
Aniridia, 2:607
Anisocytosis, 1:336, 3:1229
Anistreplase, 3:1417, 1419
Ankle
  arthroplasty, 1:116–120, 118
  arthroscopic surgery, 1:120–123
  edema, 3:1283
  nerve block, 1:231
  tendon repair, 3:1399–1400
Ankylosing spondylitis, 2:665, 692
Annual physical examination,
  3:1161–1162
Annuloplasty, 2:979–980
Anorectal anomalies, 3:1116
Anorectal manometry, 1:126
Anorectal ultrasound, 1:126
Anorexia nervosa, 3:1560
Ansaid. *See* Flurbiprofen
Antabuse. *See* Disulfiram
Antacids
  bisacodyl and, 2:866
  fluoroquinolones and, 1:547
  vs. gastric acid inhibitors, 2:567
  for heartburn, 2:583
  magnesium-based, 1:447
  for peptic ulcers, 1:98
  tetracyclines and, 1:83
Anterior capsulotomy, 2:854

Anterior cruciate ligament (ACL) injuries

Anterior cruciate ligament (ACL) injuries
  arthroscopic surgery for, 1:121, 2:791–792, 793
  demographics of, 2:791, 798
  knee osteotomy for, 2:797, 799
Anterior pelvic exenteration, 1:504
Anterior rectal resection, 3:1223, 1224
Anterior temporal lobectomy, **1:75–78**
Anterolateral thoracotomy, 3:1414
Anthropology, 1:362
Anti-arrhythmia versus implantable defibrillators trial, 2:940
Anti-HLA antibodies, 2:692
Anti-inflammatory drugs
  after wrist replacement, 3:1573
  for bunions, 1:233
  for carpal tunnel syndrome, 1:260
  eye drops, 3:1143
  hip replacement and, 2:668
  knee replacement and, 2:805
  for shoulder pain, 3:1314
  for toe abnormalities, 2:618
  wound healing and, 1:403
  See also Nonsteroidal anti-inflammatory drugs
Anti-inflammatory eye drops, 3:1433
Antianxiety drugs, **1:61, 78–80**, 79*t*, 2:772
Antiarrhythmia drugs
  for cardioversion, 1:249
  electrophysiology study and, 1:449
  for Maze procedure, 2:939, 940
Antibacterial-coated catheters, 2:687
Antibacterial soap, 2:829
Antibiotic chips, 2:600
Antibiotic eye drops, 1:344, 2:1049–1050, 3:1143–1144, 1160, 1269–1270, 1433
Antibiotic prophylaxis, **3:1206–1207**
  cephalosporins for, 1:268–269, 3:1206
  for colorectal surgery, 1:319, 320
  for colostomy, 1:323
  for rectal resection, 3:1227
Antibiotic resistance
  antibiotic susceptibility profile for, 1:49
  causes of, 3:1206
  to fluoroquinolones, 1:546
  hospital-acquired infections and, 2:687
  sulfonamides and, 3:1377
  to topical antibiotics, 1:84
Antibiotics, **1:81–84**, 82, 2:1036
  for abscesses, 1:18
  after tympanoplasty, 3:1476
  after ureterosigmoidoscopy, 3:1494
  for bedsores, 1:157
  beta-lactam, 1:81
  for bowel resection, 1:207
  broad-spectrum, 1:48, 83, 529, 2:873, 3:1331
  for cholecystectomy, 1:296

  for colonoscopy, 1:314
  for corneal transplantation, 1:344
  for cystoscopy, 1:400
  for diverticulitis, 1:208, 2:946, 949
  electrolyte balance and, 1:448
  for endoscopic sinus surgery, 1:461
  for esophageal atresia/tracheoesophageal fistula, 1:489
  for extracapsular cataract extraction, 1:513
  for face lift, 1:522
  for fetal surgery, 1:532
  for finger reattachment, 1:542, 543, 544
  for heart transplantation, 2:639, 642
  hemoglobin test and, 2:651
  for hip osteotomy, 2:662
  for hip replacement, 2:670
  for hip revision surgery, 2:676
  hospital-acquired infections and, 2:686
  immunosuppressant drugs and, 2:735
  interactions with, 3:1207
  for kidney transplantation, 2:789
  for limb salvage, 2:874
  lipid tests and, 2:876
  for mastoidectomy, 2:935
  for meningocele repair, 2:966
  for middle ear infections, 2:934, 1004
  for mitral valve disorders, 2:982, 986
  for mitral valve repair, 2:980
  Mohs surgery and, 2:991
  for nephrostomy, 2:1022
  for oophorectomy, 2:1039
  for ophthalmologic surgery, 2:1049
  for orbital exenteration, 1:505
  for pacemakers, 3:1081
  for peptic ulcers, 1:98
  for peripheral vascular bypass surgery, 3:1136
  for photorefractive keratectomy, 3:1160
  for premature labor, 1:280
  for scar revision, 3:1266
  side effects of, 3:1207
  for sling procedure, 3:1332
  for small bowel resection, 3:1335–1336
  for stapedectomy, 3:1366
  for tonsillectomy, 3:1424
  for tooth replantation, 3:1430
  topical, **1:84–86**, 1:407, 2:818
  urinary anti-infectives, 3:1502
  for urinary catheterization, 1:267
  for wounds, 3:1569–1570
Antibodies, 1:337, 2:726
Antibody-antigen complex, 2:726
Antibody screen test, 2:693, 3:1482
Anticholinergics, 1:61
Anticoagulants, **1:86–89**
  anesthesia evaluation and, 1:58

  for angioplasty, 1:74
  for aortic aneurysm repair, 1:101
  for aortic valve replacement, 1:105–106
  aspirin and, 1:132
  barbiturates and, 1:153
  for cardiac catheterization, 1:238
  for cardioversion, 1:249
  carotid endarterectomy and, 1:255
  cephalosporins and, 1:270
  colonoscopy after, 1:314
  for coronary artery bypass graft surgery, 1:348
  for coronary stenting, 1:354, 355
  craniotomy and, 1:370
  for endovascular stent surgery, 1:468
  erythromycins and, 1:485
  eye muscle surgery and, 1:518
  face lift and, 1:521
  fluoroquinolones and, 1:547
  for heart-lung transplantation, 2:632
  incisional hernia repair and, 2:749
  inguinal hernia repair and, 2:755
  laparoscopy and, 2:828
  for limb salvage, 2:873
  lymphadenectomy and, 2:923
  for Maze procedure, 2:938, 939
  for mechanical circulation support, 2:843
  microsurgery and, 2:973
  for minimally invasive heart surgery, 2:976
  for mitral valve disorders, 2:982
  for mitral valve repair, 2:979, 980
  for mitral valve replacement, 2:983, 984
  nephrostomy and, 2:1022
  NSAIDs and, 2:1028
  ophthalmologic surgery and, 2:1049
  opioid analgesics and, 1:55
  for peripheral artery disease, 3:1130, 1131
  for peripheral vascular bypass surgery, 3:1136
  phacoemulsification and, 3:1143
  prochlorperazine and, 1:93
  sulfonamides and, 3:1380
  for venous thrombosis, 3:1539
  after ventricular assist device surgery, 3:1541
Anticonvulsant drugs. *See* Antiseizure drugs
Antidepressants
  for anxiety, 1:78
  closed-angle glaucoma from, 2:772
  myelography and, 2:996
  for pain, 3:1084
  for urinary incontinence, 3:1237
  See also Tricyclic antidepressants
Antidiarrhea drugs, 1:270
Antiemetic drugs, 1:91–93, 3:1286–1288
Antifungal drugs, 2:687

Antigens, 1:337
   prostate specific, 2:1044, 1054,
      3:1454, 1455, 3:1470
   tumor marker tests, 3:1469–1470
Antiglaucoma drugs, 3:1433
Antihepatitis C antibody, 2:893
Antihistamines
   erythromycins and, 1:485
   for middle ear infections, 2:1004
   for nausea and vomiting, 1:92,
      3:1287
   opioid analgesics and, 1:55
Antihypertensive drugs, **1:89–91,** 90*t*
Antilipemics, 2:876
Antimicrobial mouthwash, 2:600
Antimitochondrial antibodies, 2:891
Antinausea drugs, **1:91–93,** 92*t*, 3:1287
Antineoplastic agents, 2:651
Antioxidants
   for atherosclerosis prevention,
      1:469, 3:1132, 1136
   for coronary artery disease, 1:356,
      472
Antiplatelet drugs, **1:86–89,** 1:352, 472
Antipsychotic drugs, 2:876, 996
Antipyretics, 2:1028
Antirejection drugs. *See* Immunosup-
   pressant drugs
Antiseizure drugs
   aspirin and, 1:133
   barbiturates and, 1:153
   cephalosporins and, 1:270
   for corpus callosotomy, 1:359
   for epilepsy, 1:77, 2:1026, 3:1513
   erythromycins and, 1:485
   gastric acid inhibitors and, 2:569
   opioid analgesics and, 1:55
   for pain, 3:1084
   prochlorperazine and, 1:93
   sulfonamides and, 3:1380
Antiseptics, **1:93–95,** 3:1570
Antispasmodic drugs, 3:1237, 1255
Antithyroid drugs, 3:1421
Antivert. *See* Mechzine; Meclizine
Antiviral capsid antigen test, 2:893
Antiviral drugs, 1:485, 2:687
Antrectomy, **1:95–100,** 2:564, 579
Antrostomy, middle meatal, 1:460
Antrum, 1:95–100
Anus, imperforate, 2:1035
Anxiety
   antianxiety drugs for, 1:78–80
   pain and, 3:1082
   preoperative, 3:1192, 1201
AOA (American Obesity Association),
   2:572, 3:1547
Aonioscopic lens, 2:851
AORN (Association of Perioperative
   Registered Nurses), 1:128
Aorta, coarctation of, 2:634, *2:635,*
   2:636, 637
Aorta CT scans, 1:382, 384
Aortic aneurysm
   arch, 1:101, 102, 103

ascending, 1:101, 102, 103
   CT scans for, 1:382, 384
   defined, 3:1519, 1520
   endovascular stent surgery for,
      1:466–467, 468
   essential surgery for, 1:501
   mortality rates for, 1:469
   ruptured, 1:384, 469
   vascular surgery for, 3:1522–1523
   See also Abdominal aortic aneurysm
Aortic aneurysm repair, **1:100–104,**
   101, 2:627
Aortic arch aneurysm, 1:101, 102, 103
Aortic insufficiency, 1:104–107
Aortic stent/graft placements, 3:1519
Aortic valve replacement, **1:104–107,**
   105
Aortic valve stenosis
   aortic valve replacement for,
      1:104–107, *1:105*
   balloon valvuloplasty for,
      1:141–143
   congenital, 2:637
Aortobifemoral bypass surgery, 3:1132,
   1135, 1136
Apert syndrome, 1:362–363, 3:1557
Aphakic patients, 2:850–851
Apheresis, 1:173, 3:1441
Apicoectomy, 3:1246
Aplastic anemia, 1:337
Apligraf, 3:1327, 1568
Apnea
   CPR for, 1:244, 246
   monitoring, 2:760
   See also Sleep apnea
Appendectomy, **1:107–110,** *108,* 1:501,
   2:579, 580–581
Appendicitis
   abdominal ultrasound for, 1:2
   appendectomy for, 1:107–110,
      1:108, 2:579, 580–581
   in children, 3:1117–1118
   demographics of, 2:580
   essential surgery for, 1:501
   laxatives and, 2:865
Appendix, ruptured, 1:109
Apraclonidine, 2:851, 852, 855
Apresoline. *See* Isoxsuprine
Aprotinin, 1:537
Aquaflow collagen wick, 3:1275
Aqueous fluid, 2:848, 849, 851, 3:1272,
   1431, 1433
Arachnoiditis, 2:997
Aramine. *See* Metaraminol
Arch supports, 1:525
Arcus tendineus, 1:395
Areflexia, 1:162
Areola reconstruction, 1:217, 220,
   3:1321, 1322
Argon lasers, 2:860
   coagulation, 1:98, 182
   iridectomy, 2:773
   iridotomy, 2:849, 851
   peripheral iridoplasty, 2:853

photocoagulation therapy, 3:1153
   plasma coagulation, 1:388
   spider veins, 3:1284
Arm artery peripheral endarterectomy,
   3:1128–1131
Armpit dissection. *See* Axillary dissection
Arnica, 1:262
Aromatase, 3:1458
Aromatherapy, 3:1348
Arrhythmia
   adrenergic drugs for, 1:33
   cardioversion for, 1:248–252
   defibrillation for, 1:411–413
   diagnosis of, 1:248–249, 2:937–938,
      998
   electrocardiography for, 1:442–442
   electrophysiology study for,
      1:449–452
   emergency surgery for, 1:453
   implantable cardioverter-defibrilla-
      tor for, 2:736–740
   Maze procedure for, 2:936–942
   myocardial resection for, 2:997–999
   non-surgical treatment of, 1:251,
      2:939, 940
   pacemakers for, 3:1079–1082
   from stress tests, 3:1376
   supraventricular, 2:977
ART (Assisted reproductive techniques), 2:740, 742
Artecoll, 1:552
Arterial blood gases test, 2:920
Arterial bypass surgery, 3:1522–1523
Arterial oxygen saturation, 1:243, 244
Arterial switch, 2:636
Arteriography
   craniotomy, 1:370
   microsurgery, 2:974
   stroke, 1:255
Arteriovenous fistula, **1:111–115,**
   1:467, 2:1019
Arteriovenous malformations (AVM)
   antrectomy for, 1:95, 97, 98
   cerebral aneurysm and, 1:271
   craniotomy for, 1:369
   stereotactic radiosurgery for,
      3:1369–1371
Arthritis
   arthroplasty for, 1:116
   demographics of, 1:507, 2:798
   knee osteotomy for, 2:797
   kneecap removal for, 2:814, 815
   non-surgical treatment of,
      1:119–120, 2:671, 796, 3:1311
   patellar, 2:814
   shoulder, 3:1310
   See also Rheumatoid arthritis
Arthrodesis, 3:1574
   hip, 2:663, 672
   knee, 2:812–813
   See also Spinal fusion
Arthrography, **1:115–116,** 2:668,
   3:1249

Arthroplasty, **1:116–120**, *117*
  bone x rays for, 1:203
  derotation, 2:617
  implant, 2:617
  non-surgical treatment of, 2:999
  shoulder, 3:1308–1312, 1314
  shoulder resection, 1:116–120,
    3:1312–1315
  surgeon skill level for, 1:540
  for toe abnormalities, 2:617
  total, 1:116–120, 507
  See also Joint replacement; Revi-
    sion surgery
Arthroscopic surgery, **1:120–123,**
  2:595, 3:1387
  Bankart procedure, 1:147
  diagnostic, 1:148–149, 2:798, 804
  knee, 1:120–123, **2:791–797**, *792,*
    2:807, 812
  microdiskectomy, 1:425
  second-look, 3:1288, 1289
Artificial disk implants, 1:425
Artificial heart, 2:637, 644, 843, 999
Artificial limbs, 2:1064
Artificial skin, 3:1264–1265,
  1326–1327
Artificial sphincter insertion,
  1:123–128, *124*
Artificial urethra, 2:703
Asbestos, 3:1175
ASBS (American Society for Bariatric
  Surgery), 3:1547, 1549
Ascending aortic aneurysm, 1:101, 102,
  103
Ascending colon, 1:204
Ascites
  causes of, 2:896, 3:1137
  liver biopsy for, 2:888
  non-surgical treatment of, 3:1139
  paracentesis for, 3:1095–1096
  peritoneovenous shunts for,
    3:1137–1140
  portal vein bypass surgery for,
    3:1179, 1181
Ascorbic acid. *See* Vitamin C
Aseptic meningitis, 2:650
Aseptic necrosis, 1:555, 2:751–752
Aseptic technique, **1:128–131**, *129*
  for anaerobic bacterial cultures,
    1:47
  for hospital-acquired infection con-
    trol, 2:687
  medical, 1:130–131
  surgical, 1:128–130
  for syringe and needle assembly,
    3:1393
  for urinary catheterization, 1:264,
    267
Asherman's syndrome, 1:421
Aspartate aminotransferase (AST),
  2:890–895
Aspiration
  biopsy, 1:211, 3:1473
  bone marrow, **1:189–193**

fine-needle, 2:951, 989, 3:1146
  for ganglion cyst removal,
    2:560–563
  for hydrocelectomy, 2:695
  joint, 2:668
  vacuum, 1:15–16, 420
Aspiration pneumonia, 2:593
Aspirin, **1:131–134**
  vs. acetaminophen, 1:21
  allergy to, 1:51, 132
  anticoagulants and, 1:87
  antiplatelet activity of, 1:86
  antrectomy and, 1:97
  for aortic valve replacement, 1:106
  cardiac catheterization and, 1:237
  carotid endarterectomy and, 1:255
  colonoscopy and, 1:314
  for colorectal polyps, 1:315
  for coronary artery bypass graft
    surgery, 1:352
  for coronary artery disease, 1:349,
    356, 472
  for coronary stenting, 1:354, 355
  craniotomy and, 1:370
  for endovascular stent surgery, 1:468
  esophagogastroduodenoscopy and,
    1:500
  eye muscle surgery and, 1:518
  face lift and, 1:521
  hemoglobin test and, 2:651
  hip replacement and, 2:668
  incision care and, 2:745
  incisional hernia repair and, 2:749
  inguinal hernia repair and, 2:755
  knee replacement and, 2:804, 805
  laminectomy and, 2:823
  laparoscopy and, 2:828
  liver biopsy and, 2:888, 889
  for low back pain, 2:824
  lymphadenectomy and, 2:923
  for Maze procedure, 2:939
  mentoplasty and, 2:968
  microsurgery and, 2:973
  for mitral valve replacement, 2:984
  ophthalmologic surgery and, 2:1049
  in opioid analgesics, 1:53
  for pain, 3:1084
  percutaneous nephrolithotomy and,
    2:1019
  for peripheral artery disease, 3:1130
  phacoemulsification and, 3:1143
  plastic surgery and, 3:1173
  pneumonectomy and, 3:1176
  pulmonary lobectomy and, 2:904
  sclerotherapy and, 3:1283
  for shoulder pain, 3:1314
  sigmoidoscopy and, 3:1316
  for tooth replantation, 3:1430
  for vasectomy, 3:1526
  for vein ligation and stripping,
    3:1534
  for wrist replacement, 3:1573
Aspirin-Free Anacin. *See* Acetaminophen

ASPRS. *See* American Society of Plas-
  tic and Reconstructive Surgeons
Assisted living facilities, 2:907,
  908–909
Assisted reproductive techniques
  (ART), 2:740, 742
Assistive devices
  for hip pain, 2:671
  hip revision surgery and, 2:670, 676
  for limb salvage, 2:873–874
Associated Jehovah's Witnesses for Re-
  form on Blood (AJWRB), 1:180
Association of Perioperative Registered
  Nurses (AORN), 1:128
AST (Aspartate aminotransferase),
  2:890–895
Astemizole, 1:485
Asthma
  adrenergic drugs for, 1:32, 33
  laparoscopy for, 2:829
  prednisone for, 2:751–752
  spirometry tests for, 3:1358
Astigmatic keratotomy, 2:848, 3:1160
Astigmatism
  from corneal transplantation, 1:344
  LASIK for, 2:841–848
  photorefractive keratectomy for,
    3:1157–1161
Atacand. *See* Candesartan
Atarax. *See* Hydroxyzine hydrochloride
Atelectasis, 2:904
Atenolol, 1:89, 90*t*, 91
Atherectomy, 1:356
Atherosclerosis
  angioplasty for, 1:72
  aortic aneurysm repair for, 1:100
  carotid endarterectomy for,
    1:252–257
  coronary stenting for, 1:353–357
  demographics of, 3:1128
  endovascular stent surgery for,
    1:465–470
  homocysteine and, 1:241
  lipid tests for, 2:875
  peripheral endarterectomy for,
    3:1128–1132
  peripheral vascular bypass surgery
    for, 3:1132–1137
  prevention of, 1:256, 469–470,
    3:1131–1132, 1135, 1136–1137
  risk factors for, 3:1129, 1134
  vascular surgery for, 3:1519–1520
Ativan. *See* Lorazepam
Atonic seizures, 1:358, 359
ATP (Adenosine triphosphate), 1:240
Atrial fibrillation
  cardioversion for, 1:248
  defibrillation for, 1:411–413, 2:982,
    986
  demographics of, 2:937
  electrocardiography of, 1:441
  implantable cardioverter-defibrilla-
    tor for, 2:739
  Maze procedure for, 2:936–942

minimally invasive heart surgery and, 2:977
non-surgical treatment of, 1:251
Atrial flutter, 1:251, 411, 412
Atrial septal defects, 2:636
Atrial shunts, 1:239
Atrioventricular canal defect, 2:637
Atrioventricular node, 1:441, 450
Atropa belladonna, 3:1286
Atropine, 1:389, 391
Attached flaps, 1:219–220
Attention-deficit/hyperactivity disorder, 3:1342
Auditory nerve, 1:308
Augmentation cystoplasty. *See* Bladder augmentation
Auricular avulsion, 2:1067, 1069
Auscultation
    for aortic stenosis, 1:106
    for mitral valve disorders, 2:980, 984
    physical examinations and, 3:1161
    stethoscope for, 3:1371–1373
Autografts, 1:185, 186–187, 3:1323, 1325
Autoimmune disorders
    from breast implants, 1:220–221
    hemolytic, 3:1362
    human leukocyte antigen test for, 2:692
    immunosuppressant drugs for, 2:733
Autologous blood donation, **1:134–136**, 1:172, 175, 3:1441, 1483
    for blood salvage, 1:178
    for hip replacement, 2:668
    for knee replacement, 2:804
    for laparoscopy, 2:829
    organ transplants, 3:1447
    preadmission, 3:1168
    preoperative, 1:134–135, 3:1196–1197, 1202
Autologous bone marrow transplantation, 1:194, 196, 197, 202
Autolytic debridement, 1:407
Automated blood cell counters, 1:335, 2:648, 3:1229
Automated endoscope reprocessing (AER) system, 1:228
Automated external defibrillators (AEDS), 1:412
Automated hematology analyzers, 1:334, 335
Automobile accidents, 1:363, 372
Autonomy, patient, 1:430, 431, 3:1190
Autotransplantation, testicular, 2:1060
Avapro. *See* Irbesartan
Avascular necrosis, 2:664–665, 667, 870
Avelox. *See* Moxifloxacin
Average reference montage, 1:445
Aversion techniques, 3:1339–1340
AVM. *See* Arteriovenous malformations
Avulsed teeth, 3:1429–1431

Awareness during surgery, 1:61–62, 162–163
Axenfeld-Reiger's syndrome, 2:607
Axenfeld's syndrome, 2:607
Axid. *See* Nizatidine
Axillary dissection, **1:136–139**, *137*, 2:923–924
    lumpectomy and, 2:910–913
    modified radical mastectomy and, 2:987
    quadrantectomy and, 3:1213–1214
    sentinel lymph node biopsy and, 3:1301
Axillary thermometers, 3:1409
Axillary thoracotomy, 3:1414
Ayurvedic medicine, 1:99
Azathioprine
    allopurinol and, 2:736
    for immunosuppression, 2:733
    for kidney transplantation, 2:789
    for liver transplantation, 2:899
    pregnancy and, 2:734
    red blood cell indices and, 3:1229
Azithromycin, 1:81, 83, 483, 484
AZT. *See* Zidovudine

B

B-mode ultrasound, 1:3
Babesiosis, 1:180
Babies. *See* Infants
Baby teeth, 3:1429–1430
Bacitracin, 1:84
Back pain
    disk removal for, 1:424–427
    laminectomy for, 2:819–827
    myelography for, 2:996
    neurosurgery for, 2:1026
    spinal fusion for, 3:1352–1355
Baclofen, 2:994, 3:1242
Bacterial cultures, anaerobic, **1:47–50**
Bacterial graft contamination, 1:187
Bacterial infections, 1:48
    antibiotic prophylaxis for, 3:1206–1207
    antibiotics for, 1:81–84
    cephalosporins for, 1:268–271
    erythromycins for, 1:483–485
    fluoroquinolones for, 1:545–548
    from heart transplantation, 2:642
    hospital-acquired, 1:130–131, 403, 2:685–688
    from lung transplantation, 3:1413
    from splenectomy, 3:1363–1364
    sulfonamides for, 3:1377–1380
    topical antibiotics for, 1:84–86
    from transplantation, 3:1413
Bacterial resistance. *See* Antibiotic resistance
Bactericides infections, 1:94
Bacteriostatics, 1:94
Bacteroides infections, 1:48, 49, 406

Bactrim. *See* Trimethoprim/sulfamethoxazole
Bactroban, 1:84
Baking soda, 2:583
Balance disorders, 3:1089
Balance tests, 1:454
Balanced anesthesia, 1:162
Baldness, 2:613–616
Ballistic chisel, 2:675
Balloon angioplasty. *See* Angioplasty
Balloon atrial septostomy, 2:636
Balloon tamponade, 3:1278
Balloon-type expanders, 3:1320–1321
Balloon valvotomy, 1:107
Balloon valvuloplasty, **1:141–143**, 2:636
Bandages, **1:143–147**, *145*, 2:744, 879
Bankart procedure, **1:147–150**, *148*
Barber service, 3:1166
Barbita. *See* Phenobarbital
Barbiturates, **1:150–153**
    anesthetics and, 1:63
    epidural anesthesia and, 1:478
    general anesthesia and, 1:60
    overdoses of, 1:151, 2:652
Bariatric surgeons, 1:437
Bariatric surgery
    vertical banded gastroplasty, 3:1544–1551
Barium enema, **1:153–155**
    colonoscopy after, 1:313
    for colorectal cancer screening, 1:154–155, 315, 3:1317
    colorectal surgery after, 1:319
    for intussusception reduction, 2:769
    for Meckel's diverticulectomy, 2:948
    for rectal resection, 3:1225
Barium esophagography, 2:583, 584
Barium sulfate, 1:154, 383, 491
Barium swallow, 1:97, 496, 2:577, 3:1489
Barotitis media, 2:1004
Barotrauma, 2:1004
Barrett's esophagus, 1:493–494, 498, 2:582, 583, 589
Bars, support, 3:1111–1112
Basal cell carcinoma
    cryotherapy for, 1:377, 378, 2:992
    curettage and electrosurgery for, 1:385
    Mohs surgery for, 2:990, 992
Base-Smith, V., 1:332
Basil, 3:1380
Basiliximab
    for immunosuppression, 2:733
    for kidney transplantation, 2:789
    pregnancy and, 2:734
Basophils, 1:336, 338
Bates, David, 2:959
Baths and incision care, 2:744–745
Batteries
    pacemaker, 3:1079, 1081

Bayer Select Maximum Strength Headache Pain Relief. *See* Acetaminophen
BDD (Body dysmorphic disorder), 1:550, 3:1173
Bearberry, 3:1380
Beauticians, 3:1166
Becaplermin, 1:46
Beckwith-Wiedemann syndrome, 2:1035
Bed rest, 1:280, 2:824
Bedsores, **1:155–159**, *157,* 1:408
Behavior weight loss therapy, 2:574–575
Belladonna alkaloid scopolamine, 3:1286
Bell's palsy, 3:1397
Belly button. *See* Umbilicus
Benazepril, 1:89, 90*t,* 429
Bendroflumethiazide, 1:91
Benign prostatic hyperplasia, 1:125, 2:1041–1045, 3:1454, 1457–1458, 1506–1507
Benzalkonium chloride, 1:94
Benzocaine, 1:65
Benzodiazepines, 1:78–80
    for conscious sedation, 3:1292
    pregnancy and, 2:994
    for premedication, 1:61
Benzothiazide, 1:91
Berger, Hans, 1:163
Bernstein test, 1:491, 492
Berry aneurysm, 1:271
Beta-adrenergic blockers, 1:89, 91
Beta blockers
    after cardioversion, 1:249
    for angina, 1:352
    aspirin and, 1:133
    for coronary artery disease, 1:472
    for intraocular pressure, 2:851
    for Maze procedure, 2:939
    for portal hypertension, 3:1181
    uses of, 1:91
Beta-carotene, 1:356, 472
Beta globulin, 2:893
Beta-lactam antibiotics, 1:81
Beta receptors, 1:33
Beta waves, 1:444, 445
Betadine, 2:659, 744, 3:1325
Betamethasone, 1:360, 532
Bezoars, 1:98
BIA. *See* Bioelectrical impedance analysis
Biaxin. *See* Clarithromycin
Bicarbonate tests, 1:446–449
Bicuspid aortic defects, 1:104
Bifidobacterium infections, 1:48
Big toe bunionectomy, 1:229–233
Bikini incision, 2:1001, 3:1258
Bilateral cleft lip, 1:303
Bilateral knee replacement, 2:802, 806
Bilateral oophorectomy, 2:1038, 1040
Bilateral orchiectomy, 2:1052
Bilateral pallidotomy, 3:1088

Bilateral salpingo-oophorectomy, 2:1038, 3:1256–1259
Bilberry extract, 3:1275
Bile, 1:159, 456, 2:557
Bile acid tests, 2:891
Bile duct cancer, 1:159, 2:657
Bile duct injuries, 2:831
Bile duct stricture
    biliary stenting for, 1:159–161
    endoscopic retrograde cholangiopancreatography for, 1:456
Bile reflux gastritis, 2:566
Bile salts, 1:297
Bilevel positive airway pressure (BiPAP), 2:945
Biliary atresia, 3:1118
Biliary colic, 1:293, 295, 2:558–559
Biliary disease
    in children, 3:1118
    demographics of, 2:900
    endoscopic retrograde cholangiopancreatography for, 1:456–459
    liver transplantation for, 2:895
Biliary obstruction
    abdominal ultrasound for, 1:1
    liver biopsy for, 2:888
Biliary stenting, **1:159–161**
Biliopancreatic diversion, 2:571
Bilirubin, 1:295, 2:890–895
    in urinalysis, 3:1499–1500, 1501
Bill of rights
    patient's, 3:1108–1109
Billroth I procedure, **2:575–579**, *576*
Billroth II procedure, 2:571, 575, 576
Bill's Island, 1:454
Binaural stethoscope, 3:1371
Binge eating disorder, 3:1560
Biobrane®, 3:1568–1569
Bioelectrical impedance analysis (BIA), 3:1546, 1558–1560
Biofeedback
    for interstitial cystitis, 3:1255
    for pain, 3:1084
    for urinary incontinence, 3:1237
Biological debridement, 1:407
Biological therapy. *See* Immunologic therapies
Biological tissue valves, 1:106, 2:984
Biomechanics, 2:801
Biomicroscopy ultrasound, 3:1274
Biopsy
    aspiration, 3:1473
    bone, 1:203
    bone marrow, **1:189–193**
    breast, **1:209–213**, *210*
    bronchoscopy for, 1:226
    complications from, 1:404
    cone, 1:329, **1:339–342**
    core-needle, 2:951
    cystoscopy for, 1:399
    endometrial, 1:421–422
    endomyocardial, 2:642
    excisional, 1:210–211, 3:1473
    fine-needle, 2:951, 989, 3:1146

image-directed, 1:404, 2:1025
    incisional, 1:210–211, 3:1473
    large-core needle, 1:211
    liver, **2:886–890**, *887*
    lung, **2:914–918**
    needle, 1:211, 2:914, 915–916, 917, 918, 3:1473
    needles for, 1:190
    percutaneous needle, 1:211
    skin, 1:437
    thoracotomy for, 3:1414, 1416
    See also Aspiration; Sentinel lymph node biopsy
Biosynthetic dressings, 1:144, 145
BiPAP (Bilevel positive airway pressure), 2:945
BIRADS (Breast Imaging Reporting and Data System), 2:931
Birth control pills. *See* Oral contraceptives
Birth defects
    abdominal wall, 1:5–7, 3:1116–1117
    amniocentesis for, 1:40–43, 532, 2:965
    amputation for, 1:44
    from anticoagulants, 1:87
    antihypertensive drugs and, 1:91
    aortic aneurysm repair for, 1:100
    aortic valve replacement for, 1:104
    craniofacial reconstruction for, 1:362–363, 365
    CT scans for, 1:384
    diagnosis of, 1:532
    from epoetin, 2:729–730
    esophageal atresia/tracheoesophageal fistula and, 1:487
    external ear, 2:1066, 1068–1069
    family planning for, 1:43
    fetal surgery for, 1:530–533, 534
    gastrointestinal, 1:487
    gastroschisis and, 1:6
    hernia, 2:753–754
    kidney, 1:487
    magnetic resonance imaging for, 2:925–926
    maternal age and, 1:41
    maternal blood screening for, 1:42
    musculoskeletal, 1:487
    neurosurgery for, 2:1026
    omphaloceles and, 1:6, 2:1035, 1037
    plastic surgery for, 3:1173
    skull x rays for, 3:1328
    therapeutic abortion for, 1:13
    urinary tract, 1:487
    VATER, 1:487
    See also Congenital heart defects
Birthmarks, strawberry, 2:644
Bisacodyl, 2:865, 866
Bismuth subsalicylate, 1:98, 2:583
Bispectral index, 1:61–62, **1:161–166**
Bite injuries
    craniofacial reconstruction for, 1:363, 367

hand surgery for, 2:621
laceration repair for, 2:818
otoplasty for, 2:1067
Biventricular pacemaker, 2:643
Bladder
    diversion, 1:166
    prolapse, 1:325, 327, 395–398
    spasms, 2:704
    ultrasound, 3:1120
Bladder augmentation, **1:166–169**, *167*
    collagen periurethral injection of,
        1:311
    for interstitial cystitis, 3:1255
Bladder cancer
    cystectomy for, 1:391–395
    demographics of, 1:391–392,
        3:1383
    ileal conduit surgery for, 2:713–716
    mortality and morbidity from,
        3:1452
    nephrostomy for, 2:1022, 1023
    pelvic exenteration for, 1:504
    transurethral bladder resections,
        3:1450–1453
    transurethral resection for, 1:394
    ureterosigmoidoscopy, 3:1493
Bladder disorders
    bladder augmentation for,
        1:166–169, *1:167*
    cystectomy for, 1:391
    cystoscopy for, 1:398–402
    ileal conduit surgery for, 2:713–716
Bladder injuries
    from needle bladder neck suspen-
        sion, 2:1012
    from open prostatectomy, 2:1044
    from urinary catheterization, 1:264
Bladder neck suspension, needle,
    2:1010–1012
Bladder stones, 1:399, 400
Bladder training
    for interstitial cystitis, 3:1255
    after meningocele repair, 2:966
    for urinary incontinence, 1:127,
        3:1237, 1332
Blebitis, 3:1274
Blebs, filtration, 3:1272, 1275
Bleeding
    adrenergic drugs for, 1:32, 33
    anemia from, 1:336, 3:1228
    from angiography, 1:72
    from anticoagulants, 1:87
    aspirin and, 1:132
    blood salvage and, 1:178, 182
    cephalosporins and, 1:270
    from cesarean section, 1:286
    from coronary stenting, 1:355
    from myomectomy, 2:1001
    from needle bladder neck suspen-
        sion, 2:1012
    from oophorectomy, 2:1040
    from pancreatectomy, 3:1093
    postoperative, 1:403–404
    reducing, 1:181–182

    from surgical procedures, 1:136
    from tracheotomy, 3:1436
    from ventricular shunts, 3:1543
    from webbed finger/toe repair,
        3:1557
    See also Gastrointestinal bleeding;
        Hemorrhage
Bleeding disorders, 1:500
Blepharoplasty, **1:169–172**, *170,* 1:549
Blepharospasm, 2:608
Blindness
    from cataracts, 1:511, 515
    from endoscopic sinus surgery,
        1:461
    from glaucoma, 3:1272
    LASIK and, 2:847
    monocular, 1:475
    from ophthalmologic surgery,
        2:1051
    See also Vision loss
Block resection techniques, 3:1474
Blood
    oxygen, 3:*1553*
    in urinalysis, 3:1499, 1501
Blood analyzers, point-of-care, 2:761,
    762
Blood banking. *See* Blood registry
Blood-borne diseases, 1:180, 3:1393
Blood cell counters, automated, 1:335,
    2:648, 3:1229
Blood chemistry tests
    for anesthesia evaluation, 1:58
    cardiac, 1:240–242
    point-of-care analyzers for, 2:761
Blood clots
    from anesthetics, 1:66
    anticoagulants and antiplatelet drugs
        for, 1:86–89
    from hepatectomy, 2:659–660
    from liposuction, 2:880
    magnetic resonance angiography of,
        2:927
    thrombolytic therapy for,
        3:1417–1419
    See also Thrombosis
Blood collection
    intraoperative, 3:1168, 1196, 1202,
        1447
    postoperative, 3:1168, 1197, 1202,
        1447
    preoperative hemodilution, 3:1447
    transfusions, 3:1439–1444
    transplants, 3:1447
Blood donation, **1:172–175**, 1:181,
    3:1168, 1440
    See also Autologous blood dona-
        tion; Transfusion
Blood groups. *See* Blood typing and
    screening
Blood loss. *See* Bleeding
Blood pH, 1:447
Blood poisoning. *See* Septicemia
Blood pressure
    adrenergic drugs for, 1:32, 33

    amputation and, 1:45
    antihypertensive drugs for, 1:89–91
    cardiac monitor for, 1:243
    smoking and, 3:1338
Blood pressure measurement,
    1:175–177, *176*
    sphygmomanometers, 3:1350–1353
    stethoscopes, 3:1552, 1553, *1553,*
        3:1371–1372
    stress test for, 3:1375–1377
Blood registry, **1:172–175**, *173*
Blood salvage, 1:135, **1:178–179**, 1:182
Blood substitutes, 1:136, 182, 3:1443
Blood tests
    for anesthesia evaluation, 1:57
    for arthroplasty, 1:118
    for colorectal cancer screening,
        1:315
    for dialysis, 2:782, 783
    for kidney function, 2:784–786
    for kidney/liver function, 3:1447
    for lung transplantation, 2:920
    for peripheral artery disease, 3:1130
    for peripheral vascular disease,
        3:1135
    phlebotomy for, 3:1150–1152
    for thyroid-stimulating hormones,
        3:1421
    See also Complete blood count
Blood-thinning drugs. *See* Anticoagu-
    lants
Blood transfusion. *See* Transfusion
Blood typing and screening,
    3:1440–1441, **3:1479–1484**, 3:*1481*
    blood donation and, 1:174
    for tissue compatibility testing,
        2:691
    transfusion reaction and, 1:180
Blood urea nitrogen (BUN)
    for kidney function, 1:113, 2:784,
        785–786
    for liver disease, 2:892
Blood vessel surgery. *See* Vascular
    surgery
Blood viscosity-reducing drugs, 1:270
Bloodless surgery, 1:136, **1:179–184,**
    3:1443
    See also Laser surgery
Bloom, David, 3:1538
Blunt dissectors, 3:1381
Blunt trauma, 1:100, 3:1362
BMI. *See* Body mass index
BMP (Bone morphogenetic proteins),
    1:187, 3:1354
Board certification, 1:540, 3:1165,
    1194–1195, 1387
Body dysmorphic disorder (BDD),
    1:550, 3:1173
Body mass index (BMI), 1:508, 2:572,
    574, 3:1545, 1546, 1559
Body temperature, 1:243, 3:1408–1411,
    1551–1552
Body weight, 1:506–507, 2:747
    See also Obesity; Weight loss

Bone

flaps, 1:274
heterotropic, 2:670, 806, 812
injuries, 1:203
loss, 2:599
markers, 3:1405
matrix, 1:184, 187
morselized, 2:675
robot-assisted cutting, 3:1243
tissue, 1:184
See also Fractures

Bone biopsy, 1:203
Bone cement, *2:665*, 2:666, 675, 811
Bone densitometry, 1:203, 2:668, 3:1111
Bone disease

bone marrow aspiration for, 1:192
oophorectomy and, 2:1040
x rays for, 1:203–204

Bone grafting, **1:184–189**, *185, 186*

craniofacial reconstruction, 1:365
dental implants, 1:415
hip revision surgery, 2:673, 675
knee revision surgery, 2:809
leg lengthening, 2:867
limb salvage, 2:872

Bone lengthening, **2:866–872**, *867, 868*
Bone marrow aspiration, **1:189–193**
Bone marrow biopsy, **1:189–193**
Bone marrow disorders, 1:339
Bone marrow fibrosis, 1:189, 337
Bone marrow transplantation, 1:189, **1:193–203**, *194, 195*, 3:1448

aftercare for, 1:200
allogenic, 1:194, 195, 197, 202
alternatives to, 1:202
autologous, 1:194, 196, 197, 202
demographics of, 1:194
human leukocyte antigen test for, 2:692
mortality and morbidity from, 1:202
preparation for, 1:198–199
procedure for, 1:196–198
risks of, 1:200–201
transfusion for, 1:181
types of, 1:194–196

Bone morphogenetic proteins (BMP), 1:187, 3:1354
Bone shortening, **2:866–872**, *867*
Bone spur, 1:230, 2:616, 822
Bone stabilization and fixation, 1:542–543
Bone tumors

bone x rays for, 1:203
limb salvage for, 2:872–875
magnetic resonance imaging for, 2:926

Bone x rays, **1:203–204**, 3:1176
Bonine. *See* Meclizine
Boots, Venodyne, 2:572
Borborygmi, 3:1372
Boric acid, 1:94
Botox, 1:523, 552
Botulinum toxin, 1:523, 552, 3:1242

Bovie, suction, 1:24
Bovine spongiform encephalopathy, 1:311
Bowel. *See* Intestines
Bowel cleansing. *See* Cleansing enema
Bowel incontinence. *See* Fecal incontinence
Bowel obstruction. *See* Intestinal obstruction
Bowel resection, **1:204–209**, *205*

for endometriosis, 2:835
for hernias, 1:529, 2:754
small bowel, **3:1333–1337**, *1334*

Bowel sounds, 3:1189
Bowel training, 2:966
Bowlegs, 2:797
BPH. *See* Benign prostatic hyperplasia
Bracelets, medical alert, 1:247
Braces

carpal tunnel syndrome, 1:260
club foot repair, 1:306
knee osteotomy, 2:798
knee stability, 2:807
limb salvage, 2:873
pectus excavatum repair, 3:1111, 1112
scoliosis, 3:1353, 1355
spinal instrumentation, 3:1356, 1357
tooth extraction, 3:1428

Brachytherapy, 1:356
Bradycardia, 1:451, 3:1079–1082
Brain abscess, 1:369, 483, 2:1026
Brain aneurysm. *See* Cerebral aneurysm
Brain damage

from aortic aneurysm repair, 1:103
electroencephalography for, 1:442
emergency surgery for, 1:452

Brain death, 1:442
Brain disorders, degenerative, 1:442
Brain hemorrhage, 2:1024–1025
Brain imaging

CT scans, 1:382, *1:382*, 1:384
magnetic resonance, 2:925–926
magnetic spectroscopy, 2:927

Brain mapping, 1:444
Brain tumors

cerebral aneurysm and, 1:271
craniotomy for, 1:369–372
cryotherapy for, 1:377
CT scans for, 1:384
demographics of, 1:369
magnetic resonance imaging for, 2:925
neurosurgery for, 2:1025–1026
stereotactic radiosurgery for, 3:1369–1371
whole-brain radiation therapy for, 3:1370

Brain wave patterns, 1:442–446
BRCA1 gene, 2:1038–1039, 3:1256
BRCA2 gene, 2:1038–1039, 3:1256
Breach rhythm, 1:445

Breast

fibrosis, 1:211
lift, 1:9, 217
mound, 1:217
prosthesis, 1:216, 3:1321

Breast augmentation

abdominoplasty and, 1:9
breast implants for, 1:213–216
for breast reconstruction, 1:220
demographics of, 1:217
non-surgical alternatives for, 1:213–216, 221

Breast biopsy, **1:209–213**, *210*
Breast cancer

axillary dissection for, 1:136–139, *1:137*
biopsy for, 1:209–213
cryotherapy for, 1:377
demographics of, 1:210, 2:912, 932, 986, 3:1213, 1294, 1319–1320, 1383
diagnosis of, 2:929, 987–989, 3:1214, 1295
estrogen-sensitive, 2:1038
male, 2:1052
mammography for, 1:210, 2:929–932, *2:930*, 2:987
metastasis, 1:137–138, 2:988, 3:1213
mortality and morbidity from, 3:1296–1297, 1322
non-surgical treatment of, 2:989
oophorectomy for, 2:1038–1039
peritoneovenous shunts for, 3:1137
quadrantectomy for, 3:1213–1215
radiation therapy for, 3:1214
recurrence of, 1:138, 2:913, 3:1214
reoperation for, 3:1230
risks with, 2:1038–1039
second opinions for, 3:1290
segmentectomy for, 3:1294–1298
sentinel lymph node biopsy for, 1:138, 2:913, 988, 3:1215, 1300
stages of, 2:987–988, 989
See also Breast reconstruction; Lumpectomy; Mastectomy

Breast conservation surgery. *See* Lumpectomy; Quadrantectomy
Breast Imaging Reporting and Data System (BIRADS), 2:931
Breast Implant Safety (FDA report), 1:221
Breast implants, *1:213*, **213–216**, *214*

abdominoplasty and, 1:9
autoimmune disorders from, 1:220–221
for breast reconstruction, 1:213, 215, 219, 220–221
silicone gel, 1:213–216, 219, 220–221, 3:1174
simple mastectomy and, 3:1321

Breast reconstruction, **1:216–222**, *217, 218*

abdominoplasty and, 1:9

breast implants for, 1:213, 215, 219, 220–221
insurance coverage of, 1:502
modified radical mastectomy and, 2:986, 987, 989
for sex reassignment surgery, 3:1306
simple mastectomy and, 3:1320–1321, 1322
Breast reduction, 1:9, **1:222–225**, *223*
Breastfeeding
antibiotics and, 1:82
anticoagulants and, 1:87
antihypertensive drugs and, 1:91
antiseptics and, 1:94
aspirin and, 1:132
barbiturates and, 1:152
breast cancer and, 2:986
breast implants and, 1:215
buspirone and, 1:80
cephalosporins and, 1:270
cesarean section and, 1:286–287
corticosteroids and, 1:360
diuretics and, 1:429
erythromycins and, 1:484
fluoroquinolones and, 1:546
immunosuppressant drugs and, 2:734–735
interferons and, 2:730
laxatives and, 2:866
middle ear infections and, 2:1006
morphine and, 3:1104
muscle relaxants and, 2:994
NSAIDs and, 2:1028
opioid analgesics and, 1:54
sclerotherapy and, 3:1282
sulfonamides and, 3:1378
tetracyclines and, 3:1407
topical antibiotics and, 1:85
Breath, shortness of, 3:1177
Breathing
exercises, 2:904, 3:1189, 1548
postoperative techniques, 3:1185
rescue, 1:244, 246–247
tubes, 3:1541
Breathing disorders
esophageal atresia/tracheo-esophageal fistula and, 1:489
snoring and, 3:1342
spirometry tests for, 3:1358–1360
Breech presentation, 1:283, 287, 480
See also Childbirth
Brevital. *See* Methohexital
Bridges, dental, 1:413, 3:1246
Brint, Stephen, 2:842
Bris Milah ceremony, 1:299, 300
Bristow procedure, 1:149–150
British National Formulary, 2:734
Broad-spectrum antibiotics, 1:48, 83, 529, 2:873, 3:1331
See also specific antibiotics
Broca-Perthes-Bankart procedure, **1:147–150**, *148*
Broken bones. *See* Fractures

Bronchial brush, 1:226, 227
Bronchial cancer, 1:226
Bronchial pneumonia, 1:292
Bronchiectasis, 2:904, 3:1358
Bronchiolitis, 2:633, 3:1413
Bronchitis, 2:903, 904, 3:1175, 1358
Bronchoalveolar lavage, 1:226–227
Bronchodilators
fluoroquinolones and, 1:547
gastric acid inhibitors and, 2:569
spirometry tests and, 3:1359
Bronchopleural fistula, 3:1177
Bronchoscopy, *1:225*, **225–229**, *227*
with esophagoscopy and laryngoscopy, 1:434
laser, 2:1075
lung biopsy and, 2:914, 917
Brooke ileostomy, 2:725
Brow lift. *See* Forehead lift
Bruit, 1:255
Brush, bronchial, 1:226, 227
Bu-Spar. *See* Buspirone
Bubble oxygenators, 2:629
Buck's skin traction, 3:1437
Buddhism, 2:683
Buerger's disease, 3:1128
Bulimia nervosa, 3:1560
Bulk-producing laxatives, 2:865
Bulking agents, 1:311, 3:1332
Bullectomy, 2:905, 3:1178
Bumetanide, 1:428
Bumex. *See* Bumetanide
BUN. *See* Blood urea nitrogen
Bunionectomy, **1:229–233**, *230*
Bunions, 1:229–233, *1:230*, 2:616
Bunke, Harry, 2:970
Buphthalmos, 2:608
Bupivacaine, 1:65, 477, 542
Buprenorphine, 1:50
Burch procedure, 1:397, 2:1011, 3:1234–1238, 1331, 1332
Burns
craniofacial reconstruction for, 1:363
cricothyroidotomy for, 1:374
from defibrillation, 1:413
demographics of, 3:1326
dressings for, 2:744
ear injuries from, 2:1069
from electrocautery, 1:404
electrolyte balance and, 1:447
emergency surgery for, 1:452
hematocrit and, 2:647
pain from, 3:1083
psychotherapy for, 3:1326
rehabilitation for, 3:1326
scar revision for, 1:1266
silver sulfadiazine for, 3:1377
skin grafting for, 3:1322–1328
third-degree, 3:1323
Burr holes, 1:410, 3:1088
Buscopan. *See* Hyoscine butylbromide
Bush, George W., 2:963
Buspirone, 1:79, 79*t*, 80

Butorphanol, 1:53*t*
Bypass surgery
aortobifemoral, 3:1132, 1135, 1136
femoropopliteal, 3:1132, *3:1133*, 3:1135, 1136
femorotibial, 3:1132, 1135, 1136
peripheral vascular, 3:1132–1137, *3:1133*
portal vein, **3:1179–1182**, *1180*
See also Coronary artery bypass graft surgery

C

C-Arm Image Intensifier, 2:882
C-peptide, 2:604
C-reactive protein, 1:240, 241, 242
C-section. *See* Cesarean section
CA-125, 3:1470, 1471
Cadaveric donors, 3:1445, 1446
Caffeine
arrhythmia and, 2:940
fluoroquinolones and, 1:547
in opioid analgesics, 1:53
Calan. *See* Verapamil
Calcitonin, 3:1083
Calcium
antibiotics and, 1:83
antrectomy and, 1:97
in bone tissue, 1:184
electrolyte balance and, 1:446, 447, 448
fracture repair and, 1:555
hyperparathyroidism and, 3:1098, 1099
reference range for, 1:448
thyroidectomy and, 3:1098–1099
Calcium alginate, 1:144
Calcium bilirubinate, 1:293
Calcium channel blockers, 1:74, 89, 249, 2:939
Calcium deposits, 2:979
Calcium hydroxylapatite, 1:552
Calcium oxalate calculi, 2:1016, 1020, 1021
Calcium sulfate grafts, 1:187
Calcium supplements
gastrectomy, 2:566
hypoparathyroidism, 3:1098
leg lengthening and shortening, 2:870
otosclerosis, 3:1367
pharyngectomy, 3:1146–1147
Calculi. *See* Stones
Caldwell-Luc procedure, 1:461–462
Calendula, 3:1430
Calipers, 3:1120
Callus, 1:555
Cameras, laparoscopic, 2:828
Canadian health care, 1:538–539
Cancer
bone marrow biopsy for, 1:189

Cancer metastasis

complementary and alternative medicine for, 1:202
demographics of, 3:1383–1384
exploratory laparotomy for, 2:836, 838
hormone therapy for, 1:202
hospice care for, 2:684
immunoprevention for, 2:731
immunotherapy for, 1:202
laparoscopy for, 2:828
obesity and, 1:507
pain, 1:67
positron emission tomography for, 3:1182
recurrence of, 3:1288, 1383
reoperation for, 3:1230
second-look surgery for, 3:1288–1290
second opinions for, 3:1290
smoking cessation and, 3:1338
surgical oncology and, 3:1382–1385
See also specific types of cancer
Cancer metastasis. *See* Metastasis
Cancer screening, 3:1469–1472
Cancer staging, 2:836, 3:1300, 1384, 1473
Cancer vaccines, 2:731
Candesartan, 1:89
Candida infections, 2:686
Canes. *See* Assistive devices
Cannabinoids, 3:1275
Cannulation sites, 2:629
CAPD (Continuous ambulatory peritoneal dialysis), 2:781, 3:1317
Capillaries, 3:1280
Capoten. *See* Captopril
Capsaicin, 1:233, 3:1255
Capsular contraction, 1:215, 221
Capsulorrhexis, 1:512
Capsulotomy
anterior, 2:854
laser posterior, 1:513, **2:854–857**
Nd:YAG, 3:1144
surgical, 2:856–857
for toe abnormalities, 2:617
Captopril, 1:89, 90*t*, 429
Car accidents, 1:363, 372
Carafate. *See* Sucralfate
Carbamazepine
barbiturates and, 1:153
opioid analgesics and, 1:55
overdoses of, 2:652
for pain, 3:1084
prochlorperazine and, 1:93
Carbapenems, 1:81
Carbocaine. *See* Mepivacaine
Carbolic anhydrase inhibitors, 1:428
Carbon dioxide lasers, 2:860
cone biopsy, 1:341
laser skin resurfacing, 2:858, 859
myringotomy, 2:1005
skin resurfacing, 1:418
snoring surgery, 3:1344
Carbon monoxide inhalation, 2:1075

Carbon sorbents, 2:652
Carboxymethylcellulose fibers, 1:144, 145
Carcinoembryonic antigens (CEA), 2:892 3:1470, 1471
Carcinoid tumors, small intestine, 3:1333, 1335
Cardene. *See* Nicardipine hydrochloride
Cardiac arrest
cardioplegia solution and, 2:627
cardiopulmonary resuscitation for, 1:246
defibrillation for, 1:411–413
from stress tests, 3:1376
sudden, 1:449
See also Heart attacks; Heart failure
Cardiac catheterization, **1:235–250**, 237
for aortic aneurysm repair, 1:103
for arrhythmia, 2:998
for congenital heart defects, 2:636, 637
endovascular stent surgery and, 1:467, 468
heart-lung machines for, 2:628
for mitral valve disorders, 2:980
PTCA and, 1:74
Cardiac compressions, 3:1414
Cardiac disease. *See* Heart disease
Cardiac mapping, 1:449–452, 450
Cardiac marker tests, **1:240–242**
Cardiac monitor, **1:242–244**, 243
Cardiac nuclear medicine scans, 1:240
Cardiac output
blood pressure measurement and, 1:176
cardiac monitor for, 1:243
mechanical circulation support for, 2:942
mitral valve repair for, 2:981
Cardiac tamponade, 3:1125–1128, 1414
Cardiac transplantation. *See* Heart transplantation
Cardiac ultrasound, 1:239–240
Cardiomegaly, 1:436
Cardiomyopathy, hypertrophic, 1:436
Cardioplegia solution, 2:627, 629, 976
Cardiopulmonary bypass
for aortic aneurysm repair, 1:101, 102, 103
for aortic valve replacement, 1:104–105
blood salvage and, 1:178
for congenital heart defects, 2:636
ECMO for, 2:942
emergency, 1:453
for heart-lung transplantation, 2:632
for heart transplantation, 2:639
for lung transplantation, 2:920
for Maze procedure, 2:937
for minimally invasive heart surgery, 2:976, 977

for mitral valve repair, 2:979
for mitral valve replacement, 2:983
for myocardial resection, 2:997, 998
See also Heart-lung machines
Cardiopulmonary bypass pump. *See* Heart-lung machines
Cardiopulmonary resuscitation, **1:244–248**, *245*
See also Do-not-resuscitate (DNR) orders
Cardiothoracic surgery, 3:1386
Cardiotomy, 2:629–630
Cardiovascular disease
echocardiography for, 1:435–437
electrocardiography for, 1:439–442
mortality from, 1:442
salpingo-oophorectomy and, 3:1258, 1259
See also Heart disease
Cardiovascular surgery, 1:438, 2:690, 3:1386
Cardioversion, **1:248–252**
See also Implantable cardioverter-defibrillator
Cardizem. *See* Diltiazem
Cardura. *See* Doxazosin mesylate
Care plans, 2:956, 1029–1030
Care quality, 2:1031, 3:1108
Caregivers, 2:906, 3:1167
Caring *vs.* curing, 2:682
Carisoprodol, 2:994
Carotid artery stenosis, 1:252–257, 466, 3:1519, 1520
Carotid endarterectomy, **1:252–257**, *253*, 1:466
Carpal boss, 2:562
Carpal tunnel release, **1:257–262**, *258*
Carpal tunnel syndrome, 1:257–262, *1:258*
arthroscopic surgery for, 1:121
from axillary dissection, 1:138
Carteolol, 1:91
Cartilage injuries
age factors in, 2:801
arthroscopic surgery for, 1:121
hip osteotomy for, 2:661, 662
knee arthroscopic surgery for, 2:791
knee replacement for, 2:800
non-surgical treatment of, 3:1311
Cartilage transplantation, 2:807, 3:1302
Cartridge syringes, 3:1392
Carts, crash, 2:760, 1046
Carvedilol, 1:89
Casanthranol, 2:866
Cascara, 2:865, 866
Case managers, 1:423, 2:679, 933
Castor oil, 2:865
Castration, male, 2:1052
Casts
club foot, 1:306, 307
fracture repair, 1:555
spinal instrumentation, 3:1356
tendon repair, 3:1400
tenotomy, 3:1404

Casual plasma glucose test, 2:606
CAT scans. *See* CT scans
Catapres, 1:90*t*
Cataract surgery
    closed-angle glaucoma from, 2:772
    cost of, 1:39
    cryotherapy, 1:377, 379–381
    demographics of, 1:510–511,
        2:1048
    extracapsular extraction, 1:381,
        509–516, 3:1140, 1144
    intracapsular extraction, 1:509, 515,
        3:1144
    iridectomy and, 2:771
    lens opacification from, 2:854
    mortality and morbidity from, 1:514
    retinal detachment from, 1:514,
        3:1152, 1268
    See also Phacoemulsification
Cataracts
    aging and, 1:510, 511
    classification of, 1:510
    congenital, 3:1140
    cortical, 1:510, 512
    from cyclocryotherapy, 1:390
    demographics of, 1:380, 3:1140
    diagnosis of, 1:512–513,
        3:1142–1143
    from laser iridotomy, 2:853
    non-surgical treatment of,
        1:514–515
    nuclear, 1:510, 512
    posterior subcapsular, 1:510, 512,
        513
    risk factors for, 1:511–512
    secondary, 3:1144
Cathartic colon, 2:865
Catheter-related infections, 2:685
Catheterization. *See* Cardiac catheterization; Urinary catheterization
Catheters
    ablating electrode, 1:450
    ablation, 1:449, 450, 451
    antibacterial-coated, 2:687
    central venous, 1:199, 404, 2:685
    complications from, 1:404
    disposable, 2:761
    Foley, 1:262, 265
    for hemodialysis, 1:112
    hydrogel-coated latex, 1:263, 266
    latex, 1:263, 266
    PTFE, 1:263, 266
    pulmonary artery, 1:243
    silastic, 1:263, 266
    silicone, 1:263, 266
    silver alloy-coated, 2:687
    size of, 1:263, 266
    after ureterosigmoidoscopy, 3:1494
Cations, 1:447
Cauda equina syndrome, 2:819, 820,
    824
CBC. *See* Complete blood count
CBE (Charting by exception), 2:957

CBT (Cognitive-behavioral therapy),
    3:1562
CCAM (Congenital cystic adenomatoid
    malformation of the lung), 1:531,
    532, 533
CCPD (Continuous cyclic peritoneal
    dialysis), 2:781
CCU (Coronary intensive care units),
    2:759
CDH (Congenital diaphragmatic hernia), 1:531
CDS-1 (Cell Density Signal-1), 3:1402
CEA (Carcinoembryonic antigens),
    3:1470, 1471
Ceclor. *See* Cefaclor
Cecum, 1:204
Cefaclor, 1:269
Cefadroxil, 1:269
Cefamandole, 3:1206
Cefazolin, 1:269, 3:1206
Cefixime, 1:269
Cefmetazole, 1:82
Cefoperazone, 1:82
Cefotaxime, 1:81, 3:1206
Cefotetan, 1:82
Cefoxitin, 1:81, 269, 529, 3:1206
Cefprozil, 1:269
Ceftazidime, 1:269
Ceftriaxone, 1:81, 82
Cefuroxime, 1:269
Cefzil. *See* Cefprozil
Celecoxib, 1:50, 2:1028
Celiac angiography, 1:70
Cell counters, automated, 1:335, 2:648,
    3:1229
Cell Density Signal-1 (CDS-1), 3:1402
Cell-free hemoglobin, 1:182
CellCept. *See* Mycophenolate
Cellular phones, 3:1081, 1167
Cellular wound dressings, 3:1568–1569
Cellulite, 2:878
Cellulitis, 1:406–407
Celsus, 2:701
Cement
    bone, *2:665*, 2:666, 675, 811
    sealer, 3:1245
Census Bureau
    on the elderly, 2:906
    on uninsured persons, 3:1204
Center for Bloodless Medicine and
    Surgery, 1:180
Center for Molecular and Cellular
    Therapy, 1:181
Centers for Disease Control and Prevention (CDC)
    on ambulatory surgery, 1:438
    on arthritis, 2:798
    on bladder cancer, 1:392
    on cervical cancer, 1:340
    on colorectal cancer screening,
        1:315
    on electrocardiography, 1:440
    on exercise, 1:506
    on gum disease, 2:598

    on hospices, 2:683
    on hospital-acquired infections,
        2:685
    on hypospadias, 2:701, 703
    on infection control programs,
        2:687
    on inpatient surgery, 1:438
    on low back pain, 2:822
    on peptic ulcers, 1:96
    on stomach ulcers, 2:580
    on surgical procedures, 1:128
    on surgical scrubs, 1:128–129
    on transfusion safety, 1:180
    on uninsured persons, 3:1204
Centers for Medicare and Medicaid
    Services (CMS), 1:541, 2:963
Central islands, 2:846
Central nervous system, 3:1083
Central nervous system depressants,
    1:55, 150–153
Central nervous system disorders,
    1:276–278, 2:1024–1027
Central nervous system infections,
    2:1026
Central venous catheters, 1:199, 404,
    2:685
Centrax. *See* Prazepam
Centrifugal pumps, 2:629, 843
Cephalexin, 1:269
Cephalopelvic disproportion, 1:283
Cephalosporins, 1:81, 82, 83,
    1:268–271
    allergies to, 1:269, 3:1206
    for antibiotic prophylaxis,
        1:268–269, 3:1206
    for hospital-acquired infections,
        2:687
Cephamycins, 1:81, 269
Ceptaz, 1:269
Ceramic grafts, 1:187
Ceramic prosthesis, 2:666
Cerclage, cervical, **1:278–281,** 2:1033
Cerebral aneurysm, 1:271–276, 369
Cerebral aneurysm repair, **1:271–276,**
    272
Cerebral angiography, 1:69, *1:69,*
    1:273
Cerebral edema, 1:427, 428
Cerebral hemispheres, 2:648
Cerebral palsy, 3:1242, 1352
Cerebrospinal fluid (CSF) analysis,
    1:276–278
    for glucose, 2:604, 606
    immunoassay tests, 2:727
    for subarachnoid hemorrhage,
        2:1025
Cerebrospinal fluid (CSF) leak
    from endoscopic sinus surgery,
        1:461
    from epidural anesthesia, 1:479
    from hypophysectomy, 2:699
    from septoplasty, 3:1304
    ventricular shunt for, 3:1542–1544

Cerebrovascular accident (CVA). *See* Stroke

Certificate of Need laws, 2:689

Certification, board, 1:540, 3:1165, 1194–1195, 1291, 1387

Certified nurse anesthetists (CRNA), *1:60,* 3:1387, 1388

Cervical cancer
  colposcopy for, 1:330
  cone biopsy for, 1:339–342
  cryotherapy for, 1:281–283, 378
  demographics of, 1:339–340, 3:1383
  hysterectomy for, 1:341, 2:706, 708
  pelvic exenteration for, 1:503

Cervical caps. *See* Diaphragm (Contraceptive)

Cervical cerclage, **1:278–281,** 2:1033

Cervical cryotherapy, **1:281–283,** 1:378, 2:1034

Cervical dysplasia, 1:281–283, 329–331

Cervical spinal fusion, 1:185–186

Cervical stenosis, 1:341

Cervical warts, 1:330

Cervicofacial rhytidectomy. *See* Face lift

Cervix, incompetent, 1:278–279

Cesarean section, **1:283–288,** *284, 285,* 2:1033
  cervical cerclage and, 1:279
  epidural anesthesia for, 1:284, 286, 477–479
  fetal surgery and, 1:532
  On-Q analgesics for, 3:1185
  regional anesthesia for, 1:63, 284, 286
  scopolamine patch for, 3:1287
  vaginal birth after, 1:283, 287
  See also Childbirth

Chaga's disease, 1:180

Channel blockers. *See* Calcium channel blockers

Charcoal, 2:652

Charcot's arthropathy, 3:1310

Charcot's triad, 2:559

Charity hospitals, 2:689

Charnley, John, 2:666

Charnley pillow, 2:666

Charnley prosthesis, 2:666

Charting by exception (CBE), 2:957

Charts, medical, **2:955–959,** 3:1106–1108, 1109

Cheiloplasty, **1:300–305,** *302*

Chelation therapy, 1:256, 470, 3:1132, 1136

Chemical debridement, 1:407

Chemical peels
  vs. dermabrasion, 1:418
  vs. laser skin resurfacing, 2:859
  for scar revision, 3:1267

Chemiluminescent immunoassay, 2:727

Chemotherapy
  bone marrow biopsy and, 1:189

bone marrow transplantation and, 1:193, 199
  for breast cancer, 2:989
  complete blood count for, 1:334
  for head and neck cancer, 3:1218
  incisional hernia repair and, 2:747
  for laryngeal cancer, 2:841
  lumpectomy and, 2:910, 913
  for lung cancer, 3:1177, 1412
  for neuroblastoma, 3:1233
  non-myeloablative allogeneic transplantation and, 1:195
  pancreatectomy and, 3:1093
  with radiotherapy, 1:202
  See also Cancer

Chest compressions, 1:244, 247

Chest deformity repair, **3:1109–1113**

Chest injuries, 3:1175, 1412

Chest pain. *See* Angina

Chest physiotherapy, 1:348–349, 2:939

Chest shells, 2:945

Chest tube insertion, **1:288–290,** 1:291

Chest x ray, *1:291,* **291–293**
  for anesthesia evaluation, 1:57
  CT scans, 1:382, 384
  for esophageal cancer, 1:496
  for lung transplantation, 2:920
  for mitral valve disorders, 2:980, 984
  serial, 1:293
  for tracheotomy, 3:1435

Child abuse, 1:362

Child day care, 2:1006

Childbirth
  anesthesiologists and, 1:67
  breech presentation, 1:283, 287, 480
  colpotomy and, 1:331
  dilation and curettage for, 1:419
  epidural anesthesia for, 1:67, 477–479, 2:1034
  episiotomy for, 1:479–483, *1:481*
  urinary incontinence and, 3:1235
  See also Cesarean section; Pregnancy

Children, 2:845
  abdominal wall defects in, 3:1116–1117
  in accidents, 3:1118–1119
  alimentary tract obstruction in, 3:1116
  anorectal anomalies in, 3:1116
  apnea in, 1:246
  appendicitis in, 3:1117–1118
  aspirin and, 1:132
  barbiturates and, 1:152
  biliary disease in, 3:1118
  bladder augmentation for, 1:168
  blood pressure measurement for, 1:176, 177, 3:1351
  bone marrow aspiration and biopsy in, 1:190–191
  brain tumors in, 1:369
  cerebral aneurysm and, 1:271
  cochlear implants for, 1:310

conscious sedation for, 3:1293
  corpus callostomy for, 1:358
  craniofacial reconstruction for, *1:362,* 1:362–363, 365, 366–367
  cricothyroidotomy for, 1:374
  Crohn's disease in, 3:1118
  cyclocryotherapy for, 1:390
  dialysis for, 2:779–780
  ear, nose and throat surgery for, 1:433
  ear infections in, 2:935
  electrophysiology study for, 1:450
  emergency surgery for, 1:453
  end-stage renal disease in, 2:779–780, 786–787
  eye enucleation for, 1:475
  eye muscle surgery for, 1:518, 519
  femoral hernia repair for, 1:527, 528
  fluoroquinolones for, 1:546
  fractures in, 1:553, 555
  gastroesophageal reflux disease in, 3:1117
  goniotomy for, 2:606–611
  gum disease in, 2:599
  head injuries in, 3:1118
  hemangiomas in, 2:644
  hemispherectomy for, 2:649
  hernia in, 3:1119
  hospices for, 2:683
  hospital-acquired infections and, 2:685
  hospital admission of, 1:27
  inflammatory bowel disease in, 3:1118
  informed consent and, 3:1193
  inguinal hernias in, 2:753
  intestinal obstruction in, 2:764, 3:1116
  intussusception reduction for, 2:767–769
  kidney transplantation for, 2:786–787
  laser posterior capsulotomy for, 2:854
  latex allergies in, 3:1192
  leg lengthening and shortening for, 2:866, 870
  liver transplantation for, 2:900
  local anesthesia for, 1:63
  Meckel's diverticulum in, 2:948, 3:1117
  Medicaid for, 2:953
  morphine for, 3:1104
  myringotomy for, 2:1002–1007
  necrotizing enterocolitis in, 3:1116
  needles and, 3:1113
  orchiopexy for, 2:1057–1063
  pain in, 3:1113
  patient-controlled analgesia for, 3:1104
  peptic ulcers in, 3:1209
  post-traumatic stress disorder in, 1:366–367
  power of attorney and, 3:1193

preoperative care for, 3:1192
preparing for surgery, 3:1113–1114
recovery room and, 3:1114, 1222
retinoblastoma in, 3:1232–1233
rhizotomy for, 3:1242
scopolamine patch for, 3:1286
septoplasty for, 3:1303
skull x rays for, 3:1329
snoring in, 3:1342, 1343, 1345
special concerns for, **3:1113–1114**
splenectomy for, 3:1364
strabismus in, 1:517
tetracyclines and, 3:1406
trauma in, 3:1118–1119
ulcerative colitis in, 3:1118
See also Adolescents; Infants; Pediatric surgery
Chili peppers, 1:233, 3:1255
Chin augmentation, 2:967–969
Chin implants, 2:967–968, 969
Chin reduction, 2:967–969
Chinplasty, **2:967–970**
Chips, antibiotic, 2:600
Chiropractic
for back pain, 2:826
Chisel, ballistic, 2:675
Chlamydia trichomatis, 2:727
Chlorambucil, 2:736
Chloramphenicol, 2:647
Chlordiazepoxide, 1:79t
Chlorhexidine, 1:94
Chloride tests, 1:446–449
Chloroprocaine, 1:477
Chlorothiazide, 1:90t, 91, 428
Chlorphenesin, 2:994
Chlortetracycline, 3:1405
Chlorthalidone, 1:90t, 91, 428
Chlorzoxazone, 2:994
Cholangiography, percutaneous transhepatic, 1:160, 458
Cholangiopancreatography
endoscopic retrograde, 1:160, **1:456–459**, *457,* 2:558, 559
magnetic resonance, 1:458
Cholangitis
endoscopic retrograde cholangiopancreatography for, 1:458
gallstone removal for, 2:558–559
primary sclerosing, 1:159, 457
Cholecystectomy, **1:293–297,** *294,* 2:558, 559, 579
for children, 3:1118
complications from, 2:581
demographics of, 2:580
telesurgery and, 3:1399
Cholecystitis
acute, 1:295, 296–297, 2:558–559
cholecystectomy for, 1:293–297
endoscopic retrograde cholangiopancreatography for, 1:458
Choledochojejunostomy, 1:161
Choledocholithiasis, 2:558–559
Choledyl. *See* Oxtriphylline
Cholelithiasis. *See* Gallstones

Cholelithotomy, **2:557–560**
Cholestasis, 2:889
Cholesteatoma, 2:934, 935, 1005, 3:1288
Cholesterol levels
atherosclerosis prevention and, 1:469
lipid tests for, 2:875–878
liver function tests for, 2:890–895
surgical risk and, 1:403
Cholesterol-lowering drugs, 1:429
Cholestyramine, 1:22, 429
Choline salicylate, 1:131
Chondroitin sulfate
for arthritis, 3:1311
for osteoarthritis, 1:119
Chondrolysis, 2:870
Chondromalacia patellae, 2:814
Chordae tendineae repair, 2:979
Chordee, 2:701, 703, 704
Chorionic villus sampling (CVS), 1:42, 43, 532, 3:1120
Chorioretinal scar, 3:1231
Choroidal detachment, 3:1464
Chromium implants, 3:1310
Chronic bronchitis, 2:903, 904, 3:1175, 1358
Chronic disease, insurance for, 2:906–910
Chronic obstructive pulmonary disease (COPD)
hospital-acquired infections and, 2:686
lung transplantation for, 2:919
mortality and morbidity from, 3:1336
non-surgical treatment of, 1:32, 33, 2:905, 3:1177–1178
pulmonary lobectomy for, 2:903
risk factors for, 3:1175
spirometry tests for, 3:1358
Chronic pain, 1:50–51, 67, 3:1083, 1086
Chronic pancreatitis, 3:1092, 1094
Chronulac. *See* Lactulose
Cigarettes. *See* Smoking
Ciliary body removal, **1:387–391**
Cilostazol, 2:570
Cimetidine
alprazolam and, 1:80
cyclosporins and, 2:736
diazepam and, 2:995
gastric acid inhibitors and, 2:568
Cinobac. *See* Cinoxacin
Cinoxacin, 1:547
Cipro. *See* Ciprofloxacin
Ciprofloxacin, 1:546, 547, 3:1206
Circulation, collateral, 3:1129, 1134
Circulation disorders, 1:70
Circulation support, mechanical, **2:942–944,** 2:999
Circumcision, **1:297–300,** *298,* 2:704
Cirrhosis
abdominal ultrasound for, 1:1

causes of, 3:1179
demographics of, 3:1137
hemoglobin test and, 2:651
hepatectomy and, 2:659
liver cancer and, 2:657
liver function tests for, 2:892–894
liver transplantation for, 2:895–901
peritoneovenous shunts for, 3:1137–1140
portal vein bypass surgery for, 3:1179–1182
primary biliary, 1:456
Cis-retinoic acid, 1:418, 2:858
Citalopram, 1:78
Citrucel. *See* Methylcellulose
CK-MB forms, 1:240–241, 242
Claforan. *See* Cefotaxime
Clamps (Surgical), 1:299–300, 3:1381
Clarithromycin, 1:81, 483, 484
Classic forehead lift, 1:549, 551
Clathrates, 1:59
Claustrophobia, 1:382, 2:927
Claw toes, 2:616–618
Cleaning, 1:128
Cleansing enema
bowel resection, 1:207
colonoscopy, 1:315
colorectal surgery, 1:319
colostomy, 1:323
rectal prolapse, 3:1224
rectal resection, 3:1225, 1227
sigmoidoscopy, 3:1316
Cleft lip repair, **1:300–305,** *301, 302*
Cleft palate, 1:301, 362
Clindamycin, 1:49, 82
Clinical interview, 2:625
Clinical nurse managers, 3:1167
Clinical obesity, 1:508
Clinical pain, 3:1183
Clinical trials, 2:918, 3:1448
Clips
for cerebral aneurysm repair, 1:274, 275
for finger reattachment, 1:543
magnetic resonance imaging and, 2:928
titanium, 1:274
Clitoris, 1:297
Clopidogrel
antiplatelet activity of, 1:86
for coronary artery bypass graft surgery, 1:352
for coronary artery disease, 1:356, 472
Clorazepate dipotassium, 1:79t
Closed-angle glaucoma, 3:1433
Clostridium infections, 1:48
Clostridium botulinum, 1:523, 552
Clostridium perfingens, 1:406
Clot formation. *See* Blood clots
Clothing, sterile surgical, 1:129
Clotting factors, 1:86
Club foot, 1:300–301, 305–307, 3:1404–1405

Club foot repair, **1:305–307**
CME (Cystoid macular edema), 1:514
CMG (Cystometrogram), 1:167–168
CMS (Centers for Medicare and Medicaid Services), 1:541, 2:963
Co-trimoxazole, 2:735
Coagulation
    argon beam lasers for, 1:98, 182
    infrared, 2:655
    myelography and, 2:996
    platelets and, 1:337
    See also Blood clots
Coarctation of the aorta, 2:634, *2:635,*
    2:636, 637
Coat's disease, 3:1153, 1231–1234
Cobalt chrome alloys, 2:666
Cobalt implants, 3:1310
Cocaine, 1:63, 460
Coccyx, 2:819
Cochlear implants, **1:308–311**, *309,*
    1:434
Cocoa butter, 3:1266
Code carts, 2:760
Code of Hammurabi, 1:510
Codeine
    acetaminophen with, 1:21, 359
    activity of, 1:53*t*
    for analgesia, 1:51, 52
    for craniotomy, 1:370
Coffee, 1:240
Coffin-Siris syndrome, 1:301
Cognitive-behavioral therapy (CBT),
    3:1562
Cognitive impairment, 1:411
Coherent ultrapulse carbon dioxide
    laser treatments, 1:523
Colace. *See* Docusate
Cold compresses
    tooth extraction, 3:1427
    tooth replantation, 3:1430
Cold intolerance, 1:545
Cold-knife conization, 1:340–341
Cold sores, 1:418, 2:858
Colds, 1:32, 33, 489
Colectomy, 1:206, 2:717
Colic, biliary, 1:293, 295, 2:558–559
Colitis
    cephalosporins and, 1:270
    colonoscopy after, 1:314
    ischemic, 2:763
    pseudomembranous, 1:82
    sigmoidoscopy and, 3:1317
    See also Ulcerative colitis
Collaborative Corneal Transplantation
    Study, 1:344
Collagen
    bone grafts and, 1:187
    in bone tissue, 1:184
    scar formation and, 3:1264
    seals, 1:236
    in skin, 3:1323
    in tendon repair, 3:1402–1403
    wicks, 3:1275
    for wrinkles, 1:552

Collagen dressings, 1:144, 145
Collagen periurethral injection,
    1:311–313
Collagenase, 1:407, 3:1273
Collapsed lung, 2:904, 916–917
Collateral circulation, 3:1129, 1134
College of American Pathologists,
    1:172
Colon
    anatomy of, 1:204–205
    cathartic, 2:865
    retraction of, 1:207
Colon cancer
    barium enema for, 1:154–155
    bowel resection for, 1:205, 208
    ileoanal anastomosis for, 2:717
    intestinal obstruction repair for,
        2:763, 764
    mortality rates for, 2:580
    peritoneovenous shunts for, 3:1137
    reoperation for, 3:1230
Colon resection. *See* Bowel resection
Colonectomy, 2:723
Colonic obstruction, 2:763–765, 3:1116
Colonoscopy, **1:313–317**, *314*
    advances in, 2:581
    for colorectal cancer screening,
        1:154, 313–317, 2:581
    colorectal surgery after, 1:319
    costs of, 1:39
    for ileoanal reservoir surgery, 2:721
    for rectal resection, 3:1225
    vs. sigmoidoscopy, 3:1315
    virtual, 1:316
Colony stimulating factors, 1:199,
    2:728, 729, 731
Colorectal cancer
    barium enema for, 1:154–155, 315,
        3:1317
    bowel resection for, 1:208
    colonoscopy for, 1:154, 313–317,
        2:581
    colorectal surgery for, 1:317–321
    colostomy for, 1:321–325
    costs of, 2:580
    demographics of, 1:317–318,
        3:1225, 1315, 1383
    diagnosis of, 2:581
    mortality and morbidity from, 1:315
    rectal resection for, 3:1225–1228
    screening for, 1:154, 315, 2:581,
        3:1317
    second-look surgery for, 3:1288
    sigmoidoscopy for, 1:315, 2:581,
        3:1315–1318
    surgical procedures for, 2:579
    x ray imaging for, 3:1317
Colorectal polyps, 1:206, 313–317,
    1:314
Colorectal surgeons, 1:206
Colorectal surgery, **1:317–321,** 2:579
Colostomy, **1:321–325,** *322,* 2:579
    bowel resection and, 1:206

for intestinal obstruction repair,
    2:764
for pelvic exenteration, 1:504
pouches, 1:318, 320, 324
rectal resection and, 3:1227
Colporrhaphy, **1:325–329**, *326,*
    1:395–397, 2:1033
Colposcopy, 1:282, **1:329–331,** 1:341,
    2:1033
Colposuspension, 1:312, 3:1236
Colpotomy, **1:331–334,** 2:1033
Colyte, 1:207, 319, 323, 3:1227
Coma, 1:445, 2:1025
Combitube, esophageal tracheal, 1:463,
    465
Comfort Care Only document, 1:431
Commissurotomy
    direct, 1:107
    mitral, 2:979, 981
Committee on Quality of Health Care
    in America, 2:959
Committee on Transfusion Medicine,
    1:180
Common bile duct, 2:557, 559, 831
Common cold, 1:32, 33, 489
Common iliac arteries, 3:1129,
    1132–1136
Communication
    errors, 2:960
    in nursing homes, 2:1031
    in physician-patient relations,
        3:1395–1396
Community home care services, 2:679
Community hospitals, 2:688
Compatibility testing, 2:789
Compazine. *See* Prochlorperazine
Complementary and alternative medicine
    anesthesia evaluation and, 1:57
    for back pain, 2:826
    for bedsores, 1:158
    for bladder cancers, 3:1452–1453
    for cancer, 1:202
    for hip replacement surgery,
        2:671–672
    hospices and, 2:684
    in hospitals, 3:1166
    for joint disorders, 1:122
    for kidney stones, 2:1021
    for knee injuries, 2:812
    for osteoarthritis, 2:807
    for snoring, 3:1348
    for spider veins, 3:1284–1285
    for stomach ulcers, 1:98–99
    for transplant recipients, 3:1448
    for TURP syndrome, 3:1457–1458
    for varicose veins, 3:1536
    for weight management,
        3:1562–1563
Complete blood count (CBC), 1:189,
    1:334–339
Complications, postoperative. *See* Postoperative complications
Composite dressings, 1:144, 145

Composite grafts, 3:1325
Compound fractures, 1:555
Compressed oxygen, 2:1074
Compression dressings, 1:543
Compression garments, 2:879, 880
Compression injuries, 1:525,
  2:619–620, 621
Compression stockings
  for blood clot prevention, 1:86
  for deep vein thrombosis, 2:669,
    670, 805, 3:1539
  Jobst, 3:1325
  for liposuction, 2:879
  purpose of, 1:144, 2:761, 3:1188
  for sclerotherapy, 3:1283
  for spider veins, 3:1284
  thromboembolic deterrent, 2:669,
    670, 805, 806
  for vein ligation and stripping,
    3:1534, 1536
Compression wrapping products,
  1:144, 145
Computed tomography scan. See CT
  scans
Computer-assisted robotic surgery,
  3:1243, 1399
Computer-assisted surgery, 3:1398–1399
Computerized axial tomography. See
  CT scans
Computerized drug order systems,
  2:690
Computerized tomographic angiogra-
  phy (CTA), 1:70, 71
Conditioning, bone marrow, 1:199
Condoms
  female, 3:1462
  male, 3:1462
Conductive hearing loss, 3:1366
Conductive keratoplasty, 2:847
Cone biopsy, 1:329, **1:339–342,** *340*
Confidentiality, **3:1106–1108**
  hospital rules for, 3:1167
  medical charts and, 2:955, 958
  patient rights and, 3:1108, 1109
Congenital cystic adenomatoid malformation of the lung (CCAM), 1:531,
  532, 533
Congenital defects. See Birth defects
Congenital diaphragmatic hernia
  (CDH), 1:531, 534, 3:1117
Congenital glaucoma, 1:388–389,
  2:606–611
Congenital heart defects
  cardiac catheterization for, 1:235
  demographics of, 2:634, *2:635*
  emergency surgery for, 1:453
  esophageal atresia/tracheoe-
    sophageal fistula and, 1:487
  heart surgery for, 2:634–638
  heart valve, 1:141–142, 143
  mitral valve, 2:979, 983
  pacemakers for, 3:1079
  septal, 1:239, 2:634, *2:635,* 2:636,
    637

Congestion, nasal. See Nasal congestion
Congestive heart failure
  chest x ray for, 1:291, 293
  diagnosis of, 2:998
  echocardiography for, 1:436
  enhanced external counterpulsation
    for, 1:470
  myocardial resection for, 2:997
  peritoneovenous shunts for, 3:1137
Conization
  cervical, 1:329, 339–342
  cold-knife, 1:340–341
  laser, 1:341
Conjugated bilirubin tests, 2:891
Connective tissue disorders, 1:220–221
Conscious sedation, 1:521, 2:858,
  3:1292–1294
Consciousness, 1:162–163
Consensus Development Conference
  Statement on Physical Activity and
  Cardiovascular Health, 1:506
Consent forms, 1:27, 2:956
  See also Informed consent
Constipation, **2:864–866**
Consultations, 2:956, 3:1200
  See also Communication
Contact dissolution therapy, 2:558
Contact lenses
  gas-permeable, 3:1161
  LASIK and, 2:844, 845, 846, 847
  photorefractive keratectomy and,
    3:1159
  for refractive vision errors,
    3:1160–1161
Continent catheterizable stomal reser-
  voir, 2:713
Continent cutaneous diversion, 1:392
Continent ileostomy, 2:725
Continent urinary diversion, 2:713, 716
Continuous ambulatory peritoneal dial-
  ysis (CAPD), 2:781, 3:1317
Continuous cyclic peritoneal dialysis
  (CCPD), 2:781
Continuous passive motion machine,
  2:798, 805, 806, 873
Continuous positive airway pressure
  (CPAP), 2:945, 3:1347
Continuous quality improvement model
  (CQI), 2:961
Contraceptives. See Oral contracep-
  tives; specific types of contraceptives
Contracted toes, 2:616
Contraction stress test (CST), 3:1509
Contractures
  joint, 2:870
  scar revision surgery for,
    3:1263–1268
  tenotomy for, 3:1404–1405
Contrast medium
  allergies to, 1:72, 237, 238, 3:1150
  for angiography, 1:68, 69, 70, 72
  for arthrography, 1:115–116

  for cardiac catheterization, 1:236,
    237
  for CT scans, 1:383
  for endoscopic retrograde cholan-
    giopancreatography, 1:457
  for magnetic resonance imaging,
    2:926, 927, 928
  for myelography, 2:996–997
  non-ionic, 1:74
  for phlebography, 3:1149
Contrast phlebography. See Phlebogra-
  phy
Contrast sensitivity
  LASIK and, 2:842, 844, 846
  ophthalmologic surgery and, 2:1050
  testing, 2:855
Copaxone. See Glatiramer acetate
COPD. See Chronic obstructive pul-
  monary disease
Cor pulmonales, 2:916
Coral grafts, 1:187
Cordis CYPHER, 1:353
Core-needle biopsy, 2:951
Corectomy, **2:770–776,** *771,* 2:853
Coreg. See Carvedilol
Corgard. See Nadolol
Cornea, 3:1152, 1273
Corneal edema, 2:851, 856
Corneal implants, 2:847
Corneal injuries, 2:846, 852
Corneal mapping, 2:842, 844, 3:1158
Corneal rings, 1:345, 2:847
Corneal stromal dystrophy, 1:344
Corneal swelling
  from cataract surgery, 1:514
  from congenital glaucoma, 2:608
  tarsorrhaphy for, 3:1397
Corneal transplantation, **1:342–346,**
  343, 2:847, 848
Corneal ulcers, 3:1397
Corns, 2:618
Coronal/glandular hypospadias,
  2:701–706
Coronal incision, 1:549
Coronary angiography, 1:69–70, 235,
  236, 348, 2:976
Coronary artery angioplasty, **1:72–75**
Coronary artery bypass graft surgery,
  1:346–353, *347*
  vs. enhanced external counterpulsa-
    tion, 1:473
  heart-lung machines for, 1:346,
    1:347, 1:348, 2:627
  minimally invasive, 2:974–978
  mortality and morbidity from,
    1:350–351, 403
  off-pump, 1:347, 2:975–978
  reoperation rates, 1:357, 3:1230
  robot-assisted, 3:1244
Coronary artery disease
  cardiac catheterization for,
    1:235–240
  coronary stenting for, 1:353–357

diagnosis of, 1:239–240, 348, 353, 435–437, 3:1375–1377
endovascular stent surgery for, 1:465–470
enhanced external counterpulsation for, 1:470–474
heart transplantation and, 2:643
lipid tests for, 2:875
Maze procedure for, 2:937
minimally invasive heart surgery for, **2:974–978**
MUGA scan for, 2:992
non-surgical treatment of, 1:349, 350, 352–353, 355, 356–357, 472
oophorectomy and, 2:1040
prevention of, 1:469–470, 471–473
reoperation for, 1:357, 3:1230
revascularization, 1:466
salpingo-oophorectomy and, 3:1258, 1259
stress test for, 3:1375–1377
ultrasound for, 1:239–240
See also Coronary artery bypass graft surgery
Coronary intensive care units (CCU), 2:759
Coronary stenting, **1:353–357**, *354*, 2:977–978
Corpus callosotomy, 1:77, **1:358–359**, 2:650, 3:1514
Corrective lenses
LASIK and, 2:841–842, 845, 846, 847
phacoemulsification and, 3:1143–1144
photorefractive keratectomy and, 3:1157, 1160
Cortical cataracts, 1:510, 512
Corticosteroids, **1:359–361**
for carpal tunnel syndrome, 1:260
for corneal transplantation, 1:344
for ganglion cyst removal, 2:562
immunosuppression and, 2:733, 736
incision care and, 2:745
for laser iridotomy, 2:852
lipid tests and, 2:876
for low back pain, 2:824
for nausea and vomiting, 1:92, 3:1287
pregnancy and, 1:360, 2:734
for scar revision, 3:1266
for scleral buckling, 3:1270
for ulcerative colitis, 2:580, 726
Corticotropins, **1:359–361**
Cortisol replacement, 2:700
Cortisone
for arthritis, 2:671, 3:1311
fracture repair and, 1:555
for osteoarthritis, 3:1314
replacement therapy, 1:359–360
for rotator cuff syndrome, 3:1250
Corzide, 1:90*t*
Cosmetic surgery, **3:1171–1175**
costs of, 1:550

demographics of, 1:521
ear, nose and throat, 1:433
elective, 1:437–439
Cosmetics, 3:1267, 1284
Costello, R.T., 2:697
Costs
of health care, 3:1204
of health insurance, 3:1204
of hospital services, 2:689
managed care plans and, 2:932
of Medicaid, 2:953–954
of nursing homes, 2:1030, 1032
of sclerotherapy, 3:1280
of second opinions, 3:1290
See also specific diseases and procedures
Cotrel-Dubousset instrumentation, 3:1356
Cotrim. *See* Trimethoprim/sulfamethoxazole
Couching, 1:510
Cough, 1:489
Cough assist devices, 2:946
Coumadin. *See* Warfarin
Counseling
postoperative, 3:1173, 1220
for smoking cessation, 3:1340
Counterpulsation, enhanced external, **1:470–474**
Cox, James L., 2:937
COX-2 inhibitors, 1:50, 2:1028, 3:1186
Cox-Maze procedure, **2:936–942**
Cozaar. *See* Losartan
CPAP (Continuous positive airway pressure), 2:945, 3:1347
CPR. *See* Cardiopulmonary resuscitation
CQI (Continuous quality improvement model), 2:961
Craniocaudal position, 2:929, 930
Craniofacial reconstruction, **1:361–369**, *362, 364*
incision care for, 2:745
mentoplasty and, 2:967
robot-assisted, 3:1244
Craniofacial surgeons, 1:184
Craniopharyngioma, 2:697–701
Craniotomy, **1:369–372**, *370*
brain tumors, 2:1025–1026
cerebral aneurysm repair, *1:272,* 1:273–274
hypophysectomy, 2:697
subarachnoid hemorrhage, 2:1025
temporal lobectomy, 1:76
Crash carts, 2:760, 1046
Creatine kinase, 1:240–241, 242
Creatinine clearance test, 2:784, 785, 786
Creatinine test, 2:784–785, 786
Cremasteric reflex, 2:1060
Creutzfeldt-Jakob disease, 1:180, 344
Cricothyroid membrane, 1:374
Cricothyroidotomy, **1:372–377**, *373,* 3:1434

Critical care, 1:67
Critical care nurses, 2:762
Critical care units. *See* Intensive care units
CRNA (Certified nurse anesthetists), *1:60,* 3:1387, 1388
Crohn's disease
in children, 3:1118
colonoscopy for, 1:313, 315
colorectal surgery for, 1:317–321, 2:579
complications from, 2:581
demographics of, 2:723, 3:1225, 1335
essential surgery for, 1:501–502
intestinal obstruction repair for, 2:763
rectal resection for, 3:1225–1228
reoperation for, 3:1230
sigmoidoscopy for, 3:1315, 1317
small bowel resection for, 3:1333
Cross-allergenicity, 1:81, 82
Cross infections. *See* Hospital-acquired infections
Crossmatching, 2:692, 3:1482–1483
Crouzon syndrome, 1:362–363
Crowns (Dental), 1:413, 415, 3:1245, 1246
Crutches. *See* Assistive devices
Cryoablation. *See* Cryotherapy
Cryoanesthesia, 1:417
Cryocautery. *See* Cryotherapy
Cryogens, 1:377, 378, 380
Cryopexy. *See* Cryotherapy
Cryoprecipitated antihemophilic factor plasma, 1:173, 174
Cryoprobes, 1:515
Cryosurgery. *See* Cryotherapy
Cryotherapy, **1:377–379**
for basal cell carcinoma, 1:377, 378, 2:992
for cataracts, 1:377, **1:379–381**
cervical, **1:281–283,** 1:329, 341, 378, 2:1034
for ciliary body removal, 1:387–391
vs. curettage and electrosurgery, 1:385, 386
for Maze procedure, 2:937
retinal, 3:1156, **3:1231–1234,** 3:1269
for skin cancer, 1:387
See also Cyclocryotherapy
Cryptococcus infections, 2:727
Cryptorchidism
demographics of, 2:1058–1059, 3:1119
diagnosis of, 2:1060–1061
hypospadias and, 2:704
non-surgical treatment of, 2:1063
orchiopexy for, 2:1058–1063, *2:1059*
testicular cancer and, 2:1053
Crystalline lens, 1:510
CSF. *See* Cerebrospinal fluid

CSF analysis. *See* Cerebrospinal fluid (CSF) analysis
CT scans, **1:381–385**, *382*
  for adrenalectomy, 1:30–31
  for chest tube insertion, 1:289
  for cholelithiasis, 1:297
  cochlear implants and, 1:310
  for craniotomy, 1:369
  for dental implants, 1:415
  for endoscopic sinus surgery, 1:461
  for gastroenterologic surgery, 2:581
  for head injuries, 2:1025
  helical, 1:383, 384, 2:918, 3:1130, 1135
  for hip replacement, 2:668
  for hip revision surgery, 2:676
  for intestinal obstruction repair, 2:764
  for intussusception reduction, 2:769
  for knee replacement, 2:804
  for leg lengthening and shortening, 2:869
  for liver biopsy, 2:886
  for lung biopsy, 2:914
  for lung cancer, 2:918, 3:1176
  for lung transplantation, 2:920
  vs. mediastinoscopy, 2:951
  myelography and, 2:996
  for peripheral artery disease, 3:1130
  for peripheral vascular disease, 3:1135
  vs. positron emission tomography, 3:1182
  for retinal cryopexy, 3:1232
  robot-assisted surgery and, 3:1243
  for rotator cuff repair, 3:1249
  for septoplasty, 3:1303
  for shoulder joint replacement, 3:1310
  spiral, 1:383, 384
  for stomach cancer, 2:577
  for stroke, 1:255
  for subarachnoid hemorrhage, 1:272–273, 2:1025
  for throat cancer, 3:1146
  for thyroid disorders, 3:1421
  for ureteral obstruction, 3:1491
  virtual colonoscopy and, 1:316–317
CTA (Computerized tomographic angiography), 1:70, 71
Culpocentesis, 3:1096
Culture (Social), 1:404–405, 2:683, 3:1082
Cultured skin substitutes, 3:1327
Cultures
  bacterial, **1:47–50**
  wound, **3:1570–1572**
Cumulative trauma disorders, 1:259
Cupid's bow, 1:303
Curettage, **1:385–387**, 2:598
  See also Dilation and curettage
Curing *vs.* caring, 2:682
Cushingoid syndrome, 1:360

Cushing's disease, 1:447, 448, 2:697–701
Custodial care, 2:908
Custom LASIK, 2:844
Cutaneous pain, 3:1083
CVS (Chorionic villus sampling), 1:42, 43, 532, 3:1120
Cyanoacrylates, 1:537, 2:744
Cyclobenzaprine, 1:55, 2:824, 994
Cyclocryotherapy, **1:387–391**, *388*, 2:610
Cyclodestruction, 3:1465
Cyclophosphamide, 2:736
Cyclophotocoagulation, 1:388, 390, 2:610
Cycloplegic refraction, 2:844, 855–856
Cyclosporine, 2:789, 898, 899, 900
Cyclosporins
  diuretics and, 1:429–430
  for immunosuppression, 2:733
  interactions with, 2:736
  for ulcerative colitis, 2:726
Cyclotrons, 3:1182
Cystectomy, **1:391–395**, *393*
  ileal conduit surgery and, 2:714, 715
  ovarian, 2:1034
  partial, 1:391, 392, 394
  radical, 1:391, 392, 394, 2:713
Cystic fibrosis
  electrolyte balance and, 1:447
  lung transplantation for, 2:918
  meconium ileus and, 3:1116
Cystine calculi, 2:1016
Cystitis, interstitial, 1:391, 400, 3:1253
Cystocele
  colporrhaphy for, 1:325, 327
  needle bladder neck suspension and, 2:1011
  non-surgical treatment of, 1:398
  recurrence of, 1:397
Cystocele repair, **1:395–398**, *396*
Cystoid macular edema (CME), 1:514
Cystometrogram (CMG), 1:167–168
Cystometry, subtracted, 3:1331
Cystoplasty, augmentation. *See* Bladder augmentation
Cystoprostatectomy, 1:504
Cystoscopy, **1:398–402**, *400*, 3:1387
  artificial sphincter insertion evaluation, 1:126
  bladder cancers, 3:1450–1451
  bladder/urethra disorders, 3:1507
  needle bladder neck suspension, 2:1011
  open prostatectomy, 2:1042
  sling procedure, 3:1331
  ureteral obstruction, 3:1491
  urinary incontinence, 3:1254
Cystostomy, 3:1497
Cystotomy, 2:1044
Cystourethroscopy. *See* Cystoscopy
Cysts
  abdominal ultrasound for, 1:1

ganglion, 2:560–563, *2:561*, 2:619
  ovarian, 2:1034, 1038
  pelvic, 1:331
Cytokines, 1:337
Cytomegalovirus, 2:633, 732, 893, 899
Cytoreduction, 3:1288
Cytotec. *See* Misoprostol
Cytoxan. *See* Cyclophosphamide

D

D & C. *See* Dilatation and curettage
D & E (Dilatation and evacuation), 1:16
Daclizumab, 2:733, 789
Dacron grafts, 1:102, 2:637, 998
Damus-Kaye-Stancel procedure, 2:636–637
Dandelion leaf, 3:1380
Danthron, 2:866
Dantrolene, 2:995
Darvocet N. *See* Propoxyphene-acetaminophen
Darvon. *See* Propoxyphene
Databases, medical error, 2:961
Daviel, Jacques, 1:510
Day care
  adult, **1:35–37**, 2:908
  child, 2:1006
Day-surgery centers. *See* Ambulatory surgery centers
Daypro. *See* Oxaprozin
DCCT (Diabetes Control and Complications Trail), 2:603
DCIS (Ductal carcinoma in situ), 2:987–988
Deadly nightshade, 3:1286
Deafness, 1:308, 310
  See also Hearing loss
Death and dying, **1:403–406**
  brain, 1:442
  culture and, 2:683
  with dignity, 2:682
  maternal, 1:16–17, 3:1262
  See also specific conditions and procedures
Debridement, **1:406–409**
  for bedsores, 1:158
  dental, 2:598
  for finger reattachment, 1:542
  knee arthroscopic surgery and, 2:794, 796, 798
  for laceration repair, 2:818
  for osteoarthritis, 2:807
  for skin grafting, 3:1325
  of wounds, 3:1567
Debulking surgery, 3:1288
Decadron. *See* Dexamethasone
Decision making
  health care proxy for, 2:622–623
  living will and, 2:901
  in nursing homes, 2:1030

power of attorney and, 3:1190
second opinions and, 3:1290
Declomycin. *See* Demeclocycline
Decompression, intestinal, 2:764, 765, 769
Decongestants, 2:1004
Decubitus ulcers. *See* Bedsores
Deep brain stimulation, **1:409–411,** 3:1089
Deep breathing techniques, 3:1185
Deep hypothermic circulatory arrest (DHCA), 2:636
Deep vein thrombosis (DVT)
from cesarean section, 1:287
compression stockings for, 2:669, 670, 805
defined, 3:1538
from knee replacement, 2:805, 806
from knee revision surgery, 2:812
from laminectomy, 2:823
phlebography for, **3:1149–1150**
from sclerotherapy, 3:1283, 1284
stockings, 2:669, 805
Defibrillation, **1:411–413**, *412*
for atrial fibrillation, 2:982, 986
for heart transplantation, 2:641
See also Implantable cardioverter-defibrillator
Defibrillators, automated external, 1:412
Degenerative brain disorders, 1:442
Dehiscence, 2:704, 745, 3:1548, 1549, 1570
Dehydration
cataracts and, 1:512
elderly and, 2:1029
electrolyte balance and, 1:447
hematocrit and, 2:647
hemoglobin test for, 2:650, 651
intravenous rehydration for, 2:766–767
kidney stones and, 2:1016
red blood cell count and, 1:335
Delayed gastric emptying, 2:583, 3:1093, 1211
Delivery. *See* Cesarean section; Childbirth; Labor
Delorme procedure, 3:1223, 1224
Delta waves, 1:444, 445
Demagraft, 3:1568
Demeclocycline, 1:81, 83, 3:1405
Demerol. *See* Meperidine
Demineralized bone matrix, 1:187
Dental anesthetics, 1:64, 65
Dental care, 1:61, 2:598, 668, 805, 968
Dental debridement, 2:598
Dental implants, **1:413–416**, *414*
Dental surgery, 3:1405, 1429
Dentures, 3:1246
Denver shunts, 3:1138
Deoxyhemoglobin, 3:1208
Depakene. *See* Valproic acid
Depakote. *See* Divalproex
Department of Defense, 1:181

Department of Health and Human Services
on blood availability, 1:181
on hospital-acquired infections, 2:685
Ombudsmen Program, 2:908–909
Department of Labor, 1:35
Dependence. *See* Drug dependence
Depression, pain and, 3:1082
See also specific conditions and procedures
Depth perception, 1:518
Dermabrasion, **1:416–419**, *417*
for actinic keratoses, 1:387
demographics of, 1:416, 3:1263
vs. laser skin resurfacing, 2:859
for scar revision, 3:1265
Dermagraft, 3:1327
Dermal regeneration templates, 3:1264–1265, 1266, 1326–1327
Dermatologists, 1:437
Dermis, 3:1323, 1326
Derotation arthroplasty, 2:617
Descending colon, 1:204
Desflurane, 1:60
Desmethyldiazepam, 1:79
Destination therapy, 2:843
Desyrel. *See* Trazodone
Detorsion, manual, 2:1063
Detrol, 3:1456
Developmental disorders, tenotomy for, 3:1404
Deviated nasal septum
septoplasty for, 1:434, 435, **3:1302–1305**, *1303*
snoring surgery for, 3:1342, 1345
Dexamethasone, 1:92, 360
Dextrose, 2:766
DHCA (Deep hypothermic circulatory arrest), 2:636
Diabetes
amputation for, 1:45, 46
body weight and, 1:506
cardiac catheterization and, 1:237
cardiovascular disease and, 1:442
carpal tunnel release and, 1:257
cataracts and, 1:512
causes of, 2:604
cephalosporins and, 1:269
cleft lip and, 1:301
congenital heart defects and, 2:634
cryotherapy and, 1:378
cyclocryotherapy and, 1:390
debridement and, 1:408
electrolyte balance and, 1:447
end-stage renal disease and, 2:786
fainting and, 1:246, 247
gallstones and, 2:557
gestational, 2:603, 604, 605, 606
glaucoma, 3:1431
glucose tests for, 2:602–606
heart-lung transplantation and, 2:633
homocysteine and, 1:240

incisional hernia repair and, 2:750
kidney failure and, 2:783
laparoscopy and, 2:829
obesity and, 1:507
periodontitis and, 2:599
peripheral artery disease and, 3:1131
retinopathy from, 2:855
scleral buckling and, 3:1271
sclerotherapy and, 3:1282
type 1, 2:604, 776–778, 3:1089–1091
type 2, 1:507, 2:604, 3:1545
urinary incontinence from, 3:1330
Diabetes & Digestive & Kidney Diseases (NIDDK), 3:1507
Diabetes Control and Complications Trail (DCCT), 2:603
Diabetes insipidus, 2:699
Diabetes medications
myelography and, 2:996
nephrostomy and, 2:1022
ophthalmologic surgery and, 2:1050
sulfonamides and, 3:1380
Diabetic retinopathy, 2:855, 3:1153
Diagnosis, nursing, 2:957–958
See also specific diseases and disorders
Diagnosis-related groups (DRG), 2:679
Diagnostic and Statistical Manual of Mental Disorders, 2:1054
Diagnostic equipment, 2:760–761, 1046
Diagnostic errors, 2:960
Diagnostic tests, preoperative, 3:1192, **3:1200–1203**
Dialysate, 2:779, 780, 781
Dialysis. *See* Kidney dialysis
Dialyzers, hollow fiber, 2:780
Diamond fraises, 1:416–417
Diamox. *See* Acetazolamide
Diaphragm (Contraceptive), 3:1462
Diarrhea
from antrectomy, 1:97, 98
cataracts and, 1:512
costs of, 2:580
electrolyte balance and, 1:447, 448
from erythromycins, 1:483
hematocrit and, 2:647
laxatives and, 2:865
mortality and morbidity from, 2:767
Diastolic pressure, 1:176, 177, 3:1350, 1351
Diathermy, 1:329, 411
Diazepam, 1:78–79, 79*t*, 2:994, 995
epidural anesthesia and, 1:478
for low back pain, 2:824
for Ménière's disease, 1:455
prochlorperazine and, 1:93
Diazoxide, 1:90
DIC (Disseminated intravascular coagulation), 1:337, 2:649–650
Diclofenac, 2:1028
Dicoumarol, 1:88

Dicumarol, 1:133
Didanosine, 1:547
Diet
  abdominoplasty and, 1:7
  anticoagulants and, 1:88–89
  antrectomy and, 1:97
  for arrhythmia, 2:939
  for atherosclerosis prevention,
    1:469–470
  cataracts and, 1:514
  for cholelithiasis, 1:297
  for colostomy, 1:324
  for coronary artery disease, 1:349,
    355, 471
  esophageal cancer and, 1:494
  for fecal incontinence, 1:127
  fracture repair and, 1:555
  gastric bypass and, 2:573
  for hemorrhoids, 2:656
  high-fiber, 2:750, 949
  ileoanal anastomosis and, 2:719
  for incisional hernias, 2:750
  for interstitial cystitis, 3:1255
  for kidney stones, 2:1016, 1020,
    1021
  kidney transplantation and,
    2:789–790
  liquid, 1:208
  low-fiber, 1:494
  low-salt, 1:455, 2:750
  for Ménière's disease, 1:455
  pharyngectomy and, 3:1146–1147
  preadmission instructions for,
    3:1168
  preoperative, 3:1197
  for rectal prolapse, 3:1224
  triglycerides and, 2:875
  for urinary incontinence, 1:127
  vegetarian, 1:470, 2:1021
  vertical banded gastroplasty and,
    3:1548
  for weight loss, 2:574
Diethylstilbestrol (DES), 1:279, 329,
  2:703, 1053
Differential stethoscope, 3:1371
Diffuse esophageal spasm, 1:490
Diffusion (Dialysis), 2:780
Digestive disease demographics,
  2:579–580
Digestive enzyme replacement, 3:1093
Digestive system surgery, 2:690,
  3:1386
Digestive tract cancer, 1:95
Digital angiography, 1:236
Digital mammography, 2:929
Digital rectal examination, 2:1044
Digital subtraction angiography, 1:69,
  255, 2:980
Digital thermometers. See Electronic
  thermometers
Digital x ray imaging, 1:203
Digitalis
  for cardioversion, 1:249
  diuretics and, 1:430

electrolyte balance and, 1:447
  for Maze procedure, 2:939
  NSAIDs and, 2:1028
  overdoses of, 2:652
Digoxin, 1:80, 430
Dihydrotestosterone, 2:1041
1,25-Dihydroxycholecalciferol,
  3:1146–1147
Dilantin. See Phenytoin
Dilatation and curettage (D & C), 1:14,
  1:16, 1:419–422, 420, 2:711, 1034
Dilatation and evacuation (D & E),
  1:16
Dilating eye drops, 2:1050, 3:1143
Dilating instruments, 3:1381
Dilaudid. See Hydromorphone
Diltiazem, 1:89, 90t
Dimenhydrinate, 1:92, 455
Diovan. See Valsartan
Diphenhydramine, 3:1287
Diphenoxylate-atropine, 1:270
Diplopia, 1:516, 518, 2:846, 1050,
  3:1144
Diprivan. See Propofol
Direct bilirubin test, 2:891, 892
Direct commissurotomy, 1:107
Directed blood donors, 3:1441
Disabled persons, 2:682, 953, 963
Discharge from the hospital,
  1:422–424, 3:1188, 1220
Discharge planning, 1:423, 2:956
Disciplinary history, physicians, 1:540
Disease-modifying antirheumatic drugs
  (DMARDS), 2:807
Disinfection. See Aseptic technique;
  Sterilization
Disk removal (Diskectomy),
  1:424–427, 425
Disks, spinal. See Intervertebral disk
Dislocations
  arthroscopic surgery for, 1:121
  Bankart procedure for, 1:147–150
  intraocular lens, 3:1144
  knee, 2:792–793, 795
  kneecap, 2:814, 815
  prosthesis, 2:670, 676
  shoulder, 1:147–150, 1:148
Disposable medical equipment, 2:761
Disposable thermometers, 3:1409
Dissecting instruments, 3:1381
Disseminated intravascular coagulation
  (DIC), 1:337, 2:649–650
Dissolution therapy, 2:558, 559
Distal pancreatectomy, 3:1092, 1093
Disulfiram
  alprazolam and, 1:80
  diazepam and, 2:995
  erythromycins and, 1:485
  sulfonamides and, 3:1380
Diucardin. See Hydroflumethiazide
Diuretics, 1:427–430
  for aortic stenosis, 1:107
  for ascites, 3:1139
  aspirin and, 1:133

for kidney stones, 2:1020
  lipid tests and, 2:876
  loop, 1:428
  for Maze procedure, 2:939, 940
  for for Ménière's disease, 1:455
  ophthalmologic surgery and, 2:1050
  osmotic, 1:428
  overuse of, 1:447, 448
  potassium-sparing, 1:428, 429, 430
  sulfonamides and, 3:1378, 1380
  thiazide, 1:89–90, 91, 428, 429,
    2:1020
Diuril. See Chlorothiazide
Divalproex, 1:270
Diverticulectomy, Meckel's,
  2:946–949, 947
Diverticulitis
  antibiotics for, 1:208, 2:946, 949
  barium enema for, 1:154–155
  bowel resection for, 1:205
  colonoscopy for, 1:315
  colorectal surgery for, 1:317–321
  intestinal obstruction repair for,
    2:763
  Meckel's diverticulectomy for,
    2:946, 948
  non-surgical treatment of, 1:208,
    2:949
  peritoneal dialysis and, 2:781
Diverticulosis, 1:318
DMARDS (Disease-modifying an-
  tirheumatic drugs), 2:807
DNA analysis, 1:368, 2:890
Do-not-resuscitate (DNR) orders,
  1:404, 1:430–432, 3:1171, 1198,
  1201
Dobutamine, 1:33
Dobutrex. See Dobutamine
DocInfo, 1:540
Doctors. See Physicians
Docusate, 2:865, 866
Dofetilide, 2:569
Dog bites. See Bite injuries
Dolasetron, 3:1287
Dolene. See Propoxyphene
Dolophine. See Methadone
Domestic violence, 1:363, 3:1429
Dong quai. See Angelica
Donor Deferral Register, 1:172, 174,
  175, 181
Donors. See Blood donation; Organ
  donors
Dopamine, 1:33, 409, 3:1087–1088
Dopaminergic, 3:1287
Doppler flowmeter examination, 2:621
Doppler ultrasound
  abdominal, 1:3
  echocardiography, 1:436
  for fetal monitoring, 1:534, 535–536
  for microsurgery, 2:974
  for mitral valve disorders, 2:980,
    984
  pelvic, 3:1120
  for peripheral artery disease, 3:1130

for peripheral vascular disease, 3:1135
for stroke, 1:255
for sympathectomy, 3:1390
for valvular disease, 1:240
Dornier MedTech Urowave, 3:1458
Dorsal rhizotomy, 3:1241
Doryx. *See* Doxycycline
Dot-matrix thermometers. *See* Disposable thermometers
Double-barrel colostomy, 1:323
Double-contrast barium enema, 1:97, 154–155
Double vision, 1:516, 518, 2:846, 1050, 3:1144
Down syndrome
achalasia and, 1:492
amniocentesis for, 1:41, 43
congenital heart defects and, 2:634
craniofacial reconstruction for, 1:362, 366
Doxapram, 2:651
Doxazosin mesylate, 1:90*t*
Doxycycline, 1:83, 3:1405–1406
Drainage
abscess, 1:18–21
aseptic technique for, 1:130
for incision care, 2:744
for pharyngectomy, 3:1147
sinus, 1:459–463
tubes, *1:19,* 1:20, 130
for urinary catheterization, 1:263, 266
Drainage tubes, *1:19,* 1:20, 130
Dramamine. *See* Dimenhydrinate
Drapes, sterile, 1:129
Drawing blood. *See* Phlebotomy
Dressings, **1:143–147,** *145,* 3:1567–1568
alginate, 1:144, 145
for bedsores, 1:157
biosynthetic, 1:144, 145
for burns, 2:744
change of, 1:130
collagen, 1:144, 145
composite, 1:144, 145
compression, 1:543
for debridement, 1:407
for dermabrasion, 1:418
Glassock, 1:454
hydrocolloid, 1:144, 145
hydrogel, 1:144, 145, 2:859
for incision care, 2:744
for laser skin resurfacing, 2:858–859
moist, 1:407
OpSite, 2:744
polyurethane, 1:144, 145, 2:744
saline-moistened, 1:407
superabsorbent, 1:144, 145
DRG (Diagnosis-related groups), 2:679
Drop attacks, 1:358, 359
Droperidol, 3:1287
Drops, eye. *See* Eye drops

Drug dependence
barbiturates and, 1:152
opioid analgesics and, 1:52, 53, 3:1087
See also Addiction
Drug-eluting stents, 1:467
Drug errors, 2:960, 961
Drugs
for abortions, 1:13, 15
computerized order systems for, 2:690
incision care and, 2:745
Medicare and, 2:963
preadmission instructions for, 3:1168
preoperative period, 3:1197, 1202
weight gain from, 3:1561
See also specific drugs and classes of drugs
Dry eye syndrome, 1:171, 2:1050
Dual-chamber pacemakers, 3:1081
Duane syndrome, 1:517
Duchenne muscular dystrophy, 3:1352, 1353
Ductal carcinoma in situ (DCIS), 2:987–988
Ductus arteriosis, 2:1075
Dulcolax. *See* Bisacodyl
Dumping syndrome
antrectomy, 1:97, 98
gastrectomy, 1:97, 98, 2:566
gastric bypass, 2:573
gastroduodenostomy, 2:577
Dunlop's traction, 3:1437
Duodenal ulcers, 3:1517
causes of, 2:579, 3:1209
demographics of, 1:96
gastrectomy for, 2:564
small bowel resection for, 3:1333
Duodenectomy, 3:1333–1337
Duodenogastric reflux, 2:577
Duodenum
esophagogastroduodenoscopy of, 1:499–501
gastroduodenostomy and, 2:575–579
small bowel resection of, 3:1333–1337
Duphalac. *See* Lactulose
Durable power of attorney. *See* Power of attorney
Duragesic. *See* Fentanyl
Duramorph. *See* Morphine
Duricef. *See* Cefadroxil
DVT. *See* Deep vein thrombosis
Dyazide. *See* Hydrochlorothiazide-triamterene
Dying. *See* Death and dying
DynaCirc. *See* Isradipine
Dyrenium. *See* Triamterene
Dyskinesias
deep brain stimulation and, 1:410, 411
pallidotomy and, 3:1087, 1088, 1089

Dysmenorrhea, 1:331
Dysphagia
from antrectomy, 1:98
esophageal atresia/tracheoesophageal fistula and, 1:489
esophageal function tests for, 1:490–493
esophageal resection for, 1:493
from fundoplication, 2:590
mechanical ventilation and, 2:945
from pharyngectomy, 3:1147
from snoring surgery, 3:1347
Dysplasia
acetabular, 2:661, 662
cervical, 1:281–283, 329–331
esophageal, 1:493, 494, 498
hip, 2:661, 662
squamous, 1:282
Dyspnea, 3:1358
Dysrhythmia. *See* Arrhythmia
Dystocia, 1:283
Dystonia, 1:409–411

E

E-Mycin, 1:483
Ear, nose and throat surgeons, 1:25
Ear, nose and throat surgery, **1:433–435**
Ear deformity otoplasty, 1:434, **2:1066–1071,** *1067*
Ear infections, 2:934–936, 3:1409
Ear injuries, 2:1067, 1069
Ear molding, 2:1068, 1070
Ear tubes, **2:1002–1007,** *1003*
Earache, pressure-related, 2:1004
Eardrums, tympanoplasty, 3:1475–1479, *1477*
Ears, protruding, 2:1066–1067, 1068, 1069, 1070
ECC (Extracorporeal circuit), 2:780
Eccentric nozzles, 3:1392
ECG. *See* Electrocardiography
Echocardiography, **1:435–437**
Doppler, 1:436
electrocardiography and, 1:442
exercise, 1:436–437
for lung transplantation, 2:920
for pectus excavatum repair, 3:1111
for pericardiocentesis, 3:1126
stress test and, 3:1375
transesophageal, 1:102, 248, 2:979, 983
ECMO (Extracorporeal membrane oxygenation), 2:628, 942–943
ECST study, 1:256
Ectopic beats, 1:441
Ectopic parathyroid, 3:1098
Ectopic pregnancy
demographics of, 3:1260
diagnosis of, 3:1261
in vitro fertilization and, 2:741, 742

mortality and morbidity from, 3:1261

non-surgical treatment of, 3:1260, 1262

pelvic ultrasound for, 3:1120

salpingostomy for, 3:1260–1263, *3:1261*

Ectopic testicles, 2:1060

Edema
cerebral, 1:427, 428
corneal, 2:851, 856
cystoid macular, 1:514
electrolyte balance and, 1:447
foot/ankle, 3:1283
macular, 1:514, 2:852, 856
pulmonary, 1:291, 2:997, 3:1150–1151

Edmonton Protocol, 3:1091

EDTA, 1:334

Education
anesthesiologists, 1:66–67
for cardiopulmonary resuscitation, 1:246
for intensive care unit equipment, 2:762–763
for microsurgery, 2:972
See also Patient education

EECP (Enhanced external counterpulsation), 1:352, 357, **1:470–474**

EEG. *See* Electroencephalography

Ehlers-Danlos syndrome, 1:100, 271

Ehrlich's diazo reagent, 2:891

Ejaculation, 2:1044, 3:1122

Ejection fraction
cardiac catheterization for, 1:238, 239
mitral valve replacement and, 2:984
MUGA scan for, 2:992–994

EKG. *See* Electrocardiography

Elastic bandages, 1:143, 2:879

Elavil. *See* Amitriptyline

Elbow
arthroplasty, 1:116–120
arthroscopic surgery, 1:120–123
tendon repair, 3:1399–1400

Elbow fractures, *1:554*

Elbow immobilizers, 1:304

Elderly
abuse of, 2:1031–1032
adult day care for, 1:35–37
anesthesia and, 1:162
barbiturates and, 1:152
dehydration in, 2:1029
demographics of, 2:906
frail, 1:35
hospital-acquired infections and, 2:685
intestinal obstruction in, 2:764
laparoscopy for, 2:829, 830
local anesthesia for, 1:63
malnutrition in, 2:1029
Medicaid for, 2:953
patient-controlled analgesia and, 3:1105

scopolamine patch for, 3:1286
sulfonamides for, 3:1378

Elective surgery, **1:437–439,** 1:538
vs. essential surgery, 1:501, 502
preparation for, 3:1194–1200
second opinions for, 3:1290, 1291

Electric fields, 2:928

Electrical stimulation
cochlear implants and, 1:308, 310
for debridement, 1:408
deep brain, **1:409–411,** 3:1089
for fracture repair, 1:553
for pain, 3:1085
pallidotomy for, 3:1088
sacral nerve, **3:1253–1256**
transcutaneous, 2:825, 3:1085
for urinary incontinence, 3:1237

Electrocardiography, **1:439–442**, *440*
for anesthesia evaluation, 1:57
cardiac monitor for, 1:242–244
electrophysiology study and, 1:449–452
for endovascular stent surgery, 1:467–468
intensive care unit equipment for, 2:760
for lung transplantation, 2:920
for mitral valve disorders, 2:980
MUGA scan and, 2:993
for pectus excavatum repair, 3:1111
stress test and, 3:1375–1377

Electrocautery
for adenoidectomy, 1:24
burns from, 1:404
for endometriosis, 2:834
in exploratory laparotomy, 2:836–837
for hemangiomas, 2:646
open prostatectomy and, 2:1044
for reducing blood loss, 1:182

Electrocoagulation, 1:386, 3:1461

Electrodes, implanted, 1:411, 443

Electrodesiccation
for skin cancer, 1:386, 2:992
for spider nevi, 3:1282
for spider veins, 3:1284

Electroencephalography (EEG), **1:442–446**, *443*
for anesthesia measurement, 1:163–164
anterior temporal lobectomy and, 1:76
for corpus callosomy, 1:358
for hemispherectomy, 2:649

Electrolyte tests, **1:446–449**

Electrolytes, 1:446–449
gastrostomy and, 2:593
for intravenous rehydration, 2:766
for kidney function, 1:113
laxatives and, 2:865

Electromagnetic fields
for leg lengthening, 2:870
pacemakers and, 3:1081

Electromagnetic pumps, 2:942

Electromyography, anal, 1:126

Electronic cell counters, 1:335, 2:648, 3:1229

Electronic thermometers, 3:1408–1409

Electrophoresis, 1:241, 276, 2:891, 893

Electrophysiologists, 2:738

Electrophysiology study of the heart, **1:449–452**

Electrosection, 1:386

Electrosurgery, **1:385–387**

Electrosurgical wire loop, 2:710

Electrotherapy. *See* Electrical stimulation

Elevating the legs, vein surgery, 3:1536

Elliptocytosis, hereditary, 3:1362

Elmiron. *See* Pentosan polysulfate sodium

Elschnig's pearls, 2:854, 856

Embolism, pulmonary, 1:384, 2:660, 894, 3:1149
See also Thrombosis

Embolization
spleen, 3:1365
uterine artery, 2:710
for uterine fibroids, 2:1002

Emergency airway puncture, **1:372–377**, *373*

Emergency surgery, 1:438, **1:452–453,** 2:973

Emergency thoracotomy, 3:1414

Emergent cerclages, 1:279

Eminase. *See* Anistreplase

EMLA cream, 1:299

Emollient laxatives, 2:865

Emphysema, 3:1412
chest x ray for, 1:291, 292
demographics of, 3:1175
lung biopsy and, 2:916
lung transplantation for, 2:918, 919
pulmonary lobectomy for, 2:903, 904
spirometry tests for, 3:1358

Employer-based health insurance, 3:1203, 1204, 1205

Empyema, 1:288, 289

Enalapril, 1:89, 90*t*, 429

Encephalopathy
bovine spongiform, 1:311
electroencephalography and, 1:445
liver, 2:892, 895

End colostomy, 1:323

End-of-life decision making, 2:622–623, 901

End-of-life hospice care, 2:682–685

End-stage glaucoma, 1:388

End-stage heart failure, 2:639, 643–644

End-stage renal disease (ESRD)
dialysis for, 1:111, 2:779–783
kidney transplantation for, 2:786–791, 3:1091

End-to-end anastomosis, 2:764, 769, 972

End-to-side anastomosis, 2:972

Endarterectomy
carotid, **1:252–257,** *253,* 1:466

peripheral, **3:1128–1132**
Endocardial resection, 2:643,
  2:997–999
Endocrine disrupters, 2:703
Endocrinologists, 1:30, 2:699
Endocrinology, reproductive, 2:1033
Endodontic treatment, **3:1244–1247**
Endodontists, 3:1429
Endolymphatic hydrops, 1:453–456
Endolymphatic sack, 1:454
Endolymphatic shunt, **1:453–456**
Endometrial ablation, 2:710
Endometrial biopsy, 1:421–422
Endometrial cancer
  D & C for, 1:419
  hysterectomy for, 2:708
  pelvic exenteration for, 1:503
Endometrial hyperplasia, 1:419
Endometrial polyps, 1:419
Endometrial resection, 2:710
Endometriosis
  causes of, 2:833
  cystectomy for, 1:391
  demographics of, 2:833, 3:1256
  diagnosis of, 2:834
  exploratory laparotomy for, 2:836
  hysterectomy for, 1:422, 2:706
  in vitro fertilization and, 2:740
  laparoscopy for, 2:831, 833–835,
    2:834
  non-surgical treatment of, 2:835,
    3:1259
  oophorectomy for, 2:835, 1038
  pregnancy and, 2:835
  salpingo-oophorectomy for, 3:1256
  second-look surgery for, 3:1288
Endomyocardial biopsy, 2:642
Endophthalmitis, 1:514, 3:1144, 1274
Endorectal pullthrough, 2:579,
  2:720–723
Endorphins, 3:1083, 1084, 1085, 1339
Endoscopic retrograde cholangiopancreatography (ERCP), 1:160,
  1:456–459, *457*, 2:558, 559
Endoscopic sinus surgery, 1:384,
  1:459–463, *460*
Endoscopy
  advances in, 2:581, 594–595
  AESOP, 3:1398
  benefits of, 2:595
  for carpal tunnel release, 1:260–262
  complications from, 1:404
  costs of, 1:39
  esophageal function tests and, 1:490
  fasciotomy, 1:525
  fetal surgery, 1:534
  fetoscopy, 1:533, 534
  forehead lift, 1:549, 550, 551
  for gastroesophageal reflux disease,
    2:589
  image-guided, 1:461
  infections from, 1:228
  miniaturized, 1:181–182
  nasal, 1:434

obstetrical, 1:535
  for peptic ulcers, 1:98
  robot-assisted, 3:1243
  for sclerotherapy, 3:1277
  second-look, 3:1288
  for shoulder resection arthroplasty,
    3:1313
  for stomach cancer, 2:577
  for stomach diseases, 1:97
  triple, 1:434
  upper esophagogastroduodenal,
    2:581
  upper gastrointestinal, 1:499–501,
    2:583, 584
  uses for, 3:1387
Endosteal implants, 1:415
Endotracheal intubation, **1:463–465**,
  464
    vs. cricothyroidotomy, 1:375
    hospital-acquired infections from,
      2:685, 687
Endovaginal scan, 3:1121
Endovascular grafts, 1:103, 466–467
Endovascular neuroradiology, 1:275
Endovascular stent surgery, **1:465–470**
Endovenous ablation, 3:1536
Endovenous laser treatment (EVLT),
  3:1536
Enema. *See* Barium enema; Cleansing
  enema
Enflurane, 1:60
Enhanced external counterpulsation
  (EECP), 1:352, 357, **1:470–474**
Enophthalmos, 3:1397
Enoxacin, 1:546
ENT surgeons, 1:25
ENT surgery, **1:433–435**
Enteral nutrition, 2:591–594, 3:1093,
  1466–1469
Enterocele, 1:327
Enterocolitis, necrotizing, 3:1116
Enterostomy, 2:769
Entrapment neuropathy, 1:260
Enucleation, eye, **1:474–477**, *475*
Environmental Protection Agency
  (EPA), 3:1410
Enzymatic sclerostomy, 3:1272–1273
Enzyme function tests, 2:891
Enzyme immunoassay, 2:727
Enzyme replacement therapy, 3:1093
Enzymes, tumor marker tests, **3:**1469
Eosinophils, 1:336, 337, 338
EPA. *See* Environmental Protection
  Agency
Ephedra, 1:34
Ephedrine, 1:460, 478
Epidermis, 3:1323, 1326
Epididymis, 2:693
Epididymitis, 2:695
Epidural therapy, 1:65, 66, **1:477–479**,
  478
  for cesarean section, 1:284, 286,
    477–479

for childbirth, 1:67, 477–479,
    2:1034
  cost of, 1:39
  for low back pain, 2:824
  for obstetric and gynecologic
    surgery, 2:1034
  preoperative, 3:1184
Epikeratophakia, 1:343
Epilepsy
  anterior temporal lobectomy for,
    1:75–78
  corpus callostomy for, 1:358–359
  demographics of, 2:649
  electroencephalography for,
    1:442–446
  focal, 1:359, 445
  hemispherectomy for, **2:648–650**
  neurosurgery for, 2:1026–1027
  temporal lobe, 1:75–78, 2:1026
  vagal nerve stimulation,
    3:1513–1515
Epinephrine
  anesthetics and, 1:65
  for laceration repair, 2:817
  for liposuction, 2:878
  for Mohs surgery, 2:990
  for skin grafting, 3:1325
  uses of, 1:33
Epineurium, 2:973
Epiphysiodesis, 2:866, 867–868, 869,
  870
Episiotomy, **1:479–483**, *481*, 2:1033
Epithelial ingrowth, 2:846
Epithelialization, 1:20
EPO. *See* Erythropoietin
Epoetin, 2:728, 729–730, 731, 782
Epogen. *See* Epoetin
Eprosartan, 1:89
Epsom salts. *See* Magnesium sulfate
Eptifibatide, 1:86
Epworth Sleepiness Scale (ESS),
  3:1345–1346
Equanil. *See* Meprobamate
Equilibrium, after tympanoplasty,
  3:1478
Equipment. *See* Medical equipment
ER. *See* Estrogen receptors
Erbium lasers, 1:418
ERCP (Endoscopic retrograde cholan-
  giopancreatography), 1:160,
  1:456–459, *457*, 2:558, 559
Erectile dysfunction
  non-surgical treatment of,
    3:1124–1125
  from open prostatectomy, 2:1044
  penile implants for, 3:1122–1125,
    3:1123
Ergonomics, 1:259
Ergot alkaloids, 3:1510, 1511
Errors. *See* Medical errors
Ery-C. *See* Erythromycins
Er:YAG lasers
  laser skin resurfacing, 2:858, 859,
    3:1265

sclerostomy, 3:1272
Erythrocin, 1:483
Erythrocytes. *See* Red blood cells
Erythromycins, 1:81, 83, **1:483–485**
  for bowel resection, 1:207
  buspirone and, 1:80
  for colorectal surgery, 1:319
  for colostomy, 1:323
  cyclosporins and, 2:736
  for hospital-acquired infections,
    2:687
  for rectal resection, 3:1227
  for small bowel resection, 3:1335
Erythropoietin, 1:183, 2:728
Eschar debridement, 1:406
Escherichia coli, 3:1569–1570
Esidrex. *See* Hydrochlorothiazide
Esomeprazole, 2:568
Esophageal atresia, 1:485–490, 3:1116
Esophageal atresia repair, **1:485–490,**
  486
Esophageal cancer
  adenocarcinoma, 1:493, 494, 2:580
  demographics of, 1:493–494, 2:580
  diagnosis of, 1:496, 2:589
  esophageal resection for, 1:493–499
  gastroesophageal reflux disease and,
    1:493–494
  metastatic, 1:496, 497
  squamous cell, 1:493, 494, 2:580
  thoracic surgery for, 3:1412
  throat cancer and, 3:1147
Esophageal clearance, 2:583
Esophageal diverticula, 1:500
Esophageal dysplasia, 1:493, 494, 498
Esophageal function tests, **1:490–493**
Esophageal injuries, medication-in-
  duced, 1:501
Esophageal manometry, 1:490–493,
  2:583–584
Esophageal perforation, 1:500
Esophageal pH monitoring, 1:490–493,
  2:583, 584, 589
Esophageal resection, **1:493–499**
Esophageal spasm, diffuse, 1:490
Esophageal speech, 2:840
Esophageal sphincters, 1:490–493,
  2:582, 586–590
Esophageal strictures, 2:582, 583
Esophageal tracheal combitube (ETC),
  1:463, 465
Esophageal varices, 3:1277–1279
Esophageal webs, 1:494
Esophagectomy, **1:493–499**
Esophagitis, 2:582, 589
Esophagogastrectomy, **1:493–499**
Esophagogastroduodenoscopy,
  1:499–501, 2:583, 584
Esophagography, barium, 2:583, 584
Esophagoscopy, 1:434, 496
ESRD (End-stage renal disease). *See*
  End-stage renal disease
ESS (Epworth Sleepiness Scale),
  3:1345–1346

Essential fatty acids, 1:256, 470,
  3:1132, 1136
Essential surgery, **1:501–502**
Essential tremor, 1:409–411
Estrogen receptors, **3:**1470, 1471
Estrogen therapy
  cyclosporins and, 2:736
  cystocele repair and, 1:397
  dantrolene and, 2:995
  erythromycins and, 1:485
  for gender reassignment, 3:1307
  hysterectomy and, 2:709
  lipid tests and, 2:876
  for oophorectomy, 2:1040
  oophorectomy and, 2:1038
  for salpingo-oophorectomy, 3:1258
  sulfonamides and, 3:1380
  for urinary incontinence, 3:1237
ESWL (Extracorporeal shock wave
  lithotripsy), **2:882–886,** *883,* 2:1019,
  1020, 1023
ETC (Esophageal tracheal combitube),
  1:463, 465
Ethanolamine, 3:1278
Ethchlorvynol overdose, 2:652
Ethics, 2:680, 3:1108
Ethics consulting, 3:1166
Ethmoid air cells, 1:460, 461
Ethmoidectomy, 3:1302, 1303
Ethnic groups and mourning, 1:405
Etodolac, 2:1028
Etomidate, 1:60–61
Eustachian tubes, 2:1004
Ewart's sign, 3:1127
Excessive sweating, 3:1389,
  1390–1391
Excimer lasers, 1:345, 2:1049, 3:1157
Excisional biopsy, 1:210–211, 3:1473
Exenteration, **1:502–506,** *503*
Exercise, **1:506–509,** *507*
  abdominoplasty and, 1:7
  aerobic, 1:508, 2:574
  for arrhythmia, 2:939
  for atherosclerosis prevention, 1:469
  breathing, 2:904, 3:1189
  for carpal tunnel syndrome, 1:262
  closed-angle glaucoma from, 2:772
  after coronary artery bypass graft
    surgery, 1:349
  for coronary artery disease, 1:349,
    355, 471
  eye, 1:518, 519
  for fecal incontinence, 1:127
  for hand surgery, 2:621
  high-impact, 3:1330
  high-intensity, 1:508
  for hip replacement, 2:669
  incision care and, 2:745
  for incisional hernias, 2:750
  isometric, 1:523
  for joint disorders, 1:119–120
  Kegel, 1:328, 398, 482, 3:1237
  for knee injuries, 2:796
  knee injuries from, 2:801–802, 812

for knee replacement, 2:804, 806
  for limb salvage, 2:873
  for low back pain, 2:825
  for Maze procedure, 2:939
  muscle-strengthening, 2:873
  for pain, 3:1084
  for pectus excavatum repair, 3:1112
  pelvic muscle, 1:127, 3:1255, 1332
  preoperation, 2:668
  after sclerotherapy, 3:1283
  for shoulder dislocations, 1:149, 150
  snoring and, 3:1343
  for spider veins, 3:1284
  for toe abnormalities, 2:617
  after vein ligation and stripping,
    3:1535–1536
  for venous thrombosis, 3:1539
  after ventricular assist device
    surgery, 3:1541
  for weight loss, 2:574
  weight management and,
    3:1561–1562
  See also Range of motion exercises
Exercise echocardiography, 1:436–437
Exercise test. *See* Stress test
Exophthalmos, 3:1397
Expanders, balloon-type, 3:1320–1321
Exploratory laparotomy, **2:836–839,**
  837
Exploratory surgery, 1:438
Extended simple mastectomy, 3:1318
External cephalic version, 1:287
External ear deformity otoplasty,
  2:1066–1071
External fetoscopy, 1:533, 534
External fixation. *See* Fixation devices
External hemorrhoids, 2:655
Extracapsular cataract extraction,
  1:381, **1:509–516,** 3:1140, 1144
Extracorporeal circuit (ECC), 2:780
Extracorporeal membrane oxygenation
  (ECMO), 2:628, 942–943
Extracorporeal shock wave lithotripsy
  (ESWL), **2:882–886,** *883*
  gallstones, 2:558, 559
  kidney stones, 2:1019, 1020
  ureteral stones, 2:1023
Extraocular muscles, 1:516–520
Exudative retinal detachment, 3:1153
Eye
  alignment, 1:516–520
  anatomy of, 3:1152
  appearance, 1:169–172
  plastic, 1:476, 504
Eye Bank Association of America,
  1:342, 344
Eye banks, 1:342
Eye cancer. *See* Eye tumors
Eye disease, 3:1397
  See also specific diseases
Eye drops
  anesthetic, 1:64, 65, 389, 2:1050,
    3:1158
  anti-inflammatory, 3:1143

for cataract cryotherapy, 1:380
for closed-angle glaucoma, 2:773
for cyclocryotherapy, 1:389
dilating, 2:1050, 3:1143
for extracapsular cataract extraction, 1:513
for eye muscle surgery, 1:518
for glaucoma, 1:388
for laser posterior capsulotomy, 2:855
for LASIK, 2:842, 844
for orbital exenteration, 1:505
for tarsorrhaphy, 3:1397
for trabeculectomy, 3:1433
See also Antibiotic eye drops
Eye enucleation, **1:474–477**, *475*
Eye examination, 3:1154–1155, 1159
Eye exercises, 1:518, 519
Eye infections
from cataract surgery, 1:514
from sclerostomy, 3:1274
topical antibiotics for, 1:85
Eye injuries
closed-angle glaucoma from, 2:772
eye enucleation for, 1:474, 475
from laser surgery, 2:864
photocoagulation therapy for, 3:1155
Eye movements, 1:516–520
Eye muscle surgery, **1:516–520**, *517*
Eye muscle training, 1:519
Eye patch, 1:344, 518
Eye shields, 3:1143
Eye surgery, 2:690, **2:1048–1051**, 3:1386
Eye tumors
demographics of, 1:475
eye enucleation for, 1:474
orbital exenteration for, 1:502–506
stereotactic radiosurgery for, 3:1369–1371
Eyeball removal, **1:474–477**
Eyebrow drooping, 1:548
Eyegear, protective, 2:862–863
Eyeglasses
LASIK and, 2:841–842, 845, 846, 847
for refractive vision errors, 3:1160–1161
See also Corrective lenses
Eyelid cancer exenteration, 1:503
Eyelids
blepharoplasty for, 1:169–172
drooping, 1:548
paralysis of, 3:1397
tarsorrhaphy of, 3:1396–1398

F

Face lift, **1:521–524**, *522*
forehead lift and, 1:549
mentoplasty and, 2:967
multiple, 1:439

Face washes, 1:94
Facial asymmetry, 2:967
Facial cancer, 1:362, 366, 3:1328
Facial fractures, 1:363, 3:1328, 1329
Facial injuries
adjustment to, 1:367
craniofacial reconstruction for, 1:362, 363, 365–366
cricothyroidotomy for, 1:374
Facial nerve paralysis, 2:934, 3:1100, 1101
Facial reconstruction. *See* Craniofacial reconstruction
Facial skin resurfacing, 2:857–859
Facioplasty. *See* Face lift
FACS (Fellow of the American College of Surgeons), 3:1195, 1291, 1387
Factor I, 2:893
Factor II, 2:893
Factor IX, 2:893
Factor VII, 2:893
Factor X, 2:893
Factor XIII, 1:537
Facultative anaerobes, 1:47
Fainting, 1:246, 247
Fallopian tube incision, 2:1034, **3:1260–1263**, *1261*
Fallopian tube ligation, 1:331, 332–333, 439, 2:1034
Fallopian tube obstruction, 2:740
Fallopian tube removal. *See* Salpingo-oophorectomy; Salpingostomy
Falope ring technique, 3:1461
False negative results
immunoassay tests, 2:727–728
mammography, 2:931
pap tests, 1:330
sentinel lymph node biopsy, 3:1301
stress tests, 3:1375
False positive results
mammography, 2:931
mediastinoscopy, 2:949
stress tests, 3:1375
Familial adenomatous polyposis
bowel resection for, 1:206
demographics of, 2:720
ileoanal anastomosis for, 2:717–720
ileoanal reservoir surgery for, 2:720–723
Family
hospices and, 2:684
hospitals and, 3:1167–1168
nursing homes and, 2:1031
preoperative preparation for, 3:1199
Family planning, 1:43
Famotidine, 2:568
Fanconi syndrome, 1:337
Farsightedness. *See* Hyperopia
FASA (Federated Ambulatory Surgery Association), 1:37
Fascial slings, 3:1329, 1331, 1332
Fascicles, 2:973
Fasciitis, plantar, 1:524–526
Fasciotomy, **1:524–526**

Fasting plasma glucose test, 2:603, 604, 605, 606
Fat deposit liposuction, 1:521, 2:878–882, *2:879, 880*
Fat injections, 1:552, 2:969
Fat rebalancing, 1:523
Fatigue and pain, 3:1082
Fatty acids, essential, 1:256, 470, 3:1132, 1136
Fatty liver, 2:889
FDA. *See* Food and Drug Administration
Fear, 3:1113, 1192, 1395
Fecal impaction, 2:865
Fecal incontinence
artificial sphincter insertion for, 1:123–128
colorectal surgery for, 1:318
demographics of, 1:125, 3:1253
sacral nerve stimulation for, 3:1253–1256
Fecal occult blood test, 1:315, 3:1317
Federated Ambulatory Surgery Association (FASA), 1:37
Federation of State Medical Boards, 1:540
FEF (Forced expiratory flow), 3:1358–1360
Fellow of the American College of Surgeons (FACS), 3:1195, 1291, 1387
Felodipine, 1:90*t*
Felon, 2:619
Female circumcision, 1:297
Female genital mutilation, 1:297
Female hormone therapy. *See* Estrogen therapy
Femoral artery, 1:236, 3:1132–1136
Femoral head, 2:661, 662, 663, 664, 666
Femoral hernia, 1:527–530, 2:754
Femoral hernia repair, **1:527–530**, *528*
Femoropopliteal bypass surgery, 3:1132, *3:1133*, 3:1135, 1136
Femorotibial bypass surgery, 3:1132, 1135, 1136
Femur
anatomy of, 2:661, 664, 800
hip revision surgery and, 2:675
knee replacement and, 2:802
lengthening and shortening of, 2:866
robot-assisted bone cutting, 3:1243
Fenfluramine, 3:1545, 1562
Fenoprofen, 1:132
Fentanyl
for conscious sedation, 3:1293–1294
for epidural anesthesia, 1:478
for pain, 1:53*t*, 3:1084
for premedication, 1:61
Fertility drugs, 2:741
See also Infertility
Fetal abnormalities. *See* Birth defects
Fetal alcohol syndrome, 1:301

Fetal death, 1:535
Fetal distress
    cesarean section for, 1:283, 286
    epidural anesthesia and, 1:478–479
    episiotomy and, 1:480
Fetal lung maturity tests, 2:875, 876,
    877
Fetal monitoring, 1:286, 533–536
Fetal surgery, **1:530–533**, 1:534, 535,
    536
Fetal ultrasound, 1:534, 535–536,
    3:1120–1122, *1121*
Fetoscopic temporary tracheal occlu-
    sion procedure, 1:531–532
Fetoscopy, **1:533–536**
FEV (Forced expiratory volume),
    3:1358–1360
Fever
    acetaminophen for, 1:21–23
    aspirin for, 1:131–134
    bone marrow biopsy for, 1:189
    defined, 3:1410
    NSAIDs for, 2:1028
    from oophorectomy, 2:1040
    from percutaneous nephrolithotomy,
        2:1019
Fever of unknown origin, 2:886
Fiber optics, 1:120–121
Fibrillation
    electrocardiography of, 1:441
    paroxysmal atrial, 2:937
    ventricular, 1:411–413, 441, 451,
        2:736–740
    See also Atrial fibrillation
Fibrin sealants, **1:536–538**
Fibrinogen, 1:537, 2:890–895
Fibroadenoma, 1:211
Fibroblasts, 3:1403, 1429
Fibroids, uterine. *See* Uterine fibroids
Fibromatosis, hereditary gingival,
    2:599
Fibrosis
    bone marrow, 1:189, 337
    breast, 1:211
    lens opacification, 2:854
    lung, 2:914, 918, 919, 3:1358, 1359
Fibula, 2:800, 866
Filgrastim, 1:198, 2:728
Film, transparent, 1:144, 145
Film dressings, 3:1568
Filtering shunts, 2:610
Filtration blebs, 3:1272, 1275
Filtration surgery, 1:388, 2:853,
    3:1271–1277
Financial incentives, 2:932, 933
Finasteride, 2:615
Finding a surgeon, **1:538–542**
Fine-needle aspiration, 2:951, 989,
    3:1146
Finger amputation, 1:542–545, *1:543,
    544,* 2:620, 621
Finger arthroplasty, 1:116–120
Finger reattachment, **1:542–545**, *543,
    544*

Fingers, webbed, 2:619, 3:*1556*
Fingertip injuries, 2:620
Fistula
    arteriovenous, 1:111–115, 467,
        2:1019
    bronchopleural, 3:1177
    from colporrhaphy, 1:327
    from glossectomy, 2:601
    from hypospadias repair, 2:704
    pharyngocutaneous, 3:1147
    salivary, 3:1100
5HT3 inhibitors, 1:92
Fixation devices
    for fracture repair, 1:553
    Ilizarov, 2:867
    for leg lengthening and shortening,
        2:867, 869, 870
    tacks, 1:550, 551
Fixed-tissue technique, 2:991
Flaps (Surgical)
    attached, 1:219–220
    bone, 1:274
    for breast reconstruction, 1:219–220
    failure of, 1:221
    free, 1:219–220, 3:1147
    gluteus maximus free, 1:220
    LASIK and, 2:844, 845, 846
    latissimus dorsi, 1:220, 221
    modified radical mastectomy and,
        2:987
    myocutaneous, 1:9, 219, 3:1147
    radial forearm free, 2:601
    for scar revision surgery,
        3:1264–1265, 1266
    transverse rectus abdominis myocu-
        taneous (TRAM), 1:9
    tummy tuck, 1:220, 221
Flashing, 3:1144, 1154
Flat feet, 1:231, 2:616
Flax seed, 3:1132, 1136
Flexeril. *See* Cyclobenzaprine
Flexible cystoscopy, 1:399
Flexible sigmoidoscopy, 1:319
Floaters (Ocular), 3:1154
Florical, 3:1367
Florinef. *See* Fludrocortisone
Flow records, 2:956, 957
Fluconazole, 2:687
Fludrocortisone, 1:360
Fluid accumulation, pleural. *See* Pleural
    effusion
Fluid balance
    diuretics for, 1:427–430
    gastrostomy and, 2:593
    hemodialysis for, 1:114
    for kidney stones, 2:1020
    overload, 1:404
Fluid replacement, 2:766–767
Fluid retention, 2:940
Fluid volume, 2:647, 651
Fluorescein angiography, 1:70, 71, 72,
    2:774, 855
Fluorescent immunoassay, 2:727

Fluorescent treponemal antibody-ab-
    sorption (FTA-ABS) test, 1:277
Fluoride, 3:1367
Fluoroquinolones, 1:81, 82, **1:545–548**,
    3:1206
Fluoroscopy
    for angiography, 1:69, 273, 275
    for angioplasty, 1:74–75
    for arthrography, 1:115–116
    for cardiac catheterization, 1:236
    electrophysiology study and, 1:450
    esophageal function tests and, 1:491
    for lung biopsy, 2:914
    for microsurgery, 2:974
    myelography and, 2:996
    roadmap, 1:74
    See also Upper GI exams
Fluorouracil, 3:1272
Fluoxetine, 3:1562
    alprazolam and, 1:80
    for anxiety, 1:78
    diazepam and, 2:995
Flurbiprofen, 2:1028
Flush solution, 3:1104
Flutter, atrial, 1:251, 411, 412
Fluvoxamine, 1:78
Foam dressings, 3:1568
Fobi gastric bypass, 2:571
Focal epilepsy, 1:359, 445
Focus charting, 2:957
Folate deficiency, 1:97, 336, 3:1228
Foley catheters, 1:262, 265
Folic acid
    atherosclerosis prevention, 1:256,
        469, 3:1132, 1136
    coronary artery disease, 1:352, 356,
        472
    neural tube defect prevention, 2:966
Folic acid deficiency, 1:335, 339
Fontan procedure, 2:637
Fontanelle, sunken, 2:766
Food and Drug Administration (FDA)
    on Aquaflow collagen wicks, 3:1275
    on the Bispectral index, 1:62
    on blood collection, 3:1439
    on blood registries, 1:172
    on Botox, 1:523, 552
    on breast implants, 1:215, 219, 221
    on cochlear implants, 1:310
    on coronary stents, 1:353
    on dermal regeneration templates,
        3:1264–1265
    on enhanced external counterpulsa-
        tion, 1:470
    on fenfluramine, 3:1545, 1562
    on fibrin sealants, 1:536
    on INFUSE Bone Grafts, 1:187–188
    on Lap-Band, 3:1549
    on laser surgery, 2:862–863
    on LASIK, 2:844
    on mammography, 2:930
    on medical errors, 2:960
    on mifepristone, 1:15
    on Repose system, 3:1345

on sacral nerve stimulation, 3:1253
on somnoplasty, 3:1344
on tumor marker tests, **3:**1470
on vagus nerve stimulation, 3:1513
on ventricular assist devices, 3:1540
on weight loss drugs, 2:575
on ZEUS Surgical System, 3:1398
Foot
club, 1:300–301, 305–307
edema, 3:1283
flat, 1:231, 2:616
ganglion cyst removal for,
2:560–563
over-pronation of, 1:233
Foot artery bypass, 3:1132–1136
Foot-in-foot prosthesis, 2:871
Foot tendon release. *See* Club foot repair
Foot ulcers, 1:46, 408
For-profit hospitals, 2:688, 689, 690
Forced expiratory flow (FEF),
3:1358–1360
Forced expiratory volume (FEV),
3:1358–1360
Forced vital capacity (FVC),
3:1358–1360
Forceps
bronchoscopy, 1:226, 227
Magill, 1:23
surgical, 3:1381
Forehead lift, **1:548–553**
Foreign bodies
chest x ray for, 1:291, 293
colonoscopy for, 1:313
CT scans for, 1:384
intestinal obstruction repair for,
2:763–764
Forensic medicine, 1:362, 363, 365,
368, 3:1479
Foreskin
phimosis, 1:267
removal of, 1:297–300, *1:298*
Fortaz. *See* Ceptaz
Foscarnet, 2:687
Fosinopril sodium, 1:90*t*
Foundation for the Accreditation of
Cellular Therapy, 1:196
Fourier transform algorithm, 1:444
Fowler-Stephens technique, 2:1060
Fracture repair, 1:184–189, **1:553–556**,
554
Fractures
aging and, 1:553, 555
bone x rays for, 1:203, 204
chest x ray for, 1:293
in children, 1:553, 555
compound, 1:555
demographics of, 1:553
distal phalangeal, 2:620
elbow, *1:554*
facial, 1:363, 3:1328, 1329
hand, 2:620
humerus, 3:1310, 1313
from knee revision surgery, 2:812

kneecap, 2:814, 815
laryngeal, 1:374
Le Fort, 1:363, 365–366
rib, 1:293, 2:977
spinal, 2:566
sternum, 1:293
Frail elderly, 1:35
Framingham Heart Study, 2:940
Fraud, Medicare, 2:963
Free flaps, 1:219–220, 3:1147
Free-tissue transfers, 2:973–974
Freestanding surgery centers. *See* Ambulatory surgery centers
Freezing, therapeutic. *See* Cryotherapy
French treatment, 1:307
Fresh frozen plasma transfusion, 1:173,
174
Fresh-tissue technique, 2:990–991
Frey's syndrome, 3:1100, 1101
Frown lines, 1:548–553
Fructosamine assay, 2:605, 606
Fryns syndrome, 1:301
FTA-ABS (Fluorescent treponemal antibody-absorption) test, 1:277
Fuch's dystrophy, 1:342
Fujita, S., 3:1344
Fulguration, 1:386
Full-face masks, 2:945
Full patellectomy, 2:814
Full-thickness grafts, 3:1325
Full-thickness wounds, 1:386
Fulminant liver failure, 2:895
Functional endoscopic sinus surgery
(FESS), **1:459–463**
Functional hemispherectomy, 2:649
Functional neurosurgery, 2:1026
Fundoplication, 2:579, **2:586–591**
for Barrett's esophagus, 1:498
laparoscopic, 2:580, 586–591,
588–589, 590
Nissen, 2:586–591, 3:1399
reoperation for, 3:1230
Fundus examination, 2:844, 1049
Fungal infections
gram stain for, 1:277
hospital-acquired, 2:685, 686, 687
Funnel chest repair, **3:1109–1113**
Furazolidone, 1:34
Furosemide, 1:90*t*, 428
Furoxone. *See* Furazolidone
Fusobacterium infections, 1:48
FVC (Forced vital capacity),
3:1358–1360

Gag reflex, 1:65, 228, 500
Gait patterns, 2:798, 801
Gait retraining, 2:873
Galen, 2:701
Gallbladder cancer, 1:159, 457
Gallbladder disease
costs of, 2:580
demographics of, 1:457
endoscopic retrograde cholangiopancreatography for,
1:456–459
obesity and, 1:508
Gallbladder removal. *See* Cholecystectomy
Gallstone removal, **2:557–560**
Gallstones
abdominal ultrasound for, 1:1
biliary stenting for, 1:159
in children, 3:1118
cholecystectomy for, 1:293–297
demographics of, 1:457, 2:557, 580
endoscopic retrograde cholangiopancreatography for, 1:456
extracorporeal shock wave lithotripsy for, 2:558, 559
from gastric bypass, 2:573
liver function tests for, 2:894
non-surgical treatment of, 1:297
obesity and, 1:508
removal of, **2:557–560**
ultrasound for, 1:295, 2:559
Gamete intrafallopian tube transfer
(GIFT), 2:742
Gamma-glutamyl transferase (GGT),
2:890–895
Gamma knife treatment, 3:1369, 1370
Gamma rays, 3:1182
Ganciclovir, 2:687
Ganglion cyst removal (Ganglionectomy), **2:560–563**, *561*, 2:619
Ganglion sympathectomy,
3:1389–1390
Ganglionic blockade, 1:65
Gangrene, 1:406, 527
Gantrisin. *See* Sulfisoxazole
Garlic, 1:470, 3:1457
Gas exchange, 2:944
Gas gangrene, 1:406
Gas-permeable contact lens, 3:1161
Gastrectomy, 1:97, **2:563–567**, *565*
partial, 1:95–100, 2:564
for stomach ulcers, 2:563–564, 576
Gastric acid. *See* Stomach acid
Gastric acid inhibitors, **2:567–570**,
2:578
Gastric antral vascular ectasia (GAVE)
syndrome, 1:95, 96, 98
Gastric bypass, 1:437, **2:570–575**,
2:896
Gastric emptying, delayed, 2:583,
3:1093, 1211
Gastric outlet obstruction, 1:95, 2:575,
578
Gastric ulcers. *See* Stomach ulcers

G

G-CSF. *See* Filgrastim
G-Hgb (Glycated hemoglobin) test,
2:603, 604, 605, 606
G-tubes, 2:591–594
Gabapentin, 1:50
Gadolinium, 1:115, 2:926

Gastrin, 1:95
Gastritis, 2:566, 577
Gastroduodenostomy, **2:575–579**, *576*
Gastroenterologic disease, 2:579–580
Gastroenterologic surgery, 1:37, **2:579–582**
Gastroenterologists, 1:499
Gastroesophageal reflux disease (GERD)
   causes of, 2:582–583, 586–587
   in children, 3:1117
   demographics of, 2:580
   diagnosis of, 2:589
   esophageal atresia/tracheoe-
     sophageal fistula and, 1:489
   esophageal cancer and, 1:493–494
   esophageal function tests for,
     1:490–493
   fundoplication for, 1:498
   gastrectomy for, 2:563–567
   gastric acid inhibitors for,
     2:567–570
   medication-induced esophageal in-
     juries and, 1:501
   non-surgical treatment of, 2:588
   obesity and, 1:508
   recurrence of, 2:590
   reoperation for, 3:1230
   scan for, 2:582–585
   surgery for, 1:498, 2:586–591,
     2:587
Gastroesophageal reflux scan,
  2:582–585
Gastroesophageal reflux surgery, 1:498,
  2:586–591, *587*
Gastrointestinal birth defects, 1:487
Gastrointestinal bleeding
   esophagogastroduodenoscopy and,
     1:500
   from GAVE syndrome, 1:96
   from laparoscopy, 2:830
   from NSAIDs, 2:1028
   second-look surgery for, 3:1288
Gastrointestinal cancer, 1:499
Gastrointestinal disorders
   demographics of, 2:563
   emergency surgery for, 1:453
   reoperation for, 3:1230
   second-look surgery for, 3:1288
Gastrointestinal surgery, 3:1515, 1517
Gastrojejunostomy, 2:571, 575, 576
Gastroplasty, vertical banded, 2:574
Gastroschisis, 1:5–7, 3:1116–1117
Gastroschisis repair, **1:5–7**
Gastroscopy, 2:595, 3:1517
Gastrostomy, **2:591–594**
   esophageal atresia/tracheoe-
     sophageal fistula and, 1:488
   gastric bypass and, 2:572
   pancreatectomy and, 3:1092
   for pharyngectomy, 3:1147
Gatifloxacin, 1:546
Gauze, 1:144, 145, 2:744

GAVE (Gastric antral vascular ectasia)
  syndrome, 1:95, 96, 98
GBLC (Geometric broken line closure),
  3:1265
Gelatin dressings, 3:1568
Gender differences
   adjustment to facial trauma, 1:367
   anesthesia, 1:162
   cataracts, 1:511
   forehead lift, 1:549
   heart attacks, 1:440
   hip revision surgery, 2:676
   kidney stones, 2:1017–1018
   knee injuries, 2:801
   knee replacement, 2:802
   knee revision surgery, 2:810
   omphaloceles, 2:1035
   open-angle glaucoma, 3:1272
   recovery at home, 3:1221
   scar revision surgery, 3:1263
   spider veins, 3:1280
   urinary incontinence, 2:1011,
     3:1253, 1330
Gender identity, 2:701, 703, 3:1306
Gender identity disorders, 2:1053,
  3:1305–1308
Gender reassignment surgery. *See* Sex
reassignment surgery
General anesthesia, **1:59–63**, *60,*
  3:1387
   for cesarean section, 1:284, 286
   hypothermia from, 3:1221
   vs. nerve blockades, 3:1184
   for obstetric and gynecologic
     surgery, 2:1034
General Internal Medicine, 2:690
General surgeons, 1:539
General surgery, **2:594–597**, 2:827,
  3:1386
Generalized infections, 2:685
Genetic factors
   cataracts and, 1:511
   hip revision surgery and, 2:676
   hypospadias and, 2:702
   low back pain and, 2:820
Genetic mutations, 3:1412
Genioplasty, sliding, 2:968, 969
Genital mutilation, female, 1:297
Genital warts, 1:329, 385, 386
Genitalia, ambiguous, 3:1305
Gentian violet, 1:418
Genuine stress urinary incontinence,
  2:1010–1011, 3:1330, 1331
Geometric broken line closure (GBLC),
  3:1265
GERD. *See* Gastroesophageal reflux
disease
Germ cell tumors, 2:894
Gestational diabetes, 2:603, 604, 605,
  606
GGT (Gamma-glutamyl transferase),
  2:890–895
Ghodoussi, Moji, 3:1399
Giant cell tumors, 2:619

Giemsa stain, 1:190
GIFT (Gamete intrafallopian tube
  transfer), 2:742
Gillies, Harold, 1:365
Gingivectomy, **2:597–600**
Gingivitis, 2:597–600
Gingko, 1:57
Ginseng, 1:34, 57
Girdlestone operation, 2:663, 672
Glanzmann's thrombasthenia, 1:337
Glare
   cataracts and, 1:512
   LASIK and, 2:844, 846
   from ophthalmologic surgery,
     2:1050
Glasgow Coma Scale, 1:162, 163, 164,
  2:1025
Glasses, eye, 2:841–842, 845, 846, 847
Glassock dressings, 1:454
Glatiramer acetate, 2:733
Glaucoma
   angle closure, 2:770–776, 848–854,
     3:1287
   carbolic anhydrase inhibitors for,
     1:428
   congenital, 1:388–389, 2:606–611
   cyclocryotherapy for, 1:388–389
   demographics of, 3:1272
   end-stage, 1:388
   juvenile-onset open angle, 2:607, 608
   from laser posterior capsulotomy,
     2:856
   malignant, 2:849, 850
   neovascular, 1:388–389, 390–391
   neurovascular, 2:849
   non-surgical treatment of, 1:428,
     2:773, 1051
   open-angle, 2:772, 849,
     3:1271–1277
   phacolytic, 2:849, 850
   pigmentary, 2:850
   pseudoexfoliation, 2:850
   refractory, 1:388–389
   risk factors for, 3:1273
   secondary, 1:515
   tests for, 2:844
   trabeculectomy, 2:1049,
     3:1431–1434, *1432*
   tube-shunt surgery, 3:1463–1466
   uveitic, 2:607
Glaucoma Research Foundation, 3:1275
Glenohumeral joint. *See* Shoulder
Glenoid component implants, 3:1310
Glioma, 2:1025
Globus pallidus internus, 1:409,
  3:1087–1088, 1089
Glomerulonephritis, 2:779, 786–787
Glossectomy, **2:600–602**, 2:840
Gloves, 1:129, *1:129*
Glucocorticoids, **1:359–361**
Gluconeogenesis, 2:604
Glucosamine for arthritis, 1:119,
  3:1311
Glucose, in urinalysis, 3:1499, 1501

Glucose regulation, 3:1091
Glucose tests, 1:276, 277, **2:602–606**, *603*
Glucose tolerance test, 2:603, *2:603*
Glues
   fibrin, 1:536–538
   tissue, 2:703, 744
Glutethimide, 2:652
Gluteus maximus free flaps, 1:220
Glyburide, 3:1380
Glycated hemoglobin test, 2:603, 604, 605, 606
Glycerin, 2:851, 865
Glycogen, 2:604
Glycogenolysis, 2:604
Glycolysis, reverse, 2:604
Glycosuria, 2:603
Glypressin, 3:1278
GnRHa (Gonadotropin-releasing hormone agonists), 2:741
Gold
   for shoulder pain, 3:1314
GoLytely, 1:207, 319, 323, 3:1227
Gomco clamps, 1:300
Gonadotropin-releasing hormone agonists (GnRHa), 2:741
Gonioscopy, 2:608, 773, 774, 851, 3:1274
Goniotomy, 1:388, **2:606–611**
Gore-Tex slings, 3:1329
Gott shunts, 1:102
Gout, 2:804
Government-supported hospitals, 2:688
Gowns, sterile, 1:130
Graefe, Albrecht von, 1:510
Graft rejection. *See* Transplant rejection
Graft *versus* host disease (GVHD), 1:201, 2:691
Grafts
   allografts, 1:185, 187, 3:1325
   autografts, 1:185, 186–187, 3:1323, 1325
   bacterial contamination of, 1:187
   ceramic, 1:187
   composite, 3:1325
   coral, 1:187
   Dacron, 1:102, 2:637, 998
   endovascular, 1:103, 466–467
   full-thickness, 3:1325
   for hemodialysis, 1:112
   impaction, 2:675, 811
   ligament, 2:793, 795, 796
   nerve, 2:973
   polymer, 1:188
   saphenous vein, 1:346, *1:347*, 1:349, 3:1135, 1136
   skin, 3:1264–1265, 1322–1328, *3:1323*
   split-thickness, 3:1325
   synthetic, 1:187
   tendon, 3:1400
   vein, 2:972
   xenografts, 2:777, 3:1325
   See also Bone grafting

Grains, whole, 1:470
Gram negative bacteria, 1:48
Gram positive bacteria, 1:48–49
Gram stain, 1:48, 277, 278
Grand mal seizures, 1:358
Granisetron, 1:92, 3:1287
Granulocytes, 1:335, 336
Granulocytic leukemia, 1:337
Granulomas, 1:192
Grave's disease, 2:692
Greenbottle fly maggots, 1:407
Grieving, 1:404–405, 2:682, 684
Groin hernia. *See* Inguinal hernia
Group health insurance, 3:1203
Group Model, 2:933
Growth factors, 1:144, 145
Guanabenz acetate, 1:90t
Guanethidine, 1:34
Guanfacine hydrochloride, 1:90*t*
Gubernaculum, 2:1058
Guglielmi detachable coils, 1:275
Guided imagery, 3:1196, 1201
Guilt, 3:1395
Gum, Nicorette, 3:1340
Gum disease
   from eating disorders, 3:1560
   gingivectomy for, 2:597–600
   immunosuppressant drugs and, 2:734
   non-surgical treatment of, 2:600
Gum injuries, 3:1430
Gunshot wounds, 1:372
Gutta percha, 3:1245
GVHD (Graft *versus* host disease), 1:201, 2:691
Gynecologic oncology, 2:1033
Gynecological surgery. *See* Obstetric and gynecologic surgery
Gynecomastia, 1:222, 223

H

H$_2$-receptor blockers, 1:98, 2:568–569, 578, 588, 590
Habitrol. *See* Nicotine replacement therapy
Haemophilus influenzae, 2:1005
Hair follicle transplants, 2:613
Hair transplantation, **2:613–616**, *614*
Hairpieces, 2:615
Halcion. *See* Triazolam
Hallux valgus, 1:232
Haloalkene, 1:62
Haloperidol, 2:876
Halos (Ocular), 2:845, 846, 1050
Halothane, 1:60, 62
Hammer, claw, and mallet toe surgery, **2:616–618**
Hammer toes, 2:616–618
Hammock procedure. *See* Sling procedure
Hand
   abnormalities, 2:619

   amputation, 2:620, 621
   fractures, 2:620
   ganglion cysts, 2:560–563
   tumors, 2:619
Hand arthroplasty, 1:118
Hand-assisted laparoscopic nephrectomy, 2:788, 1013
Hand surgery, **2:619–622**
Handwashing
   antiseptics for, 1:94
   for clinical settings, 1:128
   for hospital-acquired infection control, 2:687
   surgical scrub for, 1:128–129
Haplotypes, 2:692
Harmonic scalpels, 1:182
Harrington rods, 3:1356
Harry Benjamin International Gender Dysphoria Association, 2:1053, 1054
Hashimoto's thyroiditis, 2:692
Hazardous waste, 1:130
Haze, 3:1160
HBOC-201, 1:136, 3:1443
HCFA (Health Care Financing Administration), 2:963
hCG. *See* Human chorionic gonadotropin
HCUP Nationwide Inpatient Sample, 2:1013–1014
HDN. *See* Hemolytic disease of the newborn
Head cancer
   craniofacial reconstruction for, 1:362, 363, 366
   from dialysis, 2:782
   non-surgical treatment of, 3:1218
   radical neck dissection for, 3:1217–1219
   from smoking, 3:1241
   surgery for, 1:434
Head injuries
   in children, 3:1118
   craniofacial reconstruction for, 1:362, 363
   neurosurgery for, 2:1025
Head nurses, 3:1167
Head reconstruction. *See* Craniofacial reconstruction
Head surgery, 1:404, 433, 434, 2:1025
Headache
   from forehead lift, 1:551
   from lumbar puncture, 1:277
   from myelography, 2:996
   from snoring, 3:1342
   spinal, 1:66, 479
Health assessment, 3:1161
Health Care Financing Administration (HCFA), 2:963
Health care proxy, **2:622–623**, 3:1190
Health care system, 1:538–539
   commercialization of, 1:39
   costs of, 3:1204
   managed care plans and, 2:932–933
   medical errors and, 2:960

national, 1:538–539

Health care team. *See* Patient care teams

Health history, 1:56–57, **2:623–627**, *624*

Health insurance
confidentiality and, 3:1106
costs of, 3:1204
employer-based, 3:1203, 1204, 1205
essential surgery and, 1:502
finding surgeons, 1:538–539
group, 3:1203
for heart transplantation, 2:641
for hip replacement, 2:668
home care and, 2:679
for hospital services, 3:1165
indemnity plans, 3:1203
long-term care, **2:906–910**, 2:953, 1030, 3:1203
medical charts and, 2:956
for nursing homes, 2:1030
for outpatient surgery, 2:1071
for oxygen therapy, 2:1075
for physical examinations, 3:1162
private, **3:1203–1206**, 3:1316
for second opinions, 1:541, 3:1291
for sigmoidoscopy, 3:1316
tax credit proposals for, 3:1205
vertical banded gastroplasty and, 3:1547
See also Health maintenance organizations; Medicare

Health Insurance Association of American (HIAA), 2:907, 908

Health Insurance Portability and Accountability Act (HIPAA), 3:1106, 1107, 1204

Health maintenance organizations (HMOs), 2:932–933
description of, 3:1203
home care and, 2:679
hospital services and, 2:689
organ transplants and, 3:1446
patient rights and, 3:1108
surgeon referrals and, 1:538
See also Health insurance

Health People 2000, Final Review, 2:798

Healthy Aging Project, 2:963

Hearing aids, 3:1367

Hearing loss
cochlear implants for, 1:308–311
conductive, 3:1366
diagnosis of, 3:1366
from Ménière's disease, 1:454
sensorineural, 1:308, 3:1366
from stapedectomy, 3:1367
stapedectomy for, 3:1365–1368
surgery for, 1:433–434

Hearing tests, 1:454

Heart
anatomy of, 1:236
artificial, 2:637, 644, 843, 999
electrical impulses, 1:441–442, 449–450

electrophysiology study of, 1:449–452
enlarged, 1:436
mapping, 1:449–452
perforation of, 3:1081
See also terms beginning with Cardiac

Heart attacks
from angiography, 1:72
aspirin prophylaxis for, 1:132
cardiac catheterization for, 1:235
cardiac marker tests for, 1:240–242
coronary artery bypass graft surgery and, 1:346, 348
demographics of, 1:440
emergency surgery for, 1:452, 453
fundoplication for, 2:586
gender differences in, 1:440
liver function tests for, 2:892, 894
pacemakers for, 3:1079
prevention of, 1:256, 469–470
smoking cessation and, 3:1338
from stress tests, 3:1376
thrombolytic therapy for, 3:1417–1419

Heart birth defects. *See* Congenital heart defects

Heart catheterization. *See* Cardiac catheterization

Heart disease
anesthesia evaluation and, 1:56
body weight and, 1:506
cardiac catheterization for, 1:235–240
chest x ray for, 1:291
echocardiography for, 1:435–437
electrocardiography for, 1:439–442
electrophysiology study for, 1:449–452
endovascular stent surgery for, 1:466
hysterectomy and, 2:709
intensive care units and, 2:759
obesity and, 1:507
prevention of, 1:471–473
risk factors for, 1:247
spirometry tests for, 3:1359
thoracotomy for, 3:1414
See also Cardiovascular disease

Heart failure
ascites from, 3:1096
end-stage, 2:639, 643–644
heart transplantation for, 2:639–644
mechanical circulation support for, 2:942–944
NYHA heart failure classification for, 2:980, 984, 986
See also Cardiac arrest; Congestive heart failure

Heart-lung machines, **2:627–630**, *628*
for congenital heart defects, 2:636
for coronary artery bypass, 1:346, *1:347*, 1:348, 2:627

for heart-lung transplantation, *2:631, 2:632*
for heart transplantation, 2:639
for Maze procedure, 2:937
in operating rooms, 2:1045

Heart-lung transplantation, **2:630–634**, *631*, 2:918, 920, 921, 3:1444
See also Heart transplantation

Heart murmurs, 1:436

Heart muscle activity scan, **2:992–994**

Heart rate
exercise, 2:739
fetal, 1:534, 535
resting, 1:508
smoking and, 3:1338
stress test for, 3:1375–1377

Heart rhythm, irregular. *See* Arrhythmia

Heart sonogram. *See* Echocardiography

Heart sounds, 3:1371–1372

Heart stimulants, 1:32, 33

Heart surgery, **2:634–638**
for birth defects, *2:635*
heart-lung machines for, 2:627
minimally invasive, **2:974–978**, *975*
myocardial resection, 2:643, 997–999
open heart, 1:103, 2:627, 975

Heart transplantation, **2:638–644**, *640*, 3:1444, 1445, 1448
for congenital heart defects, 2:637
mechanical circulation support for, 2:942
vs. myocardial resection, 2:999
pacemakers for, 2:641, 3:1079
smoking cessation and, 3:1340–1341
ventricular assist devices and, 3:1540
See also Heart-lung transplantation

Heart valve disorders
birth defects, 1:141–142, 143
cardiac catheterization for, 1:235
Doppler ultrasound for, 1:240
echocardiography for, 1:435–437
Maze procedure for, 2:937

Heart valve repair
minimally invasive surgical procedures for, 2:975
mitral, **2:978–983**, *981*
valvotomy, 1:107, 2:986
valvuloplasty, **1:141–143**, 2:636

Heart valve replacement
aortic, **1:104–107**, *105*
mitral, 2:979, **2:983–986**
robot-assisted, 3:1244

Heart valve stenosis
aortic, 1:104–107, *1:105*, 1:141–143, 2:637
balloon valvuloplasty for, 1:141–143
Doppler ultrasound for, 1:240
echocardiography for, 1:437
mitral, 1:141–143, 2:978–986
pulmonary, 1:141–143
tricuspid, 1:141–143

Heart valves
  biological tissue, 1:106, 2:984
  leaflets, 1:143
  mechanical, 1:106, 2:984
Heartbeat. *See* Pulse
Heartburn, 1:491, 2:563, 582–583, 588, 3:1549
  See also Gastroesophageal reflux disease
Heat exchangers, 2:628
Heel-cord release. *See* Tenotomies
Heel pain, 1:525
Hefner cerclage, 1:279
Heidelberg retinal tomography (HRT), 3:1274
Helical CT scans, 1:383, 384, 2:918, 3:1130, 1135
Helicobacter pylori, 1:81, 97–98, 2:578–580, 3:1209–1211, 1212, 1515
Heliox therapy, 2:1074
Hemangioma excision, **2:644–647**
Hematocrit, 1:335–336, **2:647–648**
  for anemia, 3:1228–1229
  blood salvage and, 1:179
  critical values for, 1:339
  definition of, 1:334
  dialysis and, 2:781–782
  normal values for, 1:338, 2:648
Hematology analyzers, automated, 1:334, 335
Hematoma
  from angiography, 1:71
  from face lifts, 1:523
  intracerebral, 2:1024
  from lithotripsy, 2:885
  from otoplasty, 2:1069
  from parathyroidectomy, 3:1098
  from pharyngectomy, 3:1147
  from thyroidectomy, 3:1422
  vulvar, 2:1034
  from wounds, 3:1569
Hematoxylin-eosin stain, 1:190
Hemiarthroplasty, 3:1314
Hemifacial microsomia, 2:1066
Hemimegalencephaly, 2:649
Hemispherectomy, 1:359, **2:648–650**
Hemochromatosis
  hereditary, 2:692
  liver biopsy for, 2:886
  phlebotomy for, 3:1150, 1151
Hemodialysis, **1:111–115,** 2:779–783
Hemodilution
  acute normo-volemic, 1:135
  immediate preoperative, 3:1168, 1196, 1202
  for reducing blood loss, 1:182
Hemoglobin, 1:58
  blood salvage and, 1:179
  cell-free, 1:182
  transfusion and, 1:181
Hemoglobin test, 1:335, **2:650–652**
  for anemia, 3:1228–1229
  critical values for, 1:339
  glycated, 2:603, 604, 605, 606

normal values for, 1:338, 2:651
  postoperative anemia and, 1:182
  pulse oximetry, 2:760
Hemolysis, 1:339, 2:985
Hemolytic anemia, 1:447, 2:604, 892
Hemolytic disease of the newborn (HDN), 2:894, 3:1479, 1480, 1481
Hemolytic disorders, autoimmune, 3:1362
Hemolytic reactions, 3:1442
Hemolytic-uremic syndrome (HUS), 1:337
Hemoperfusion, **2:652–653**
Hemophilia, 1:116
Hemophilus infections, 2:727
Hemopure, 1:136, 3:1443
Hemorrhage
  after thrombolytic therapy, 3:1418
  from angiography, 1:72
  from aortic aneurysm repair, 1:103
  brain, 2:1024–1025
  colonoscopy for, 1:313
  intracranial, 2:1024–1025
  from pallidotomy, 3:1089
  retinal, 2:847
  subarachnoid, 1:271–276, 2:1024–1025
  suprachoroidal, 3:1274
  See also Bleeding
Hemorrhagic strokes, 3:1418
Hemorrhoidectomy, **2:653–657**
Hemorrhoids
  colorectal surgery for, 1:318
  demographics of, 2:654–655
  hemorrhoidectomy for, 2:653–657
  non-surgical treatment of, 2:656
  sclerotherapy for, 3:1280
Hemosiderin, 3:1283, 1284
Hemostasis, 1:536–538
Hemothorax, 1:288, 289, 2:904
Heparin
  activity of, 1:86
  for aortic aneurysm repair, 1:101
  for coronary artery bypass graft surgery, 1:348
  craniotomy and, 1:370
  for finger reattachment, 1:543, 545
  lymphadenectomy and, 2:923
  NSAIDs and, 2:1028
  platelet count and, 1:337
  for venous thrombosis, 3:1539
Hepatectomy, **2:657–661,** *658*
Hepaticojejunostomy, 1:161
Hepatitis
  blood collection, 3:1442
  blood donation and, 1:174
  dermabrasion and, 1:418
  fibrin sealants and, 1:536
  hepatectomy and, 2:659
  immunoassay tests for, 2:727
  liver function tests for, 2:892–894
  liver transplantation for, 2:895
  muscle relaxants and, 2:994

Hepatitis B
  from dialysis, 2:782
  immunoassay tests for, 2:727, 893
  liver cancer and, 3:1137–1138
  phlebotomy for, 3:1150
Hepatitis B surface antigen test, 2:893
Hepatitis C
  cirrhosis from, 3:1179
  from dialysis, 2:782
  liver biopsy for, 2:886
  liver cancer and, 2:657, 3:1137
  liver function tests for, 2:893
  liver transplantation for, 2:900
Hepatocellular carcinoma, 2:657
Hepatoma, 2:657
Hepatotoxicity. *See* Liver damage
Herbs
  adrenergic drugs and, 1:34
  anesthesia evaluation and, 1:57
  for atherosclerosis prevention, 1:470
  for stomach ulcers, 1:99
  sulfonamides and, 3:1380
  for weight management, 3:1562–1563
  See also specific herbs
Hereditary elliptocytosis, 3:1362
Hereditary gingival fibromatosis, 2:599
Hereditary hemochromatosis, 2:692
Hereditary spherocytosis, 3:1229, 1362, 1364
Hernia
  abdominal, 2:573
  acquired, 2:753–755
  in children, 3:1119
  congenital, 2:753–754
  congenital diaphragmatic, 1:531, 534, 3:1117
  demographics of, 2:753
  femoral, 1:527–530, *1:528,* 2:754
  hiatal, 2:583, 586, 588, 589
  incarcerated, 1:527–529, 2:748, 754, 756
  incisional, 2:746–750, 3:1336
  indirect *vs.* direct, 2:753–755, 756
  Littre's, 2:948
  parastomal, 1:320, 325
  perianal, 1:318
  peritoneal dialysis and, 2:781
  strangulated, 1:527, 528, 529, 2:748, 756
  umbilical, 3:1119
  ventral, 2:746–750
  See also Inguinal hernia
Hernia repair
  femoral, **1:527–530,** *528*
  incisional, **2:746–750,** *747*
  inguinal, **2:752–757,** *753*
  for intestinal obstruction, 2:764
Herniated intervertebral disk
  causes of, 2:820
  disk removal for, 1:424–427
  laminectomy for, 2:822
  myelography for, 2:995–997
  neurosurgery for, 2:1026
  spinal fusion for, 3:1353–1354

Herniorrhaphy. *See* Hernia repair
Heroin, 1:63
Herpes simplex infections, 2:858
Herpes virus infections, 1:342
Herpes zoster, 2:735
Heterotropic bone, 2:670, 806, 812
Heterotropic liver transplantation, 2:896
Hexachlorophane, 1:94
Hexadrol. *See* Dexamethasone
HIAA (Health Insurance Association of America), 2:907, 908
Hiatal hernia, 2:583, 586, 588, 589
Hibiscrub, 2:659
Hibiscus, 1:34
High blood pressure. *See* Hypertension
High-density lipoproteins, 2:875–878
High-fiber diet, 2:750, 949
High-heeled shoes, 3:1536
High-impact exercise, 3:1330
High tibia osteotomy (HTO), 2:797, 798–799
Highly selective vagotomy, 2:566, 3:1515, 1517
Hip and Knee Center, 2:811–812
Hip arthrodesis, 2:663, 672
Hip arthroplasty. *See* Hip replacement
Hip arthroscopic surgery, 1:120–123
Hip bone grafts, 1:187
Hip dysplasia, 2:661, 662
Hip injuries, 2:664
Hip joint, 2:661, 664, 666–668, 671–672, 673
Hip osteotomy, **2:661–664,** 2:672
Hip prosthesis, 2:664–678, *2:674*
Hip replacement, 1:116–120, 2:663, **2:664–673**, *665, 667*
    aftercare, 2:669, 3:1221
    description of, 2:666
    legal and financial considerations for, 2:668
    life expectancy of, 2:670, 677
    life style changes for, 2:668–669
    mortality and morbidity from, 2:670–671
    non-surgical alternatives for, 2:671–672
    vs. osteotomy, 2:663
    purpose of, 2:664–665
    risks of, 2:670
    total, 2:663, 664–665, 673
Hip revision surgery, 2:666, 670, **2:673–678,** *674*
HIPAA (Health Insurance Portability and Accountability Act), 3:1106, 1107, 1204
Hippocrates, 2:560
Hippocratic Oath, 3:1106
Hirschsprung's disease, 1:206, 208, 3:1116
Hirsutism, 3:1283
Hismanal. *See* Astemizole
Histamine, 1:337, 2:568
Histocompatibility antigens, 1:344

Histocompatibility complex (MHC), 2:691–692
Histocompatibility tests, **2:691–693**
Histologic technicians, 1:190
History of present illness (HPI), 2:625
HIV (Human immunodeficiency virus)
    blood collection, 3:1439, 1442, 1443
    blood donation and, 1:174, 3:1482
    dermabrasion and, 1:418
    from dialysis, 2:782
    fibrin sealants and, 1:536
    immunoassay tests for, 2:727
HLA (Human leukocyte antigen) test, 1:194, 196, **2:691–693,** 2:789
HMOs. *See* Health maintenance organizations
Hodgkin's lymphoma
    bone marrow biopsy for, 1:189
    cancer staging, 3:1473
    liver function tests for, 2:894
    mediastinoscopy for, 2:951
    splenectomy for, 3:1362
Hoffman, Felix, 1:131
Holding and voiding urine test (VCUG), 1:167
Holism, 2:680
Hollow fiber dialyzers, 2:780
Holter monitors, 2:998
Home care, **2:678–681**
    for hip replacement, 2:669
    hospice, 2:682, 683
    hospital services and, 3:1166
    of incisions, 2:744–745
    for knee replacement, 2:806
    long-term care insurance for, 2:907
    Medicare for, 2:679, 963
    oxygen therapy and, 2:1073, 1075
    patient education for, 3:1188
    preoperative preparation for, 3:1197
    recovery at home, **3:1219–1221**
Home care agencies, 2:678–679
Home health aides, 2:678
Homeopathy, 2:1006, 3:1348
Homocysteine
    atherosclerosis and, 1:256, 356, 469, 3:1131–1132, 1136–1137
    cardiac marker tests for, 1:240, 241, 242
    coronary artery disease and, 1:352
Hooks, spinal instrumentation, 3:1355–1357
Hormone creams, breast augmentation, 1:215, 221
Hormone replacement
    cyclosporins and, 2:736
    for cystocele, 1:398
    for endometriosis, 2:835
    face lift and, 1:521
    for gender reassignment, 2:1054–1055
    for hypophysectomy, 2:699
    mammography and, 2:931
    for oophorectomy, 2:1040

    for salpingo-oophorectomy, 3:1258
    See also Estrogen therapy
Hormone therapy
    for cancer, 1:202
    for cryptorchidism, 2:1063
    for gender reassignment, 2:1057
    for hypospadias repair, 2:704
    lumpectomy and, 2:913
    for prostate cancer, 2:1056
Hormones
    adrenal gland, 1:28, 30
    imbalance, 1:30, 31
    pain and, 3:1083
    steroid, 3:1561
    tumor marker tests, **3:**1470
    See also Androgens; Estrogen therapy
Horner's syndrome, 3:1390
Horse chestnut extract, 3:1284–1285
Hospices, **2:682–685,** 2:908, 963
Hospital-acquired infections, 1:130–131, 403, **2:685–688**
Hospital rooms, 1:27, 3:1167
Hospital services, **2:688–691,** 3:1166–1167
    health insurance for, 3:1165
    managed care plans and, 3:1165
    Medicaid for, 2:952
    Medicare for, 2:963, 3:1165
Hospitals
    accreditation of, 1:540, 3:1195
    admission to, **1:26–28,** 2:757, 956, 3:1169–1171
    ambulatory surgery centers and, 1:39
    charity, 2:689
    community, 2:688
    demographics of, 2:688
    discharge from, **1:422–424,** 2:956, 3:1188, 1220
    government-supported, 2:688
    health maintenance organizations, 2:689
    hospice care in, 2:683
    items to bring to, 3:1169, 1197
    length of stay in, 2:679, 689
    pediatric, 3:1113, 1114
    planning a stay in, 3:1165–1171
    proprietary (for-profit), 2:688, 689, 690
    registration, 3:1169–1171
    research, 2:689
    selecting, 3:1195
    specialty, 2:689
    teaching, 2:688, 689, 3:1388
    visiting, 3:1167–1168
Houdini jackets, 2:761
House, William, 1:454
HPI (History of present illness), 2:625
HRT (Heidelberg retinal tomography), 3:1274
HSV. *See* Highly selective vagotomy
HTO (High tibia osteotomy), 2:797, 798–799

Hulka clips, for tubal ligation, 3:1461

Human bites. *See* Bite injuries

Human chorionic gonadotropin (hCG), 2:726, 741, **3:1471–1472**

Human error, 2:960

Human experimentation, 2:751

Human immunodeficiency virus. *See* HIV

Human leukocyte antigen test, 1:194, 196, **2:691–693,** 2:789

Human papillomavirus (HPV), 1:298, 330, 385, 3:1147

Human recombinant bone morphogenetic protein-2, 3:1354

Humerus fractures, 3:1310, 1313

HUS (Hemolytic-uremic syndrome), 1:337

Hutchinson v. United States, 2:751–752

Hyaluronic acid, 1:552

Hycodan, 1:53*t*

Hyde shunts, 3:1138

Hydralazine, 1:91

Hydration therapy, 2:1020

Hydrocele, 1:299, 2:693–697, *2:694*

Hydrocelectomy, **2:693–697***, 694*

Hydrocephalus, 1:384, 2:650, 965, 966, 3:1542–1544

Hydrochloric acid, 1:491

Hydrochlorothiazide, 1:89, 90*t*, 91, 428, 3:1380

Hydrochlorothiazide-triamterene, 1:428, 429, 430

Hydrocodone, 1:53*t*

Hydrocodone-acetaminophen, 1:52

Hydrocolloid dressings, 1:144, 145

Hydrocortisone, 1:359–360, 2:726

Hydrodiuril. *See* Hydrochlorothiazide

Hydrofibers, 1:144, 145

Hydroflumethiazide, 1:89, 91

Hydrogel-coated latex catheters, 1:263, 266

Hydrogel dressings, 1:144, 145, 2:859

Hydrogen peroxide, 1:94

Hydrogen/potassium adenosine triphosphate, 2:568

Hydromorphone, 1:52, 53*t*

Hydropolymers, 1:144, 145

Hydrosalpinx, 3:1260, 1261

Hydroxyapatite, 1:184, 187

Hydroxyzine hydrochloride, 1:79*t*

Hygroton. *See* Chlorthalidone

Hyoscine butylbromide, 3:1277

Hyperaldosteronism, 1:31

Hyperbaric oxygen therapy, 2:1073, 1074

Hyperglycemia tests, 2:602–606

Hyperhidrosis, 3:1389, 1390–1391

Hyperkalemia, 1:447

Hyperlipidemia, 2:633

Hypermagnesemia, 2:866

Hypermetabolism, 3:1420

Hypermobile urethra. *See* Urethral hypermobility

Hypernatremia, 1:447

Hyperopia
    LASIK for, 2:841–848
    non-surgical treatment of, 2:1051
    photorefractive keratectomy for, 3:1157–1161

Hyperosmotic drugs, 2:851

Hyperosmotic laxatives, 2:865

Hyperparathyroidism
    electrolyte balance and, 1:447
    parathyroidectomy for, 3:1097–1099

Hyperpigmentation
    cryotherapy, 1:378
    laser skin resurfacing, 2:859
    laser surgery, 2:864

Hyperplasia
    benign prostatic, 3:1454, 1457–1458, 1506–1507
    endometrial, 1:419

Hypersplenism, 3:1360–1365

Hyperstat. *See* Diazoxide

Hypertension
    antihypertensive drugs for, 1:89–91
    blood pressure measurement for, 1:176, 177
    body weight and, 1:506–507
    diuretics for, 1:427
    electrolyte balance and, 1:448
    end-stage renal disease and, 2:779, 786
    heart-lung transplantation and, 2:633
    intracranial, 1:369, 2:760, 1046
    laparoscopy and, 2:829
    from liver failure, 2:895
    ocular, 3:1273
    portal, 3:1137, 1179–1182, 1277
    pulmonary, 2:916, 919, 980, 981, 984
    spontaneous intracranial hemorrhage and, 2:1025

Hyperthermia, malignant, 1:59, 62, 63, 2:994

Hyperthyroidism, 3:1420

Hypertrophic cardiomyopathy, 1:436

Hypertrophic scars, 1:305, 3:1263–1267

Hyphema
    cataract surgery, 1:514
    goniotomy, 2:609
    sclerostomy, 3:1274

Hypnosis
    during anesthesia, 1:162
    for post-surgical pain, 3:1185
    for smoking cessation, 3:1339

Hypoalbuminemia, 3:1137

Hypochromic anemia, 1:339, 3:1229

Hypodermic needles, **3:1392–1394***, 1393*

Hypodermoclysis, 2:767

Hypoglycemia
    from gastroduodenostomy, 2:577
    glucose tests for, 2:602–606
    laparoscopy and, 2:829
    reactive, 2:566

Hypokalemia, 1:447

Hypokinesis, 2:993

Hyponatremia, 1:447

Hypoparathyroidism
    electrolyte balance and, 1:447, 448
    from parathyroidectomy, 3:1098
    surgical risks of, 3:1421

Hypopharyngeal carcinoma, 3:1145–1149

Hypophysectomy, **2:697–701***, 698*

Hypopigmentation
    cryotherapy, 1:378
    laser skin resurfacing, 2:859
    laser surgery, 2:864

Hypopituitarism, 2:699

Hypoplasia, pulmonary, 1:531, 534

Hypoplastic left heart syndrome, 2:634, *2:635*

Hypospadias, 1:299, 2:701–706, *2:702*

Hypospadias repair, **2:701–706***, 702*

Hypotension
    adrenergic drugs for, 1:33
    blood pressure measurement for, 1:176, 177
    from dialysis, 2:782
    from epidural anesthesia, 1:477, 478–479
    from general anesthesia, 1:59
    orthostatic, 1:91
    in surgery, 1:182

Hypothalamic-anterior pituitary-adrenocortical axis, 1:359

Hypothermia
    for cerebral aneurysm repair, 1:274
    defined, 3:1410
    from general anesthesia, 3:1221
    heart-lung machines for, 2:628

Hypothyroidism, 3:1421–1422

Hypotony, 1:390, 3:1275, 1465

Hypoxia, 1:335, 2:647, 650

Hysterectomy, **2:706–710***, 707,* 2:1034
    abdominal, 1:332, 333, 2:708, 709, 3:1259
    for cervical cancer, 1:341, 2:706, 708
    colpotomy and, 1:331
    complications from, 3:1259
    vs. cone biopsy, 1:340
    cystocele repair and, 1:395
    demographics of, 1:332, 2:706, 1000
    vs. dilation and curettage, 1:422
    for endometriosis, 1:422, 2:706, 835
    mortality and morbidity from, 1:333, 2:1040
    vs. myomectomy, 2:1001–1002
    On-Q analgesics for, 3:1185
    oophorectomy and, 2:1038, 1040
    radical, 1:341, 2:706, 708
    salpingo-oophorectomy and, 2:706, 708, 709, 3:1256
    for sex reassignment surgery, 3:1306
    subtotal, 1:341, 2:706, 708

total, 2:708
for uterine fibroids, 2:706, 708, 711–712, 1001–1002
vaginal, 1:332, 333, 2:708–709, 3:1259
Hysterosalpingography, 3:1261
Hysteroscopic myomectomy, 2:710
Hysteroscopy, **2:710–712**
vs. dilatation and curettage, 1:422, 2:711
myomectomy and, 2:999, 1000, 1001
second-look, 3:1289
Hysterosonography, 3:1121
Hysterotomy, 1:16, 536
Hytrin. *See* Terazosin hydrochloride

I

IABP (Intra-aorta balloon pump), 2:760, 843, 1046
IBSR (International Bariatric Surgery Registry), 3:1545
Ibuprofen
activity of, 2:1028
aspirin and, 1:132
for cervical cryotherapy, 1:282
for colposcopy, 1:330
craniotomy and, 1:370
for fever, 2:1028
for gingivectomy, 2:599
for hip pain, 2:671
liver biopsy and, 2:888, 889
for pain, 3:1084
pneumonectomy and, 3:1176
pulmonary lobectomy and, 2:904
for root canal treatment, 3:1246
for shoulder pain, 3:1314
wrist replacement and, 3:1573
ICCE (Intracapsular cataract extraction), 1:509, 515, 3:1144
ICD storm, 2:739
Ice packs. *See* Cold compresses
ICSI (Intracytoplasmic sperm injection), 2:742, 3:1530
Ictal electroencephalography (EEG), 1:444
Idiopathic scoliosis, 3:1353, 1356
Idiopathic thrombocytic purpura (ITP), 1:337, 3:1364–1365
IgM antibody test, 2:893
Ileal conduit surgery, 1:504, **2:713–716**, *715*, 3:1497
Ileal resection, 3:1333–1337
Ileectomy, 3:1333–1337
Ileoanal anastomosis, 1:318, **2:717–720**, *718*, 2:725, 726
Ileoanal reservoir surgery, 2:579, **2:720–723**
Ileostomy, 1:318, 2:579, **2:723–726**, *724*
Brooke, 2:725

continent, 2:725
vs. ileoanal anastomosis, 2:717, 719, 725
ileoanal reservoir surgery and, 2:720, 721, 722
for intestinal obstruction repair, 2:764
Kock, 2:725
loop, 2:717
Iliac crest, 1:190, 196–197
Ilizarov fixator, 2:867
Image-directed stereotactic needle biopsy, 2:1025
Image-guided endoscopy, 1:461
Imaging techniques. *See* specific technique
Imipenem, 2:687
Imipramine, 3:1084
Immediate preoperative hemodilution, 3:1168, 1196, 1202
Immigrants, 2:953
Immobility and bedsores, 1:156–157
Immobilizers, 1:304, 555
Immune response
immunologic therapies for, 2:728–732
lymphocytes and, 1:337
to transfusion errors, 1:181
Immune thrombocytopenic purpura (ITP), 3:1362
Immunizations, 2:734
Immunoassay tests, 1:241, **2:726–728**
Immunoglobulin, 1:276, 3:1440
Immunologic therapies, 1:202, **2:728–732**, 3:1091
Immunonephelometry, 2:727
Immunoprecipitation, 2:727
Immunoprevention, 2:731
Immunosuppressant drugs, **2:732–736**
for heart transplantation, 2:641, 642
for islet cell transplantation, 2:777
for kidney transplantation, 2:789, 790
for liver transplantation, 2:898–899, 900
for lung transplantation, 2:921, 3:1413
for pancreas transplantation, 3:1091
side effects of, 2:633
Immunotherapy. *See* Immunologic therapies
Impaction grafting, 2:675, 811
Imperforate anus, 2:1035
Impingement syndrome, 1:121
Implant arthroplasty, 2:617
Implantable cardioverter-defibrillator, **2:736–740**, *737*, 2:998
Implants
acrylic, 2:855, 856
alloplastic, 2:968
artificial disk, 1:425
chin, 2:967–968, 969
chromium, 3:1310
cobalt, 3:1310

corneal, 2:847
dental, **1:413–416**, *414*
electrodes, 1:411, 443
endosteal, 1:415
glenoid component, 3:1310
intervertebral disk, 1:425
multi-component inflatable, 3:1124
penile, **3:1122–1125**, *1123*
PMMA, 2:855, 856
shoulder, 3:1310
silicone gel, 1:213–216, 219, 220–221, 3:1174
silicone lens, 2:855, 856
silicone rubber, 2:617
subperiosteal, 1:415
See also Breast implants; Intraocular lens implants
Impotence
from cystectomy, 1:392–393
penile prosthesis for, 3:1122–1125, *3:1123*
Imuran. *See* Azathioprine
In vitro fertilization, 2:703, **2:740–743**, *742*, 3:1530
Incentives, financial, 2:932, 933
Incision care, 1:349, **2:743–746**
Incisional biopsy, 1:210–211, 3:1473
Incisional hernia, 2:746–750, 3:1336, 1548
Incisional hernia repair, **2:746–750**, *747*
Incompetent cervix, 1:278–279
Incomplete cleft lip, 1:302–303
Incontinence
bedsores from, 1:156, 158
demographics, 3:1507
demographics of, 1:124–125
See also Fecal incontinence; Urinary incontinence
Incontinent urinary diversion, 2:713
Indapamide, 1:89, 90*t*, 91
Indemnity plans and programs, 2:908, 3:1203
Independent Practice Association (IPA), 2:933
Inderal. *See* Propranolol
Inderide, 1:90*t*
Indiana pouch, for ureteral obstruction, 3:1497
Indirect ophthalmoscopes, 3:1232
Indocin, 1:532
Indomethacin
aspirin and, 1:132
hemoglobin test and, 2:651
for heterotropic bone, 2:670
for low back pain, 2:824
Induced abortion, **1:12–18**, 2:1034
Indwelling urinary catheterization, 1:262, 263, 264, 265–266, 267
Infant-parent bonding, 2:1037
Infants
bone marrow aspiration and biopsy in, 1:190, 192
circumcision of, 1:297–300

esophageal atresia/tracheoe-
sophageal fistula repair for,
1:485–490
femoral hernia repair for, 1:527
hemangiomas in, 2:644
hip dysplasia in, 2:662
intravenous rehydration for, 2:766
low birth weight, 2:702–703, 753
meningocele repair for, 2:964–967
patent urachus repair for,
3:1101–1103
physical examination for, 3:1162
premature, 1:299, 2:644, 753, 1075
preparing for surgery, 3:1113
sulfonamides for, 3:1378
See also Newborns
Infection control programs, 2:687
Infections
amputation and, 1:46
burn-related, 3:1326
catheter-related, 2:685
central nervous system, 2:1026
from cesarean section, 1:286, 287
from compound fractures, 1:555
from cryotherapy, 1:378
from dialysis, 2:782
from dilation and curettage, 1:421
from endoscopes, 1:228
fungal, 1:277, 2:685, 686, 687
generalized, 2:685
hand surgery for, 2:619
heart-lung transplantation and,
2:633
from heart transplantation, 2:642
from hip replacement, 2:670
from hip revision surgery, 2:676
from hypophysectomy, 2:699
immunosuppressant drugs and,
2:734, 735
incision care and, 2:745
from kidney transplantation, 2:790
from knee replacement, 2:806
from knee revision surgery, 2:812
from laceration repair, 2:817, 818
from LASIK, 2:846–847
from leg lengthening and shortening, 2:870
from limb salvage, 2:874
from liposuction, 2:881
from liver transplantation, 2:899
localized, 2:685, 686
from lung transplantation, 2:921
middle ear, 2:934–936, 1002–1007
from oophorectomy, 2:1040
opportunistic, 2:899
from pacemakers, 3:1081
parasitic, 1:180, 2:685
from phacoemulsification, 3:1144
from pharyngectomy, 3:1147
from photorefractive keratectomy,
3:1160
postoperative, 1:128, 130, 269,
403–404
pulmonary, 3:1413

from spinal fusion, 3:1355
from urinary catheterization, 1:264,
267
viral, 2:642, 685, 687
white blood cell count and, 1:339
from wounds, 3:1569–1570
See also Bacterial infections; Hospital-acquired infections; Surgical
site infections; Urinary tract infections
Infectious disease markers, 3:1482
Infectious mononucleosis, 2:892–894
Infertility
from cryptorchidism, 2:1058
from cystectomy, 1:393
hysteroscopy for, 2:711
hysterosonography for, 3:1121
in vitro fertilization for, 2:740–743
myomectomy for, 2:999
obstetric and gynecologic surgery
for, 2:1033
from oophorectomy, 2:1040
salpingo-oophorectomy for, 3:1256
salpingostomy for, 3:1260, 1261
Inflammation
aspirin for, 1:132
from hip replacement, 2:670
NSAIDs for, 2:1027–1028
orthopedic surgery and, 2:1065
scar formation and, 3:1263
from sclerotherapy, 3:1283
Inflammatory bowel disease
in children, 3:1118
colorectal surgery for, 1:317–321,
2:579
colostomy for, 1:323
ileoanal reservoir surgery for, 2:720,
721
sigmoidoscopy for, 3:1315, 1317
Inflatable sphincter insertion,
1:123–128, *124*
Informed consent, **2:750–752**
children and, 3:1193
confidentiality and, 3:1106
for elective surgery, 1:439
for general anesthesia, 1:61
hospital admissions and, 3:1170
medical charts and, 2:956
patient rights and, 3:1108
preoperative, 3:1193, 1197–1198
for presurgical testing, 3:1201
second opinions and, 3:1290
Infrared coagulation, 2:655
Infraspinatus muscle, 3:1247
INFUSE Bone Graft, 1:187–188
Infusion pumps, 2:760, 1046
Inguinal hernia, **2:752–757**
in children, 2:753, 3:1119
cryptorchidism and, 2:704, 1058
hydrocelectomy and, 2:695
hypospadias repair and, 2:704
Inguinal hernia repair, **2:752–757**, *753*
Inguinal orchiectomy, 2:1053, 1054
Inhalation anesthetics, 1:60, 162

Inhalation injuries, 3:1326
Injection snoreplasty, 3:1345
Injections
for local anesthesia, 1:64, 65
syringe and needle assembly for,
3:1392–1394
Injuries. *See* Trauma; specific types of
injuries
Inner ear drainage, 1:453–456
Inotropic agents, 2:980
Inpatient surgery
aftercare for, 2:690
demographics of, 1:438, 2:689–690,
3:1200, 1386
Medicaid for, 2:952
INR values, 2:984, 985
Inspiratory flow system, 2:1074
Institute of Medicine, 2:959, 961,
3:1388
Instruments. *See* Surgical instruments
Insufflation, 2:828, 830
Insulin
cardiac catheterization and, 1:237
islet cell transplantation for,
2:776–778
measurement of, 2:604
nephrostomy and, 2:1022
ophthalmologic surgery and, 2:1050
pancreas transplantation for,
3:1089–1091
production of, 2:604
Insulin-dependent diabetes. *See* Type 1
diabetes
Insurance. *See* Health insurance
Integra, 3:1326
Integra Dermal Regeneration Template,
3:1569
Integrilin. *See* Eptifibatide
Integumentary system. *See* Skin
Intense pulsed light (IPL) systems,
3:1284
Intensive care unit equipment,
2:759–763, *761*
Intensive care units, **2:757–759**
admission to, 1:27, 3:1188
coronary, 2:759
medical errors in, 2:690
neonatal, 2:759, 760
neuromedical, 2:760
pediatric, 2:758, 759
physiologic monitoring in, 2:758,
760, 762
purpose of, 2:690
surgical, 2:759
trauma/burn, 2:760
Intensivists, 2:690, 757, 758, 762
Intercostal thoracotomy, 3:1414
Intercourse, urinary catheterization and,
1:264, 267
Interferon alfa-n1, 2:729
Interferon alfa-n3, 2:729
Interferons, 1:387, 2:728–729, 730, 731
Interleukin-2, 2:728
Interleukin-2 receptor antibodies, 2:899

Intermittent claudication, 3:1129, 1134
Intermittent peritoneal dialysis (IPD), 2:781
Intermittent urinary catheterization, 1:262, 263, 265, 267
Internal hemorrhoids, 2:655
International Bariatric Surgery Registry (IBSR), 3:1545
International Islet Transplant Registry, 2:776
Interns, 3:1167, 1388
Interpositional reconstruction, 1:116–120
Interpreters, 3:1166
Interstitial cystitis
    bladder augmentation for, 3:1255
    cystectomy for, 1:391
    cystoscopy for, 1:400
    sacral nerve stimulation for, 3:1253–1256
Intervertebral disk
    compression, 2:819–820
    degeneration of, 3:1353–1354
    disk removal for, 1:424–427
    herniated, 2:820, 822, 995–997, 1026, 3:1353–1354
    implants, 1:425
    myelography of, 2:995–997
    spinal fusion for, 3:1353–1355
Interview, clinical, 2:625
Intestinal bleeding, 2:948
Intestinal cancer, 2:763, 3:1333
    See also Colorectal cancer
Intestinal decompression, 2:764, 765, 769
Intestinal obstruction
    bowel resection for, 1:205–206
    in children, 3:1116
    intussusception reduction for, **2:767–770**
    laxatives and, 2:865
    repair, 2:763–765
    small bowel resection for, 3:1333–1334, 1336
Intestinal obstruction repair, **2:763–765**
Intestinal polyps
    in children, 3:1117
    demographics of, 3:1335
    sigmoidoscopy for, 3:1317
    small bowel resection for, 3:1334–1335
Intestinal resection. See Bowel resection
Intestines
    clearance of, 3:1192
    incarcerated/strangulated, 2:749
    inguinal hernia and, 2:754
    intussusception of, 2:763, 764, **2:767–770,** 3:1116
    leakage, 2:573
    strangulated, 2:765
    transplants, 3:1444
    See also Large intestines
Intra-aorta balloon pump (IABP), 2:760, 843, 1046

Intracapsular cataract extraction (ICCE), 1:509, 515, 3:1144
Intracardiac pressure measurement, 1:238, 239, 243
Intracerebral hematoma, 2:1024
Intracranial aneurysm, 1:70, 2:1024–1025
Intracranial hypertension, 1:369, 2:760, 1046
Intracytoplasmic sperm injection (ICSI), 2:742, 3:1530
Intraocular eye melanoma, 1:474
Intraocular lens implants
    dislocation of, 3:1144
    extracapsular extraction for, 1:509–516
    foldable, 3:1140, 1141
    laser posterior capsulotomy for, 2:854, 855, 856
Intraocular lens opacification, 2:852–853, 854–857
Intraocular pressure (IOP)
    aquaflow collagen wick for, 3:1275
    from cataract surgery, 1:514
    cataracts and, 1:512
    closed-angle glaucoma and, 2:773
    cyclocryotherapy for, 1:388–391
    glaucoma, 3:1431, 1433
    goniotomy for, 2:607, 608, 609
    laser iridotomy for, 2:848–854
    laser posterior capsulotomy for, 2:855–856
    melanoma of the iris and, 2:774
    non-surgical treatment of, 2:851, 3:1275
    nonpenetrating deep sclerectomy for, 3:1275
    peripheral iridoplasty for, 2:742
    sclerostomy for, 3:1271–1277
    tests for, 3:1154
    tube-shunt surgery, 3:1463–1466
    viscocanalostomy for, 3:1275
Intraoperative blood collection, 3:1168, 1196, 1202
Intraoperative blood salvage, 1:135
Intraoperative period
    aseptic technique for, 1:129–130
    complications from, 1:404
    pain management for, 3:1185
    surgical team for, 3:1385
Intraperitoneal fluid, 2:838
Intrastromal corneal rings, 1:345
Intrauterine devices (IUD), 1:240, 2:711
Intrauterine growth retardation (IUGR), 3:1509
Intravenous anesthetics, 1:60–61, 162
Intravenous pyelogram, 2:884, 1018
Intravenous rehydration, **2:766–767**
Intravesical medications, 3:1255
Intrinsic sphincter deficiency (ISD)
    needle bladder neck suspension for, 2:1010–1011, 1012
    non-surgical treatment of, 3:1332

retropubic suspension for, 3:1234, 1236
    sling procedure for, 2:1011, 3:1237, 1330, 1331
Intron A, 2:729
Intropin. See Dopamine
Intubation
    for anesthesia, 1:62
    complications from, 1:404
    endotracheal, 1:375, **1:463–465,** 464, 2:685, 687
Intussusception
    intestinal, 2:763, 764, 767–770, 3:1116
    rectal, 3:1222
Intussusception reduction, 2:767–769, **2:767–770,** 768
Inventional neuroradiology, 1:275
Involution process, 2:644–645, 646
Iodine
    allergies to, 1:115, 237, 2:659
    for angiography, 1:68
    for arthrography, 1:115–116
    for CT scans, 1:383
Iodine tincture, 1:94
Iontophoresis, pilocarpine, 1:448
IOP. See Intraocular pressure
Iowa system, 1:303
IPD (Intermittent peritoneal dialysis), 2:781
IPL systems, 3:1284
IPO (Independent Practice Association), 2:933
Irbesartan, 1:89
Iridectomy, **2:770–776,** 771, 2:853, 3:1432–1433
Iridoplasty, argon laser peripheral, 2:853
Iridotomy, laser, 2:772–773, 2:775, **848–854,** 849
Iris capture, 2:854
Iris melanoma, 2:770–776
Iris plateau, 2:849, 850
Iritis, 2:856
Iron deficiency
    blood tests for, 1:335, 339
    fluoroquinolones and, 1:547
    from phlebotomy, 3:1151
Iron-deficiency anemia, 1:97, 336, 3:1228–1229
Iron lung, 2:945
Iron supplements
    colonoscopy and, 1:315
    sigmoidoscopy and, 3:1316
Iron surplus, 3:1150–1152
Irradiation. See Radiation therapy
Irregular heart rhythm. See Arrhythmia
Irrigation
    bladder, 3:1451
    wound, 2:817
Ischemic colitis, 2:763
Ischemic stroke, 1:254

Ischemic stroke

ISHLT (Registry of the International Society for Heart and Lung Transplantation), 2:643
Islam and circumcision, 1:297
Islet cell transplantation, **2:776–778,** 3:1091
Ismelin. *See* Guanethidine
Isoflurane, 1:60
Isolation units
  aseptic technique for, 1:130
  for bone marrow transplantation, *1:194,* 1:200
  for hospital-acquired infection control, 2:687
Isometric exercise, 1:523
Isoniazid
  acetaminophen and, 1:22
  alprazolam and, 1:80
  diazepam and, 2:995
Isoproterenol, 1:33
Isoptin. *See* Verapamil
Isosulfan blue, 2:988
Isotretinoin, 3:1266
Isoxsuprine, 1:89
Isradipine, 1:90*t*
ITP (Immune thrombocytopenic purpura), 3:1362, 1364–1365
Itraconazole
  buspirone and, 1:80
  gastric acid inhibitors and, 2:569
  for hospital-acquired infections, 2:687
IUD (Intrauterine devices), 1:240, 2:711
IUGR (Intrauterine growth retardation), 3:1509
IV rehydration, **2:766–767**
IVF. *See* In vitro fertilization
Ivor-Lewis esophagectomy, 1:495

J

J-pouch, 2:720
Jacobson, Jules, 2:970
Jamshidi needles, 1:190, 2:886
Jarcho-Levin syndrome, 3:1557
Jaundice
  from liver failure, 2:895
  liver function tests for, 2:892–894
  neonatal, 3:1118
Jaw injuries, 1:374
Jawbone, *1:413,* 1:414, 415, 2:967
JCAHO. *See* Joint Commission on Accreditation of Healthcare Organizations
Jehovah's Witnesses, 1:178, 180
Jejunectomy, 3:1333–1337
Jejunostomy, 3:1092
Jejunum, 2:572, 3:1333–1337
JOAG (Juvenile-onset open angle glaucoma), 2:607, 608
Jobst stockings, 3:1325

Jogging, 2:801–802
Johns, Murray, 3:1345
Joint aspiration, 2:668
Joint Commission on Accreditation of Healthcare Organizations (JCAHO)
  accreditation by, 3:1195
  on ambulatory surgery centers, 1:38, 2:595, 1047, 1072
  on blood registries, 1:172
  on complications, 3:1388
  on confidentiality, 3:1106
  on hospital accreditation, 1:540
  on nursing homes, 2:1030
  on patient rights, 3:1109
  on postoperative complications, 1:404
Joint contractures, 2:870
Joint disorders
  arthrography for, 1:115–116
  bone x rays for, 1:203–204
  magnetic resonance imaging for, 1:115, 2:926
  non-surgical treatment of, 1:119–120, 122
  See also Arthroplasty; Arthroscopic surgery; Dislocations
Joint pain
  arthroplasty for, 1:116–120
  hip, 2:664, 666–668, 671–672, 673
  shoulder, 3:1247–1251, 1308–1312, 1314
  See also Knee pain
Joint radiography. *See* Arthrography
Joint replacement
  shoulder, **3:1308–1312,** 3:1314
  surgeon skill level for, 1:540
  total, 1:116–120, 507
  See also Hip replacement; Knee replacement; Revision surgery
Joint resection. *See* Arthroplasty
Joint x rays. *See* Arthrography
Joints, tendon repair and, 3:1399–1403
Judaism
  circumcision and, 1:297, 299, 300
  hospices and, 2:683
Juvenile diabetes. *See* Type 1 diabetes
Juvenile-onset open angle glaucoma (JOAG), 2:607, 608

K

K/DOQI (Kidney Disease Outcomes Quality Initiative), 2:783
K-ras mutations, in lung cancer, 3:1412
K-wires, 1:543
Kabikinase. *See* Streptokinase
Kamami, Yves-Victor, 3:1344
Kanamycin
  for bowel resection, 1:207
  for colorectal surgery, 1:319
  for colostomy, 1:323
  for rectal resection, 3:1227
  for small bowel resection, 3:1335

Kaposi's sarcoma, 2:729
Kava kava, 1:57
Keflex. *See* Cephalexin
Kefzol. *See* Cefazolin
Kegel exercises, 1:328, 398, 482, 3:1237
Kelman, Charles, 3:1140
Keloid scars
  from cleft lip repair, 1:305
  from dermabrasion, 1:418
  vs. hypertrophic scars, 3:1264
  laser skin resurfacing for, 3:1265
  from mastectomy, 2:989
  non-surgical treatment of, 3:1266
  scar revision surgery for, 3:1263–1267
  from wounds, 3:1570
Kenalog, 2:1069
Keratectomy, photorefractive, 1:345, 2:848, **3:1157–1161,** *1158*
Keratinocytes, 3:1323
Keratitis, nonspecific diffuse intralamellar, 2:846
Keratoconus, 1:342, 344, 345
Keratometer, 1:513, 2:844, 1049
Keratopathy, pseudophakic bullous, 1:342, 344
Keratoplasty, **1:342–346,** *343*
  conductive, 2:847
  lamellar, 1:343
  laser thermal, 2:848
  penetrating, 1:343
Keratotomy
  astigmatic, 2:848, 3:1160
  radial, 2:848, 3:1160
Ketamine, 1:60, 61, 164
Ketoconazole
  alprazolam and, 1:80
  for cortisol production, 2:700
  diazepam and, 2:995
  gastric acid inhibitors and, 2:569
  for hospital-acquired infections, 2:687
Ketones, 2:604, 3:1499, 1501
Ketoprofen, 1:282, 3:1084
Ketorolac
  for acute pain, 2:1027–1028
  for analgesia, 1:51
  side effects of, 3:1186
  for sling procedure, 3:1332
Keyhole incision, 3:1320
Kidney angiography, 1:70
Kidney cancer, 2:1014, 1015, 3:1506
Kidney defects, 1:487
  See also Kidney failure; Kidney injuries
Kidney dialysis, **2:779–783,** *780*
  arteriovenous fistula for, **1:111–115**
  hemodialysis, **1:111–115,** 2:779–783
  mortality from, 1:114
  peritoneal, 1:112, 2:779–783, 3:1317
Kidney disease
  abdominal ultrasound for, 1:2, *1:2*

anemia from, 1:339
anesthesia evaluation and, 1:57, 58
ascites from, 3:1095–1096
cephalosporins and, 1:270
hemoperfusion for, 2:652–653
ileal conduit surgery and, 2:713
immunosuppressant drugs and,
2:735
from immunosuppressive agents,
2:633
peritoneovenous shunts for, 3:1137
tests for, 2:783–786
See also End-stage renal disease
Kidney Disease Outcomes Quality Initiative (K/DOQI), 2:783
Kidney failure
demographics of, 1:114
diabetes and, 2:783
dialysis for, 2:779–783
electrolyte balance and, 1:447
hemodialysis for, 1:111–115
kidney transplantation for,
2:786–791, 3:1091
Medicare for, 2:963
mortality rates for, 1:453
nephrectomy for, 2:1013–1016
from nonsteroidal anti-inflammatory
drugs (NSAIDs), 3:1186
thoracic aneurysms and, 1:103
Kidney function tests, 1:112–113,
2:783–786
Kidney injuries, 1:166, 168
Kidney removal. *See* Nephrectomy
Kidney stones
cystoscopy for, 1:399
demographics of, 2:1017–1018,
1022
diagnosis of, 2:1018
lithotripsy for, 2:882–886, *2:883,*
2:1019, 1020
non-surgical treatment of, 2:885,
1020
percutaneous nephrolithotomy for,
2:1016–1021, *2:1017,* 3:1289
risk factors for, 2:1016
Kidney surgery, laparoscopic, 3:1507
See also Kidney transplantation;
Nephrectomy
Kidney transplantation, **2:786–791,**
787, 3:1444, 1445, 1448
dialysis and, 2:779
human leukocyte antigen test for,
2:692
living donors for, 2:789, 790, 1013,
1015
nephrectomy for, 2:788, 1013, 1014
with pancreas transplantation,
3:1090, 1091
surgical team for, 3:1386
waiting list for, 2:783
Knee
amputation above, *1:44,* 1:46
anatomy of, 2:800
bone grafts, 1:187

dislocations, 2:792–793, 795
instability, 2:797–799, 800, 807
Knee arthrodesis, 2:812–813
Knee arthroplasty. *See* Knee replacement
Knee arthroscopic surgery, 1:120–123,
2:791–797, *792, 794*
Knee injuries
arthroscopic surgery for, 2:791–797
causes of, 2:800–802, 812
knee replacement for, 2:800
non-surgical treatment of, 2:796,
812
Knee ligaments, 2:791–792, 793, 795,
800, 815
Knee osteotomy, **2:797–799**
Knee pain
arthroscopic surgery for, 2:791–797
knee osteotomy for, 2:797–799
knee replacement for, 2:799–809
knee revision surgery for,
2:809–814
non-surgical treatment of, 2:807
Knee prosthesis, **2:799–809,** 2:809–814
Knee replacement, 1:116–120,
2:799–809, *801*
aftercare for, 2:805–806
bilateral, 2:802, 806
costs of, 2:804
demographics of, 2:802, 810
description of, 2:802
knee revision surgery after, 2:806,
809–814
mortality and morbidity from,
2:806–807
preparation for, 2:802–805
purpose of, 2:800–803
risks of, 2:806
total, 2:800, *2:803,* 2:814
Knee revision surgery, 2:806,
2:809–814
Kneecap, 2:800, 802, 811
dislocations, 2:814, 815
fractures, 2:814, 815
tendons, 2:814, 815
Kneecap removal, **2:814–816**
Knees, tendon repair, 3:1399–1400
Knife wounds, 1:372
Kock ileostomy, 2:725
Konsil. *See* Psyllium
Kt/V test, 2:783
KTP 532nm lasers, 3:1284
Kübler-Ross, Elisabeth, 2:682
Kyphosis, 3:1355
Kytril. *See* Granisetron

L

Labetalol, 1:89, 90*t,* 91
Labia minora, 1:263
Labor
epidural anesthesia for, 1:477–479

episiotomy and, 1:479–483, *1:481*
induced, 1:16
non-progressive, 1:283, 287
trial of, 1:287
See also Childbirth; Premature labor
Laboratory tests
for anesthesia evaluation, 1:57–58
Medicare for, 2:963
preoperative, 3:1192, 1198,
1200–1203
See also specific types of tests
Labyrinthectomy, 1:455
Laceration repair, **2:817–819**
Lactate, 1:276, 277
Lactate dehydrogenase (LDH), 1:276,
277, 2:890–895
Lactation. *See* Breastfeeding
Lactulose, 2:865, 866
Laënnec, René, 3:1373
Lamellar keratoplasty, 1:343
Laminectomy, **2:819–827,** *821*
Laminotomy, 2:825–826
Lanoxin. *See* Digoxin
Lansoprazole, 1:98, 2:568
Lap-band gastric restrictive procedure,
2:574, 3:1549
Laparoscopic vertical banded gastroplasty (LVBG), 3:1545–1546
Laparoscopy, *2:827,* **827–833,** *829,*
3:1387
adrenalectomy, 1:28, 30, 31
advances in, 2:580–581
antrectomy, 1:96
appendectomy, 1:107, 108
benefits of, 2:594
bowel resection, 1:206–207, 208
cholecystectomy, 1:293–297, 2:558,
580, 3:1118, 1399
colonoscopy, 1:325
colorectal, 1:318–319
cystocele repair, 1:397
for endometriosis, **2:833–835,** *834*
esophagectomy, 1:495
femoral hernia repair, 1:527,
529–530
fundoplication, 2:580, 586–591
gallstone removal, 2:558
gastrectomy, 2:564
gastric bypass, 2:571, 572
hydrocelectomy, 2:695
hysterectomy, 2:708–709, 3:1259
hysteroscopy, 2:712
ileoanal reservoir surgery,
2:720–721
in vitro fertilization, 2:741
incisional hernia repair, 2:748, 749,
750
inguinal hernia repair, 2:755, 756
intestinal obstruction repair, 2:764
intussusception reduction, 2:769
iridectomy, 2:772–773
vs. laparotomy, 2:832, 838
local anesthesia for, 1:64
lymphadenectomy, 2:923

Meckel's diverticulectomy, 2:948
myomectomy, 2:710, 999, 1000, 1001
needle bladder neck suspension, 2:1011
nephrectomy, 2:788, 1013, 1015
oophorectomy, 2:1039
pain management for, 3:1185
pancreatectomy, 3:1092
parathyroidectomy, 2:828
radiofrequency ablation, 2:828
rectal prolapse repair, 3:1223, 1224
retropubic suspension, 3:1234, 1236, 1237
robot-assisted, 2:1046, 3:1243–1244
salpingo-oophorectomy, 3:1258
salpingostomy, 3:1260–1261
second-look, 3:1289
small bowel resection, 3:1335
splenectomy, 3:1363
for stomach cancer, 2:577
surgical mesh in, 3:1487
telesurgery and, 3:1398
thyroidectomy, 2:828
tubal ligation, 1:333, 3:1461
Laparotomy
exploratory, **2:836–839**, *837*
for intestinal obstruction repair, 2:764
for intussusception reduction, 2:768
vs. laparoscopy, 2:832, 838
for salpingostomy, 3:1260, 1261
second-look, 3:1289
Large bowels. *See* Large intestines
Large-core needle biopsy, 1:211
Large intestine cancer, 1:159
See also Colorectal cancer
Large intestine obstruction. *See* Intestinal obstruction
Large intestine resection. *See* Bowel resection
Large intestines
anatomy of, 1:204–205
barium enema of, 1:153–155
See also Colon
Laryngeal cancer, 2:839–841, 3:1145
Laryngeal injuries, 1:374
Laryngeal mask airway, 1:62, 465
Laryngeal nerve damage, 2:917, 3:1098
Laryngectomy, 1:433, **2:839–841,** 3:1146
Laryngopharyngectomy, 3:1145, 1146
Laryngoscope, McCoy, 1:62
Laryngoscopy
for endotracheal intubation, 1:463–465
esophagectomy and, 1:495
with esophagoscopy and bronchoscopy, 1:434
for pharyngectomy, 3:1146
Laser-assisted myringotomy, 2:1005
Laser-assisted uvulopalatoplasty (LAUP), 1:434, 3:1344, 1345, 1347
Laser doppler measurements, 1:45

Laser in-situ keratomileusis (LASIK), **2:841–848**, *842, 843*, 2:1048
retinal detachment from, 3:1153
vs. photorefractive keratectomy, 2:848, 3:1157–1158, 1160
Laser iridotomy, 2:772–773, 775, **2:848–854**, *849*
Laser photocoagulation. *See* Photocoagulation therapy
Laser posterior capsulotomy, 1:513, **2:854–857**
Laser skin resurfacing, **2:857–859**
costs of, 3:1263
demographics of, 3:1263
vs. dermabrasion, 1:416, 418
for scar revision, 3:1265
Laser surgery, **2:859–864**, *861*
for actinic keratoses, 1:387
for adenoidectomy, 1:24
for cervical dysplasia, 1:282, 329
coherent ultrapulse carbon dioxide, 1:523
conization, 1:341
cost of, 1:39
for esophageal cancer, 1:498
goniotomy, 2:610
for hemangiomas, 2:646
for hemorrhoids, 2:655
hot spots from, 2:846
iridectomy, 2:771, 775
for peptic ulcers, 1:98
for skin cancer, 1:387
for smoking cessation, 3:1339
for spider nevi, 3:1282
for spider veins, 3:1284
trabeculoplasty, 1:388, 2:850
for vision loss, 1:438
Laser thermal keratoplasty, 2:848
Laser trabeculoplasty, 3:1433
Lasers, 2:1046–1047
alexandrite, 3:1284
arthroscopic surgery and, 1:121
for bronchoscopy, 2:1075
erbium, 1:418
Er:YAG, 2:858, 859, 3:1265, 1272
excimer, 1:345, 2:1049, 3:1157
KTP 532nm, 3:1284
pulsed dye, 3:1265
See also Argon lasers; Carbon dioxide lasers; Nd:YAG lasers
Lash cerclage, 1:279
LASIK (Laser in-situ keratomileusis), 1:160, **2:841–848**, *842, 843*, 2:1048, 3:1157–1158
Lasix. *See* Furosemide
Lateral collateral ligament (LCL), 2:791–792, 793
Lateral release. *See* Knee arthroscopic surgery
Latex allergies, 3:1192
Latex catheters, 1:263, 266
Latissimus dorsi flaps, 1:220, 221
Laughing gas. *See* Nitrous oxide

LAUP (Laser-assisted uvulopalatoplasty), 1:434, 3:1344, 1345, 1347
Lavage
bronchioalveolar, 1:226–227
knee arthroscopic surgery and, 2:794, 796
LaVeen shunts, 3:1138
Lavender, 3:1348
Laxatives, **2:864–866**
after transurethral resection of the prostate, 3:1456
bulk-producing, 2:865
for colonoscopy, 1:315
emollient, 2:865
hyperosmotic, 2:865
nitrofurantoin and, 3:1504–1505
for rectal prolapse, 3:1224
for sigmoidoscopy, 3:1316
stimulant, 2:865
vitamin K and, 1:89
LCL (Lateral collateral ligament), 2:791–792, 793
LDH (Lactate dehydrogenase), 1:276, 277, 2:890–895
Le Fort, René, 1:363
Le Fort fractures, 1:363, 365, 366
Lead points, 2:767
Leak point pressure test, 3:1332
Leape, Lucian, 2:959
Lecithin tests, 2:875, 877
LED (Light-emitting diodes), 3:1207–1208
Leech therapy, 2:974
LEEP (Loop electrocautery excision procedure), 1:282, 341
Left heart syndrome, hypoplastic, 2:634, *2:635*
Left-to-right atrial shunts, 1:239
Left-to-right ventricular shunts, 1:239
Left ventricular assist devices (LVAD), 3:1540, 1541
Leg amputation, 1:43–47
Leg arteries, 3:1128–1131, 1132–1136
Leg length
hip replacement and, 2:670
hip revision surgery and, 2:676
knee revision surgery and, 2:812
Leg lengthening, **2:866–872**, *867, 868*
Leg pain, 1:426
Leg pumps, 3:1539
Leg shortening, **2:866–872**, *867*
Leg vein phlebography, **3:1149–1150**
Legal issues
Certificate of Need laws, 2:689
in confidentiality, 3:1106–1108
in home care, 2:680
medical charts and, 2:955–959
patient rights and, 3:1108–1109
See also Informed consent; Living wills; Power of attorney
Leiomyomas, 1:419
Leiomyosarcoma, 2:564, 3:1336
Length of stay, 2:679, 689
Lengthening, leg, **2:866–872**, *867, 868*

Lens, crystalline, 1:510
Lens opacification
    from laser iridotomy, 2:852–853
    laser posterior capsulotomy for,
        2:854–857
    See also Intraocular lens implants
Leonard, Alfred, 3:1111
Leonard procedure, 3:1111
Lepirudin, 1:86
Leukemia
    anemia from, 1:339
    bone marrow aspiration for, 1:192
    bone marrow biopsy for, 1:189
    granulocytic, 1:337, 2:742
    gum disease and, 2:599
    liver function tests for, 2:892
    thrombocytopenia from, 1:337
    white blood cell count and, 1:339
Leukeran. *See* Chlorambucil
Leukine. *See* Sargramostim
Leukocyte count. *See* White blood cell
    count
Leuprolide, 2:1001
Levaquin. *See* Ofloxacin
Levo-Dromoran. *See* Levorphanol
Levodopa
    benzodiazepines and, 1:80
    deep brain stimulation and, 1:410,
        411
Levophed. *See* Norepinephrine
Levorphanol, 1:53*t*
Liability, informed consent and, 2:752
    See also Legal issues
Libritabs. *See* Chlordiazepoxide
Librium. *See* Chlordiazepoxide
Licensure
    nursing homes, 2:1030
    surgeons, 1:539, 540
Lidocaine
    for bone marrow aspiration and
        biopsy, 1:190
    for circumcision, 1:299
    for curettage and electrosurgery,
        1:386
    elderly and, 1:63
    for epidural anesthesia, 1:477
    for laceration repair, 2:817
    for Mohs surgery, 2:990
    for pericardiocentesis, 3:1126
    for topical anesthesia, 1:65
Life, quality of, 2:623, 907, 3:1342
Life expectancy, 3:1204, 1338
Life support equipment, 2:760
Life-sustaining treatment, 1:430–432,
    2:901–902
Life-threatening medical conditions,
    2:1009
Lifestyle, 1:507, 508, 2:820
Lifestyle changes
    arrhythmia, 2:939, 940
    coronary artery bypass graft surgery,
        1:352
    coronary artery disease, 1:349, 350,
        355, 471–473

knee replacement, 2:805, 807
    snoring, 3:1347–1348
Lifting, 2:750, 820, 822
Ligaments
    grafting, 2:793, 795, 796
    knee, 2:791–792, 793, 795, 800, 815
    toe, 2:617
Ligamentum flavum, 2:822
Light-emitting diodes (LED),
    3:1207–1208
Limb length discrepancy, 2:866–872,
    2:867, 868
Limb salvage, **2:872–875**
Limbs, artificial, 2:1064
Lincomycin, 1:82
Lincosamindes, 1:82
Linear accelerator-based machine,
    3:1369
Linear salpingostomy, 3:1260
Linkage analysis, 2:691–692
Lioresal. *See* Baclofen
Lip, cleft, 1:300–305, *1:302*
Lip cancer, 2:633
Lip reading, 1:310
Lipectomy, suction-assisted. *See* Lipo-
    suction
Lipid tests, **2:875–878**
Lipoma, 2:619
Lipoplasty. *See* Abdominoplasty; Lipo-
    suction
Lipoprotein levels
    coronary artery disease and, 1:352,
        472
    lipid tests for, 2:875–878
    liver function tests for, 2:893
Liposhaving, 2:878, 879
Liposuction, **2:878–882**, *879, 880*
    abdominoplasty and, 1:9, 12
    for breast reduction, 1:223
    face lift and, 1:521
    facial, 2:967, 969
Liquid diet, 1:208
Liquid-in-glass thermometers,
    3:1409–1410
Liquid nitrogen, 1:377, 380
Liquid oxygen, 2:1074
Liquid tissue glues, 2:744
Lisinopril, 1:90t
Lisinopril hydrochlorothiazide, 1:90t
Lithium, 1:430, 2:1028
Litholysis, oral bile acid, 2:558
Lithotripsy, extracorporeal shock wave,
    2:558, 559, **2:882–886**, *883*, 2:1019,
    1020
Littre's hernia, 2:948
Liver biopsy, **2:886–890**, *887*
Liver cancer
    angioma, 2:888
    biliary stenting for, 1:159
    cryotherapy for, 1:377, 378
    demographics of, 2:657,
        3:1137–1138, 1294
    hepatectomy for, 2:657–661
    liver biopsy for, 2:886, 888, 889

liver function tests for, 2:891,
    892–894
    localized resectable, 2:657
    mortality and morbidity from,
        2:660, 3:1297
    segmentectomy for, 3:1294
Liver damage, 1:404, 2:994
Liver disease
    abdominal ultrasound for, 1:1
    anemia and, 1:336, 339, 3:1228
    anesthesia evaluation and, 1:57, 58
    ascites from, 3:1095
    cephalosporins and, 1:270
    costs of, 2:580
    demographics of, 2:900
    endoscopic retrograde cholan-
        giopancreatography for,
        1:456–459
    esophageal varices from, 3:1277,
        1278
    immunosuppressant drugs and,
        2:735
    laxatives and, 2:865
    liver biopsy for, 2:886–890, *2:887*
    liver function tests for, 2:890–895
    obstructive, 2:891–894
    peritoneovenous shunts for,
        3:1137–1140
Liver encephalopathy, 2:892, 895
Liver failure
    after hepatectomy, 2:660
    fulminant, 2:895
    hemoperfusion for, 2:652
    liver function tests for, 2:893
    liver transplantation for, 2:895–901
    portal vein bypass surgery for,
        3:1179
Liver function tests, **2:890–895**
Liver transplantation, **2:895–901**,
    3:1444, 1445, 1448
    angiography for, 1:70
    for ascites, 3:1139
    for biliary atresia, 3:1118
    for esophageal varices, 3:1279
    hepatectomy and, 2:657, 659
    heterotopic, 2:896
    human leukocyte antigen test for,
        2:692
    liver biopsy for, 2:886
    orthotopic, 2:896
    for portal hypertension, 3:1181
    reduced-size, 2:896
    transfusion for, 1:181
Living organ donors, 2:789, 790, 1013,
    1015
Living wills, **2:901–902**
    DNR orders and, 1:431
    emergency surgery and, 1:453
    health care proxy and, 2:622–623
    hospital admissions and, 1:27
    purpose of, 1:404
Load and shift test, 1:148
Lobectomy
    anterior temporal, 1:75–78

hepatic, 2:657–661, *2:658*
lung, 3:1414
partial anterior temporal, 2:1026
pulmonary, **2:902–906,** 3:1295
temporal, 1:359, 2:1026
Local anesthesia, **1:63–66,** 3:1387
for circumcision, 1:299
for dermabrasion, 1:417
for hair transplantation, 2:614
informed consent and, 1:61
for phacoemulsification, 3:1143,
1144
tumescent (wet), 2:878, 880
Localization procedures, 2:912
Localized infections, 2:685, 686
Localized resectable liver cancer, 2:657
Lodine. *See* Etodolac
Lomefloxacin, 1:82, 546
Lomotil. *See* Diphenoxylate-atropine
Long QT syndrome, 2:736
Long Term Care Accreditation Pro-
gram, 2:1030
Long-term care insurance, **2:906–910,**
2:953, 1030, 3:1203
Longevity, 3:1204
Loniten. *See* Minoxidil
Loop colostomy, 1:323
Loop diuretics, 1:428
Loop electrocautery excision procedure
(LEEP), 1:282, 341
Loop ileostomy, 2:717
Loose skin abdominoplasty, 1:7
Lopressor. *See* Metoprolol
Lorazepam, 1:78, 79, 79*t*
Lordosis, 3:1355
Lortab. *See* Hydrocodone-aceta-
minophen
Losartan, 1:89
Lotensin. *See* Benazepril
Loupes, surgical, 1:543, 2:971
Low back pain
causes of, 2:820
demographics of, 2:822
diagnosis of, 2:822–823
laminectomy for, 2:819–827
non-surgical treatment of,
2:824–825
Low birth weight infants, 2:702–703,
753
Low blood pressure. *See* Hypotension
Low-density lipoproteins, 2:875–878,
893
Low-fiber diet, 1:494
Low laser irradiation, 1:408
Low-salt diet, 1:455, 2:750
Low transverse incision, 1:283, 285
Lower esophageal sphincters,
2:586–590
Lower extremity amputation, **1:43–47**
Lower GI exam. *See* Barium enema
Lower urinary tract symptoms (LUTS),
2:1041, 1042
Lozenges, nicotine, 3:1340
Lozol. *See* Indapamide

Lubricating gels, 1:263, 266
Lucilia sericata, 1:407
Luer-lock nozzles, 3:1392
Lumbar laminectomy, 2:820, 824
Lumbar puncture, 1:273, 276, 277,
2:1025
See also Cerebrospinal fluid (CSF)
analysis
Lumbar spine, 2:819, 820
Lumpectomy, **2:910–913,** *911*
axillary dissection and, 1:138,
2:910–913
radiation therapy and, 2:910–911,
913, 3:1319
vs. simple mastectomy, 2:913,
3:1318, 1320
Lung
abscess, *1:19,* 2:904
collapsed, 2:904, 916–917
congenital cystic adenomatoid malformation of, 1:531, 532, 533
fibrosis, 2:914, 918, 919, 3:1358,
1359
infections, 2:914–918
See also Pneumothorax
Lung biopsy, **2:914–918**
Lung cancer
bronchoscopy for, 1:225
chest x ray for, 1:291, 292–293
cryotherapy for, 1:377
CT scans for, 1:384, 2:918
demographics of, 1:226, 2:903, 914,
3:1175, 1294, 1383
diagnosis of, 3:1295
liver function tests for, 2:894
lung biopsy for, 2:914–918
mediastinoscopy for, 2:949–952
metastatic, 3:1176
mortality and morbidity from,
3:1297–1298
non-small cell, 3:1177, 1295
non-surgical treatment of, 2:905,
3:1177
pneumonectomy for, 3:1175–1179
positron emission tomography for,
3:1176
pulmonary lobectomy for,
2:902–906
segmentectomy for, 3:1294–1298
small cell, 3:1177, 1295
from smoking, 3:1241
soft tissue sarcoma, 2:873
thoracic surgery for, 3:1411–1412
thoracotomy for, 3:1413, 1414
throat cancer and, 3:1147
Lung disease
anesthesia evaluation and, 1:56
angiography for, 1:70
bronchoscopy for, 1:225–229
chest x ray for, 1:291–293
demographics of, 3:1175
intensive care units and, 2:759
smoking and, 3:1338
Lung function tests, 3:1358–1360, 1372

Lung maturity tests, fetal, 2:875, 876,
877
Lung transplantation, 2:905,
2:918–922, *919,* 3:1178, 1412–1413,
1444, 1445, 1448
Lung volume reduction surgery
(LVRS), 2:905, 3:1177, 1178, 1412
Lupron. *See* Leuprolide
Lupus, systemic erythematosus, 1:271
Luque rods, 3:1356
LUTS (Lower urinary tract symptoms),
2:1041, 1042
LVAD. *See* Left ventricular assist devices
LVBG. *See* Laparoscopic vertical banded gastroplasty
LVRS. *See* Lung volume reduction
surgery
Lyme disease, 1:180, 2:727
Lymph node biopsy. *See* Sentinel
lymph node biopsy
Lymph node dissection
esophageal resection and,
1:493–499
gastrectomy and, 2:564
lumpectomy and, 2:910–913
lymphadenectomy, 2:922–924
prophylactic, 3:1301
radical neck dissection and, 3:1217
regional, 3:1383
See also Axillary dissection; Sentinel lymph node biopsy
Lymph nodes
breast cancer and, 2:988
cancer invasion and, 3:1473
CT scans of, 1:384
tongue cancer and, 2:600, 602
Lymphadenectomy, **2:922–924**
Lymphadenitis, 3:1119
Lymphedema
from axillary dissection, 1:138,
2:913, 3:1214
from lymphadenectomy, 2:923–924
from sentinel lymph node biopsy,
3:1301
from simple mastectomy, 3:1321
surgery for, 3:1523
Lymphocyte crossmatch test, 2:692
Lymphocytes, 1:335, 336, 337
Lymphoma
bone marrow aspiration for, 1:192
CT scans for, 1:384
demographics of, 3:1383
heart-lung transplantation and,
2:633
Hodgkin's, 1:189, 2:894, 951,
3:1362
liver function tests for, 2:892, 894
mediastinoscopy for, 2:949–952
non-Hodgkin's, 1:189, 3:1383
small intestine, 3:1333, 1335
stomach, 2:564
thrombocytopenia from, 1:337
Lymphoscintigraphy, 3:1300

Lysis, 2:764
Lysodren. *See* Mitotane

M

M-mode ultrasound, 1:3
Macrobid, 3:1456
Macrocytic anemia, 1:336, 339, 3:1228–1229
Macrolides, 1:81–82, 83
Macromastia, 1:222–225
Macroplastique, 1:311
Macula, 3:1152
Macular edema, 1:514, 2:852, 856
Macular holes, 2:856
Maggot therapy, 1:407
Magill forceps, 1:23
Magnesium, 1:447–448
Magnesium-based antacids, 1:447
Magnesium citrate, 2:865
Magnesium salicylate, 1:131
Magnesium sulfate, 1:280, 532, 2:865, 866
Magnesium supplements, 3:1146–1147
Magnetic fields, 2:928
Magnetic resonance angiography (MRA), 1:70–71, 2:925, 927, 3:1130, 1135
Magnetic resonance cholangiopancreatography, 1:458
Magnetic resonance imaging (MRI), **2:925–929**, *926*
    for adrenalectomy, 1:30–31
    angiography, 1:70–71, 2:925, 927, 3:1130, 1135
    for anterior temporal lobectomy, 1:76
    brain, 2:925–926, 927
    for breast cancer, 2:929
    cochlear implants and, 1:310
    for colorectal cancer, 1:319
    coronary stenting and, 1:355
    for craniotomy, 1:369
    endovascular stent surgery and, 1:468
    for hip replacement, 2:668
    for hypophysectomy, 2:697
    for joint disorders, 1:115, 2:926
    for knee replacement, 2:804
    for low back pain, 2:823
    vs. mediastinoscopy, 2:951
    pacemakers and, 3:1081
    for peripheral artery disease, 3:1130
    for peripheral vascular disease, 3:1135
    vs. positron emission tomography, 3:1182
    for rectal resection, 3:1225
    for retinal cryopexy, 3:1232
    robot-assisted surgery and, 3:1243
    for rotator cuff repair, 3:1249
    for shoulder resection arthroplasty, 3:1313
    spinal, 2:926
    for stroke, 1:255
    for subarachnoid hemorrhage, 1:273
    virtual colonoscopy and, 1:316
Magnetic resonance spectroscopy (MRS), 2:925, 927
MAGPI (Metal advancement and glanuloplasty), 2:703
Maine Woman's Health Study, 2:709
Mainz II pouch, 3:1493
Malabsorption, 1:97, 2:577
Malabsorptive procedures, 2:571
Malaria, 1:180, 3:1362
Male hormones. *See* Androgens
Male urinary catheterization, **1:265–268**
Malignant glaucoma, 2:849, 850
Malignant hyperthermia, 1:59, 62, 63, 2:994
Malignant pleural effusion, 1:290
Mallet toes, 2:616–618
Malnutrition, 1:512, 2:1029
Malocclusion, 2:968
Malpractice, 1:540
    See also Legal issues
Mammary artery, 1:346, *1:347*, 1:347–348, 2:976
Mammary hyperplasia, 1:222–225
Mammography, 1:210, **2:929–932**, *930*, 2:987
Managed care plans, **2:932–934**
    hospital services and, 2:689, 3:1165
    Medicare and, 2:963
    patient rights and, 3:1108
    surgeon referrals and, 1:538
    See also Health insurance
Mandol. *See* Cefamandole
Manipulation
    for club foot, 1:307
    osteopathic, 2:825
Mannitol, 1:427, 428, 2:851
Manometry
    anorectal, 1:126
    esophageal, 1:490–493, 2:583–584
Manual detorsion, 2:1063
Manual vacuum aspiration, 1:15–16
Manufacturing errors, 2:960
MAO (Monoamine oxidase) inhibitors, 1:55, 80
Maolate. *See* Chlorphenesin
Mapping
    brain, 1:444
    cardiac, 1:449–452
    cochlear implants, 1:309
    corneal, 2:842, 844, 3:1158
    statistical probability, 1:444
Marcaine. *See* Bupivacaine
Marescaux, Jacques, 3:1399
Marfan syndrome
    aortic aneurysm repair for, 1:100
    goniotomy for, 2:607
    pectus excavatum repair for, 3:1110
scleral buckling and, 3:1271
Marijuana, 1:63, 3:1275
Marjoram oil, 3:1348
Marrow ablation, 1:199
Marshall-Marchetti-Krantz procedure, 3:1234–1238
Maryland Center for Limb Lengthening and Reconstruction, 2:867
Masks
    laryngeal anesthetic, 1:62
    oxygen therapy, 2:1074
    sterile, 1:130
    ventilator, 2:945, 946
Mason, Edward E., 3:1544
Massachusetts State Board of Registration in Pharmacy, 2:960
Massage, for scar revision, 3:1266
    See also Complementary and alternative medicine
Mastectomy
    abdominoplasty and, 1:9
    axillary dissection and, 1:138
    breast implants for, 1:213
    vs. lumpectomy, 2:913
    modified radical, **2:986–990**, *987*, 3:1318, 1320, 1322
    nipple-sparing, 3:1320, 1322
    partial, 3:1320
    prophylactic, 3:1319
    vs. quadrantectomy, 3:1214–1215
    radical, 3:1215, 1320
    simple, 3:1214–1215, **3:1318–1322**, *1319*
    skin-sparing, 3:1320, 1322
    See also Breast reconstruction
Mastoidectomy (Mastoid tympanoplasty), **2:934–936**, 3:1289
Mastoiditis, **2:934–936**
Mastoidoscopy, second-look, 3:1288
Mastopexy, 1:9, 217
Maternal age, 1:41
Maternal blood screening, 1:42
Maternal-fetal medicine, 2:1033
Maternal mortality, 1:16–17, 286, 287, 3:1262
Mattresses and bedsores, 1:158–159
Maxaquin. *See* Lomefloxacin
Maxillofacial surgery, 3:1386
Maximal voluntary ventilation (MVV), 3:1358–1360
Maxzide. *See* Hydrochlorothiazide-triamterene
Mayo clinic, 2:807
Maze procedure, **2:936–942**
McComb nasal tip plasty, 1:303
McCoy laryngoscope, 1:62
McDonald cerclage, 1:279
McGill Questionnaire, Short-Form, 3:1184
MCL (Medial collateral ligament), 2:791–792, 793
M:E ratio, 1:189, 192

Mean corpuscular hemoglobin concentration (MCHC)

Mean corpuscular hemoglobin concentration (MCHC), 1:336, 338, 3:1228–1229
Mean corpuscular hemoglobin (MCH), 1:336, 339, 3:1228–1229
Mean corpuscular volume (MCV), 1:336, 338, 3:1228–1229
Measles, 3:1365
Mechanical circulation support, **2:942–944,** 2:999
Mechanical debridement, 1:407
Mechanical leg pumps, 3:1539
Mechanical rings, 3:1125
Mechanical valves, 1:106, 2:984
Mechanical ventilation, **2:944–946**
  for ALS, 3:1436
  hospital-acquired infections and, 2:685, 686
  for muscular dystrophy, 3:1436
  for omphalocele repair, 2:1036
Mechzine, 1:455
Meckel's diverticulectomy, **2:946–949,** 947
Meckel's diverticulum, **2:946–949,** 3:1117
Meclizine, 1:92
Meconium ileus, 3:1116
Meconium plug syndrome, 3:1116
Medial collateral ligament (MCL), 2:791–792, 793
Median nerve compression, 1:259, 260, 2:619–620
Median sternotomy, 3:1414
Mediastinitis, 2:917
Mediastinoscopy, 2:914, 915, 916, 917, **2:949–952**
Mediation, for weight management, 3:1562
Medicaid, **2:952–955,** 2:963
  adult day care and, 1:36
  costs of, 2:953–954
  for heart-lung transplantation, 2:632
  for heart transplantation, 2:641
  home care and, 2:679, 907
  hospital services and, 2:689
  kidney transplantation and, 2:788
  nursing homes and, 2:907, 952, 953, 1030
  for sigmoidoscopy, 3:1316
  See also Health insurance
Medical abortion, 1:13–14
Medical alert tags, 1:247
Medical aseptic technique, 1:130–131
Medical charts, **2:955–959,** 3:1106–1108, 1109
Medical equipment
  aseptic technique for, 1:129
  diagnostic, 2:760–761, 1046
  disposable, 2:761
  errors and, 2:960, 961
  intensive care unit, 2:759–763
  life support, 2:760
  for microsurgery, 2:971–972
  for operating rooms, 2:1045–1047

for physiologic monitoring, 2:1046
provision of, 2:690
resuscitative, 2:760, 1045–1046
standards for, 2:961
See also specific equipment
Medical errors, 1:180–181, 2:690, **2:959–962**
Medical history, 1:56–57, **2:623–627,** 624, 2:956, 3:1192
Medical records, **2:955–959,** 3:1106–1108, 1109
Medical savings accounts (MSA), 3:1204
Medical specialties. *See* Specialties
Medically necessary surgical procedures, 1:502
Medicare, **2:962–964**
  adult day care and, 1:36
  ambulatory surgery centers and, 1:38, 39–40
  for cataract surgery, 3:1140
  for corneal transplantation, 1:342
  for enhanced external counterpulsation, 1:470
  for gastrostomy, 2:593
  for heart-lung transplantation, 2:632
  for heart transplantation, 2:641
  for hip revision surgery, 2:673
  home care and, 2:679, 907
  hospices and, 2:683
  hospital services and, 2:689, 3:1165
  kidney transplantation and, 2:788
  for knee replacement, 2:804
  for mammography, 2:931
  Medigap and, 2:1030, 3:1203
  nursing homes and, 2:1030
  for oxygen therapy, 2:1075
  for risk factors for surgery, 3:1388
  for second opinions, 3:1291
  for sigmoidoscopy, 3:1316
Medicare Payment Advisory Commission, 1:39
Medicare Supplemental Insurance, 2:907
Medication errors, 2:960, 961
Medications. *See* Drugs
Medigap, 2:1030, 3:1203
Mediolateral position, 2:929, 930
Medionecrosis, 1:100
Meditation for pain, 3:1084, 1185
Mefoxin. *See* Cefoxitin
Megacolon, 3:1116, 1317
Megakaryocytes, 1:192, 337
Megaloblastic anemia, 2:892
Meig's syndrome, 3:1095
Melanoma
  alfa interferons for, 2:729
  demographics of, 2:990
  intraocular eye, 1:474
  iris, 2:770–776
  Mohs surgery for, 2:990
  sentinel lymph node biopsy and, 3:1300, 1301
Membrane oxygenators, 2:629

Memory loss, 3:1541
Menghini needles, 2:886
Ménière's disease, 1:453–456
Meningitis
  aseptic, 2:650
  from cochlear implants, 1:310
  immunoassay tests for, 2:727
  neurosurgery for, 2:1026
Meningocele repair, **2:964–967**
Meniscectomy, 2:796
Meniscus, 2:800
Meniscus injuries, 1:121, 2:794, *2:794,* 2:796
Menopause
  breast cancer and, 2:986
  oophorectomy and, 2:1040
  surgical, 3:1258, 1259
  urinary catheterization and, 1:264
Menstrual extraction, 1:15–16
Mentoplasty, **2:967–970**
Meperidine
  for analgesia, 1:51, 52, 53t
  for cholecystectomy, 1:297
  for endolymphatic shunt, 1:454
  opioid analgesics and, 1:55
  for pain, 3:1084
  patient-controlled analgesia and, 3:1104
Mepivacaine, 1:65
Meprobamate, 1:79t, 2:652
Mercaptopurine, 2:736
Mercury, environment and, 3:1410
Mercury compounds, 1:94
Mercury thermometers, 3:1408–1410
Meridia. *See* Sibutramine
Mersol. *See* Thimerosal
Mesalamine, 2:726
Mesenteric angiography, 1:70
Mesenteric arteries, 1:207, 3:1129, 1131
Mesh
  for incisional hernia repair, 2:748, 750
  for inguinal hernia repair, 2:755
Mesocaval shunts, 3:1179
Metabolic alkalosis, 1:447
Metabolic disorders, 2:1016
Metal advancement and glanuloplasty (MAGPI), 2:703
Metamucil. *See* Psyllium
Metaphysis, 2:675
Metaraminol, 1:33
Metastasis
  to bone, 2:872
  bone marrow aspiration for, 1:192
  breast cancer, 1:137–138, 2:988, 3:1213
  exploratory laparotomy for, 2:838
  lung cancer, 3:1176
  lymphadenectomy for, 2:923–924
  radical neck dissection and, 3:1217
  sentinel lymph node biopsy for, 3:1298–1302
  surgical oncology for, 3:1383
  tumors and, 3:1473

Metaxalone, 2:994
Metformin, 1:237, 2:1022
Methadone, 1:53*t*, 3:1084
Methenamine, 3:1502, 1503, 1504
Methicillin, 1:81
Methocarbamol, 2:824, 994
Methohexital, 1:60
Methotrexate
    for abortions, 1:15
    aspirin and, 1:133
    for ectopic pregnancy, 3:1260, 1262
    overdoses of, 2:652
    for shoulder pain, 3:1314
    sulfonamides and, 3:1380
Methyclothiazide, 1:91
Methyl salicylate, 1:94
Methyl tertiary-butyl ether (MTBE),
    2:558
Methylcellulose, 2:851, 865
Methyldopa, 1:34, 90*t*
Metoclopramide hydrochloride, 1:92*t*
Metolazone, 1:90t, 91
Metoprolol, 1:80, 90*t*, 2:995
Meyer-Overton theory, 1:59
MFPR (Multifetal pregnancy reduc-
    tion), 1:13
MHC (Histocompatibility complex),
    2:691–692
Micardis. *See* Telmisartan
Microcytic anemia, 1:339
Microcytotoxicity test, 2:692
Microdermabrasion, 1:24, 3:1263,
    1266–1267
Microdiskectomy, 1:425, 2:825–826
Microgenia, 2:967–969
Micrografts, 2:613
Microkeratomes, 2:843, 844, 846, 1049
Microlaparoscopy, 2:827, 828
Micronase. *See* Glyburide
Microphones, cochlear implant, 1:308,
    1:309
Microscopes, microsurgery, 2:971
Microsurgery, 2:594, **2:970–974**, *971*
    craniofacial reconstruction and,
        1:366
    ear, nose and throat, 1:434
    for free flap procedures, 1:219, 220
Microtia, 2:1066, 1067–1068
Microwave Maze procedure, 2:937
Microwave ovens and pacemakers,
    2:739
Midamor. *See* Amiloride
Midazolam, 1:78, 79, 3:1293
MIDCAB (Minimally invasive direct
    coronary artery bypass), 2:975–978
Middle ear infections
    mastoidectomy for, 2:934–936
    myringotomy for, 2:1002–1007
    prevention of, 2:1006
Middle meatal antrostomy, 1:460
Middle turbinate, 1:460, 461
Midwives, 1:480
Mifeprex. *See* Mifepristone
Mifepristone, 1:15

Milia, 2:859
Millard rotation advancement (RA)
    technique, 1:303
Miller Roux-en-Y (RNY) gastric by-
    pass, 2:571
Milliman and Robertson obesity guide-
    lines, 3:1546, 1547
Miltown. *See* Meprobamate
Mineral oil, 2:865, 866
Mineralocorticoids, **1:359–361**
Mini-percutaneous nephrolithotomy
    (MPCNL), 2:1018
Mini-suction, 1:15–16
Minigrafts, 2:613
Minimally invasive direct coronary
    artery bypass (MIDCAB), 2:975–978
Minimally invasive surgical procedures
    in ambulatory surgery centers, 1:37,
        38
    coronary artery bypass graft surgery,
        1:347
    disk removal, 1:425
    for endovascular grafts, 1:103
    heart surgery, **2:974–978**, *975*
    for heart valve repair, 2:975
    hip replacement, 2:666
    surgical team for, 3:1386–1387
    See also Endoscopy; Laparoscopy
Minipress. *See* Prazosin hydrochloride
Minocin. *See* Minocycline
Minocycline, 1:83, 3:1405–1406
Minor tranquilizers. *See* Antianxiety
    drugs
Minoxidil, 1:89, 2:615
Miotics, 1:389
Miscarriage
    vs. abortion, 1:12
    from amniocentesis, 1:43
    cervical cerclage for, 1:278
    from cone biopsy, 1:341
    dilatation and curettage for, 1:419,
        421
    smoking and, 3:1338
Misoprostol, 1:15, 98
Mitomycin C, 2:1005, 3:1272
Mitotane, 2:700
Mitral commissurotomy, 2:979, 981
Mitral valve insufficiency
    diagnosis of, 2:980, 984
    mitral valve repair for, 2:978–983
    mitral valve replacement for,
        2:983–986
Mitral valve prolapse
    diagnosis of, 2:980, 984
    mitral valve repair for, 2:978–983
    mitral valve replacement for,
        2:983–986
Mitral valve repair, **2:978–983**, *981*
Mitral valve replacement, 2:979,
    2:983–986
Mitral valve stenosis
    balloon valvuloplasty for,
        1:141–143
    diagnosis of, 2:980, 984

mitral valve repair for, 2:978–983
mitral valve replacement for,
    2:983–986
Mixed urinary incontinence, 3:1235,
    1330
Mobile x ray imaging, 2:760, 1046
Mobility, impaired, 1:156–157
Modified radical mastectomy,
    2:986–990, *987, 988,* 3:1318, 1320,
    1322
Modified radical mastoidectomy, 2:935
Moduretic, 1:90t
Mogen clamps, 1:300
Mohs surgery, 1:387, **2:990–992**
Molding, ear, 2:1068, 1070
Moles, 1:437
Monitoring. *See* Physiologic monitor-
    ing
Monoamine oxidase (MAO) inhibitors,
    1:55, 80
Monoclonal antibodies, 2:733, 777
Monocular blindness, 1:475
Monocyte count, 1:335–338
Mononucleosis, infectious, 2:892–894
Monopril. *See* Fosinopril sodium
Monovision, 2:845
Monsel's solution, 1:330
Montage, average reference, 1:445
Mood swings, 3:1541
Moraxella catarrhalis, 2:1005
Morbid obesity, 1:7–8, 508, 2:793
Morphine
    for analgesia, 1:51, 52, 53*t*
    breastfeeding and, 3:1104
    for children, 3:1104
    for epidural anesthesia, 1:478
    for open prostatectomy, 2:1044
    patient-controlled analgesia and,
        3:1104
    for premedication, 1:61
Morselized bone, 2:675
Motion sickness, 1:92
Motrin. *See* Ibuprofen
Mourning, 1:404–405, 2:684
Mouth cancer, 1:363, 2:600–601,
    3:1147, 1339
Mouthpieces, 3:1347
Mouthwash, 2:600, 3:1340, 1430
Movement disorders, 1:411
Movement therapy
    for back pain, 2:826
    for weight management, 3:1562
    See also Complementary and alter-
        native medicine
Moxifloxacin, 1:546
MPCNL (Mini-percutaneous
    nephrolithotomy), 2:1018
MRA (Magnetic resonance angiogra-
    phy), 2:925, 927
MRI. *See* Magnetic resonance imaging
MRS (Magnetic resonance spec-
    troscopy), 2:925, 927
MSA (Medical savings accounts),
    3:1204

MTBE (Methyl tertiary-butyl ether), 2:558

Mucosal proctectomy, 2:717

Mucous membranes, 1:93–95, 204

MUGA scan. *See* Multiple-gated acquisition (MUGA) scan

Multi-component inflatable implants, 3:1124

Multicentre Aneurysm Screening Group, 1:103

Multidisciplinary team, 2:757, 762, 3:1166

Multifetal pregnancy reduction (MFPR), 1:13

Multimodal analgesia, 3:1185–1186

Multiple-gated acquisition (MUGA) scan, **2:992–994**

Multiple myeloma, 1:189

Multiple pregnancy, 1:7, 284, 2:741, 742

Multiple subpial transection, 2:650

Mupirocin, 1:84

Murmur, heart, 1:436

Muromonab, 2:733, 736

Murphy's sign, 2:559

Muscle relaxants, 1:55, 2:824, **2:994–995**

Muscle-strengthening exercise, 2:873

Muscle wasting diseases, 2:892

Muscles
    atrophy, 1:261
    mass, 1:508
    shortening of, 3:1403–1404
    spasms, 2:994

Muscular dystrophy, 3:1436

Muscularis propria, 1:204

Musculoskeletal defects, 1:487
    See also specific anatomical terms

Musculoskeletal surgery. *See* Orthopedic surgery

Mushroom poisoning, 2:895

MVV (Maximal voluntary ventilation), 3:1358–1360

Myasthenia gravis, 3:1397

Mycobacterium tuberculosis, 1:277

Mycophenolate mofetil
    for immunosuppression, 2:733
    for kidney transplantation, 2:789
    for liver transplantation, 2:899
    pregnancy and, 2:734

Myelin basic protein, 1:276

Myelofibrosis, 1:192, 3:1362

Myelography, 2:823, **2:995–997**

Myeloma, 1:189, 192

Myelomeningocele, 1:531, 532, 533, 2:964–966

Myocardial infarction. *See* Heart attacks

Myocardial resection, 2:643, **2:997–999**

Myocardium, 2:992–994, 3:1182

Myocutaneous flaps, 1:9, 219, 3:1147

Myoglobin, 1:241, 242

Myomas, 1:331, 332

Myomectomy, 2:710, **2:999–1002**, *1000*, 2:1033

Myopia
    glaucoma and, 3:1273
    LASIK for, 2:841–848
    non-surgical treatment of, 2:1051
    phacoemulsification for, 3:1144
    photorefractive keratectomy for, 3:1157–1161
    retinal detachment and, 3:1152
    from scleral buckling, 3:1270

Myopic shift, 1:512

Myringotomy, 1:303, 434, **2:1002–1007**, *1003*

Myringotomy tubes, 1:303

N

Nabumetone, 2:1028

Nadolol, 1:90*t*, 3:1278

NADSA (National Adult Day Services Association), 1:36

Nalbuphine, 1:50, 53*t*

Nalidixic acid, 1:547, 3:1503, 1504

Naloxone, 3:1293–1294

Naltrexone, 1:55

Nanophthalmos, 2:850

Naprelan. *See* Naproxen

Naproxen
    for cervical cryotherapy, 1:282
    for fever, 2:1028
    for pain, 3:1084
    for root canal treatment, 3:1246

Narcotics. *See* Opioid analgesics

Nardil. *See* Phenelzine

Narrow-angle glaucoma. *See* Angle closure glaucoma

Nasal bleeding. *See* Nosebleeds

Nasal cannula, 2:1074, 1075

Nasal congestion
    adrenergic drugs for, 1:32, 33
    snoring and, 3:1345
    surgery for, 1:434, 435

Nasal deformity, 1:303

Nasal endoscopy, 1:434

Nasal excision, adenoidectomy, 1:24

Nasal masks, 2:945

Nasal obstruction septoplasty, 3:1302–1305

Nasal polyps, 3:1302, 1303

Nasal regurgitation, 3:1347

Nasal septum
    deviated, 1:434, 435, 3:1302–1305, *3:1303*, 3:1342, 1345
    perforation of, 2:699, 1075
    septoplasty of, 1:434, 3:1302–1305
    snoring and, 3:1345

Nasal septum surgery, 1:434, **3:1302–1305**, *1303*

Nasal sprays, 3:1305, 1340

Nasal steroids, topical, 1:24

Nasal surgery. *See* Nose surgery

NASCET (North American Symptomatic Carotid Endarterectomy Trial), 1:256

Nasogastric decompression, 2:764, 765, 769

Nasogastric tubes
    complications from, 1:404
    hospital-acquired infections from, 2:687
    for omphalocele repair, 2:1036
    purpose of, 1:207, 323

National Adult Day Services Association (NADSA), 1:36

National Ambulatory Medical Care Survey, 3:1313

National Blood Data Resource Center, 1:172

National Cancer Institute (NCI)
    on bone tumors, 2:872
    on bronchial cancer, 1:226
    on colorectal cancer, 1:317–318
    on colorectal polyps, 1:315
    on liver cancer, 2:657, 660
    on lung cancer, 1:226
    on mastectomy, 3:1320
    on retinoblastoma, 3:1231
    on skin cancer, 2:990
    on small intestine cancer, 3:1335, 1336

National Center for Health Statistics
    on hospices, 2:683
    on inguinal hernia repair, 2:753
    on inpatient surgery, 1:438, 2:689–690, 3:1200, 1386
    on outpatient surgery, 3:1200, 1386
    on teeth replantation, 3:1429

National Cholesterol Education Program (NCEP), 2:876, 877

National Citizen's Coalition for Nursing Home Reform, 2:1031

National Committee for Quality Assurance (NCQA), 2:932

National Council on the Aging, 1:36

National Diabetic and Digestive Diseases (NDDK), 2:580

National Digestive Diseases Clearinghouse, 2:580

National Eye Institute
    on cataracts, 2:1048, 3:1140
    on enucleation, 1:476
    on glaucoma, 3:1272, 1273

National Health and Nutrition Survey, 1:457

National health care system, 1:538–539

National Heart, Lung and Blood Institute (NHLBI), 1:182

National Hospice and Palliative Care Organization (NHPCO), 2:683

National Hospital Discharge Survey, 1:226

National Institute of Diabetes, Digestive and Kidney Diseases (NIDDK), 1:125

National Institute of Environmental Health Sciences, 2:1000
National Institute of Neurological Disorders and Stroke (NINDS), 1:252
National Institute on Deafness and Other Communication Disorders (NIDCD), 1:454
National Institutes of Health (NIH), 3:1448
    clinical trials, 2:918, 3:1448
    Consensus Development Conference Statement on Physical Activity and Cardiovascular Health, 1:506
    on gastric bypass, 2:571
    on obesity, 3:1545
    on pectus excavatum repair, 3:1112
    on scleral buckling, 3:1271
    on vasectomy, 3:1526
National Institutes of Mental Health (NIMH), 3:1560
National Kidney Foundation, 1:111, 2:783, 3:1506
National Lung Health Education Program, 3:1358
National Marrow Donor Program (NMDP), 1:194, 196
National Nosocomial Infection Surveillance System, 2:685
National Organ Transplant Act, 1:194
National Pressure Ulcer Advisory Panel (NPUAP), 1:157, 158
National Prison Hospice Association, 2:683
National Stroke Association, 1:252, 256
National Survey of Ambulatory Surgery Reports, 1:226
National Veterans Affairs Surgical Risk Study, 1:403
Nausea
    antinausea drugs for, 1:91–93
    from dialysis, 2:782
    postoperative, 1:62, 3:1286–1288
    scopolamine patch for, 3:1286–1288
    after vertical banded gastroplasty, 3:1548
NCEP (National Cholesterol Education Program), 2:876, 877
NCI. See National Cancer Institute
NCQA (National Committee for Quality Assurance), 2:932
NDDK (National Diabetic and Digestive Diseases), 2:580
Nd:YAG lasers, 2:860
    adenoidectomy, 1:24
    capsulotomy, 3:1144
    goniotomy, 2:610
    laser iridotomy, 2:773, 849, 851, 852
    laser posterior capsulotomy, 2:854–857
    peptic ulcers, 1:98
Nearsightedness. See Myopia
Necessary surgery, **2:1009–1010**

Neck cancer
    craniofacial reconstruction for, 1:363, 366
    non-surgical treatment of, 3:1218
    radical neck dissection for, 3:1217–1219
    from smoking, 3:1241
    surgery for, 1:434
Neck dissection
    complications of, 1:404
    modified, 3:1217
    radical, 1:434, 435, **3:1217–1219**
Neck injury cricothyroidotomy, 1:372–377
Neck tumors, 3:1119
Necrosis
    aseptic, 1:555, 2:751–752
    avascular, 2:664–665, 667, 870
    debridement of, 1:406–409
    liver function tests and, 2:893
Necrotizing enterocolitis, 3:1116
Needle aspiration, wounds, 3:1570–1571
Needle biopsy, 1:190
    breast, 1:211
    core-needle, 2:951
    fine-needle, 2:951, 989, 3:1146
    large-core needle, 1:211
    lung, 2:914, 915–916, 917, 918
    tumors, 3:1473
Needle bladder neck suspension, 1:312, **2:1010–1012,** 3:1332
Needle core biopsy. See Bone marrow biopsy
Needle cricothyroidotomy, 1:372, 374, 375
Needle-stick injuries, 3:1392, 1393
Needles
    bronchoscopy, 1:227
    children and, 3:1113
    hypodermic, 3:1392–1394, *3:1393*
    Jamshidi, 1:190, 2:886
    Menghini, 2:886
    suture, 2:972, 3:1374
    Veses, 2:831
    Westerman-Jensen trephine, 1:190
Nefazodone, 1:80
Negative-pressure airflow, 1:130
NegGram. See Nalidixic acid
Nembutal. See Pentobarbital
Neo-Synephrine. See Phenylephrine
Neobladders, 1:392, 2:716, 3:1494
Neodymium:yttrium-aluminum-garnet lasers. See Nd:YAG lasers
Neomycin
    for bowel resection, 1:207
    for colorectal surgery, 1:319
    for colostomy, 1:323
    for rectal resection, 3:1227
    for small bowel resection, 3:1335
    topical antibiotics, 1:84
Neonatal intensive care units (NICU), 2:759, 760
Neonatal jaundice, 3:1118

Neonates. See Newborns
Neoral. See Cyclosporins
Neosalpingostomy, 3:1260
Neosporin, 1:84
Neovascular glaucoma, 1:388–389, 390–391
Nephrectomy, 2:*1013*, **2:1013–1016**
    kidney transplantation and, 2:788, 1013, 1014
    laparoscopic, 2:788, 1013, 1015
    open, 2:788
Nephroblastoma, 3:1119
Nephrolithotomy
    mini-percutaneous, 2:1018
    percutaneous, **2:1016–1021**, *1017,* 3:1289
Nephrologists, 1:112, 2:783
Nephroscopy, 2:1018
Nephrostomy, 2:1018, 1019, **2:1021–1024**, 3:1491
Nephrotoxic drugs, 2:652
Nerve anastomosis. See Nerve repair
Nerve blockades, 1:64, 65
    for bunionectomy, 1:231
    for carpal tunnel release, 1:261
    for circumcision, 1:299
    for finger reattachment, 1:542, 545
    penile, 1:299, 2:704
    peripheral, 3:1184
    subcutaneous ring, 1:299
Nerve compression syndrome, 1:259, 260, 2:619–620, 621
Nerve damage
    from cerebral aneurysm repair, 1:272, 274, 275
    from cryotherapy, 1:378
    from face lift, 1:523
    from hip replacement, 2:670
    from liposuction, 2:881
    from lithotripsy, 2:885
    from lymphadenectomy, 2:924
    pain from, 3:1084
    from radical neck dissection, 3:1218
    from spinal fusion, 3:1355
    from spinal instrumentation, 3:1357
    from wrist replacement, 3:1574
Nerve grafts, 2:973
Nerve repair, 1:543, 2:972–973
Nerve root rhizotomy, **3:1241–1242**
Nervous system
    adrenergic drugs and, 1:32
    central, 3:1083
    pain and, 3:1083
    peripheral, 3:1083
    sympathetic, 1:32, 3:1389–1392
Nesacaine. See Chloroprocaine
Network Model, 2:933
Neupogen. See Filgrastim
Neural tube defects, 2:964, 965, 966
Neurectomy, vestibular, 1:455
Neuroblastoma, 1:30
Neurofibromatosis, 2:607
Neuroimaging, 1:369–370, 2:649
Neurologic examination, 3:1162

Neurological damage. *See* Nerve damage
Neurological disorders, 2:759, 3:1182
Neuromedical intensive care units, 2:760
Neuromuscular diseases, 3:1404
Neuropathic arthropathy, 3:1310
Neuropsychological tests, 1:358, 2:649
Neuroradiology, inventional, 1:275
Neurorrhaphy. *See* Nerve repair
Neurosurgeons, 1:184, 358
Neurosurgery, **2:1024–1027,** 3:1243, 1386
Neurosyphilis, 1:277
Neurotransmitters, 2:850, 3:1083, 1184
Neurovascular glaucoma, 2:849
Neutropenia, 1:189
Neutrophils, 1:336, 337, 338
Nevi, spider, 3:1282
Newborns
    antiseptics and, 1:94
    club foot repair for, 1:306
    esophageal atresia/tracheoe-
        sophageal fistula repair for,
        1:485–490
    hemolytic disease of, 2:894
    sex reassignment surgery for,
        3:1305
    surgery for, 3:1115–1116
    See also Infants
Nexium. *See* Esomeprazole
NHLBI (National Heart, Lung and
    Blood Institute), 1:182
NHPCO (National Hospice and Pallia-
    tive Care Organization), 2:683
Niacin and lipid tests, 2:876
Nicardipine hydrochloride, 1:90*t*
Nicoderm. *See* Nicotine replacement
    therapy
Nicorette gum, 3:1340
Nicotine, 3:1241, 1338–1342
    See also Smoking
Nicotine replacement therapy, 3:1339,
    1340
Nicotrol, 3:1340
NICU (Neonatal intensive care units),
    2:759, 760
NIDCD (National Institute on Deafness
    and Other Communication Disor-
    ders), 1:454
NIDDK (National Institute of Diabetes,
    Digestive and Kidney Diseases),
    1:125 3:1507
Nifedipine, 1:89, 90*t*
Night vision
    bilberry extract for, 3:1275
    LASIK and, 2:844, 846
    ophthalmologic surgery and, 2:1050
NIH. *See* National Institutes of Health
NIH Consensus Statement on dental
    anesthesia, 1:61
NIMH (National Institutes of Mental
    Health), 3:1560

NINDS (National Institute of Neuro-
    logical Disorders and Stroke), 1:252
Nipple-sparing mastectomy, 3:1320,
    1322
Nipples
    breast reconstruction and, 1:217,
        220, 3:1321, 1322
    breast reduction and, 1:224
NISHOT (Noninfectious serious haz-
    ards of transfusion), 1:180–181
Nissen fundoplication, 2:586–591,
    3:1399
Nitrates
    angina, 1:352
    angioplasty, 1:74
    coronary artery disease, 1:472
Nitrites, in urinalysis, 3:1500, 1501
Nitrofurantoin, 3:1503–1504, 1504
Nitrogen, liquid, 1:377, 380
Nitroglycerin, 1:133, 3:1278
Nitropress. *See* Sodium nitroprusside
Nitrous oxide, 1:60, 164
Nizatidine, 2:568
Nizoral. *See* Ketoconazole
NMDP (National Marrow Donor Pro-
    gram), 1:194, 196
NMP22. *See* Nuclear matrix proteins
Nociceptors, 3:1083
Nomograms, 2:843
Non-absorbable sutures, 2:743, 748,
    818, 972, 3:1374
Non-Hodgkin's lymphoma, 1:189,
    3:1383
Non-insulin-dependent diabetes, 1:507
Non-ionic contrast medium, 1:74
Non-myeloablative allogeneic trans-
    plantation, 1:195
Non-small cell lung cancer, 3:1177,
    1295
Noninfectious serious hazards of trans-
    fusion (NISHOT), 1:180–181
Noninvasive mechanical ventilation,
    2:946
Nonpenetrating deep sclerectomy,
    3:1275
Nonproductive pain, 1:50
Nonselective beta blockers, 3:1181
Nonselective nonsteroidal anti-inflam-
    matory drugs, 2:1028
Nonspecific diffuse intralamellar ker-
    atitis, 2:846
Nonsteroidal anti-inflammatory drugs
    (NSAIDs), **2:1027–1029**
    acetaminophen and, 1:22
    for analgesia, 1:50, 51
    for arthritis, 1:119, 3:1311
    C-reactive protein and, 1:240
    cardiac catheterization and, 1:237
    complications of, 3:1086
    COX-2 specific, 2:1028
    craniotomy and, 1:370
    esophagogastroduodenoscopy and,
        1:500
    for hip pain, 2:671

hip replacement and, 2:668
    interactions with, 1:133, 2:1028
    kidney failure from, 3:1186
    for knee pain, 2:807
    knee replacement and, 2:805
    laparoscopy and, 2:828
    for low back pain, 2:824
    mentoplasty and, 2:968
    microsurgery and, 2:973
    nonselective, 2:1028
    opioid analgesics and, 3:1186
    for pain, 3:1084
    peptic ulcers and, 1:98, 3:1211
    for plantar fasciitis, 1:525, 526
    for post-surgical pain, 3:1185
    for rotator cuff syndrome, 3:1250
    side effects of, 2:1028, 3:1186
    for spider veins, 3:1284
    stomach ulcers from, 2:567
    after vein ligation and stripping,
        3:1536
Nontreponemal antibodies, 1:277
Norepinephrine, 1:33, 3:1087–1088
Norflex. *See* Orphenadrine
Norfloxacin, 1:546, 547
Normocytic anemia, 1:339,
    3:1228–1229
Normodyne. *See* Labetalol
Noroxin. *See* Norfloxacin
North American Symptomatic Carotid
    Endarterectomy Trial (NASCET),
    1:256
Nose surgery, **1:433–435,** 3:1406
    See also Rhinoplasty
Nosebleeds
    from hypophysectomy, 2:699
    non-surgical treatment of, 3:1305
    septoplasty for, 3:1302
Nosocomial infections. *See* Hospital-
    acquired infections; Surgical site in-
    fections
Nothing by mouth (NPO), 3:1188,
    1193
Nozzles, syringe, 3:1392
NPUAP (National Pressure Ulcer Advi-
    sory Panel), 1:157
NSAIDs. *See* Nonsteroidal anti-inflam-
    matory drugs
Nubian. *See* Nalbuphine
Nuclear cataracts, 1:510, 512
Nuclear magnetic resonance. *See* Mag-
    netic resonance imaging (MRI)
Nuclear matrix proteins (NMP22),
    3:1471
Nuclear medicine scans
    cardiac, 1:240
    esophageal, 1:491
    thyroid, 3:1421
Numorphan. *See* Oxymorphone
Nuremberg Trials, 2:751
Nurse anesthetists, *1:60,* 3:1387, 1388
Nurses
    critical care, 2:762
    hospital, 3:1167

informed consent and, 2:752
in intensive care units, 2:757
managed care plans and, 2:933
operating, 3:1387
pain evaluation by, 3:1082–1083
patient-controlled analgesia and,
3:1104–1105
postoperative care by, 3:1187–1188
workload of, 2:960, 961
wound ostomy continence, 2:1022,
3:1495
Nursing care
in adult day care, 1:36
home care, 2:678, 679–680
in intensive care units, 2:758
medical charts and, 2:955
wound, 1:146, 2:1022
Nursing diagnosis, 2:957–958
Nursing homes, **2:1029–1032**
bedsores in, 1:156
costs of, 2:1030, 1032
long-term care insurance for, 2:907
Medicaid for, 2:907, 952, 953, 954,
1030
Medicare for, 1:1, 2:963
obesity and, 1:508
Ombudsmen Program and,
2:908–909
Nuss, Donald, 3:1111
Nuss procedure, 3:1111, 1112
Nutrition
enteral, 3:1466–1469
weight management and, 3:1561
See also Diet
Nutrition-related disorders, 3:1561
Nutritional supplements
for atherosclerosis prevention,
1:256, 3:1131–1132
for osteoarthritis, 1:119
preoperative, 3:1192
See also Diet; specific supplements
Nuttall, Gregory, 1:180
NYHA heart failure classification,
2:980, 984, 986
Nystagmus, 1:517
Nystagmus Network, 1:517
Nystatin, 2:687

O

OA. *See* Overeaters Anonymous
OAA/SS (Observer's Assessment of
Alertness/Sedation Scale), 1:162–163
Obesity
abdominoplasty and, 1:7–8
clinical, 1:508
demographics of, 1:507, 2:570–571
diagnosis of, 2:572
fracture repair and, 1:555
gallstones and, 2:557
gastric bypass for, 2:570–575

guidelines for, 3:1545, 1546, 1547,
1558–1560
hip replacement and, 2:666, 668
hip revision surgery and, 2:676
laparoscopy and, 2:829, 830
low back pain and, 2:820
morbid, 1:7–8, 508, 2:793
mortality and morbidity from,
1:508, 2:574
non-surgical alternatives for,
2:574–575
risks of, 1:507–508
sleep apnea from, 3:1343
snoring and, 3:1345
spider veins from, 3:1280
support groups, 3:1547
surgery for, 3:1544–1551, 1549
urinary incontinence from, 3:1330
Obligate anaerobes, 1:47
Observer's Assessment of Alertness/Se-
dation Scale (OAA/SS), 1:162–163
Obsessive-compulsive disorder, 2:865
Obstetric and gynecologic surgery,
2:1033–1035
ambulatory surgery centers and,
1:37
elective, 1:438
endoscopic, 1:535
laparoscopic, 2:827
microsurgery, 2:970
See also Pregnancy
Obstetricians, 1:480, 2:1033
Obstructive liver disease, 2:891–894
Obstructive sleep apnea, 3:1302, 1305,
1342–1349
Occult rectal prolapse, 3:1222
Occupational injuries
hand, 2:619
low back pain from, 2:820, 822,
823, 825
spider veins from, 3:1280
Occupational rehabilitation, 1:261
Octreotide, 3:1278, 1279
Ocular hypertension, 3:1273
Ocular pain, 1:388, 389, 390–391
Ocular prosthesis, 1:476, 504
Oculoplethysmography (OPG), 1:255
Off-pump CABG (OPCAB), 1:347,
2:975–978
Off-pump MIDCAB, 2:975–978
Office-Based Surgery Accreditation
program, 1:38
Office-based surgical practices, 1:39,
2:1072
*The Official ABMS Directory of Board-
Certified Medical Specialists*, 3:1166,
1195
Ofloxacin, 1:546, 547
OGTT (Oral glucose tolerance test),
2:603, 605, 606
Older Americans Act, 2:908–909
Oligohydramnios, 1:533
Olsalazine, 2:726

Ombudsmen Program, 2:908–909,
3:1166
Omeprazole, 1:98, 2:568, 578, 589, 590
Omphalocele repair, 1:5–7,
2:1035–1038
On-Q administration, 3:1185
Oncogenes, 3:1470
Oncology, surgical, **3:1382–1385**
See also Cancer
Ondansetron, 1:92, 92*t*, 3:1287
Oophorectomy, 2:1034, **2:1038–1041**
bilateral, 2:1040
for endometriosis, 2:835
for sex reassignment surgery,
3:1306
Opacification. *See* Lens opacification
OPCAB (Off-pump CABG), 1:347,
2:975–978
Open adrenalectomy, 1:30
Open-angle glaucoma, 2:772, 849,
3:1271–1277, 1433
Open bowel patch, 1:167
Open cholecystectomy, 1:293, 295,
296, 2:558
Open fetal surgery, 1:532, 533, 535,
536
Open heart surgery
for aortic aneurysm repair, 1:103
heart-lung machines for, 2:627
minimally invasive, *2:975*
See also Myocardial resection
Open nephrectomy, 2:788, 1013, 1015
Open prostatectomy, **2:1041–1045**,
1043
Open tenotomy, 3:1404
Open vertical banded gastroplasty,
3:1545
Operating nurses, 3:1387
Operating rooms, **2:1045–1048**
in ambulatory surgery centers, 1:38
aseptic technique for, 1:128–130
positive-pressure airflow for, 1:129
Operation Lindbergh, 3:1398–1399
Operations. *See* Surgery
OPG. *See* Oculoplethysmography
(OPG)
Ophthalmic anesthetics, 1:64, 65, 389,
2:1050, 1058
Ophthalmic surgeons, 1:474
Ophthalmologic surgery, 1:37, 2:690,
2:1048–1051, 3:1386
Ophthalmologists, 1:380, 513, 2:772,
3:1431, 1463
Ophthalmoscopes, 1:380, 513, 3:1232,
1274
Opioid analgesics, 1:50–51, **1:52–55**,
1:53*t*, 3:1084
acetaminophen with, 1:21
addiction to, 1:52, 3:1087, 1185
complications of, 3:1086
for conscious sedation,
3:1292–1294
hospice care and, 2:684
NSAIDs and, 3:1186

patient-controlled analgesia and,
3:1104, 1105, 1185, 1186
tolerance to, 3:1186
Opioids. *See* Opioid analgesics
Opitz syndrome, 1:301
Opportunistic infections, 2:899
OpSite dressings, 2:744
Optic nerve cancer exenteration, 1:503
Optional surgery. *See* Elective surgery
OPTN (Organ Procurement and Transplantation Network), 2:632, 789, 790,
3:1091
Optometrists, 3:1159
Oral appliances, 3:1347
Oral bile acid litholysis, 2:558
Oral cancer, 1:363, 2:600–601, 3:1147,
1339
Oral Cancer Foundation, 2:600–601
Oral contraceptives
alprazolam and, 1:80
antibiotics and, 1:83
barbiturates and, 1:153
C-reactive protein and, 1:240
cephalosporins and, 1:270
diazepam and, 2:995
for endometriosis, 2:835
face lift and, 1:521
hip replacement and, 2:668
knee replacement and, 2:805
lipid tests and, 2:876
spider veins from, 3:1280
sulfonamides and, 3:1380
tetracyclines and, 3:1406
Oral dissolution therapy, 2:558
Oral glucose tolerance test (OGTT),
2:603, 605, 606
Oral rehydration, 2:767
Oral surgery, 2:598, 3:1386
teeth extraction, **3:1426–1429,**
3:1427
teeth replantation, 3:1429–1431
Oral thermometers, 3:1409
Orbicularis oris, 1:302
Orbital exenteration, **1:502–506**
OrCel, 3:1569
Orchiectomy, **2:1051–1058,** *1052,*
2:1058
Orchiopexy, **2:1058–1063,** *1059*
Organ donors, 3:1444–1445,
1444–1447
cadavers, 2:692
human leukocyte antigen test for,
2:691–693
living, 2:789, 790, 1013, 1015
matching, 2:632, 641
Organ harvesting, 3:1445–1446
Organ Procurement and Transplantation Network (OPTN), 2:632, 789,
790, 3:1091
Organ rejection. *See* Transplant rejection
Orlistat, 2:575
Orphenadrine, 2:994
Orthoclone OKT3. *See* Muromonab
Orthodontic appliances, 3:1428

Orthognathic surgery, 2:967
Orthokeratology, 2:847, 3:1161
Orthopedic surgeons, 1:118, 184,
2:669, 675, 1063–1064, 3:1555
Orthopedic surgery, 1:438,
2:1063–1066
ambulatory surgery centers and,
1:37
complications from, 1:404
demographics of, 2:690, 3:1386
robot-assisted, 3:1243
tendon repair, 3:1400
tetracyclines in, 3:1405–1406
Orthoptic urethral anastomosis, 2:713
Orthoptics, 1:519
Orthostatic hypotension, 1:91
Orthotics
for knee stability, 2:807
for leg lengthening and shortening,
2:670, 867, 870–871
toe abnormalities and, 2:618
Orthotopic liver transplantation, 2:896
Osmolality
plasma, 1:447, 448
urine, 2:784, 785
Osmotic diuretics, 1:428
Osteoarthritis
arthroplasty for, 1:116, 118, 507
arthroscopic surgery for, 1:121
debridement for, 2:807
demographics of, 3:1310, 1313
diagnosis of, 2:804
hip osteotomy for, 2:661
hip replacement for, 2:664, 667
knee osteotomy for, 2:797, 799
knee replacement for, 2:800, 801,
802
low back pain from, 2:820
non-surgical treatment of, 1:51, 119,
2:621, 799, 807, 3:1314
obesity and, 1:507
shoulder joint replacement for,
3:1310
shoulder resection arthroplasty for,
3:1312–1315
wrist replacement and, 3:1572
Osteoblasts, 1:184
Osteoclasts, 1:184
Osteoconduction, 1:184
Osteocytes, 1:184
Osteogenesis, 1:184
Osteoinduction, 1:184
Osteolysis, 2:810, 811
Osteomalacia, 2:865
Osteomeatal complex, 1:460
Osteomyelitis, 2:870, 3:1329
Osteonecrosis, 3:1310
Osteopathic manipulative treatment,
2:825
Osteoporosis
bone x rays for, 1:203, 204
hysterectomy and, 2:709
from immunosuppressive agents,
2:633

orchiectomy and, 2:1055
prevention of, 2:672
salpingo-oophorectomy and, 3:1259
Osteosclerosis, 3:1365–1368
Osteotomy
for bunions, 1:231
high tibia, 2:797, 798–799
hip, **2:661–664,** 2:672
knee, **2:797–799**
for leg lengthening, 2:867
pelvic, 2:662
varus derotational, 2:662
varus rotational, 2:662
Ostomy
antrostomy, 1:460
colorectal surgery and, 1:318, 319
enterostomy, 2:769
gastroduodenostomy, 2:575–579,
2:576
gastrojejunostomy, 1:541, 2:575
ileal conduit surgery and,
2:715–716
kidney stones and, 2:1016
for Meckel's diverticulectomy, 2:948
psychological complications of,
1:320
tracheostomy, 1:465, 2:945, 946
See also Colostomy; Gastrostomy;
Ileostomy
Otitis, 2:934
Otitis media with effusion
demographics of, 2:1004
diagnosis of, 2:1005
myringotomy for, 2:1002–1007
non-surgical treatment of, 2:1004
Otolaryngologists, 3:1423, 1476
See also Ear, nose and throat surgeons
Otolaryngology, 1:37, 2:970
Otoplasty, 1:434, **2:1066–1071,** *1067*
Otorhinolaryngologists, 1:433
Otorrhea, 2:1006
Outpatient surgery, 1:37–40,
2:1071–1072
accreditation of, 1:540
aftercare for, 2:690
anesthesia and, 1:61, 2:690
costs of, 1:39, 2:1071
demographics of, 1:438, 2:690,
3:1200, 1386
description of, 2:595
laser, 2:862
Medicaid for, 2:952
Medicare for, 2:963
number of, 2:1071
office-based, 1:38, 39, 2:1072
ophthalmologic surgery as, 2:1050
pain management for, 3:1184
See also Ambulatory surgery centers
Ovarian abscess, 2:1038
Ovarian cancer
demographics of, 2:1039, 3:1256,
1383
hysterectomy for, 2:706

oophorectomy for, 2:1038–1041
pelvic exenteration for, 1:503
peritoneovenous shunts for, 3:1137
salpingo-oophorectomy for,
3:1256–1259
second-look surgery for, 3:1288
Ovarian cystectomy, 2:1034
Ovarian cysts, 2:1034, 1038
Ovarian surgery, 2:1034
Ovariectomy. *See* Oophorectomy
Ovary and fallopian tube removal. *See*
Salpingo-oophorectomy
Ovary removal. *See* Oophorectomy
Overdose
acetaminophen, 1:22, 2:652, 886
anesthesia, 1:60
barbiturates, 1:151, 2:652
carbamazepine, 2:652
dialysis for, 2:779
digitalis, 2:652
ethchlorvynol, 2:652
glutethimide, 2:652
intensive care units and, 2:759
meprobamate, 2:652
methotrexate, 2:652
theophylline, 2:652
Overeaters Anonymous (OA), 3:1562
Overflow urinary incontinence, 1:123,
3:1235, 1330
Overhydration, 2:766
Overweight, defined, 3:1558–1560
See also Obesity; Weight manage-
ment
Oxacillin, 1:81
Oxalic acid, 2:1016
Oxaloacetate, 2:891
Oxaprozin, 2:1028
Oxazepam, 1:79*t*
Oximetry. *See* Pulse oximeter
Oxtriphylline, 1:547, 2:569
Oxybutynin, 3:1255
Oxycodone, 1:52, 53*t*, 454, 3:1084
Oxycodone-acetaminophen, 1:21, 52
Oxygen
compressed, 2:1074
liquid, 2:1074
after vertical banded gastroplasty,
3:1548
Oxygen concentrators, 2:1074
Oxygen conserving devices, 2:1074
Oxygen deprivation, fetal, 1:286
Oxygen saturation
cardiac monitor for, 1:243, 244
conscious sedation and,
3:1292–1293
oxygen therapy and, 2:1075
pulse oximetry for, 2:760,
3:1207–1209
Oxygen tanks, 2:1074, 1075
Oxygen tension measurements, 1:45
Oxygen therapy, **2:1072–1077**, *1073*
hyperbaric, 2:1073, 1074
vs. mechanical ventilation, 2:944
transtracheal, 2:1074

Oxygenators, 2:629
Oxyhemoglobin, 3:1208
Oxymorphone, 1:53*t*
Oxytetracycline, 3:1405
Oxytocin, 3:1509–1510
epidural anesthesia and, 1:479
for non-progressive labor, 1:287
urinary incontinence from, 3:1330

P

PABD (Preoperative autologous blood
donation), 1:134–135, 3:1196–1197,
1202
Pacemaker syndrome, 3:1081
Pacemakers, **3:1079–1082**, *1080*
batteries for, 3:1079, 1081
biventricular, 2:643
dual-chamber, 3:1081
for heart transplantation, 2:641,
3:1079
lithotripsy and, 2:884
magnetic resonance imaging and,
2:928
Maze procedure and, 2:940
microwave ovens and, 2:739
for minimally invasive heart
surgery, 2:977
temporary, 1:348, 3:1079–1080,
1081
Packed cell volume. *See* Hematocrit
PACU (Postanesthesia care units),
3:1187–1188
Paget's disease of the bone, 3:1329
Pain
abdominal, 1:1, 3, 2:884
acetaminophen for, **1:21–23**
acute, 1:50, 67, 3:1083, 1086
from amputation, 1:46
anesthesiologists and, 1:67
aspirin for, 1:131–134
from burns, 3:1083
cancer, 1:67
in children, 3:1113
chronic, 1:50–51, 67, 3:1083, 1086
from circumcision, 1:299
clinical, 3:1183
cutaneous, 3:1083
evaluation of, 3:1082–1083, *3:1085*,
3:1085–1086
experience of, 3:1082
heel, 1:525
hip joint, 2:664, 666–668, 671–672,
673
history, 3:1085–1086
leg, 1:426
nonproductive, 1:50
ocular, 1:388, 389, 390–391
perception of, 3:1184, 1185
physiologic, 3:1183
productive, 1:50
somatic, 3:1083

surgical procedures for, 3:1085
thresholds, 3:1184
tolerance of, 3:1184
visceral, 3:1083
See also Back pain; Knee pain;
Post-surgical pain
Pain management, **3:1082–1087**
analgesics for, 1:50–51
hospices and, 2:682, 684
intraoperative period, 3:1185
multimodal, 3:1185–1186
non-pharmacologic, 3:1084–1085,
1086–1087
patient-controlled analgesia for,
3:1103–1106
patient education for, 3:1193–1194
pharmaceutical, 3:1084, 1086, 1087
postoperative care and, 3:1188,
1189
preoperative, 3:1184–1186
See also Post-surgical pain
Pain medications. *See* Analgesics; Opi-
oid analgesics
"Pain relief ball," 3:1185
Pain scales, *3:1085*, 3:1085–1086,
1184
Palate, cleft, 1:301, 362
Palliative care, 3:1474
Pallidotomy, 1:411, **3:1087–1089**
Pallikari, Ioannis, 2:842
Palpation, 3:1161
PAM (Potential acuity meter), 2:855
Panadol. *See* Acetaminophen
Pancreas divisum, 1:457
Pancreas removal, 3:1091–1095
Pancreas transplantation, 2:777–778,
783, **3:1089–1091**, 3:1444, 1445,
1448
Pancreatectomy, **3:1091–1095**
Pancreatic anastomosis, 3:1093
Pancreatic cancer
biliary stenting for, 1:159
demographics of, 1:457
endoscopic retrograde cholan-
giopancreatography for, 1:457,
458
pancreatectomy for, 3:1091–1095
Pancreatic disease, 1:1, **1:456–459**
Pancreatic duct stricture, 1:457
Pancreatic enzyme replacement, 3:1093
Pancreatic insufficiency, 3:1093
Pancreatic islet cell transplantation,
2:776–778, 3:1091
Pancreatic pseudocysts, 1:457
Pancreatic stones, 1:1
Pancreaticoduodenectomy, 3:1092,
1093, 1094
Pancreatitis
acute, 2:580
ascites from, 3:1095
biliary stenting for, 1:159
chronic, 3:1092, 1094
demographics of, 1:457
electrolyte balance and, 1:448

endoscopic retrograde cholangiopancreatography for,
1:456–457
from lithotripsy, 2:885
liver function tests for, 2:894
pancreatectomy for, 3:1092
Pancytopenia, 1:189
Panel reactive antibodies (PRA) test,
2:641, 693, 789
Panniculectomy, 1:7
Pannus, 1:7
Pantoprazole, 2:568
PaO₂ (Partial pressure of oxygen),
2:1075
Pap test, 1:281–282, 329–330, 340, 341
Papillary capture, 2:854
Paracentesis, **3:1095–1096,** 3:1138
serial, 3:1139
tympanic, 1:303, 434, 2:1002–1007,
2:1003
Paraflex. *See* Chlorzoxazone
Paralysis
from Botox, 1:523
from epilepsy, 2:649
eyelid, 3:1397
from regional anesthesia, 1:65
small bowel, 1:6
from spinal fusion, 3:1355
from spinal instrumentation, 3:1357
Paralytic ileus. *See* Intestinal obstruc-
tion repair
Paraplegia, 1:103, 156
Paraquat poisoning, 2:652
Parasitic infections, 1:180, 2:685
Parastomal hernia, 1:320, 325
Parasympathetic nervous system,
3:1083
Parathyroid, ectopic, 3:1098
Parathyroid gland removal, 2:828,
3:1097–1099
Parathyroid hormone, 1:447
Parathyroidectomy, 2:828, *3:1097,*
1097–1099
Paravaginal surgery, 1:312,
2:1010–1012, 3:1332
Parents, 3:1113–1114
See also Family
Parkinson's disease
deep brain stimulation for,
1:409–411
demographics of, 1:409, 3:1088
pallidotomy for, 3:1087–1089
Parnate. *See* Pranylcypromine
Paronychia, 2:619
Parotid gland removal, **3:1100–1101**
Parotid gland tumors, 3:1100–1101
Parotidectomy, **3:1100–1101**
Paroxysmal atrial fibrillation, 2:937
Partial abdominoplasty, 1:9
Partial anterior temporal lobectomy,
2:1026
Partial cystectomy, 1:391, 392, 394
Partial gastrectomy, 1:95–100, 2:564
Partial laryngectomy, 2:839

Partial mastectomy. *See* Lumpectomy
Partial nephrectomy, 2:1013
Partial pancreatectomy, 3:1092
Partial patellectomy, 2:814
Partial pharyngectomy, 3:1145
Partial pressure of oxygen (PaO₂),
2:1075
Partial splenectomy, 3:1363
Partial-thickness wounds, 1:386
Partial thromboplastin time (PTT),
2:916
Particle immunoassay tests, 2:727
Parvovirus, 1:536
Passive immunotherapy, 2:731
Passive range of motion exercises
continuous passive motion machine
for, 2:798, 805, 806, 873
for shoulder joint replacement,
3:1311
for shoulder resection arthroplasty,
3:1313
Passive smoking, 3:1338–1339
Pastoral care, 3:1166, 1192
Patches
nicotine, 3:1340
transdermal fentanyl, 3:1084
Patella, 2:800, 802, 811
Patella-femoral syndrome, 2:791, 793,
795
Patella removal, **2:814–816**
Patellar arthritis, 2:814
Patellar tendon, 2:814, 815
Patent ductus arteriosus, 2:636, 637
Patent urachus repair, **3:1101–1103,**
1102
Paternity testing, 2:691, 3:1479
Patient autonomy, 1:430, 431, 3:1190
Patient care teams
evaluation of, 3:1166
intensive care unit, 2:757, 762
members of, 3:1195
multidisciplinary, 2:757, 762,
3:1166
in nursing homes, 2:1031
surgical, 1:452, 3:1385–1389
Patient charts. *See* Medical charts
Patient confidentiality, **3:1106–1108**
hospital rules for, 3:1167
medical charts and, 2:955, 958,
3:1106–1108
patient rights and, 3:1109
Patient-controlled analgesia (PCA),
1:52, 3:1084, **3:1103–1106,** 3:1188,
3:1447, 1548
for hip replacement, 2:669
hospice care and, 2:684
for knee replacement, 2:805
for laminectomy, 2:823
opioid analgesics and, 3:1185, 1186
patient education for, 3:1105, 1194
for spinal fusion, 3:1354
Patient discharge, **1:422–424**
Patient education
for home care, 3:1188

hospital-based, 3:1166
informed consent and, 2:751
for oxygen therapy, 2:1074–1075
for pain management, 3:1193–1194
for patient-controlled analgesia,
3:1105, 1194
for post-surgical pain, 3:1185
for postoperative care, 3:1188, 1189
preoperative, 3:1188, 1191–1192,
1193–1194, 1196, 1200
for recovery at home, 3:1220
Patient history, **2:623–627,** *624*
for anesthesia evaluation, 1:56–57
medical charts for, 2:956
preoperative, 3:1192
Patient positioning, 1:158
Patient responsibilities, 3:1167
Patient rights, 2:1030–1031, 3:1108,
3:1108–1109, 3:1167
Patient Self-Determination Act, 2:901,
3:1190
Patient State Analyzer, 1:164
Pattern baldness, 2:613
Pauling, Linus, 1:59
PBSC (Peripheral blood stem cell
transplantation), 1:195–196, 198
PCA. *See* Patient-controlled analgesia
PCL (Posterior cruciate ligament),
2:791–792, 793
PCNL (Percutaneous nephrolithotomy),
2:1016–1021, *2:1017,* 3:1289
PCP. *See* Phencyclidine
PCTA (Percutaneous transluminal coro-
nary angioplasty), 1:74, 353, 2:628,
977–978
Pectoralis major, 2:986, 987
Pectus excavatum repair, **3:1109–1113,**
1110
Pediatric concerns, **3:1113–1114**
Pediatric hospitals, 3:1113, 1114
Pediatric intensive care units (PICU),
2:758, 759
Pediatric orthopedic surgeons, 1:306
Pediatric surgeons, 1:5, 3:1115
Pediatric surgery, **3:1114–1120,** *1115,*
3:1167, 1386
Pedicle screws, 3:1356
Peer review, professional, 1:540
Pelletier, Kenneth, 2:1006, 3:1284
Pelvic cysts, 1:331
Pelvic exenteration, **1:502–506,** *503*
Pelvic floor disorders, 1:318
Pelvic inflammatory disease, 2:711
Pelvic lymphadenectomy, 2:924
Pelvic muscle exercises, 1:127, 3:1255,
1332
Pelvic organ prolapse, 1:325–329,
395–398
Pelvic osteotomy, 2:662
Pelvic pouch procedure, 2:579,
720–723
Pelvic ultrasound, **3:1120–1122,** *1121*
Pelvic washing, 2:838
Penbutolol, 1:91

Penetrating chest wounds, 3:1416
Penetrating keratoplasty, 1:343
Penetrating wounds, 1:95, 372
Penetrex. See Enoxacin
Penicillinase-resistant penicillins, 1:81
Penicillins, 1:81
  allergies to, 3:1206
  cephalosporins and, 1:269
  hematocrit and, 2:647
  for hospital-acquired infections, 2:687
  penicillinase-resistant, 1:81
  resistance to, 1:49
  side effects of, 1:82
  for splenectomy, 3:1364
Penile cancer, 1:298, 3:1300
Penile implants, **3:1122–1125**, *1123*
Penile nerve blockades, 1:299, 2:704
Penile prosthesis, **3:1122–1125**, *1123,* 3:1231, 1307
Penis
  amputation of, 1:300
  foreskin, 1:266, 267, 297–300, *1:298*
  hypospadias of, 1:299, 2:701–706
Penis construction, 3:1306, *3:1306,* 3:1307
Penoscrotal hypospadias, 2:701
Pentalogy of Cantrell, 2:1035
Pentazocine, 1:50, 53*t*
Pentobarbital, 1:151
Pentosan polysulfate sodium, 3:1255
Pentoxifylline, 1:270, 3:1284
Pepcid. See Famotidine
Peppermint oil, 1:490
Peptic ulcers
  antrectomy for, 1:95–96
  causes of, 2:1028, 3:1209–1211
  in children, 3:1209
  demographics of, 3:1209
  diagnosis of, 3:1211
  mortality and morbidity from, 3:1212
  non-surgical treatment of, 1:98
  pyloroplasty for, 3:1209–1212
  symptoms of, 3:1211
Pepto-Bismol. See Bismuth subsalicylate
Peptostreptococcus, 1:49
Perclose, 1:236
Percocet. See Oxycodone-acetaminophen
Percodan. See Oxycodone
Percussion, 3:1161
Percutaneous balloon valvuloplasty, 1:141–143, 2:636
Percutaneous liver biopsy, 2:886
Percutaneous mitral balloon valvotomy, 2:986
Percutaneous needle biopsy, 1:211
Percutaneous nephrolithotomy (PCNL), **2:1016–1021**, *1017,* 3:1289
Percutaneous nephrostomy, 3:1497
Percutaneous radiofrequency ablation, 3:1390

Percutaneous tenotomy, 3:1404
Percutaneous transhepatic cholangiography (PTC), 1:160, 458
Percutaneous transluminal coronary angioplasty (PCTA), 1:72, 74, 353, 2:628, 977–978
Perianal hernia, 1:318
Pericardial effusion, 3:1125–1128
Pericardiocentesis, **3:1125–1128**
Pericarditis, 3:1125–1128
Perineal repair, 3:1223
Perineum, episiotomy of, 1:479–483, *1:481*
Perineurium, 2:973
Periodontists, 1:184
Periodontitis, 2:597–600
Perioperative blood salvage, 1:178
Perioperative period, 1:67, 3:1385
Peripheral arterial disease. See Peripheral vascular disease
Peripheral blood stem cell transplantation, 1:195–196, 198
Peripheral bypass surgery, 3:1522–1523
Peripheral endarterectomy, **3:1128–1132**
Peripheral iridoplasty, 2:853
Peripheral nerve blockades, 3:1184
Peripheral nerve repair, 2:973
Peripheral nervous system, 3:1083
Peripheral vascular bypass surgery, **3:1132–1137**, *1133*
Peripheral vascular disease
  angioplasty for, 3:1520, 1521, 1523
  defined, 3:1519
  demographics of, 3:1128, 1132, 1134
  homocysteine and, 1:241
  minimally invasive heart surgery for, 2:975
  non-surgical treatment of, 3:1135
  peripheral endarterectomy for, 3:1128–1132
  peripheral vascular bypass surgery for, 3:1132–1137
  prevention of, 3:1131–1132, 1136–1137
Peripheral vascular stent/graft placements, 3:1519
Peripheral vasodilators, 1:89, 91, 543
Peristalsis, 2:583, 865
Peritoneal dialysis, 1:112, 2:779–783
  continuous ambulatory, 2:781, 3:1317
  continuous cyclic, 2:781
  intermittent, 2:781
Peritoneal fluid, 2:693, 695, 3:1095–1096
Peritoneal fluid analysis. See Paracentesis
Peritoneovenous shunts, **3:1137–1140**
Peritonitis
  from abdominal wall defect repair, 1:6

  ascites from, 3:1095
  from cystectomy, 1:394
  from dialysis, 2:782
  from ruptured appendix, 1:109
Permanent pacemakers. See Pacemakers
Persistent labial groove, 1:302
Personal care attendants, 2:678–679
Personal information, 3:1106–1108
Persons United Limiting Substandard and Errors in Health Care (PULSE), 3:1109
Pessary, 1:328, 398, 3:1332
PET. See Positron emission tomography
Peter's anomaly, 2:607
PGE2. See Prostaglandin
pH monitoring
  blood, 1:447
  esophageal, 1:490–493, 2:583, 584, 589
  in urinalysis, 3:1499
Phaco flip, 3:1142
Phacoemulsification, 1:381, 509–510, **3:1140–1145**, *1141, 1142*
  demographics of, 2:1048, 3:1140
  vs. extracapsular extraction, 1:512, 514
Phacolytic glaucoma, 2:849, 850
Phacomatoses, 2:607
Phagocytic cells, 1:337
Phalen test, 1:260
Phantom limb syndrome, 1:46, 3:1083
Pharmaceutical services, 2:690, 3:1168
Pharmacists, 2:758
Pharyngeal cancer, 2:600–601, 3:1145
Pharyngectomy, **3:1145–1149**
Pharyngocutaneous fistula, 3:1147
Pharynx removal. See Pharyngectomy
Phase II step-down units, 3:1222
Phencyclidine, 1:61, 63
Phenelzine, 1:55, 80
Phenergan. See Promethazine hydrochloride
Phenobarbital, 1:151
Phenol acid, 1:418
Phentermine, 2:575, 3:1545
Phenylephrine, 1:33, 3:1305
Phenylketonuria, 1:269
Phenytoin
  gastric acid inhibitors and, 2:569
  NSAIDs and, 2:1028
  for pain, 3:1084
  prochlorperazine and, 1:93
  red blood cell indices and, 3:1229
Pheochromocytoma, 1:31
Phimosis, 1:267, 297, 298
Phlebectomy, 3:1532
Phlebitis, 2:913
Phlebography, **3:1149–1150**
Phlebotomy, **3:1150–1152**
Phobia, social *vs.* specific, 1:78
Phosphate salts, 1:184
Phosphates, 3:1099

Phospho-Soda. *See* Sibasic sodium phosphate
Phosphorus
    electrolyte balance and, 1:446, 447
    pharyngectomy and, 3:1146–1147
    reference range for, 1:448
Photocoagulation therapy, 2:1049, **3:1152–1157**
    vs. retinal cryopexy, 3:1233
    scleral buckling and, 3:1268–1269, 1271
Photodetector probes, 3:1207–1208
Photodynamic therapy, 1:387, 498
Photographic equipment, laparoscopic, 2:828
Photomultiplier-scintillators, 3:1182
Photorefractive keratectomy (PRK), 1:345, 2:848, **3:1157–1161**, *1158*
Photoselective vaporization of the prostate, 3:1457
Photosensitivity
    antibiotics, 1:82, 83
    congenital glaucoma, 2:608
    diuretics, 1:428
    fluoroquinolones, 1:547
    LASIK, 2:846
    sulfonamides, 3:1378
Phototherapeutic keratectomy, 1:345
Phthisis bulbi, 1:390
Phyllanthus niruri, 2:1021
Physical activity. *See* Exercise
Physical examination, **3:1161–1165**
    for anesthesia evaluation, 1:57
    health history and, 2:625
    medical charts for, 2:956
    preoperative, 3:1198
Physical therapy
    chest, 1:348–349, 2:939
    for club foot, 1:307
    for hip replacement, 2:669
    home care and, 2:678
    for knee replacement, 2:805–806
    for kneecap removal, 2:815
    for leg lengthening and shortening, 2:869–870
    for limb length discrepancy, 2:871
    for low back pain, 2:825
    muscle relaxants for, 2:994
    for orthopedic surgery, 2:1064–1065
    for osteoarthritis, 3:1314
    for pain, 3:1084
    for pectus excavatum repair, 3:1112
    purpose of, 2:690
    for rotator cuff syndrome, 3:1248, 1250
    for shoulder dislocations, 1:149
    for shoulder joint replacement, 3:1311
    for shoulder resection arthroplasty, 3:1313
    for simple mastectomy, 3:1321
    for tendon repairs, 3:1402
    for tenotomy, 3:1404
    for urinary incontinence, 1:312

Physician-patient relations
    communication in, 3:1395–1396
    confidentiality and, 3:1106
    informed consent and, 2:751
Physicians
    board certified, 1:540, 3:1165, 1194–1195, 1291
    disciplinary history of, 1:540
    evaluating, 3:1165–1166
    Medicaid and, 2:954
    medical errors and, 2:960, 961
    in nursing homes, 2:1031
    oversupply of, 1:39
    perioperative, 1:67
    primary care, 1:538
    second opinions and, 3:1290–1292
    selecting, 3:1194–1195
    talking to, 3:1395–1396
    workload of, 2:960
    See also Surgeons
Physiologic monitoring, 2:758, 760, 762, 1046
Physiologic pain, 3:1183
Physiotherapy. *See* Physical therapy
PICU (Pediatric intensive care units), 2:758, 759
PIE charting, 2:957
Piezoelectric chips, 1:3
Pig xenografts, 2:777
Pigment dispersion, 2:850
Pigmentary glaucoma, 2:850
Pigmentation changes
    from cryotherapy, 1:378
    dermabrasion for, 1:416, 418
    laser iridotomy for, 2:850
    from laser skin resurfacing, 2:859, 3:1265
    from laser surgery, 2:860, 864
    laser trabeculoplasty for, 2:850
    from liposuction, 2:881
    from sclerotherapy, 3:1283
Piles. *See* Hemorrhoids
Pillow, Charnley, 2:666
Pilocarpine, 2:851
Pilocarpine iontophoresis, 1:448
Pinback otoplasty, 2:1066–1067, *2:1067*
Pindolol, 1:89, 90t, 91
Pins
    for leg lengthening and shortening, 2:867, 869, 870
    magnetic resonance imaging and, 2:928
    for robot-assisted surgery, 3:1243
Pitocin. *See* Oxytocin
Pituitary adenoma, 2:697
Pituitary deficiency, 1:359, 360
Pituitary gland removal. *See* Hypophysectomy
Pituitary Network Association, 2:697
Pituitary tumors, 2:697–701
Placenta previa, 1:284, 285
Placental abruption, 1:283–284
Planning a hospital stay, **3:1165–1171**

Plantar fasciitis, 1:524–526
Plantigrade, 1:305
Plaque
    carotid endarterectomy for, 1:252–257
    endovascular stent surgery for, 1:465–470
    peripheral endarterectomy for, 3:1128–1132
    peripheral vascular bypass surgery for, 3:1132–1137
    prevention of, 1:256, 469–470
    See also Atherosclerosis
Plasma
    apheresis, 1:173
    cryoprecipitated antihemophilic factor, 1:173, 174
    fresh frozen, 1:173, 174
    osmolality, 1:447, 448
    trasfusions, 3:1440
Plasma coagulation, argon beam, 1:98
Plaster casts, 1:555
Plastic eye, 1:476, 504
Plastic surgeons, 1:9, 549
Plastic surgery, **3:1171–1175**, 3:1386
    advertisements for, 1:541
    ambulatory surgery centers and, 1:37
    description of, 3:1172
    elective, 1:438
    microsurgery and, 2:970
Plateau iris, 2:849, 850
Platelet counts
    abnormal, 1:337
    for anesthesia evaluation, 1:58
    critical values for, 1:339
    for liver biopsy, 2:888
    for lung biopsy, 2:916
    normal values for, 1:338
    procedure for, 1:335
Platelet transfusion, 1:173–174
Platelets
    alloimmunization of, 1:179
    role of, 1:193
    trasfusions, 3:1440
Plates
    for leg lengthening and shortening, 2:870
    magnetic resonance imaging and, 2:928
Plavix. *See* Clopidogrel
Play, 3:1113–1114
Plendil. *See* Felodipine
Pletal. *See* Cilostazol
Pleural effusion
    chest tube insertion for, 1:288–290
    chest x ray for, 1:291
    malignant, 1:290
    paracentesis for, 3:1096
    spirometry tests for, 3:1359
PMMA implants, 2:855, 856
Pneumatic compression stockings, 3:1539
Pneumatic pumps, 2:942

Pneumatic retinopexy, 3:1156, 1233, 1271
Pneumobelt, 2:945
Pneumococcal vaccine, 3:1363
Pneumococcus infections, 2:1005
Pneumocystis carinii pneumonia (PCP), 2:899, 914, 3:1377, 1413
Pneumonectomy, **3:1175–1179,** 3:1295, 1414
Pneumonia
    aspiration, 2:593
    bronchial, 1:292
    burn-related, 3:1326
    chest x ray for, 1:291, 292
    esophageal atresia/tracheoe-sophageal fistula and, 1:489
    hospital-acquired, 2:685, 686
    from oxygen therapy, 2:1075
    after lung transplantation, 3:1413
    Penumcystis carinii, 2:899, 914, 3:1377, 1413
    spirometry tests for, 3:1359
    ventilator-associated, 2:685
Pneumothorax, 3:1416
    chest tube insertion for, 1:288, 289
    chest x ray for, 1:291
    from lung biopsy, 2:917
    from pacemakers, 3:1081
    pulmonary lobectomy for, 2:904
    spirometry tests for, 3:1359
POAG (Primary open-angle glaucoma), 3:1272
Poikilocytosis, 1:336
Point-of-care monitoring, 2:761, 762, 1046
Point-of-service (POS) plans, 2:932–933
Point pressure leak test, 3:1236
Poisoning
    dialysis for, 2:779
    hemoperfusion for, 2:652–653
Poland syndrome, 3:1110, 1557
Polidocanol, 3:1282
Pollution, 2:903, 3:1175
Polychromasia, 1:336
Polycystic kidneys, 1:271
Polycythemia vera
    complete blood count for, 1:335, 337
    hematocrit and, 2:647
    hemoglobin test for, **2:650–652**
    phlebotomy for, **3:1150–1152**
Polydactyly, 3:1555, 1557
Polyethylene cement, 2:811
Polyethylene prosthesis, 2:673, 810
Polyglycemic unawareness, 2:777
Polyhydramnios, 1:488
Polymer grafts, 1:188
Polymer sorbents, 2:652
Polymyxin B, 1:84
Polypectomy
    colorectal, *1:314,* 1:317
    nasal, 3:1302, 1303
Polypropylene mesh, 2:748, 755

Polyps
    barium enema for, 1:154–155
    colorectal, 1:206, **1:313–317**
    endometrial, 1:419
    intestinal, 3:1117, 1317, 1334–1335
    nasal, 3:1302, 1303
    uterine, 2:711, 712
Polysporin, 1:84
Polystyrene injections, 3:1365
Polythiazide, 1:89
Polyurethane dressings, 1:144, 145, 2:744
Polyurethane membrane, 2:744
Polyvinyl alcohol, 2:710, 3:1365
Ponseti, Ignacio, 1:307
Ponseti treatment, 1:307
Pool-of-money contracts, 2:908
Porphyromonas infections, 1:48
Portacaval shunts, 3:1139, 1179
Portal hypertension
    esophageal varices from, 3:1277
    non-surgical treatment of, 3:1181
    peritoneovenous shunts for, 3:1137
    portal vein bypass surgery for, 3:1179–1182
    sclerotherapy for, 3:1181
Portal vein angiography, 1:70
Portal vein bypass surgery, **3:1179–1182,** *1180*
POS plans, 2:932–933
Posey vests, 2:761
Positions, patient, 1:158
Positive-pressure airflow, 1:129
Positron emission tomography (PET), **3:1182–1183**
    for anterior temporal lobectomy, 1:76
    for breast cancer, 2:929
    for lung cancer, 3:1176
Post-cholecystectomy syndrome, 1:296
Post-surgical pain, **3:1183–1187**
    acetaminophen for, 1:21
    anesthesiologists and, 1:67
    opioid analgesics for, 1:52, 3:1185
Post-traumatic stress disorder, 1:162, 366–367, 3:1326
Postanesthesia care units (PACU), 3:1187–1188
    See also Recovery room
Posterior cruciate ligament (PCL), 2:791–792, 793
Posterior pelvic exenteration, 1:504
Posterior subcapsular cataracts, 1:510, 512, 513
Posterior synechia, 2:852
Posterior vitreous detachment, 3:1153
Posterolateral thoracotomy, 3:1176, 1414
Postlaparoscopy syndrome, 2:830
Postoperative blood collection, 3:1168, 1197, 1202
Postoperative blood salvage, 1:135, 178, 179
Postoperative care, **3:1187–1190**
    anesthesiologists and, 1:67

    exercise and, 1:506, 508
    at home, 3:1219–1221
    in intensive care units, 2:759
    recovery room for, 3:1221–1222
    surgical team for, 3:1385, 1388
    See also Post-surgical pain
Postoperative complications
    bleeding, 1:403–404
    from cataract surgery, 1:514
    in for-profit *vs.* non-profit hospitals, 2:690
    from laparoscopy, 2:827, 830–831
    post-discharge, 1:424
    scopolamine patch for, 3:1286–1288
    surgical oncology and, 3:1384–1385
Postoperative infections, 1:128–130, 269
    See also Surgical site infections
Postpartum depression, 1:286
Postsplenectomy sepsis, 3:1363–1364
Potassium-sparing diuretics, 1:428, 429, 430
Potassium supplements, 1:91
    for cardioplegia, 2:629
    diuretics and, 1:428, 430
    for Maze procedure, 2:939
Potassium tests, 1:446–449
Potential acuity meter (PAM), 2:855
Potentiometry, 1:448
Pouch
    for bladder augmentation, 1:166–168
    colostomy, 1:318, 320, 324
    for ileoanal anastomosis, 2:717–719, *2:718*
    for ileoanal reservoir surgery, 2:720, 722
    for interstitial cystitis, 3:1255
    J-pouch, 2:720
    for urinary diversion, 1:392, *1:393,* 1:393–394
Pouchitis, 2:719, 722
Poverty level, 2:953
Povidone iodine, 1:94
Power of attorney, **3:1190–1191**
    children and, 3:1193
    DNR orders and, 1:431
    hospital admissions and, 1:27
    living will and, 2:901
    nursing homes and, 2:1030
    purpose of, 1:404
PPO (Preferred provider organizations), 2:932–933, 3:1203
    See also Health insurance
PR. *See* Progesterone receptors
PRA test, 2:641, 693, 789
Pranylcypromine, 1:55
Pravaz, Charles, 3:1392
Prazepam, 1:79*t*
Prazosin hydrochloride, 1:90*t*
Pre-eclampsia, 3:1271
Pre-hospital Medical Care Directive, 1:431

Preadmission instructions, 3:1168–1169
Preadmission testing, 3:1168
Prealbumin tests, 2:891, 893
Precancerous conditions, 1:329–331, 340
  See also Cancer
Prednisolone, 1:360, 2:733
Prednisone
  for asthma, 2:751–752
  for eye enucleation, 1:476
  immunosuppressant drugs and, 2:736
  for liver transplantation, 2:899
  for Ménière's disease, 1:455
  uses of, 1:360
Preemptive analgesia, 3:1184
Preferred provider organizations (PPO), 2:932–933, 3:1203
  See also Health insurance
Pregnancy
  abdominoplasty and, 1:7, 8
  antianxiety drugs and, 1:79–80
  antibiotics and, 1:82–83
  anticoagulants and, 1:87
  antihypertensive drugs and, 1:91
  antinausea drugs and, 1:93
  antiseptics and, 1:94
  aspirin and, 1:132
  barbiturates and, 1:152
  benzodiazepines and, 2:994
  carpal tunnel release and, 1:257, 261
  cephalosporins and, 1:269
  colpotomy and, 1:331
  cone biopsy and, 1:341
  corticosteroids and, 1:360
  CT scans and, 1:383
  delivery weights, 3:1437
  diuretics and, 1:429
  electrophysiology study and, 1:449
  endometriosis and, 2:835
  epoetin and, 2:729–730
  erythromycins and, 1:484
  fluoroquinolones and, 1:546
  gallstones and, 2:557
  gestational diabetes and, 2:603
  immunoassay tests for, 2:726
  immunosuppressant drugs and, 2:734
  interferons and, 2:730
  laser surgery and, 2:860
  laxatives and, 2:866
  lithotripsy and, 2:884
  lumpectomy and, 2:910–911
  magnetic resonance imaging and, 2:928
  multiple, 1:7, 2:741, 742
  muscle relaxants and, 2:994
  myomectomy and, 2:1001
  NSAIDs and, 2:1028
  opioid analgesics and, 1:53
  otosclerosis and, 3:1365
  pelvic ultrasound for, **3:1120–1122**

sclerotherapy and, 3:1282
skull x rays and, 3:1329
smoking and, 3:1338
spider veins from, 3:1280
spirometry tests for, 3:1359
sulfonamides and, 3:1378
tetracyclines and, 3:1406–1407
thrombolytic therapy and, 3:1418
topical antibiotics and, 1:85
  See also Childbirth; Ectopic pregnancy
Pregnancy tests, 1:92
Premature infants
  circumcision of, 1:299
  hemangioma in, 2:644
  inguinal hernias in, 2:753
  oxygen therapy for, 2:1075
Premature labor
  cervical cerclage for, 1:278–281
  demographics of, 1:279, 280
  fetal surgery and, 1:533
  from fetoscopy, 1:535
  non-surgical delaying of, 1:280
  tocolytics for, 1:532, 2:876
Premedication, 1:61
Premiums, climbing, 2:907–908
Prenatal screening
  for abdominal wall defect repair, 1:5, 6
  chorionic villus sampling, 1:42, 43, 532, 3:1120
  lipid tests for, 2:875
  for omphaloceles, 2:1036
  pelvic ultrasound for, 3:1120–1122
  for spina bifida, 2:965
  See also Amniocentesis
Preoperation, exercise, 2:668
Preoperative autologous blood donation (PABD), 1:134–135, 3:1196–1197, 1202
Preoperative blood salvage, 1:178
Preoperative care, **3:1191–1194**
  patient education for, 3:1188, 1191–1192, 1193–1194, 1196, 1200
  surgical team for, 3:1385, 1387–1388
  tests for, 3:1196
Preoperative period, 3:1194–1200
  anxiety during, 3:1192, 1201
  aseptic technique for, 1:128–129
  drug use during, 3:1197, 1202
  exercise and, 2:668
  instructions for, 3:1196–1197
  pain management for, 3:1184–1186
  presurgical testing, **3:1200–1203**
Preoperative testing, 3:1192, **3:1200–1203**
Preparing for surgery, **3:1194–1200**
Presbyopia, 2:845, 1051, 3:1160
Preschool children, 3:1113
Prescriptions
  computerized order systems for, 2:690

errors in, 2:960
Medicare and, 2:963
  See also Drugs
Pressure-related ear pain, 2:1004
Pressure sores/ulcers, **1:155–159**, *157*, 1:408
Pressure ventilators, 2:945
Presurgical testing, 3:1192, **3:1200–1203**
Pretracheal incision, 1:549
Prevacid. *See* Lansoprazole
Preventive medicine, 2:963
Prevotella infections, 1:48
Prilocaine, 1:299, 386
Prilosec. *See* Omeprazole
Primaquine, 2:651
Primary biliary cirrhosis, 1:456
Primary care nurses, 2:933
Primary care physicians, 1:538
Primary open-angle glaucoma (POAG), 3:1272
Primary sclerosing cholangitis, 1:159, 457
Primary snoring, 3:1342, 1345
Primary teeth, 3:1429–1430
Privacy, 3:1109
Private insurance plans, **3:1203–1206,** 3:1316
  See also Health insurance
PRK. *See* Photorefractive keratectomy
Probing instruments, 3:1381
Probucol, 1:356, 472
Procardia. *See* Nifedipine
Processus vaginalis, 2:695
Prochlorperazine, 1:92, 92*t*, 93
Procollagen, 3:1402
Procrit. *See* Epoetin
Proctectomy, mucosal, 2:717
Proctocolectomy, 2:720, 723
Proctosigmoidectomy, 3:1223
ProDisc, total, 1:425
Productive pain, 1:50
Professional organizations, 3:1165–1166, 1195
Professional peer review, 1:540
Profound deafness, 1:310
Progesterone receptors, 3:1471, 1472
Prograf. *See* Tacrolimus
Progress notes, 2:956, 957
Prolapse
  bladder, 1:325, 327, 395–398
  mitral valve, 2:978–986
  pelvic organ, 1:325–329, 395–398
  rectal, 1:318, 325, 327, 395, 3:1222–1225
  small intestine, 1:327
  stoma, 1:320, 325
  urethral, 1:327
  uterine, 1:327
Proleukin. *See* Aldesleukin
Prolonged prothrombin time (PT), 2:916
Prolotherapy, 3:1402–1403
Prolymphocytes, 1:335

Promethazine hydrochloride, 1:92*t*, 3:1287
Prophylactic antibiotics. *See* Antibiotic prophylaxis
Prophylactic mastectomy, 3:1319
Prophylactic oophorectomy, 2:1039, 1040
Propionibacterium infections, 1:49
Propofol, 1:61
Propoxyphene, 1:80
  for analgesia, 1:51, 53*t*
  diazepam and, 2:995
  opioid analgesics and, 1:55
Propoxyphene-acetaminophen, 1:52, 55
Propranolol
  alprazolam and, 1:80
  diazepam and, 2:995
  for esophageal varices, 3:1278
  for hypertension, 1:89, 90*t*
Proprietary (for-profit) hospitals, 2:688, 689, 690
Prostaglandin E2, 2:1028
Prostaglandin synthetase, 2:1028
Prostaglandins, 3:1509
  aspirin and, 1:132
  cyclocryotherapy and, 1:389
  pain and, 3:1083
  peptic ulcers and, 1:98
  uterine stimulants, 3:1510–1511
Prostate cancer
  cryotherapy for, 1:377, 378
  cystoscopy for, 1:400
  demographics, 3:1506
  demographics of, 2:1052, 3:1383
  diagnosis of, 2:1054
  non-surgical treatment of, 2:1056–1057
  orchiectomy for, 2:1052, 1054
  pelvic exenteration for, 1:503, 504
Prostate disorders, 1:125, 398–402, 2:1041–1045
Prostate specific antigen (PSA), 2:1044, 1054, 3:1454, 1455, 1470, 1472
Prostate transurethral resection, 2:1042
Prostatectomy
  fecal incontinence from, 1:125
  open, **2:1041–1045**, *1043*
  retropubic, 2:1042, 1044
  robot-assisted, 3:1243
  suprapubic (transvesical), 2:1044
  surgeon skill level for, 1:540
Prostatic stents, 3:1458
Prostep. *See* Nicotine replacement therapy
Prosthesis
  advances in, 2:1064
  breast, 1:216, 3:1321
  cementless, 2:802
  ceramic, 2:666
  Charnley, 2:666
  dislocations, 2:670, 676
  foot-in-foot, 2:871
  hip, 2:664–678, *2:674*

knee, **2:799–809**, 2:809–814
  life expectancy of, 2:670, 677
  for limb salvage, 2:872
  ocular, 1:476, 504
  penile, **3:1122–1125**, *1123*, 3:1231, 1307
  polyethylene, 2:673, 810
  in reconstructive surgery, 3:1172
  shoulder, 3:1308–1312, 1314
  teeth, 1:415
  tongue, 2:602
  See also Joint replacement; Revision surgery
Protective devices
  for laser surgery, 2:862–863
  sterile surgical, 1:129
Protein
  cerebrospinal fluid analysis of, 1:276, 277
  liver function tests for, 2:890–895
  myelin basic, 1:276
  in urinalysis, 2:784, 785, 786, 3:1499, 1501
Protein electrophoresis, 1:276, 2:893
Protein intoxication, 3:1278
Prothrombin time
  for liver biopsy, 2:888
  liver function tests for, 2:890–895
Proton pump inhibitors, 1:98, 2:568, 569, 578, 588, 590
Protozoal infections, 1:81
Protruding ears, 2:1066–1067, 1068, 1069, 1070
Proxy, health care, **2:622–623**, 2:902, 3:1190
Prozac. *See* Fluoxetine
Prune belly syndrome, 2:1059, 3:1103
Prussian blue stain, 1:190
PSA. *See* Prostate specific antigen
PSA 4000, 1:164
Pseudoarthrosis, 2:663, 672, 3:1355
Pseudocysts, 1:1
Pseudoexfoliation glaucoma, 2:850
Pseudomembranous colitis, 1:82
Pseudomonas aeruginosa infections, 1: 81, 82, 83
  after lung transplantation, 3:1413
  wounds and, 3:1569–1570
Pseudophakic bullous keratopathy, 1:342, 344
Psychiatric evaluation
  for gender reassignment, 2:1054, 1055
  for low back pain, 2:823
  for plastic surgery, 3:1173
  for scar revision surgery, 3:1265–1266
  for vertical banded gastroplasty, 3:1546
Psychological complications
  of colostomy, 1:324
  of craniofacial reconstruction, 1:366–367
  of ostomy, 1:320

Psychotherapy
  for burns, 3:1326
  for orchiectomy, 2:1055
  for plastic surgery, 3:1173
  postoperative, 3:1220
  sex reassignment surgery and, 3:1306
Psyllium, 2:656, 865, 949
PT (Prolonged prothrombin time), 2:916
PTA (Percutaneous transluminal angioplasty), 1:72, 74, 353, 2:628, 977–978
Pterygium, 1:342
PTFE catheters, 1:263, 266
Ptosis, 1:548
PTT (Partial thromboplastin time), 2:916
Public Health Service, 1:283
Pubocervical fascia, 1:395, 397
Pubovaginal sling. *See* Sling procedure
Pulmonary angiography, 1:70
Pulmonary artery banding, 2:637
Pulmonary artery catheters, 1:243
Pulmonary atresia, 2:637
Pulmonary disease. *See* Lung disease
Pulmonary edema
  chest x ray for, 1:291
  myocardial resection for, 2:997
  phlebotomy for, 3:1150–1151
Pulmonary embolism, 1:384, 2:660, 894, 3:1149, 1538
Pulmonary fibrosis, 2:914, 918, 3:1358, 1359
Pulmonary function tests, 2:904, 920
Pulmonary hypertension
  lung biopsy and, 2:916
  lung transplantation and, 2:919
  mitral valve repair and, 2:980, 981
  mitral valve replacement and, 2:984
Pulmonary hypoplasia, 1:531, 534
Pulmonary infections, 3:1413
Pulmonary lobectomy, **2:902–906**, 3:1295
Pulmonary resection, 3:1412
Pulmonary surfactants. *See* Surfactants
Pulmonary valve stenosis, 1:141–143
Pulmonologists, 1:226
Pulpitis, 3:1244–1247
Pulsatile paracorporeal mechanical circulatory support, 2:843
Pulse, 1:244, 246, 3:1130, 1135, 1552, *1553*, 1554
  See also Arrhythmia
Pulse generators, 1:410, 411
Pulse oximeter, **3:1207–1209**, *1208*
  for conscious sedation, 3:1292–1293
  in intensive care units, 2:760
  for microsurgery, 2:974
  in operating rooms, 2:1046
PULSE (Persons United Limiting Substandard and Errors in Health Care), 3:1109
Pulsed dye lasers, 3:1265

Pumpkin seed oil, 3:1458
Pumps
    infusion, 2:1046
    intra-aorta balloon, 2:760, 843, 1046
    for mechanical circulation support, 2:942
    for patient-controlled analgesia, 3:1104
    for venous thrombosis, 3:1539
    See also Heart-lung machines
Punch instruments, adenoid, 1:23
Puncture wounds, 1:1
    See also Penetrating wounds
Pupillary block, 2:849–850, 853
Pupillary block glaucoma. *See* Angle closure glaucoma
Pupillary reaction, 3:1154
Pupillometer, 2:844
Purinethol. *See* Mercaptopurine
Purpura, idiopathic thrombocytic, 1:337, 3:1364–1365
Purse-string stitch, 1:279
Pus, 1:18
    See also Infections
PVD. *See* Peripheral vascular disease
PVP. *See* Photoselective vaporization of the prostate
Pyelogram
    intravenous, 2:884, 1018
    retrograde, 1:399
    for ureteral obstruction, 3:1491
Pyelonephritis, 2:716
Pygeum bark, 3:1458
Pyloric atresia, 3:1116
Pyloric stenosis, 3:1117
Pyloric valve disorders, 2:575
Pyloroplasty, 2:566, 579, **3:1209–1212**, *1210*, 3:1515
Pyridium, 3:1456

Q

Quadrantectomy, **3:1213–1215**
    See also Lumpectomy
Quadriceps tendon, 2:814, 815
Quadriplegia, 1:156
Qualitative immunoassay tests, 2:726, 727
Quality improvement, 2:961
Quality Interagency Coordination Task Force (QuIC), 2:959, 960, 961
Quality of care, 2:1031, 3:1108
Quality of life, 2:623, 907, 3:1342
Quantitative EEG, 1:444
Quantitative immunoassay tests, 2:726, 727
Quantitative ventilation/perfusion (V/Q) scan, 2:904, 920
Questions to Ask Your Doctor Before You Have Surgery, 1:539
Questran. *See* Cholestyramine

QuIC (Quality Interagency Coordination Task Force), 2:959, 960, 961
Quinapril, 1:89, 90*t*

R

Rabeprazole, 2:568
RACE study, 1:250–251
Radial artery, 1:346
Radial forearm free flaps, 2:601
Radial keratotomy, 2:848, 3:1160
Radiance, 1:552
Radiation, ultraviolet, 1:511
Radiation exposure
    angiography, 1:72
    bone x rays, 1:203–204
    cardiac catheterization, 1:238
    CT scans, 1:383
    electrophysiology study, 1:449
    nuclear medicine scans, 1:240
    phlebography, 3:1149
    pituitary tumors treatment, 2:699–700
    skull x rays, 3:1329
Radiation therapy
    for basal cell carcinoma, 2:992
    bone marrow transplantation and, 1:193, 199
    for breast cancer, 2:989, 3:1214
    for cancer, 1:202
    complete blood count for, 1:334
    for head and neck cancer, 3:1218
    for heterotropic bone, 2:670
    for laryngeal cancer, 2:841
    limb salvage and, 2:873
    low laser, 1:408
    lumpectomy and, 2:910–911, 913, 3:1319
    for lung cancer, 3:1177
    for neuroblastoma, 3:1233
    non-myeloablative allogeneic transplantation and, 1:195
    pancreatectomy and, 3:1093
    for pituitary tumors, 2:699–700
    segmentectomy and, 3:1295, 1296
    for skin cancer, 1:387
    whole-brain, 3:1370
Radical cystectomy, 1:391, 392, 394, 2:713
Radical hysterectomy, 1:341, 2:706, 708
Radical mastectomy, 3:1215, 1320
Radical mastoidectomy, 2:935
Radical neck dissection, 1:434, 435, **3:1217–1219**
Radical nephrectomy, 2:1013, 1015
Radical orchiectomy, 2:1054
Radioactive wire therapy, 2:602
Radiofrequency ablation
    for arrhythmia, 2:999
    laparoscopic, 2:828
    for Maze procedure, 2:937
    for sympathectomy, 3:1390

Radiofrequency volumetric tissue reduction (RFVTR), 3:1344
Radioimmunoassay, 2:727
    See also Immunoassay tests
Radiologic technologists, 2:762
Radiopharmaceuticals, 3:1182
Radiosurgery, stereotactic, **3:1369–1371**
Radiotherapy. *See* Radiation therapy
Radon, 2:903, 3:1175
Ramipril, 1:90*t*
Ramsey Sedation Score, 1:162–163
Range of motion
    arthroplasty for, 1:116–120
    finger reattachment and, 1:545
    hip revision surgery and, 2:677
    knee arthroscopic surgery and, 2:796
    knee osteotomy and, 2:798
    shoulder joint replacement and, 3:1311
    after tendon repairs, 3:1402
    tenotomy for, 3:1404–1405
Range of motion exercises
    continuous passive, 2:798, 805, 806, 873
    for knee injuries, 2:796
    for leg lengthening, 2:870
    for limb salvage, 2:873
    for shoulder joint replacement, 3:1311
    for shoulder resection arthroplasty, 3:1313
    for simple mastectomy, 3:1321
Ranitidine, 2:568
Rapamune. *See* Sirolimus
Rapamycin, 2:899
Rash. *See* Skin lesions
Rasmussen disease, 2:649, 650
Rate Control *vs.* Electrical Cardioversion for Persistent Atrial Fibrillation study, 1:250–251
Raynaud's disease, 2:583, 3:1128, 1389
RBCs. *See* Red blood cells
RDW (Red cell distribution width), 1:339, 3:1229
Reactive hypoglycemia, 2:566
Reasonable patient standard, 2:751
Receiver-stimulators, cochlear, 1:308, *1:309*
Recombinant interferon alfa-2a, 2:729
Recombinant interferon alfa-2b, 2:729
Reconstructive surgery, **3:1171–1175,** 3:1386
    for bedsores, 1:158
    bladder augmentation for, 1:166
    bone grafts for, 1:184
    craniofacial, **1:361–369,** 2:745, 967, 3:1244
    description of, 3:1172
    ear, nose and throat, 1:433
    elective, 1:437–439
    microsurgery for, 2:973–974
    See also Breast reconstruction

Records, medical, **2:955–959,** 3:1106–1108, 1109

Recovery at home, 1:506, 508, **3:1219–1221**

Recovery room, 2:690, 3:1114, 1187–1188, **3:1221–1222**

Recreational drugs. *See* Street drugs

Rectal anastomosis, 3:1225

Rectal artificial sphincter, **1:123–128,** *124*

Rectal bleeding, **3:1315–1318**

Rectal cancer
    barium enema for, 1:154–155
    bowel resection for, 1:208
    pelvic exenteration for, 1:503, 504

Rectal intussusception, 3:1222

Rectal prolapse
    colorectal surgery for, 1:318
    colporrhaphy for, 1:325, 327
    cystocele repair for, 1:395
    demographics of, 3:1223
    non-surgical treatment of, 3:1224
    repair, 1:395, 3:1222–1225

Rectal resection, **3:1225–1228,** *1226*
    See also Colorectal surgery

Rectal thermometers, 3:1409–1410

Rectocele, 1:318, 325, 327, 3:1222

Rectopexy, 3:1223–1224

Rectovaginal fascia, 1:327

Recurrent laryngeal nerve damage, 3:1098

Red blood cell indices, 1:334, 336, **3:1228–1230**
    See also Hematocrit; Hemoglobin test

Red blood cell transfusion, 1:173, 179, 3:1439–1440

Red blood cells, 1:277, 278, 335, 338
    alloimmunization of, 1:179
    bone marrow aspiration for, 1:189
    morphology of, 1:336
    role of, 1:193
    substitutes for, 1:182
    in urinalysis, 3:1502
    washed packed, 1:179
    white blood cell counts and, 3:1565

Red cell distribution width (RDW), 1:339, 3:1229

Red Cross. *See* American Red Cross

Reduced-size liver transplantation, 2:896

Reduction mammoplasty. *See* Breast reduction

Referrals, 1:40, 538–539

Reflex sympathetic dystrophy, 3:1389, 1390

Reflexia, 1:166

Refludan. *See* Lepirudin

Reflux. *See* Gastroesophageal reflux disease

Reflux esophagitis, 2:582

Refractive vision errors
    LASIK for, 2:841–848

non-surgical treatment of, 3:1160–1161
    ophthalmologic surgery for, 1:438, 2:1048, 1049, 1050
    photorefractive keratectomy for, 3:1157–1161

Refractory glaucoma, 1:388–389

Refractory periodontitis, 2:599

Refusal of treatment, 3:1108

Regional anesthesia, 1:63–66, 3:1387
    for cervical cerclage, 1:279
    for cesarean section, 1:63, 284, 286
    for obstetric and gynecologic surgery, 2:1034

Regional lymph node dissection, 3:1383

Registration, hospital, 3:1169–1171

Registry of the International Society for Heart and Lung Transplantation (ISHLT), 2:643

Reglan. *See* Metoclopramide hydrochloride

Regranex, 1:46

Regurgitation, 1:494

Rehabilitation
    for amputation, 1:46
    for burns, 3:1326
    for knee arthroscopic surgery, 2:795
    for knee injuries, 2:796
    for limb salvage, 2:873–874
    for microsurgery, 2:974
    occupational, 1:261
    for orthopedic surgery, 2:1064–1065
    recovery at home for, 3:1221

Rehydration therapy, 2:766–767

Reiger's anomaly, 2:607

Reimbursement, 2:1032

Rejection, graft. *See* Transplant rejection

Relafen. *See* Nabumetone

Relaxation techniques
    for pain, 3:1084
    preoperative, 3:1196, 1201
    See also Complementary and alternative medicine

Religions
    hospices and, 2:683
    orchiectomy and, 2:1052

REM stage, 1:60

REMATCH trial, 2:643

Remote surgery, **3:1398–1399**

Renal angiography, 1:70

Renal arteries, 1:466, 3:1129

Renal cell carcinoma, 2:1014, 1015

Renal failure. *See* Kidney failure

Renal pelvis tumors, 2:1022, 1023

Renal transplantation. *See* Kidney transplantation

Renese. *See* Polythiazide

Reoperation, **3:1230–1231**
    aortic valve replacement, 1:106–107
    artificial sphincter insertion, 1:126
    breast cancer, 3:1230
    cancer, 3:1230

colon cancer, 3:1230
    coronary artery disease, 1:357, 3:1230
    Crohn's disease, 3:1230
    fundoplication, 3:1230
    gastroesophageal reflux disease, 3:1230
    gastrointestinal disorders, 3:1230
    vasectomy, 3:1231

Repeated large-volume paracentesis, 3:1139

Repetitive stress injury, 1:257, 2:619, 3:1400

Replantation surgery, 2:973

Report to the President on Medical Errors, 2:959

Repose system, 3:1345

Reproductive endocrinology, 2:1033

Rescue breathing, 1:244, 246–247

Research hospitals, 2:689

Residents, 2:960, 3:1167, 1388

Residual volume (RV), 3:1358–1360

Resiniferatoxin, 3:1255

Resins, 2:652

Respirators, 2:760

Respiratory arrest, 1:246

Respiratory distress syndrome, 2:876, 3:1412

Respiratory failure, 2:760, 944–946

Respiratory rate, 3:1552, *1553,* 1553–1554

Respiratory syncytial virus, 2:1005

Respiratory therapists, 2:758–759, 762

Respiratory therapy, 2:678, 690, 904
    See also Oxygen therapy

Respiratory tract infections, upper, 1:460, 489

Responsibilities, patients', 3:1167

Restenosis
    balloon valvuloplasty and, 1:143
    coronary stenting and, 1:353, 355, 356
    minimally invasive heart surgery and, 2:977
    peripheral endarterectomy and, 3:1131
    peripheral vascular bypass surgery and, 3:1136

Resting heart rate, 1:508

Restraints, 2:1030

Resuscitation. *See* Cardiopulmonary resuscitation

Resuscitation carts, 2:760

Resuscitative medical equipment, 2:1045–1046

Resuscitative thoracotomy. *See* Emergency thoracotomy

Reticulocytes, 1:335, 338

Retinal cancer exeneration, 1:503

Retinal cryopexy, **3:1231–1234,** 3:1269, 1271

Retinal detachment
    from cataract surgery, 1:514, 3:1152, 1268

Retinal hemorrhage

cryopexy for, 3:1231–1234, 1269
demographics of, 3:1152, 1231, 1268
diagnosis of, 3:1154–1155, 1270
exudative, 3:1153
fluorescein angiography for, 1:70
from laser posterior capsulotomy, 2:856
from LASIK, 3:1153
from phacoemulsification, 3:1144
photocoagulation therapy for, 3:1152–1157, 1271
pneumatic retinopexy for, 3:1156
rhegmatogenous, 3:1152–1153, 1156
risk factors for, 3:1153
scleral buckling for, 3:1156, 1233, 1268–1271
from surgical capsulotomy, 2:857
traction, 3:1153
vitrectomy for, 3:1156–1157, 1268, 1270, 1271
Retinal hemorrhage, 2:847
Retinal tear
from cataract surgery, 1:514
photocoagulation therapy for, 3:1152–1157
scleral buckling for, 3:1268–1271
Retinoblastoma, 1:474, 3:1231–1234
Retinoic acid, 1:418
Retinopathy
diabetic, 2:855, 3:1153
of prematurity, 2:1075, 3:1153, 1156
Retinopexy, pneumatic, 3:1156, 1233, 1271
Retractile testicles, 2:1060
Retractors, 3:1381
Retrograde ejaculation, 2:1044
Retrograde pyelogram, 1:399
Retropubic colposuspension, 1:397, 3:1236
Retropubic prostatectomy, 2:1042, 1044
Retropubic suspension, 3:1234–1238, 1235, 3:1331
Retrovir. See Zidovudine
Revascularization, 1:466, 3:1128, 1132
Reverse glycolysis, 2:604
Revia. See Naltrexone
Revision surgery
for craniofacial reconstruction, 1:366
hip, 2:666, 670, 2:673–678, 674
knee, 2:806, 2:809–814
Reye's syndrome, 1:132, 2:892–894
RFVTR (Radiofrequency volumetric tissue reduction), 3:1344
Rh blood group, 1:174, 180, 3:1441, 1480–1481, 1483
Rh immune globulin, 1:16
RhBMP-2, 1:187–188
Rhegmatogenous retinal detachment, 3:1152–1153, 1156

Rheumatic fever, 1:142, 2:979, 982–983, 986
Rheumatoid arthritis
arthroplasty for, 1:116, 118, 119
arthroscopic surgery for, 1:121
bunions and, 1:231
carpal tunnel release and, 1:257
complementary and alternative medicine for, 2:672
hip replacement for, 2:664
knee replacement for, 2:800, 801
non-surgical treatment of, 1:119, 2:621, 807
shoulder joint replacement for, 3:1310
toe abnormalities and, 2:616
wrist replacement and, 3:1572
Rheumatrex. See Methotrexate
Rhinitis, allergic, 3:1305
Rhinophyma, 1:416
Rhinoplasty, 2:967, 3:1238–1241, 1239, 3:1302
See also Nose surgery
Rhizotomy, 3:1241–1242
RhoGAM. See Rh immune globulin
Rhytides, 2:858
Rhytidoplasty. See Face lift
Rib fractures, 1:293, 2:977
RICE (Rest, ice, compression, elevation), 2:796
Rickets, vitamin D dependent, 1:447
Ridley, Harold, 1:510
Rifadin. See Rifampin
Rifampin, 1:55, 2:651
Right ventricular assist devices (RVAD), 3:1540, 1541
Rights of patients, 2:1030–1031, 3:1108–1109, 3:1167
Rigid cystoscopy, 1:399
Rigid fixation, 1:365
Ringer's lactate, 1:477, 543
Rinne's test, 3:1366
Ritodrine, 1:280
Roadmap fluoroscopy, 1:74
Robaxin. See Methocarbamol
Robot-assisted surgery, 2:828, 1046, 3:1242–1244, 1:1399
Rods
Harrington, 3:1356
for leg lengthening and shortening, 2:870
Luque, 3:1356
magnetic resonance imaging and, 2:928
semi-rigid, 3:1124
for spinal instrumentation, 3:1355–1357
Rofecoxib, 1:50, 2:1028
Roferon, 2:729
Roller pumps, 2:629
Rooms, hospital, 1:27, 3:1167
Root canal treatment, 3:1244–1247, 1245
Root resectioning, 3:1246

Ross procedure, 2:637
Rotablation, 1:356
Rotary pumps, 2:942
Rotator cuff repair, 1:121, 2:926, 3:1247–1251, 1249
Rounded shoulders, 3:1112
Routine urinalysis. See Urinalysis
Roux, Cesar, 3:1549
Roux-en-Y gastric bypass, 2:571, 2:571–572, 3:1549
Roux limb, 2:572
Roxicet. See Oxycodone-acetaminophen
RU-486. See Mifepristone
Rubber band ligation, 2:655, 656
Rubber dam, 3:1245
Rubell syndrome, 2:607
Rufen. See Ibuprofen
Ruptured appendix, 1:109
RV (Residual volume), 3:1358–1360
RVAD. See Right ventricular assist devices

S

Sacral nerve stimulation, 3:1253–1256
Sacrococcygeal teratoma (SCT), 1:531, 532, 533
Sacrum, 2:819
St. John's wort, 1:34, 57, 3:1407–1408
Salicylates
for analgesia, 1:50, 131
C-reactive protein and, 1:240
for fever, 1:131, 2:1028
for ulcerative colitis, 1:208
Salicylic acid, 1:378
Saline cathartics, 2:865
Saline solution
bedsores, 1:157
breast implants, 1:213, 1:213–216, 1:214, 1:219
hysterosonography, 3:1121
laser skin resurfacing, 2:859
mechanical debridement dressings, 1:407
sclerotherapy, 3:1282
Saliva, 2:583
Salivary fistula, 3:1100
Salivary gland tumors, 3:1100
Salpingectomy, 2:1034, 3:1262
Salpingo-oophorectomy, 3:1256–1259, 1257
bilateral, 2:1038, 3:1256–1259
for endometriosis, 2:835
hysterectomy and, 2:706, 708, 709, 3:1256
unilateral, 3:1256–1259
Salpingostomy, 2:1034, 3:1260–1263, 1261
Salts
for Ménière's disease, 1:455
oral rehydration, 2:767

Sandimmune. *See* Cyclosporins
Sands of the Sahara, 2:846
Sandwich therapy, 2:1020
SangCya. *See* Cyclosporins
Sanitization, 1:128
Saphenous vein grafts, 1:346, *1:347,*
  1:349, 3:1135, 1136
  See also Peripheral vascular bypass
    surgery
Sarcoidosis
  liver biopsy for, 2:886
  lung biopsy for, 2:914
  mediastinoscopy for, 2:949
Sarcoma
  Kaposi's, 2:729
  small intestine, 3:1333, 1335
  soft tissue, 2:872–875
Sargramostim, 2:728
Sarsaparilla, 3:1380
Saunders, Cicely, 2:682
Saw palmetto, 3:1457
SB Chariet III, 1:425
SBFT. *See* Small bowel follow-through
Scalp reduction, 2:613
Scalpels, 1:182, 3:1381
Scar revision surgery, **3:1263–1268**
Scars
  acne, 3:1266
  from breast implants, 1:215, 221
  from breast reduction, 1:224
  burn, 3:1266
  from carpal tunnel release, 1:261
  cigarettes and, 1:224
  from cleft lip repair, 1:303, 304, 305
  cosmetics for, 3:1267
  from craniofacial reconstruction,
    1:366
  dermabrasion for, 1:416–419,
    3:1265
  dermal regeneration templates for,
    3:1264–1265, 1266
  from dilation and curettage, 1:421
  flaps for, 3:1264–1265, 1266
  formation of, 3:1263–1264
  from hemangioma excision, 2:645,
    646
  hypertrophic, 1:305, 3:1263–1267
  incisional hernia repair and, 2:746,
    747
  from laceration repair, 2:818
  laser skin resurfacing and, 2:858,
    859, 3:1265
  from liposuction, 2:881
  maturation of, 3:1263
  from mediastinoscopy, 2:951
  microdermabrasion for, 3:1263,
    1267
  myocardial resection for, 2:997
  non-surgical treatment of,
    3:1266–1267
  from otoplasty, 2:1069
  scar revision surgery for,
    3:1263–1268
  from scleral buckling, 3:1270
  shoulder resection arthroplasty and,
    3:1313
  silicone gel sheeting for, 3:1266
  skin grafts for, 3:1264–1265, 1266
  from staples, 2:744
  surgical excision of, 3:1264
  from sutures, 2:744
  from tendon repairs, 3:1402
  uterine, 1:421
  See also Keloid scars
Schiotz tonometry, 2:608
Schistosomiasis, 3:1362
Schlemm's canal, 2:609–610, 3:1275
Schwarz, Richard, 3:1402
Sciatica, 2:820
SCID (Severe combined immunodeficiency disease), 1:194
Scientific Registry of Transplant Recipients (SRTR), 2:789, 921, 3:1448
Scintigraphy, 1:30–31
Scissors, 3:1381
Sclera, 2:853, 3:1152
Scleral buckling, 2:772, 3:1156, 1233,
  3:1268–1271, *1269*
Sclerectomy, nonpenetrating deep,
  3:1275
Scleroderma, 2:583
Sclerosing agents, 3:1277–1278, 1279,
  1281, 1282, 1283
Sclerostomy, **3:1271–1277**
Sclerotherapy
  esophageal varices, 3:1277–1279
  hemorrhoids, 2:655
  hydrocelectomy, 2:695
  portal hypertension, 3:1181
  varicose veins, **3:1279–1286**, *1281,*
    3:1536
Scoliosis
  idiopathic, 3:1353, 1356
  physical therapy for, 2:871
  spinal fusion for, 3:1352–1353, 1355
  spinal instrumentation for, 3:1355
Scopolamine patch, **3:1286–1288**
Screws
  for fracture repair, 1:553, *1:554*
  for leg lengthening and shortening,
    2:867, 870
  magnetic resonance imaging and,
    2:928
  pedicle, 3:1356
Scrotal hematoma, 3:1529
Scrotum hydroceles, 2:693–697
Scrubs, 2:1045
SCT. *See* Sacrococcygeal teratoma
Secobarbital, 1:93, 151
Seconal. *See* Secobarbital
Second hand smoke, 3:1338–1339
Second-look surgery, **3:1288–1290**
Second opinions, 3:1196, 1200,
  3:1290–1292
  for elective surgery, 1:438
  health insurance for, 1:541
  for necessary surgery, 2:1009
  surgical team and, 3:1388
Sectral. *See* Acebutolol
Sedation
  anesthesia evaluation and, 1:57
  beta waves and, 1:445
  bispectral index for, 1:161–166
  conscious, 1:521, 2:858,
    3:1292–1294
  direct measurement of, 1:163
  indirect measurement of, 1:162–163
  level of, 1:161–166
  muscle relaxants for, 2:994
Sedentary life style, 1:507
SEF (Spectral edge frequency), 1:163
Segmental excision. *See* Lumpectomy
Segmental resection. *See* Segmentectomy
Segmentectomy, **3:1294–1298**, 3:1414
Seiler, Theo, 2:842
Seizures
  anterior temporal lobectomy for,
    1:75–78
  from antibiotics, 1:82
  atonic, 1:358, 359
  barbiturates for, 1:150–153
  corpus callostomy for, 1:358–359
  electroencephalography for,
    1:442–446
  grand mal, 1:358
  hemispherectomy for, 2:648–650
  from myelography, 2:997
  temporal lobe, 1:75–78, 2:1026
  tonic-clonic, 1:358
Selective dorsal rhizotomy, 3:1241
Selective posterior rhizotomy, 3:1241
Selective serotonin reuptake inhibitors
  (SSRIs), 2:772
Selective vestibular neurectomy, 1:455
Self-care skills, 3:1220
Self-catheterization, 1:263, 3:1332
Semi-rigid rods, 3:1124
Senna, 1:319, 2:866, 3:1227
Sensorcaine. *See* Bupivacaine
Sensorineural hearing loss, 1:308,
  3:1366
Sensory changes
  deep brain stimulation and, 1:410
  hemispherectomy and, 2:649
Sentinel lymph node biopsy,
  3:1298–1302, *1299*
  for breast cancer, 1:138, 2:913, 988,
    3:1215, 1300
  vs. lymphadenectomy, 2:924
Sepsis, 1:407, 2:685, 3:1363–1364
Septal defects (Cardiac), 1:239, 2:634,
  2:635, 2:636, 637
Septicemia, 1:264, 267, 3:1428
Septoplasty, 1:434, **3:1302–1305**, *1303*
Septostomy, balloon atrial, 2:636
Septra. *See* Trimethoprim/sulfamethox-
  azole (TMP-SMZ)
Septum, nasal. *See* Nasal septum
Ser-Ap-Es, 1:90*t*
Serax. *See* Oxazepam
Serial paracentesis, 3:1139

Serosa, 1:204
Serotonin receptor antagonists, 3:1287
Serotonin-specific reuptake inhibitors
(SSRIs), 1:78, 2:772
Serous fluid glucose test, 2:606
Serrated wheel dermabrasion, 1:416,
417
Serum electrolyte tests. See Electrolyte
tests
Serum glutamic pyruvic transaminase
(SGPT), 2:891
Setback otoplasty, 2:1066–1067,
2:1067, 2:1068–1069, 1069
Seton tube implants. See Tube shunt
surgery
Severe combined immunodeficiency
disease (SCID), 1:194
Sevoflurane, 1:60, 62
Sex change surgery. See Sex reassign-
ment surgery
Sex differences. See Gender differences
Sex reassignment surgery,
3:1305–1308, *1306, 1307*
demographics of, 2:1053, 3:1305
mentoplasty and, 2:967
non-surgical alternatives for,
2:1057, 3:1307
orchiectomy for, 2:1052, 1054–1055
Sexual activity and urinary catheterization, 1:264, 267
Sexual assault, 1:329
SGPT (Serum glutamic pyruvic
transaminase), 2:891
Shapiro, James, 3:1091
Sharp debridement, 1:406–407
Sharps, 3:1381, 1393
Shingles, 2:735
SHIP (State health insurance assistance
program), 2:907, 908
Shirodkar cerclage, 1:279
Shock
adrenergic drugs for, 1:33
cardiopulmonary resuscitation for,
1:246
hematocrit and, 2:647
liver function tests for, 2:894
Shoes
bunions and, 1:230–231, 233
for club foot, 1:307
high-heeled, 3:1536
knee injuries from, 2:801
for leg lengthening and shortening,
2:670, 870–871
spider veins from, 3:1284
toe abnormalities and, 2:616, 618
Short bowel syndrome, 1:6
Short-Form McGill Questionnaire,
3:1184
Shortening, leg, **2:866–872**, *867*
Shortness of breath, 3:1177
Shoulder joint
arthritis, 3:1310
arthroplasty, 1:116–120, *1:117,*
1:118

arthroscopic surgery, 1:120–123
implants, 3:1310
instability, 1:147, 3:1313
magnetic resonance imaging of,
2:926
rounded, 3:1112
tendons, 3:1247, 1399–1400
Shoulder joint dislocations
Bankart procedure for, 1:147–150,
1:148
Bristow procedure for, 1:149–150
non-surgical treatment of, 1:150
Shoulder joint replacement,
3:1308–1312, *3:1309,* 1314
Shoulder pain
non-surgical treatment of, 3:1314
rotator cuff repair for, 3:1247–1251
shoulder joint replacement for,
3:1308–1312
Shoulder prosthesis, 3:1308–1312, 1314
Shoulder resection arthroplasty,
3:1312–1315
Showers and incision care, 2:744–745
Shunts
for congenital heart defects, 2:637
Denver, 3:1138
endolymphatic, **1:453–456**
filtering, 2:610
Gott, 1:102
Hyde, 3:1138
LaVeen, 3:1138
left-right atrial, 1:239
left-to-right ventricular, 1:239
mesocaval, 3:1179
peritoneovenous, **3:1137–1140**
portacaval, 3:1139, 1179
splenorenal, 3:1179
transjugular portosystemic, 3:1139
transvenous portosystemic, 3:1179,
1181, 1279
SIADH (Syndrome of inappropriate antidiuretic hormone secretion), 1:81, 447
Sibasic sodium phosphate, 2:865
Sibling organ donors, 2:692
Sibutramine, 2:575, 3:1562
Sickle cell anemia, 1:175, 339, 3:1362
SICU (Surgical intensive care units),
2:759
SIDS (Sudden infant death syndrome),
3:1338
Sigmoid colon, 1:204
Sigmoidoscopy, **3:1315–1318,** 3:1387
advances in, 2:581
for colorectal cancer screening,
1:315, 2:581, 3:1315–1317
flexible, 1:319
for ileoanal reservoir surgery, 2:721
for rectal resection, 3:1225
Silastic catheters, 1:263, 266
Sildenafil citrate, 3:1124
Silicon bulking agents, 1:311
Silicone
buckles, 3:1269–1270
catheters, 1:263, 266

dermal regeneration templates,
3:1264–1265
injection, 3:1365
lens implants, 2:855, 856
rubber implants, 2:617
Silicone gel
breast implants, 1:213–216, 219,
220–221, 3:1174
for scar revision, 3:1266
Silicone rubber bands, 3:1461
Silicosis, 2:919
Silo pouch, 1:6
Silver alloy-coated catheters, 2:687
Silver sulfadiazine, 3:1377
Simlect. See Basiliximab
Simple mastectomy, 3:1214–1215,
3:1318–1322, *1319*
Simple mastoidectomy, 2:935
Simple nephrectomy, 2:1013
Simple orchiectomy, 2:1053
Single photon emission tomography
(SPECT), 1:76
Sinoatrial node, 1:449–450
Sinus CT scans, 1:382, 384
Sinus disorders, 1:433, 434, 435,
459–463
Sinus drainage, **1:459–463**
Sinus node, 1:441
Sinus surgery, endoscopic, **1:459–463**,
460
Sinus tumors, 1:384, 3:1328
Sinus x rays, **3:1328–1329**
Sinusitis
demographics of, 1:460
endoscopic sinus surgery for, 1:384,
459–463
non-surgical treatment of, 3:1305
second-look surgery for, 3:1288
septoplasty for, 3:1302
skull x rays for, 3:1328–1329
Sirolimus
immunosuppression, 2:733, 736
kidney transplantation, 2:789
liver transplantation, 2:899
Sjögren's syndrome, 2:583, 3:1397
Skelaxin. See Metaxalone
Skeletal imaging, 2:926
Skeletal muscle relaxants, 1:55, 2:824,
2:994–995
Skeletal traction, 1:553, 3:1437
Skiing, 2:791, 798
Skill level, surgeons, 1:539–540
Skilled nursing facilities, 2:908
Skin
anatomy of, 3:1323
artificial, 3:1264–1265, 1326–1327
equivalents, 1:144, 145, 3:1327
infections, 1:84–86
loose, 1:7
preoperative preparation of,
1:93–95, 3:1192
sagging, 1:169, *1:170,* 1:521
thickness, 3:1323
traction, 3:1437

Skin biopsy, 1:437
Skin cancer
    cryotherapy for, 1:377–379
    curettage and electrosurgery for,
        1:385–387
    demographics of, 2:990
    electrodesiccation for, 1:386, 2:992
    heart-lung transplantation and,
        2:633
    immunosuppressant drugs and,
        2:735
    Mohs surgery for, 1:387, 2:990–992
Skin discoloration. *See* Pigmentation
    changes
Skin fluorescent studies, 1:45
Skin grafting, **3:1322–1328**, *1323,
    1324*
    for scar revision surgery,
        3:1264–1265, 1266
    skin substitutes for, 1:144, 145,
        3:1327
Skin lesions
    cryotherapy for, 1:377–379
    curettage and electrosurgery for,
        1:385
    dermabrasion of, 1:416–419
    from gastric acid inhibitors, 2:569
Skin perfusion measurements, 1:45
Skin resurfacing, laser, 1:416, 418,
    2:857–859, 3:1263, 1265
Skin smoothing. *See* Dermabrasion
Skin-sparing mastectomy, 3:1320, 1322
Skin temperature measurements, 1:45,
    543–544
Skin ulcers
    bedsores, 1:155–159, *1:157*, 1:408
    from sclerotherapy, 3:1283, 1284
Skull x rays, **3:1328–1329**
Sleep apnea, 1:434, 435
    diagnosis of, 3:1345–1346
    mechanical ventilation for, 2:944
    non-surgical treatment of, 3:1305
    obstructive, 3:1302, 1305,
        1342–1349
    septoplasty for, 3:1302
Sleep disorder surgery, 1:434
Sleep testing, 3:1346
Sleep theta wave patterns, 1:445
Sleepiness, 3:1345–1346
Sleeping pills, 1:55, 3:1345
Sleeping position, 3:1347–1348
Sliding genioplasty, 2:968, 969
Sling procedure, 1:312, **3:1329–1333**
    vs. artificial sphincter insertion,
        1:127
    for intrinsic sphincter deficiency,
        2:1011, 3:1237, 1330
    tension-free vaginal tape, 3:1329
    for urethral hypermobility, 1:127,
        3:1330, 1331–1332
Slings
    fascial, 3:1329, 1331, 1332
    Gore-Tex, 3:1329
    teflon, 3:1329

Slip tip nozzles, 3:1392
Slit lamp examination
    cataracts, 1:380, 513
    glaucoma, 1:390
    laser iridotomy, 2:851
    laser posterior capsulotomy, 2:855
    LASIK, 2:844
    ophthalmologic surgery, 2:1049
    retinal detachment, 3:1154–1155,
        1232
Small bowel follow-through (SBFT),
    3:1489
Small bowel resection, **3:1333–1337**,
    1334
Small cell lung cancer, 3:1177, 1295,
    1411
Small eyes, 2:850
Small intestine cancer
    demographics of, 3:1335
    mortality and morbidity from,
        3:1336
    sarcomas, 3:1333, 1335
    small bowel resection for, 3:1333
Small intestine obstruction, 2:725,
    763–765
Small intestine paralysis, 1:6, 529
Small intestine prolapse, 1:327
Smoke, second hand, 3:1338–1339
Smokeless tobacco, 3:1339
Smoking
    acetaminophen and, 1:22
    anesthesia evaluation and, 1:57
    arrhythmias and, 1:251
    bladder cancers, 3:1450
    cataracts and, 1:511
    coronary artery bypass graft surgery
        and, 1:348
    dental implants and, 1:415
    effects of, 3:1338
    esophageal cancer and, 1:494
    health problems from, 3:1241,
        1338–1339
    homocysteine and, 1:240
    laryngeal cancer from, 2:839
    lung cancer from, 2:903, 3:1175,
        1341
    middle ear infections and, 2:1006
    organ transplants and, 3:1446
    passive, 3:1338–1339
    premature labor and, 1:279
    scars and, 1:224
    snoring and, 3:1343
    throat cancer from, 3:1147
    tongue cancer and, 2:601
    vascular diseases from, 3:1519
    withdrawal symptoms, 3:1340
Smoking cessation, **3:1338–1342**
    for arrhythmia, 2:939, 940
    for atherosclerosis prevention, 1:469
    coronary artery bypass graft surgery
        and, 1:348
    for coronary artery disease, 1:349,
        353, 355, 471

enhanced external counterpulsation
    and, 1:471
    face lift and, 1:521–522
    fracture repair and, 1:555
    for hip replacement, 2:668
    knee replacement and, 2:804
    for lung biopsy, 2:915
    preadmission instructions for,
        3:1168
    preoperative, 1:508, 3:1197, 1201
Snake bites, 1:525, 526
Snellen test, 1:512
Snoreplasty, 3:1345
Snoring
    demographics of, 3:1343–1344
    diagnosis of, 3:1345–1346
    non-surgical treatment of,
        3:1347–1348
    risk factors for, 3:1342–1343
Snoring surgery, 1:434, **3:1342–1349**,
    1343
Soap, antibacterial, 2:829
SOAP notes, 2:957
Social phobia, 1:78
Social Security Act Amendment, 2:952,
    963
Social workers, 3:1167
Society for Pediatric Urology, 2:703
Society of American Gastrointestinal
    Endoscopic Surgeons, 2:580
Sodium
    electrolyte tests for, 1:446–449
    urine test for, 2:785
Sodium bicarbonate, 1:65, 447
Sodium biphosphate, 2:865
Sodium chloride solution, 1:121, 2:766
Sodium loss, 1:90
Sodium nitroprusside, 1:90
Sodium salicylate, 1:131
Sodium Tc-pertechnetate, 2:948
Sodium tetradecyl sulfate, 3:1278,
    1282, 1345
Soemmering's ring, 2:854
Soft palate, 3:1344, 1345
Soft tissue fillers, 1:552
Soft tissue sarcomas, 2:872–875
Soft tissue tumors, 2:562
Soma. *See* Carisoprodol
Somatic pain, 3:1083
Somatostatin, 3:1278
Somnoplasty, 3:1344
Sonography. *See* Ultrasound
Sorbents, 2:652
Sores, pressure, **1:155–159**, *157*, 1:408
Sotalol, 1:91
Sparfloxacin, 1:546
Spasms, 2:994
Spasticity, **3:1241–1242**, 3:1242
Specialties, board certification for,
    1:540, 3:1165–1166, 1194–1195
    See also specific specialties
Specialty hospitals, 2:689
Specific gravity, in urinalysis, 3:1499,
    1500, 1501

Specific phobia disorder, 1:78
SPECT (Single photon emission to-
mography), 1:76
Spectral edge frequency (SEF), 1:163
Spectroscopy, magnetic resonance,
2:925, 927
Speculum, 1:327
Speech
esophageal, 2:840
mechanical ventilation and, 2:945
pharyngectomy and, 3:1145
tracheoesophageal, 2:840
Speech disorders, postoperative, 3:1347
Speech-language therapy, 2:678, 840
Speech processors, 1:308
Speech reading, 1:310
Sperm banking, 2:1054
Sperm count, 2:740
Spermatic ducts, 2:693
Sphenoidal electrodes, 1:443
Spherocytosis, hereditary, 3:1229,
1362, 1364
Sphincter hyperflexia, 1:123
Sphincter insertion, artificial,
1:123–128, *124*
Sphincter insufficiency, 1:125
Sphincter muscle tightening, 1:318
Sphincters
anal, 1:123–128
esophageal, 1:490–493, 2:582
lower esophageal, 2:586–590
urinary, 1:123–128
Sphingomyelin, 2:876
Sphygmomanometer, 1:176,
3:1350–1352
See also Blood pressure measure-
ment
Sphygmomanometers, 3:1553
Spicules, 1:190
Spider angioma, 3:1282
Spider nevi, 3:1282
Spider veins, 3:1279–1286
Spina bifida
latex allergies and, 3:1192
meningocele repair for, 2:964–967
myelomeningocele and, 1:531, 532,
533, 2:964–966
Spina Bifida Association of America,
2:964, 966
Spina bifida manifesta, 2:964–965
Spina bifida occulta, 2:965
Spinal abnormalities, congenital, 2:996
Spinal anatomy, 2:819, 3:1352
Spinal anesthesia
for cervical cerclage, 1:279
for cesarean section, 1:284, 286
for childbirth, 1:67
for obstetric and gynecologic
surgery, 2:1034
risks of, 1:65–66
Spinal canal myelography, 2:995–997
Spinal cancer, 2:996
Spinal cord, 1:102, 103, 3:1083
Spinal cord cancer myelography, 2:996

Spinal degeneration, 1:184, 2:1026
Spinal disorders
neurosurgery for, 2:1024–1027
spinal fusion for, 3:1352–1355
spinal instrumentation for,
3:1355–1358
Spinal epidural abscess, 2:1026
Spinal fluid analysis. *See* Cerebrospinal
fluid (CSF) analysis
Spinal fractures, 2:566
Spinal fusion, **3:1352–1355**, *1353*
bone grafts for, 1:185–186
cervical, 1:185–186
disk removal and, 1:424
laminectomy and, 2:822, 824
spinal instrumentation and,
3:1355–1358
Spinal headache, 1:66, 479
Spinal imaging, 2:926
Spinal instrumentation, 3:1354,
3:1355–1358
Spinal tap. *See* Lumbar puncture
Spiral CT scans, 1:383, 384
Spirograms, 3:1358
Spirometry tests, **3:1358–1360**
Spironolactone, 1:90*t*
Spleen
abscess, 3:1362
embolization, 3:1365
rupture, 3:1363
vertical banded gastroplasty and,
3:1548
Spleen cancer, 3:1362
Spleen disease
abdominal ultrasound for, 1:2
angiography for, 1:70
splenectomy for, 3:1360–1365
Splenectomy, 2:604, **3:1360–1365**, *1361*
Splenic artery rupture, 3:1362
Splenomegaly, 3:1362
Splenoportography, 1:70
Splenorenal shunts, 3:1179
Splints
for carpal tunnel syndrome, 1:260
for club foot, 1:307
for fracture repair, 1:555
for septoplasty, 3:1302, 1304
after tendon repairs, 3:1400, 1402
for toe abnormalities, 2:618
See also Braces
Split-thickness grafts, 3:1325
SPM (Statistical probability mapping),
1:444
Spock ear, 2:1066
Spondylitis, ankylosing, 2:665, 692
Spontaneous abortion. *See* Miscarriage
Spontaneous intracranial hemorrhage,
2:1024–1025
Sporanox. *See* Itraconazole
Spores, 1:48
Sports
avulsed teeth, 3:1429
injuries, 3:1313
tendon repair and, 3:1400

Sports medicine, 2:1064
Sprains, 2:994
Squamous cell carcinoma
cryotherapy for, 1:377, 378
curettage and electrosurgery for,
1:385
esophageal, 1:493, 494, 2:580, 3:1412
lung, 3:1411
Mohs surgery for, 2:990
Squamous dysplasia, 1:282
Squatting, 2:802
SRTR (Scientific Registry of Trans-
plant Recipients), 2:789, 921, 3:1448
SSI (Supplemental Security Income),
2:953
SSRI (Selective serotonin reuptake in-
hibitors), 1:78, 2:772
ST segment, 2:977, 3:1376
Stadol. *See* Butorphanol
Staff Model, 2:933
Staff ratios, 2:1031
Staghorn calculi, 2:1016
Stahl's ear, 2:1066, 1070
Stainless steel instruments, 3:1380
Stainless steel mesh, 2:748, 755
Stainless steel staples, 2:744, 3:1374
Standard LASIK, 2:842–844
Standard open esophagectomy, 1:495
Standards
for adult day care, 1:36
for blood registries, 1:172, 175
for informed consent, 2:751
for medical equipment, 2:961
for medical error rates, 2:961
for nursing homes, 2:1030
reasonable patient, 2:751
*Standards of the American Association
of Blood Banks,* 1:172, 175
Stapedectomy, 1:434, **3:1365–1368**
Stapedotomy, 3:1367
Staphylococcus aureus, 3:1569–1570,
1571
Staphylococcus infections, 1:555
Staples, 2:744, **3:1373–1375**
State health insurance assistance program (SHIP), 2:907, 908
Statistical probability mapping (SPM),
1:444
Steatorrhea, 2:865
Stelazine. *See* Trifluoperazine hydrochloride
Stem cells, 1:193
See also Peripheral blood stem cell
transplantation
Stenosis
angioplasty for, 1:72–75
carotid arteries, 1:252–257, 466
cervical, 1:341
recurrence of, 1:75
stoma, 1:320, 325
urethral, 2:704
vertical banded gastroplasty and,
3:1548
See also Heart valve stenosis

Stenting
vs. thrombolytic therapy, 3:1417
for vascular diseases, 3:1519
Stents
biliary, **1:159–161**
coated, 1:353
coronary, **1:353–357**, *354*,
2:977–978
drug-eluting, 1:467
endovascular, **1:465–470**
heart-lung machines for, 2:628
prostatic, 3:1458
ureteral, 2:714, 715, 716
Step-down units, 3:1222
Stereopsis. *See* Depth perception
Stereotactic imaging
breast biopsy guidance, 1:211
deep brain stimulation, 1:409–410
hypophysectomy, 2:697
neurosurgery, 2:1026
pallidotomy, 3:1088
Stereotactic radiosurgery, **3:1369–1371**
Steri-strips, 1:529, 2:744
Sterilization
for hospital-acquired infection control, 2:687
of instruments, 3:1381
of intensive care unit equipment,
2:762
for operating rooms, 2:1045
purpose of, 1:439
Sterilization, female, 1:331, 332–333,
439, 2:1034
Sterilization, male, 3:1231
Sternotomy, 3:1413
aortic valve replacement, 1:104
minimally invasive heart surgery,
2:975, 976, 977
mitral valve repair, 2:979
mitral valve replacement, 2:983
Sternum, 1:190
Sternum fractures, 1:293
Steroids, 3:1561
aspirin and, 1:133
avascular necrosis from, 2:667
for bunions, 1:233
C-reactive protein and, 1:240
cataracts and, 1:512
cyclocryotherapy and, 1:389
for endoscopic sinus surgery, 1:461
for extracapsular cataract extraction,
1:513
for eye enucleation, 1:476
for face lift, 1:522
fracture repair and, 1:555
for glaucoma, 1:391
for hemangiomas, 2:646
incisional hernia repair and, 2:747
for Ménière's disease, 1:455
for middle ear infections, 2:1004
for orbital exenteration, 1:505
stomach ulcers from, 2:567
topical nasal, 1:24
after tube-shunt surgery, 3:1464

Stethoscope, 1:177, 255, 3:1350,
3:1371–1373, 3:1552, 1553
Stevens-Johnson syndrome, 1:342,
3:1378
Stimulant laxatives, 2:865
Stimulants, 1:251
Stitches, **3:1373–1375**
absorbable, 2:743, 972, 3:1374
incisional hernia repair and, 2:747,
748, 750
for laceration repair, 2:818
for microsurgery, 2:972
needles for, 2:972, 3:1374
non-absorbable, 2:743, 748, 818,
972, 3:1374
Stockings, compression. *See* Compression stockings
Stoma
care techniques, 1:318, 324, 2:719
for colostomy, 1:323
complications from, 1:320, 324–325
for gastric bypass, 2:572, 573
for ileal conduit surgery, 2:716
for ileoanal reservoir surgery, 2:721
for ileostomy, 2:723, 725
for laryngectomy, 2:839, 840
for Meckel's diverticulectomy,
2:948
prolapsed, 1:320, 325
for urinary diversion, 1:392, 394
See also Ostomy
Stomach
leakage, 2:573
perforation, 1:500
watermelon, 1:95, 96, 98
Stomach acid, 1:97
gastric acid inhibitors for,
2:567–570
irritation from, 2:582–583
peptic ulcers and, 3:1209
Stomach bypass. *See* Gastric bypass
Stomach cancer
adenocarcinoma, 2:566, 576
antrectomy for, 1:96, 98
demographics of, 2:567, 576
diagnosis of, 2:577
esophageal resection for, 1:493–499
gastrectomy for, 2:563–567
gastroduodenostomy for,
2:575–579, *2:576*
mortality rates for, 2:566
Stomach diseases
antrectomy for, 1:95–100
diagnosis of, 1:96–97
esophagogastroduodenoscopy for,
1:499–501
Stomach resection. *See* Gastrectomy
Stomach stapling. *See* Vertical banded
gastroplasty (VBG)
Stomach tubes. *See* Gastrostomy
Stomach ulcers
antibiotics for, 1:81
antrectomy for, 1:96, 98–99
aspirin and, 1:132

causes of, 2:567, 579
costs of, 2:580
demographics of, 2:580
gastrectomy for, 2:563–567, 576
gastric acid inhibitors for,
2:567–570, 578
gastroduodenostomy for, 2:575, 576
non-surgical treatment of, 2:578
from NSAIDs, 2:1028
pyloroplasty for, 3:1209–1212
recurrence of, 2:566
surgical procedures for, 2:579, 581
symptoms of, 3:1211
Stones
bladder, 1:399, 400
pancreatic, 1:1
ureteral, 2:1021, 1023
See also Gallstones; Kidney stones
Stool bulking agents, 2:656
Stool softeners, 2:865, 3:1224
Strabismus, 1:516, 518, 519
Strawberry hemangioma, 2:644
Street drugs, 1:63, 247, 460
Strength training, 1:508
Streptase. *See* Streptokinase
Streptococcus infections, 1:555, 2:727,
3:1418
Streptococcus pneumoniae, 1:241
Streptokinase, 3:1417–1419
Streptomyces coelicolor, 3:1405
Streptomyces infections, 1:81
Stress
adrenergic drugs for, 1:32
pain and, 3:1082
preoperative, 3:1201
Stress test, **3:1375–1377**, *1376*
echocardiography and, 1:436–437
electrocardiography and, 1:440,
441, 442
for endovascular stent surgery,
1:468
for mitral valve disorders, 2:980,
984
MUGA scan and, 2:992, 993
Stress ulcers, 2:568
Stress urinary incontinence
artificial sphincter insertion for,
1:123–125
collagen periurethral injection for,
1:311–313
colporrhaphy for, 1:328
cystocele repair and, 1:397
demographics of, 2:1011
diagnosis of, 2:1011–1012, 3:1236
genuine, 2:1010–1011, 3:1330,
1331
needle bladder neck suspension for,
2:1010–1012
non-surgical treatment of, 3:1237,
1332
obesity and, 1:508
recurrence of, 3:1332
retropubic suspension for,
3:1234–1238

sacral nerve stimulation for, 3:1253
sling procedure for, 3:1330
Striae, 2:846
Strictureplasty, 1:318
Strohl, Kingman, 3:1342
Stroke
    from angiography, 1:72
    aspirin for prevention of, 1:132
    carotid endarterectomy for prevention of, 1:252–257
    CT scans for, 1:384
    demographics of, 1:252
    emergency surgery for, 1:453
    endovascular stent surgery for, 1:466
    gastrostomy and, 2:593
    homocysteine and, 1:241
    ischemic, 1:254
    magnetic resonance imaging for, 2:925
    from Maze procedure, 2:940
    minimally invasive heart surgery for, 2:975
    obesity and, 1:507
    prevention of, 1:256, 469–470
    smoking and, 3:1338
    thrombolytic therapy for, 3:1417–1419
Stroke Council (American Heart Association), 1:256
Struvite calculi, 2:1016
Sturge-Weber syndrome, 2:607, 649
Subarachnoid hemorrhage, 1:271–276, 2:1024–1025
Subarachnoid space, 1:63
Subcapsular orchiectomy, 2:1053, 1054
Subcutaneous ring nerve blockades, 1:299
Subdural hematoma, 3:1543
Subdural strip electrodes, 1:443
Subjective standard, 2:751
Sublimaze. See Fentanyl
Sublingual thermometers. See Oral thermometers
Subluxations, 3:1404–1405
Submucosa, 1:204
Subperiosteal implants, 1:415
Subscapularis muscle, 3:1247
Subspecialties, 1:539, 3:1115
Substance abuse, 3:1106–1107
    See also Addiction
Substance P, 3:1083
Substantia nigra, 1:409
Subthalamic nucleus, 1:409, 410, 3:1089
Subtotal gastrectomy, 2:564, 567
Subtotal hysterectomy, 1:341, 2:706, 708
Subtracted cystometry, 3:1331
Sucralfate, 1:98, 547
Suction-assisted lipectomy. See Liposuction
Suction Bovie, 1:24
Suction devices, 3:1381

Sudden cardiac arrest, 1:449
Sudden infant death syndrome (SIDS), 3:1338
Sulfa drugs. See Sulfonamides
Sulfapyridine, 1:208
Sulfasalazine, 2:726, 3:1314
Sulfisoxazole, 3:1377
Sulfonamides, 1:81, 3:1377–1380
    allergies to, 1:429, 3:1378
    hemoglobin test and, 2:651
    for ulcerative colitis, 1:208
    urinary anti-infectives, 3:1502
Sulindac, 1:132
Sun exposure
    cataracts and, 1:511, 3:1140
    immunosuppressant drugs and, 2:735
    incision care and, 2:745
    scar revision surgery and, 3:1266
    tetracyclines and, 3:1406
Sunlight sensitivity. See Photosensitivity
Superabsorbent dressings, 1:144, 145
Superficial parotidectomy, 3:1100
Superior mesenteric artery endarterectomy, 3:1129
Supplemental Security Income (SSI), 2:953
Support garments, 2:879, 880
Support groups
    for orchiectomy, 2:1055
    postoperative recovery and, 3:1220
    for simple mastectomy, 3:1321
    for smoking cessation, 3:1340
    vertical banded gastroplasty, 3:1547, 1548
Support hose. See Compression stockings
Suprachoroidal hemorrhage, 3:1274
Suprapubic prostatectomy, 2:1044
Supraspinatus muscle, 3:1247
Supraventricular arrhythmia, 2:977
Supraventricular tachycardia, 1:451
Suprax. See Cefixime
Surfactants, 2:875, 876, 877
Surgeon General, 1:506
Surgeon-guided robot-assisted surgery, 3:1243
Surgeons
    board certified, 1:540, 3:1165, 1194–1195, 1291, 1387
    experience of, 2:831
    finding, 1:538–542
    licensure, 1:539, 540
    personality of, 1:540
    recommendations for, 1:541
    referrals and, 1:40, 538–539
    second opinions and, 3:1290–1292
    selecting, 3:1194–1195
    skill level of, 1:539–540
    surgical team and, 3:1387
    talking to, 3:1395–1396
    See also Surgical specialties
Surgery
    awareness during, 1:61–62, 162–163

bloodless, 1:136, 1:179–184, 3:1443
    computer-assisted, 3:1398–1399
    elective, 1:437–439, 1:501, 502, 538, 3:1290–1291
    emergency, 1:438, 1:452–453, 2:913
    essential, 1:501–502
    general, 2:594–597, 2:827, 3:1386
    inpatient, 1:438, 2:689–690, 952, 3:1200, 1386
    necessary, 2:1009–1010
    postoperative recall of, 1:162
    preparation for, 3:1192, 1194–1200
    remote, 3:1398–1399
    robot-assisted, 2:823, 1046, 3:1242–1244, 1399
    scheduling, 3:1195–1196, 1201
    second-look, 3:1288–1290
    See also specific procedures and conditions
Surgery centers. See Ambulatory surgery centers
Surgical abortion, 1:15–16
Surgical adhesive, 2:703
Surgical clamps. See Clamps (Surgical)
Surgical cricothyroidotomy, 1:374
Surgical debridement, 1:406–407
Surgical field, 1:129–130
Surgical flaps. See Flaps (Surgical)
Surgical instruments, 3:1380–1382
    aseptic technique for, 1:129
    microsurgery, 2:971–972
    for reducing blood loss, 1:181–182
Surgical intensive care units (SICU), 2:759
Surgical loupes, 1:543, 2:971
Surgical oncology, 3:1382–1385
    See also Cancer
Surgical scrub, 1:128–129
Surgical site infections
    aseptic technique for prevention of, 1:128–131
    causes of, 2:686, 1012
    risks of, 1:403, 2:685
Surgical specialties, 1:539, 540, 3:1115, 1386
Surgical subspecialties, 1:539
Surgical sutures. See Stitches
Surgical team, 1:452, 3:1385–1389
Surgicenters. See Ambulatory surgery centers
Surrogates, 2:622–623, 2:902, 3:1190
Susruta, 1:510
Suture needles, 2:972, 3:1374
Sutures. See Stitches
Swabs, 1:48
Swallowing disorders. See Dysphagia
Sweat samples, 1:448
Sweating, excessive, 3:1389, 1390–1391
Sympathectomy, 3:1389–1392
Sympathetic nervous system, 1:32, 3:1389–1392

Syndactyly, 2:619, **3:1555–1558,** 3:*1556*

Syndrome of inappropriate antidiuretic hormone secretion (SIADH), 1:81, 447

Synechia, posterior, 2:852

Synovial fluid, 2:560, 606

Synovial joint, 1:116

Synovitis, 1:116, 121

Syphilis, 1:100, 277, 278

Syringe and needle assembly, **3:1392–1394,** *1393*

Systemic lupus erythematosus (SLE), 1:271

Systems analysis, 2:961

Systolic pressure, 1:176, 177, 3:1350, 1351

T

T-lymphocytes, 2:691

Tables, operating room, 1:130

Tachycardia
    electrolyte balance and, 1:448
    electrophysiology study for, 1:449, 450
    pacemakers for, 3:1079–1082
    supraventricular, 1:451
    ventricular, 1:412, 451, 2:736, 737, 739, 740

Tacrolimus, 2:733
    for liver transplantation, 2:898–899, 900
    pregnancy and, 2:734
    side effects of, 2:736

Tagamet. *See* Cimetidine

Tai chi, for weight management, 3:1562

Take Off Pounds Sensibly (TOPS), 3:1562

Talipes equinovarus. See Club foot

Talking to the doctor, **3:1395–1396**

Talwin. *See* Pentazocine

Tamponade, balloon, 3:1278

Tardive dyskinesia, 1:92

Tarsoconjunctival blepharoplasty, 1:170

Tarsorrhaphy, **3:1396–1398**

Tartrazine, 1:132

Task Force on Preanesthesia Evaluation, 1:56

Taste disorders, 3:1367

Tax credit proposals, 3:1205

Tay-Sachs disease, 1:41

Tazicef. *See* Ceptaz

Tazidime. *See* Ceptaz

Teaching hospitals, 2:688, 689, 3:1388

Teams. *See* Patient care teams

Technetium 99, 2:988, 993, 3:1300

Technology, home care and, 2:680

Teenagers. *See* Adolescents

Teeth
    decay, 3:1428
    eating disorders and, 3:1560

extraction, **3:1426–1429,** 3:*1427*
    prosthetic, 1:415
    replacement, 1:413–416
    replantation, **3:1429–1431**

TEF (Tracheoesophageal fistula) repair, **1:485–490**

Tefla gauze, 3:1302

Teflon paste, 1:311

Teflon slings, 3:1329

Tegretol. *See* Carbamazepine

Telangiectasia, 1:418, 3:1279–1280, 1282

Telangiectatic matting, 3:1284

Telecare, 2:680

Telerobotic surgery, 3:1399

Telesurgery, **3:1398–1399**

Telethermometers, 1:543–544

Telmisartan, 1:89

Temperature, body. *See* Body temperature

Templating review, 2:676

Temporal lobe seizures, 1:75–78, 2:1026

Temporal lobectomy, 1:359, 2:1026, 3:1514

Temporary colostomy, 1:321

Tenacula, 3:1381

Tendinitis, 2:619

Tendon lengthening. *See* Tenotomies

Tendon release. *See* Tenotomies

Tendons
    ganglion cyst removal and, 2:560, 2:*561*
    imbalance, 2:616, 617
    injuries, 1:546
    kneecap, 2:814, 815
    repair of, **3:1399–1403,** 3:*1401*
    shoulder, 3:1247
    tenotomies, **3:1403–1405**

Tenex. *See* Guanfacine hydrochloride

Tennis elbow, 3:1400

Tenoplasty, 2:617

Tenoretic, 1:90*t*

Tenormin. *See* Atenolol

Tenotomies, 1:307, **3:1403–1405**

TENS (Transcutaneous electrical nerve stimulation), 2:825, 3:1085

Tension-free repair (Hernia), 2:755

Tension-free vaginal tape sling procedure (TVT), 3:1329

Tequin. *See* Gatifloxacin

Teratoma, sacrococcygeal, 1:531

Terazosin hydrochloride, 1:90*t*

Terbutaline, 1:280, 532

Teres minor, 3:1247

Terlipressin, 3:1279

Terminally ill patients
    hospices for, 2:682–685
    power of attorney and, 3:1190

Terramycin. *See* Oxytetracycline

Testicles
    development of, 2:1058
    ectopic, 2:1060

hydrocelectomy for, 2:693–697, 2:*694*
    retractile, 2:1060
    undescended, 2:704, 1053, 1058–1063, 2:*1059,* 3:1119

Testicular autotransplantation, 2:1060

Testicular cancer
    demographics of, 2:1052–1053, 1058
    diagnosis of, 2:1054
    hypospadias repair and, 2:701
    non-surgical treatment of, 2:1056
    orchiectomy for, 2:1051–1058
    sentinel lymph node biopsy for, 3:1300

Testicular torsion, 2:1058–1063

Testosterone, 2:1052

Tetanus, 1:542, 2:994

Tetany, 1:446, 448

Tetracaine, 1:65, 2:817

Tetracyclines, 1:81, **3:1405–1409**
    for hospital-acquired infections, 2:687
    NSAIDs and, 2:1028
    side effects of, 1:83

Tetralogy of Fallot, 2:636, 637

Teveten. *See* Eprosartan

Thalamotomy, 1:411, 3:1089

Thalassemia, 1:335–336, 339, 3:1228–1229, 1362

Thalassemia minor, 2:647, 3:1229

Thallium scans, 3:1375

Theo-Dur. *See* Theophylline

Theophylline
    fluoroquinolones and, 1:547
    gastric acid inhibitors and, 2:569
    overdoses of, 2:652

Therapeutic abortion, 1:13, 533

Therapeutic phlebotomy, 3:1150–1152

Thermometers, **3:1408–1411**

Thermoscalpels, 2:646

Theta waves, 1:444, 445

Thiazide diuretics, 1:89–90, 91, 428, 429, 2:1020

Thiersch procedure, 3:1223

Thimerosal, 1:94

Thiopental, 1:60

Third-degree burns, 3:1323

Thoracic aneurysm, 1:101, 102, 103, 469

Thoracic spine, 2:819

Thoracic surgeons, 2:738

Thoracic surgery, 1:404, **3:1411–1413**

Thoracoscopic surgery, video-assisted, 2:914–915, 916

Thoracoscopy. *See* Video assisted thoracoscopic surgery

Thoracotomy, 3:1413, **3:1414–1417,** 3:*1415*
    for analgesia, 2:920
    for aortic valve replacement, 1:104
    esophagectomy and, 1:495
    for lung biopsy, 2:914

for minimally invasive heart
surgery, 2:976
posterolateral, 3:1176
for pulmonary lobectomy, 2:903
Thoratec Heart-Mate VE, 2:644
Thought stopping, 3:1339–1340
Three-hole esophagectomy, 1:495
Throat cancer
chest x ray for, 1:291
craniofacial reconstruction for,
1:363
pharyngectomy for, 3:1145–1149
risk factors for, 3:1147
Throat surgery, **1:433–435**
Thrombin, 1:537
Thrombin inhibitors, 1:86
Thrombocytopenia, 1:189, 337, 2:568
Thrombocytosis, 1:337, 3:1151
Thromboembolic deterrent (TED)
stockings, 2:669, 670, 805, 806
Thromboembolism. *See* Thrombosis
Thromboendarterectomy, 3:1129–1130
Thrombolysis, 3:1519
Thrombolytic agents, 3:1417
Thrombolytic therapy, **3:1417–1419**
vs. angioplasty, 1:72–73
for blood clots, 1:86
for peripheral artery disease, 3:1130
Thrombopoietin, 2:728
Thrombosed hemorrhoids, 2:655
Thrombosis
C-reactive protein and, 1:241
deep vein, 2:670
peripheral endarterectomy and,
3:1131
thromboendarterectomy for,
3:1129–1130
See also Deep vein thrombosis
Thumb amputation, 1:542
Thyroid-stimulating hormones, 3:1421
Thyroid storm, 3:1422
Thyroidectomy, 2:828, 3:1098–1099,
3:1419–1423, 3:*1420*
Thyroiditis, Hashimoto's, 2:692
TIA (Transient ischemic attacks),
1:254, 255
Tibia
anatomy of, 2:800
knee replacement and, 2:802
lengthening and shortening of,
2:866, 868
Tibial traction, 3:*1438*
Ticlid. *See* Ticlopidine
Ticlopidine, 1:86
Tigan. *See* Trimethobenzamide hy-
drochloride
Tikosyn. *See* Dofetilide
Timoptic, 2:855
Tinel's sign, 1:260
Tinnitus, 3:1478
TIPP (Transilluminated powered phle-
bectomy), 3:1532–1533
TIPS (Transvenous portosystemic
shunts), 3:1179, 1181, 1279

Tirofiban, 1:86
Tissue Adhesive Center, 1:537
Tissue adhesives, 1:536–538
Tissue compatibility testing, 2:691
Tissue glues, 2:703, 744
Tissue plasminogen activator (TPA),
3:1417
Tissue receptors, 3:1469
Titanium
clips, 1:274
dental implants, 1:415
miniplates, 1:365
pins, 2:867
staples, 2:744
Tizanidine, 2:994
TMP-SMZ (Trimethoprim/sul-
famethoxazole), 3:1377
TNF-238A gene, 2:676
TNM system, 3:1473
Tobacco, smokeless, 3:1339
See also Smoking
Tocolytics, 1:280, 532, 2:876
Toe abnormalities, 2:616–618
Toe bunionectomy, 1:229–233
Toe injuries, 2:616
Tofranil. *See* Imipramine
TOL. *See* Trial of labor
Tolmetin, 1:132
Tomography, 1:76, 3:1274
See also CT scans; Positron emis-
sion tomography
Tongue cancer surgery, 2:600–602
Tongue prosthesis, 2:602
Tongue suspension procedure, 3:1345,
1347
Tonic-clonic seizures, 1:358
Tonometry
for closed-angle glaucoma, 2:773
for open-angle glaucoma,
3:1273–1274
Schiotz, 2:608
TonoPen, 2:608
Tonsillectomy, 1:433, 434, 435,
3:1423–1425, 3:*1424*
adenoidectomy and, 1:23
snoring surgery and, 3:1344, 1345
tongue suspension procedure and,
3:1345
Tooth decay, 3:1428
Tooth extraction, 3:1246, **3:1426–1429,**
3:*1427*
Tooth migration, 1:414
Toothache, 3:1244–1247
Toothpick weed, 2:1021
Topical anesthetics, 1:64, 65, 2:656,
817
Topical antibiotics, **1:84–86,** 1:407,
2:818, 3:1464
Topical nasal steroids, 1:24
TOPS. *See* Take Off Pounds Sensibly
Toradol. *See* Ketorolac
Total arthroplasty, 1:116–120, 507
Total artificial heart, 2:843, 999
Total bilirubin test, 2:891, 892

Total body sodium excess, 1:447
Total cholesterol test, 2:875–878
Total disk removal, 1:425
Total gastrectomy, 2:564
Total glossectomy, 2:601, 602, 664–665
Total hepatectomy, 2:659
Total hip replacement, 2:663, 664–665,
673
Total hysterectomy, 2:708
Total joint replacement, 1:116–120,
507
Total knee replacement, 2:800, 2:*803,*
2:814
Total laryngectomy, 2:839
Total mastectomy, 3:1214–1215,
3:1318–1322, *1319*
Total pancreatectomy, 3:1093
Total parotidectomy, 3:1100
Total pelvic exenteration, 1:504
Total pharyngectomy, 3:1145, 1146,
1147
Total protein levels
cerebrospinal fluid analysis of,
1:276, 277
liver function tests for, 2:890–895
Total shoulder joint replacement,
3:1309, 1310, 1314
Toxic megacolon, 1:314, 3:1317
Toxins. *See* Poisoning
TPA. *See* Tissue plasminogen activator
Trabecular meshwork, 2:607, 610, 848,
849, 850
Trabeculectomy, 2:610, 1049,
3:1431–1434, 3:*1432,* 1463
Trabeculoplasty, laser, 1:388, 2:850
Trabeculotomy, 2:609–610
Tracheal bronchoscopy, 1:225–229
See also Endotracheal intubation
Tracheal injuries, 1:372–377
Tracheoesophageal fistula, 1:485–490,
3:1116
Tracheoesophageal fistula repair,
1:485–490
Tracheoesophageal speech, 2:840
Tracheostomy, 1:465, 2:945, 946
Tracheotomy, **3:1434–1437,** 3:*1435*
for ear, nose and throat surgery,
1:434
for laryngectomy, 2:839
for pharyngectomy, 3:1146
See also Cricothyroidotomy
Traction, 1:553, **3:1437–1439,** 3:*1438*
Traction retinal detachment, 3:1153
Traditional open appendectomy, 1:107,
108
Trager work, 3:1562
Training. *See* Education
TRAM flap reconstruction, 1:9
Tranquilizers, 1:543, 3:1345, 1561
See also Antianxiety drugs
Transcutaneous electrical nerve stimu-
lation (TENS), 2:825, 3:1085
Transcyte, 3:1327, 1569
Transderm-V. *See* Scopolamine patch

Transdermal fentanyl patches, 3:1084

Transdermal Scop. *See* Scopolamine patch

Transducers, 1:2–3, 243, 436, 3:1120

Transected Roux-en-Y (RNY) gastric bypass, 2:571

Transesophageal echocardiography, 1:102, 248, 2:979, 983

Transfusion, **3:1439–1444**
 allogenic, 1:134, 136
 alternatives to, 1:136
 autologous blood donation for, 1:28, **1:134–136**
 availability of, 1:181
 for bone marrow transplantation, 1:181
 cryoprecipitated antihemophilic factor, 1:174
 fresh frozen plasma, 1:173, 174
 for liver transplantation, 1:181
 need for, 1:181, 182
 noninfectious serious hazards of, 1:180–181
 platelet, 1:173–174
 preadmission, 3:1168
 red blood cell, 1:173, 179
 safety of, 1:180–181
 whole blood, 1:173
 See also Blood donation

Transfusion reaction
 blood salvage and, 1:178, 179
 liver function tests for, 2:894
 from medical errors, 1:180–181

Transhiatal esophagectomy, 1:495

Transient ischemic attacks (TIA), 1:254, 255

Transilluminated powered phlebectomy (TIPP), 3:1532–1533

Transillumination, 2:695

Transitional repair, 3:1263

Transjugular portosystemic shunts, 3:1139

Transmitters, cochlear, 1:308

Transparent film, 1:144, 145

Transplant physicians, 1:196

Transplant rejection
 bone marrow transplantation and, 1:201
 causes of, 2:691
 corneal transplantation and, 1:344
 heart-lung transplantation and, 2:633
 heart transplantation and, 2:641, 642
 immunosuppressant drugs for, 2:732–736
 kidney transplantation and, 2:790
 liver transplantation and, 2:899
 lung transplantation and, 2:921

Transplant surgery, **3:1444–1450**

Transplantation
 cartilage, 2:807, 3:1302
 corneal, **1:342–346**, *343*
 hair, **2:613–616**, *614*
 heart-lung, **2:630–634**, *631*, 2:918, 920, 921
 human leukocyte antigen test for, 2:691–693
 immunosuppressant drugs for, 2:732–736
 islet cell, **2:776–778**, 3:1091
 lung, 2:905, **2:918–922**, *919*, 3:1178, 1412–1413
 microsurgery for, 2:973
 non-myeloablative allogeneic, 1:195
 pancreas, 2:777–778, 783, **3:1089–1091**
 peripheral blood stem cell, 1:195–196, 198
 surgical team for, 3:1386
 umbilical cord blood, 1:196
 See also specific types of transplantation

Transportation, 3:1169, 1197, 1202

Transposition of the great vessels, 2:634, *2:635*, 2:636–637

Transrectal ultrasound, 2:1054

Transscleral cyclophotocoagulation, 3:1433

Transsexuals, 1:213
 See also Sex reassignment surgery

Transthoracic esophagectomy, 1:495

Transthyretin tests, 2:891, 893

Transtracheal jet ventilation (TTJV), 1:375–376

Transtracheal oxygen therapy, 2:1074

Transuretero ureterostomy (TUU), 3:1495, 1496

Transurethral alcohol treatment, 3:1458

Transurethral bladder resections, 1:394, **3:1450–1453**

Transurethral electrovaporization, 3:1457

Transurethral incision of the prostate (TUIP), 3:1454, 1457

Transurethral microwave thermotherapy (TUMT), 3:1457

Transurethral needle ablation (TUNA), 3:1457

Transurethral resection of the prostate (TURP), 2:1042, **3:1453–1459**, 3:*1455*

Transvaginal ultrasound, 2:832

Transvenous portosystemic shunts (TIPS), 3:1179, 1181, 1279

Transverse colon, 1:204

Transverse rectus abdominis myocutaneous (TRAM) flap reconstruction, 1:9

Transvesical prostatectomy, 2:1044

Tranxene. *See* Clorazepate dipotassium

Tranylcypromine, 1:80

Trauma
 amputation for, 1:44
 anesthesiologists and, 1:67
 avulsed teeth, 3:1429, 1430
 blunt, 1:100, 3:1362
 chest, 3:1412

in children, 3:1118–1119
 cricothyroidotomy for, 1:372
 emergency surgery for, 1:452–453
 low back pain and, 2:820
 post-traumatic stress disorder and, 1:366–367

Trauma/burn intensive care units, 2:760

Trauma centers, 1:452, 2:628

Trauma surgery, essential, 1:501

Trazodone, 3:1084

Treacher Collins syndrome, 1:362, 366, 2:1066

Treatment refusal, 3:1108

Treatment withholding, 1:431

Tremor, essential, 1:409–411

Trendar. *See* Pentoxifylline

Trental. *See* Pentoxifylline

Trexan. *See* Naltrexone

Triage nurses, 2:933

Trial of labor (TOL), 1:287

Trials, clinical. *See* Clinical trials

Triamcinolone, 1:360

Triamterene, 1:428

Triazolam, 1:55

Trichlormethiazide, 1:91

Trichloroacetic acid, 1:418, 2:991

Tricuspid atresia, 2:637

Tricuspid valve stenosis, 1:141–143

Tricyclic antidepressants
 adrenergic drugs and, 1:34
 for analgesia, 1:50
 closed-angle glaucoma from, 2:772
 hemoperfusion for, 2:653
 for interstitial cystitis, 3:1255
 opioid analgesics and, 1:55

Trifluoperazine hydrochloride, 1:79t

Triglycerides
 gallstones and, 2:557
 lipid tests for, 2:875–878
 liver function tests for, 2:890–895

Trilostane, 2:700

Trimethadione, 2:651

Trimethobenzamide hydrochloride, 1:92t

Trimethoprim/sulfamethoxazole (TMP-SMZ), 3:1377

Triple antibiotic ointment, 1:84

Triple endoscopy, 1:434

Triple lumen central venous catheters, 1:199

Trisomy 21. *See* Down syndrome

Trocar injuries, 2:831

Tropisetron, 3:1287

Troponin C, 1:241

Troponin I, 1:241, 242

Troponin T, 1:241, 242

Trovafloxacin, 3:1206

Trovan. *See* Trovafloxacin

Trust, 3:1395

TSH. *See* Thyroid-stimulating hormones

TTJV (Transtracheal jet ventilation), 1:375–376

TTTS (Twin/Twin transfusion syndrome)

TTTS (Twin/twin transfusion syndrome), 1:531, 532, 534
Tubal ligation, 1:331, 332–333, 439, 2:1034, **3:1459–1462**, 3:*1460*, 1526
Tubal pregnancy. *See* Ectopic pregnancy
Tube insertion. *See* Intubation
Tube shunt surgery, 3:1433, **3:1463–1466**
Tuberculosis
   ascites from, 3:1095
   chest x ray for, 1:291
   CT scans for, 1:384
   liver biopsy for, 2:886
   lung biopsy for, 2:914, 917
   pulmonary lobectomy for, 2:903
Tubes
   chest, **1:288–290**, 1:291
   disposable, 2:761
   drainage, 1:*19*, 1:20, 130
   ear, 2:1002–1007, 2:*1003*
   gastrostomy or "g," 2:591–594
   myringotomy, 1:303
   See also Endotracheal intubation; Nasogastric tubes
Tucks pads, 1:481
TUIP (Transurethral incision of the prostate), 3:1454, 1457
Tumescent local anesthesia, 2:878, 880
Tummy tuck flaps, 1:220, 221
Tumor marker tests, **3:1469–1472**
Tumor removal, **3:1472–1475**
TUMT (Transurethral microwave thermotherapy), 3:1457
TUNA (Transurethral needle ablation), 3:1457
Tunica vaginalis, 2:693, 695
Turbinate surgery, 3:1302, 1303
TURP. *See* Transurethral resection of the prostate
TUU (Transuretero ureterostomy), 3:1495, 1496
TVT (Tension-free vaginal tape sling procedure), 3:1329
Twilight anesthesia, 1:521, 2:858, **3:1292–1294**
Twin/twin transfusion syndrome (TTTS), 1:531, 532, 534
Twins, 1:511, 534
Tylectomy. *See* Lumpectomy
Tylenol. *See* Acetaminophen
Tylosis, 1:494
Tympanic thermometers, 3:1409–1410
Tympanoplasty, 1:434, **3:1475–1479**, 3:*1477*
   See also Mastoidectomy
Tympanosclerosis, 2:1006
Tympanostomy, 1:303, 434, **2:1002–1007**, *1003*
Type 1 diabetes
   glucose tests for, 2:604
   islet cell transplantation for, 2:776–778
   pancreas transplantation for, 3:1089–1091

Type 2 diabetes, 1:507, 2:604
Typing and screening, blood, 3:1440–1441, **3:1479–1484**, 3:*1481*

U

Ulcerative colitis
   barium enema and, 1:155
   bowel resection for, 1:206, 208
   in children, 3:1118
   colonoscopy for, 1:313, 315
   colorectal surgery for, 1:317–321, 2:579
   demographics of, 2:580, 720, 723, 3:1225
   ileoanal anastomosis for, 2:717–720
   ileoanal reservoir surgery for, 2:720–723
   ileostomy for, 2:723–726
   non-surgical treatment of, 1:208, 2:580, 725–726
   rectal resection for, 3:1225–1228
   sigmoidoscopy for, 3:1315, 1317
Ulcers
   corneal, 3:1397
   decubitus (pressure), **1:155–159**, *157*, 1:408
   duodenal, 1:96, 2:564, 579, 3:1209, 1333
   foot, 1:46, 408
   skin, 1:155–159, *1:157*, 1:408, 3:1283, 1284
   stress, 2:568
   vagotomy, 3:1515, 1517
   See also Peptic ulcers; Stomach ulcers
Ulnar nerve compression, 2:620
Ultrasound
   A-mode, 1:3
   abdominal, **1:1–5**, *2*
   for amniocentesis, 2:876, 3:1120
   anorectal, 1:126
   B-mode, 1:3
   biomicroscopy, 3:1274
   for birth defects, 1:532
   bladder, 3:1120
   for breast biopsy guidance, 1:211
   for breast cancer, 2:929
   cardiac, 1:239–240
   for cesarean section, 1:285–286
   for coronary artery disease, 1:239–240
   for endometriosis, 2:835
   for esophageal cancer, 1:496
   fetal, 1:534, 535–536, **3:1120–1122**, *1121*
   for gallstones, 1:295, 2:559
   for ganglion cyst removal, 2:562
   for glaucoma, 1:390
   for hip dysplasia, 2:662
   for hypospadias, 2:704
   for inguinal hernia repair, 2:755

   for intussusception reduction, 2:769
   for laser iridotomy, 2:851
   for leg lengthening, 2:870
   for liposhaving, 2:879
   for lithotripsy, 2:884
   for liver biopsy, 2:886
   M-mode, 1:3
   vs. mediastinoscopy, 2:951
   for omphaloceles, 2:1036
   pelvic, **3:1120–1122**, *1121*
   for phacoemulsification, 1:509, 512, 3:1140
   phlebography and, 3:1149
   for retinal cryopexy, 3:1232
   for retinal detachment, 3:1155
   for shoulder resection arthroplasty, 3:1313
   sound waves in, 1:2–3
   for spina bifida, 2:965
   for stomach cancer, 2:577
   transrectal, 2:1054
   transvaginal, 2:832
   for ureteral obstruction, 3:1491
   See also Doppler ultrasound
Ultraviolet radiation, 1:511
Umbilical cord, 1:5, 283
Umbilical cord blood transplantation, 1:196
Umbilical hernia, 3:1119
Umbilical hernia repair, **3:1485–1488**, 3:*1486*
Umbilicus
   abdominoplasty and, 1:8–9
   bowel resection and, 1:207
   laparoscopy and, 2:829
   patent urachus repair and, 3:1103
Unconjugated bilirubin tests, 2:891
Undescended testicles
   demographics of, 2:1058–1059, 3:1119
   hypospadias and, 2:704
   orchiopexy for, 2:1053, 1058–1063, 2:*1059*
UNICEF (United Nations Children's Fund), 2:767
Unilateral cleft lip, 1:301
Unilateral pallidotomy, 3:1088
Unilateral salpingo-oophorectomy, 3:1256–1259
Uninsured patients, 2:689, 3:1165, 1204
United Nations Children's Fund (UNICEF), 2:767
United Network for Organ Sharing (UNOS), 3:1446
   on heart-lung transplantation, 2:633
   on heart transplantation, 2:639, 641
   on histocompatability tests, 2:693
   on kidney transplants, 2:783, 788–789, 1014
   on liver transplantation, 2:896, 900
   on lung transplantation, 2:920
   on pancreas/kidney transplantation, 3:1090–1091

United Ostomy Association, 2:723
United States Renal Data System (USRDS), 2:779–780, 783, 786–787, 790
UNOS. *See* United Network for Organ Sharing
Upper esophagogastroduodenal endoscopy, 2:581
Upper extremity amputation, 1:44
Upper gastrointestinal endoscopy, **1:499–501,** 2:583, 584
Upper GI exams, 1:97, 496, 2:577, 3:*1486,* **3:1489–1490**
Upper motor neuron syndrome, 3:1404
Upper respiratory tract infections, 1:460, 489, 3:1343
UPPP (Uvulopalatopharyngoplasty), *3:1343,* 3:1344, 1345, 1346
Urachus tube defects, 3:1101–1103
Urea clearance test, 2:784, 786
Urea reduction ratio (URR), 2:783
Urease breath test, 1:97
Ureteral injuries, 2:830, 831
Ureteral obstruction, 2:1021–1024
Ureteral stenting, 2:714, 715, 716, **3:1490–1492**
Ureteral stones, 2:1021, 1022, 1023
Ureteroscopy, 2:1021
Ureterosigmoidoscopy, **3:1492–1495**
Ureterostomy, cutaneous, **3:1495–1498**
Urethra
    artificial, 2:703
    collagen periurethral injection of, 1:311
    injuries, 2:1012
    inserts, 3:1332
    instability, 3:1330
    plugs, 3:1237
    prolapse, 1:327
    stenosis, 2:704
    strictures, 1:400
    urinary catheterization and, 1:262–263, 264, 265, 266
Urethral anastomosis, 2:713
Urethral cancer exenteration, 1:504
Urethral hypermobility
    artificial sphincter insertion for, 1:125–126
    diagnosis of, 3:1236
    needle bladder neck suspension for, 2:1010–1012
    retropubic suspension for, 3:1234–1238
    sling procedure for, 1:127, 3:1330, 1331–1332
    Valsalva leak test for, 3:1236
Urethral meatus hypospadias repair, 2:701–706
Urethral obstructions, 1:531
Urethrocele, 1:327
Urethroscopes, 1:399
Urge urinary incontinence
    artificial sphincter insertion for, 1:123

retropubic suspension for, 3:1234–1238
sacral nerve stimulation for, 3:1253
sling procedure for, 3:1330
Uric acid calculi, 2:1016
Uric acid levels, 2:785
Urinalysis, **3:1498–1502**
    for anesthesia evaluation, 1:57–58
    for glucose, 2:606
    for kidney function, 1:113, 2:784, 785
    osmolality, 2:784, 785
    pH, 2:885
    physical examination and, 3:1162
    protein, 2:784, 785, 786
Urinary anti-infectives, **3:1502–1506**
Urinary bladder cancer. *See* Bladder cancer
Urinary catheterization
    clean intermittent, 2:713
    drainage for, 1:263, 266
    female, 1:262–265
    hospital-acquired infections and, 2:685, 687
    indwelling, 1:262, 263, 264, 265–266, 267
    intermittent, 1:262, 263, 265, 267
    male, 1:265–268
    self, 1:263, 3:1332
    urinary tract infections and, 1:263
Urinary diversion
    for bedsores, 1:158
    continent, 2:713, 716
    cystectomy and, 1:392, *1:393,* 1:393–394
    ileal conduit surgery for, 2:713–716
    incontinent, 2:713
    for interstitial cystitis, 3:1255
    for pelvic exenteration, 1:504
Urinary incontinence
    artificial sphincter insertion for, 1:123–128
    bladder augmentation for, 1:166–169
    catheterization for, 1:263, 267
    causes of, 3:1330
    childbirth and, 3:1235
    colporrhaphy for, 1:325–329
    cystocele repair for, 1:395–398
    demographics of, 1:124–125, 327, 2:1011, 3:1235, 1253, 1330
    diagnosis of, 3:1236, 1254, 1331–1332
    gender differences in, 2:1011, 3:1253, 1330
    genuine stress, 2:1010–1011, 3:1330, 1331
    from intrinsic sphincter deficiency, 2:1010–1011, 1012
    mixed, 3:1235, 1330
    needle bladder neck suspension for, 2:1010–1012
    non-surgical treatment of, 1:127, 312, 328, 398, 3:1237, 1332

overflow, 1:123, 3:1235, 1330
    retropubic colposuspension for, 1:397
    retropubic suspension for, 3:1234–1238
    sacral nerve stimulation for, 3:1253–1256
    sling procedure for, 3:1329–1333
    urge, 1:123, 3:1234–1238, 1253, 1330
    See also Stress urinary incontinence
Urinary meatus, 1:263, 266
Urinary osmolality test, 1:113
Urinary output, 1:113, 427
Urinary retention, 2:1012
Urinary sphincter hyperreflexia, 3:1253
Urinary tract defects, 1:487
Urinary tract infections (UTI)
    from cesarean section, 1:287
    circumcision and, 1:298
    hospital-acquired, 2:685, 686
    hypospadias repair for, 2:701
    from laparoscopy, 2:830
    urinary catheterization and, 1:263, 267
Urinary tract obstructions, fetal, 1:531, 534
Urine leakage, 2:716
Urine tests. *See* Urinalysis
Urobilinogen, 3:1500, 1502
Urogynecologists, 3:1450
Urogynecology, 2:1033
Urokinase, 3:1417–1418
Urolithiasis, 2:1016, 1017–1018
Urologic surgery, **3:1506–1509**
Urological Foundation, 3:1506
Urologists, 2:703, 970, 3:1450
Urologix Targis TM System, 3:1458
Urostomy bags, 3:1496
URR (Urea reduction ratio), 2:783
USRDS (United States Renal Data System), 2:779–780, 783, 786–787, 790
Uterine artery embolization, 2:710
Uterine bleeding, 1:419–422, 2:711
Uterine cancer
    colpotomy for, 1:331
    demographics of, 3:1383
    hysterectomy for, 2:706, 708
Uterine fibroids
    demographics of, 2:999–1000
    dilation and curettage for, 1:419, 422
    embolization for, 2:1002
    endometrial ablation for, 2:710
    hysterectomy for, 2:706, 708, 1001–1002
    hysteroscopy for, 2:711, 712
    myomectomy for, 2:710, 999–1002, *2:1000*
    recurrence of, 2:1001
    second-look surgery for, 3:1288
Uterine perforation, 2:712
Uterine polyps, 2:711, 712
Uterine prolapse, 1:327

Uterine rupture, 1:287
Uterine scars, 1:421
Uterine staplers, 1:532
Uterine stimulants, **3:1509–1512**
UTI. *See* Urinary tract infections
Utilization review, 2:933
Uveitic glaucoma, 2:607
Uveitis, 1:514, 2:772, 852
Uvula, 3:1344, 1345
Uvulopalatopharyngoplasty (UPPP),
    3:1343, 3:1344, 1345, 1346
Uvulopalatoplasty
    laser-assisted, 3:1344, 1345, 1347

V

V/Q scan, 2:904, 920
Vaccines
    cancer, 2:731
    immunosuppressant drugs and,
        2:734
    pneumococcal, 3:1363
VACTRRL syndrome, 1:487
Vacuum aspiration, 1:15–16, 420
Vacuum scraping, 1:422
VAD. *See* Ventricular assist device
Vagal nerve stimulation, **3:1513–1515**
Vagal-sparing esophagectomy, 1:495
Vaginal birth after a cesarean (VBAC),
    1:283, 287
Vaginal cancer exenteration, 1:503
Vaginal cones, 3:1237
Vaginal delivery, 1:286
Vaginal disorders
    colposcopy for, 1:329–331
    hysterectomy for, 2:706, 708
    surgery for, 2:1033
Vaginal hysterectomy, 1:332, 333,
    2:708–709, 3:1259
Vaginal paravaginal repair, 1:397
Vaginal surgery, 1:312, 331–334, 2:1033
Vaginal wall defects, 1:325–329,
    395–397
Vaginotomy, **1:331–334**, 2:1033
Vagotomy, **3:1515–1518**, *3:1516*
    antrectomy and, 1:96
    demographics of, 2:579
    gastrectomy and, 2:564
    highly selective, 2:566
    pyloroplasty and, 3:1211
Vagus nerve stimulation, 1:359
Valerian, 1:57
Valgus osteotomy, 2:797–799
Valium. *See* Diazepam
Valproic acid
    alprazolam and, 1:80
    aspirin and, 1:133
    barbiturates and, 1:153
    cephalosporins and, 1:270
    diazepam and, 2:995
    erythromycins and, 1:485
    sulfonamides and, 3:1380

Valsalva leak test, 3:1236
Valsartan, 1:89
Valve repair. *See* Heart valve repair
Valves, heart. *See* Heart valves
Valvotomy, 1:107, 2:986
Valvular angioplasty, 1:141
Valvuloplasty, balloon, **1:141–143**,
    2:636
Van der Woude syndrome, 1:301
Vancomycin, 2:687
Variceal band ligation, 3:1181
Varicose vein sclerotherapy,
    3:1279–1286, *3:1281*
Varicose veins
    ambulatory phlebectomy for, 3:1532
    causes of, 3:1531–1532
    demographics, 3:1531, *1531*
    ligation and stripping of, 3:*1533*
    transilluminated powered phlebecto-
        my for, 3:1532–1533
Varus derotational osteotomy (VDO),
    2:662
Varus osteotomy, 2:797–799
Varus rotational osteotomy (VRO),
    2:662
Vascular access, 1:111–115
Vascular magnetic resonance angiogra-
    phy, 2:927
Vascular malformation, 2:645–646
Vascular surgery, **3:1518–1524**
    vs. endovascular stent surgery, 1:467
    microsurgery, 2:970, 972
    surgical team for, 3:1386
Vasectomy, 3:1231, 1462,
    3:1524–1527, 3:*1525*
Vasoconstriction, 1:65, 3:1389
Vasodilan. *See* Isoxsuprine
Vasodilators
    for aortic stenosis, 1:107
    for finger reattachment, 1:543, 545
    peripheral, 1:89, 91, 543
Vasopressin, 3:1278, 1279
VasoSeal, 1:236
Vasospasm, 1:273, 274, 543
Vasotec. *See* Enalapril
Vasovagal response, 1:135, 136
Vasovasostomy, 3:1525–1526,
    3:1527–1530, 3:*1528*
VATER syndrome, 1:487
VATS. *See* Video assisted thoracoscopic
    surgery
VBAC (Vaginal birth after a cesarean),
    1:283, 287
VBG. *See* Vertical banded gastroplasty
VC (Vital capacity), 3:1358–1360
VCUG (Holding and voiding urine
    test), 1:167
VDO (Varus derotational osteotomy),
    2:662
VDRL test, 1:277
Vegetarian diet, 1:470, 2:1021
Vein grafts, 2:972
Vein ligation and stripping, 3:*1528*,
    3:1530–1538, 3:*1531, 1533*

Venipuncture, 3:1392–1394
Venlafaxine, 3:1562
Venodyne boots, 2:572
Venography, **3:1149–1150**
Venous switch, 2:637
Venous system anatomy, 3:1280
Venous thromboembolism. *See* Deep
    vein thrombosis
Venous thrombosis prevention,
    3:1538–1540
Ventilation, transtracheal jet,
    1:375–376
Ventilation/perfusion (V/Q) scan,
    2:904, 920
Ventilator-associated pneumonia, 2:685
Ventilator masks, 2:945, 946
Ventilators, 2:760, 945, 961,
    1045–1046
    See also Mechanical ventilation
Ventolin. *See* Albuterol
Ventral hernia, **2:746–750**
Ventricular assist device, 2:637, 643,
    843, 999, **3:1540–1542**
Ventricular fibrillation
    defibrillation for, 1:411–413
    electrocardiography for, 1:441
    electrophysiology study for, 1:451
    implantable cardioverter-defibrilla-
        tor for, 2:736–740
Ventricular restoration, 2:643, 997–998,
    999
Ventricular septal defects, 2:634, *2:635*,
    2:637
Ventricular shunts, 1:239, **3:1542–1544**
Ventricular tachycardia
    defibrillation for, 1:412
    electrophysiology study for, 1:451
    implantable cardioverter-defibrilla-
        tor for, 2:736, 737, 739, 740
Verapamil, 1:89
Verapamil hydrochloride, 1:90*t*
Vermilion notch, 1:303
Versed. *See* Midazolam
Vertebrae, 2:819
Vertical banded gastroplasty (VBG),
    2:574, **3:1544–1551**, 3:1562
Vertical (Fobi) gastric bypass, 2:571
Vertigo, 1:454, 455
Veseretic, 1:90*t*
Veses needle, 2:831
Vestibular neurectomy, 1:455
Vestibular suppressants, 1:455
Veterans Administration, 2:961
Vfend. *See* Voriconazole
Viagra. *See* Sildenafil citrate
Vibramycin. *See* Doxycycline
Vibration, 1:259
Video-assisted arthroscopic mi-
    crodiskectomy, 1:425
Video assisted thoracoscopic surgery
    (VATS), 2:914–915, 916, 3:1413, 1416
Video equipment, laparoscopic, 2:828
Videostroboscopy, 1:434
Videx. *See* Didanosine

Vigilon, 1:418
Viral infections, 2:642, 685, 687
Virginity, 1:297
Virtual colonoscopy, 1:316
Visceral pain, 3:1083
Viscocanalostomy, 3:1275
Viscoelastic material, 1:512
Vision
    double, 1:516, 518, 2:846, 1050,
      3:1144
    night, 2:844, 846, 1050, 3:1275
Vision loss
    from cataracts, 1:512
    from congenital glaucoma, 2:608,
      609
    from cyclocryotherapy, 1:390
    demographics of, 1:475
    from hypophysectomy, 2:699
    laser surgery for, 1:438
    ophthalmologic surgery for,
      2:1048–1051
Vision therapy, 1:518, 519
Visiting hospitals, 3:1167–1168
Visiting nurse associations, 2:679
Visken. See Pindolol
Visual acuity, 2:846
    cataracts and, 1:512
    laser posterior capsulotomy for,
      2:854, 855, 856
    phacoemulsification for, 3:1144
    retinal cryopexy and, 3:1232
    tests for, 2:1049, 3:1154
Visual field tests, 2:608, 852, 3:1089,
    1274
Visualization, 3:1185
Vital capacity (VC), 3:1358–1360
Vital signs, **3:1551–1554**, 3:*1553*
Vitamin A, 1:514
Vitamin A deficiency, 3:1147
Vitamin B$_6$
    for atherosclerosis prevention,
      1:256, 469, 3:1132, 1136
    for coronary artery disease, 1:352,
      356, 472
Vitamin B$_{12}$
    for atherosclerosis prevention,
      1:256, 469, 3:1132, 1136
    for coronary artery disease, 1:352,
      356, 472
Vitamin B$_{12}$ deficiency, 1:335, 336,
    339, 3:1228
Vitamin C
    for atherosclerosis prevention,
      1:256, 469, 3:1132, 1136
    cataracts and, 1:514
    for coronary artery disease, 1:356,
      472
    for spider veins, 3:1284
    after vein ligation and stripping,
      3:1536
Vitamin D dependent rickets, 1:447
Vitamin E
    for atherosclerosis prevention,
      1:256, 469, 3:1132, 1136

cataracts and, 1:514
for coronary artery disease, 1:352,
    356, 472
for scar revision, 3:1266
for spider veins, 3:1284
thrombolytic agents and, 3:1419
after vein ligation and stripping,
    3:1536
Vitamin K
    anticoagulants and, 1:88–89
    liver function tests for, 2:893
Vitamins
    after gastrectomy, 2:566
    after gastric bypass, 2:573
Vitelline duct, 2:946
Vitrectomy
    closed-angle glaucoma from, 2:772
    for retinal detachment,
      3:1156–1157, 1268, 1270, 1271
Vitreous body, 3:1152
Vitreous detachment, posterior, 3:1153
Vivox. See Doxycycline
Vocal cords, 2:839
Voice box cancer. See Laryngeal cancer
Voltaren. See Diclofenac
Volume expanders, 1:136, 3:1443
Volvulus, 2:763, 765
Vomiting
    antinausea drugs for, 1:91–93
    bilious, 2:566
    from dialysis, 2:782
    electrolyte balance and, 1:447
    from general anesthesia, 1:62
    postoperative, 3:1286–1288
    scopolamine patch for, 3:1286–1288
    after vertical banded gastroplasty,
      3:1548, 1549
Voriconazole, 2:570
VRO (Varus rotational osteotomy),
    2:662
Vulcan ear, 2:1066
Vulvar hematoma, 2:1034
Vulvectomy, 2:1034

W

W-plasty, 3:1265
Waardenburg syndrome, 1:301
Wada test, 1:358, 2:649
Wagner technique, 2:867
Waist circumference measurements,
    2:572
Walkers. See Assistive devices
Warfarin
    acetaminophen and, 1:22
    activity of, 1:86
    for aortic valve replacement, 1:106
    aspirin and, 1:132, 133
    for atherosclerosis prevention,
      3:1132
    for cardioversion, 1:249
    cephalosporins and, 1:270

    fluoroquinolones and, 1:547
    gastric acid inhibitors and, 2:569
    laparoscopy and, 2:828
    lymphadenectomy and, 2:923
    for Maze procedure, 2:939
    microsurgery and, 2:973
    for mitral valve repair, 2:980
    for mitral valve replacement, 2:984
    NSAIDs and, 2:1028
    opioid analgesics and, 1:55
    phacoemulsification and, 3:1143
    prochlorperazine and, 1:93
    sulfonamides and, 3:1380
    for tooth extraction, 3:1426
    vitamin K and, 1:88
Warts
    cervical, 1:330
    cryotherapy for, 1:377, 378
    genital, 1:329, 385, 386
Washed packed red blood cells, 1:179
Watchful waiting, 3:1290
Water-induced thermotherapy (WIT),
    3:1457
Water pills. See Diuretics
Watermelon stomach, 1:95, 96, 98
Wavefront analyzer, 2:844
WBC count. See White blood cell count
WBRT (Whole-brain radiation thera-
    py), 3:1370
Webbed finger/toe repair, 2:619,
    3:1555–1558, 3:*1556*
Weber's test, 3:1366
Weight Information Network of the Na-
    tional Institutes of Health, 3:1561
Weight loss
    abdominoplasty and, 1:7, 8, 12
    from antrectomy, 1:97
    for arrhythmia, 2:939
    for atherosclerosis prevention, 1:469
    from bowel resection, 1:208
    for coronary artery disease, 1:349,
      355, 471
    gallstones and, 2:557
    gastric bypass for, 2:570–575
    for incisional hernias, 2:750
    for low back pain, 2:825
    non-surgical alternatives for,
      2:574–575
    for urinary incontinence, 3:1332
    See also Body weight; Obesity;
      Weight management
Weight loss drugs, 2:575
Weight Loss for Life, 3:1561
Weight management, **3:1558–1564,**
    3:*1559*
    See also Body weight; Obesity;
      Weight loss
*Weight Management and Health Insur-
    ance,* 3:1547
Weight traction, 3:1437
Weizmann Institute of Science, 3:1273
Westerman-Jensen trephine needle,
    1:190
Wheelchairs and bedsores, 1:158

Whipple's procedure, 3:1092
Whirlpool baths, 1:157
White blood cell count, 1:336–337,
  3:1564–1566
  alloimmunization of, 1:179
  bone marrow aspiration for, 1:189
  cerebrospinal fluid analysis of,
    1:276–277
  critical values for, 1:339
  differential, 1:276–277, 278,
    336–337, 3:1564–1565
  infection, 3:1571
  normal values for, 1:338
  role of, 1:193
  transfusions, 3:1439, 1440
  in urinalysis, 3:1500, 1502
WHO. *See* World Health Organization
Whole blood glucose tests, 2:604, 605
Whole blood transfusion, 1:173, 3:1439
Whole-brain radiation therapy
  (WBRT), 3:1370
Whole grains, 1:470
Wigs, 2:615
Wills, living. *See* Living wills
Wilm's tumor, 3:1119
Wilson's disease, 2:886
Wire brushes, dermabrasion, 1:416, 417
Wire spinal instrumentation,
  3:1355–1357
Wires
  fixation, 1:553
  localization, 1:211
  radioactive, 2:602
Wiskott-Aldrich syndrome, 1:337
WIT (Water-induced thermotherapy),
  3:1457
Witch hazel, 1:481, 2:656
WOCN (Wound ostomy continence
  nurses), 2:1022, 3:1495
Wolf-Hirschhorn syndrome, 2:702
Women's Health and Cancer Rights
  Act, 1:220, 502
Wood, Alexander, 3:1392
Worker's compensation, 2:822
Workload, 2:960, 961
World Health Organization (WHO)
  on cataracts, 1:511
  on glaucoma, 3:1272
  on leg venous disorders, 3:1531
  on pain management, 3:1084
  on vasectomy, 3:1526
Wound care, **3:1566–1570**
  amputation and, 1:46
  anti-inflammatory drugs and, 1:403
  bandages and dressings for,
    1:143–147
  debridement, 1:406–409
  fracture repair and, 1:555
  incision care for, 2:743–746
  irrigation, 2:817
  for laser skin resurfacing, 2:858–859
  scar formation and, 3:1263
  skin grafting for, 3:1323
  smoking cessation and, 3:1338

topical antibiotics and, 1:84
Wound-care nursing, 1:146
Wound closure
  fibrin sealants for, 1:536–538
  incision care for, 2:743–744
  laceration repair for, 2:817–819
  stitches and staples for,
    3:1373–1375
Wound culture, **3:1570–1572**
Wound dehiscence. *See* Dehiscence
Wound fillers, 1:144, 145–146
Wound ostomy continence nurses
  (WOCN), 2:1022, 3:1495
Wound pouches, 1:144, 146
Wounds
  full-thickness, 1:386
  gunshot, 1:372
  knife, 1:372
  partial-thickness, 1:386
  penetrating, 1:95, 372, 3:1416
  puncture, 1:1
  See also Wound care
Wright-Giemsa stain, 1:190
Wright stain, 1:190, 336
Wrinkles
  face lift and, 1:521, 523
  forehead lift for, 1:548–553
  laser skin resurfacing for, 2:857–859
  non-surgical treatment of, 1:552
Wrist
  arthroplasty of, 1:118
  arthroscopic surgery for, 1:120–123
  ganglion cyst removal for,
    2:560–563
  repetitive stress injury, 1:257
Wrist replacement, **3:1572–1575**
Wurm cerclage, 1:279
Wytensin. *See* Guanabenz acetate

X

X ray imaging
  vs. abdominal ultrasound, 1:1
  for arthroplasty, 1:118
  for artificial sphincter insertion eval-
    uation, 1:126
  bone, **1:203–204**, 3:1176
  for breast biopsy guidance, 1:211
  for colorectal cancer, 3:1317
  dental, 3:1430
  digital, 1:203
  esophageal, 1:490–493
  for ganglion cyst removal, 2:562
  for hand injuries, 2:621
  for hip dysplasia, 2:662
  for hip revision surgery, 2:676
  for ileoanal reservoir surgery, 2:721
  for intussusception reduction, 2:769
  for kidney stones, 2:1018
  for knee replacement, 2:804
  for leg lengthening and shortening,
    2:869

for low back pain, 2:823
for mentoplasty, 2:968
mobile, 2:760, 1046
for rotator cuff repair, 3:1249
for shoulder joint replacement,
  3:1310
for shoulder resection arthroplasty,
  3:1313
sinus, **3:1328–1329**
skull, **3:1328–1329**
for syndactyly, 3:1557
for traction, 3:1438
for ulcers, 3:1517
See also specific types of x rays
Xanax. *See* Alprazolam
Xenical. *See* Orlistat
Xenografts, 2:777, 3:1325
Xenon 133 studies, 1:45
Xylocaine. *See* Lidocaine

Y

YAG lasers. *See* Nd:YAG lasers
Yoga
  for back pain, 2:826
  for pain, 3:1084
  for weight management, 3:1562
Yohimbe, 1:34
YSI telethermometers, 1:543–544

Z

Z-plasty, 3:1265, 1266, 1404
Zagam. *See* Sparfloxacin
Zantac. *See* Ranitidine
Zaroxolyn. *See* Metolazone
Zen Hospice Project, 2:683
Zenapax. *See* Daclizumab
Zestoretic. *See* Lisinopril hy-
  drochlorothiazide
Zestril. *See* Lisinopril
ZEUS Surgical System, 3:1398, 1399
Zidovudine
  acetaminophen and, 1:22
  aspirin and, 1:132
  erythromycins and, 1:485
  NSAIDs and, 2:1028
  opioid analgesics and, 1:55
  red blood cell indices and, 3:1229
ZIFT (Zygote intrafallopian tube trans-
  fer), 2:742
Zinc, 1:547, 3:1457
Zithromax. *See* Azithromycin
Zofran. *See* Ondansetron
Zolicef. *See* Cefazolin
Zollinger-Ellison syndrome, 2:567–570
Zubieta, Jon-Kar, 3:1184
Zyban, 3:1339, 1340
Zygote intrafallopian tube transfer
  (ZIFT), 2:742

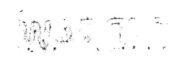